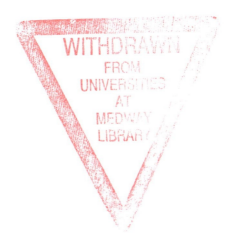

CANCER DRUG RESISTANCE

CANCER DRUG DISCOVERY AND DEVELOPMENT

BEVERLY A. TEICHER, SERIES EDITOR

CANCER DRUG RESISTANCE

Edited by

BEVERLY A. TEICHER, PhD

Genzyme Corporation
Framingham, MA

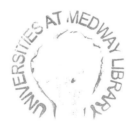

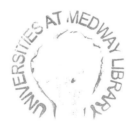

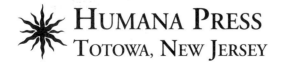

HUMANA PRESS
TOTOWA, NEW JERSEY

© 2006 Humana Press Inc.
999 Riverview Drive, Suite 208
Totowa, New Jersey 07512

www.humanapress.com

Cover illustration: Fig. 3 in Chapter 1, "The Cycle Between Angiogenesis, Perfusion, and Hypoxia in Tumors," by Mark W. Dewhirst, Yiting Cao, Benjamin Moeller, and Chuan-Yuan Li.

Cover design by Patricia F. Cleary

This publication is printed on acid-free paper. ⊚
ANSI Z39.48-1984 (American National Standards Institute)
Permanence of Paper for Printed Library Materials

For additional copies, pricing for bulk purchases, and/or information about other Humana titles, contact Humana at the above address or at any of the following numbers: Tel.: 973-256-1699; Fax: 973-256-8341; E-mail: orders@humanapr.com; or visit our Website: www.humanapress.com

Printed in the United States of America. 10 9 8 7 6 5 4 3 2 1

eISBN 1-59745-035-9

Library of Congress Cataloging-in-Publication Data

Cancer drug resistance / edited by Beverly A. Teicher.
    p. ; cm. -- (Cancer drug discovery and development)
  Includes bibliographical references and index.
  ISBN 1-58829-530-3 (alk. paper)
  1. Drug resistance in cancer cells. [DNLM: 1. Drug Resistance,
Neoplasm. 2. Antineoplastic Agents--therapeutic use. QZ 267 C2187
2006] I. Teicher, Beverly A., 1952- II. Series.
  RC271.C5C3225 2006
  616.99'4061--dc22
                      2005052500

For the Beautiful Ones,

Joseph and Emily

PREFACE

As genomic techniques allow us a closer and closer look at malignant disease, the ability of cells to respond to chemical and biological insults with remarkable flexibility of phenotype makes it clear that, despite some small successes, there is much to be done to control and eliminate malignant disease. The recruitment of a wide variety of host 'normal' cells into the malignant disease process is critical to disease progression. And so, the difficulties in discovering and/or designing highly effective anticancer therapeutics have been clarified. First, malignant cells can respond with epigenetic, as well as genetic, alterations to escape therapeutic attack. Second, there is a continuum of abnormalities and deregulated behaviors between host "normal" cells and neoplastic cells. To address the resistance of solid tumors to anticancer therapeutics, mechanisms that involve alterations in genetics and epigenetics, cellular biochemistry, properties related to physiology of the solid tumor mass, and alterations in host metabolic and immune status induced by the presence of malignant disease must be considered. Owing to the efforts and expertise of each contributor, *Cancer Drug Resistance* describes the current state of knowledge in these numerous areas and relates to resistance to cancer chemotherapy, radiation therapy, and immunotherapies.

This volume represents a point on the path of the long journey toward understanding the complex interactions between host, tumor, and cytotoxic or immunomodulatory agents. Classically, antitumor therapy sensitivity studies were carried out in tumor-bearing animals. Two observations were made during the course of these early studies. One was that tumors repeatedly treated with a drug could become nonresponsive, that is, resistant to that agent. The other observation was that the pharmacology and pharmaco-kinetics of drugs were different in tumor-bearing animals compared with normal animals. The advent of cell culture techniques allowed studies of therapeutic resistance to focus on the tumor cell. Critical changes in cellular biochemistry and molecular biology that confer resistance to specific therapeutic agents and treatments have been identified.

Techniques for examining the physiology of solid tumors and host normal tissues have been devised and refined. Abnormalities in solid tumor oxygenation, pH, interstitial pressure, perfusion, and vascular structure have been documented. Evidence continues to support the notion that the abnormal physiology of solid tumors protects these masses from therapeutic attack by chemotherapy, radiation therapy, and biological therapies based on protein molecules that include antibodies, cytokines, and growth factors.

The enormous growth of knowledge in the areas of protein effector molecules, cytokines, growth factors, and hormones has brought the study of therapeutic resistance back to the tumor/host as an interactive system with a new insight. The paracrine and autocrine effects of these secreted peptides, proteins, and small molecules continue to be elucidated. Defining a relationship between levels of these factors in a host and response of a tumor in that host to cancer therapies is only beginning to be realized.

Cancer Drug Resistance will serve as a resource to scientists of diverse specialties with interests relating to the response of malignant disease to current and experimental therapies.

Beverly A. Teicher, PhD

CONTENTS

CONTRIBUTORS

ENRIQUE ALVAREZ, DVM, MA • *Mechanism of Action, Pharmamar USA, Cambridge, MA*

ANIBAL A. ARJONA, PhD • *Pharmacology Department, CuraGen Corporation, Branford, CT*

CARLOS L. ARTEAGA, MD • *Breast Cancer Research Program, Departments of Medicine and Cancer Biology, Vanderbilt-Ingram Comprehensive Cancer Center, Vanderbilt University School of Medicine, Nashville, Tennessee*

MENASHE BAR-ELI, PhD • *Department of Cancer Biology, The University of Texas MD Anderson Cancer Center, Houston, Texas*

SUSAN E. BATES, MD • *Cancer Therapeutics Branch, National Cancer Institute, Bethesda, MD*

ROBERT BROWN, PhD • *Cancer Research UK Beatson Laboratories, Glasgow University, Glasgow, Scotland*

YITING CAO, MD, PhD • *Department of Radiation Oncology, Duke University Medical Center, Durham, NC*

BRENDA COOMBER, PhD • *Department of Biomedical Sciences, University of Guelph, Ontario, Canada*

WILLIAM S. DALTON, MD, PhD • *H. Lee Moffitt Cancer Center and Research Institute, Tampa, FL*

JOHN DEEKEN, MD • *Cancer Therapeutics Branch, National Cancer Institute, Bethesda, MD*

ALBERT B. DELEO, PhD • *University of Pittsburgh Cancer Institute, Hillman Cancer Center, Pittsburgh, PA*

PAUL DENT, PhD • *Department of Radiation Oncology, Virginia Commonwealth University, Richmond, VA*

MARK W. DEWHIRST, DVM, PhD • *Department of Radiation Oncology, Duke University Medical Center, Durham, NC*

GABRIELA DONTU, PhD • *University of Michigan Comprehensive Cancer Center, Ann Arbor, MI*

CHAOHONG FAN, MD, PhD • *Cancer Therapeutics Branch, National Cancer Institute, Bethesda, MD*

VICTORIA J. FINDLAY, PhD • *Department of Pharmacology, Medical University of South Carolina, Charleston, SC*

VARSHA GANDHI, PhD • *Experimental Therapeutics, The University of Texas MD Anderson Cancer Center, Houston, Texas*

M. LUZ GARCÍA-HERNÁNDEZ, PhD • *Norris Comprehensive Cancer Center, University of Southern California, Los Angeles, CA*

STEVEN GRANT, MD • *Department of Radiation Oncology, Virginia Commonwealth University, Richmond, VA*

JEFFREY E. GREEN, MD • *Transgenic Oncogenesis Group, Laboratory of Cell Regulation and Carcinogenesis, National Cancer Institute, Bethesda, MD*

LEE M. GREENBERGER, PhD • *Cancer Therapeutics Research, Johnson & Johnson, Raritan, NJ*

ROBERT GRIFFIN, PhD • *Department of Therapeutic Radiology/Radiation Oncology, University of Minnesota Medical School, Minneapolis, MN*

MICHAEL P. HAGAN, MD, PhD • *Department of Radiation Oncology, Virginia Commonwealth University, Richmond, VA*

LORI A. HAZLEHURST, PhD • *H. Lee Moffitt Cancer Center and Research Institute, Tampa, FL*

RICHARD P. HILL, PhD • *Applied Molecular Oncology, Ontario Cancer Institute/ Princess Margaret Hospital; Departments of Medical Biophysics and Radiation Oncology, University of Toronto, Ontario, Canada*

STEPHEN B. HOWELL, MD • *Department of Medicine and the Rebecca and John Moores Cancer Center, University of California, San Diego, La Jolla, CA*

W. MARTIN KAST, PhD • *Norris Comprehensive Cancer Center, University of Southern California, Los Angeles, CA*

KRISTIN KEE, PhD • *Transgenic Oncogenesis Group, Laboratory of Cell Regulation and Carcinogenesis, National Cancer Institute, Bethesda, MD*

YI TING KOH, BSc • *Norris Comprehensive Cancer Center, University of Southern California, Los Angeles, CA*

D. JAMES KOROPATNICK, PhD • *Cancer Research Laboratories, London Regional Cancer Centre, Ontario, Canada*

KENNETH A. KROHN, PhD • *Nuclear Medicine, Radiation Oncology and Chemistry, University of Washington Medical Center, Seattle, WA*

CHUAN-YUAN LI, PhD • *Department of Radiation Oncology, Duke University Medical Center, Durham, NC*

SULING LIU, PhD • *University of Michigan Comprehensive Cancer Center, Ann Arbor, MI*

SARAH JANE LUNT, PhD • *Applied Molecular Oncology, Ontario Cancer Institute/ Princess Margaret Hospital; Departments of Medical Biophysics, University of Toronto, Ontario, Canada*

DAVID A. MANKOFF, MD, PhD • *Division of Nuclear Medicine, University of Washington Medical Center; Seattle Cancer Care Alliance, Seattle, WA*

ILIA MANTLE, PhD • *University of Michigan Comprehensive Cancer Center, Ann Arbor, MI*

INGRID A. MAYER, MD • *Division of Hematology/Oncology, Department of Medicine, Vanderbilt-Ingram Comprehensive Cancer Center, Vanderbilt University School of Medicine, Nashville, TN*

VLADISLAVA O. MELNIKOVA, PhD • *Department of Cancer Biology, The University of Texas MD Anderson Cancer Center, Houston, TX*

KATHY D. MILLER, MD • *Division of Hematology and Oncology, Department of Medicine, Indiana Cancer Pavilion, Indianapolis, IN*

BENJAMIN MOELLER, PhD • *Department of Radiation Oncology, Duke University Medical Center, Durham, NC*

ELENA MONTI, PhD • *Section of Pharmacology, Department of Structural and Functional Biology, University of Insubria, Varese, Italy*

PATRICE J. MORIN, PhD • *Laboratory of Cellular and Molecular Biology, National Institute on Aging, National Institutes of Health, Baltimore, MD*

FAIYAZ NOTTA, MSc • *Cancer Research Laboratories, London Regional Cancer Centre, Ontario, Canada*

RUTH M. O'REGAN, MD • *Translational Breast Cancer Research Program, Winship Cancer Institute, Atlanta, GA*

CLODIA OSIPO, PhD • *The Robert H. Lurie Comprehensive Cancer Center, Feinberg School of Medicine of Northwestern University, Chicago, IL*

HEON JOO PARK, MD, PhD • *Department of Therapeutic Radiology/Radiation Oncology, University of Minnesota Medical School, Minneapolis, MN; Department of Microbiology, Medical School, Inha University, Inchon, Korea*

JAN PINKAS, PhD • *Genzyme Corporation, Framingham, MA*

JANUSZ W. RAK, MD, PhD • *Henderson Research Centre, McMaster University, Ontario, Canada*

ROBERT W. ROBEY, BChE • *Cancer Therapeutics Branch, National Cancer Institute, Bethesda, MD*

ROOHANGIZ SAFAEI, PhD • *Department of Medicine and the Rebecca and John Moores Cancer Center, University of California, San Diego, La Jolla, CA*

DEEPAK SAMPATH, PhD • *Oncology Research, Wyeth Research, Pearl River, NY*

BEATRIZ SANCHEZ-VEGA, PhD • *Experimental Therapeutics, The University of Texas MD Anderson Cancer Center, Houston, TX*

BRYAN SCHNEIDER, MD • *Division of Hematology and Oncology, Department of Medicine, Indiana Cancer Pavilion, Indiana University, Indianapolis, IN*

IE-MING SHIH, MD, PhD • *Departments of Gynecology/Obstetrics, Oncology, and Pathology, Johns Hopkins Medical Institutions, Baltimore, MD*

ZAHID H. SIDDIK, PhD • *Department of Experimental Therapeutics, The University of Texas MD Anderson Cancer Center, Houston, TX*

GEORGE W. SLEDGE, JR., MD • *Division of Hematology and Oncology, Department of Medicine, Indiana Cancer Pavilion, Indianapolis, IN*

CHANG W. SONG, PhD • *Department of Therapeutic Radiology/Radiation Oncology, University of Minnesota Medical School, Minneapolis, MN*

MIKA A. SOVAK, MD, PhD • *Department of Medical Oncology, The Cancer Institute of New Jersey, New Brunswick, NJ*

DAVID R. SPRIGGS, MD • *Memorial Sloan-Kettering Cancer Center, New York, NY*

CHRISTOPHER J. SWEENEY, MBBS • *Division of Hematology and Oncology, Department of Medicine, Indiana Cancer Pavilion, Indianapolis, IN*

BEVERLY A. TEICHER, PhD • *Genzyme Corporation, Framingham, MA*

JENS M. TEODORIDIS, PhD • *Cancer Research UK Beatson Laboratories, Glasgow University, Glasgow, Scotland*

KENNETH D. TEW, PhD • *Department of Pharmacology, Medical University of South Carolina, Charleston, SC*

DANYELLE M. TOWNSEND, PhD • *Department of Pharmacology, Medical University of South Carolina, Charleston, SC*

VICTOR E. VELCULESCU, MD, PhD • *Department of Oncology, Johns Hopkins Medical Institutions, Baltimore, MD*

TIAN-LI WANG, PhD • *Department of Oncology, Johns Hopkins Medical Institutions, Baltimore, MD*

WILLIAM R. WAUD, PhD • *Cancer Therapeutics, Southern Research Institute, Birmingham, AL*

MAX S. WICHA, MD • *University of Michigan Comprehensive Cancer Center, Ann Arbor, MI*

ADLY YACOUB, PhD • *Department of Radiation Oncology, Virginia Commonwealth University, Richmond, VA*

M. JIM YEN • *Departments of Gynecology/Obstetrics, Oncology, and Pathology, Johns Hopkins Medical Institutions, Baltimore, MD*

JOANNE L. YU, PhD • *Henderson Research Centre, McMaster University, Ontario, Canada*

I | PHYSIOLOGICAL RESISTANCE

1

The Cycle Between Angiogenesis, Perfusion, and Hypoxia in Tumors

Mark W. Dewhirst, DVM, PhD, Yiting Cao, MD, PhD Benjamin Moeller, PhD, and Chuan-Yuan Li, PhD

CONTENTS

SUMMARY

This chapter will present a pathophysiologic paradigm that occurs in solid tumors that is characterized by a self-propagating cycle of abnormally regulated angiogenesis, instability in perfusion, and hypoxia. Interactions between tumor and endothelial cells occur during tumor growth and in response to therapy. These interactions are of central importance in establishing codependence that contributes to promotion of cell survival, treatment resistance, enhanced invasion, and metastasis. Results indicate that concurrent targeting of both tumor and endothelial cells may be of central importance in improving treatment responses to both radiation and chemotherapy.

Key Words: Angiogenesis; perfusion; hypoxia; vasculature; diffusion.

1. INTRODUCTION

The objective of this chapter is to examine the interrelationships between tumor hypoxia, angiogenesis, and perfusion in tumors. These three features of tumor growth are inextricably linked and contribute collectively to maintaining a microenvironment typified by unstable oxygenation, hypoxia, and acidosis, promoting treatment resistance, and

From: *Cancer Drug Discovery and Development: Cancer Drug Resistance*
Edited by: B. Teicher © Humana Press Inc., Totowa, NJ

Table 1
Direct and Indirect Proangiogenic Factors Upregulated by Hypoxia

Direct-acting factors	Indirect-acting factors
Vascular endothelial growth factor[a]	Hypoxia-inducible factor 1
Basic fibroblast growth factor[a]	Nuclear factor-κB
Angiopoietin 2[a]	AP-1
Platelet-derived growth factor	Pyruvate[a]
Placental growth factor	Lactate[a]
Transforming growth factors[a]	
Plasminogen activator inhibitor 1[a]	
Thrombospondins	
Matrix metalloproteinases	[a]Factors directly or indirectly influenced by hypoxia-inducible factor 1 activity.
Endothelins	
Adrenomedullin	
Angiogenin	
Endoglin	
Placental growth factor	
Fractalkine	
Connective tissue growth factor	
Interleukin 8	
Macrophage migration inhibitory factor	
Leptina	

increased propensity for invasion and metastasis. This chapter will emphasize the process of vascular angiogenesis. Lymphangiogenesis is also important in tumor growth, but will not be discussed here. Readers are referred to other excellent reviews on this subject.

2. THE ANGIOGENIC SWITCH

Angiogenesis is the process by which new vascular segments are added to an existing vascular system. This process is largely quiescent in the normal adult, with the exception of processes such as the menstrual cycle and exercise adaptation (1). On the other hand, angiogenesis is a prominent feature of pathologic conditions, such as wound healing, chronic inflammation, diabetic retinopathy (2), and cancer. The initiation of angiogenesis in a nascent tumor is often referred to as the "angiogenic switch," a term initially coined by Folkman (3). There are at least two stimuli that can be involved in triggering the angiogenic switch, hypoxia (4) and/or alterations in oncogene or tumor suppressor gene function (5). Although there are numerous molecular signals that mediate this switch (Table 1), there are some master regulators that play predominant roles, hypoxia-inducible factor (HIF)-1 being the best-studied example. HIF-1 is activated directly by hypoxia as well as by overactivity in certain signaling pathways. It is a transcriptional activator that serves to enhance the expression of dozens of genes, including those for a number of important proangiogenic cytokines (4).

The regulatory mechanisms controlling HIF-1 stability are important in this context (Fig. 1). The protein is a heterodimer consisting of an α- and a β-subunit; these are constitutively expressed in nearly all cells. However, in aerobic conditions HIF-1α is constantly targeted for degradation via ubiquitylation (6). This process depends on modification of HIF-1α's oxygen-dependent degradation domain by a family of hy-

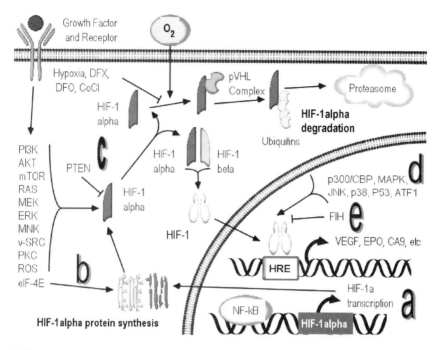

Fig. 1. Different regulatory points of hypoxia-inducible factor 1 (HIF)-1 signaling. HIF-1 promoter activity is regulated in at least five ways: **(A)** Transcription of HIF-1α: nuclear factor (NF)-κB, and so on, can upregulate the transcription of HIF-1α. **(B)** Translation of HIF-1α: both the phosphatidylinositol 3 kinase (PI3K)–Akt–mammalian target of rapamycin pathway and RAS–mitogen-activated protein kinase kinase (MEK)–extracellular signal-related kinase (ERK) pathway can upregulate eIF-4E-mediated HIF-1α protein synthesis. **(C)** Posttranslational modification: phosphokinase C (*PKC*), phosphatase and tensin homolog deleted on chromosome ten (*PTEN*), and potentially other suppressor genes can control posttranslational modification of HIF-1α, which is important for its heterodimerization with HIF-1β. **(D)** Degradation of HIF-1α: oxygen controls the binding of HIF-1α to von Hippel Lindau (pVHL) protein complex, which is responsible for HIF-1α degradation. **(E)** Transcriptional activity of HIF-1 by other transcriptional regulators or cofactors: mitogen-activated protein kinase (MAPK) family members such as p38, p42/p44 can phosphorylate HIF-1α. Factor inhibiting hypoxia-inducible factor (FIH) can hydroxylate HIF-1α. Those modifications directly affects the binding of HIF-1 to other transcriptional coactivators such as p300/CBP. P53 controls the degradation of HIF-1 and might affect the binding of HIF-1 and p300.

droxylases, using elemental oxygen as a cofactor, rendering it recognizable by the ubiquitin ligase von Hippel Lindau (VHL) complex *(6)*. Therefore, when a cell is normally oxygenated, the heterodimer does not form. Although the most powerful inducer of HIF-1 stabilization is hypoxia, there are circumstances wherein the heterodimer can form under normoxic conditions. For example, overexpression of oncogenes such as *Her-2* can lead to increased HIF-1α synthesis, which can outpace the degradation machinery *(7)*. In addition, mutations in tumor suppressor genes such as phosphatase and tensin homolog deleted on chromosome ten can block the degradation of HIF-1α by VHL *(8)*. Once the heterodimer is formed, there are other points of regulation including cofactors such as p300/CBP that influence binding to DNA *(9)*. It has also been reported that reactive oxygen and nitrogen species may also prevent the degradation of HIF-1α *(10,11)*. Because tumors tend to have elevated levels of reactive oxygen/nitrogen species *(12)*, this may serve as another source of proangiogenic stimulus in tumors. Reactive oxygen

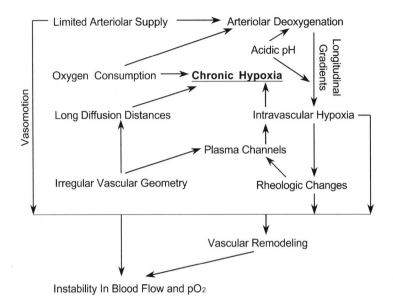

Fig. 2. Factors that contribute to chronic and cyclic hypoxia in tumors. Multiple factors influence oxygen delivery to tumors, including oxygen consumption, vascular geometry (including inadequate vascular density), limited number and orientation of feeding arterioles, longitudinal oxygen gradients that result from inadequate arteriolar input, and rheologic changes that occur in microvessels as a result of intravascular hypoxia and acidosis. Superimposed on the basic limitations of oxygen delivery is instability in microvessel red cell flux (perfusion). The underlying cause for this well-described phenomenon is not defined currently, but could be related to arteriolar vasomotion, vascular remodeling, and angiogenesis as well as rheological effects that influence the distribution of red cells at bifurcation points. (Adapted from ref. *19*.)

species formation may in fact be stimulated by hypoxia–reoxygenation injury, which may occur in tumors as a result of instabilities in perfusion *(13,14)*. To date, there have not been any reports showing whether genetic alterations can be sufficient to initiate angiogenesis without causing tumor hypoxia first in vivo, although it is well established that proangiogenic factors, such as vascular endothelial growth factor (VEGF), are upregulated in some tumor lines with a variety of oncogene and suppressor gene mutations, in the absence of hypoxia in vitro *(5,7)*.

Angiogenesis occurs through two physically different pathways, sprouting and intussusception *(15,16)*. Sprouting is mediated primarily by VEGF and begins with vasodilation of existing vessels *(17)*. The hypoxic trigger for HIF-1-mediated VEGF upregulation is thought to be caused by limitations in oxygen diffusion into the interior of a tumor as it grows *in situ* or collapse of preexisting coopted host vessels, leading to a hypoxic crisis *(18)*. Once angiogenesis has been established, however, hypoxia persists as a result of aberrancies in tumor microvascular geometry and function, as well as imbalances between oxygen consumption rates and supply (Fig. 2) *(19,20)*. The resultant persistent hypoxia maintains a constant proangiogenic stimulus as the tumor continues to grow. Clinically, hypoxia is a prominent pathophysiologic feature of solid tumors. It has been observed in nearly all solid-tumor histologies in which it has been examined. It is important to note, however, that some human tumors appear to rely exclusively on cooption of preexisting host vasculature for growth, as opposed to stimulation of angiogenesis. This phenotype has been observed in early-stage gliomas *(21)*, primary non-small cell lung cancers *(22)*, and in metastatic breast cancer of the liver *(23)*. Some information is emerging about how tumors mediate this type of growth.

Specific blockade of VEGF receptor 2 (VEGFR-2) with antibody *(24)*, VEGF trap *(25)*, or antibody to VEGF *(26)* have been reported to reduce intratumoral microvessel density and inhibit tumor growth. Interestingly, however, use of a VEGFR-2 antibody has been reported to effectively inhibit angiogenesis in primary tumors of an intracerebral glioma model, yet it exacerbates vascular cooption, leading to increased formation of satellite tumor recurrences removed from the primary site *(24)*. Both angiopoietin 2 and VEGF are upregulated at the margin of these tumors, suggesting that they play a role in the cooption process *(27)*. However, these same factors are involved in regulation of angiogenesis as well. Thus, the underlying mechanisms that regulate angiogenesis vs vessel cooption remain undefined.

3. REGULATION OF NEW BLOOD VESSEL GROWTH (ANGIOGENESIS)

Angiogenesis is initiated by a combination of molecular and environmental signals. To initiate the process, VEGF increases vascular permeability, partly via stimulating endothelial cell production of nitric oxide *(28)*. The VEGF receptor VEGFR-2 is also upregulated in response to hypoxia, which increases vascular responsiveness to VEGF within the tumor *(29)*. The resulting hyperpermeability permits extravasation of plasma proteins into the extravascular space. One of these proteins, fibrinogen, is rapidly converted to fibrin and crosslinked through the actions of thrombin and tissue transglutaminase, respectively *(30)*. The fibrin matrix promotes angiogenesis by providing scaffolding for endothelial cell migration and proliferation *(30)*. Transglutaminase upregulation has been observed in breast and pancreatic cancer *(31,32)* and is affiliated with poor prognosis in breast cancer and may be associated with poorer overall prognosis *(33)*. Transforming growth factor-β) and basic fibroblast growth factor (bFGF), which are also HIF-1-mediated proangiogenic factors, work with tissue transglutaminase and VEGF to promote angiogenesis *(30)*.

In order for angiogenesis to be fully activated, appropriate signaling through the Tie2 receptor is required. Tie2 is an endothelial cell-specific tyrosine kinase receptor that is regulated by two primary ligands, angiopoietin 1 (Ang1) and angiopoietin 2 (Ang2) *(34,35)*. Angiopoietin 1 is expressed constitutively and activates the receptor, promoting stable intercellular junctions and tight association with basement membrane and vascular-supporting cells, such as pericytes and smooth muscle cells *(36)*. Vessels that show high levels of Ang1 binding to Tie2 are relatively refractory to VEGF signaling *(37)*. Ang2, on the other hand, competes with Ang1 for binding to Tie2, promoting disassociation of endothelial cells from basement membrane and pericytes, and priming vessels to respond to VEGF and promote angiogenesis (Fig. 3) *(38)*. Hypoxia plays an angiogenesis-stimulating role in this pathway as well, downregulating Ang1 *(39)* and upregulating Ang2 *(40,41)*. The effect of Ang2 in vessel remodeling depends on the context in which it is expressed. Ang2 upregulation leads to vessel remodeling in the presence of VEGF. In contrast, Ang2 acts as a destabilizing factor and results in vessel regression in the absence of VEGF *(42)*. These results suggest that the relative ratio of VEGF to Ang2 could determine whether these factors contribute to either vessel remodeling or regression.

The actual process of angiogenesis involves migration and proliferation of endothelial cells in cords, which join other cords and then form a lumen *(30)*. Under normal circum-

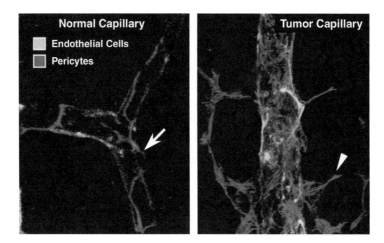

Fig. 3. Morphologic differences in pericyte–endothelial contacts: normal vs tumor tissues. Pericytes of normal capillaries have skeletal shapes and are closely attach to endothelial cells. In contrast, pericytes in a tumor model (MCa-IV) show irregular shapes and are attached loosely to endothelial cells. Many projections are observed from the pericyte into the interstitial space. Arrow: pericytes of normal capillary. Arrowhead: pericytes of tumor capillary. (Adapted with permission from ref. *38.*)

stances, this process is tightly regulated. As new vessels are formed, normal pO_2 is restored, leading to a reduction in hypoxia-mediated proangiogenic cytokines and reestablishment of a mature vasculature, as Ang1 once again dominates binding to Tie2. It has been demonstrated experimentally and theoretically in a corneal pocket angiogenesis model that the nature of this vascular bed (in terms of vessel lengths, branching patterns and overall density that is formed) is highly dependent on the relative concentration of VEGF at the tips of the vascular sprouts *(43)*.

4. ANGIOGENESIS IN METASTASES—EVIDENCE FOR PARACRINE SIGNALS BETWEEN TUMOR CELLS AND HOST VASCULATURE

It is generally believed that host vessels tend to be coopted by tumor cells before the onset of overt angiogenesis. It has been shown that this process involves selective invasion and proliferation of tumor cells toward host vessels, followed by formation of tumor cell cuffs around such vessels. It has been suggested that vascular collapse leads to a hypoxic catastrophe following vascular cuff formation, and this event triggers new vessel formation *(18)*. We have evidence against this theory, at least for metastatic tumors. Using tumor cell lines transduced stably with green fluorescence protein, we serially monitored tumor cell behavior and growth following transplantation into a window chamber model *(44,45)*. Both of the tumor types studied expressed VEGF at baseline in the absence of hypoxia—a scenario that would often be typical of a metastatic tumor. The 4T1 tumor line, a mammary carcinoma, underwent the epithelial–mesenchymal cell transition, typified by a change in shape to a fibroblastic-appearing cell. This adaptation has been linked to hypoxia-regulated expression of cell surface receptors such as autocrine motility factor, metalloproteinase, and keratin subtype expression that facilitates cell fluidity *(46)*. Perivascular cuffs formed, but we saw no evidence for vascular shut down before the onset of new vessel formation.

Interestingly, when VEGF signaling was blocked in this model, the epithelial–mesenchymal cell transition failed to materialize. Instead, the tumor cells underwent apoptosis and failed engraftment before the onset of angiogenesis. This observation suggested the existence of a paracrine relationship between tumor and host microvessels. Recently, we have shown that this putative paracrine relationship is modulated by bFGF (promotes better tumor cell survival) and Tie2 function (blockade of Tie2 tends to reduce tumor cell survival) *(45)*. It has not been reported whether hypoxia plays a role in this preangiogenic behavior, but we have observed that tumor cells farthest removed from host vasculature tend not to make the epithelial–mesenchymal cell transition and instead undergo apoptosis.

The metastatic behavior of lung metastases is not consistent with this paradigm. These metastases have been reported to adhere to and proliferate inside lung vasculature until they break down the vessel wall, allowing the tumor cells to escape and grow in the interstitial space *(47,48)*. It is not known whether paracrine relationships exist between host vasculature and tumor cells in primary sites or in this model of pulmonary metastasis.

5.VASCULAR REMODELING—INTUSSUSCEPTION AND PRUNING

Intussusception is the formation of new vessels by insertion of transcapillary tissue posts into an existing vessel, using a mechanism that does not involve sprouting or endothelial cell proliferation. The first step in intussusceptive growth is creation of a contact point in the lumen between endothelial cells from opposing capillary walls. The intercellular junctions of the endothelial layer are then reorganized to create central perforations, and an interstitial pillar core is formed from invading endothelial support cells. These pillars then enlarge, stabilized by the migration of pericytes and the laying down of interstitial matrix proteins to form a thicker wall between the vessels *(49)*. Although intussusception has been reported to occur in tumors *(15,50)*, it has been most extensively studied in the chorioallantoic membrane and in a variety of developing organs *(51)*. At least three different types of intussusception occur: intussusceptive microvascular growth, which expands the capillary plexus; intussusceptive arborization, which develops arterial and venous feeding vessels; and intussusceptive branching remodeling, which alters arterial and venous bifurcations (Fig. 4) *(49,52)*. Intussusception does not require VEGF, and in fact in one tumor line the process was most active in tumor regions devoid of VEGF expression *(50)*. However, studies in the chicken chorioallantoic membrane have indicated that VEGF can stimulate this process, depending on how it is presented to the tissue (acute vs chronic exposure) *(16)*. In addition to creating new segments through sprouting and intussusception, vessels also eliminate unnecessary segments of vasculature through vessel pruning *(52)*.

The mechanisms regulating intussusceptive angiogenesis are much less well characterized than those for sprouting angiogenesis. There is clear evidence that shear stress is involved. If shear stress is acutely modified, ion channels within endothelial cells are activated, resulting in rearrangements in cytoskeleton and gap junctions within minutes to hours *(49)*. Mature (stable) formation of intussusceptive angiogenesis involves interactions between endothelial cells and pericytes, which leads to the hypothesis that Tie2 and the angiopoietins may be involved *(42,49)*. The relative lack of pericytes in tumors could be influential in the stability of this process in tumors. Currently, it is not known whether hypoxia alters vascular intussusception. However, it has been hypothesized that pruning can be regulated by vessel shear stress as well as hypoxia *(42)*. Pries et al. have

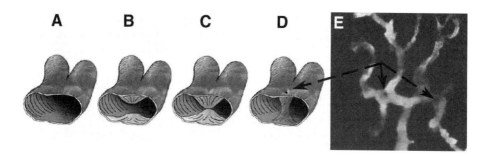

Fig. 4. Intussusceptive angiogenesis—the alternative to capillary sprouting. Three-dimensional representation of discrete steps in intussusceptive angiogenesis: **(A)** A capillary before intussusceptive angiogenesis. **(B)** Endothelial cells opposite of each other in the capillary wall protrude into the lumen and form a pillar. **(C)** Direct contact of the protruded endothelial cells. **(D)** Perforation of the endothelial pillar forms a cylindrical bridge extending across the capillary lumen. **(E)** A confocal microscopic image of intussusceptive angiogenesis. Arrows: Cylindrical endothelial bridges during intussusceptive angiogenesis. ([A]–[D]: Reproduced with permission from ref. *16*. [E]: Unpublished data from Dr. Dewhirst and Matthew Dreher.)

modeled structural responses of microcirculatory networks to small changes in demand and have compared the predictions to experimental observations. Their conclusion was that the primary mode of control was via shear stress, as compared with transmural wall pressure and oxygenation *(53)*. The molecular signaling processes that govern intussusception are not well understood, but it is speculated that many of the ligands and receptors involved in sprouting angiogenesis may play a role (Table 2). Additionally, theoretical analyses based on experimental observations indicate that the initiation of vascular adaptation may involve information transfer up and down the vascular network by as yet clearly defined mechanisms. In a region where acute changes in shear stress occur, it is speculated that information transfer occurs via transmission up and down the vascular network or via metabolic changes. For example, if a particular segment experiences a change in diameter, then the resultant shear stress change will alter the flow properties of the contiguous segments up- and down-stream, leading to vascular responses.

In tumors, hypoxia may influence intussusception in an indirect way. One of the hallmarks of tumor microvasculature is the presence of microvascular hypoxia *(54,55)*. Although some have speculated that this is because of temporary flow stasis, we have shown that it is because of: (1) longitudinal tissue oxygen gradients that result from inadequate arteriolar supply *(56)*, (2) relatively low vascular density with disorganized vascular geometry *(57)*, and (3) oxygen demand that is out of balance with supply *(58)*. Importantly, hypoxia occurs in microvessels that are actively perfused. The combination of low pO_2 and acidosis decreases the deformability of red cells by causing them to shrink, thereby losing optimal volume to surface area ratio. The crenation of these cells increases red cell suspension viscosity, leading to increased flow resistance and rouleaux formation *(59)*. The increase in blood viscosity alters shear stress, thereby creating a scenario that is primed for stimulation of vascular adaptation (*see* Fig. 2).

6. TUMORS ARE "WOUNDS THAT DO NOT HEAL"

Wound healing presents a unique paradigm regarding angiogenesis as a mechanism to reestablish homeostasis. It is well established that neovasculature is present only to

Table 2

Putative Factors Regulating Intussusceptive Angiogenesis

Category	Regulating factors	Effects
Physical factors	Hemodynamic forces, shear stress (in endothelial cells), wall stress (in smooth muscle cells).	Activation of ion channel, rearrangements of cytoskeletal system, changes in gap-junction complex.
Environmental factors	Hypoxia, normoxia, hyperoxia.	Induce multiple growth factors involved in vessel destabilization, angiogenesis, and remodeling; adjust vascular endothelial growth factor expression to proangiogenic, maintenance and submaintenance levels to cooperate with other growth factors.
Growth factors	Angiopoietin-1, angiopoietin-2, Tie-receptors, platelet-derived growth factor-B, monocyte chemotactic protein 1, ephrins, Eph-B receptors.	Recruitment of pericytes in type I and type IV pillars, stabilize intussusceptive endothelial meshes.

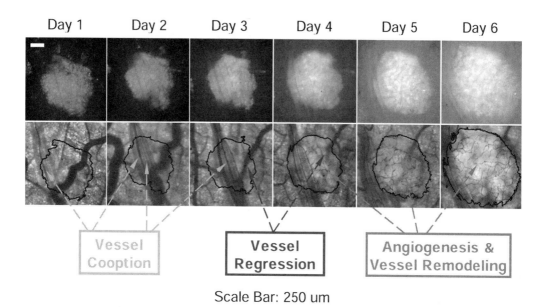

Scale Bar: 250 um

Fig. 5. Tumor vessel cooption, regression and angiogenesis. Human colon cancer cells (HCT116 with a constitutively expressed red fluorescence protein gene) were inoculated into a nude mouse dorsal skin-fold window chamber on day 0. Cooption of host vessels occurred first. With continued tumor growth, preexisting vessels destabilized. Vessel regression, angiogenesis and vessel remodeling reveal dynamic day-to-day changes in this developing tumor vasculature (black closed curves). Bar = 250 μm. (Unpublished data of Y. Cao and M. W. Dewhirst)

facilitate the closure of the wound. Once that occurs, the neovasculature regresses, leaving in its wake an avascular scar *(60)*. We studied serially punch biopsy wounds of rats to monitor angiogenesis, growth factor expression, and hypoxia. Surprisingly, the initial surge of VEGF, bFGF, and tumor growth factor-β, occurring 24 h after the wound was created, was not associated with hypoxia; it likely came from tissue stores of these cytokines as well as from platelets. The greatest level of hypoxia was observed at a point in time where the wound surface had reepithelialized and there was active proliferation in many cells of the maturing wound. The hypoxia at this time point was ubiquitous, involving endothelial cells, macrophages, and fibroblasts. It was hypothesized that the hypoxia was induced as a result of high oxygen consumption by the granulating wound. Concomitant with the hypoxia, there was widespread apoptosis of endothelial cells *(60)*. In the following days, the vasculature continued to regress, eventually leaving a fibrous, avascular scar. It is interesting to speculate that the signal for wound vessel regression may have been hypoxia, because upregulation of factors such as p53 in response to hypoxia could lead to apoptosis *(61)*.

Tumor microvasculature can demonstrate a similar behavior, exemplified by the onset of new vessel formation followed by vascular regression and/or pruning (Fig. 5). The difference with tumors, of course, is that the signals for new vessel formation do not cease, leading to the paradigm coined by Dvorak *(62)*, that "tumors are wounds that do not heal." Thus, when vessels regress, there remains a stimulus for a new wave of angiogenesis. Whether or not vessels undergo regression is also dependent on the maturity of the vessel and the balance of factors that favor survival vs apoptosis. In this regard,

VEGF is believed to be an important survival signal for immature vasculature, whereas Ang1 is believed to be an important signal for maintenance of mature vessels *(42)*.

7. EFFECTS OF CANCER THERAPY ON ANGIOGENESIS

Teicher was the first investigator to show that the combination of angiogenesis inhibition with either chemotherapy or radiation therapy yielded superior antitumor effects, compared with either treatment alone *(63)*. This occurred while tumor oxygenation was improved, and it was speculated that the improvement in oxygenation favored increased radiosensitivity *(64)*. This result was surprising to many, who speculated that use of antiangiogenic therapies would lead to reduction in vascular density and increased tumor hypoxia. However, it put important emphasis on the role of the endothelial cell in controlling treatment response. This result, along with the suggestion that selective killing of endothelial cells would be a very efficient means for killing tumor cells as a result of ischemia, led to the development of therapies that selectively target tumor vascular endothelium *(65)*.

It has been speculated that the key target cell for radiotherapy is the endothelial cell. Garcia-Barros and coworkers studied the role of the endothelial cell in tumor response to radiotherapy by using a sphingomyelinase-deficient knockout mouse *(66)*. Endothelial cells of this mouse are resistant to radiation-induced apoptosis because of the deficiency in this enzyme. Identical tumor lines transplanted into wild type vs the knockout strain showed remarkable resistance to radiation treatment in the latter. Whereas this paper stimulated significant controversy *(67)*, there is other emerging evidence supporting the importance of the endothelial cell in governing treatment response.

Forty years ago, Rubin and Cassarett described a "supervascularized" state after radiotherapy, using a microangiographic technique in a murine tumor model *(68)*. In fact, this phenomenon was thought for many years to be responsible for the process of tumor "reoxygenation," which provides logic for using fractionated radiotherapy to take advantage of improved oxygenation in subsequent treatments. Since that time, others have reported on this same type of phenomenon using a variety of preclinical models *(69,70)*.

We have recently reported, however, that tumor reoxygenation may have negative consequences for treatment efficacy *(71)*. Using a fluorescent reporter of HIF-1 activity, we found that HIF-1 signaling increased twofold after radiotherapy, peaking 48 h after the last treatment fraction (Fig. 6A). This activation was associated with increased HIF-1 protein levels, as well as increased expression of several downstream proteins that are important for stabilizing tumor endothelium, such as VEGF and bFGF. Therefore, it was reasoned that radiation-induced HIF-1 activation might contribute to treatment resistance by minimizing radiation damage to the tumor vasculature. This hypothesis was proven correct in experiments using RNA interference and YC-1, a drug recently found to inhibit HIF-1, which were both able to significantly interfere with the ability of tumors to protect endothelial cells from radiation damage. The HIF-1 pathway, then, may serve as a critical "node" for radiation resistance whose targeting could significantly improve radiotherapy.

Mechanistically, radiation-induced HIF-1 overactivity was found to be attributable to two separate events: (1) HIF-1α stabilization in aerobic tumor regions via production of free radicals and (2) dissolution of hypoxia-induced stress granules during reoxygenation. We demonstrated the relative importance of free radicals in stabilizing HIF-1 in several ways. First, we showed that free radicals were produced in tumors after radiation treat-

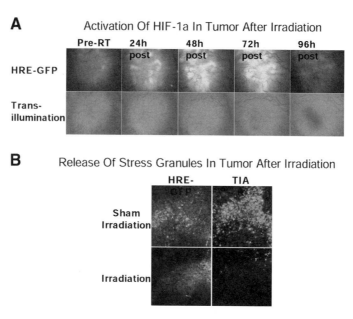

Fig. 6. Increased hypoxia-inducible factor 1 (HIF-1) activity and release of stress granules postirradiation. **(A)** A representative time course of HIF-1-driven green fluorescent protein (GFP) reporter activity following radiation. 4T1 murine mammary carcinomas, expressing stably an hormone response element (HRE)–GFP construct, were grown in dorsal skin-fold window chambers implanted onto Balb/c mice. Tumors were irradiated (2 × 5 Gy) and monitored with serial intravital fluorescence microscopy to determine relative HIF-1 activity levels. HIF-1 signaling typically peaked 48 h after treatment. **(B)** 4T1 mouse mammary carcinoma tumor sections were stained with an anti-TIAR antibody to visualize stress granules. In sham-irradiated tumors, these granules demonstrated tight colocalization with hypoxia, as marked by an endogenous HIF-1-driven GFP reporter. In irradiated tumors, examined 48 h after treatment, stress granules were much less abundant.

ment, and that scavenging of these free radicals with a small molecule superoxide dismutase mimetic blocked both the upregulation of HIF-1 protein levels and signaling activity after radiation treatment. Importantly, we demonstrated that when the superoxide dismutase mimetic was given after radiotherapy, it led to significant vascular regression, supporting the theory that HIF-1 is a critical targetable molecule regulating vascular radiosensitivity.

Stress granules are a recently recognized defense mechanism identified in a wide variety of eukaryotic cells *(72,73)*. They are composed of several mRNA-binding proteins and stress-responsive proteins that coalesce in the cytoplasm and sequester transcripts so that they cannot enter the endoplasmic reticulum to be translated to protein. They assemble when the cell is exposed to a stressor (e.g., heat shock, osmotic shock), and disassemble when the stress is alleviated. Teleologically, stress granules are believed to function to prevent cells from expending crucial energy unnecessarily during potentially lethal stress conditions. We found that hypoxia is amongst the stressors which can stimulate stress granule polymerization, and that stress granules are abundant in hypoxic regions of tumor tissue *(see* Fig. 6B). Moreover, HIF-1-regulated transcripts, in particular, appear to associate with stress granules during hypoxia. Disrupting stress granule polymerization, by expressing a mutant form of a stress granule scaffolding protein,

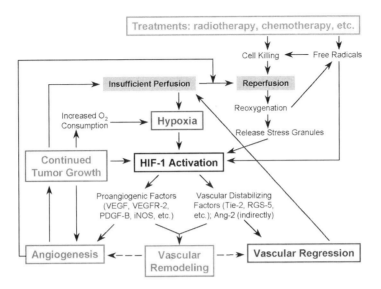

Fig. 7. Cycle between angiogenesis, perfusion, and hypoxia in tumors. The network of interactions between tumor growth, perfusion, angiogenesis, and hypoxia. The process of tumor reoxygenation, occurring as a result of instabilities in perfusion (causes depicted in more detail in Fig. 2) and/or as a result of therapeutic interventions, serves to initiate hypoxia-inducible factor 1 (HIF-1) promoter activity, promoting angiogenesis and tumor cell survival.

significantly increased the ability of tumor cells to upregulate downstream HIF-1 targets during hypoxia. When tumors reoxygenate, as occurs during treatment, these stress granules depolymerize and allow their previously sequestered hypoxia-induced transcripts, including those stimulated by HIF-1 activity, to be translated.

These two mechanisms contributed, therefore, to a HIF-1-dependent proangiogenic stimulus after radiotherapy that, in turn, protected tumors from radiation damage to their vasculature. This mechanism is likely to occur following any treatment that leads to tumor cell apoptosis and reoxygenation, but it is predicated on a preexisting condition of hypoxia (in vitro, we observed stress granule formation after a few hours at 0.5% O_2). For example, Taxol™ has been reported to induce apoptosis and increase tumor oxygenation *(74)*. Hyperthermia treatment has also been reported to cause reoxygenation in preclinical models and in clinical trials *(75,76)*. Because we have previously shown that VEGF is important for tumor cell survival post transplant by a yet-to-be-defined paracrine mechanism, one can conclude that therapies that cause reoxygenation will favor endothelial cell, and indirectly, tumor cell, survival. It is also important to note that the instability in tumor oxygenation at baseline, discussed here, could also contribute to stabilization of HIF-1-mediated transcripts, via the same mechanisms described for irradiated tumors.

8. SUMMARY AND CONCLUSIONS

In this chapter, we have emphasized the dynamic nature of tumor angiogenesis, which interplays with the fundamental limitations of oxygen delivery to create a tumor microenvironment that is typified by cycles of hypoxia and reoxygenation. This type of injury leads to increased concentrations of free radicals, which in turn contribute to upregulation of HIF-1, propagation of angiogenesis, and alterations in other cellular functions that promote survival of both tumor and endothelial cells (Fig. 7). Tumor therapies that cause reoxygenation can further exacerbate this prosurvival interdependence between tumor and endothelial cells. The results suggest that successful therapies should selectively target HIF-1 and/or its downstream target genes, such as VEGF, in order to break this cycle of interdependency.

ACKNOWLEDGMENTS

This work was supported by grants from the NCI (CA40355) and the Duke SPORE for breast cancer. The authors appreciate the editorial review of this manuscript by Catherine Sullivan and the confocal image of tumor microvascular intussusception provided by Matthew Dreher for Fig. 3.

REFERENCES

1. Kraus RM, Stallings HW III, Yeager RC, Gavin, TP. Circulating plasma VEGF response to exercise in sedentary and endurance-trained men. J Appl Physiol 2004; 96:1445–1450.
2. Wilkinson-Berka JL. Vasoactive factors and diabetic retinopathy: vascular endothelial growth factor, cycoloxygenase-2 and nitric oxide. Curr Pharm Des 2004; 10:3331–3348.
3. Folkman J, Hanahan D. Switch to the angiogenic phenotype during tumorigenesis. Princess Takamatsu Symp 1991; 22:339–347.
4. Semenza GL. Targeting HIF-1 for cancer therapy. Nat Rev Cancer 2003; 3:721–732.
5. Rak J, Mitsuhashi Y, Bayko L, et al. Mutant ras oncogenes upregulate VEGF/VPF expression: implications for induction and inhibition of tumor angiogenesis. Cancer Res 1995; 55:4575–4580.
6. Ohh M, Park CW, Ivan M, et al. Ubiquitination of hypoxia-inducible factor requires direct binding to the beta-domain of the von Hippel-Lindau protein. Nat Cell Biol 2000; 2:423–427.
7. Laughner E, Taghavi P, Chiles K, Mahon PC, Semenza GL. HER2 (neu) signaling increases the rate of hypoxia-inducible factor 1alpha (HIF-1alpha) synthesis: novel mechanism for HIF-1-mediated vascular endothelial growth factor expression. Mol Cell Biol 2001; 21:3995–4004.
8. Zundel W, Schindler C, Haas-Kogan D, et al. Loss of PTEN facilitates HIF-1-mediated gene expression. Genes Dev 2000; 14:391–396.
9. Arany Z, Huang LE, Eckner R, et al. An essential role for p300/CBP in the cellular response to hypoxia. Proc Natl Acad Sci U S A 1996; 93:12,969–12,973.
10. Zhou J, Fandrey J, Schumann J, Tiegs G, Brune B. NO and TNF-alpha released from activated macrophages stabilize HIF-1alpha in resting tubular LLC-PK1 cells. Am J Physiol 2003; 284:C439–C446.
11. Yang ZZ, Zhang AY, Yi FX, Li PL, Zou AP. Redox regulation of HIF-1alpha levels and HO-1 expression in renal medullary interstitial cells. Am J Physiol Renal Physiol 2003; 284: F1207–F1215.
12. Kuppusamy P, Li H, Ilangovan G, et al. Noninvasive imaging of tumor redox status and its modification by tissue glutathione levels. Cancer Res 2002; 62:307–312.
13. Kimura H, Braun RD, Ong ET, et al. Fluctuations in red cell flux in tumor microvessels can lead to transient hypoxia and reoxygenation in tumor parenchyma. Cancer Res 1996; 56:5522–5528.
14. Braun RD, Lanzen JL, Dewhirst MW. Fourier analysis of fluctuations of oxygen tension and blood flow in R3230Ac tumors and muscle in rats. Am J Physiol 1999; 277(2 Pt 2):H551–H568.
15. Patan S, Munn LL, Jain RK. Intussusceptive microvascular growth in a human colon adenocarcinoma xenograft: a novel mechanism of tumor angiogenesis. Microvasc Res 1996; 51:260–272.
16. Burri PH, Hlushchuk R, Djonov V. Intussusceptive angiogenesis: its emergence, its characteristics, and its significance. Dev Dyn 2004; 231:474–488.
17. Folkman J. Angiogenesis and angiogenesis inhibition: an overview. EXS 1997; 79:1–8.
18. Holash J, Wiegand SJ, Yancopoulos GD. New model of tumor angiogenesis: dynamic balance between vessel regression and growth mediated by angiopoietins and VEGF. Oncogene 1999; 18:5356–5362.
19. Dewhirst MW. Concepts of oxygen transport at the microcirculatory level. Semin Radiat Onco, 1998; 8:143–150.
20. Gulledge CJ, Dewhirst MW. Tumor oxygenation: a matter of supply and demand. Anticancer Res 1996; 16:741–749.

21. Kim ES, Serur A, Huang J, et al. Potent VEGF blockade causes regression of coopted vessels in a model of neuroblastoma. Proc Natl Acad Sci U S A 2002; 99:11,399–11,404.

22. Passalidou E, Trivella M, Singh N, et al. Vascular phenotype in angiogenic and non-angiogenic lung non-small cell carcinomas. Br J Cancer 2002; 86:244–249.

23. Stessels F, Van den Eynden G, Van der Auwera I, et al. Breast adenocarcinoma liver metastases, in contrast to colorectal cancer liver metastases, display a non-angiogenic growth pattern that preserves the stroma and lacks hypoxia. Br J Cancer 2004; 90:1429–1436.

24. Kunkel P, Ulbricht U, Bohlen P, et al. Inhibition of glioma angiogenesis and growth in vivo by systemic treatment with a monoclonal antibody against vascular endothelial growth factor receptor-2. Cancer Res 2001; 61:6624–6628.

25. Holash J, Davis S, Papadopoulos N, et al. VEGF-Trap: a VEGF blocker with potent antitumor effects. Proc Natl Acad Sci U S A 2002; 99:11,393–11,398.

26. Ferrara N. Vascular endothelial growth factor: basic science and clinical progress. Endocr Rev 2004; 25:581–611.

27. Peoch M, Farion R, Hiou A, Le Bas JF, Pasquier B, Remy, C. Immunohistochemical study of VEGF, angiopoietin 2 and their receptors in the neovascularization following microinjection of C6 glioma cells into rat brain. Anticancer Res 2002; 22:2147–2151.

28. Kimura H, Esumi H. Reciprocal regulation between nitric oxide and vascular endothelial growth factor in angiogenesis. Acta Biochim Pol 2003; 50:49–59.

29. Brekken RA, Thorpe PE. VEGF-VEGF receptor complexes as markers of tumor vascular endothelium. J Control Release 2001; 74:173–181.

30. Haroon ZA, Lai TS, Hettasch JM, Lindberg RA, Dewhirst MW, Greenberg CS. Tissue transglutaminase is expressed as a host response to tumor invasion and inhibits tumor growth. Lab Invest 1999; 79:1679–1686.

31. Hettasch JM, Bandarenko N, Burchette JL, et al. Tissue transglutaminase expression in human breast cancer. Lab Invest 1996; 75:637–645.

32. Iacobuzio-Donahue CA, Ashfaq R, Maitra A, et al. Highly expressed genes in pancreatic ductal adeno-carcinomas: a comprehensive characterization and comparison of the transcription profiles obtained from three major technologies. Cancer Res 2003; 63:8614–8622.

33. Mehta K, Fok J, Miller FR, Koul D, Sahin AA. Prognostic significance of tissue transglutaminase in drug resistant and metastatic breast cancer. Clin Cancer Res 2004; 10:8068–8076.

34. Davis S, Aldrich TH, Jones PF, et al. Isolation of angiopoietin-1, a ligand for the TIE2 receptor, by secretion-trap expression cloning. Cell 1996; 87:1161–1169.

35. Maisonpierre PC, Suri C, Jones PF, et al. Angiopoietin-2, a natural antagonist for Tie2 that disrupts in vivo angiogenesis. Science 1997; 277:55–60.

36. Papapetropoulos A, Garcia-Cardena G, Dengler TJ, Maisonpierre PC, Yancopoulos GD, Sessa WC. Direct actions of angiopoietin-1 on human endothelium: evidence for network stabilization, cell survival, and interaction with other angiogenic growth factors. Lab Invest 1999; 79:213–223.

37. Thurston G, Rudge JS, Ioffe E, et al. Angiopoietin-1 protects the adult vasculature against plasma leakage. Nat Med 2000; 6:460–463.

38. Morikawa S, Baluk P, Kaidoh T, Haskell A, Jain RK, McDonald DM. Abnormalities in pericytes on blood vessels and endothelial sprouts in tumors. Am J Pathol 2002; 160:985–1000.

39. Enholm B, Paavonen K, Ristimaki A, et al. Comparison of VEGF, VEGF-B, VEGF-C and Ang-1 mRNA regulation by serum, growth factors, oncoproteins and hypoxia. Oncogene 1997; 14:2475–2483.

40. Mandriota SJ, Pepper MS. Regulation of angiopoietin-2 mRNA levels in bovine microvascular endothelial cells by cytokines and hypoxia. Circ Res 1998; 83:852–859.

41. Oh H, Takagi H, Suzuma K, Otani A, Matsumura M, Honda Y. Hypoxia and vascular endothelial growth factor selectively up-regulate angiopoietin-2 in bovine microvascular endothelial cells. J Biol Chem 1999; 274:15,732–15,739.

42. Zakrzewicz A, Secomb TW, Pries AR. Angioadaptation: keeping the vascular system in shape. News Physiol Sci 2002; 17:197–201.

43. Tong S, Yuan F. Numerical simulations of angiogenesis in the cornea. Microvasc Res 2001; 61:14–27.

44. Li CY, Shan S, Cao Y, Dewhirst MW. Role of incipient angiogenesis in cancer metastasis. Cancer Metastasis Rev 2000; 19:7–11.

45. Shan S, Robson ND, Cao Y, et al. Responses of vascular endothelial cells to angiogenic signaling are important for tumor cell survival. FASEB J 2004; 18:326–328.

46. Krishnamachary B, Berg-Dixon S, Kelly B, et al. Regulation of colon carcinoma cell invasion by hypoxia-inducible factor 1. Cancer Res 2003; 63:1138–1143.

47. Wong CW, Song C, Grimes MM, et al. Intravascular location of breast cancer cells after spontaneous metastasis to the lung. Am J Pathol 2002; 161:749–753.

48. Al-Mehdi AB, Tozawa K, Fisher AB, Shientag L, Lee A, Muschel RJ. Intravascular origin of metastasis from the proliferation of endothelium-attached tumor cells: a new model for metastasis. Nat Med 2000; 6:100–102.

49. Burri PH, Djonov, V. Intussusceptive angiogenesis—the alternative to capillary sprouting. Mol Aspects Med 2002; 23(Suppl):S1–S27.

50. Djonov V, Andres AC, Ziemiecki A. Vascular remodelling during the normal and malignant life cycle of the mammary gland. Microsc Res Tech 2001; 52:182–189.

51. Djonov VG, Kurz H, Burri PH. Optimality in the developing vascular system: branching remodeling by means of intussusception as an efficient adaptation mechanism. Dev Dyn 2002; 224:391–402.

52. Djonov V, Baum O, Burri PH. Vascular remodeling by intussusceptive angiogenesis. Cell Tissue Res 2003; 314:107–117.

53. Pries AR, Reglin B, Secomb TW. Structural response of microcirculatory networks to changes in demand: information transfer by shear stress. Am J Physiol 2003; 284:H2204–2212.

54. Dewhirst MW, Ong ET, Klitzman B, et al. Perivascular oxygen tensions in a transplantable mammary tumor growing in a dorsal flap window chamber. Radiat Res 1992; 130:171–182.

55. Helmlinger G, Yuan F, Dellian M, Jain RK. Interstitial pH and pO_2 gradients in solid tumors in vivo: high-resolution measurements reveal a lack of correlation. Nat Med 1997; 3:177–182.

56. Dewhirst MW, Ong ET, Braun RD, et al. Quantification of longitudinal tissue pO_2 gradients in window chamber tumours: impact on tumour hypoxia. Br J Cancer 1999; 79:1717–1722.

57. Secomb TW, Hsu R, Braun RD, Ross JR, Gross JF, Dewhirst MW. Theoretical simulation of oxygen transport to tumors by three-dimensional networks of microvessels. Adv Exp Med Biol 1998; 454:629–634.

58. Dewhirst MW, Secomb TW, Ong ET, Hsu R, Gross JF. Determination of local oxygen consumption rates in tumors. Cancer Res 1994; 54:3333–3336.

59. Kavanagh BD, Coffey BE, Needham D, Hochmuth RM, Dewhirst MW The effect of flunarizine on erythrocyte suspension viscosity under conditions of extreme hypoxia, low pH, and lactate treatment. Br J Cancer 1993; 67:734–741.

60. Haroon ZA, Raleigh JA, Greenberg CS, Dewhirst MW. Early wound healing exhibits cytokine surge without evidence of hypoxia. Ann Surg 2000; 231:137–147.

61. Graeber TG, Osmanian C, Jacks T, et al. Hypoxia-mediated selection of cells with diminished apoptotic potential in solid tumours. Nature 1996; 379:88–91.

62. Dvorak HF. Tumors: wounds that do not heal. Similarities between tumor stroma generation and wound healing. N Engl J Med 1986; 315:1650–1659.

63. Teicher BA, Sotomayor EA, Huang ZD. Antiangiogenic agents potentiate cytotoxic cancer therapies against primary and metastatic disease. Cancer Res 1992; 52:6702–6704.

64. Teicher BA, Holden SA, Ara G, et al. Influence of an anti-angiogenic treatment on 9L gliosarcoma: oxygenation and response to therapy. Int J Cancer 1995; 61:732–737.

65. Denekamp J. Review article: Angiogenesis, neovascular proliferation and vascular pathophysiology as targets for cancer therapy. Br J Radiol 1993; 66:181–196.

66. Garcia-Barros M, Paris F, Cordon-Cardo C, et al. Tumor response to radiotherapy regulated by endothelial cell apoptosis. Science 2003; 300:1155–1159.

67. Brown M, Bristow R, Glazer P, et al. Comment on "Tumor response to radiotherapy regulated by endothelial cell apoptosis" (II). Science 2003; 302:1894; author reply 1894.

68. Rubin P, Casarett G. Microcirculation of tumors. II. The supervascularized state of irradiated regressing tumors. Clin Radiol 1966; 17:346–355.

69. Hilmas DE, Gillette EL. Tumor microvasculature following fractionated X-irradiation. Radiology 1975; 116:165–169.

70. Dewhirst MW, Oliver R, Tso CY, Gustafson C, Secomb T, Gross JF. Heterogeneity in tumor microvascular response to radiation. Int J Radiat Oncol Biol Phys 1990; 18:559–568.

71. Moeller BJ, Cao Y, Li CY, Dewhirst MW. Radiation activates HIF-1 to regulate vascular radiosensitivity in tumors: role of reoxygenation, free radicals, and stress granules. Cancer Cell 2004; 5:429–441.

72. Gilks N, Kedersha N, Ayodele M, et al. Stress granule assembly is mediated by prion-like aggregation of TIA-1. Mol Biol Cell 2004; 15:5383–5398.

73. Kedersha N, Anderson P. Stress granules: sites of mRNA triage that regulate mRNA stability and translatability. Biochem Soc Trans 2002; 30(Pt 6):963–969.
74. Milas L, Hunter N, Mason KA, Milross C, Peters LJ. Tumor reoxygenation as a mechanism of taxol-induced enhancement of tumor radioresponse. Acta Oncol 1995; 34(3):409–412.
75. Vujaskovic Z, Song CW. Physiological mechanisms underlying heat-induced radiosensitization. Int J Hyperthermia 2004; 20:163–174.
76. Jones EL, Prosnitz LR, Dewhirst MW, et al. Thermochemoradiotherapy improves oxygenation in locally advanced breast cancer. Clin Cancer Res 2004; 10:4287–4293.

2 Influence of Tumor pH on Therapeutic Response

Chang W. Song, PhD, Robert Griffin, PhD, and Heon Joo Park, MD, PhD

Contents

SUMMARY

The intratumor microenvironment is intrinsically acidic due mainly to accumulation of lactic acid as a result of increased aerobic and anaerobic glycolysis by the tumor cells. In general, the extracellular pH (pHe) in human tumors is below 7.0, whereas the intracellular pH (pHi) is maintained at neutral range, i.e., >7.0, by powerful pHi control mechanisms. The low pHe and the significant gradients between pHe and pHi affect markedly the response of tumors to various treatments such as chemotherapy, radio-therapy and hyperthermia. For instance, the acidic pHe increases the cellular uptake of weakly acidic drugs such as cyclophosphamide and cisplatin and thus increases the effect of the drugs, whereas the acidic pHe retards the uptake of weakly basic drug such as doxorubicin and vinblastine, thereby reducing the effect of the drugs. The radiation-induced apoptosis is suppressed by an acidic environment, whereas the hyperthermia-induced cell death is potentiated by an acidic environment. Better understanding of the control mechanisms of pHe and pHi in tumors may lead to device effective treatment strategy of human tumors.

From: *Cancer Drug Discovery and Development: Cancer Drug Resistance*
Edited by: B. Teicher © Humana Press Inc., Totowa, NJ

Key Words: Intratumor pH; extracellular pH; intracellular pH; intratumor pH control mechanism; chemotherapy; radiotherapy; hyperthermia.

1. INTRODUCTION

The environmental acidity or pH of living cells and tissues is one of the major factors that influence molecular processes involved in cell cycle progression, cell proliferation, and differentiation. Likewise, oncogenesis, malignant transformation, metastasis, and angiogenesis are greatly influenced by environmental acidity. The environmental acidity also greatly influences the response of cancer cells to various treatments. The vascular network in tumors is inhomogeneous, causing insufficient oxygen supply to parts of tumors. The resultant hypoxia forces glucose metabolism through the glycolytic pathway instead of respiration, thereby resulting in the formation of lactic acid *(1–7)*. In addition, tumor cells convert glucose and other substrates preferentially to lactic acid and other acidic metabolites even under aerobic conditions, leading to acidification of the intratumor environment *(5,8,9)*. Whereas the interstitial or extracellular environment in tumors is acidic, the intracellular pH (pHi) in tumors has been found to be at neutral range, i.e., < 7.0, similar to the pHi of normal tissues *(1,2,5–12)*. This intracellular and extracellular pH (pHe) gradient in tumor cells is maintained by sophisticated biophysical mechanisms *(1,2,13)*. It has been demonstrated that the gradient between pHe and pHi of tumor cells renders the cells resistant to weakly basic drugs by hindering the cellular uptake of the drugs, whereas the same pH gradient increases the uptake of weakly acidic drugs. The influence of tumor acidity on the thermosensitivity of tumor cells has been extensively investigated. On the other hand, relatively little has been revealed on the effect of acidic intratumor environment on the response of tumor cells to radiotherapy. In this chapter, we review the pHi control mechanisms and the implications of tumor pH and that of the pH gradient between the outside and inside of tumor cells on the response of tumor cells to various treatments.

2. TUMOR pH

It has long been known that the microenvironment in tumors of both animal and human is acidic as compared with that in normal tissues because of elevated in anaerobic as well as aerobic glycolysis in tumors *(1–6)*. As tumor nodules are formed, neovascularization begins from host venules stimulated by a number of angiogenic factors secreted by the tumor cells as well as adjacent normal cells. The newly formed tumor vascular beds are characterized by a heterogeneous distribution of dilated, irregularly bulged, constricted, twisted, and sharply bent capillary-like blood vessels *(14–23)*. Consequently, tumor blood perfusion is sluggish, resulting insufficient supply of various nutrients, including oxygen, to tumor cells. As the tumor grows larger, the intercapillary distance progressively increases, and areas beyond oxygen diffusion distance from capillaries, i.e., about 150 µm, become hypoxic *(24)*. In addition, probably because of progressively increasing interstitial pressure caused by the increasing tumor cell population *(25)*, tumor blood vessels are compressed, and the blood perfusion ceases intermittently or permanently resulting in intermittent or permanent hypoxia *(20–23)*. Hypoxia upregulates various transcription factors including hypoxia-inducible factor-1 (HIF-1), which activates the transcription of numerous genes whose protein products facilitate adaptation to hypoxia, driving the tumor toward a more malignant phenotype *(26–28)*. A well-known response of cells to hypoxia is an increase in hyperglycolytic activity characterized by increased

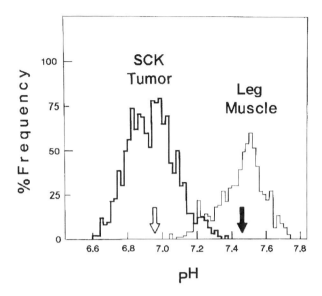

Fig. 1. Histograms of interstitial pH in the leg muscle of A/J mice and that in SCK tumors grown subcutaneously in the leg of A/J mice. The tumor diameters were 7–9 mm. The pH was measured with glass microelectrodes 50–80 mm in diameter *(3)*.

glucose uptake and formation of lactic acid, resulting in acidification of intratumor environment *(5–7)*. It has also been demonstrated that hypoxia activates carbonic anhydrase, thereby causing hydration of CO_2 molecules to carbonic acid *(7)*. Hulikova et al. *(29)* reported that tumor-associated carbonic anhydrase IX isoform is the most likely candidate involved in the formation of carbonic acid under hypoxic conditions. Hydrolysis of ATP is also a significant contributor to acidosis in tumors during acute hypoxia *(30)*. It should be pointed out, however, that tumor acidification can occur independent of hypoxia. It was shown in the early part of the last century that tumor cells metabolize glucose preferentially through glycolysis, even in the presence of oxygen *(8)*. It is believed that the endogenous acidification is an integral property of tumor cells that may have evolved to provide tumor cells with a competitive advantage over stromal cells *(5,8)*. Elstrom et al. *(31)* reported that the high rate of aerobic glycolysis in cancer cells is because of upregulation of the serine/threonine kinase Akt *(9)*.

2.1. pH in Tumors vs Normal Tissues

Until recent years, pH of animal and human tumors was determined by glass or fiber optic pH electrodes *(3,4,32–35)*. Because the diameters of the electrodes are larger than the diameters of cells and the tissue damage caused by the electrodes can be substantial, the pH values obtained with microelectrodes represent mainly pHe. Despite the technical difficulties, important information on tumor pH has been accumulated during the last several decades. Figure 1 shows histograms of pHe in SCK mammary carcinoma and that of the leg muscle of A/J mice obtained with glass microelectrodes *(3)*. It is demonstrated that the pHe in SCK tumors ranged from 6.60 to 7.38, with a mean value of 6.96, whereas that of the muscle ranged from 7.05 to 7.72, with a mean value of 7.45. This difference between mean tumor pH and mean muscle pH of as much as 0.5 pH units means that the concentration of the active H^+ ions in the interstitial space in SCK tumors was five times greater than that in the muscle. Wike-Hooley et al. *(4)* reviewed a number of reports on the pHe value in tumors and normal tissues of animals and concluded that the tumor pHe ranged from 5.8 to 7.68, with an average of 7.09, and that the pHe in normal tissues such as muscle and liver was about 0.5 pH units higher than that in tumors. Vaupel et al. *(36)* reported that whereas average pHe in a C3H murine mammary carcinoma was 6.7, the pHe in some microareas was as low as 5.8–6.3. On the other hand, the pHe measured in extensively necrotic areas was higher than that in normal tissues, probably because of lack of formation of acidic metabolites as a consequence of previous cell death. Jahde et al. *(37)* observed that the pHe in neuroectodermal TV1A tumors grown subcutaneously in the flank of BDIX rats ranged from 6.8 to 7.1, with a mean of 7.0. Interestingly, the pHe values in the brain and kidney of BDIX rats were similar to that measured in brain tumors of the same animal.

Meyer et al. *(38)* reported as early as 1948 that the pHe of human tumors was lower than that in normal tissues, and other investigators subsequently reported similar results *(4,32,39–49)*. Wike-Hooley et al. *(4)* also reviewed the distribution of pHe in human tumors and normal tissues. The tumor pHe ranged 6.0–7.6, with a median pHe of 7.1, whereas the subcutis/muscle pHe ranged 7.3–7.8, with a median pHe of 7.55. It has been reported that, in general, the range of pH values in tumors is much greater than that the normal tissues, probably because the distribution of the vascular supply and blood perfusion in tumors are heterogeneous *(3,4)*. In this regard, the intertumor pHe variance was more striking than the intratumor pHe variance *(4)*. Based on numerous reports, Wike-Hooley et al. *(4)* concluded that the pH values in human tumors were not related to the tumor histology, degree of differentiation, tumor size, patient age, or treatment histology. However, the pHe values in metastases were higher than those in the primary tumors of a given patent.

2.2. Intracellular pH

It has become increasingly evident in recent years that pHi is not equal to pHe in tumor cells. We have studied the pHi of tumor cells in vitro using the pH-sensitive dye BCECF *(1,2)*, as shown in Fig. 2. The pHi remained at about 7.4 when the medium pH, i.e., pHe, was in the 7.0–7.4 range. As the pHe was lowered, the pHi also decreased, but only slightly. For example, at pHe 7.0 and 6.0, the pHi was 7.4 and 6.7, respectively. This in vitro study demonstrated clearly that pHi of tumor cells in a low-pHe environment remains near the neutral pH range. It has become possible in recent years to determine pHi of tumor cells *in situ* by virtue of impressive progress in magnetic resonance spectroscopy (MRS) technology. The pHi of tumors has been measured with ^{31}P-nuclear magnetic resonance (NMR), which determines the shifts in intracellular inorganic phosphate and phosphocreatine *(10,50–54)*. It is now possible to determine pHe using ^{1}H-MRS and also simultaneously determine pHi and pHe by incorporating a pHe indicator, 3-aminopropyl phosphonate, into ^{31}P-NMR *(6)*. The pHe and pHi in the same tumor cells can also be determined with ^{19}F-MRS using 6-fluropyridoxol, a vitamin B6 analog (6-fluoro-pyridoxol and 6-fluoropyridoxamine) or 3-[N-(4-fluor-2-trifluoromethyl-phenyl)-sulphamoyl]propionic acid (ZK-150471). Gillis et al. *(6)* reviewed reports on the differences between pHi and pHe in animal and human tumors determined with MRS methods and reported that the pHi was usually higher than pHe in human tumors *in situ*. In Fig. 3, we further analyzed the relationship between the pHe and pHi in human, murine,

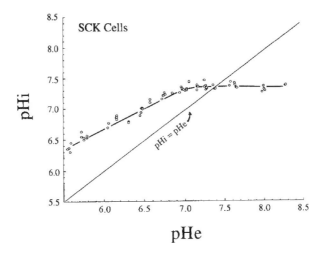

Fig. 2. Relationship between extracellular pH (pHe) and intracellular pH (pHi) of SCK tumor cells in vitro. The cells were maintained at pHe 7.2 before exposure to a new pHe. The pHi was measured using the pH-sensitive dye BCECF method 20–30 min after exposure to new pHe.

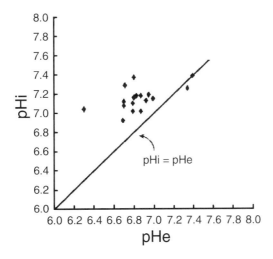

Fig. 3. The relationship between extracellular pH (pHe) and intracellular pH (pHi) in human, rat and mouse tumors *in situ*. Both pHe and pHi in the same tumors were determined with magnetic resonance imaging/magnetic resonance spectroscopy method. Data reported by ref. *6* were used to construct this figure.

and rat tumors determined with MRS/magnetic resonance imaging method and reviewed by Gilles *(6)*. It can be seen that the pHi values are higher than the pHe values in the same tumors in all tumors studied. The pHe values were correlated with phenotype, and the pHe values in larger tumors were lower than that in smaller tumors, probably because of poorer blood perfusion in larger tumors and more accumulation of acidic byproducts of glycolysis *(6)*. In conclusion, all available evidence indicates that the intracellular environment in tumor cells is less acidic as compared with extracellular environment in vitro as well as in vivo.

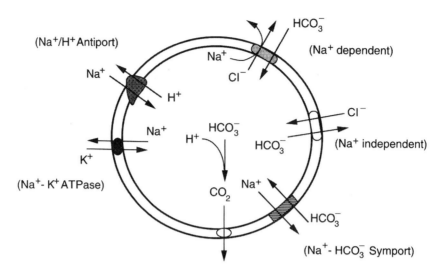

Fig. 4. Most common membrane-based intracellular pH regulatory mechanisms in mammalian cells.

3. MECHANISM OF pHi CONTROL

The fact that pHi is significantly higher than pHe in tumors demonstrates the existence of powerful mechanisms to prevent acidification of the intracellular environment *(13,55–61)*. Such significant gradient between pHe and pHi has been attributed to existence of short-term and long-term mechanisms for pHi control *(13)*. The short-term mechanisms are essentially rapid buffering responses against an acute acid load in the cytosol of cells. The most important short-term regulatory mechanism is the physiochemical buffering of the acids. Other rapid mechanisms include metabolic consumption of nonvolatile acids and transfer of acids from the cytosol to the organelles. These three mechanisms are only for rapid consumption of H^+ ions to minimize rapid acidification in the cells; therefore, their capacity to maintain the intracellular environment at neutral pH for a prolonged period is limited. Almost all mammalian cells that have been investigated thus far possess powerful systems to regulate pHi using several long-term mechanisms *(13)*. The most important mechanism for long-term pHi regulation is the exchange of Na^+ ions for H^+ ions using the Na^+/H^+ antiport, an ion exchanger in the plasma membrane (Fig. 4) *(56,57)*. This process is believed to occur by the binding of intracellular H^+ ions to the cytoplasmic surface of the exchanger and the binding of Na^+ ions to the cell surface of the exchanger. However, indications are that the exchange of Na^+ ions and H^+ ions is not a simple one-for-one exchange. It has been postulated that there might be a second cytoplasmic H^+ binding site that allosterically activates the antiport *(56,59)*. The influx of Na^+ ions and efflux of H^+ ions by this antiport is driven by a Na^+ gradient across the cell membrane. However, even in the presence of large Na^+ gradient energy, the exudation of H^+ ions from the cells is limited, and the pHi is stabilized at neutral values. This fact indicates that although the Na^+ gradient is important for the Na^+/H^+ exchange, it is not the only factor that controls the pHi. The antiport may become inactive when the pHi reaches a certain level, even though the Na^+ gradient remains large *(56)*. When the extracellular Na^+ ion concentration is low, the Na^+ gradient is reversed, and H^+ ions will enter the cells *(56)*. The Na^+ ions that enter the cells are extruded from cells driven by ATP hydrolysis. The activity of the Na^+/H^+ antiport is partially reduced under hypoxic conditions, which may be attributed to the reduction of ATP content *(13,60)*. There is evidence that the Na^+/H^+ antiport system is secondarily dependent on the Na^+/K^+-ATPase *(60)*. A number of compounds have been demonstrated to interfere with the Na^+/H^+ antiport. Amiloride, a diuretic drug and weak base, and many of its analogs inhibit the Na^+/H^+ antiport activity by competing with Na^+ ions for the Na^+ channel *(9,11,13,57,58,61)*. Ethylisopropylamiloride, an analog of amiloride, is a more specific inhibitor of Na^+/H^+ antiport than amiloride, and as such, ethylisopropylamiloride is a much more potent inhibitor of Na^+/H^+ antiport than amiloride *(12,57)*.

The intracellular acidity is also regulated by bicarbonate-linked mechanisms, namely (1) Na^+-dependent Cl^-/HCO_3^- exchange, (2) Na^+-independent Cl^-/HCO_3^- exchange, and (3) Na^+/HCO_3^- symport (*see* Fig. 4) *(11,13,55,57,58)*. All three mechanisms are not always present in all types of cells. Usually, various combinations of the three mechanisms are found in different cell types. Among these, Na^+-dependent Cl^-/HCO_3^- exchange is probably the most important bicarbonate-linked mechanism for pHi control in mammalian cells. It responds only to acid challenge and neutralizes the intracellular environment by exchanging the negatively charged intracellular Cl^- with the extracellular Na^+/HCO_3^- complex *(62,63)*. The exchange is believed to be driven by Na^+ gradient and in some circumstances, by an additional inward-directed HCO_3^- gradient. The Na^+-independent Cl^-/HCO_3^- exchange is involved in protecting the cells from relatively rare occurrences of cell alkalinization. In this case, HCO_3^- ions are extruded from the cells, and Cl^- ions are transported into the cells to prevent the pHi from rising to an abnormally high level *(62,63)*. The Na^+/HCO_3^- symport is electrogenic, unlike the other two mechanisms *(64,65)*. A sudden reduction of Na^+ and Cl^- ions activates this mechanism to transport these two ions. Whereas this mechanism may be important for specialized acid-secreting cells, its role in regulating pHi in other mammalian cells is uncertain. All of the bicarbonate-dependent transporting mechanisms are inhibited by 4,4'-diisothiocyanostilbene 2,2'-disulfonic acids (DIDS), and 4-acetamindo-4'-isothiocyantostilbene 2,2'-disulfonic acids *(13,57,66–68)*. Ethacarynic acid inhibits the Na^+-independent Cl^-/HCO_3^- antiporter without affecting the Na^+-independent one, and picrylsulfonic acid has the opposite effect *(69)*. The Na^+-coupled Cl^-/HCO_3^- exchange is also inhibited by depletion of ATP, and the Na^+-independent Cl^-/HCO_3^- exchange is inactivated by a low-pH environment *(62,70)*.

The relative importance in maintaining pHi at neutral range of the different mechanisms mentioned varies markedly in different cell types and under different conditions. The lactate /H^+ symport, which is inhibited by the bioflavionoids quercetin and others, is one of the most active exchange in the regulation of pHi in tumor cells *(71,72)*. However, under hypoxic conditions the lactate extrusion is reduced, and so this exchange has little effect on resting pHi in the hypoxic cells *(5)*. In the gastric glands, the Na^+/H^+ antiporter plays the dominant role, whereas in the neighboring oxyntic cells, the Cl^-/HCO_3^- exchange plays the dominant role for the pHi regulation *(57)*. Three types of ATP-driven H^+ pumps have also been identified *(57)*. One of these is an ATPase-linked H^+ pump found in some specialized epithelial cells. It has been reported that one of the mechanisms to maintain the cytosolic pH at physiological level is sequestration of cytosolic protons into acidic cellular vesicles such as endoplasmic reticulum, endosomes, and lysosomes. Interestingly, the ATPase-linked H^+ pump has been identified in a number of intracellular organelles, indicating that the ATPase-linked H^+ pump plays an important role in regulating pH in the vesicles and cytosol. The other two mechanisms are a H^+-translocating

Table 1
Genes Activated by Low pH

AP-1	VEGF
NFκB	bFGF
p53	PDECGF
p21	IL-8
MTIIA	Cyclines
GRPs	HSPs
Bax	NQO1

ATPase and a K^+/H^+ exchange ATPase, which can be suppressed by nigericin. Further understanding of the pHi control mechanisms may enable us to control the response of cells to internal as well as external stresses including various cancer treatments.

4. EFFECT OF pH ON ANGIOGENESIS AND METASTASIS

It has been established that hypoxic environment upregulates a number of transcription factors such as HIF-1, nuclear factor κB, and activator protein 1 (73–76). HIF-1 has been demonstrated to activate transcription of as many as 70 genes including glucose transporters and glycolytic enzymes, which may account for the increased anaerobic glycolysis and resultant acidification of tumors under a hypoxic environment (26–28). Like hypoxia, acidosis also upregulates transcription factors and activates a number of genes (77–79). We have observed that exposure of tumor cells to a low pH medium elevates significantly p53 expression and p21 expression (77). When the low pH medium was replaced with neutral pH medium, the expression of p53 and p21 promptly returned to normal level. Table 1 shows some of the genes or their products upregulated by an acidic environment. Note that many of the genes activated by acidosis are the same genes activated by hypoxia. For example, the angiogenic factors such as vascular endothelial growth factor, basic fibroblast growth factor, platelet-derived endothelial cell growth factor, and interleukin 8 are upregulated by both hypoxia and acidosis. In view of the fact that many hypoxic cells in tumors are in an acidic environment, how the hypoxia and acidosis interact in promoting the angiogenic process remains an important avenue to be elucidated.

The metastatic potential of tumors has been demonstrated to be related closely to the environmental acidity. The ability of murine tumor cells to form lung metastases after intravenous injection increased significantly when the cells were cultured in acidic medium before the injection (79,80). Deliberate exposure of mice bearing tumors to cyclic low-oxygen breathing (12 cycles of 5% oxygen breathing for 10 min interspersed with 10 min of air breathing) every day doubled the incidence of lung metastases (81). It appeared that acidosis in combination with hypoxia induced by the low-oxygen breathing enhanced the incidence of metastasis. However, acidification of murine tumors by daily administration of metaiodobenzylguanidine and/or glucose without lowering tumor pO_2 did not enhance the spontaneous metastasis potential of tumor cells in the same model (82). In addition to angiogenesis, induction of genomic instability or epigenetic regulation of gene expression may be involved in the increase in metastasis in acidic and hypoxic environments (83). It is likely that the cells that survive the acidic and hypoxic hostile intratumor environment are more aggressive and metastatic as compared with

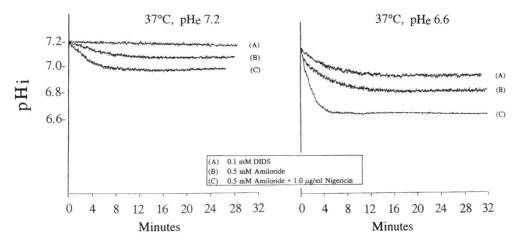

Fig. 5. Changes in pHi (BCECF intensity) in SCK tumor cells upon treating the cells with inhibitors of intracellular pH (pHi) regulatory mechanisms in extracellular pH (pHe) 7.2 or pHe 6.6. The decline in pHi caused by the inhibitors was much greater at pHe 6.6 than that at pHe.7.2.

cells in a less hostile environment. We have observed that when cells in culture were exposed to relatively mild acidic medium, cell cycle progression is slowed and thus, cell proliferation is slowed initially *(84)*. However, cells adapt eventually to the low-pH environment, and the proliferation rate is restored. It is conceivable that cells adapted to low pH are able to survive and form metastatic foci on distributing to other potentially suboptimal locations in the body.

5. THERAPEUTIC POTENTIAL OF INTRACELLULAR ACIDIFICATION

Indications are that acidification of intracellular environment is cytotoxic to tumor cells *(1,2,58,85–88)*. We have reported that the magnitude of decrease in pHi by inhibitors of pHi regulation is significantly greater in an acidic pHe environment than in neutral pHe environment. For instance, as shown in Fig. 5, a combination of amiloride, DIDS, and nigericin reduced pHi of SCK tumor cells to 6.9 and 6.4 in pH 7.2 and pH 6.6 media, respectively. Rotin et al. *(85)* reported that lowering pHi of tumor cells to 6.5 or lower with nigericin, a K^+/H^+ ionophore, was cytotoxic. Inhibition of the Na^+/H^+ antiport with amiloride or inhibition of the Cl^-/HCO_3^- exchange with DIDS alone was not toxic to the cells, even when the pHe was as low as 6.0. However, combination of amiloride or DIDS with nigericin was toxic to cells at pHe 6.5–6.8. Likewise, carbonylcyanide-3-chlorophenylhydrazine, which transports H^+ into cells, was toxic to tumor cells at pHe lower than 6.5, and its toxicity was greatly enhanced by amiloride or DIDS *(88)*. Apoptosis occurred in human leukemia HL-60 cells when pHi was lowered to 7.2–6.7 by inhibiting pHi regulation *(86,87)*. Increasing in intracellular Ca^{2+} with 4 μM ionomycin, a Ca^{2+} ionophore, further increased the acid-induced apoptosis of HL-60 human leukemia cells. Importantly, the toxicity of various inhibitors of pHi regulation was observed to markedly increase when the cells were heated at 42–44°C *(1,2,9,11,89–97)*.

The direct mechanisms responsible for the cell death caused by low pHi is unclear. We have observed that an exposure of HL-60 human leukemia cells and other tumor cells to an acidic medium induces cell death through apoptosis of cells in G_1 phase *(86,87)*. The acid-induced apoptosis could be further increased when the pHi regulatory mechanisms were inhibited *(86)*. Detailed analysis indicated that a low-pHi environment first upregulates proapoptotic protein Bax, thereby activating caspases followed by poly(ADP-ribose) polymerase cleavage and DNA fragmentation *(87)*. Interestingly, exposing cells to pH 6.2 medium was less effective than exposing to pH 6.4 or pH 6.6 medium in causing apoptosis in HL-60 cells *(87)*. It was concluded that there are optimal pH values for the major events in the apoptosis cascade such as Bax activation, caspase activation and activity, poly(ADP-ribose) polymerase cleavage, and DNA fragmentation so that an extremely acidic environment such as pH 6.2 was less effective than a pH 6.4–6.6 environment in inducing cell death via apoptosis. Recent studies *(98,99)* have indicated that cell death caused by certain chemotherapy drugs was attributable to an acidification of cells as a result of inhibition of pHi regulation mechanisms caused by H_2O_2 produced by mitochondria. These results demonstrate that the pHi regulatory mechanism may be an effective therapy target, because inhibition of pHi regulation will cause a reduction of pHi preferentially in tumor cells in acidic extracellular environment relative to normal cells and thus cause damage preferentially in tumor cells.

6. EFFECT OF pH ON RADIATION DAMAGE

Unlike extensive studies on the effects of hypoxia on radiosensitivity in the past, little has been studied in regard to the effects of acidic pH on radiosensitivity. In a series of studies, we observed that acidic environments markedly prolong radiation-induced G_2 arrest in cancer cells *(84,100–103)*. For example, when RKO human colorectal cancer cells were irradiated with 12 Gy in pH 7.5 medium, the G_2 arrest peaked at 12–16 h, and then the cells progressed into G_1 phase or died of apoptosis. On the other hand, when RKO cells were irradiated with 12 Gy and maintained in pH 6.6 medium, significant portions of cells were still in G_2 arrest 72 h after irradiation (Fig. 6). Interestingly, the radiation-induced G_2 arrest in acidic pH medium rapidly decayed as soon as the acidic pH medium was replaced with neutral pH medium *(100)*. Importantly, the apoptosis and clonogenic cell death caused by irradiation were significantly less in acidic medium than in neutral pH medium (Fig. 7). It appeared that the increase in radioresistance in acidic pH environment resulted from an increased DNA damage repair during the prolonged G_2 arrest. Similar increases in radioresistance in low extracellular pH environment have been reported by others *(104–106)*. Importantly, the environmental pH had to be reduced after treatment in order to confer resistance *(104)*.

Our studies indicate that the prolonged G_2 arrest after irradiation in an acidic pH medium was due, at least in part, to activation of CDC2, which is known to inhibit cyclin B1-CDC2 kinase activity responsible for the progression of cells through G_2/M phase *(101)*. Because the radiation-induced changes in cell cycle progression, apoptosis, and clonogenic cell death are intimately related to p53 expression, we have investigated the effect of pH on the kinetics of p53 expression *(107)*. We found that acidic environments significantly enhance the radiation-induced expression of p53, partly by increasing the formation of p53 and also partly by slowing down the degradation of p53 through inhibition of p53–murine double minute 2 (p53–MdM2) complex formation.

7. EFFECTS OF pH ON HYPERTHERMIA DAMAGE

It is well established that an acidic environment markedly increases thermal damage *(108–114)*. Detailed studies by a number of investigators using different cell lines dem-

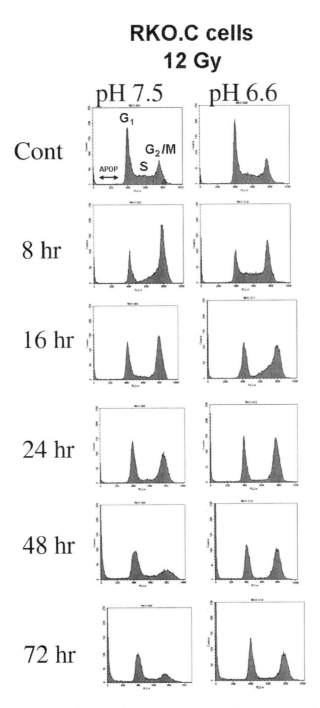

Fig. 6. Cell cycle progression and apoptosis, as demonstrated with flow cytometry, of RKO human colorectal cancer cells after irradiation with 12 Gy in pH 7.5 or pH 6.6 medium. The cell cycle progression was delayed particularly at G_2/M phase after irradiation in pH 6.6 medium compared to the delay caused in pH 7.5 medium.

HL60 cells
4h after 12 Gy in different pHe

pH 7.9 7.5 7.3 7.1 6.9 6.7 6.6 6.6

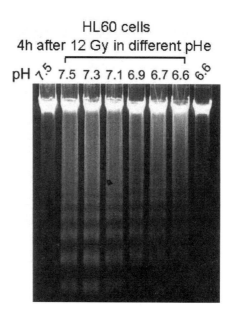

Fig. 7. Apoptotic fragmentation of DNA from HL-60 cells 4 h after irradiation with 12 Gy in different pH media. The radiation-induced apoptosis was markedly suppressed as the medium pH was lowered.

onstrated that pHi, and not pHe, is the determinant of the thermosensitivity *(113,114)*. Hahn and Shiu *(115)* reported that Chinese hamster ovary cells maintained in acidic medium for prolonged periods were not as heat-sensitive as the cells exposed to acidic medium shortly before heating, and concluded that adaptation to a low-pH environment rendered the cells resistant to heat. Cook and Fox *(116)*, and Chu and Dewey *(114)* found that the pHi of the cells that adapted to a low pH environment was significantly higher than the pHi of the unadapted cells. Furthermore, the thermal survival curves of cells adapted and unadapted to a low-pH environment were identical when the survival curves were plotted against pHi instead of pHe. Chu and Dewey *(114)* therefore concluded that the increase in pHi was the reason why cells that adapted to a low-pH environment were resistant to heat at low pHe relative to the unadapted cells. van der Berg et al. *(117)* reported that the thermosensitivity of human tumors showing an acidic interstitial pH was not necessarily greater than the thermosensitivity of tumors showing neutral interstitial pH. They concluded, therefore, that the cells in human tumors adapted to an acidic environment, and thus, the tumor cells were not heat-sensitive despite the low intratumor pH. Conceivably, an acute acid loading to cells adapted to a certain pHe would still render the areas heat-sensitive.

The intratumor pH has been observed to decrease markedly during heating of tumors, probably owing to vascular damage *(3,14,15,20,118)* and to the resultant increase in the accumulation of lactic acid *(119)*. Acute build-up of acidity during heating, particularly in the nonacidic areas, would be expected to sensitize tumor cells to heat. We observed that tumor cells in vivo were far more thermosensitive than the same cells in vitro, and we concluded that the acidic intratumor environment and the further increase in acidity during heating enhanced the thermal damage to the tumor cells *(14,119)*. The vasculature in human tumors has been reported to be more heat-resistant than the vasculature in rodent tumors, and thus, the pH in human tumors may not drop as severely as in animal tumors on heating *(32,120)*. However, it is also quite possible that the human tumors in these previous studies were not adequately heated, and thus, the blood flow as well as the tumor pH remained unchanged. It is likely that both in human tumors or animal tumors, the pH will decrease on application of hyperthermia if heating temperature is high enough to cause vascular damage and induce hypoxia. Along these lines, attempts are being made to sensitize human tumors to hyperthermia by acidifying the tumors using hyperglycemia *(121)*.

8. EFFECT OF pH ON CHEMOTHERAPY

It is known that the influx of drugs into tumor cells will be greatly affected by the pK_a value of the drugs. The acidic extracellular environment in tumors traps weakly basic drugs, thereby hindering the influx of the drugs into cells, whereas it enhances the influx of weakly acidic drugs into cells. Furthermore, the pH gradient between the vesicular compartments and the cytosol of cells has been known to be considerable. Therefore, it is conceivable that weakly basic drugs may be trapped inside the acidic compartments, thereby limiting their cytotoxicity *(122,123)*. It follows that cells containing a larger number of acidic vesicles may be resistant to weakly basic drugs, whereas they may be sensitive to weakly acidic drugs. In addition, intracellular pH may affect the molecular interaction between drugs and their targets such as various intracellular organelles, DNA, RNA, proteins involved in cell cycle progression and cell division, and signals involved in apoptosis. The effect of pH on commonly used anticancer drugs is briefly addressed in this section.

8.1. At Normal Temperatures

Table 2 shows the relative cytotoxicity of various anticancer drugs in acidic (pH < 7.0), neutral (pH 7.0–7.4), and alkaline (pH >7.4) environments. The cytotoxicity of *bis*-chloroethylating agents such as cyclophosphamide and its derivatives, e.g. mafosfamide, nor-nitrogen mustard, melphalan, and chlorambucil, was reported to be significantly increased in acidic pH environments *(124,125)*. Cyclophosphamide is a prodrug, and a low-pH environment accelerated its bioactivation. On the other hand, the cytotoxicity of ifosfamide, an oxazaphosphorine analog of cyclophosphamide, was unaffected by the environmental acidity *(124)*. In ifosfamide, one of the chloroethryl side chains is shifted from an amino nitrogen to a ring nitrogen. Therefore, it was concluded that the *bis*-chloroethyl amine group may be a critical determinant for the H^+ ion-mediated enhancement of cytotoxicity in this group of agents *(124)*. The cytotoxicity of mafosfamide could be enhanced markedly by increasing intracellular acidity with nigericin (K^+/H^+ ionophore) in acidic medium *(124,125)*. Jahde et al. *(124)* concluded that the increase in the cytotoxicity of cyclophospamide and its derivatives in an acidic pH environments were because of an increase in the cellular uptake of the drugs and also to an increase in the monofunctional alkalinization of DNA. It was further concluded that the phase of DNA crosslink formation and that of crosslink removal were relatively independent of the environmental pH. Skarsgard et al. *(126)* reported that a low-pH environment potentiated the cytotoxicity of melphalan and chlorambucil by increasing the uptake of the drugs. Methylmethane sulphonate, a monofunctional alkylate, was reported to be independent of environmental acidity *(115)*. The alkylating potency of *bis*-chloroethylnitrosurea (BCNU) was also independent of environmental acidity *(115)*, whereas that of cyclohexyl-chloroethylnitrosourea was reported to decrease in acidic environment *(127)*.

Table 2
Activity of Drugs Under Various Acidities (pH) and Temperatures

Compounds	37°C			Hyperthermia[a]			Ref.
	<7.0	7.0–7.4	>7.4	<7.0	7.0–7.4	>7.4	
Cyclophosphamide	++	+					122, 124, 125
4-Hydroperoxycyclophosphamide	++	+					124
Mafosamide	++	+					124, 125
Mechlorethamine	++	+					124
Melphalan	++	+					124, 126
Chlorambucil	++	–					122, 124, 126
nor-Nitrogen mustard	++	+					124
Ifosfamide	+	+					124
Triethylenemelamine	++	+					129
Thiophosphamide	++	+					130
MMS	+	+	+	+++	++		115
BCNU	+	+	+	++++	++	+	115, 131
CCNU	+	++					127
Thiotepa	++	+					127
Methotrexate	+	+	+	++	+	+	131
5-Flourouracil	++	+					122
Bleomycin	+	+	+	++++	++	+	115, 131, 134
Mitomycin C	++	+					133
Amphotericin B	+	+	+	+++	++	+++	4, 115, 131
Doxorubicin	+	++					122, 134
Mitoxantrone	+	++					122
Vinblastine	+	++					137
PtCl$_4$(Fast Black)$_2$	++	+		+++	++		141
Cisplatin	+++	+		++++	++	+	115, 139, 141
Plato	+	+		+	++		139
Plant	++	+		++	+		139
Paclitaxel	+	+		+	++		122

MMS, methylmethane sulfonate; BCNU, bis-chloroethylnitrosourea; CCNU, cyclophexylcholroethyl-nitrosourea; Plato, (1,2,-diamino-r-nitrobenzene) dichloroplatinum(II); Plant, trans-bis(2-amino-5-nitrothiazole)dichloroplatinum(II).

[a]The hyperthermia was 42°–44°C.

34

The cytotoxicity of thiotepa, another alkylating agent, increased when the environment was made acidic *(128)*. The cytotoxicity of both triethylenemelamine *(129)* and thiophosphamide *(130)*, alkylating agents, against transplanted rodent tumors was found to be increased when the intratumor environment was made acidic by induction of hyperglycemic. On the other hand, the effect of methotrexate, an antimetabolite known to be very effective against certain cancers, was independent of pH in vitro *(131)*. 5-Fluorouracil is a prodrug and becomes an antimetabolite after intracellular conversion. 5-fluorouracil is a weak acid, and thus, acidic pH environment increases its cellular uptake *(132)*. Mitomycin C, bleomycin, amphotericin B, and doxorubicin (Adriamycin™) are naturally occurring anticancer agents. The cytotoxicity of mitomycin C, a bioreductive alkylating agent, slightly increased when the environmental pH was lowered *(133)*. The increase in mitomycin C cytotoxicity in an acidic environment appeared to be because of an increase in the DNA crosslinking. The cytotoxicity of bleomycin *(115,131,134)* and amphotericin B *(115,131,135)* was unchanged, whereas doxorubicine toxicity declined in an acidic pH environment *(134,136)*. Doxorubicin has a primary amine with a basic pK_a, and thus, its cellular uptake may be reduced in an acidic medium. Indeed, the uptake of doxorubicin at pH 6.6 environment was only one half of that at a pH 7.4 environment *(122,123)*. Furthermore, doxorubicin is trapped and sequestrated in acidic vesicles within the cytoplasm, which prevents the interaction of the drug with its target. A number of agents have been used to enhance the cytotoxicity of doxorubicin by inhibiting the formation of acidic vesicles, thereby releasing the doxorubicin into the cytoplasm *(122,123)*. Vinblastine and vincristine are also naturally occurring anticancer drugs. The uptake of these alkaloids has been reported to decline in an acidic environment *(137)*. The pK_a of vinblastine and vincristine are 5.0–5.5 and 7.4 at physiological pH, respectively. We have reported previously that intracellular acidification alone is able to activate caspases, thereby triggering apoptosis *(86,87)*. Interestingly, apoptosis in cancer cells caused by certain chemotherapy drugs has been attributed to intracellular acidosis caused by the drugs. As mentioned previously, Hirpara et al. *(98)* reported recently that chemotherapy drugs trigger production of H_2O_2 by mitochondria, which then inhibit the Na^+/H^+ exchanger, resulting in intracellular acidification. The resultant intracellular acidification causes mitochondrial recruitment of Bax and release of cytochrome *c* from mitochondria, thereby activating the caspase cascade leading to apoptosis *(98,99)*. Lastly, paclitaxel is one of the taxanes extracted from yew trees and a common chemotherapeutic. It is highly lipophilic and devoid of any ionizable groups, with pK_a values in the physiological range *(139)*. Therefore, the cellular uptake of this drug is independent of pHe. In all, these results clearly indicate that efficacy of many, but not all, anticancer drugs may be significantly increased by altering intratumor pH based on the pK_a value of the drugs.

8.2. At Elevated Temperatures

Although the effect of methylmethane sulphonate *(115)*, BCNU *(115,131)*, methotrexate *(137)*, bleomycin *(115,131,134)*, and amphotericin B *(4,115,131)* were independent of the environmental pH at 37°C, their cytotoxicity increased in a low-pH environment if the cells were heated (*see* Table 2). Interestingly, the cytotoxicity of amphotericin B also increased when the environment was made alkaline at elevated temperatures *(4,115)*. Hahn *(138)* suggested that heat may increase the cellular uptake of certain drugs or inhibit the repair of damage caused by drugs, and the acidic environment accentuates these processes. Related to this, Hahn and Shiu *(115)* reported that the low-pH-adapted cells were resistant to thermochemotherapy with bleomycin, amphotericin B, and cisplatin, but not with BCNU. Thus, it was concluded that the pH dependence of cytotoxicity for some drugs at elevated temperature is affected by the pH history of the target cells.

Cisplatin is platinum complex with potent anticancer activity. The cytotoxicity of this drug increases with an increase in the environmental acidity *(115,139,140)*. Herman et al. *(84)* demonstrated that heating caused a greater increase in the cytotoxicity of cisplatin in an acidic pH environment than in a neutral pH environment. At 37°C and pHe 7.4, no difference in the sensitivity to cisplatin was observed between oxic cells and hypoxic cells. When cells were heated in pH 7.4 medium, the sensitivity of oxic cells to cisplatin markedly increased, whereas that of hypoxic cells remained unchanged. On the other hand, in pH 6.45 medium, the sensitivity of both oxic and hypoxic cells to cisplatin increased on heating. Herman et al. *(139)* also studied the cytotoxicity of analogs of cisplatin such as (1,2-diamino-4-nitrobenzene)dichloroplatinum(II) (Plato) and *trans-bis*-(2-amino-5-nitro-thiazole)dichloroplatinum(II) (Plant) under various conditions. When the environmental acidity was increased, the cytotoxicity of Plato decreased and that of Plant increased. Unlike cisplatin, Plato and Plant were more toxic toward hypoxic cells than oxic cells, but the cytotoxicity of these drugs did not increase with an increase in temperature. Teicher et al. *(140)* reported that the cytotoxicity of $PtCl4(Fast Black)_2$, an analog of cisplatin, was greater in an acidic than in a neutral environment at 37°C, and heating increased the cytotoxicity of this drug in both acidic and neutral pH environments. Oxic cells and hypoxic cells were equally sensitive to this drug at 37°C. However, when heated, oxic cells were slightly more sensitive to this drug in pH 7.4 medium, whereas hypoxic cells were slightly more sensitive to this drug in pH 6.45 medium. Teicher et al. *(141)* observed that the changes in the concentration of cisplatin and $PtCl_4(Fast Black)_2$ in the cells after the environmental pH and temperature were changed did not correlate with the changes in the cytotoxicity, and concluded that an increase in the reaction of the drugs with DNA was the direct cause of the increase in the cytotoxicity of the drugs in a low-pH medium at elevated temperatures. It was also suggested that metabolic changes that must occur to maintain neutral pHi in acidic environment may increase directly or indirectly the response of the cells in an acidic environment to the drugs.

9. ACIDIFICATION AND ALKALINIZATION OF TUMORS

Because an acidic intratumor environment increases the response of tumors to certain chemotherapeutic drugs and also to hyperthermic treatment, various attempts have been made to acidify the intratumor environment. It has long been known that tumors can be acidified by induction of hyperglycemia by administration of excess glucose *(10,142–144)*. It was initially proposed that the decline in the intratumor pH by hyperglycemia resulted from an increase in glucose metabolism by aerobic glycolysis *(144)*. However, indications are that the decline in intratumor pH by hyperglycemia results not only from an increase in aerobic glycolysis, but also from an increase in anaerobic glycolysis as a consequence of blood flow decline and ensuing hypoxia. The mechanisms for the decline in tumor blood flow by hyperglycemia are complicated. A serious problem in using hyperglycemia for induction of acidosis in human tumors is that tumor acidification requires a large dose of glucose exceeding the tolerable level for most patients. Furthermore, the reduction in blood flow by hyperglycemia may decrease the drug delivery to tumor cells. Acidification of rodent tumors by hyperglycemia could be enhanced by concomitant administration of metaiodobenzylguanidine *(82,121)*, which inhibits mito-chondrial respiration at complex I of the electron transport chain, resulting in an increase in lactic acid formation.

Hydralazine, a vasodilator, also decreases tumor blood flow *(145–147)*, and thus, it may increase tumor acidity. As with hyperglycemia, tumor acidification by hydralazine may not be useful to enhance the effects of drugs, because drug delivery to tumors will be reduced owing to the decrease in tumor blood flow that occurs. Furthermore, the effect of hydralazine is strongly dependent on the location of the tumor in the body, and it can reduce blood flow in many normal tissues as well *(146,147)*.

Conversely, the cellular uptake of weakly basic chemotherapy drugs may be enhanced if pHe is raised to alkaline range. Indeed, treatment of tumor-bearing mice with sodium bicarbonate has been demonstrated to cause tumor-specific alkalinization of extracellular pH and increase the antitumor effect of the weakly basic drug, mitoxantrone, which has two ionizable amines with pK_a values of 8.3–8.6 *(123)*. This strategy appears to have limited use because of the dangers of affecting blood chemistry and pH with buffering agents.

10. CONCLUSION

The intratumor environment is acidic because of elevated production of lactic acid and other acidic metabolities as a result of high aerobic and anaerobic glycolysis. However, the pHi of tumor cells is maintained at neutral range despite the acidic pHe by virtue of powerful pHi regulatory mechanisms. Lowering the pHi by inhibitors of pHi regulation is cytotoxic, particularly in a low-pHe environment. The acidic pHe and the gradient between pHe and pHi greatly affect the response of tumor cells to chemotherapy drugs, radiotherapy, and hyperthermia. The feasibility of controlling pHe and pHi by various means with the goal of increasing the response of tumor cells to various treatments is being investigated.

ACKNOWLEDGMENTS

This work was supported by RO1CA-44114 from NIH/NCI awarded to C.W.S and the 2003 Korean National Cancer Grant 03203002-2 and the National Nuclear Technology Program grant from KISTEP awarded to H.J.P. We thank Mr. Brent Williams for his help arranging the figures and tables.

REFERENCES

1. Song CW, Lyon JC, Luo Y. Intra- and extracellular pH in solid tumors: influence on therapeutic response. In: Teicher BV, ed. Drug resistance in oncology. New York: Marcel Dekker, 1993:25–51.
2. Song CW, Park HJ, Ross BD. Intra- and extracellular pH in solid tumors. In Teicher BV, ed. Antiangiogenic adnets in cancer therapy. Totowa: Humana Press, 1998:51–64.
3. Rhee JG, Kim TH, Levitt SH, Song CW. Changes in acidity of mouse tumors by hyperthermia. Int J Radiat Oncol Biol Phys 1985; 10:393–399.
4. Wike-Hooley JL, Haveman J, Reinhold HS. The relevance of tumour pH to the treatment of malignant disease. Radiother Oncol 1984; 2:343–366.
5. Webb SD, Sherratt JA, Fish RG. Mathematical modeling of tumour acidity: regulation of intracellular pH. J Theor Biol 1999; 196:237–250.
6. Gilles RJ, Raghunand N, Karczmar GS, et al. MRI of the tumor microenvironment. J Magn Reson Imaging 2002; 16:430–450.
7. Svastove E, Hulikova A, Rafajova M, et al. Hypoxia activates the capacity of tumor-associated carbonic anhydrase IX to acidify extracellular pH. FEBS Lett 2004; 19:439–435.

8. Aisenberg AC. The glycolysis and respiration of tumors. New York: Academic, 1961.
9. Kim GE, Lyons JC, Levitt SH, Song CW. Effects of amiloride on intracellular pH and thermosensitivity. Int J Radiat Oncol Biol Phys 1991; 20:541–549.
10. Gerweck LE, Rhee JG, Koutcher JA, Song CW, Urano M. Regulation of pH in murine tumor and muscle. Radiat Res 1991; 126:206–209.
11. Lyons JC, Kim GE, Song CW. Modification of intracellular pH and thermosensitivity. Radiat Res 1992; 129:79–87.
12. Lyons JC, Ross B, Song CW. Enhancement of hyperthermia effect in vivo by amiloride and DIDS. Int J Radiat Oncol Biol Phys 1993; 25:95–103.
13. Roos A, Baron WF. Intracellular pH. Physiol Rev 1981; 61:296–434.
14. Song, CW. Effect of local hyperthermia in blood flow and microenvironment: a review. Cancer Res 1984; 44(Suppl):4721s–4730s.
15. Vaupel P, Muller Klieser W, Otte J, Manz R, Kallinowski F. Blood flow, tissue oxygenation and pH distribution in malignant tumors upon localized hyperthermia. Strahlentherapie 1983; 159:73–81.
16. Hetzel FW. Biological rationale for hyperthermia. Radiol Clin North Am 1987; 27:499–508.
17. Dewhirst MW, Gross JF, Sim D, Arnold P, Boyer D. The effect of rate of heating or cooling prior to heating on tumor and normal tissue microcirculatory blood flow. Biorheology 1984; 21:539–558.
18. Jain RK, Ward-Hartely K. Tumor blood flow: characterization, modifications and role in hyperthermia. IEEE Trans Son Ultrason 1984; SU-31:504–526.
19. Song CW. Tumor blood flow response to heat. Funktionsanal Biol Syst 1991; 20:123–141.
20. Reinhold HS, Endrich B. Tumour microcirculation as a target for hyperthermia. Int J Hypertherm 1986; 2:111–137.
21. Jain RK. Determinant of tumor blood flow. A review. Cancer Res 1988; 48:2641–2658.
22. Eddy HA. Microangiographic techniques in the study of normal and tumor tissue vascular systems. Microvasc Res 1976; 11:391–413.
23. Peterson HI. Tumor blood circulation: Angiogenesis, vascular morphology and blood flow of experimental and human tumors. Boca Raton: CRC Press, 1978.
24. Thomlinson RH, Gray LH. The histological structure of some human lung cancers and possible implications for radiotherapy. Br J Cancer 1955; 9:539–549.
25. Jain RK. Physiological barriers to delivery of monoclonal antibodies and other macromolecules in tumors. Cancer Res 1990; 50(Suppl):814s–819s.
26. Hong SS, Lee H, Kim KW. HIF-1a: a valid therapeutic target for tumor therapy. Cancer Res Treat 2004; 36:344–353.
27. Mazure NM, Brahimi-Horn MC, Berta MA, et al. HIF-1: master and commander of the hypoxic world. A pharmacological approach to its regulation by siRNAs. Biochem Pharmacol 2004; 68:971–980.
28. Semenza GL. Targeting HIF-1 for cancer therapy. Nat Rev Cancer 2003; 3:721–732.
29. Griffiths JR, McIntyre DJ, Howe FA, Stubbs M. Why are cancers acidic? A carrier-mediated diffusion model for H+ transport in the interstitial fluid. Novartis Found Symp 2001; 240:46–62.
30. Busa WB, Nuccitelli R. Metabolic regulation via intracellular pH. Am J Physiol 1984; 246:R409–R438.
31. Schornack PA, Gillies RJ. Contribution of cell metabolisms and H+ diffusion to the acidic pH of tumors. Neoplasia 2002; 5:135–145.
32. van der Berg AP. Tissue pH of human tumors and its variation upon therapy in tumor blood supply and metabolic microenvironment. Funktionsanal Biol Syst 1991; 20:234–235.
33. Hinke JA. Ction-selective microelectrodes for intracellular use. In: Eiserman G, ed. Glass electrodes for hydrogen and other cations. New York: Marcel Dekker, 1967:474–477.
34. Thomas RC. New design of a sodium-sensitive glass microelectrode. J Physiol 1970; 210:829–839.
35. Lin J-C, Levitt SH, Song CW. Relationship between vascular thermotolerance and intratumor pH. Int J Radiat Oncol Biol Phys 1991; 22:123–129.
36. Vaupel PW, Frinak S, Bicher HI. Heterogenous oxygen partial pressure and pH distribution in C3H mouse mammary adenocarcinoma. Cancer Res 1981; 41:2008–2013.
37. Ja'hde E, Rajewsky MF, Ba'umgart H. pH distribution in transplanted neural tumors and normal tissues of BDIX rats as measured with pH microelectrodes. Cancer Res 1982; 42:1498–1504.
38. Meyer KA, Kammerling EM, Amtan L, et al. pH studies of malignant tissues in human being. 1948; 8:513–518.
39. Pampus F. Die Wasserstoffionenkonzentration des Hirngewebes bei raumfordernden intracraniellen Prozessen. Acta Neurochir 1963; 11:305–318.

40. Ashby BS. pH studies in human malignant tumours. Lancet 1966; 2:312–315.
41. Thistlethwaite AJ, Leeper DB, Moylan DJ, et al. pH distribution in human tumors. Int J Radiat Oncol Biol Phys 1985; 11:1647–1652.
42. Wike-Hooley JL, van den Berg AP, van der Zee J, Reinhold HS. Human tumour pH and its variation. Eur J Cancer Clin Oncol 1985; 21:785–791.
43. van den Berg AP, Wike-Hooley JL, van den Berg-Blok AE, et al. Tumour pH in human mammary carcinoma. Eur J Cancer Clin Oncol 1982; 18:457–462.
44. Inch WR, Direct current potential and pH of several varieties of skin neoplasms. Can J Biochem Physiol 1954; 32:519–525.
45. Millet H. Measurements of the pH of normal, fetal, and neoplastic tissues by means of the glass electrode. J Biol Chem 1923; 78:281–288.
46. Naeslund J, Senson KE. Investigations on the pH of malignant tumors in mice and humans after the administration of glucose. Acta Obstet Gynecol Scand 1953; 32:359–367.
47. Vaupel P, Kallinowski F, Okunieff P. Blood flow, oxygen and nutrient supply, and metabolic microenvironment of human tumours: a review. Cancer Res 1989; 49:6449–6465.
48. Griffiths JR. Are cancer cells acidic? Br J Cancer 1991; 64:425–427.
49. Engin K, Leeper DB, Cater JR, et al. Extracellular pH distribution in human tumours. Int J Hyperthermia 1995; 11:211–216.
50. Eden M, Haines B, Kahler H. The pH of rat tumors measured in vivo. J Natl Cancer Inst 1955; 16:541–556.
51. Evanochko WT, Ng TC, Lilly, MB, et al. In vivo ^{31}P-NMR study of the metabolism of murine mammary 16/C adenocarcinoma and its response to chemotherapy, x-irradiation and hyperthermia. Proc Natl Acad Sci U S A 1983; 80:334–338.
52. Gillies RJ, Ogina T, Shulman RG, Ward DC. ^{31}P nuclear magnetic resonance evidence for the regulation of intracellular pH by Ehrlich ascites tumor cells. J Cell Biol 1982; 95:24–28.
53. Evelhoch JL, Sapareto SA, Jick DEL, Ackerman JJH. In vivo metabolic effects of hyperglycemia in murine radiation induced fibrosarcoma: a ^{31}P-NMR investigation. Proc Natl Acad Sci U S A 1984; 81:6496–6500.
54. Okunieff PG, Koutcher JA, Gerweck L, et al. Tumor size dependent metabolic changes in a murine fibrosarcoma: use of Fourier transformed ^{31}P-NMR to evaluate energy metabolism. Int J Radiat Oncol Biol Phys 1986; 12:793–799.
55. Madshus IH. Regulation of intracellular pH in eukaryotic cells. J Biochem 1988; 250:1–8.
56. Grinstien S, Rothstein S. Mechanisms of regulation of the Na^+/H^+ exchanger. J Membrane Biol 1986; 90:1–12.
57. Frelin C, Vigne P, Ladoux A, Lazdunski M. The regulation of the intracellular pH in cells from vertebrates. Eur J Biochem 1988; 174: 3–14.
58. Tannock, IF, Rotin D. Acid pH in tumors and its potential for therapeutic exploitation. Cancer Res 1989; 49:4373–4384.
59. Aronson PS. Kinetic properties of the plasma membrane Na^+/H^+ exchange. Annu Rev Physiol 1985; 47:545–560.
60. Cassel D, Katz M, Rotman M. Depletion of cellular ATP inhibits Na^+/H^+ antiport in cultured human cells. Modulation of the regulatory effect of intracellular protons on the antiporter activity. J Biol Chem 1986; 261:5460–5466.
61. Zhung YX, Cragoe EJ Jr, Glaser L, Cassel D. Characterization of potent Na^+/H^+ exchange inhibitor from the aniloride series in A431 cells. Biochemistry 1984; 23:4481–4488.
62. Cassel D, Scharf O, Rotman M, et al. Characterization of Na^+-linked and Na^+-independent Cl^-/HCO_3^- exchange systems in Chinese hamster lung fibroblasts. J Biol Chem 1988; 263:6122–6127.
63. Boron WF. Intracellular pH regulation in epithelial cells. Am Rev Physiol 1986; 43:377–388.
64. Jentsch TJ, Matthes H, Keller SK, Wiederholt M. Carrier-mediated reabsorption of small peptides in renal proximal tribute. Am J Physiol 1986; 251:F945–F968.
65. Grassl SM, Aronson PS. Na^+/CHO_3^- Co-transport in basolateral membrane vesicles isolated from rabbit renal cortex. J Biol Chem 1986; 26:8778–8783.
66. Hutton JC. The internal pH and membrane potential of the insulin-secretory granule. J Biochem 1982; 204:171–178.
67. Thomas RC. Ionic mechanism of the H^+ pump in a snail neurone. Nature 1976; 262: 54–55.
68. Russell JM, Boron WF. Role of chloride transport in regulation of intracellular pH. Nature 1976; 264:73–74.

69. Boron WF, Hogan E., Russell JM. pH-sensitive activation of the intracellular-pH regulation system in squid axons by ATP-γ-S. Nature 1988: 332:2672–265.
70. Moolenaar WH, Tertoolen LGL, de Laat SW. The regulation of cytoplasmic pH in human fibroblasts. J Biol Chem 1984; 259:7563–7569.
71. Belt JA, Thomas JA, Buchsbaum RN, Racker E. Inhibition of lactate transport and glycolysis in Ehrlich ascites tumor cells by bioflavanoids. Biochemistry 1979; 18:3506–3511.
72. Kim JH, Kim SH, ALdieri AA, Young CW. Quercetin, an inhibitor of lactate transport and hyperthermic sensitizer of HeLa cells. Cancer Res 1984; 44:102–106.
73. Turpaev KT. Reactive oxygen species and regulation of gene expression. Biochemistry (Mosc) 2002; 67:281–292.
74. Subarsky P, Hill RP. The hypoxic tumour microencironment and metastatic progression. Clin Exp Metastasis 2003; 20:237–250.
75. Le QT, Denko NC, Giaccia AJ. Hypoxic gene expression and metastasis. Cancer Metastasis Rev 2004; 23:293–310.
76. Vaupel P, Kelleher DK, Hockel M. Oxygen status of malignant tumors: pathogenesis of hypoxia and significance for tumor therapy. Semin Oncol 2001; 28:29–35.
77. Ohtsubo T, Wang X, Takahashi A, et al. p53-dependent induction of WAF1 by low pH culture condition in human glioblastoma cells. Cancer Res 1997; 57:3910–3913.
78. Griffiths L, Dachs GU, Bicknell R, et al. Influence of oxygen tension and pH on the expression of platelet-derived endothelial cells growth factor/thymidine phosphorylase in human breast tumor cells growth in vitro and in vitro. Cancer Res 1997; 57:570–572.
79. Schlappack OK, Zimmermann A, Hill RP. Glucose starvation and acidosis: effect on experimental metastatic potential, DNA content and MTX resistance of murine tumour cells. Br J Cancer 1991; 64:663–670.
80. Jang A, Hill RP. An examination of the effects of hypoxia, acidosis, and glucose starvation on the expression of metastasis-associated genes in murine tumor cells. Clin Exp Metastasis 1997; 15:469–483
81. Hill RP, Jaeger KD. Jang A, Cairns R. pH, hypoxia and metastasis. The tumor microenvironment: causes and consequences of hypoxia and acidity. Chichester: Wiley, 2001:154–168.
82. Kalliomaki T, Hill RP. Effects of tumour acidification with glucose+MIBG on the spontaneous metastatic potential of two murine cell lines. Br J Cancer 2004: 90:1842–1849
83. Rofstad EK. Microenvironment-induced cancer metastasis. Int J Radiat Biol 2000; 76:589–605.
84. Park HJ, Lyons JC, Griffin RJ, Lim BU, Song CW. Apoptosis and cell cycle progression in an acidic environment after irradiation. Radiat Res 2000; 153:295–304.
85. Rotin D, Wan P, Grinstien S, Tannock I. Cytotoxicity of compounds that interfere with the regulation of intracellular pH: a potential new class of anticancer drugs. Cancer Res 1987; 47:1497–1505.
86. Park HJ, Makepeace CM, Lyons JC, Song CW. Effect of intracellular acidity and ionomycin on apoptosis in HL-60 cells. Eur J Cancer 1996; 32A:540–546.
87. Park HJ, Lyons JC, Ohtsubo T, Song CW. Acidic environment causes apoptosis by increasing caspase activity. Br J Cancer 1999; 80:1892–1897.
88. Newell KT, Tannock I. Reduction of intracellular pH as a possible mechanism for killing cells in acidic regions of solid tumors: effect of carbonylcyanide03-chrophgenylhydrazone. Cancer Res 1989; 49:4477–4482.
89. Haveman J. The pH of the cytoplasm as an important factor in the survival of vitro cultured malignant cells after hyperthermia. Effects of carbonylcyanide-3-chlorophenylhyrazone. Eur J Cancer 1979; 15:1281–1288.
90. Miyakoshi J, Oda W, Harata M, et al. Effects of amiloride on thermosensitivity of Chinese hamster cells under neutral and acidic pH. Cancer Res 1986; 46:1840–1843.
91. Ruifrok ACC, Konings AWTR. Effects of amiloride on hyperthermic cell killing of normal and thermotolerant mouse fibroblast LM cells. Int J Radiat Biol 1987; 52:385–392.
92. Varnes Me, Glazver KG, Gray C. pH-dependent effects of the ionophore nigericin on response of mammalian cells to radiation and heat treatment. Radiat Res 1989; 117:285–292.
93. Song CW, Lyons JC, Griffin RJ, et al. Increase in thermosensitivity of tumor cells by lowering intracellular pH. Cancer Res 1993; 53:1599–1601.
94. Song CW, Lyons JC, Griffin RJ, Makepeace CM. Thermosensitization by lowering intracellular pH with EIPA. Radiother Oncol 1993; 27:252–258.
95. Song CW, Lyons JC, Makepeace CM, et al. Effects of HMA, an analog of amiloride, on the thermosensitivity of tumors in vivo. Int J Radiat Oncol Biol Phys 1994; 30:133–139.

96. Song CW, Kim GE, Lyons JC, et al. Thermosensitization by increasing intracellular acidity with amiloride and its analogs. Int. J Radiat Oncol Biol Phys 1994; 30:1161–1169.

97. Takasu T, Lyons JC, Park HJ, Song CW. Apoptosis and perturbation of cell cycle progression by hyperthermia in an acidic environment. Cancer Res 1998; 58:2504–2508.

98. Hirpara JL, Clements MV, Pervaiz A. Intracellular acidification triggered by mitochondrial-derived hydrogen peroxide is an effector mechanism for drug-induced apoptosis in tumor cells. J Biol Chem 2001; 276:514–521.

99. Ahmad KS, Iskandar KB, Hirpara JL, et al. Hydrogen peroxide-mediated cytosolic acidification is a signal for mitochondrial translocation of Bax during drug-induced apoptosis of tumor cells. Cancer Res 2004; 64:7867–7878.

100. Lee H-S, Park HJ, Lyons JC, et al. Radiation-induced apoptosis in different pH environments in vitro. Int J Radiat Oncol Biol Phys 1997; 38:1079–1087.

101. Park HJ, Lyons JC, Ohtsubo T, Song CW. Cell cycle progression and apoptosis after irradiation in an acidic environment. Cell Death Differ 2000; 7:729–738.

102. Ohtsubo T, Igawa H, Saito T, et al. Acidic environment modifies heat- or radiation-induced apoptosis in human maxillary cancer cells. Int J Radiation Oncology Biol Phys 2001; 49:1391–1399.

103. Park HJ, Lee SH, Chung H, et al. Influence of environmental pH on G2-phase arrest caused by ionizing radiation. Radiat Res 2003; 159:86–93.

104. Freeman ML, Sierra E. An acidic extracellular environment reduces the fixation of DNA damage. Radiat Res 1984; 97:154–161.

105. Holahan EV. Stuart PK, Dewey WC. Enhancement of survival of CHO cells by acidic pH after X-irradiation. Radiat Res 1982; 89:433–435.

106. Haveman J. The influence of pH on the survival after X-irradiation of cultured malignant cells. Effects of carbonylbyanide 3-chlorophenylhydrazone. Int J Radiat Biol 1980; 37:201–205.

107. Choi EK, Robert K, Gfiffin RJ, et al. Effect of pH on radiation-induced p53 expression. Int J Radiat Oncol Biol Phys 2004; 60:1264–1271.

108. Freeman ML, Dewey WC, Hopewood LE. Effect of pH on hyperthermic cell killing: brief communication. J Natl Cancer Inst 1977; 58:1837–1839.

109. Gerweck LE. Modification of cell lethality at elevated temperatures. Radiat Res 1977; 70:224–235.

110. Gerweck LE, Dahlberg WK, Greco B. Effect of pH on single or fractionated heat treatment at 42–45°C. Cancer Res 1983; 43:1163–1167.

111. Nlsen OS, Overgaard J. Effect of extracellular pH on thermotolerance and recovery of hyperthermia damage in vitro. Cancer Res 1979; 39:2772–2778.

112. Goldin EM, Leeper DB. The effect of reduced pH on the induction of thermotolerance. Radiology 1981; 141:505–508.

113. KG Hofer, Mivichi NF. Tumor cell sensitivity to hyperthermia as a function of extracellular and intracellular pH. J Natl Cancer Inst 1980; 65:621–625.

114. Chu GL, Dewey WC. The role of low intracellular or extracellular pH in sensitization of hyperthermia. Radiat Res 1988; 11:4154–167.

115 Hahn GM, Shiu E. Adaptation of low pH modified thermal and thermochemical response of mammalian cells. Int J Hypertherm 1986; 2:379–387.

116. Cook JA, Fox MH. Effects of acute pH 6.6 and 42.0°C heating on the intracellular pH of Chinese hamster cells. Cancer Res 1988; 48:497–502.

117. van den Berg A, Wike-Hooley JL, Broekmayer-Reurink MP, van der Zee J, Reinhold HS. The relationship between the unmodified initial tissue pH of human tumors and the response to combined radiotherapy and local hyperthermia treatment. Eur J Cancer Clin Oncol 1989; 25:73–78.

118. Hetzel FW, Avery K, Chopp M. Hyperthermic "dose" dependent changes in intralesional pH. Int J Radiat Oncol Biol Phys 1989; 16:183–186.

119. Kang, MS, Song CW, Levitt SH. The role of vascular function in the response of tumors in vivo to hyperthermia. Cancer Res 1980; 40:1130–1135.

120. Thistlethwaite AJ, Leeper DB, Moylan DJ, Nerlinger RE. pH distribution in human tumors. Int J Radiat Oncol Biol Phys 1985; 11:1647–1652.

121. Canter RJ, Zhou R, Kesmodel SB, et al. Metaiodobenzylguanidine and hyperglycemia augment tumor response to isolated limb perfusion in a rodent model of human melanoma. Ann Surg Oncol 2004; 11:265–273.

122. Mahoney BP, Raghunand N, Baggett B, et al. Tumor acidity, ion trapping and chemotherapeutics. I. Acid pH affects the distribution of chemotherapeutic agents in vitro. Biochem Pharmacol 2003; 66:1207–1218.

123. Raghunand N, Mahoney BP, Gilles RJ. Tumor acidity, ion trapping and chemotherapeutics. II. pH-dependent partition coefficients predict importance of ion trapping on pharmacokinetics of weakly basic chemotherapeutic agents. Biochem Pharmacol 2003; 66:1219–1229.
124. Jahde E, Glusenkamp KH, Klunder I, Hulser DF, Tietze LF, Rajewsky MF. Hydrogen ion-mediated enhancement of cytotoxicity of bis-chlorethylating drugs in rat mammary carcinoma cells in vitro. Cancer Res 1989; 49:2965–2972.
125. Jahde E, Glusenkamp KH, Rajewsky MF. Nigericin enhances mafosfamide cytotoxicity at a low extracellular pH. Cancer Chemother Pharmcol 1991; 27:440–444.
126. Skarsgard LD, Chaplin DJ, Wilson DJ, et al. The effect of hypoxia and low pH on the cytotoxicity of melphalan and chlorambucil in vitro (abstract 23). Proceedings of the 7th International Conference on Chemical Modifiers of Cancer Treatment, Clearwarter, Florida, 2–5 Feb 1992.
127. Kwok TT, Twentyman PR. Effects of changes in oxygen tension, pH and glucose concentration on the response to CCNU and EMT6 mouse tumor monolayer cells and multicellular spheroids. Int J Radiat Oncol Biol Phys 1988; 14:1221–1229.
128. Euler J, Sauerman G, Priesching A. Wirkung von temperature, pH und thiotepa auf angehraten und thymodineinbau von aszitestumorzellen. Wien Klin Wocheschr 1974; 86:211–219.
129. Connors TA, Mitchley BCV, Rosenoer VM, Ross WCJ. The effect of glucose pretreatment on the cardinostatic and toxic activities of some alkylating agents. Biochem Pharm 1964; 13:395–400.
130. Oskinsky S, Bubnovskyja L, Sergienko T. Tumor pH under induced hyperglycemia and efficacy of chemotherapy. Anticancer Res 1987; 7:199–202.
131. Hahn GM, Shiu EC. Effect of pH and elevated temperatures on cytotoxicity of some chemotherapeutic agents on Chinese hamster cells in vitro. Cancer Res 1983; 43:5789–5791.
132. Ojugo AS, McSheehy PM, Stubbs M, et al. Influence of pH on the uptake of 5-fluorouracil into isolated tumour cells. Br J Cancer 1998; 77:873–879.
133. Kennedy KA, McGurl JD, Leondaridis L, Alabaster O. pH dependent of mitomycin C-induced cross linking activity in MET6 tumor cells. Cancer Res 1985; 45:3541–3547.
134. Urano M, Kahn J, Kenton LA. Effect of bleomycin on murine tumor cells at elevated temperatures and two different pH values. Cancer Res 1988; 48:616–619.
135. Born R, Eicholtz-Wirth H. Effect of different physiological conditions on the action of Adriamycin on Chinese hamster cells in vitro. Br J Cancer 1981; 44:241–246.
136. Hindenberg AA, Stewart VJ, Baker MA, Taub RN. Effect of pH on cellular accumulation of duanorubicvin. Am Assoc Cancer Res 1987; 28:261 (abstract no. 1031).
137. Ferguson PJ, Phillips JR, Selner M, Case CE. Differential activity of vincristine and vinblastine against cultured cells. Cancer Res 1984; 44:3307–3312.
138. Vukovic V, Tannock IF. Influence of low pH on cytotoxicity of paclitaxel mitoxantrone and topotecan. Br J Cancer 1997; 75:1167–1172.
139. Hahn GM. Hyperthermia to enhance drug delivery. In: Rational basis for chemotherapy. New York: Alan R. Liss, 1983:427–436.
140. Herman TS, Teicher BA, Collins LS. Effect of hypoxia and acidosis on the cytotoxicity of four platinum complexes at normal and hyperthermic temperatures. Cancer Res 1988; 48:2342–2347.
141. Teicher BA, Herman TS, Pfeffer MR, et al. Interaction of $PtCl_4(Fast Black)_2$ with hyperthermia. Cancer Res 1989; 49:6208–6219.
142. Ward JH, DipPette DJ, Held TN, Jain RK. Effect of intravenous versus intraperitoneal glucose injection on systemic hemodynamics and blood flow rate in normal and tumor tissues in rats. Cancer Res 1991; 51:3612–3616.
143. Vaupel PW, Okunieff PG. Role of hypovolemic hemoconcentration in dose-dependent flow decline observed in murine tumors after interperitoneal administration of glucose or mannitol. Cancer Res 1988; 48:7102–7106.
144. Calderwood SK, Dickson JA. Effect of hyperglycemia on blood flow, pH and response to hyperthermia (42°C) of the Yoshida sarcoma in the rat. Cancer Res 1980; 40:4728–4733.
145. Voorhees WD, Babbs CF. Hydralazine-enhanced selective heating of transmissible venereal tumor implanted in dogs. Eur J Cancer Clin Oncol 1982; 19:1027–1033.
146. Lin J-C, Song CW. Effects of hydralazine on the blood flow in RIF-1 tumors and normal tissues of mice. Radiat Res 1990; 124:171–177.
147. Hasegawa T, Song CW. Effect of hydralazine on the blood flow in tumors and normal tissues of rats. Int J Radiat Oncol Biol Phys 1991; 20:1001–1007.

3 Tumor Oxygenation and Treatment Response

Sarah Jane Lunt, PhD and Richard P. Hill, PhD

CONTENTS

INTRODUCTION
HYPOXIA IN TUMORS
MARKERS OF HYPOXIA
TUMOR HYPOXIA AND DISEASE PROGRESSION
TUMOR HYPOXIA AND GENOMIC INSTABILITY
HYPOXIA-MEDIATED GENE EXPRESSION
HYPOXIA-TARGETED THERAPY
SUMMARY
REFERENCES

SUMMARY

Solid tumor oxygenation is highly heterogeneous, often showing regions of hypoxia that demonstrate oxygen concentrations much lower than those encountered in normal tissues. Tumor hypoxia can cause treatment resistance, resulting in a poorer treatment outcome. In addition, hypoxia forms a part of the pathophysiologic microenvironment that characterizes solid tumors and is involved in disease progression, possibly through alterations in gene expression. This chapter discusses recent research focused on methods of measuring tumor hypoxia accurately and extensively, with the aim of tailoring treatment on an individual patient basis. Examples of therapeutic approaches designed to exploit tumor hypoxia directly or indirectly, are discussed.

Key Words: Tumor hypoxia; HIF-1; hypoxic markers; bioreductive drugs; gene-directed enzyme prodrug therapy.

1. INTRODUCTION

Tissue oxygenation is the result of a balance between oxygen supply and consumption, a balance that is finely regulated in normal tissues. In solid tumors this balance is disturbed, such that the supply is no longer adequate, resulting in hypoxia. The definition of hypoxia varies between studies, and the term has been used to describe severe oxygen deprivation, near 0 mmHg, or oxygen levels (~15–20 mmHg) approaching those of

From: *Cancer Drug Discovery and Development: Cancer Drug Resistance*
Edited by: B. Teicher © Humana Press Inc., Totowa, NJ

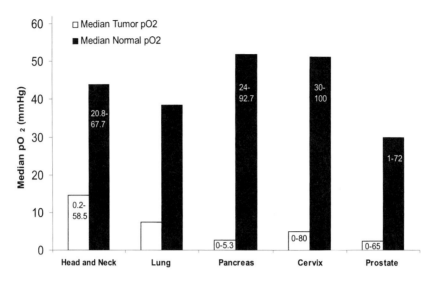

Fig. 1. Differences in median pO_2 of normal tissue (black bar) vs tumor tissue (white bar). The range of pO_2 values are shown within the bars for head and neck *(118)*, pancreas *(119)*, cervix *(120)*, and prostate cancers *(58)*. The median values for the lung samples were taken from Brown and Wilson *(6)*, and no range was available.

normal, well-oxygenated tissue. Experimentally, hypoxia is often used to describe pO_2 values below ~7.5 mmHg. Solid tumors demonstrate a low median pO_2 of ~5–20 mmHg, as compared to most normal tissues (median pO_2 of ~20–95 mmHg). Representative values for human tumors are shown in Fig. 1. Tumor oxygenation is highly heterogeneous, both within an individual tumor and between tumors *(1)*. Hypoxia in tumors has long been known to induce resistance to both radiation and chemotherapy, and clinically median oxygen partial pressures (pO_2) below ~10 mmHg are generally found to be associated with poorer treatment outcome. There is also mounting evidence of a role for tumor hypoxia in tumor progression *(2)*. As a consequence of the negative impact of tumor hypoxia on treatment outcome, recent research has focused on further elucidating the role of hypoxia in disease progression *(2,3)*, on methods of measuring tumor hypoxia accurately and extensively *(4,5)*, and on exploiting tumor hypoxia to improve treatment response *(6,7)*. This chapter provides an overview of each of these three areas.

2. HYPOXIA IN TUMORS

The tumor microenvironment is characterized by several pathophysiologic conditions including tumor hypoxia, reduced pH, and elevated interstitial fluid pressure, all of which are, to varying extents, a consequence of the disorganized structure and function of the abnormal vasculature that characterizes solid tumors *(8)*. Tumor growth and development is supported by both the pre-existing host vasculature and by neovasculature generated through the process of angiogenesis. Studies using tumors growing in window chambers have shown that this process may be initiated early in tumor growth when the tumor comprises 60–80 cells *(9)*. The host vessels do not increase in number during tumor growth (initially they may actually regress) *(10)*, and consequently, the number of preexisting vessels is reduced in comparison to the area they supply. Furthermore, the host venules undergo morphological changes including elongation and dilation, and may become obstructed or compressed by the surrounding tumor cells *(11)*. The arterioles remain largely intact, but are restricted to the fascial surface of the tumor, resulting in longer transport distances through the arteriolar tumor supply vessels *(12)*. The neovasculature that develops through angiogenesis is highly chaotic, resulting in further spatial heterogeneity. The vessels formed are immature and demonstrate several abnormalities, being dilated, tortuous, and lacking in enervation. They often have an incomplete or missing endothelial cell layer and basement membrane that makes them more permeable *(13)*. In addition, they are prone to excessive branching, blind ends and neovascular shunts (Fig. 2). These abnormalities result in increased geometric resistance, plasma channels containing few or no red blood cells, and longitudinal pO_2 gradients, all of which contribute to aberrant flow and the development of a pathophysiologic tumor microenvironment that is extremely heterogeneous, both within an individual tumor and between different tumor types *(1,8,11)*.

The existence of hypoxic cells in tumors was highlighted in 1955 by Thomlinson and Gray, who noted that regions of necrosis were often observed in human lung cancers at distances of 160–200 μm away from the supporting vasculature. As these distances were consistent with the calculated diffusion distances of oxygen from the capillary network, it was suggested that viable chronically hypoxic cells alongside regions of necrosis were a feature of solid tumors as a consequence of oxygen diffusion limitations *(14)*. The diffusion radius of oxygen depends on the rate of oxygen consumption by the cells and the pO_2 in the adjacent vessel(s); thus, the distance from the blood vessels to the edge of the necrotic region (sometimes called the tumor cord radius) may vary from tumor to tumor and within tumors because of declining levels of oxygen and pO_2 in the vasculature as it progresses through the tumor parenchyma. In addition, the existence of a highly chaotic vascular network and plasma channels as well as rheologic effects, such as altered blood viscosity and subsequent slow flow rates, can lead to the development of regions of hypoxia in areas that would appear to have an adequate vascular network, possibly through a reduction in the intravessel blood oxyhemoglobin saturation. Oxyhemoglobin saturation levels in a tumor can be much lower than those in normal vessels, possibly because of increased oxygen consumption to facilitate rapid proliferation or through an increase in extraction of oxygen from hemoglobin at low pO_2 as a result of sluggish flow *(8)*.

Oxygen diffusion limitations may be expected to give rise to tumor cells that are hypoxic over extended periods of time, referred to as chronically hypoxic cells. However, there are also regions in tumors that fluctuate between normoxic and hypoxic states, and this is referred to as acute, transient, or perfusion-limited hypoxia. The existence of transiently hypoxic tumor cells was investigated in studies using fluorescent dyes that stain cells adjacent to functional vasculature. The administration of two dyes either simultaneously or sequentially showed colocalization only for simultaneous administration. With sequential administration, there was mismatch in the staining patterns of these dyes, consistent with variations in perfusion *(15)*. This study went on to demonstrate that differences in vascular flow were reflective of differences in viable hypoxic cells in the tumors over time. Fluctuations in tumor blood flow were also observed by direct measurements of regional blood flow using laser Doppler techniques *(16)*, and indirectly by measuring temporal changes in tumor temperature *(17)*.

However, the situation is at once more complex and more subtle. The dye mismatch studies could only identify fluctuating flow and acute hypoxia as a result of complete

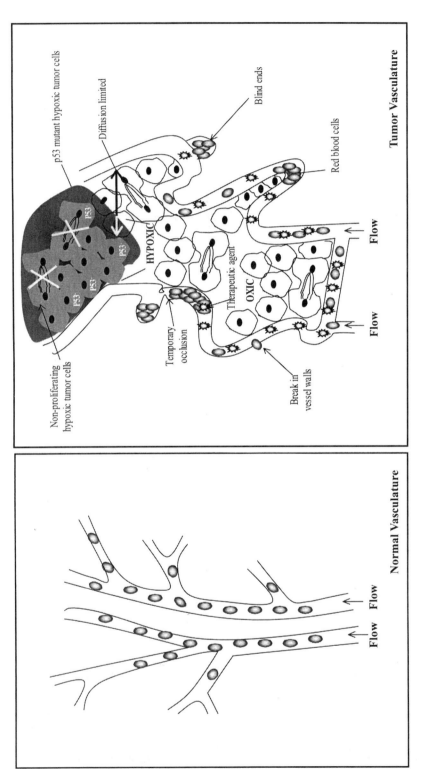

Fig. 2 Schematic representation of normal vasculature versus tumor vasculature, illustrating the development of tumor hypoxia and potential methods of drug resistance. Normal vasculature shows several structural abnormalities as indicated on the figure. Tumor vasculature is evenly spaced and organized, ensuring a sufficient supply of oxygen and nutrients. Tumor vasculature shows several structural abnormalities as indicated on the figure. These abnormalities lead to functional deficiencies, which result in regions of hypoxia and drug resistance. Temporary occlusions in the vasculature may lead to perfusion limited hypoxia. They may also block the delivery of therapeutic agents. The tortuous nature of the vasculature and abnormalities such as blind ends combined with sluggish blood flow can lead to diffusion limited hypoxia. These diffusion limitations may reduce the efficacy of many conventional drugs. Hypoxia may also select for nutrients. Hypoxia *per se* may reduce cell proliferation, which reduces the efficacy of many conventional drugs. Hypoxia may also select for p53 mutant cell lines with increased apoptotic resistance and consequently increased resistance to some drugs. (Modified from ref. 6.)

occlusion and subsequent reopening of the vessels, whereas studies measuring red cell flux over a two hour period demonstrated that complete occlusion may be a relatively rare event *(18)*. More recent data from studies focused on measuring changes in tissue pO_2 continuously over 30- to 90-min periods demonstrated frequent fluctuations above and below 5 mmHg *(19,20)*. This is suggestive of a higher frequency of tumor cell exposure to cyclic hypoxia-reoxygenation than previously anticipated. The impact of this cyclic hypoxia on tumor progression and therapeutic response is not well established, although a major product of hypoxia-reoxygenation is the reactive oxygen species, superoxide anion, which could result in enhanced mutagenic frequency, potentially contributing to tumor progression.

Hypoxic cells are known to be approximately three times more resistant to ionizing radiation than oxygenated cells, because oxygen can chemically modify, and thus prevent, direct chemical repair of the damage caused by the initial radiation-induced radicals *(21)*. The oxygen level required for half-maximal sensitization to radiation is widely reported to be about 3 mmHg for mammalian cells, but recent work has suggested that the value may be higher in tumors (~7.5 mmHg) because of higher levels of nonprotein sulphydryls, particularly cysteine *(22)*.

The role of hypoxia in resistance to chemotherapeutic drugs is less well defined, but there are several proposed mechanisms. Hypoxic areas distant from functional vasculature will have limited diffusion of therapeutic agents, as will cells surrounding chaotic vasculature and plasma channels where perfusion may be limited. Reduced drug delivery is likely to be associated with reduced efficacy. Furthermore, many traditional chemotherapeutic agents were designed to target dividing cells. Under hypoxic conditions cellular proliferation is reduced, impacting negatively on the cytotoxic effects of these agents. Additionally, some drugs require oxygen to modify DNA damage, similar to radiotherapy *(6,23)*. As well as these physiological constraints, hypoxia contributes to genetic and epigenetic changes *(2)* including the upregulation of several genes involved in drug resistance and the selection of cells with p53 mutations, which can increase cellular resistance to apoptosis and reduce drug sensitivity (*see* Fig. 2) *(6)*.

3. MARKERS OF HYPOXIA

The link between solid tumor hypoxia and both treatment resistance and disease progression makes the ability to measure tumor hypoxia accurately and extensively extremely desirable. As such, different approaches have been, and are being, examined to achieve this aim and thus tailor treatment accordingly. The majority of clinical data relating tumor hypoxia to treatment resistance and/or disease progression is based currently on pO_2 measurements taken using the Eppendorf polarographic electrode system *(5,24)*. This system involves a fine-needle probe with a sampling volume of approximately 500 cells that automatically progresses through the tissue in a stepping motion, thereby measuring pO_2 at multiple points within a tumor *(25)*. However, the system is limited to easily accessible tumors and does not distinguish regions of necrosis, or even normal cells. Furthermore, the Eppendorf electrode gives no information as to the location or kinetics of tumor hypoxia, in relation to proximity to the vasculature or the acute versus chronic hypoxia status of the cells in the hypoxic region. To overcome these limitations, there have been numerous studies into alternative methods of measuring tumor hypoxia, with particular attention paid to the use of exogenous and endogenous markers that can be used with biopsy specimens. Alternative mechanisms of measuring tumor hypoxia would need to fulfill certain criteria for successful application in the clinic, in particular that they are associated with prognosis. Ideally, the degree of hypoxia would also correlate to results obtained using the Eppendorf electrode, the current gold standard. In addition, some method of standardization, both in the biopsy procedure and subsequent analyses would be required to validate widespread use.

3.1. Exogenous Markers

Three alternative possibilities for evaluating tumor hypoxia are exogenous markers (2-nitroimidazoles), endogenous markers (genes upregulated by hypoxia), and noninvasive imaging. Each of these methods has potential advantages and limitations. The 2-nitroimidazole compounds used as exogenous markers were developed originally as radiosensitizers for use in conjunction with conventional radiotherapy. They are metabolized in, and bind strictly to, hypoxic cells. The most commonly used 2-nitroimidazoles are pimonidazole (1-(2-nitro-1-imidazolyl)-3-N-piperidino-2-propanol) and EF-5 (nitroimidazole [2-(2-nitro-1H-imidazol-1-yl)-N-(2,2,3,3,3-pentafluoro-propyl)acetamide]). These markers exhibit comparable mechanisms of activation, and are reduced by viable hypoxic cells to generate reduction products that form adducts in the cells that are easily detectable through immunohistochemistry *(26)*. Both markers are reduced at oxygen concentrations below ~10 mmHg, and they tend to mark regions more distant from the vasculature than the endogenous markers CA-IX or glucose transporter (Glut)-1 (*see* Subheading 3.2.).

Tumor hypoxia as marked by pimonidazole has been shown to correlate with other methods of hypoxic detection known to indicate levels of hypoxia that affect cellular radiosensitivity (radiobiologically relevant hypoxia), in both murine and human tumors. This would imply that pimonidazole labeling is representative of radiobiologically relevant hypoxia *(5)*. However, pimonidazole labeling was found to show only a weak, nonsignificant correlation with tumor hypoxia assessed using the Eppendorf electrode method in human tumors *(27)*. A similar result was seen for EF-5 in squamous cell carcinomas *(28)*, and in brain tumors *(29)*. One possible explanation for this disparity may be the inherent differences in the techniques; the Eppendorf electrode measures discrete volumes of cells in a stepping method through the tumor before amalgamating the results to give an overall definition of the hypoxic nature of the tumor. In contrast, the use of exogenous markers specifies hypoxia on an individual cell basis and is dependent on the level of hypoxia and exposure time to the markers. Furthermore, the heterogeneity of tumor oxygenation requires the examination of multiple tissue sections to provide an overall picture of the hypoxic status of a tumor. Such analyses have rarely been performed to date.

Nevertheless, current data would suggest that exogenous markers can indicate radiobiologically relevant hypoxia in tumors accessible for biopsy, thereby overcoming a major difficulty of the Eppendorf electrode method. In addition, they can provide information on hypoxia at a cellular level and allow hypoxia to be assessed in relation to other parameters such as vascular density or regions of necrosis. Both pimonidazole and EF-5 have been successfully applied in the clinic. One study measured tumor hypoxia using pimonidazole binding in patients selected for a clinical trial of *a*ccelerated *r*adiotherapy, *c*arbogen, *n*icotinamide (ARCON), a therapeutic approach aimed at improving the response of hypoxic regions to radiotherapy. Pimonidazole binding was found to correlate with poor prognosis, primarily in patients that did not receive ARCON, suggesting that ARCON was successful in reducing the impact of hypoxia on treatment response *(30)*.

3.2. Endogenous Markers

Endogenous markers share the advantages of the exogenous markers, with the further benefit that there is no need to administer any agents before obtaining a tissue biopsy. This enables retrospective analyses as well as current evaluation, provided that the biopsy material has been stored adequately. This method of marking hypoxia is focused on the hypoxia-specific expression of proteins. Hypoxic gene expression is primarily regulated by a heterodimeric transcription factor, hypoxia inducible factor (HIF)-1. HIF-1 is responsible for the hypoxia-mediated transcriptional regulation of a wide selection of genes initiated through a cognate recognition sequence, to which HIF-1 binds upstream of the coding region (*see* Subheading 6.). This is termed the hypoxia response element (HRE), and all the known HIF-1-responsive genes have been found to contain HREs of 50 bp or less, with a conserved region functionally essential for HIF-1 binding *(7,31)*. Thus, studies of endogenous markers of hypoxia have considered the use of HIF-1α, the hypoxia-regulated element of HIF-1, or genes upregulated by HIF-1, most commonly carbonic anhydrase 9 (*CA-IX*) or *Glut-1*. HIF-1α is targeted for rapid degradation by the proteasome under normoxic conditions (*see* Subheading 3.4.) *(32)*. Thus, CA-IX and Glut-1 have an advantage over HIF-1α in that they are neither rapidly degraded on exposure to oxygen, nor stabilized in response to hypoxia, potential problems in the removal and preparation of biopsy specimens for analysis. However, if the specimens are prepared correctly and rapidly, HIF-1α should be indicative of the hypoxic state of cells at the specific time of the biopsy, whereas CA-IX and Glut-1 may be more representative of long term or diffusion limited hypoxia *(4)*. The simultaneous analysis of these markers with differing expression profiles could potentially distinguish between areas of diffusion limited and transient perfusion limited hypoxia, providing HIF-1α is not constitutively expressed, as appears to be the case in some tumors *(33)*.

Endogenous markers have been linked with outcome. HIF-1α expression has been demonstrated as indicative of a worse prognosis *(34–36)*, as has CA-IX *(37–40)* and, to a lesser degree, Glut-1 *(41)*. However, the published results are not consistent, as HIF-1α expression was also correlated with significantly improved disease-free and overall survival in head and neck squamous cell carcinoma patients *(42)*. Likewise, CA-IX expression in renal carcinoma was indicative of an improved prognosis in one study *(43)*. It is possible that this difference could be because of differences in HIF-1 activity, as renal carcinomas have demonstrated defective regulation of HIF-1α *(33)*. In the previously mentioned ARCON study (*see* Subheading 3.1.), a greater hypoxic fraction as revealed by CA-IX expression did not correlate with outcome, despite a good correlation between CA-IX expression and pimonidazole binding *(30)*. Thus, the current data are not conclusive and, to date, potential limitations of these studies associated with the handling of the biopsies and with heterogeneity in labeling from one region of the tumor to another have not been adequately addressed. A further potential limitation of these markers is that their expression may also have alternative mechanisms of regulation distinct from that of hypoxia, and thus they may not necessarily be specific markers of tumor oxygenation, but may also reflect other changes within the tumor microenvironment *(7,44,45)*. This does not rule out the future use of these markers, but rather suggests that further study is required to elucidate the most appropriate approach.

3.3. Noninvasive Imaging

Noninvasive imaging methods of quantifying tumor hypoxia would be of great therapeutic benefit, as they are not restricted to accessible tumors, although they are not applicable to retrospective studies. A major advantage of noninvasive imaging is the potential to measure hypoxia dynamically and to monitor the activity of therapeutic agents in relation to tumor hypoxia, thus verifying whether hypoxia is influencing drug delivery or whether resistance is the result of alternative causes *(46)*. Such methods can potentially enable real-time imaging of fluctuations in flow and hypoxia, possibly allowing for measurement of both diffusion-limited and transient perfusion-limited hypoxia. Two imaging mechanisms that have been widely studied are positron emission tomography (PET) and single-photon emission computed tomography (SPECT) *(47)*. Both PET and SPECT involve the introduction of isotope-labeled hypoxia-targeted drugs and the emitted radiation is used to generate an image. However, the results obtained to date do not correlate well with those generated using the Eppendorf electrode method *(26)*.

A further imaging method that is being investigated is blood-oxygenation level-dependent (BOLD) imaging, a functional magnetic resonance technique. Unlike PET and SPECT, isotope-labeled agents are not required. Instead, BOLD imaging relies on the inherent magnetic properties of hemoglobin, which vary according to its oxygenation state *(26)*. Thus, BOLD imaging permits a direct measurement of (blood) oxygenation without the use of any other agents, similar to endogenous markers. However, this method also has limited spatial resolution, and the linkage between blood oxygenation levels and tissue oxygenation levels is likely indirect because of the heterogeneous and chaotically organized vasculature in tumors. The same concern also applies to other magnetic resonance and computed tomography techniques for measuring blood perfusion in tumors. The use of noninvasive imaging methods to measure tumor hypoxia is still at a relatively early stage of application *(48)*. Results to date are promising but further work is needed to determine their true potential.

4. TUMOR HYPOXIA AND DISEASE PROGRESSION

The advent of the Eppendorf electrode as a reliable and reproducible method of measuring tumor pO_2 in the clinic permitted widespread clinical studies focused on both the incidence of hypoxia in solid tumors and consequent treatment outcome, primarily over the past decade. These studies have revealed substantial levels of hypoxia in cervical carcinoma *(49–51)*, head and neck carcinoma *(52–54)*, soft tissue sarcoma *(55,56)*, and prostate carcinoma *(57–59)*. Furthermore, tumor hypoxia has been linked with a poorer prognosis/reduced survival outcome in cervix carcinoma, head and neck carcinoma and soft tissue sarcoma *(49–52,56)* (Table 1). Current data are suggestive of a similar link in prostate carcinoma *(59)*. There are several potential explanations for this link. As discussed above, hypoxic tumor cells are known to be refractory to radiotherapy, and common chemotherapeutic drugs and this may reduce treatment efficacy. However, the effect of hypoxia on treatment outcome was apparent in patients treated with radiotherapy, chemotherapy, or surgical resection. In addition, there was a correlation between tumor hypoxia and distant spread as well as local failure. Both of these observations imply that hypoxia is associated with more aggressive disease as well as being involved in treatment resistance *(49,50)*.

Experimental data are indicative of a role for tumor hypoxia in disease progression. Early work demonstrated that a 24-h exposure of three murine tumor cell lines to hypoxia

Table 1
Clinical Studies Showing a Correlation Between Tumor pO$_2$ Measured Using the Eppendorf Electrode and Treatment Outcome

Tumor type	Treatment	Patient number	Association	Reference
Cervical carcinoma	Radiation	106	DFS, DMFS	Fyles et al. 2002 (49)
	Radiation	40	DFS, LRC	Sundfor et al. 2000 (121)
	Radiation	51	DFS	Knocke et al. 1999 (122)
	Radiation or surgery	89	DFS	Hockel et al. 1999 (123)
Head and neck carcinoma	Radiation and/or chemotherapy	194	DSS	Rudat et al. 2001 (124)
	Radiation and chemotherapy	41	DFS	Rudat et al. 2000 (125)
	Radiation	35	LRC	Nordsmark et al. 2000 (54)
	Radiation or radiochemotherapy	59	DFS	Stadler et al. 1999 (126)
	Radiation and/or chemotherapy	63	DFS, LRC	Brizel et al. 1999 (52)
	Radiation	35	LRC	Nordsmark et al. 1996 (53)
Soft tissue	Surgery and/or radiation	28	DSS	Nordsmark et al. 2001 (55)
Sarcoma	Radiation, surgery and hyperthermia	22	DMFS	Brizel et al. 1996 (56)

DFS, disease-free survival; DSS, disease-specific survival: LRC, locoregional control; DMFS, distant metastases-free survival.

in vitro, before intravenous injection in vivo, resulted in enhanced metastatic ability *(60)*. Interestingly, this effect was transient, suggesting a potential role for hypoxia-mediated alterations in gene expression. Concomitant with this, a significant correlation between hypoxic fraction, as measured using the Eppendorf electrodes, and micrometastases in the lungs was demonstrated for one of the cell lines (murine fibrosarcoma) *(61)*. Similarly, a correlation between the formation of macroscopic metastases and tumor hypoxia has been demonstrated using an orthotopic pancreatic xenograft model *(62)*. Comparable results have been seen in a human melanoma cell line, in accord with its level of expression of vascular endothelial growth factor (*VEGF*), a hypoxia-regulated gene. An increase in the number of metastases following hypoxic exposure, and consequent induction of *VEGF*, was seen only in a cell line with low constitutive expression of *VEGF*. A melanoma cell line with high constitutive expression of *VEGF* did not demonstrate increased metastatic potential, despite similar hypoxic induction. Thus, hypoxia-enhanced metastases would appear to occur in a manner specific to individual tumor cells *(63)*.

Experimentally induced acute hypoxia (12 cycles 5–7% O_2 for 10 min, followed by 10 min of air each day) in murine fibrosarcoma-bearing mice significantly increased the formation of micrometastases in the lung relative to both control (air breathing) and chronic hypoxia (5–7% O_2 for 120 min each day) treatment groups *(64)*. Similarly, mice bearing orthotopically implanted cervix carcinoma xenografts exposed to the same acute hypoxia treatment demonstrated an increase in lymph node metastases. These data are indicative of a causal role for acute hypoxia in metastases formation, both in blood borne and lymphatic metastases *(65)*. The exact mechanisms through which this occurs remain to be elucidated, but a possibility is that regions of acute hypoxia may contribute to metastatic disease because of their increased cell viability and proximity to tumor vasculature.

5. TUMOR HYPOXIA AND GENOMIC INSTABILITY

There is no definitive explanation for how hypoxia might contribute to a more aggressive phenotype, but experimental studies suggest an assortment of genetic alterations endowing hypoxic cells with a survival advantage. These phenotypic changes could arise from hypoxia-mediated upregulation of gene transcription or via hypoxia-mediated genomic instability *(2,66)*. The tumor suppressor gene *p53* is involved in the apoptotic response to DNA damage and accumulates under hypoxic conditions. It is commonly mutated in many cancers, resulting in a survival advantage under conditions characteristic of the tumor microenvironment. Oncogenically transformed p53$^{+/+}$ and p53$^{-/-}$ murine embryonic fibroblasts demonstrated a clear survival advantage for p53-deficient cells following hypoxic exposure. The p53-deficient line was extremely resistant to apoptosis. In addition, if the two cell populations were mixed at a ratio of 1:1000 of p53$^{-/-}$:p53$^{+/+}$ and cultured under repeated rounds of hypoxia, the percentage of p53$^{-/-}$ cells increased following each treatment until they became the predominant cells in the culture. Consistent with this result, tumors grown from the p53$^{+/+}$ cells in vivo demonstrated a substantially higher apoptotic frequency as compared to tumors from the p53$^{-/-}$ cells despite similar hypoxic profiles *(67)*. This provides evidence for hypoxia-mediated selection of mutant variants.

Transient inactivation of p53 under hypoxic conditions may also lead to increased resistance to stress-induced apoptosis. Recent studies in a murine fibrosarcoma model have demonstrated that hypoxia can upregulate the expression of murine double minute 2 (mdm2), a negative regulator of p53 that targets p53 protein for degradation by the proteasomal degradation pathway, consequently downregulating p53 protein levels. The tumor cells with increased mdm2 expression were found to be more efficient at forming lung metastases following intravenous injection, because they were more resistant to apoptosis induced by the stress of being arrested in the lung environment *(68)*.

Hypoxic tumors have also been reported to demonstrate a higher incidence of mutations than the same tumor cell line grown under oxic conditions in vitro, and studies involving intermittent exposure to hypoxia and reoxygenation in vitro resulted in increased mutation frequency relative to the number of exposures *(69)*. This suggests that in vivo exposure to fluctuating levels of hypoxia can result in increased mutation levels and possibly genomic instability. In addition, tumor hypoxia has been found to reduce the expression of genes involved in DNA mismatch repair *(70)*. These hypoxia-mediated effects could contribute to treatment resistance as well as disease progression *per se*, potentially through reduced drug efficacy as a consequence of decreased apoptotic ability or deregulated expression of genes involved in drug resistance.

6. HYPOXIA-MEDIATED GENE EXPRESSION

Hypoxia imposes a stress on cells, thereby inducing a response to improve survival. High throughput screens, such as microarray analysis and differential display, have enabled the discovery of a large number of genes that respond to hypoxia, including proapoptotic and antiapoptotic genes, genes involved in invasion, metabolism, growth arrest and differentiation, and synthesis of DNA, RNA, and proteins. Apart from HIF-1, hypoxia-mediated gene expression can also be regulated through several transcription factors such as the cyclic AMP-response-element-binding (CREB) protein, the activator protein 1 (AP-1), the nuclear factor-κB (NFκB), the early growth response-1 protein (EGR-1), and p53 *(2,3)*. HIF-1 has been the most extensively studied, and is responsible for the transcriptional regulation of over 60 genes involved in survival mechanisms, including angiogenesis (e.g., *VEGF*, endoglin, leptin, transforming growth factor-β3), metabolism (e.g., hexokinases 1 and 2, *Glut-1*, lactate dehydrogenase A, phosphoglycerate kinase 1, triosephosphate isomerase), and proliferation (e.g., cyclin G2, insulin-like growth factor [IGF]-2, IGF-binding protein [BP]-1, *TGF-α*, *TGF-β3*), many of which are classically associated with cancer *(7,71)*. HIF-1 is a heterodimer composed of two subunits, HIF-1α and HIF-1β. HIF-1β is constitutively expressed such that HIF-1α is the regulatory subunit of HIF-1, undergoing rapid posttranslational oxygen dependent degradation *(32)* with a half-life of about 5 min following reoxygenation *(72–75)*. The ubiquitin-proteasome pathway is known to be involved through the interaction of HIF-1α with the von Hippel Lindau protein (pVHL), the product of the VHL tumor suppressor gene *(33,76)*. pVHL interacts physically with HIF-1α via its β-domain and targets it for degradation *(77)*. This interaction is regulated through hydroxylation of conserved proline residues 402 and 564 on HIF-1α by prolyl hydroxylase proteins 1–3 *(7,78,79)*. These HIF-1α prolyl hydroxylase proteins require molecular oxygen as a substrate, providing a mechanism through which oxygen dependent degradation of HIF-1α is achieved *(7)*.

Under hypoxic conditions, there is an instantaneous and strong stabilization of HIF-1α protein, and thus, the HIF-1 dimer is formed and induces expression of its downstream genes. HIF-1 activation occurs only when there is nuclear translocation of HIF-1α protein, allowing it to dimerize with HIF-1β *(73,77)* and its coactivator CBP/p300. CBP/p300 is a general transcriptional coactivator that binds to the HIF-1α transactivation domain, an interaction that is also oxygen dependent, as factor inhibiting HIF-1(FIH) mediates hydroxylation of asparagine residue 803 and acts to inhibit this interaction under normoxia *(80)*.

There is a variety of both clinical and experimental data to suggest a role for HIF-1 in tumor progression, although not all reports support such a role *(42)*. Clinically, evidence of HIF-1α overexpression is found in many human tumors *(34,35,81–84)*, such that HIF-1α is reported to be expressed in over 90% of all colon, lung and prostate cancers, whereas there is no corresponding expression in normal tissue *(31,71)*. Clinical studies have linked this overexpression with subsequent poor prognosis in carcinoma of the head and neck, ovaries, oesophagus, brain, breast, cervix, and uterus *(7)*. Experimentally, it has been demonstrated that by disrupting the ability of HIF-1α to interact with its transcriptional coactivator CBP/p300, thereby inhibiting HIF-1 activation in a dominant negative manner, tumor growth could be restricted *(85)*. A study of naturally occurring pancreatic cell lines with constitutive expression of HIF-1α, alongside corresponding low-expressing variants, demonstrated better tumor growth of those expressing HIF-1α. Furthermore, the cell lines expressing HIF-1α demonstrated improved survival in response to hypoxia and glucose deprivation in vitro, a result that could be replicated in the low-expressing cell lines by stable transfection of HIF-1α *(86)*.

Together, the clinical and experimental data suggest that HIF-1 is involved in potentiating tumor growth, although the precise mechanisms through which this may be achieved remain unclear. One possibility is that HIF-1 may enhance the ability of the tumor cells to utilize the restricted nutrients of the microenvironment most efficiently. The introduction of an HIF-1α expression vector into a human colon carcinoma line, thereby upregulating HIF-1α expression, demonstrated a significantly enhanced ability to invade through Matrigel under hypoxic conditions. Correspondingly, inhibition of HIF-1α through targeted degradation with small-interfering RNA (siRNA) reduced the invasive-capacity of this cell line. Subsequent analyses of gene expression in both murine embryonic stem cells and human VHL-deficient tumor cells demonstrated HIF-1-dependent induction of genes such as urokinase-type plasminogen activator receptor and matrix metalloproteinase 2, both of which are involved in the degradation of the basement membrane. Specific inhibition of urokinase-type plasminogen activator receptor inhibited invasion. Taken together, these data provide evidence for a role for HIF-1 in enhanced tumor cell invasion, a vital characteristic of tumor metastasis *(87)*.

7. HYPOXIA-TARGETED THERAPY

In view of its effect on progression, coupled with its negative implications for both radiotherapy and common chemotherapy agents, tumor hypoxia has traditionally been viewed as a therapeutic obstacle. However, because it is predominantly a tumor-specific condition, recent work focused on its potential for targeted therapeutic approaches. Traditionally, attempts were made to reoxygenate the tumor cells, thereby rendering them susceptible to conventional therapies; however, current work has concentrated on the development of drugs designed to elicit a cytotoxic response selectively under hypoxic conditions, or to target genes upregulated by the hypoxic environment (Table 2; Fig. 3).

7.1. Bioreductive Drugs

Bioreductive prodrugs represent a group of drugs that are enzymatically reduced to yield a cytotoxic moiety, a process that is facilitated under hypoxic conditions. This reduction is catalyzed by a variety of reductases, most commonly cytochrome P450 reductase and the cytochrome P450 family. In general, there is an initial formation of a one-electron-reduced intermediate, which is further reduced to elicit toxicity. This inter-

Table 2

Hypoxia-Targeted Therapies: Examples of Promising Studies for Different Hypoxia-Directed Therapies Along With an Outline of Their Mechanism of Hypoxia-Selective Toxicity

Therapy	Name	Mechanism of toxicity	Reference
Bioreductive prodrugs	Tirapazamine (TPZ) AQ4N	Reduced to form an oxidizing radical. Acts as a topoisomerase poison. Has a bystander effect.	Brown 1993 (review) (127) Patterson et al. 2000 (128)
	NLCQ-1	DNA-targeted reactive electrophile.	Papadopoulou and Bloomer 2003 (review) (129)
GDEPT studies	LDH/cytosine deaminase with 5-FC	Facilitates activation of 5-FC to its toxic form 5-FU by producing the bacterial enzyme cytosine deaminase	Dachs et al. 1997 (108)
	LDH/P450R with RB6145	Enhances tumor response by increasing levels of required reductase enzyme, P450R	Patterson et al. 2002 (109)
	LDH/P450R with TPZ and radiation	Enhances tumor response by increasing levels of required reductase enzyme, P450R	Cowen et al. 2004 (112)
HIF-1-targeted studies	Topotecan	Inhibits HIF-1α translation in a topoisomerase I-dependent manner.	Rapisarda et al. 2002, 2004 (115,117)
	YC-1	Inhibits HIF-1α at posttranscriptional level.	Yeo et al. 2003 (116)
	Dominant-negative variant of HIF-1α	Inhibits functional HIF-1 formation in a dominant-negative manner.	Chen et al. 2003 (130)
	Antisense HIF-1α- and B7-1–mediated immunotherapy	Inhibits HIF-1α expression potentiating the antitumor effects of B7-1–mediated immunotherapy	Sun et al. 2001 (131)
	Antisense HIF-1α and VHL protein	Inhibits HIF-1α expression potentiating the antitumor effects of overexpression of the tumor suppressor pVHL	Sun et al. 2003 (132)

TPZ, tirapazamine; GDEPT, gene-directed enzyme prodrug therapy; LDH, lactate dehydrogenase; P450R, P450 reductase; 5-FC, 5-fluorocytosine, 5-FU, 5-fluorouracil; YC-1, 3-(5¢-hydroxymethyl-2¢-furyl)-1-benzylindazole; VHL, von Hippel Lindau; pVHL, von Hippel Lindau protein.

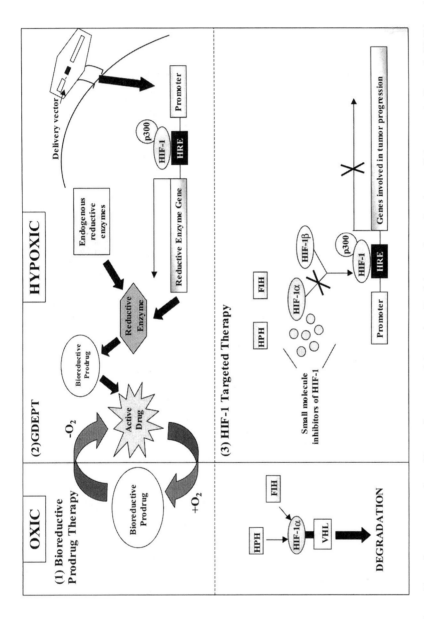

Fig. 3. Schematic outline of some examples of hypoxia-targeted therapies. Both hypoxic and oxic conditions are indicated. (1) Bioreductive prodrugs are reduced by specific reductive enzymes under hypoxic conditions to form an active drug able to elicit a cytotoxic response. Under oxic conditions these drugs undergo a process of futile cycling where they are back-oxidized into their nontoxic form. (2) Gene directed enzyme prodrug therapy (GDEPT) can be used to target expression of the reductive enzymes required for prodrug activation to hypoxic regions, thus enhancing prodrug efficacy. This is commonly achieved through use of the hypoxia inducible factor (HIF)-1/hypoxia response element (HRE) system. (3) As HIF-1, a transcription factor responsible for the regulation of many target genes, is normally only formed under hypoxic conditions it also represents a hypoxia-specific target. HIF-1-directed therapy generally targets HIF-1α. Targeting approaches have included the use of small molecule inhibitors, or dominant negative, small interfering RNA or antisense variants, thereby inhibiting the transcriptional regulation of downstream target genes involved in tumor progression.

56

mediate can be back-oxidized in the presence of oxygen in a process known as futile cycling, thereby preventing the production of the toxic species (*see* Fig. 3). However, futile cycling produces a superoxide radical that can induce aerobic toxicity to varying extents *(88–90)*. Because cytotoxic bioreductive drugs selectively target hypoxic tumor cells, combination therapy in conjunction with radiation or classic chemotherapeutic drugs, which are more effective against well oxygenated cells, should result in a greatly enhanced response through the complimentary killing of the cells refractory to the different treatment modalities *(6,91)*. However, the stringent hypoxic requirement of many of these drugs represents a potential problem, in that bioreductive drugs generally elicit a cytotoxic response at oxygen concentrations only below ~3 mmHg. In contrast, cellular radioresistance becomes apparent below ~20 mmHg. Thus, combined treatment with a bioreductive drug and radiotherapy might result in a survival advantage for cells at intermediate oxygen concentrations *(92)*.

Clinically, the most widely studied bioreductive drug is tirapazamine (TPZ), a benzotriazine di-*N*-oxide that elicits cytotoxicity through a nitroxide radical intermediate that causes single- and double-stranded DNA breaks *(90,93)*. Unlike most bioreductive drugs, the toxicity range of TPZ extends to intermediate oxygen concentrations. Thus, TPZ can target those cells that are radioresistant but too well oxygenated to represent a suitable target for the majority of bioreductive drugs. Furthermore, TPZ enhances the toxicity of cisplatin *(94)*. It has achieved some success in clinical trials in combination with cisplatin *(95–98)*, and/or with radiotherapy *(99–102)* (*see* Table 3). The combination of TPZ and cisplatin was found to improve significantly median survival and response rate in a phase III trial of patients presenting with non-small cell lung cancer *(98)*. Further studies began in 2004 with this drug in combination with radiation and cisplatin in head and neck cancers *(102a)*. However, despite the success achieved to date in the clinic, there is evidence for dose-limiting toxicity and the development of analogs that may have a better therapeutic ratio is in progress *(6)*.

Aside from TPZ, we are aware of only one other bioreductive prodrug that underwent clinical trials in 2004, AQ4N. AQ4N is a di-N-oxide prodrug that is reduced under conditions of low-oxygen tension to form the active species, AQ4, an alkylamino-anthraquinone metabolite *(103)*. The process of futile cycling, in which the active drug is back-oxidized into its nontoxic form on the reintroduction of oxygen, typical of most bioreductive drugs, does not occur. Instead, oxygen completely inhibits the reducing enzyme, cytochrome P450 (isoform 3A; CYP3A), and once formed, AQ4 is highly stable. AQ4 is a DNA affinic, topoisomerase II poison and, as such, targets predominantly cycling cells, a potential drawback when targeting hypoxic tumor cells, which generally demonstrate substantially reduced proliferation rates. However, the stability of AQ4 enables cytotoxic targeting of transiently hypoxic tumor cells as they become oxic, thus facilitating an improved response when combined with fractionated radiotherapy, which can cause reoxygenation of hypoxic cells in tumors *(21)*. AQ4 is also able to diffuse into surrounding oxygenated tumor cells and elicit a cytotoxic response, thus causing a bystander effect *(6,104–107)*. Interim results have been released recently of a phase I clinical trial examining the safety of AQ4N in patients with advanced esophageal carcinoma undergoing palliative radiotherapy. The current results, in 13 of an anticipated 22 patients, are promising (KuDOS Pharmaceuticals 2004; http://www.kudospharma.co.uk/news/current_item.php?time=1092673109&page_id=44).

Table 3
Clinical Trials With Tirapazamine

Treatment	Tumor type	Patient number	Reference
Phase I			
TPZ and cyclophosphamide	Pediatric solid tumors	23	Aquino et al. 2004 (133)
	Advanced malignant solid tumors	28	Hoff et al. 2001 (134)
TPZ, carboplatin, and paclitaxel	Advanced malignant solid tumors	42	Lara et al. 2003 (135)
TPZ, cisplatin, and radiotherapy	Advanced head and neck carcinoma	16	Rischin et al. 2001 (102)
TPZ and radiotherapy	Advanced malignant solid tumors	43	Shulman et al. 1999 (136)
TPZ and cisplatin	Recurrent cervical carcinoma	12	Aghajanian et al. 1997 (137)
	Advanced malignant solid tumors	13	Johnson et al. 1997 (95)
TPZ	Advanced malignant solid tumors	28	Senan et al. 1997 (138)
Phase I/II			
TPZ, cisplatin, and radiotherapy	Locally advanced cervix carcinoma	15	Craighead et al. 2000 (100)
Phase II			
TPZ and radiotherapy	Glioblastoma multiforme	124	Del Rowe et al. 2000 (101)
	Advanced head and neck carcinoma	40	Lee et al 1998 (99)
TPZ and cisplatin	Malignant melanoma	48, 48	Bedikian et al. 1997, 1999 (97,139)
			Richin et al. 2005 (102a)
	Advanced non-small cell lung carcinoma	44	Treat et al 1998 (140)
		20	Miller et al 1997 (96)
Phase III			
TPZ and cisplatin	Non-small cell lung carcinoma	446	von Pawel et al. 2000 (98)

Phase I, II, and III clinical trials are indicated alongside tumor type and the patient numbers involved. TPZ, tirapazamine.

7.2. Gene-Directed Enzyme Prodrug Therapy

One limitation of bioreductive drug therapy is the requirement for specific reductase enzymes for cytotoxic activation *(88,90)*. The presence and level of reductase enzymes is highly heterogeneous in tumors, and thus, the efficiency of a drug will demonstrate a corresponding degree of tumor-specific variability. This has led to the development of gene-directed enzyme prodrug therapy approaches, which can be used to develop a further degree of selectivity through conferment of specificity in the expression of the drug metabolizing enzyme. This was originally demonstrated through the exploitation of the HIF-1/HRE system to drive the expression of the enzyme cytosine deaminase. This enzyme is required for reduction of the prodrug 5-fluorocytosine (5-FC) to its active form, 5-fluorouracil. Mammalian cells are resistant to 5-FC, because the enzyme cytosine deaminase is not produced at sufficiently high levels to elicit significant reduction of the drug. The use of HRE-driven expression of cytosine deaminase was shown to selectively sensitize hypoxic tumor cells to 5-FC in vitro *(108)*.

More recently, the generation of a tumor cell line stably expressing HRE-mediated cytochrome P450 reductase was used to demonstrate a 30-fold increase, both in vitro and in vivo, in the toxic effect of the bioreductive drug RSU1069 *(109)*, a 2-nitroimidazole that achieves toxicity under hypoxic conditions through an alkylating aziridine group as its active species *(110,111)*. A similar effect was observed in a separate study using the HIF-1/HRE system to drive expression of human P450 reductase in hypoxic tumor regions. To facilitate delivery of the gene to these regions, an adenoviral vector was generated, allowing infection of both dividing and quiescent tumor cells on intratumoral injection of the virus. Administration of this viral vector before combined TPZ and radiation treatment resulted in cure in 85% of treated mice, irrespective of tumor size on treatment, a significant improvement on TPZ and radiation treatment alone *(112)*. There are a substantial number of gene-directed enzyme prodrug therapy-based studies examining a variety of different reductive enzymes, prodrugs, and delivery methods; some promising examples are shown in Table 2. A key difficulty with regard to this type of approach is delivery of these vectors to all the tumor cells, particularly as regions of hypoxia are a requisite for activation. Thus, this strategy does not circumvent one of the problems tumor hypoxia presents for conventional therapeutic approaches, namely that hypoxic tumor cells are either distant from vasculature or proximal to faulty vasculature, limiting the diffusion of therapeutic agents.

7.3. Inhibition of HIF-1

Another therapeutic approach is to target HIF-1 specifically and thus reduce or eliminate its expression. Recent data have shown HIF-1 to be upregulated in response to radiation, potentiating endothelial cell radioresistance through upregulation of VEGF and bFGF *(113)*. There is also evidence to suggest that HIF-1 can render cells resistant to chemotherapy. Exposure of HIF-1α-positive (HIF-1α+/+$^{+/+}$) and negative (HIF-1$\alpha^{-/-}$) murine embryonic fibroblast cell lines to two chemotherapeutic agents revealed a substantially lower IC$_{50}$ (concentration that yields a 50% inhibition of growth) in the HIF-1$\alpha^{-/-}$ line, an effect that was mimicked in vivo. There was an increased incidence of apoptosis in the HIF-1$\alpha^{-/-}$ line, in accord with a decreased ability to repair double-stranded DNA breaks *(114)*.

One potential strategy to target HIF-1 is the use of small molecule inhibitors*(115,116)*. A high-throughput screen identified four potential small molecule inhibitors of HIF-1α, and studies of one of these agents, the Camptothecin analogue, Topotecan, demonstrated a dose-dependent reduction in hypoxia-regulated expression of VEGF mRNA and protein *(115)*, and of HIF-1α protein *(117)*. Further studies showed the effect of Topotecan on inhibition of HIF-1α protein accumulation to occur at the translational level and to be dependent on the presence of topoisomerase I, the target of this drug. The exact mechanism remains unclear *(117)*.

Another small molecule inhibitor of HIF-1α, 3-(5'-hydroxymethyl-2'-furyl)-1-benzylindazole (YC-1), has been shown to delay tumor growth in vivo. YC-1 was originally developed to treat circulatory disorders and it inhibits platelet aggregation and vascular contraction through the activation of soluble guanylyl cyclase. YC-1 has also been found to completely inhibit HIF-1α at the posttranscriptional level. Similar to Topotecan, exposure to YC-1 under hypoxia in vitro was found to reduce HIF-1α protein, and HIF-1 regulated genes, in a dose-dependent manner in a selection of cell lines. Furthermore, treatment of tumors in vivo with YC-1 induced a growth delay. Immunohistochemical analysis demonstrated no HIF-1α staining in tumors from mice that had received YC-1, in contrast to the detection of HIF-1α in untreated tumors *(116)*. The investigators attributed the reduced growth of the tumors to the inhibition of angiogenesis, because there was reduced immunostaining for the endothelial marker CD31 and concordant reduction in VEGF protein expression.

The use of HIF-1 inhibitors is still relatively unexplored. Current data are promising and imply a potential role for the use of these drugs in cancer therapy *(7)*. It is of note that the small molecule inhibitors so far identified act to inhibit HIF-1 through indirect mechanisms, and as such may have effects distinct from those of HIF-1α inhibition. Also, HIF-1α protein levels, although principally regulated through hypoxia-inhibited proteasomal degradation, are also affected by growth factors and cytokines *(7)*, and by tumor suppressor mutations and oncogene activation *(71)*, both of which are common occurrences in solid tumors. Thus, therapeutics targeted at HIF-1α have the potential for a broader spectrum of efficacy than more specific hypoxia-targeted therapeutics. Direct inhibition of HIF-1α has been achieved experimentally through siRNA approaches or the use of dominant negative variants and antisense DNA (*see* Table 2), although the practicalities of such applications in the clinic require further study. A greater degree of specificity than that achieved with the small molecule inhibitors would allow for analysis of the specific role of HIF-1α *per se* in tumor progression, and thus the potential for subsequent development of more directed therapeutics.

8. SUMMARY

Tumor hypoxia results in resistance to common therapeutic regimens, and has also been shown to be associated with disease progression. Tumor hypoxia is extremely heterogeneous both spatially and temporally, and thus, the ability to assess the hypoxic status of tumors in individual patients and tailor treatment accordingly is desirable. Methods of measuring tumor hypoxia have been, and are being, developed with the eventual aim of measuring the overall hypoxic fraction, and preferably the nature of hypoxia (chronic vs transient), in all tumors, irrespective of location. Noninvasive methods are most desirable but are currently at an early stage of testing. Endogenous markers have the potential to indicate the nature of hypoxia, with the added benefit of allowing retrospective analysis of stored patient samples, a useful research tool. In line with this, the impact of tumor hypoxia on treatment outcome and disease progression is being evaluated to improve prognosis, and in addition, drug development through improved understanding of the causal relationships. Finally, therapeutic methods designed to target hypoxic tumor cells are being explored for use in combination with conventional therapies to improve treatment response and reduce local failure and metastatic dissemination. At present, few of these approaches are in clinical trials. However, an increasing level of information on all aspects of tumor hypoxia is developing from recent research that should enable the development of improved therapeutic strategies that are more effective in their methods of delivery and targeting of hypoxia. Targeting tumor hypoxia is a dynamic and promising area of therapeutic study.

REFERENCES

1. Vaupel P, Kelleher DK, Höckel M. Oxygen status of malignant tumors: pathogenesis of hypoxia and significance for tumor therapy. Semin Oncol 2001; 28:29–35.
2. Subarsky P, Hill RP. The hypoxic tumour microenvironment and metastatic progression. Clin Exp Metastasis 2003; 20:237–250.
3. Le QT, Denko NC, Giaccia AJ. Hypoxic gene expression and metastasis. Cancer Metastasis Rev 2004; 23:293–310.
4. Bussink J, Kaanders JH, van der Kogel AJ. Tumor hypoxia at the micro-regional level: clinical relevance and predictive value of exogenous and endogenous hypoxic cell markers. Radiother Oncol 2003; 67:3–15.
5. Olive PL, Banath JP, Aquino-Parsons C. Measuring hypoxia in solid tumours—is there a gold standard? Acta Oncol 2001; 40:917–923.
6. Brown JM, Wilson WR. Exploiting tumour hypoxia in cancer treatment. Nat Rev Cancer 2004; 4:437–447.
7. Semenza GL. Targeting HIF-1 for cancer therapy. Nat Rev Cancer 2003; 3:721–732.
8. Dewhirst MW. Concepts of oxygen transport at the microcirculatory level. Semin Radiat Oncol 1998; 8:143–150.
9. Li CY, Shan S, Huang Q, et al. Initial stages of tumor cell-induced angiogenesis: evaluation via skin window chambers in rodent models. J Natl Cancer Inst 2000; 92:143–147.
10. Yancopoulos GD, Davis S, Gale NW, Rudge JS, Wiegand SJ, Holash J. Vascular-specific growth factors and blood vessel formation. Nature 2000; 407:242–248.
11. Vaupel P, Kallinowski F, Okunieff P. Blood flow, oxygen and nutrient supply, and metabolic microenvironment of human tumors: a review. Cancer Res 1989; 49:6449–6465.
12. Dewhirst MW, Ong ET, Braun RD, et al. Quantification of longitudinal tissue pO_2 gradients in window chamber tumours: impact on tumour hypoxia. Br J Cancer 1999; 79:1717–1722.
13. Baluk P, Morikawa S, Haskell A, Mancuso M, McDonald DM. Abnormalities of basement membrane on blood vessels and endothelial sprouts in tumors. Am J Pathol 2003; 163:1801–1815.
14. Thomlinson RH, Gray LH. The histological structure of some human lung cancers and the possible implications for radiotherapy. Br J Cancer 1955; 9:539–549.
15. Chaplin DJ, Olive PL, Durand RE. Intermittent blood flow in a murine tumor: radiobiological effects. Cancer Res 1987; 47:597–601.
16. Pigott KH, Hill SA, Chaplin DJ, Saunders MI. Microregional fluctuations in perfusion within human tumours detected using laser Doppler flowmetry. Radiother Oncol 1996; 40:45–50.
17. Li X, Brown SL, Hill RP. Factors influencing the thermosensitivity of two rodent tumors. Radiat Res 1992; 130:211–219.
18. Kimura H, Braun RD, Ong ET, et al. Fluctuations in red cell flux in tumor microvessels can lead to transient hypoxia and reoxygenation in tumor parenchyma. Cancer Res 1996; 56:5522–5528.
19. Dewhirst MW, Braun RD, Lanzen JL. Temporal changes in pO_2 of R3230AC tumors in Fischer-344 rats. Int J Radiat Oncol Biol Phys 1998; 42:723–726.
20. Brurberg KG, Graff BA, Rofstad EK. Temporal heterogeneity in oxygen tension in human melanoma xenografts. Br J Cancer 2003; 89:350–356.
21. Hall EJ. Radiobiology for the Radiologist. Philadelphia: Lippincott Williams & Wilkins, 2000.
22. Horan AD, Koch CJ. The K_m for radiosensitization of human tumor cells by oxygen is much greater than 3 mmHg and is further increased by elevated levels of cysteine. Radiat Res 2001; 156:388–398.
23. Teicher BA. Hypoxia and drug resistance. Cancer Metastasis Rev 1994; 13:139–168.

24. Kallinowski F, Zander R, Hoeckel M, Vaupel P. Tumor tissue oxygenation as evaluated by computerized-pO_2-histography. Int J Radiat Oncol Biol Phys 1990; 19:953–961.

25. Milosevic M, Fyles A, Hedley D, Hill R. The human tumor microenvironment: Invasive (needle) measurement of oxygen and interstitial fluid pressure. Semin Radiat Oncol 2004; 14:249–258.

26. Evans SM, Koch CJ. Prognostic significance of tumor oxygenation in humans. Cancer Lett 2003; 195:1–16.

27. Nordsmark M, Loncaster J, Chou SC, et al. Invasive oxygen measurements and pimonidazole labeling in human cervix carcinoma. Int J Radiat Oncol Biol Phys 2001; 49:581–586.

28. Evans SM, Hahn S, Pook DR, et al. Detection of hypoxia in human squamous cell carcinoma by EF5 binding. Cancer Res 2000; 60:2018–2024.

29. Evans SM, Judy KD, Dunphy I, et al. Comparative measurements of hypoxia in human brain tumors using needle electrodes and EF5 binding. Cancer Res 2004; 64:1886–1892.

30. Kaanders JH, Wijffels KI, Marres HA, et al. Pimonidazole binding and tumor vascularity predict for treatment outcome in head and neck cancer. Cancer Res 2002; 62:7066–7074.

31. Semenza GL. Expression of hypoxia-inducible factor 1: mechanisms and consequences. Biochem Pharmacol 2000; 59:47–53.

32. Huang LE, Arany Z, Livingston DM, Bunn HF. Activation of hypoxia-inducible transcription factor depends primarily upon redox-sensitive stabilization of its alpha subunit. J Biol Chem 1996; 271:32,253–32,259.

33. Maxwell PH, Wiesener MS, Chang GW, et al. The tumour suppressor protein VHL targets hypoxia-inducible factors for oxygen-dependent proteolysis. Nature 1999; 399:271–275.

34. Zhong H, De Marzo AM, Laughner E, et al. Overexpression of hypoxia-inducible factor 1alpha in common human cancers and their metastases. Cancer Res 1999; 59:5830–5835.

35. Birner P, Schindl M, Obermair A, et al. Overexpression of hypoxia-inducible factor 1alpha is a marker for an unfavorable prognosis in early-stage invasive cervical cancer. Cancer Res 2000; 60:4693–4596.

36. Aebersold DM, Burri P, Beer KT, et al. Expression of hypoxia-inducible factor-1alpha: a novel predictive and prognostic parameter in the radiotherapy of oropharyngeal cancer. Cancer Res 2001; 61:2911–2916.

37. Chia SK, Wykoff CC, Watson PH, et al. Prognostic significance of a novel hypoxia-regulated marker, carbonic anhydrase IX, in invasive breast carcinoma. J Clin Oncol 2001; 19:3660–3688.

38. Koukourakis MI, Giatromanolaki A, Sivridis E, et al. Hypoxia-regulated carbonic anhydrase-9 (CA9) relates to poor vascularization and resistance of squamous cell head and neck cancer to chemoradiotherapy. Clin Cancer Res 2001; 7:3399–3403.

39. Loncaster JA, Harris AL, Davidson SE, et al. Carbonic anhydrase (CA IX) expression, a potential new intrinsic marker of hypoxia: correlations with tumor oxygen measurements and prognosis in locally advanced carcinoma of the cervix. Cancer Res 2001; 61:6394–6399.

40. Maseide K, Kandel RA, Bell RS, et al. Carbonic anhydrase IX as a marker for poor prognosis in soft tissue sarcoma. Clin Cancer Res 2004; 10:4464–4471.

41. Airley R, Loncaster J, Davidson S, et al. Glucose transporter glut-1 expression correlates with tumor hypoxia and predicts metastasis-free survival in advanced carcinoma of the cervix. Clin Cancer Res 2001; 7:928–934.

42. Beasley NJ, Leek R, Alam M, et al. Hypoxia-inducible factors HIF-1alpha and HIF-2alpha in head and neck cancer: relationship to tumor biology and treatment outcome in surgically resected patients. Cancer Res 2002; 62:2493–2497.

43. Bui MH, Seligson D, Han KR, et al. Carbonic anhydrase IX is an independent predictor of survival in advanced renal clear cell carcinoma: implications for prognosis and therapy. Clin Cancer Res 2003; 9:802–811.

44. Kaluz S, Kaluzova M, Chrastina A, et al. Lowered oxygen tension induces expression of the hypoxia marker MN/carbonic anhydrase IX in the absence of hypoxia-inducible factor 1 alpha stabilization: a role for phosphatidylinositol 3'-kinase. Cancer Res 2002; 62:4469–4477.

45. Maxwell PH, Dachs GU, Gleadle JM, et al. Hypoxia-inducible factor-1 modulates gene expression in solid tumors and influences both angiogenesis and tumor growth. Proc Natl Acad Sci U S A 1997; 94:8104–8109.

46. West CM, Jones T, Price P. The potential of positron-emission tomography to study anticancer-drug resistance. Nat Rev Cancer 2004; 4:457–469.

47. Koch CJ, Evans SM. Non-invasive PET and SPECT imaging of tissue hypoxia using isotopically labeled 2-nitroimidazoles. Adv Exp Med Biol 2003; 510:285–292.

48. Mazurchuk R, Zhou R, Straubinger RM, Chau RI, Grossman Z. Functional magnetic resonance (fMR) imaging of a rat brain tumor model: implications for evaluation of tumor microvasculature and therapeutic response. Magn Reson Imaging 1999; 17:537–548.

49. Fyles A, Milosevic M, Hedley D, et al. Tumor hypoxia has independent predictor impact only in patients with node-negative cervix cancer. J Clin Oncol 2002; 20:680–687.

50. Hockel M, Schlenger K, Mitze M, Schaffer U, Vaupel P. Hypoxia and radiation response in human tumors. Semin Radiat Oncol 1996; 6:3–9.

51. Rofstad EK, Sundfor K, Lyng H, Trope CG. Hypoxia-induced treatment failure in advanced squamous cell carcinoma of the uterine cervix is primarily due to hypoxia-induced radiation resistance rather than hypoxia-induced metastasis. Br J Cancer 2000; 83:354–359.

52. Brizel DM, Dodge RK, Clough RW, Dewhirst MW. Oxygenation of head and neck cancer: changes during radiotherapy and impact on treatment outcome. Radiother Oncol 1999; 53:113–117.

53. Nordsmark M, Overgaard M, Overgaard J. Pretreatment oxygenation predicts radiation response in advanced squamous cell carcinoma of the head and neck. Radiother Oncol 1996; 41:31–39.

54. Nordsmark M, Overgaard J. A confirmatory prognostic study on oxygenation status and loco-regional control in advanced head and neck squamous cell carcinoma treated by radiation therapy. Radiother Oncol 2000; 57:39–43.

55. Nordsmark M, Alsner J, Keller J, et al. Hypoxia in human soft tissue sarcomas: adverse impact on survival and no association with p53 mutations. Br J Cancer 2001; 84:1070–1075.

56. Brizel DM, Scully SP, Harrelson JM, et al. Tumor oxygenation predicts for the likelihood of distant metastases in human soft tissue sarcoma. Cancer Res 1996; 56:941–943.

57. Parker C, Milosevic M, Toi A, et al. Polarographic electrode study of tumor oxygenation in clinically localized prostate cancer. Int J Radiat Oncol Biol Phys 2004; 58:750–757.

58. Movsas B, Chapman JD, Hanlon AL, et al. Hypoxia in human prostate carcinoma: an Eppendorf pO_2 study. Am J Clin Oncol 2001; 24:458–461.

59. Movsas B, Chapman JD, Hanlon AL, et al. Hypoxic prostate/muscle pO_2 ratio predicts for biochemical failure in patients with prostate cancer: preliminary findings. Urology 2002; 60:634–639.

60. Young SD, Marshall RS, Hill RP. Hypoxia induces DNA overreplication and enhances metastatic potential of murine tumor cells. Proc Natl Acad Sci U S A 1988; 85:9533–9537.

61. De Jaeger K, Kavanagh MC, Hill RP. Relationship of hypoxia to metastatic ability in rodent tumours. Br J Cancer 2001; 84:1280–1285.

62. Buchler P, Reber HA, Lavey RS, et al. Tumor hypoxia correlates with metastatic tumor growth of pancreatic cancer in an orthotopic murine model. J Surg Res 2004; 120:295–303.

63. Rofstad EK, Danielsen T. Hypoxia-induced metastasis of human melanoma cells: involvement of vascular endothelial growth factor-mediated angiogenesis. Br J Cancer 1999; 80:1697–1707.

64. Cairns RA, Kalliomaki T, Hill RP. Acute (cyclic) hypoxia enhances spontaneous metastasis of KHT murine tumors. Cancer Res 2001; 61:8903–8908.

65. Cairns RA, Hill RP. Acute hypoxia enhances spontaneous lymph node metastasis in an orthotopic murine model of human cervical carcinoma. Cancer Res 2004; 64:2054–2061.

66. Rofstad EK. Microenvironment-induced cancer metastasis. Int J Radiat Biol 2000; 76:589–605.

67. Graeber TG, Osmanian C, Jacks T, et al. Hypoxia-mediated selection of cells with diminished apoptotic potential in solid tumours. Nature 1996; 379:88–91.

68. Zhang L, Hill RP. Hypoxia enhances metastatic efficiency by up regulating mdm2 in KHT cells and increasing resistance to apoptosis. Cancer Res 2004; 64:4180–4190.

69. Reynolds TY, Rockwell S, Glazer PM. Genetic instability induced by the tumor microenvironment. Cancer Res 1996; 56:5754–5757.

70. Mihaylova VT, Bindra RS, Yuan J, et al. Decreased expression of the DNA mismatch repair gene *Mlh1* under hypoxic stress in mammalian cells. Mol Cell Biol 2003; 23:3265–3573.

71. Maxwell PH, Pugh CW, Ratcliffe PJ. Activation of the HIF pathway in cancer. Curr Opin Genet Dev 2001; 11:293–299.

72. Huang LE, Gu J, Schau M, Bunn HF. Regulation of hypoxia-inducible factor 1alpha is mediated by an O_2-dependent degradation domain via the ubiquitin-proteasome pathway. Proc Natl Acad Sci USA 1998; 95:7987–7992.

73. Kallio PJ, Wilson WJ, O'Brien S, Makino Y, Poellinger L. Regulation of the hypoxia-inducible transcription factor 1alpha by the ubiquitin-proteasome pathway. J Biol Chem 1999; 274:6519–6525.

74. Salceda S, Caro J. Hypoxia-inducible factor 1alpha (HIF-1alpha) protein is rapidly degraded by the ubiquitin-proteasome system under normoxic conditions. Its stabilization by hypoxia depends on redox-induced changes. J Biol Chem 1997; 272:22,642–22,647.

75. Wang GL, Jiang BH, Rue EA, Semenza GL. Hypoxia-inducible factor 1 is a basic-helix-loop-helix-PAS heterodimer regulated by cellular O_2 tension. Proc Natl Acad Sci U S A 1995; 92:5510–5514.

76. Ohh M, Park CW, Ivan M, et al. Ubiquitination of hypoxia-inducible factor requires direct binding to the beta-domain of the von Hippel-Lindau protein. Nat Cell Biol 2000; 2:423–427.

77. Tanimoto K, Makino Y, Pereira T, Poellinger L. Mechanism of regulation of the hypoxia-inducible factor-1 alpha by the von Hippel-Lindau tumor suppressor protein. EMBO J 2000; 19:4298–4309.

78. Ivan M, Kondo K, Yang H, et al. HIFalpha targeted for VHL-mediated destruction by proline hydroxylation: implications for O_2 sensing. Science 2001; 292:464–468.

79. Jaakkola P, Mole DR, Tian YM, et al. Targeting of HIF-alpha to the von Hippel-Lindau ubiquitylation complex by O_2-regulated prolyl hydroxylation. Science 2001; 292:468–472.

80. Lando D, Gorman JJ, Whitelaw ML, Peet DJ. Oxygen-dependent regulation of hypoxia-inducible factors by prolyl and asparaginyl hydroxylation. Eur J Biochem 2003; 270:781–790.

81. Blancher C, Moore JW, Talks KL, Houlbrook S, Harris AL. Relationship of hypoxia-inducible factor (HIF)-1alpha and HIF-2alpha expression to vascular endothelial growth factor induction and hypoxia survival in human breast cancer cell lines. Cancer Res 2000; 60:7106–7113.

82. Bos R, van der Groep P, Greijer AE, et al. Levels of hypoxia-inducible factor-1alpha independently predict prognosis in patients with lymph node negative breast carcinoma. Cancer 2003; 97:1573–1581.

83. Koukourakis MI, Giatromanolaki A, Sivridis E, et al. Lactate dehydrogenase-5 (LDH-5) overexpression in non-small-cell lung cancer tissues is linked to tumour hypoxia, angiogenic factor production and poor prognosis. Br J Cancer 2003; 89:877–885.

84. Talks KL, Turley H, Gatter KC, et al. The expression and distribution of the hypoxia-inducible factors HIF-1alpha and HIF-2alpha in normal human tissues, cancers, and tumor-associated macrophages. Am J Pathol 2000; 157:411–421.

85. Kung AL, Wang S, Klco JM, Kaelin WG, Livingston DM. Suppression of tumor growth through disruption of hypoxia-inducible transcription. Nat Med 2000; 6:1335–1340.

86. Akakura N, Kobayashi M, Horiuchi I, et al. Constitutive expression of hypoxia-inducible factor-1alpha renders pancreatic cancer cells resistant to apoptosis induced by hypoxia and nutrient deprivation. Cancer Res 2001; 61:6548–6554.

87. Krishnamachary B, Berg-Dixon S, Kelly B, et al. Regulation of colon carcinoma cell invasion by hypoxia-inducible factor 1. Cancer Res 2003; 63:1138–1143.

88. Jaffar M, Williams KJ, Stratford IJ. Bioreductive and gene therapy approaches to hypoxic diseases. Adv Drug Deliv Rev 2001; 53:217–228.

89. Stratford IJ, Adams GE, Bremner JC, et al. Manipulation and exploitation of the tumour environment for therapeutic benefit. Int J Radiat Biol 1994; 65:85–94.

90. Stratford IJ, Williams KJ, Cowen RL, Jaffar M. Combining bioreductive drugs and radiation for the treatment of solid tumors. Semin Radiat Oncol 2003; 13:42–52.

91. Brown JM, Giaccia AJ. The unique physiology of solid tumors: opportunities (and problems) for cancer therapy. Cancer Res 1998; 58:1408–1416.

92. Koch CJ. Unusual oxygen concentration dependence of toxicity of SR-4233, a hypoxic cell toxin. Cancer Res 1993; 53:3992–3997.

93. Biedermann KA, Wang J, Graham RP, Brown JM. SR 4233 cytotoxicity and metabolism in DNA repair-competent and repair-deficient cell cultures. Br J Cancer 1991; 63:358–362.

94. Dorie MJ, Brown JM. Modification of the antitumor activity of chemotherapeutic drugs by the hypoxic cytotoxic agent tirapazamine. Cancer Chemother Pharmacol 1997; 39:361–366.

95. Johnson CA, Kilpatrick D, von Roemeling R, et al. Phase I trial of tirapazamine in combination with cisplatin in a single dose every 3 weeks in patients with solid tumors. J Clin Oncol 1997; 15:773–780.

96. Miller VA, Ng KK, Grant SC, et al. Phase II study of the combination of the novel bioreductive agent, tirapazamine, with cisplatin in patients with advanced non-small-cell lung cancer. Ann Oncol 1997; 8:1269–1271.

97. Bedikian AY, Legha SS, Eton O, et al. Phase II trial of tirapazamine combined with cisplatin in chemotherapy of advanced malignant melanoma. Ann Oncol 1997; 8:363–367.

98. von Pawel J, von Roemeling R, Gatzemeier U, et al. Tirapazamine plus cisplatin versus cisplatin in advanced non-small-cell lung cancer: A report of the international CATAPULT I study group. Cisplatin and Tirapazamine in Subjects with Advanced Previously Untreated Non-Small-Cell Lung Tumors. J Clin Oncol 2000; 18:1351–1359.

99. Lee DJ, Trotti A, Spencer S, et al. Concurrent tirapazamine and radiotherapy for advanced head and neck carcinomas: a Phase II study. Int J Radiat Oncol Biol Phys 1998; 42:811–815.

100. Craighead PS, Pearcey R, Stuart G. A phase I/II evaluation of tirapazamine administered intravenously concurrent with cisplatin and radiotherapy in women with locally advanced cervical cancer. Int J Radiat Oncol Biol Phys 2000; 48:791–795.

101. Del Rowe J, Scott C, Werner-Wasik M, et al. Single-arm, open-label phase II study of intravenously administered tirapazamine and radiation therapy for glioblastoma multiforme. J Clin Oncol 2000; 18:1254–1259.

102. Rischin D, Peters L, Hicks R, et al. Phase I trial of concurrent tirapazamine, cisplatin, and radiotherapy in patients with advanced head and neck cancer. J Clin Oncol 2001; 19:535–542.

102a. Rischin D, Peters L, Fisher R, et al. Tirapazamine, cisplatin, and radiation versus fluorouracil, cisplatin and radiation in patients with locally advanced head and neck cancer: a randomised phase II trial of the Trans-Tasman Radiation Oncology Group (TROG 98.02). J Clin Oncol 2005; 23(1):79–87.

103. Patterson LH. Bioreductively activated antitumor N-oxides: the case of AQ4N, a unique approach to hypoxia-activated cancer chemotherapy. Drug Metab Rev 2002; 34:581–592.

104. Hejmadi MV, McKeown SR, Friery OP, McIntyre IA, Patterson LH, Hirst DG. DNA damage following combination of radiation with the bioreductive drug AQ4N: possible selective toxicity to oxic and hypoxic tumour cells. Br J Cancer 1996; 73:499–505.

105. Loadman PM, Swaine DJ, Bibby MC, Welham KJ, Patterson LH. A preclinical pharmacokinetic study of the bioreductive drug AQ4N. Drug Metab Dispos 2001; 29:422–426.

106. Patterson LH, McKeown SR. AQ4N: a new approach to hypoxia-activated cancer chemotherapy. Br J Cancer 2000; 83:1589–1593.

107. McCarthy HO, Yakkundi A, McErlane V, et al. Bioreductive GDEPT using cytochrome P450 3A4 in combination with AQ4N. Cancer Gene Ther 2003; 10:40–48.

108. Dachs GU, Patterson AV, Firth JD, et al. Targeting gene expression to hypoxic tumor cells. Nat Med 1997; 3:515–520.

109. Patterson AV, Williams KJ, Cowen RL, et al. Oxygen-sensitive enzyme-prodrug gene therapy for the eradication of radiation-resistant solid tumours. Gene Ther 2002; 9:946–954.

110. O'Neill P, McNeil SS, Jenkins TC. Induction of DNA crosslinks in vitro upon reduction of the nitroimidazole-aziridines RSU-1069 and RSU-1131. Biochem Pharmacol 1987; 36:1787–1792.

111. Stratford IJ, Walling JM, Silver AR. The differential cytotoxicity of RSU 1069: cell survival studies indicating interaction with DNA as a possible mode of action. Br J Cancer 1986; 53:339–344.

112. Cowen RL, Williams KJ, Chinje EC, et al. Hypoxia targeted gene therapy to increase the efficacy of tirapazamine as an adjuvant to radiotherapy: reversing tumor radioresistance and effecting cure. Cancer Res 2004; 64:1396–1402.

113. Moeller BJ, Cao Y, Li CY, Dewhirst MW. Radiation activates HIF-1 to regulate vascular radiosensitivity in tumors: role of reoxygenation, free radicals, and stress granules. Cancer Cell 2004; 5:429–441.

114. Unruh A, Ressel A, Mohamed HG, et al. The hypoxia-inducible factor-1 alpha is a negative factor for tumor therapy. Oncogene 2003; 22:3213–3220.

115. Rapisarda A, Uranchimeg B, Scudiero DA, et al. Identification of small molecule inhibitors of hypoxia-inducible factor 1 transcriptional activation pathway. Cancer Res 2002; 62:4316–4324.

116. Yeo EJ, Chun YS, Cho YS, et al. YC-1: a potential anticancer drug targeting hypoxia-inducible factor 1. J Natl Cancer Inst 2003; 95:516–525.

117. Rapisarda A, Uranchimeg B, Sordet O, et al. Topoisomerase I-mediated inhibition of hypoxia-inducible factor 1: mechanism and therapeutic implications. Cancer Res 2004; 64:1475–1482.

118. Becker A, Hansgen G, Bloching M, et al. Oxygenation of squamous cell carcinoma of the head and neck: comparison of primary tumors, neck node metastases, and normal tissue. Int J Radiat Oncol Biol Phys 1998; 42:35–41.

119. Koong AC, Mehta VK, Le QT, et al. Pancreatic tumors show high levels of hypoxia. Int J Radiat Oncol Biol Phys 2000; 48:919–922.

120. Lyng H, Sundfor K, Rofstad EK. Oxygen tension in human tumours measured with polarographic needle electrodes and its relationship to vascular density, necrosis and hypoxia. Radiother Oncol 1997; 44:163–169.

121. Sundfor K, Lyng H, Trope CG, Rofstad EK. Treatment outcome in advanced squamous cell carcinoma of the uterine cervix: relationships to pretreatment tumor oxygenation and vascularization. Radiother Oncol 2000; 54:101–107.

122. Knocke TH, Weitmann HD, Feldmann HJ, Selzer E, Potter R. Intratumoral pO_2-measurements as predictive assay in the treatment of carcinoma of the uterine cervix. Radiother Oncol 1999; 53:99–104.

123. Hockel M, Schlenger K, Hockel S, Vaupel P. Hypoxic cervical cancers with low apoptotic index are highly aggressive. Cancer Res 1999; 59:4525–4528.

124. Rudat V, Stadler P, Becker A, et al. Predictive value of the tumor oxygenation by means of pO_2 histography in patients with advanced head and neck cancer. Strahlenther Onkol 2001; 177:462–468.

125. Rudat V, Vanselow B, Wollensack P, et al. Repeatability and prognostic impact of the pretreatment pO_2 histography in patients with advanced head and neck cancer. Radiother Oncol 2000; 57:31–37.

126. Stadler P, Becker A, Feldmann HJ, et al. Influence of the hypoxic subvolume on the survival of patients with head and neck cancer. Int J Radiat Oncol Biol Phys 1999; 44:749–754.

127. Brown JM. SR 4233 (tirapazamine): a new anticancer drug exploiting hypoxia in solid tumours. Br J Cancer 1993; 67:1163–1170.

128. Patterson LH, McKeown SR, Ruparelia K, et al. Enhancement of chemotherapy and radiotherapy of murine tumours by AQ4N, a bioreductively activated anti-tumour agent. Br J Cancer 2000; 82:1984–1990.

129. Papadopoulou MV, Bloomer WD. NLCQ-1 (NSC 709257): exploiting hypoxia with a weak DNA-intercalating bioreductive drug. Clin Cancer Res 2003; 9:5714–5720.

130. Chen J, Zhao S, Nakada K, et al. Dominant-negative hypoxia-inducible factor-1 alpha reduces tumorigenicity of pancreatic cancer cells through the suppression of glucose metabolism. Am J Pathol 2003; 162:1283–1291.

131. Sun X, Kanwar JR, Leung E, et al. Gene transfer of antisense hypoxia inducible factor-1 alpha enhances the therapeutic efficacy of cancer immunotherapy. Gene Ther 2001; 8:638–645.

132. Sun X, Kanwar JR, Leung E, Vale M, Krissansen GW. Regression of solid tumors by engineered overexpression of von Hippel-Lindau tumor suppressor protein and antisense hypoxia-inducible factor-1alpha. Gene Ther 2003; 10:2081–2089.

133. Aquino VM, Weitman SD, Winick NJ, et al. Phase I trial of tirapazamine and cyclophosphamide in children with refractory solid tumors: a pediatric oncology group study. J Clin Oncol 2004; 22:1413–1419.

134. Hoff PM, Saad ED, Ravandi-Kashani F, Czerny E, Pazdur R. Phase I trial of i.v. administered tirapazamine plus cyclophosphamide. Anticancer Drugs 2001; 12:499–503.

135. Lara PN, Jr., Frankel P, Mack PC, et al. Tirapazamine plus carboplatin and paclitaxel in advanced malignant solid tumors: a California cancer consortium phase I and molecular correlative study. Clin Cancer Res 2003; 9:4356–4362.

136. Shulman LN, Buswell L, Riese N, et al. Phase I trial of the hypoxic cell cytotoxin tirapazamine with concurrent radiation therapy in the treatment of refractory solid tumors. Int J Radiat Oncol Biol Phys 1999; 44:349–353.

137. Aghajanian C, Brown C, O'Flaherty C, et al. Phase I study of tirapazamine and cisplatin in patients with recurrent cervical cancer. Gynecol Oncol 1997; 67:127–130.

138. Senan S, Rampling R, Graham MA, et al. Phase I and pharmacokinetic study of tirapazamine (SR 4233) administered every three weeks. Clin Cancer Res 1997; 3:31–38.

139. Bedikian AY, Legha SS, Eton O, et al. Phase II trial of escalated dose of tirapazamine combined with cisplatin in advanced malignant melanoma. Anticancer Drugs 1999; 10:735–739.

140. Treat J, Johnson E, Langer C, et al. Tirapazamine with cisplatin in patients with advanced non-small-cell lung cancer: a phase II study. J Clin Oncol 1998; 16:3524–3527.

4 Oncogenes and Tumor Suppressor Genes in Therapeutic Resistance

The Role of Evolving Interrelationships Between Cancer Cells and Host Tissues

Janusz W. Rak, MD, PhD, Brenda Coomber, PhD, and Joanne L. Yu, PhD

CONTENTS

SUMMARY

Development of therapeutic resistance is intrinsic to the neoplasia and is associated with the complexity, plasticity, and dynamics of the process. Some aspects of drug resistance, such as the ability to repopulate the tumor mass by clonogenic/stem cell subsets or adhesion/aggregation-dependent changes in responsiveness to therapy may be related to genetic tumor progression, genetic instability, and expression of oncogenic proteins. Combinations of cytoreductive agents with oncogene-directed signal transduction inhibitors or angiogenic agents have already produced promising preclinical and clinical results. In the not-too-distant future, refinement and commercialization of pharmacogenomic tests in cancer will enable more-accurate predictions regarding responsiveness of individual patients to new and established agents. These data will also enable understanding of pathways of drug resistance and ways to overcome it.

Key Words: Oncogenes; tumor suppressor genes; drug resistance; microenvironment; tumor–host interactions.

From: *Cancer Drug Discovery and Development: Cancer Drug Resistance*
Edited by: B. Teicher © Humana Press Inc., Totowa, NJ

1. INTRODUCTION: MULTIFACETED NATURE OF THERAPEUTIC RESISTANCE IN CANCER

Despite the already large and increasing number of anticancer agents developed to date, only a handful of human tumors is currently susceptible to a curative therapeutic intervention (including germ cell, trophoblastic, and hematologic malignancies) *(1)*. The remaining majority of cancers, particularly at their advanced stages, tend to persist, progress or recur while therapy is being administered, i.e., such tumors display a behavior that could define "therapeutic resistance" *(1)*. Such an operational definition of the latter term has at least two major weaknesses, which often lead to misperceptions and confusion, especially at the boundary between preclinical and clinical analysis. First, detection of "resistance" is often based on intuitive comparisons between the *actual* and *expected* therapeutic outcomes, often without sufficient consideration as to whether the expectations themselves are reasonable and well founded (true drug resistance), or not (the agent or therapeutic schedule *per se* are simply ineffective, i.e., chosen without proper justification or sufficient knowledge of its activity in a given context). This is an important distinction as it points to the significance of a well-developed rationale for both selecting potentially active agents and defining realistic ways to bring about a reversal of bona fide therapeutic resistance. Second, the criteria for what constitutes therapeutic *response* (end points, degree, duration) may differ between clinical and preclinical studies, and in the context of different classes of agents. Consequently, what may seem as a "good" antitumor response in a battery of in vitro and in vivo assays (e.g., tumor growth delay in a xenograft model) may be *a priori* below or outside of what is viewed as therapeutic response in clinical settings *(2)*. For these reasons the question as to why many "promising" anticancer therapies depressingly often fail to save lives seems to require a more comprehensive approach to therapeutic resistance.

Resistance to anticancer agents is usually classified as either *intrinsic* (*de novo*) or *acquired (1)*. In the former case, an agent that can reasonably be expected to cause an antitumor effect (e.g., on the basis of prior experience with similar cases of malignancy of the same or different type) fails to do so at the very beginning of therapy. In this case, the cause of resistance is independent of, and precedes the timing of drug administration. In contrast, *acquired drug resistance* is apparently (and implicitly) secondary to the exposure, i.e., the impact of a given agent appears to be diminished with consecutive rounds of treatment *(1)*.

It is increasingly obvious that the apparent therapeutic ineffectiveness (resistance) that might be observed in clinical settings likely represents a compound effect of several events occurring at the cell, tissue, or organismal level. Those include specific molecular characteristics, the changing properties of molecular targets of the given agent (e.g., mutations, shift in isoform expression, polymorphisms in the patient population, i.e., host dependent susceptibility), composition of various subsets of tumor cells, paracrine, and adhesive interactions between tumor cells *(3–5)*, interactions with their stromal host counterparts, and or extracellular matrix (e.g., in the case of cell adhesion-dependent drug resistance) *(6)*, tumor cytoarchitecture (microdomain structure), the type, abundance and functional status of stromal or inflammatory infiltrates within the tumor mass, the nature and dynamic changes within the tumor vascular bed and related fluctuation in blood perfusion and oxygen supply *(7)*, circulation of interstitial fluid, tissue oxygenation and many other parameters *(3,8–11)*. Many of these diverse factors, which likely influence therapeutic resistance in cancer, remain (albeit implicitly and often indirectly) in a causal relationship with oncogenic lesions in cancer cells, the signaling consequences of which are ultimately responsible for progression of human malignancies *(12,13)*. Hence, responsiveness to therapy and genetic tumor progression are interrelated in a complex and reciprocal fashion *(14–19)*. In this context, the influence of oncogenic lesions on therapeutic resistance could occur at three different levels relative to the presumed (or actual) "target process" at which the drug/modality is directed. Thus, such resistance may be related to the *target* itself, to *pretarget* processes (e.g., drug delivery, detoxification, cellular uptake), and to *posttarget* events (execution of cell death programs induced by the treatment) *(20)*.

In view of a large spectrum of questions pertinent to genetic determinants of cancer resistance to therapy, and abundance of excellent relevant literature, this chapter focuses mainly on one particular fragment of the mosaic. In so doing we explore primarily the role transforming genes (oncogenes and tumor suppressors) may have in the development of resistance to standard cytoreductive therapies (chemotherapy and ionizing radiation) and to their own or related inhibitors (targeted agents) directed at transforming signaling pathways. We also discuss in some detail the role of oncogenes in formation of the "private" tumor microcirculation and tumor–blood interface, and we consider how this may impact responses of cancers to therapies aimed at the tumor parenchymal (e.g., anticancer therapy) or stromal/vascular compartment (e.g., antiangiogenesis, antivascular therapy).

1.1. The Linkage Between Genetic Tumor Progression and Responsiveness to Therapy

If responsiveness to traditional anticancer radio- and/or chemotherapy protocols is taken as a paradigm, two opposing processes appear to take place during the natural history of human cancers. First, the initial transformation, tumor progression, and the resulting "activated" functional status of cancer cells (e.g., increased mitogenesis), generally makes such cells potentially vulnerable to cytotoxic, antimitogenic, and proapoptotic activities of conventional anticancer agents. Indeed, this is the basis on which these agents were found to be selectively toxic for cancer cells (possibly also their "activated" supporting stroma), and without causing equivalent damage to most of the nontransformed (and quiescent/nonactivated) normal tissues. Undesired toxicity of such therapies is therefore manifested in organs where the functional status of cells resemble that of cancer cells elsewhere (e.g., toxicity of antimitotic agents against tissues with active physiological mitogenesis and ongoing self-renewal, such as bone marrow, gut epithelium, skin, and so on). Second, additional transforming events may reverse and distort this initial drug/radiation sensitivity profile of cancer cells and bring about a bona fide therapeutic resistance. Such secondary alterations may occur in cancer cells "spontaneously" during the natural course of disease progression (i.e., drug resistance being a "side effect" of tumor progression), or may be related to recurrent exposure to rounds of noncurative genotoxic and potentially mutagenic therapeutic insults separated by cycles of tumor cell selection, recovery, and change *(21)*. Thus, both acquired responsiveness and resistance to anticancer treatment can be viewed as parts of the same biological continuum the direction of which could be influenced by underlying cancer genetics *(15)*.

1.2. The Cellular Basis of Responsiveness to Anticancer Therapy

Our understanding of what constitutes an anticancer effect and lack thereof (resistance) has undergone a considerable evolution. This is largely because of a change in definition of essential attributes of the malignant process, which was traditionally linked to exuberant unlimited mitogenesis. More-recent analysis led to understanding that cancer as a disease is far more complex, heterologous, host dependent, and represented by at least six distinct functional "hallmarks" *(22)* and the multitude of their corresponding molecular pathways *(12,22)*. Still, increase in the net cell number (and their destructive influence on the organ integrity) is a fundamental problem associated with cancer growth, and the main therapeutic concern. This imbalance in cell number could originate from heterogenous defects in control of mitogenesis, physiological apoptosis, differentiation, self-renewal (clonogenicity, stem cell properties) and senescence, in a manner that is driven by both intrinsic (oncogenic) and extrinsic (microenvironment-related) regulatory abnormalities *(15,22,23)*. The latter encompass paracrine, adhesive, and microenvironmental stimuli (e.g., oxygen supply), many of which are linked to functions of "activated" host stromal cells and the vasculature *(22)*. Indeed, this emerging understanding led to several recent developments, including fundamental reevaluation of how various agents exert their anticancer effects (e.g., through induction of apoptosis, necrosis, senescence, or mitotic catastrophe rather than "growth inhibition") to realization that traditional "gold standard" assays and surrogate parameters for testing drug responsiveness and resistance when used in an indiscriminate (universal) manner may often be inadequate and misleading (e.g., in vitro testing of cellular viability, growth inhibition, clonogenicity assays, transplantable and transgenic models). This also led to conception and development of "targeted therapeutics" directed at molecules rather than properties of cancer cells. Examples of the latter include oncogene-directed agents *(24)*, drugs directed at tumor vasculature (e.g., angiogenesis inhibitors and antivascular agents) *(25,26)*, or modalities with combined activity *(27,28)*.

2. EXAMPLES OF ONCOGENIC INFLUENCE ON THERAPEUTIC RESISTANCE TO MAJOR CLASSES OF ANTICANCER AGENTS

With enormous influx of new data and evolving treatment modalities, the comprehensive coverage of all aspects of oncogene-related therapeutic resistance in cancer is daunting, if not impossible, in one chapter. However, it may be of interest to consider in a more selective manner at least some examples of how the increasing understanding of oncogenic processes helps integrate, rationalize, and ultimately refine therapeutic approaches, and leads to progress in dealing with the problem of treatment resistance in cancer. In this chapter we limit our comments to three therapeutic modalities, namely cytoreductive therapies (chemotherapy and radiation), targeted agents (directed at elements of oncogenic pathways), and antiangiogenics (broadly defined as agents targeting tumor microcirculation).

2.1. Oncogenes and Cytoreductive Therapies—Chemotherapy and Ionizing Radiation

Cytoreductive therapeutic modalities (chemotherapy and radiation) have been the main stay of nonsurgical cancer management for over 50 yr *(20)*. Their advent and development has been largely empirical and based on selection of agents or protocols that could produce a preferential tumor cell kill, while sparing normal tissues. Indeed, a degree of selectivity that was achieved was historically attributed to intrinsically higher mitotic activity of cancer cells relative to their normal counterparts. Not surprisingly therefore, highly mitogenic normal tissues (bone marrow, gut mucosa, epidermis, hair follicles) have been sites of the most severe dose limiting toxicity, and often served as surrogates of biological activity *(20)*. The reasoning centered on cellular mitogenesis has also become the basis for design of drug activity assays, mathematical models of treatment responsiveness and explanation of possible causes of therapeutic success or failure *(29)*. The latter is an issue of particular significance, as unquestionable effectiveness of chemotherapy and radiation in certain types of human malignancies (leukemias, testicular cancer, chorionepithelioma) was not matched by similar successes in major advanced human malignancies (e.g., those of the breast, lung, colon, brain, and prostate) often described as occupying higher positions on "the axis of intractability" *(30)*. In other words, management of such cancers continues to present a seemingly insurmountable problem of therapeutic resistance *(11,20,31–33)*.

The precise mechanistic (molecular) causes of the antitumor effects of various cytotoxic modalities remain unclear, even long after their introduction as standards of care. Likewise, the specific reasons for acquired and/or *de novo* therapeutic resistance in the clinic remain largely unclear. Such resistance is often explained at the operational level, by such aspects of tumor pathobiology, as the existence of the noncycling (resistant) tumor stem/clonogenic cells, which could repopulate the tumor after initial response *(34)*, specific cell cycle distribution of cancer cells, parallel transitory states of treatment susceptibility, or the numerical (asymptotic) nature of the cytotoxic effect as such ("fractional kill"), where eradication of all tumor cells could only be approached, but rarely (if ever) achieved *(33,35,36)*. Other pretarget forms of drug resistance were also put forward, such as poor drug penetration (delivery) into the tumor mass because of altered cytoarchitecture, high interstitial pressure, abnormal vascular structures, poor blood perfusion, *(37)* and related microenvironmental perturbations, such as hypoxia, which is known to impair the effects of ionizing radiation *(8,38–40)*. In the context of this discussion, it is important to point out that many if not all of these parameters could be (and probably are at least indirectly) affected by the genetic "program" of the malignant process itself, including various influences of activated oncogenes on cellular mitogenesis, survival, stroma recruitment, angiogenesis, lymphangiogenesis, immunity, three-dimensional growth patterns and tolerance to hypoxia (Table 1) *(12,28,41–44)*. One informative example of such indirect influence of transforming cellular pathways on therapeutic resistance emerged out of studies on radiosensitizing effects of farnesyl transferase inhibitors (FTIs). These agents interfere with posttranslational processing, membrane localization, and activity of mutant Ras oncoproteins (possibly also other farnesylated cellular targets), and thereby provoke an increase in intrinsic cellular radiosensitivity in vitro in affected cancer cells *(38)*. Somewhat surprisingly, FTIs exerted an even greater radiosensitizing effect in the context of corresponding experimental tumors in vivo, and this was correlated with, and possibly mediated by, improved tumor perfusion and decreased hypoxia *(38)*. This is counterintuitive as FTIs are known to diminish vascular endothelial growth factor (VEGF) expression and other proangiogenic effects associated with expression of mutant Ras *(45)*. However, if such antiangiogenic effects were limited in magnitude (e.g., because of conservative dosing regimen or limited biological activity of the drug), this could result in a phenomenon recently referred to as "vessel normalization" (i.e., diminution of structural exuberance of the tumor vasculature coupled with paradoxically improved function; *see* Section 2.3.) *(46)*, and explain the increase in tumor perfusion and radiosensitization after FTI treatment. This interpretation is consistent with another example of unexpected therapeutic synergy in cancer, observed between direct angiogenesis inhibitors (e.g., angiostatin, minocyclin, and other

Table 1
The Impact of Oncogenic Events on Different Levels of Resistance to Cytotoxic
Anticancer Therapies—Examples

- Pretarget mechanisms
  - Influence on angiogenesis, blood perfusion tissue oxygenation
    and drug delivery (ras, src, ErbB1/2).
  - Regulation of local drug metabolism (ras).
  - Regulation of P-gp and other drug efflux mechanisms
    (N-myc, H- and K-ras).
  - Regulation of mitogenic activity (ras, raf, p53).
  - Existence of stem cells (genetic determinants unknown).
- Target mechanisms
  - Influence on genetic instability and DNA repair (ras, HER-2, v-src).
  - Influence on stress response pathways (ras, HER-2, p53).
- Posttarget mechanisms
  - Regulation of apoptotic pathways (ras, Akt, phosphatase and tensin
    homologue deleted in chromosome ten, p53, bcl-2).
  - Regulation of senescence pathways (p53, ras, ARF).
  - Regulation of cell cycle checkpoints (p53, p16).

---

agents) and both radio- and chemotherapy protocols *(47–50)*. Nevertheless, data obtained with FTIs and other targeted agents strongly suggest that oncogenic pathways may influence therapeutic resistance to cytotoxic modalities through direct effects on cancer cells *(38,51)* (*see* below), but also indirectly, i.e., through changes in the complexity of the tumor microenvironment *(38)*. Indeed, in some instances therapeutic resistance to cytotoxic modalities may be manifested exclusively in vivo *(52)*.

A significant conceptual shift in understanding the variability of responsiveness to cytotoxic anticancer therapies was precipitated by the discovery of molecular mediators of multidrug resistance *(53,54)*. These studies revealed a mechanism of active drug extrusion from cancer cells through the action of an ATP-dependent transmembrane "pump" known as P-glycoprotein (multidrug resistance-1/P-gp) *(53)*. More recently, several other similar entities (ATP-binding cassette [ABC] transporters) have been identified (e.g., multidrug resistance protein [MRP]1, lung resistance protein [LRP]), and found to be upregulated in both, drug resistant cancer cell lines and tumors in vivo *(20,54–56)*. The P-gp-mediated drug resistance affects tumor cell responsiveness to a particular subset of structurally unrelated, small lipophilic compounds (vinblastive, vincristine, doxorubicin, etoposide, paclitaxel), and this effect could be reversed (at least in vitro and sometimes also in vivo) by several pharmacological antagonists (drug sensitizers, reversal agents), such as calcium channel blockers (verapamil), cyclosporine analogues (PSC-833), quinoline derivatives (MS-209) and several other agents *(54)*. Whereas ABC transporters and their reversal agents established an illuminating paradigm of molecular mechanisms of drug resistance and its pharmacological reversal *(55)*, they have also been a subject of much debate, some disappointment and unexplained paradoxes *(1,40,57)*. First, the P-gp reversal agents have not delivered on their promises to effectively combat resistance to lipophilic anticancer drugs in solid tumors *(54)*. Second, genetic and clinical tumor progression are often paralleled by mounting drug resistance of increasing severity, an observation suggesting that oncogenic lesions could be expected to upregulate the levels of ABC transporters. Whereas, in some instances such parallel was indeed observed, e.g., between MRP level and N-*myc* positivity in neuroblastoma *(58)*, in other cases the reverse was true, e.g., expression of mutant N- or K-*ras* in acute myeloid leukemia correlated with reduced expression of P-gp (with no change in MRP1 and LRP levels) *(59)*. This should also be put in the context of the physiological function of P-gp (and ABC transporters) in maintenance of tissue integrity (brain), and/or function (gut, liver, kidney) in certain organ sites, where exclusion of extracellular toxins through high expression of "pump" proteins is a natural process *(54,60)*. Therefore, it is reasonable to assume that regulation of ABC transporters by differentiation, paracrine factors, oncogenic- and stress-related signals may contribute to drug resistance in some tumor settings *(61,62)*, but the role of oncogenes in tumor responsiveness to chemotherapy would likely also include other, perhaps more robust mechanisms *(31,54,63,64)*.

Cytoreductive anticancer modalities were developed to inflict maximal and selective damage on the cellular mitotic machinery in tumor cells, and ultimately (in a direct or indirect manner) compromise the process of DNA replication and maintenance of structural and functional integrity of the cancer cell genome. Indeed, the latter could be viewed as a broadly defined direct "target" of such therapies. Consequently, several target-related forms of therapeutic resistance involve alterations in DNA synthesis and repair mechanisms *(13)*. For instance, proteins involved in nucleotide excision repair, including excision repair crosscomplementing 1 and xeroderma pigmentosum gene products have been implicated in removal of DNA adducts postcisplatinum treatment *(32)*. Interestingly, excision repair crosscomplementing 1 mRNA was recently found to be upregulated in patients with non-small cell lung cancer (NSCLC) *(32)*. It remains to be seen whether there was any relationship between this event and the oncogenic status of these patients. In another study, however, expression of v-*Src* oncogene in a gallbladder cell line resulted in a more efficient removal of interstrand crosslinks and was reversible by treatment with radicicol, but not with inhibitors of phosphoinositide 3-kinase (PI3K) and protein kinase C pathways *(65)*. On the other hand, fibroblastic cells exhibited resistance to cisplatinum and increased efficiency of DNA repair on expression of oncogenic H-*ras* and subsequent activation of the PI3K/rac/reactive oxygen species pathway *(66)*. Inactivation of the *HER-2* oncogene in breast cancer cells diminished DNA repair and survival of breast cancer cells exposed to cisplatinum *(67)*. As oncogenic pathways also influence, or modify other events related to maintenance of DNA integrity, such as cell cycle checkpoints or mismatch repair processes *(12,32,68)* further studies may reveal their additional role in responsiveness to cytotoxic therapies.

It is worthy of attention that in some instances oncogenic events actually promote responsiveness to cytotoxic agents (Table 2). For instance, inactivation of the p53 tumor suppressor gene in U87 human astrocytoma and murine glioma sensitizes these cells to the cytotoxic action of nitrosourea derivatives *(16,69)*. Expression of activated oncogenes such as *HER-2 (70)* or *E1A (71)* was also associated with increased (rather than decreased) sensitivity to cisplatinum. *HER-2* amplification was also linked to increased responsiveness of breast cancers to antracyclines, but the impact of the accompanying coamplification of other genes in the same region of chromosome 17q12, notably topoisomerase IIα, remains a possible factor in manifestation of this phenotype *(17)*. These examples illustrate the complexity of the relationship between oncogenic events and the impact various classes of chemotherapeutics may have on causing fatal DNA damage. It is conceivable that unifying explanations for these divergent effects could be found only in specific cellular, signaling, and therapeutic contexts.

Table 2
Dual Role of Oncogenes in Determining Cellular Responses to Genotoxic Therapies

- Examples of oncogenic events that may sensitize cancer cells to genotoxic therapies
  - P53 mutations and sensitivity of glioma cells to nitrosourea derivatives.
  - Overexpression of HER-2 and athracycline sensitivity in breast cancer.
  - Cisplatin sensitivity in gallbladder cancer cells expressing HER-2.
  - Chemosensitivity of experimental lymphoma expressing oncogenic myc.
- Examples of oncogenic events that may cause resistance to genotoxic therapies
  - Bcl-2 overexpression, resistance to chemotherapy.
  - Akt activation, resistance to chemotherapy.
  - Resistance to chemotherapy in cells overexpressing eIF-4E.
  - Resistance to ionizing radiation and sulindac in cells expressing activated Ras.
  - Resistance to radio- or chemotherapy in p53-deficient tumor cells.

See text for references.

Posttarget effects of chemotherapeutics and radiation involve induction of cellular growth arrest, functional paralysis and programmed cell death. The molecular control of these events has recently attracted considerable attention, owing to realization that ultimate causes of cellular demise after genotoxic or microtubule insult lie with activation of precisely controlled intracellular programs of self-destruction *(72)*. Implicitly, these death processes are controlled by signaling pathways of which transforming proto-oncogenes are an important part *(12,20)*. Whereas much of the cytotoxicity associated with anticancer treatment modalities was initially attributed to induction of apoptosis *(72)*, alternative cellular responses have recently come to light including mitotic catastrophe/necrosis and terminal growth arrest also known as cellular senescence or STASIS (*st*ress or *a*berrant *s*ignaling *i*nduced *s*enescence) *(20,73–77)*. The importance of this distinction extends beyond semantics. Indeed, drug-related activation of the apoptotic caspase cascade (mostly through mitochondrial pathway) leads to fragmentation, release and phagocytosis of the cellular material (including DNA) without inflammatory reaction, a process that ultimately results in disappearance of affected cancer cells *(74)*. In the cumulative "macroscale," such events could amount to tumor shrinkage, an established clinical criterion of therapeutic response (according to Response Evaluation Criteria in Solid Tumors protocol) *(74,57,78)*. Similarly, severe and acute drug-induced damage can result in endomitosis, cell cycle arrest, and inability of the cellular machinery to repair DNA and restore chromosomal integrity followed by cell death through a mechanism often compared to necrosis *(74)*. Again, in this case the cell is eventually eliminated and even with stromal or inflammatory reaction, tumor shrinkage could be expected *(23,74)*. When the ability of a cancer cell to execute its own physical demise through apoptotic or mitotic pathways becomes permanently compromised (e.g., because of defects in the apoptotic pathway), cytotoxic injury may result in disruption of mitotic capacity, but without destruction of physical structure and metabolic activity of the affected cell. The accompanying change in cellular phenotype is reminiscent of cellular proliferative senescence as indicated by positivity for several markers: acidic β-galactosidase and upregulation of *p16*, *p53*, *PAI-1*, and other genes *(23,73,79)*. In this case, the apparent tumor shrinkage may be less apparent, or absent, but instead the macroscopic growth is halted with the remaining tumor mass containing viable, but nondividing cancer cells continues to persist

Table 3
Oncogenic Events Associated With Changes in Resistance to Oncogene-Directed (Targeted) Agent

- Example of oncogenic mutations that sensitize cancer cells to targeted agents
  - Expression of mutant EGFR in NSCLC sensitive to gefitinib
- Examples of oncogenic events that confer resistance to targeted agents
  - Mutations and amplification of bcr-abl in CML patients treated with imatinib
  - Upregulation of VEGF in cells resistant to EGFR inhibitors
  - Overexpression of AR in androgen independent prostate cancer
  - Androgen-independent activation of AR in prostate cancer

EGFR, endothelial growth factor receptor; NSCLC, non-small cell lung cancer; CML, chronic myelogenous leukemia; VEGF, vascular endothelial growth factor: AR, androgen receptor.
See text for references.

(as apparent "disease stabilization") *(23)*. Senescent cancer cells, like their normal counterparts, may eventually die after protracted growth arrest, but they may also constitute a reservoir of occult disease, presumably because of paracrine stimulation and genetic progression of residual surviving tumor cell clones *(23)*.

Responsiveness to cytotoxic treatment modalities often declines with more clinically and genetically advanced disease. As several genes involved in growth arrest, apoptosis, and senescence possess properties of oncogenes or tumor suppressors (*see* Tables 1 and 2; Table 3), it could be expected that their contribution to the genetic tumor progression may alter the pattern of therapeutic resistance intrinsically, i.e., without prior drug exposure *(22,74)*. Conversely, some of the events associated with tumor progression could be induced, accelerated, or altered by exposure to cell death-inducing stimuli of physiological (hypoxia) or treatment-related nature *(74)*. Even such an unrelated but relevant property of cancer cells as expression of the proangiogenic phenotype could be a product of such "collateral" selection process, which favors cells able to evade apoptosis through expression of oncogenic proteins, known inducers of angiogenesis *(80)* (*see* Section 2.3.). The relationship between responsiveness to cytotoxic therapies and genetic tumor progression is epitomized by actions of *p53*, the most common genetic alteration in human cancer (reviewed in ref. *74*). Thus, DNA damage is now known to cause activation of "sensory" mechanisms including several kinases (Ataxia telangiestasia mutated protein, ataxia telangiectasia- and Rad3-related, checkpoint 1, checkpoint 2) and resultant expression/stabilization of TP53 *(20)*. Depending on the magnitude of the injury, TP53 could either activate a growth arrest pathway (p21) coupled with DNA repair (GADD45) or trigger the programs of apoptotic cell death and senescence. Consequently, loss of p53 and its integrating role is often (but not always) associated with drug resistance *(20,74)*. Interestingly, oncogenic events involving *ras*, *E1A*, *myc*, and other transforming genes are also associated with upregulation of TP53 executed through a pathway involving upregulation of p19[ARF] (also promyelocytic leukemia [PML]) and resulting in inhibition of murine double minute 2 (MDM2)-dependent TP53 degradation *(12,81)*. In the context of intact tumor suppressors (p53, p16, p19) these events may also activate apoptotic or senescence pathways and induce what is often referred to as "oncogenic stress" phenomenon *(20,74,81,82)*. It is therefore noteworthy that isolated overexpression of oncogenic proteins (e.g., Ras) may lower the apoptotic threshold and promote (rather than inhibit) tumor cells' sensitivity to genotoxic insults, a phenotype that is eventually overridden by secondary genetic events

(15,74). However, the apparent dependence of oncogenic transformation (e.g., in association with heterozygous mutations of *ras*) on preceding loss of tumor suppressor pathways (e.g., p53, p16, adenomatous polyposis coli) has recently been questioned in studies utilizing refined transgenic models in which point mutation of a single allele was used instead of overexpression *(83,84)*. Even with this in mind, it is still possible that, whereas K-ras may possess transforming properties without preceding changes in p16 or p53, such additional changes will contribute to subsequent (multigenic) resistance to genotoxic therapy observed in advanced human cancers.

The interrelationship between oncogenic events and pathways of drug-induced cellular apoptosis and senescence has been recently elegantly delineated using a murine model of spontaneous development of B-cell lymphoma under the influence of the *myc* oncogenic transgene (E-*myc*) *(15,74)*. In this model (the biology of which is reminiscent of Burkitt's lymphoma), treatment with high doses of cyclophosphamide (CTX) can produce an ostensibly curative outcome, as measured by the duration of tumor-free survival, in a large proportion of animals *(23)*. This effect was associated with massive induction of apoptotic death (intense TdT-mediated dUTP nick end labeling [TUNEL] staining), physical shrinkage of lymph nodes and clearance of green fluorescent protein-tagged tumor cell deposits from all accessible disease sites *(23)*. Additional genetic defects changed fundamentally the biology of this model disease and responsiveness to therapy. For instance, overexpression of the antiapoptotic Bcl-2 proto-oncogene in E-myc hematopoietic precursor cells obliterated the cellular responses (apoptosis) to CTX therapy, which no longer resulted in the shrinkage of the palpable tumor masses in lymph nodes *(23)*. Paradoxically, there was also a considerable prolongation of progression-free survival *(23)*. This was because of a continued responsiveness of tumor cells to therapy, albeit in a qualitatively different manner. In this case the defect in apoptotic pathway led to induction of cellular senescence-like process whereby tumor cells remained physically intact and metabolically active but were paralyzed (at least temporarily) in their ability to support the disease progression *(23)*. It is interesting to note that this state represents a form of resistance from a "clinical" standpoint, but less so from the biological perspective (as CTX-exposed senescent tumor cells would become unable to sustain their clonogenicity). Even in such a "paralyzed" state cancer cells might, however, be able to provoke growth of their less damaged or altered (stem-like) minority subsets, which may constitute a disease reservoir and a source of recurrence *(23,74)*. The behavior of the Bcl-2-expressing E-myc lymphoma could be altered further by introduction of genetic defects that compromise the senescence pathway (e.g., by removal of *p53* or *INK4a/ARF* genes) *(23)*. In such an instance, both control and Bcl-2-expressing tumors became resistant to therapy and prolongation of tumor-free survival was significantly reduced *(15,23,74)*. Again, this sequence of events (i.e., changes in failsafe, apoptotic and senescence pathways may occur under selective pressure of therapy but also spontaneously during tumor progression (because of evolving resistance to natural selective pressures, e.g., oxygen/growth factor deprivation) and result in *de novo* resistance to therapeutic modalities targeting the respective pathways of cell-loss control *(15)*.

Identification of oncogene-dependent events as a source of resistance to the genotoxic insult provided a rational basis for new strategies aimed at using oncogene-directed agents effectively as radiation- or chemosensitizers in combination with traditional treatments *(31,76)*. Several such attempts with various inhibitors of oncogenic signal transduction have shown some promise, irrespectively whether such targeted agents themselves (as monotherapy) exert a potent antitumor effect or not *(31,76)*. For instance, as mentioned earlier the complex (partially Ras-directed) action of FTIs may result in significant radiosensitization effects in vitro and particularly in vivo *(38)*. Similarly, antagonists of *ErbB* oncogenes (Herceptin, C225/erbitux and various other epithelial growth factor receptor [EGFR] inhibitors) have been shown to lower the apoptotic threshold, modulate cell cycle progression, and enhance the activity of cytoreductive modalities (e.g., radiation, cisplatinum, doxorubicin, and paclitaxel) *(67,85–93)*. It has also been noticed that some of the common survival pathways located downstream of many oncogenic pathways may be used as targets for chemosensitization (or radiosensitization) regardless of the activating genetic lesion. A case in point is the recent evidence that a pathway involving PI3K/Akt, its downstream effector mammalian target of rapamycin (mTOR) and a translation factor eIF-4E (itself a proto-oncogene) *(94)* may be involved in resistance to chemotherapeutic agents. Again, by using the aforementioned E-myc lymphoma model Wendel, Lowe, and colleagues demonstrated that when tumor cells are engineered to express the activated (oncogenic) form of Akt (or bcl-2) they become more aggressive and irresponsive to treatment with CTX or doxorubicine because of a severe defect in their ability to execute apoptotic death on genotoxic injury *(76,77)*. This could be overridden by treatment with the antagonist of mTOR rapamycin, but only if the cells did not constitutively express upregulated levels of mTOR effector eIF-4E *(76,77)*. These results exemplify how the knowledge of signaling pathways that control cell death processes may lead to derivation of a different type of targeted therapy, namely *targeted reversal agents* directed at specific forms of oncogene dependent therapeutic resistance.

It may be useful to close our remarks regarding the role of oncogenes in responsiveness to cytoreductive agents with two summarizing thoughts. First, oncogenes by definition affect cellular signaling pathways and gene expression profiles in a multifaceted and "cascade-like" manner *(12)*. The consequences of such broad influence may encompass, therefore, several putative molecular mediators that could be involved in various forms and mechanisms of drug/radiation resistance including (*see* Table 1):

1. Mechanisms that control drug delivery and tumor microenvironment (e.g., angiogenesis, lymphangiogenesis, thrombosis, vessel remodeling).
2. Expression of membrane transporters (e.g., P-gp, MRP1, LRP).
3. Cellular detoxification mechanisms (e.g., glutathione *S*-transferase, metallothioneins, bleomycin hydrolase).
4. Enzymatic activities involved in DNA synthesis and metabolism (e.g., dihydrofolate reductase).
5. Mechanisms of drug activation (e.g., DT-diaphorase, nicotinamide adenine dinucleotide phosphatase, P450 reductase).
6. DNA repair mechanisms (e.g., topoisomerase II, O^6-methyl guanine-DNA methyltransferase, human mut-L homologue 1, human mut-L homologue 2, checkpoint 1, p21^{WAF1}).
7. Mechanisms that control cell cycle progression (e.g., cell adhesion signaling, E-cadherin, p27^{Kip1}, p21^{WAF1}).
8. Mechanisms that control cellular stress response, survival, apoptosis, and senescence (e.g., p53, p73, Bcl-2, p19/ARF, bclx$_L$, cell adhesion-dependent drug resistance).

Second, in spite of the ultimate causation of clinical progression and cancer-related mortality by oncogenic lesions, their influence on therapeutic resistance to cytoreductive modalities is not unidirectional. Indeed, oncogenic events can contribute to an increase in therapeutic resistance to chemo- and/or radiotherapy in some settings*(15,19,32,51,65,100–103)*, but to a decrease (i.e., cause sensitization) in other contexts*(16,69,70,104–106)*. This dichotomy (*see* Table 2) is thought-provoking, as it suggests that at the early stages of tumor progression (at least in some cases) the incipient genetic influences may provoke a state of "oncogenic stress" and propensity to activate apoptotic program on additional cell injury, whereas at the later stages of disease and during the course of therapy-induced cellular selection, additional genetic events may emerge, and oncogenic pathways may become rewired to produce a state of increasing resistance to cytotoxic insults*(12,20,74,76)*. Moreover, genetic changes that induce drug resistance to one agent may sensitize cancer cells to another, a notion with significant unexplored therapeutic potential *(107)*.

2.2. Resistance to Oncogene-Directed Therapies

Whereas oncogenic events are often the source of therapeutic resistance to traditional anticancer agents *(31,32,38,76,108,109)*, they also have recently become targets of the new generation ("targeted") anticancer drugs *(54,110,111)*. One of the expectations associated with such oncogene-directed signal transduction inhibitors has been that they may not only block molecular mechanisms of cellular transformation *per se* but also, consistent with aforementioned considerations, act as sensitizing agents in the context of traditional cytoreductive therapies *(38,108)*. It therefore came as somewhat of a surprise (although perhaps one that should have been expected) that cancer sensitivity to these "sensitizing agents" did in fact show variation, diminished, or even disappeared over time, thereby manifesting hallmarks of a bona fide therapeutic resistance.

With regards to the nature of resistance to targeted agents, the case in point was provided early on by thus far the most successful drug in this class known as imatinib mesylate (STI571, Glivec®, Gleevec™) *(112,113)*. Imatinib is an ATP-competitive inhibitor selective for a narrow group of tyrosine kinases, most particularly c-Abl, but also platelet-derived growth factor receptor (PDGFR)-β and c-Kit. Because of these properties, the agent became a "hit" in the search for antagonists of the constitutively active and transforming bcr-abl fusion gene product that forms during the reciprocal t(9;22) translocation associated with the aberrant 22q Philadelphia chromosome. This translocation is detectable in the majority (95%) of patients with chronic myelogenous leukemia (CML) and in a subset of cases of acute lymphoblastic leukemia (ALL) *(112)*. By combining the constitutive tyrosine (possibly also serine-threonine) kinase activity of aberrant c-Abl with effects rendered by the aggregation domain of the *bcr* gene product, the bcr-abl oncogene delivers a potent transforming signal to myelogenous progenitors, presumably by altering their differentiation, mitogenesis, survival, mobility, adhesion and angiogenic properties *(112,114,115)*. This is executed through several effector pathways, including: Crkl, Src, Stat5, Fak/paxilin, Grb2/Sos/Ras/mitogen-activated protein kinase (MAPK), PI3K/Akt, and downstream apoptotic regulators such as Bad and Bclx$_L$ *(112)*. Various major isoforms of bcr-abl (p190, p210, p230) may differ in their ability to activate the respective pathways, but they represent the apparent common causal event in the clonal expansion of leukemic cells in the majority of CML patients, and thereby a prime therapeutic target *(112)*. So much so that blockade of the bcr-abl activity (e.g., by imatinib) could be viewed as tantamount to reversal of the leukemic process.

Indeed, in chronic phases of CML imatinib therapy resulted initially in a staggering 96.8% of complete hematological responses and 76.2% complete cytogenetic responses, thereby vastly outperforming the prior standard treatment with α-interferon and cytosine arabinoside (69% complete hematological response and 14.5% complete cytogenetic responses, respectively) *(112)*. However, it is now known that a fraction of CML patients treated with imatinib progress to accelerated and blast phases of the disease and begin to display reduced responsiveness (resistance) to therapy. Because of the paradigmatic role of imatinib amongst oncogene-directed agents, mechanisms of this somewhat unanticipated resistance have been subjected to considerable scrutiny. Among the possible factors that could render imatinib less/not effective in CML the levels of drug bioavailability have been considered, particularly in relation to plasma levels of α1-acid-glycoprotein, or concurrent erythromycin therapy *(112)*. It is also possible that drug metabolism, drug exclusion from cells through multidrug resistance (e.g., multidrug resistance-1/Pgp)-dependent mechanisms, and other factors may also contribute to reduced imatinib activity *(112)*. However, in advanced CML the apparent drug resistance is now attributed mainly to qualitative and quantitative changes in the bcr-abl oncogene itself *(112)*. Thus, *BCR-ABL* gene amplification, protein upregulation, mutational changes in Bcr-abl kinase activity, and deregulation of alternative signaling pathways are thought to alter the relative effectiveness of imanitib in CML patients *(112)*.

The increasing understanding of the mechanisms governing imatinib resistance precipitated a search for effective pharmacological countermeasures. In the event of the involvement of alternative kinases (e.g., Bruton's tyrosine kinase), their respective inhibitors are being contemplated as additives to imatinib therapy *(112)*. Similarly, targeting aforementioned downstream targets of bcr-abl (e.g., PI3K, MAPK kinase, mTOR) may prove useful in the context of diminished imatinib activity, as could, according to recent evidence, combining imatinib with protein farnesyl transferase inhibitors (Ras inhibitors) such as SCH66336 and L-744832, proteasome inhibitors (PS341/Velcade), trichostatin A, LAQ284 and other agents *(112)*.

However, it is unclear whether these strategies will be effective in addressing perhaps the most troublesome aspect of imatinib resistance, namely the existence of mutations within the bcr-abl kinase domain that render imatinib unable to maintain the oncogene in the autoinactivated state *(112)*. Interestingly, some of these mutant imatinib-resistant forms of Bcr-abl can still be effectively blocked by alternative inhibitors such as PD173955, or such agents developed against similar Src kinase as piridopirimidines (PD180970), trisubstituted purines (AP23464), or novel orally available compounds (BMS-354825) *(116,117)*. In some instances, different imatinib resistant alleles of *BCR-ABL* can be targeted with their specific inhibitors including PD166326 (directed at *BCR-ABL*[E255K]) *(118)*. On the other hand, imatinib found extended applications in inhibiting unrelated oncogenic tyrosine kinases such as *C-KIT* in stromal intestinal tumors *(119)* or *FLIP1L1-PDGFRA* in hypereosinophilic syndrome *(118)*. Interestingly, in the latter case another inhibitor (staurosporin derivative PKC412) was shown to overcome resistance to imatinib because of the expression of the *FLIP1L1-PDGFRA* mutant in vivo *(118)*. Even with these developments, certain Bcr-abl mutants (e.g., T315I) remain noninhibitable with presently available agents, and occult CML clones harboring such variant oncogenes are of concern as a source of disease reservoir, recurrence and progression *(116)*.

The inescapable question in this context is: What is the source of Bcr-abl mutations in CML? When do they occur, and what is their relationship to exposure to imatinib? Because multiple mutant forms of Bcr-abl kinase may be present in the same patient, it could be suggested that not only a selection process of preexisting CML clones could be facilitated during drug exposure, but also a high rate of unrepaired DNA errors in the *BCR-ABL* sequence (and elsewhere) could be generated during disease progression. It is therefore possible that constitutive or transient deregulation in DNA repair mechanisms may occur in CML during the stages of disease that precede, accompany, or follow (are because of?) expression of the *BCR-ABL* oncogene and contribute to its additional mutational changes. These questions await more-rigorous analysis, not only in relation to imatinib resistance, but also to better understand the emerging resistance to other targeted therapeutics.

In general terms, experience with imatinib has been illuminating, if not always uniformly successful, as it led to some thought provoking and generally applicable conclusions related to possible mechanisms of resistance to molecularly targeted anticancer agents. Thus, such resistance is thought to arise through three major classes of events including (1) target related changes (mutations, amplifications, overexpression); (2) pharmacokinetic changes (extracellular or cellular mechanisms, e.g., α1-acid-glycoprotein or P-gp, respectively); and (3) biological changes in the pathomechanisms of the disease (e.g., disease reservoir in molecularly distinct silent cancer stem cell population, activation of alternative transformation pathways) *(118)*.

Indeed, such forms of therapeutic resistance have been detected in the case of several agents directed at oncogenic pathways in cancer, a trend that is likely to continue with this expanding class of therapeutics. In this regard, the best-characterized cases include agents designed to inhibit oncogenenic forms of EGFR (EGFR/HER-1/ErbB1) and its related HER-2/ErbB2/*neu* kinase in various epithelial cancers, the PML-RARα oncogene in acute promyelocytic leukemia (APL) and activated androgen receptor (AR) in human prostate cancer.

Recent massive efforts to generate inhibitors of EGFR (EKIs) resulted in a diverse group of agents that entered advanced clinical trials, including ZD1839/Iressa/Gefitinib, cetuximab/erbitux/C225, CI-1033, erlotinib/OSI-774/Tarceva, PKI166, ABX-EGF, H-R3, and several others *(86)*. In this regard, gefitinib has been a frontrunner in terms of approval for clinical use in Japan and North America, and hence, this agent provided ample insights to the possible mechanisms of drug resistance. Thus, in spite of promising preclinical data, in patients with chemotherapy-resistant NSCLC, gefitinib induced heterogeneous responses with approximately 10% of cases demonstrating appreciable efficacy, whereas the reminder being more refractory *(110,120)*. To the credit of the particular group of investigators involved in these studies, this discrepancy was not treated as merely an indication of high frequency of failure or statistical inconvenience, but rather led to in-depth and rather revealing studies *(110,120–124)*. Thus, in spite of ubiquitous expression of EGFR in NSCLC, occurrence of specific deletions (e.g., E746-A750, L747-S752) and mutations (e.g., L858R) in the tyrosine kinase domain of the EGFR have been noted in a subset (10% in North America and 28% in Japan) of NSCLC cases *(120,124)*. Moreover, these genetic lesions were linked to preferential activation of the signal transduction activating transcription (STAT) and Akt-mediated pathways, but not the MAPK pathway *(121)*. This paralleled the enhanced susceptibility of NSCLC cells to EGFR inhibitors that target the ATP-binding pocket of this receptor (gefitinib and erlotinib). Strikingly, these "sensitizing" mutations were found at high frequency (75%) in NSCLC affecting nonsmokers *(122)*. Conversely, signaling through EGFR-independent pathways or through a wild-type EGFR may serve as an example of target-related resistance of NSCLC to gefitinib and similar acting agents. In this context, it is also worth considering that in certain types of human malignancies (e.g., in breast cancer) various members of the ErbB family of kinases are coexpressed and cooperate in causing cellular transformation in part by forming heteromeric complexes (e.g., EGFR/HER-2), and through mechanisms of "horizontal signaling" *(125,126)*. Therefore, whereas this is unusual in the realm of clinical drug development, it would seem reasonable to combine inhibitors of EGFR (e.g., erlotinib) and HER-2 (herceptin) to counteract the emerging resistance to blockade of each of these oncoproteins.

It is important to recognize that activated EGFR (or HER-2) may also be subject to posttarget drug-resistance mechanisms. As one of the consequences of EGFR inhibition is obliteration of the proangiogenic phenotype *(127,128)*, it may be anticipated that activation of an alternative angiogenic pathway (phenotype), e.g., through EGFR-independent oncogenic alterations, inflammatory influences, and/or hypoxia, may result in reduced responsiveness to EKIs *(27)*. For instance, it is known that tumorigenic and angiogenic capacity (in mice) of squamous cell carcinoma cells A431 depends on EGFR-dependent upregulation of VEGF *(127,129)*. We have recently demonstrated that bypassing the effects of EGFR by exogenous overexpression of VEGF under control of a strong viral promoter leads to significant reduction of the impact EKIs such as the C225 antibody has on tumor growth in vivo *(130)*. It is noteworthy that in spontaneously derived EKI-resistant variants of A431 cells the expression of VEGF is constitutively elevated. This may be because of the influence of alternative (EGFR-independent) oncogenic pathways (e.g., ras/MAPK), the activation of which could provide the cells with a selective growth/angiogenic advantage during continuous exposure to EKIs in vivo *(130,131)*. Again, these kinds of observations would suggest that simultaneous targeting VEGF/VEGF receptor (VEGFR), EGFR, and possibly other oncogenic targets (e.g., HER-2 in breast cancer) would seem to merit serious consideration, something that has only recently entered early stages of clinical evaluation *(132,133)*.

Indeed, similar paradigms of target-related or -unrelated therapeutic resistance are also applicable to more traditional targeted therapeutics such as agents directed at the PML-RARα oncogene in APL (all-*trans* retinoic acid [ATRA]) and AR in prostate cancer. With regard to the former, ATRA resistance, which is detected in 25–30% of APL patients, has been attributed to increased catabolism of ATRA through cytochrome P450-dependent pathways or mutations in the RARα sequence *(133)*. Obliteration of oncogenic AR signaling in prostate cancer is achieved by surgical (orchidectomy) or pharmacological (gonadotropin-releasing hormone analogs) androgen ablation often combined with AR antagonists (e.g., bicalutamide, hydroxyflutamide) *(133)*. In spite of initial effectiveness of this approach, androgen-independent disease often develops because of emergence of one or more of the following mechanisms *(133–137)*:

1. AR overexpression or amplification.
2. AR mutations (e.g., AR^{T877A}).
3. Androgen-independent activation of AR (e.g., by interleukin [IL]-6, protein kinase A, insulin-like growth factor 1).
4. Upregulation of alternative oncogenic pathways (EGFR, HER-2).
5. Inactivation of tumor suppressor genes (e.g., phosphatase and tensin homologue deleted in chromosome ten [PTEN]).
6. Deregulation of epithelial–stromal interactions.
7. Deregulation of apoptotic pathways.

Again, in order to produce a bona fide in vivo resistance to androgen ablation and disease progression, the impact of these various events is expected to affect not only cellular mitogenesis, but also cell survival, angiogenesis, as well as interaction with local and ectopic stroma (e.g., at the site of bone metastasis) *(136)*. It is of considerable interest that at least some of these mechanisms are directly or indirectly related (as in the case of other aforementioned targeted agents) to secondary oncogenic events known (e.g., activation of EGFR/HER-2) or unknown. In this sense, oncogenes appear to be the source of resistance to oncogene-dependent therapy. Again, this reinforces the notion that "antion-cogenic drug cocktails" should be considered strongly as the next step in the development of molecularly targeted therapies *(123)*.

2.3. Oncogenes, Tumor Suppressor Genes, and Agents Targeting Tumor Vasculature—the Balance Between Vascular Supply and Demand in Cancer

2.3.1. RATIONALE FOR ANTIANGIOGENIC THERAPY

Tumor growth, invasion, and metastasis are fundamentally dependent on the access of cancer cells to blood vessels *(138)*. This necessity is attributed to the requirement for influx of oxygen, glucose, nutrients, and metabolites, and efflux of catabolites to and from the tumor mass, respectively, but also to paracrine effects of vascular stroma (including endothelial cells) on growth, survival, motility, and other properties of cancer cells *(139–143)*. Cancer cells secure their blood vessel proximity by seeking actively preexisting vascular networks (vascular cooption and/or invasion) *(144,145)*, formation of pseudovascular channels (vasculogenic mimicry) *(146)*, or (perhaps more commonly) by recruitment of new capillaries to areas within and around the tumor. The latter scenario may be realized through several possible mechanisms, collectively designated as "tumor angiogenesis," including blood vessel sprouting, vascular intussusception, vessel splitting, vascular remodeling, and postembryonal vasculogenesis, all of which have been described in detail elsewhere *(147,148)*. We have also proposed recently that the processes of arteriogenesis *(149)*—defined as circumferential growth and remodeling of vessels "feeding" a particular vascular bed (e.g., tumor microcirculation)—is essential for expansion of the vascularized tumor masses *(150)*. Moreover, formation of lymphatic metastases has recently been linked to tumor-induced formation of new lymphatics (tumor lymphangiogenesis) *(151–154)*.

The notion of a basic dependence of the malignant process on angiogenesis *(145)*, arteriogenesis *(150)*, and lymphangiogenesis *(154)* suggests that these processes (and their distinct cellular and molecular mechanisms) could serve as therapeutic targets in cancer. Although mechanisms of these various processes are increasingly well understood *(25,148,154,155)* and have already inspired the search for new therapeutic opportunities, angiogenesis inhibition has been in focus of such efforts for the longest time *(138)*. For this reason, antiangiogenesis research is currently sufficiently advanced *(156)* to warrant a meaningful discussion of the likelihood and forms of therapeutic resistance to this modality. In this regard, it may be useful to first consider more carefully the expectations associated with this form of anticancer therapy *(26)*. Thus, in addition to the unique principle of targeting tumor vasculature (an essential host aspect supporting tumor growth and metastasis) instead of cancer cells themselves, the appeal of antiangiogenic therapy stems from several considerations related to specificity, safety, and anticancer efficacy of this modality. For instance, antiangiogenic agents would be expected to be tumor selective, as cellular and molecular properties of tumor-associated blood vessels appear to be unique owing to increased mitogenic activity, motility, and a permanent "activation" state of their constituent endothelium, and resulting morphological, architectural, and functional changes of the capillaries themselves *(147,148)*. Likewise, tumor-associated endothelial cells can be distinguished at the molecular level from their normal quiescent (or even physiologically activated) counterparts, notably by expression several unique tumor endothelial markers *(157)*, by their patterns of reexpression, utilization, and/or dependence on key molecular mediators of vascular development including VEGF, VEGR receptors (Flt-1/VEGFR-1 and Flk-1/KDR/VEGFR-2), hypoxia-inducible factor 1α, Tie-2/tek, Notch, Dll4, and several others *(148,158,159)*. More recently, other (nonendothelial) cellular elements of the tumor vasculature (e.g., pericytes) have entered the scene as possible targets for angiogenesis inhibition, again because they appear to possess distinct functional and molecular properties *(160)*. Henceforth, minimal side effects (dose limitations) are predicted to accompany angiogenesis inhibition because of the virtual absence of similar processes (active angiogenesis) in healthy adult tissues (with qualified exclusion of female reproductive organs, exercising muscle, regenerating tissues, granulation tissue, and a few other rare and/or tolerable circumstances) *(161)*. There is also a reasonable expectation that obliteration of tumor blood vessels should precipitate a catastrophic collapse of their dependent and much larger tumor cell populations because of reliance of the latter on noninterrupted passage of blood *(26,147,162)*. Selectivity and relative safety of antiangiogenesis may also be achieved by approaches that relay on blocking the onset ("angiogenic switch") *(163)* and maintenance ("angiogenesis progression") *(139,164,165)* of the angiogenic process, namely through counteracting the altered levels of various stimulators and inhibitors (*indirect* angiogenesis inhibition) at the level of their production, release, or biological activity (as in the case of bevacizumab). Functional obliteration of the activators (e.g., VEGF, fibroblast growth factors, transforming growth factors), or restoration of the endogenous inhibitors (e.g., thrombospondin [TSP]-1, -2, METH-1/2, pigment epithelium-derived factor) could be achieved by various means *(26,148,163)*, e.g., by delivery of recombinant preparations or pharmacological analogues of endogenous antiangiogenic factors to the tumor (an approach known as a *direct* mode of angiogenesis inhibition) *(26,166,167)*.

Perhaps one of the most appealing reasons to develop agents that could inhibit (antiangiogenics) or obliterate (antivascular therapeutics) the expanding tumor-associated microvasculature *(26,147,168,169)* is the prediction that such therapies could be inherently "resistant to resistance" *(170)*. This argument rests primarily on the contention that ultimately, much of the acquired resistance to traditional genotoxic anticancer therapeutics is driven by genetic instability (and indefinite phenotypic plasticity) *(171)* of target cancer cells *(170)*. As postulated by the clonal evolution hypothesis *(21)* and numerous subsequent experimental studies *(171)*, genetic instability leads to diversification of the cancer cell population, from which resistant cellular variant inevitably emerge through therapy-driven negative selection *(170)*. In contrast—it was reasoned—antiangiogenic agents affect genetically stable (nonmutable) type of cells (namely host endothelial cells), which would not be expected to give rise to significant diversity, variability, selection and resistance *(170)*.

2.3.2. The Specter of Irresponsiveness to Antiangiogenic Agents in Certain Tumor Contexts

In spite of the relatively short history of tumor angiogenesis research, it is now recognized widely that tumor blood vessels represent a validated, attractive, and unique therapeutic target in cancer. This notion led over the last two decades to development of a host of prospective antiangiogenic agents *(25,26,161)*, several recent clinical trials (listed and reviewed elsewhere in detail *[25,26]*, e.g., http://www.cancer.gov/clinicaltrials/developments/anti-angio-table, www.angio.org), and one drug (bevacizumab/Avastin®) approval for clinical use in cancer (http://www.gene.com/gene/news/press-releases/Feb26,2004). Whereas these are remarkable developments that underscore the basic correctness of the antiangiogenesis concept *(138)*, the field has reached the stage at which raising practical questions as to the inevitable limitations of this new treatment modality may be both timely and necessary, including a possibility (and indeed a reality) of irresponsiveness (resistance) to certain antiangiogenic agents and their classes in certain tumor contexts.

In 1996, we proposed that, whereas classical mechanisms of (mutational) therapeutic resistance may not apply to angiogenesis inhibition (this may still need to be qualified), there are reasons to suggest that in the broader sense, some forms of refractoriness or unresponsiveness are still to be expected *(172)*. We reasoned that sources of such resistance may, as with other agents, lie in pharmacokinetics, pharmacodynamics, bio-availability, and molecular interactions (detoxification) of antiangiogenic agents (pretarget considerations), in the status of endothelial cells themselves and that of their molecular regulators (target-related events), and—contrary to the prior dogma—treatment resistance could also reside in properties of the cancer cells ("posttarget" events) *(172)*. Further discussion of some of these possibilities has recently been undertaken in the emerging literature *(11,173)*, and therefore, we focus mainly on those aspects of therapeutic resistance to antiangiogenics that could be linked to genetic tumor progression.

There are reasons to believe that responsiveness to antiangiogenic agents can change with tumor progression *(18,172)*. Whereas tumor size, histotype, structure, vascularity, angiogenic profile, and other phenotypic features may be indicative of such emerging changes *(160,164,174,175)*, it is also worth considering an underlying causal role of genetic (oncogenic) events in the process. In theory, oncogenes could affect efficacy of antiangiogenic agents in several different ways:

1. Through changes in properties of cancer cells themselves that alter the impact and the consequences of the vascular insult (e.g., by changes in the angiogenic phenotype, increase/alteration in production of proangiogenic and survival factors, changes in sensitivity to oxygen deprivation, anaerobic metabolism, activation of survival pathways, and in several other ways) *(28,41,42)*.
2. Through indirect modification of various components of the angiogenic micromilieu (e.g., by oncogene-driven alterations in deposition and remodeling of the extracellular matrix, impact on stromal and inflammatory cell recruitment, and activation, as well as modifications of the hemostatic circuitry within and around the tumor) *(176–178)*.
3. Through secondary changes in structural and functional properties of the tumor microvasculature that may alter the likelihood of achieving a sustained antiangiogenic effect (e.g., changes in vascular architecture, patterning, stabilization, and "normalization" resulting from molecular changes set off or modified by oncogenic events).
4. Through genetic alterations within endothelial cells themselves (e.g., because of some of these cells, or their precursors originating from a transformed/aberrant progenitors in certain malignancies, "horizontal" gene transfer between tumor cells and their adjacent endothelium or else through contribution of genetically altered cancer cells to blood vessel wall—"vasculogenic mimicry") *(146,179–181)*. We discuss some of these possibilities (many still hypothetical or experimental in nature) in the remainder of this article (also, compare Fig. 1).

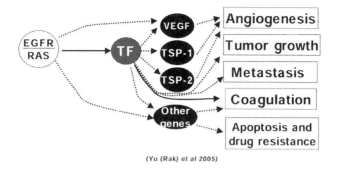

(Yu (Rak) et al 2005)

Fig. 1. The evolving interrelationship between transforming genetic events and the host vascular system. Oncogenic events affecting cancer cells alter/induce both proangiogenic and procoagulant properties in cancer cells. The latter aspect is exemplified by overexpression of the principal procoagulant receptor–tissue factor on the surface of cancer cells harboring oncogenic lesions (mutant ras, p53, activated epithelial growth factor receptor [EGFR], and several others). Tissue factor may not only trigger perivascular clotting events (on binding to factor VII or otherwise), but also transmit signals to the cellular interior thereby changing the expression of angiogenic (vascular endothelial growth factor), antiangiogenic (thrombospondin-1, -2), survival-altering, migratory, and mitogenic molecules (see references in the text).

2.3.3. ONCOGENES AND THE IMPACT OF CANCER CELL PROPERTIES ON RESPONSIVENESS TO BLOOD VESSEL-DIRECTED THERAPIES—THE QUESTION OF VASCULAR SUPPLY AND VASCULAR DEMAND

An important but often overlooked consideration in the context of the antiangiogenic therapy is that *the ultimate target of all anticancer therapies are cancer cells themselves*, and endothelial cell (vascular) inhibition/destruction is simply an intermediate step in the same process. Consequently, as with other anticancer therapies (albeit to a different extent), tumor cell heterogeneity and plasticity may have a significant bearing on the efficacy of antiangiogenic agents. For instance, withdrawal of blood vessel supply, whereas deadly in principle, may spare those cancer cells that have adapted to growth/ survival under ischemic conditions, e.g., because of alterations in hypoxia-, hypoglycemia- and growth factor-response pathways *(172)*. Changes in metabolic properties *(41)* of cancer cells are now known to be linked to oncogenic transformation. Indeed, ostensibly normal embryonic fibroblasts deficient for the *p53* tumor suppressor gene demonstrate a degree of resistance to hypoxia *(182)*. The *p53* gene product represents an interesting case because of the multiplicity of roles this tumor suppressor plays in neoplasia, including in maintaining genetic integrity ("guardian of the genome"), regulator of genotoxic stress responses *(183)*, resistance to anticancer treatments *(184,185)*, regulation of cell cycle checkpoints *(186)*, and more recently, in triggering angiogenic changes in affected cancer cells *(187)*.

In addition to these widely appreciated and fundamental properties, we have recently demonstrated that loss of p53 and at least three other types of cancer-related molecular alterations (loss of hypoxia-inducible factor 1, high levels of Ras activity, and unknown molecular defect in advanced melanoma) segregate with the ability of certain tumor cell subsets to populate poorly perfused tumor microdomains and withstand low blood vessel density (*see* Table 5, on p. 91) *(139,188–190)*. Several other independent studies recorded

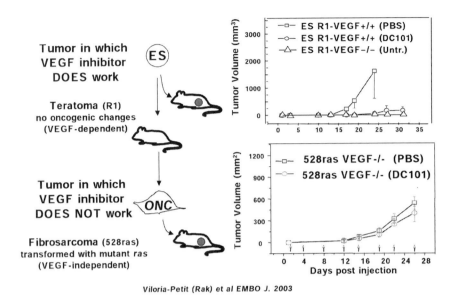

Fig. 2. Impact of vascular endothelial growth factor (VEGF) targeting in two different contexts of tumor angiogenesis. Teratoma formation by embryonic stem (ES) cells is blocked by targeting the VEGF gene (VEGF$^{-/-}$) and/or administration of the antibody (DC101) that blocks VEGF receptor (VEGFR-2) (upper panel). Isogenic cells derived from chimeric mice harboring the progeny of the aforementioned VEGF$^{-/-}$ ES cells can be used as donors of VEGF$^{-/-}$ adult dermal fibroblasts (middle section). When such fibroblasts are transformed with activated oncogenes (H-*ras*), the resulting fibrosarcoma cells (528ras1) form aggressive and angiogenic tumors in the absence of tumor-derived VEGF and are not growth-inhibited by VEGFR-2 blockade (DC101). Thus, in this setting at least two tumor-related forms of angiogenesis seem to exist, one of which (teratoma) is sensitive to VEGF/VEGR-2 inhibition, whereas the other (oncogene-driven pathway) appears to be resistant to such treatment (*see* text).

similar findings *(182,191,192)*. In spite of increasing vascular densities in certain tumor contexts, hypoxia and low (rather than high) microvascular density was associated with late stages of colorectal and pancreatic cancers where a considerable likelihood of multiple genetic defects including activation of K-ras and loss of p53 could be readily expected *(193,194)*. On the basis of these observations, we proposed that transforming events not only contribute to growth, survival, and onset of proangiogenic properties (the latter could be described as *vascular supply*) of cancer cells, but also define their relative reliance of such cells on blood vessel proximity, a property we refer to as *vascular demand (195)*. This led to a prediction that genetic defects could lower vascular demand of cancer cells and this in turn could diminish the efficacy of antiangiogenic therapies *(172)*. Indeed, in a recent study we were able to demonstrate that in the case of human colorectal cancer xenografts loss of p53 by tumor cells was associated with a reduced (though not abolished) tumor responses to a protocol combining two potent antiangiogenic agents, namely: metronomic dosing of vinblastine and intensive treatment with VEGFR-2 inhibitor (DC101) *(189)*. In fact, this finding links (at least in experimental settings) the genetic properties of cancer cells with the outcome of therapy targeting host-derived blood vessels (also *compare* Fig. 2).

Oncogenic alterations could also affect the outcome of blood vessel directed therapy through changes in the angiogenic profile of cancer cells (i.e., as a function of *vascular supply*). Thus, as mentioned earlier, the "angiogenic switch" in cancer is a function of cellular transformation and related alterations in intracellular signaling during the expression of angiogenesis related genes (*see* Fig. 1) *(28,196)*. This first came to light as a result of pioneering studies initiated by Bouck's laboratory, in which loss of p53 *(196)* was linked to down-regulation of TSP-1 (a proangiogenic event) in cultured fibroblasts isolated from patients with the Li-Fraumeni syndrome *(187,197)*. Subsequently, activated forms of K- and H-ras proto-oncogenes were shown to trigger proangiogenic processes by causing upregulation of VEGF *(45,198)*, and in some cases, also by downregulation of TSP-1 *(131,199,200)*. It is now recognized that Ras oncoproteins are able to affect tumor angiogenesis in multiple and diverse ways, for instance, by causing upregulation of IL-8 and related vascular and proinflammatory responses *(201)*, or by triggering expression of tissue factor, a change that may affect blood vessel dynamics in coagulation-related and/or -unrelated manner *(202)* (*see* Fig. 1). These observations have now been extended to a large number of transforming proteins, many of which may affect expression of several different regulators of angiogenesis, including growth factors, hormones, proteases, extracellular matrix proteins, and their antiangiogenic fragments (recently reviewed extensively in refs. *26* and *27*).

More importantly, oncogenes and tumor suppressors appear to act not only in a constitutive manner, but also through mimicking, amplifying, and modulating physiological mechanisms of angiogenesis, including the various activities of the hemostatic system *(128,202)*, hypoxia response pathways *(203,204)*, inflammatory responses *(201)*, and other microenvironmental influences to produce an increasingly abundant proangiogenic environment *(163)*. In fact, more-advanced disease that is associated with the progressive activation of various oncogenic pathways (reviewed recently in ref. *12*) may generate the level of proangiogenic stimulation, the robustness of which may be difficult to counteract by therapeutic means. For instance, increasing VEGF expression (a likely consequence of the occult oncogenic changes) was found to accompany evolving resistance to antiangiogenic effects of TSP-1 in experimental tumor models *(205)*, and conversely, VEGF knockdown achieved through RNA interference exerted a TSP-1 "sensitizing" effect *(206)*. This is important, because peptide analogues of the second type I repeat, the main antiangiogenic motif of TSP-1 known to interact with endothelial CD36 receptor, are in clinical trials as possible anticancer agents *(167)*. It is therefore of some concern, whether high levels of VEGF could render certain types of tumor (e.g., brain or renal cancers) resistant to this class of agents. In this regard, our recent study suggests that when cancer cells are rendered VEGF deficient (by VEGF gene targeting, *see* Fig. 2) TSP-1 peptides (but not VEGF antagonists) exert an appreciable anticancer effect *(176)*. A corollary to this discussion could be that inasmuch as the onset of angiogenesis in cancer depends on changes in the "angiogenic balance" *(163,196)*, the reversal/obliteration of this process may also be attainable by producing a context-dependent *antiangiogenic balance*, and not simply by delivery of a fixed amount of a given inhibitor.

It should be noted that a degree of endothelial cell stimulation is believed to be required for full manifestation of antiangiogenic effects of TSP-1 *(207)* and perhaps other angiogenesis inhibitors, as well. It is therefore necessary to assume that there may be a transition point where quantitative and/or qualitative changes in endothelial stimulation are no longer "sensitizing" these cells to the effects of angiogenesis inhibitors, but rather become a source of "angioprotection" and therapeutic resistance. The latter scenario seems to be operative when certain anticancer chemotherapeutics are tested for their

Table 4
Differential Responsiveness to Vascular Endothelial Growth Factor Inhibition
in Major Human Cancers

Avastin® trial	Cancer site	Preceding VEGF expression	Survival rate (in Avastin arm)	p-Value
AVF2107g	mCRC	+++	OS +4.7 mo	0.00003
			PFS +4.3 mo	>0.00001
AVF2119g	mBC	+++	PFS +0.5 mo	0.627

• Trial-related problem (pretreated versus untreated patients?).
• Pharmacological problem (need for better agents/regimens?).
• Biological problem (need for different agents/approaches?).

mCRC, metastatic colorectal cancer; mBC, metastatic breast cancer; OS, overall survival; PFS, progression-free survival. (Adapted from refs. *244* and *245*.)

antiendothelial effects in vitro *(208)* in the presence or absence of VEGF *(209,210)*. In such settings, VEGF triggered upregulation of survivin, *XIAP*, and other antiapoptotic genes, thereby counteracting the effects of chemotherapy in a manner operationally indistinguishable from a bona fide drug resistance *(173,209,210)*. Also in vivo, antiangiogenic (metronomic) scheduling of standard chemotherapy was relatively less effective on its own as compared to a combination of such therapy (e.g., using vinblastine) with agents blocking the activity of VEGF/VEGFR-2 pathway *(211)*. Likewise, the effects of metronomic treatment with cyclophosphamide were enhanced by addition of another antiangiogenic agent (TNP470) *(212)*. In mice deficient for TSP-1 (TSP-1$^{-/-}$), metronomic therapy with cyclophosphamide was less effective, perhaps suggesting a role for endothelial/host-derived TSP-1 in responsiveness to these vascular insults *(213)*. This observation points, albeit indirectly, to the possibility that low TSP-1 expression (whatever the mechanism) could be a cause of therapeutic resistance to metronomic angiogenesis inhibition. It is also known that a potent proangiogenic growth factor - basic fibroblast growth factor (bFGF) can alleviate antiendothelial effects of high doses of ionizing radiation through its effects on acidic sphingomyelinase/ceramide pathway *(214–217)*. Again, VEGF, bFGF, TSP-1, and many other effectors of angiogenesis that can participate in the aforementioned manifestations of therapeutic resistance to antiangiogenic therapies are targets of several known oncogenes. Future studies will show whether resistance to certain forms of antiangiogenic therapy segregates with defined stages and pathways in genetic progression of major human tumors.

2.3.4. Oncogenes and Tumor Responsiveness to Agents Targeting VEGF Pathway of Angiogenesis

In the light of this discussion, the nature of the possible resistance to VEGF inhibitors is of particular interest. This is because of the recent Food and Drug Administration approval of Avastin (bevacizumab, Genentech), a humanized neutralizing monoclonal antibody directed against human VEGF and the first antiangiogenic agent to ever enter clinical oncology. Whereas this has been a momentous development in the field of angiogenesis and antiangiogenesis research, it also signifies the need to consider the possibilities, causes and consequences of both, successes and failures (i.e., therapeutic resistance) of this strategy in the future (*compare* Table 4). With regard to the former, there are several reasons to believe that VEGF and its endothelial receptors (VEGFR-1/ Flt-1 and VEGFR-2/KDR/Flk-1) represent particularly well-suited, rational, selective, and well-validated therapeutic targets *(26,169)*. For instance, VEGF overexpression is ubiquitous in several types of cancer, preclinical data with several aforementioned inhibitory agents (including A 4.6.1 antibody, from which bevacizumab originated) revealed impressive antitumor effects in several recent studies *(218–221)* (also reviewed in ref. *222*). Amongst those compelling results, perhaps the strongest indication as to the potential effectiveness of VEGF inhibitors comes from genetic inactivation of their molecular targets—VEGF and VEGF receptors in mice. Thus, in mice harboring homozygous null mutation of either VEGFR-1 or VEGFR-2, death occurs during early gestation because of massive defects in vascular development *(223,224)*. Even more severe are the consequences of targeting the VEGF ligand, because even heterozygous mutant (VEGF$^{+/-}$) embryos die in mid-gestations of defects in vasculogenesis and angiogenesis *(225,226)*. In addition, in experimental tumors of embryonal or endocrine origin, VEGF gene inactivation led to severe impairment of angiogenic capacity and growth *(178,226–230)*. Collectively, these observations seem to indicate that the role of VEGF in blood vessel formation is essential, highly dose sensitive, and nonredundant, and hence, targeting this angiogenic pathway in cancer could hold a particularly great promise *(222)*.

Indeed, the recently concluded double-blinded, randomized phase III clinical trial (AVF2107) involving patients with metastatic colorectal cancer demonstrated that bevacizumab in combination with a version of Saltz's chemotherapy protocol (5FU/LV/ CPT-11) performed considerably better (offering 4.7 mo of an increase in overall patient survival) than chemotherapy alone *(231)* (*see* Table 4). Moreover, as a single agent, bevacizumab delayed time to progression in renal cancer, although no statistically significant increase in overall survival was noticed in that study *(232)*. In fact, whereas bevacizumab is a frontrunner of these efforts, a much larger body of inhibitory agents directed at VEGF/VEGFR-1/2 is in preclinical and clinical development offering an awesome future expansion of this important armamentarium. Those novel agents include, for example, several anti-VEGF antibodies (bevacizumab, HuMV833), antibodies against VEGF/VEGFR-2 complex (2C3), VEGF inhibiting soluble receptors (VEGF-TRAP), antibodies blocking VEGFR-2 (2C7), small molecule VEGFR inhibitors (SU11248, SU6668, PTK-787, ZD6474), anti-VEGFR-1 ribozymes (Angiozyme™) *(233)*, and many other agents.

Whereas VEGF targeting has proven to be a highly effective way of blocking angiogenic processes, there are also indications that this strategy may encounter some limitations. This is because (as mentioned earlier) the inclusion of bevacizumab into treatment of advanced colorectal cancer produced significant gains, but the effects have not been curative, i.e., tumor vasculature eventually evaded the therapy. Moreover, another phase III clinical trial (AVF2119) has been concluded recently, in which bevacizumab was administered to previously treated patients with metastatic breast cancer along with a standard regimen of capecitabine *(234)*. Unlike in the colorectal cancer cohort, this trial, however, yielded negative results, in that the arm with bevacizumab failed to meet the expected survival end points *(234)*, an outcome operationally tantamount to *de novo* therapeutic resistance (*see* Table 4). Because expression of VEGF and VEGFR (bevacizumab targets) has been described in both breast and colorectal cancers *(235)*, it could be argued that other aspects of these malignancies may have contributed to the divergent outcomes of the aforementioned clinical trials. For instance, various differences in trial design and characteristics of the corresponding patient cohorts (e.g., pretreatment in the case of breast cancer patients), subtleties of regimens, and other considerations should be taken into consideration (*see* Table 4).

However, there are reasons to believe that relative dependence of various tumors on the VEGF pathway may (contrary to common beliefs) be strikingly different (*176*), and hence, the consequences of VEGF inhibition may vary accordingly. For instance, it was noted that VEGF expression is a predominant angiogenic feature of early stage breast cancer, and this profile becomes more complex, with ever-increasing spectrum and abundance of proangiogenic growth factors (including FGF, endothelial cell growth factor, and several others) in more advanced tumors (*164*). This raises the question as to whether in the latter setting, VEGF becomes redundant rather than indispensable. Informative in this regard is a recent study where ectopic VEGF expression could be manipulated genetically in a breast cancer cell line, simply by activation/inactivation of a doxycycline-regulatable promoter (*174*). In this case, VEGF withdrawal did produce antitumor effects, but only at the early stages of breast cancer xenograft expansion in immunodeficient mice (*174*). In contrast, the same manipulation was inconsequential in more advanced (larger) tumors (*174*). Another thought-provoking preclinical study was conducted with various pharmacological inhibitors directed at VEGFR-2 specifically (SU5416), or capable of inhibition of several receptor tyrosine kinases including PDGFR, FGF receptor, and VEGFR (SU6668) (*160*). Interestingly, each of these drugs produced a different antitumor (and antiangiogenic) effect, depending on the stage in development of the same spontaneous and VEGF-dependent murine tumor (driven by expression of the same oncogenic transgene—RipTag model) (*160*). In the same model system, a tumor stage-specific pattern of therapeutic responsiveness/resistance was also observed with other antiangiogenics (*175*).

Expression of VEGF in the tumor mass may be a function of genetic (oncogenic), microenvironmental (hypoxic), or combined influences (*28,165,202,236*) (also, *see* Fig. 1). It is therefore reasonable to ask whether the efficacy of VEGF/VEGFR targeting agents would be altered by these different contexts. We have recently examined this question by comparing the impact of VEGF gene targeting and obliteration of VEGF receptors in two types of fundamentally distinct but isogenic tumors (*see* Fig. 2). Thus, in the case of ectopic (subcutaneous) injection of embryonic stem (ES) cells, highly aggressive tumors (ES cells-derived teratomas), arise as a result of aberrant differentiation and ostensibly in the absence of any stable alteration to the tumor cell genome (*176*). The same ES cells can instead be used to create healthy chimeric mice. It is from such mice that adult fibroblastic cells were isolated and subjected to oncogenic transformation by enforced expression of activated oncogenes (H-*ras*, *HER-2*, or *myc*) to produce a series of tumorigenic fibrosarcoma cell lines (*176*). We have recently employed both types (ES and oncogene-transformed) of tumorigenic cells to compare the role of the VEGF/VEGFR-2 pathway in two corresponding settings of tumor neoangiogenesis (*176*). Interestingly, VEGF gene disruption (an equivalent of inhibited VEGF production by cancer cells) resulted in dramatically different outcomes depending on the nature of the tumorigenic phenotype. In particular, whereas the growth ES-derived (VEGF$^{-/-}$) teratomas was almost completely abrogated, their VEGF$^{-/-}$ oncogene-transformed fibrosarcoma counterparts retained largely undiminished in vivo aggressiveness and angiogenic capacity (*176*). Moreover, a powerful neutralizing antibody against VEGFR-2 (DC101) blocked growth of VEGF proficient (VEGF$^{+/+}$) ES teratomas, but was relatively ineffec-

Table 5
Oncogenic Lesions Involved in Alteration
of "Vascular Dependence" of Cancer Cells

- H-Ras transformation
  See ref. *139.*
- HIF-1 a deletion
  See refs. *188, 191*, and *192.*
- Unknown lesion in human melanoma
  See ref. *188.*
- P53 loss in human colorectal cancer cells
  See ref. *189.*

HIF-1α, hypoxia-inducible factor 1α.

tive against oncogene-driven fibrosarcomas, even if the latter tumors were composed entirely of VEGF$^{-/-}$ cancer cells *(176)*. Selective inhibition of VEGFR-1 was ineffective in either case. These results suggest that activated oncogenes, whereas known to drive VEGF expression, may also render the tumor formation and blood vessel recruitment processes relatively unsusceptible to inhibition of the VEGF pathway (unlike in developmental context or in genetically unaltered isogenic teratoma, *see* Fig. 2) *(176)*. This could be because of a wider spectrum of VEGF-unrelated angiogenesis effectors deregulated by oncogenic events, including downregulation of several endogenous inhibitors (e.g., TSP-1, pigment epithelium-derived factor). In other words, the oncogene-driven ability of malignant cells to trigger sustained vascular supply may be more redundant and robust than angiogenesis in other biological contexts *(18,176,195)*. This apparent oncogene-dependent resistance to VEGF antagonists could also be attributed to diminished vascular demand of transformed cells that could withstand suboptimal conditions of blood perfusion (Table 5) *(18,195)*.

2.3.5. VASCULAR ARCHITECTURE AND RESPONSIVENESS OF TUMORS TO ANTIANGIOGENIC THERAPY

Although this can only be inferred indirectly, oncogenic events may also influence the architecture of the vascular tumor stroma and thereby the responses to antiangiogenic therapy. Indeed, because the angiogenic profile appears to be a function of genetic tumor progression *(28,165,195)*, so too could be the structural properties of the resulting neovasculature. This is exemplified by the observation that even relatively subtle changes in expression of VEGF isoforms by tumor cells can lead to significant changes in vascular architecture *(228,237)*, and likely to different consequences following antiangiogenic insults. In this regard, it was noted by Jain *(46)* that quantitative differences in magnitude of such insults may translate into qualitatively different outcomes in terms of the status of the tumor microcirculation. It was proposed that, whereas total obliteration of the angiogenic process may lead to a collapse of the tumor vascular network and cessation of blood supply, a less efficacious treatment may actually improve tumor microcirculation as a result of the removal of the structural exuberance of the vascular bed, a process named "vessel normalization" *(46)*. It is argued that the latter outcome may not be entirely negative, as it may facilitate delivery of anticancer therapeutics and improved radiation sensitivity of the tumor, both extremely important practical considerations *(46)*. Similarly, antiangiogenic effects of IL-12 were linked in a recent study with a form of vessel normalization (or "stabilization") process *(238)*, namely the treatment led to an increase in the fraction of tumor vessels associated with α-smooth muscle actin (SMA)-positive pericytes. A modest increase in α-SMA positivity was also observed when TSP-1 peptides were administered to mice harboring H-ras-driven and TSP-1-negative tumors *(176)*. Conversely, treatment of mice harboring VEGF-dependent tumors with antagonists of the VEGF/VEGFR-2 pathway (AG-013736 and VEGF-TRAP) led to preferential elimination of vascular elements with the highest expression of VEGFR-2 and to a reduction in vessel-associated α-SMA staining, an observation that points to resistance of VEGFR-2-negative/-low capillaries to such treatment, but also to (less obviously) the corresponding shift in pericyte composition *(239)*. Age-dependent alterations in responsiveness of the vasculature to changes in levels of VEGF and angiopoietin 1 signaling have also been noticed *(240)*. Our own more recent observations (Coomber, Fathers, Braithwaite, and Rak, unpublished) suggest that qualitative changes in the composition (heterogeneity) of the tumor vasculature may include decreases in the fraction of tie-2/tek-positive tumor capillaries. Again, this vascular heterogeneity may signify differential susceptibility of certain subsets of tumor blood vessels to therapeutic agents, which implies that some vascular segments may exhibit (or acquire) features of therapeutic resistance to specific antiangiogenics or their classes. Because oncogenic lesions in cancer cells affect ultimately the angiogenic environment within the tumor, including recruitment, selection, and modulation of vascular elements, it is implicit (but remains to be conclusively proven) that genetic tumor progression, vascular heterogeneity, and responsiveness to certain antiangiogenic agents are interrelated.

2.3.6. Genetic Alterations in Tumor-Associated Endothelial Cells

The genetically stable nature of tumor-associated endothelial cells has been recently challenged by several observations, albeit thus far applicable to a limited spectrum of malignancies. For instance, a recent study suggests that host cells may be susceptible to an uptake of partially intact DNA from apoptotic cancer cells *(181)*. It cannot be excluded that endothelial cells may acquire in this manner some of the oncogenic sequences, as well as expression of drug resistance and antiapoptotic properties. Even less hypothetical is a recent finding, which suggests that in a number of hematopoietic malignancies (B-cell lymphoma, CML), endothelial cell compartments contain the same chromosomal rearrangements, gains, or losses as the ones found in the hematopoietic tumor cells themselves *(179,241)*. This could be interpreted as an indication that precursors contributing to these kinds of tumors may have given rise to abnormal clones (leukemic blasts) and their associated endothelial progenitors. Consequently, differentiated endothelial cells would inherit at least some of the same oncogenic properties, genetic instability, and potential to develop therapeutic resistance as the ones present in their sister malignant leukocytes. For instance, in six patients with CML, bone marrow-derived endothelial progenitor cells were found to harbor the *BCR-ABL* oncogene, a signature genetic lesion for tumor cells in this disease *(179)*. Whereas the presence of the *BCR-ABL* oncogene in endothelial cells may render them resistant to some therapies, including angiogenesis inhibition (this needs to be examined more closely), this property may also suggest that in CML, the antitumor effects of Bcr-abl inhibitors (e.g., imatinib mesylate) could include an indirect, but also a direct antiangiogenic effect related to the blockade of bcr-abl in tumor supporting endothelial cells *(115,242)*.

It is also of considerable interest whether, and to what degree, vasculogenic mimicry by cancer cells contributes to sustained vascular supply *(146)*. As this process involves formation of vascular channels by certain types of cancer cells (e.g., ocular melanoma) rather than endothelium, targeting the latter cells may be relatively ineffective unless directed at common molecular features (e.g., VE-cadherin). Naturally, in spite of the acquisition of several endothelial properties (and function) by cancer cells in such settings they would remain genetically unstable and, at least in theory could display phenotypic plasticity and acquired drug/therapy resistance. Indeed, van der Schaft reported that unlike endothelial cells, the quasivascular networks formed by tumor cells do not respond to exposure to several angiogenesis inhibitors *(243)*. Whereas these and other observations may be applicable to a relatively narrow spectrum of tumor-related circumstances, they suggest that endothelial cells are not exempted from genetic instability and related therapeutic resistance.

3. CLOSING THOUGHTS AND PERSPECTIVES

Development of therapeutic resistance is intrinsic to the neoplastic process as such and associated with its complexity, plasticity, and dynamics. In this sense, prior predictions as to one or the other form of therapy being fundamentally outside of the problem of drug resistance (targeted agents, antiangiogenic therapies) have often been confronted with the reality of "refractory" or nonresponsive tumors (i.e., forms of *de facto* therapeutic resistance). Much debate, frustration, or even pessimism has crept into the field in relation to various novel and traditional therapeutic modalities, not because of some particular fundamental flaws, but rather because of what all too often appears to be excessive expectations. It therefore seems more practical to consider the prospect of therapeutic resistance to be a natural and indeed, inevitable, consequence of applying a therapeutic pressure (direct or indirect) on a narrow set of properties within otherwise heterogeneous and hypermutable tumor cell population. It should also be considered that some aspects of drug resistance, such as the ability to repopulate the tumor mass by clonogenic/stem cell subsets, or adhesion/aggregation dependent changes in responsiveness to therapy may be related to genetic tumor progression, genetic instability, and expression of oncogenic proteins. With this in mind, combinatorial therapeutic approaches clearly have a significant appeal and are in the forefront of clinical explorations. In these settings, not one but several mechanisms of malignancy are simultaneously targeted (intentionally or not), thereby reducing probability of therapeutic resistance. Combinations of cytoreductive agents with oncogene-directed signal transduction inhibitors *(77)* or antiangiogenics *(180)* have already produced, promising preclinical and clinical outcomes, and this process will likely undergo further refinements. The latter depends largely on our ability to incorporate into preclinical development of new anticancer agents an element of "preemptive" analysis of possible mechanisms of therapeutic resistance and ways to overcome them later on. This is relatively infrequently done at the present time in spite of considerable expense, effort, and indeed, suffering and lives that may be at stake when confronting therapeutic resistance at the stage of clinical trials and in clinical practice. Finally, it is very likely that in the not-too-distant future, refinement and commercialization of pharmacogenomics in cancer will enable not only more accurate predictions as to the responsiveness of individual patients to new and established agents, but also to provide valuable clues to understand pathways of drug resistance and suggest ways of their interruption. Thus, emerging patterns of oncogenic signaling and drug responses in cancer cells and their stroma, however complex, incomplete, and confusing, are likely to be a factor in more rational and effective design of anticancer therapies.

ACKNOWLEDGMENTS

This work was supported by grants from the National Cancer Institute of Canada (to J.R. and B.L.C.), and postdoctoral fellowship from Canadian Institutes for Health Research (J.L.Y.). We thank our colleagues and collaborators and above all our families for their continued support. Special thanks to my daughter Anna Rak for being...special.

REFERENCES

1. Goldie JH. Drug resistance in cancer: a perspective. Cancer Metastasis Rev 2001; 20:63–68.
2. McCarty MF, Liu W, Fan F, et al. Promises and pitfalls of anti-angiogenic therapy in clinical trials. Trends Mol Med 2003; 9:53–58.
3. Miller BE, Miller FR, Heppner GH. Interactions between tumor subpopulations affecting their sensitivity to the antineoplastic agents cyclophospamide and methotrexate. Cancer Res 1981; 41:4378–4381.
4. Miller BE, Miller FR, Heppner GH. Therapeutic perturbation of the tumor ecosystem in reconstructed heterogeneous mouse mammary tumors. Cancer Res 1989; 49:3747–3753.
5. Heppner GH, Miller BE. Therapeutic implications of tumor heterogeneity. Semin Oncol 1989; 16:91–105.
6. Damiano JS, Cress AE, Hazlehurst LA, Shtil AA, Dalton WS. Cell adhesion mediated drug resistance (CAM-DR): role of integrins and resistance to apoptosis in human myeloma cell lines. Blood 1999; 93:1658–1667.
7. Erler JT, Cawthorne CJ, Williams KJ, et al. Hypoxia-mediated down-regulation of Bid and Bax in tumors occurs via hypoxia-inducible factor 1-dependent and -independent mechanisms and contributes to drug resistance. Mol Cell Biol 2004; 24:2875–2889.
8. Durand RE. Intermittent blood flow in solid tumours—an under-appreciated source of "drug resistance." Cancer Metastasis Rev 2001; 20:57–61.
9. Hill BT. In vitro human tumour model systems for investigating drug resistance. Cancer Surv 1986; 5:129–149.
10. Jain RK. Delivery of novel therapeutic agents in tumors: physiological barriers and strategies. J Natl Cancer Inst 1989; 81:570–576.
11. Broxterman HJ, Lankelma J, Hoekman K. Resistance to cytotoxic and anti-angiogenic anticancer agents: similarities and differences. Drug Resist Updat 2003; 6:111–127.
12. Vogelstein B, Kinzler KW. Cancer genes and the pathways they control. Nat Med 2004; 10:789–799.
13. Kessel D. Modes of resistance to antitumor agents. in vivo 1994; 8:829–834.
14. Blagosklonny MV. Oncogenic resistance to growth-limiting conditions. Nat Rev Cancer 2002; 2:221–225.
15. Schmitt CA. Senescence, apoptosis and therapy—cutting the lifelines of cancer. Nat Rev Cancer 2003; 3:286–295.
16. Nutt CL, Chambers AF, cairncross JG. Wild-type p53 renders mouse astrocytes resistant to 1,3-*bis*(2-chloroethyl)-1-nitrosourea despite the absent of a p53-dependent cell cycle arrest. Cancer Res 1996; 56:2748–2751.
17. Jarvinen TA, Liu ET. HER-2/*neu* and topoisomerase IIα in breast cancer. Breast Cancer Res Treat 2003; 78:299–311.
18. Rak JW, Yu JL, Kerbel RS, Coomber BL. What do oncogenic mutations have to do with angiogenesis/vascular dependence of tumors. Cancer Res 2002; 62:1931–1934.
19. Samid D, Miller AC, Rimoldi D, Gafner J, Clark EP. Increased radiation resistance in transformed and nontransformed cells with elevated ras proto-oncogene expression. Radiat Res 1991; 126:244–250.
20. Johnstone RW, Ruefli AA, Lowe SW. Apoptosis: a link between cancer genetics and chemotherapy. Cell 2002; 108:153–164.
21. Nowell PC. The clonal evolution of tumor cell populations. Science 1976; 194:23–28.
22. Hanahan D, Weinberg RA. The hallmarks of cancer. Cell 2000; 100:57–70.

23. Bardin N, Moal V, Anfosso F, et al. Soluble CD146, a novel endothelial marker, is increased in physiopathological settings linked to endothelial junctional alteration. Thromb Haemost 2003; 90:915–920.

24. Rak J. Preface. In: Rak J, ed. Oncogene-directed therapies. Totowa: Humana Press, 2003; v–viii.

25. Rak J, Kerbel RS. Prospects and progress in the development of anti-angiogenic agents. Rosenberg, S. A. Principles and practice of biologic therapy of cancer—updates 3[3], 1–13. New York: Lippincott, Willams & Wilkins, 2002.

26. Kerbel RS, Folkman J. Clinical translation of angiogenesis inhibitors. Nat Rev Cancer 2002; 2:727–739.

27. Rak J, Kerbel RS. Oncogenes and tumor angiogenesis. In: Rak J, ed. Oncogene-directed therapies. Totowa: Humana Press, 2003; 171–218.

28. Rak J, Yu JL, Klement G, Kerbel RS. Oncogenes and angiogenesis: signaling three-dimensional tumor growth. J Investig Dermatol Symp Proc 2000; 5:24–33.

29. Moscow J, Morrow CS, Cowan KH. Drug resistance and its clinical circumvention. In: Kufe D, Pollock RE, Weichselbaum RR, et al., eds. Cancer medicine. Hamilton, London: Decker, 2003; 711–725.

30. Stein WD, Bates SE, Fojo T. Intractable cancers: the many faces of multidrug resistance and the many targets it presents for therapeutic attack. Curr Drug Targets 2004; 5:333–346.

31. Kim R, Toge T. Changes in therapy for solid tumors: potential for overcoming drug resistance in vivo with molecular targeting agents. Surg Today 2004; 34:293–303.

32. Wang G, Reed E, Li QQ. Molecular basis of cellular response to cisplatin chemotherapy in non-small cell lung cancer (review). Oncol Rep 2004; 12:955–965.

33. Dang C, Gilewski TA, Surbone A, Norton L. Cytokinetics. In: Kufe D, Pollock RE, Weichselbaum RR, et al, eds. Cancer medicine. London: Decker, 2003; 645–668.

34. Buick RN, Pollak MN. Perspectives on clonogenic tumor cells, stem cells, and oncogenes. Cancer Res 1984; 44:4909–4918.

35. Pittillo RF, Schabel FMJ, Skipper HE. The "sensitivity" of resting and dividing cells. Klin Oczna 1971; 41:137–142.

36. Tannock IF. Tumor growth and cell kinetics. In: Tannock IF, Hill RP, eds. The basic science of oncology. Toronto: Pergamon, 1995; 140–159.

37. Jain RK. Vascular and interstitial barriers to delivery of therapeutic agents in tumors. Cancer Metastasis Rev 1990; 9:253–266.

38. Brunner TB, Gupta AK, Shi Y, et al. Farnesyltransferase inhibitors as radiation sensitizers. Int J Radiat Biol 2003; 79:569–576.

39. Sausville EA. The challenge of pathway and environment-mediated drug resistance. Cancer Metastasis Rev 2001; 20:117–122.

40. Tannock IF. Tumor physiology and drug resistance. Cancer Metastasis Rev 2001; 20:123–132.

41. Dang CV, Semenza GL. Oncogenic alterations of metabolism. Trends Biochem Sci 1999; 24:68–72.

42. Semenza GL. Hypoxia, clonal selection, and the role of HIF-1 in tumor progression. Crit Rev Biochem Mol Biol 2000; 35:71–103.

43. Harris AL. Hypoxia—a key regulatory factor in tumour growth. Nat Rev Cancer 2002; 2:38–47.

44. Brown JM, Giaccia AJ. The unique physiology of solid tumors: opportunities (and problems) for cancer therapy. Cancer Res 1998; 58:1408–1416.

45. Rak J, Mitsuhashi Y, Bayko L, Filmus J, Sasazuki T, Kerbel RS. Mutant *ras* oncogenes upregulate VEGF/VPF expression: implications for induction and inhibition of tumor angiogenesis. Cancer Res 1995; 55:4575–4580.

46. Jain RK. Normalizing tumor vaculature with anti-angiogenic therapy: a new paradigm for combination therapy. Nature Med 2001; 7:987–989.

47. Teicher BA. Potentiation of cytotoxic cancer therapies by antiangiogenic agents. In: Teicher BA, ed. Antiangiogenic agents in cancer therapy. Totowa: Humana Press, 1999; 277–316.

48. Greenberger JS. Antitumor interaction of short course endostatin and ionizing radiation. Cancer J 2000; 6:279–281.

49. Gorski DH, Mauceri HJ, Salloum RM, et al. Potentiation of the antitumor effect of ionizing radiation by brief concomitant exposures to angiostatin. Cancer Res 1998; 58:5686–5689.

50. Mauceri HJ, Hanna NN, Beckett MA, et al. Combined effects of angiostatin and ionizing radiation in antitumour therapy. Nature 1998; 394:287–291.

51. Sklar MD. The ras oncogenes increase the intrinsic resistance of NIH 3T3 cells to ionizing radiation. Science 1988; 239:645–647.

52. Teicher BA, Herman TS, Holden SA, et al. Tumor resistance to alkylating agents conferred by mechanisms operative only in vivo. Science 1990; 247:1457–1461.

53. Bradley G, Juranka PF, Ling V. Mechanisms of multidrug resistance. Biochim Biophys Acta 1988; 948:87–128.

54. Tsuruo T, Naito M, Tomida A, et al. Molecular targeting therapy of cancer: drug resistance, apoptosis and survival signal. Cancer Sci 2003; 94:15–21.

55. Borst P. Genetic mechanisms of drug resistance. Rev Oncol 1991; 4:87–105.

56. Cole SP, Bhardwaj G, Gerlach JH, et al. Overexpression of a transporter gene in a multidrug-resistant human lung cancer cell line. Science 1992; 258:1650–1654.

57. Bates SE. Drug resistance: still on the learning curve. Clin Cancer Res 1999; 5:3346–3348.

58. Bordow SB, Haber M, Madafiglio J, Cheung B, Marshall GM, Norris MD. Expression of the multidrug resistance-associated protein (MRP) gene correlates with amplification and overexpression of the N-*myc* oncogene in childhood neuroblastoma. Cancer Res 1994; 54:5036–5040.

59. Schaich M, Ritter M, Illmer T, et al. Mutations in ras proto-oncogenes are associated with lower *mdr1* gene expression in adult acute myeloid leukaemia. Br J Haematol 2001; 112:300–307.

60. Regina A, Demeule M, Laplante A, et al. Multidrug resistance in brain tumors: roles of the blood–brain barrier. Cancer Metastasis Rev 2001; 20:13–25.

61. Labialle S, Gayet L, Marthinet E, Rigal D, Baggetto LG. Transcriptional regulators of the human multidrug resistance 1 gene: recent views. Biochem Pharmacol 2002; 64:943–948.

62. Shtil AA. Signal transduction pathways and transcriptional mechanisms as targets for prevention of emergence of multidrug resistance in human cancer cells. Curr Drug Targets 2001; 2:57–77.

63. Efferth T, Grassmann R. Impact of viral oncogenesis on responses to anti-cancer drugs and irradiation. Crit Rev Oncog 2000; 11:165–187.

64. el Deiry WS. Role of oncogenes in resistance and killing by cancer therapeutic agents. Curr Opin Oncol 1997; 9:79–87.

65. Masumoto N, Nakano S, Fujishima H, Kohno K, Niho Y. v-*src* induces cisplatin resistance by increasing the repair of cisplatin-DNA interstrand cross-links in human gallbladder adenocarcinoma cells. Int J Cancer 1999; 80:731–737.

66. Cho HJ, Jeong HG, Lee JS, et al. Oncogenic H-Ras enhances DNA repair through the Ras/phosphatidylinositol 3-kinase/Rac1 pathway in NIH3T3 cells. Evidence for association with reactive oxygen species. J Biol Chem 2002; 277:19,358–19,366.

67. Pietras RJ, Pegram MD, Finn RS, Maneval DA, Slamon DJ. Remission of human breast cancer xenografts on therapy with humanized monoclonal antibody to HER-2 receptor and DNA-reactive drugs. Oncogene 1998; 17:2235–2249.

68. El-Deiry WS. Role of oncogenes in resistance and killing by cancer therapeutic agents. Curr Opin Oncol 1997; 9:79–87.

69. Xu GW, Nutt CL, Zlatescu MC, Keeney M, Chin-Yee I, Cairncross JG. Inactivation of p53 sensitizes U87MG glioma cells to 1,3-*bis*(2-chloroethyl)-1-nitrosourea. Cancer Res 2001; 61:4155–4159.

70. Boudny V, Murakami Y, Nakano S, Niho Y. Expression of activated c-erbB-2 oncogene induces sensitivity to cisplatin in human gallbladder adenocarcinoma cells. Anticancer Res 1999; 19:5203–5206.

71. Viniegra JG, Losa JH, Sanchez-Arevalo VJ, et al. Modulation of PI3K/Akt pathway by E1a mediates sensitivity to cisplatin. Oncogene 2002; 21:7131–7136.

72. Eastman A. Activation of programmed cell death by anticancer agents: cisplatin as a model system. Cancer Cells 1990; 2:275–280.

73. Shay JW, Roninson IB. Hallmarks of senescence in carcinogenesis and cancer therapy. Oncogene 2004; 23:2919–2933.

74. Schmitt CA, Lowe SW. Apoptosis and chemoresistance in transgenic cancer models. J Mol Med 2002; 80:137–146.

75. Schmitt CA, Lowe SW. Apoptosis and therapy. J Pathol 1999; 187:127–137.

76. Wendel HG, Lowe SW. Reversing drug resistance in vivo. Cell Cycle 2004; 3:847–849.

77. Wendel HG, de Stanchina E, Fridman JS, et al. Survival signalling by Akt and eIF4E in oncogenesis and cancer therapy. Nature 2004: 428:332–337.

78. Woo RA, Poon RY. Activated oncogenes promote and cooperate with chromosomal instability for neoplastic transformation. Genes Dev 2004; 18:1317–1330.

79. Roninson IB. Tumor cell senescence in cancer treatment. Cancer Res 2003; 63:2705–2715.

80. Rak J, Mitsuhashi Y, Sheehan C, et al. Collateral expression of proangiogenic and tumorigenic properties in intestinal epithelial cell variants selected for resistance to anoikis. Neoplasia 1999; 1:23–30.

81. McCormick F. Signal transduction networks. Ras as a paradigm. In: Rak J, ed. Oncogene-directed therapies. Totowa: Humana Press, 2003; 35–46.

82. Serrano M, Lin AW, McCurrach ME, Beach D, Lowe SW. Oncogenic ras provokes premature cell senescence associated with accumulation of p53 and p16INK4a. Cell 1997; 88:593–602.

83. Guerra C, Mijimolle N, Dhawahir A, et al. Tumor induction by an endogenous K-ras oncogene is highly dependent on cellular context. Cancer Cell 2003; 4:111–120.

84. Tuveson DA, Shaw AT, Willis NA, et al. Endogenous oncogenic K-ras(G12D) stimulates proliferation and widespread neoplastic and developmental defects. Cancer Cell 2004; 5:375–387.

85. Mendelsohn J. Epidermal growth factor receptor inhibition by a monoclonal antibody as anticancer therapy. Clin Cancer Res 1997; 3:2703–2707.

86. Lin EH, Abbruzzese J. Clinical evaluation of agents targeting epidermal growth factor receptor (EGFR) in cancer. In: Rak J, ed. Oncogene-directed therapies. Totowa: Humana Press, 2003; 313–330.

87. Pegram MD, Lipton A, Hayes DF, et al. Phase II study of receptor-enhanced chemosensitivity using recombinant humanized anti-p185HER2/neu monoclonal antibody plus cisplatin in patients with HER2/neu-overexpressing metastatic breast cancer refractory to chemotherapy treatment. J Clin Oncol 1998; 16:2659–2671.

88. Konecny GE, Arboleda J, Slamon D, Pegram M. Inhibition of the *HER-2* oncogene: A translational research model for the development of future targeted therapies. In: Rak J, ed. Oncogene-directed therapies. Totowa: Humana Press, 2003; 331–352.

89. Liang K, Lu Y, Jin W, Ang KK, Milas L, Fan Z. Sensitization of breast cancer cells to radiation by trastuzumab. Mol Cancer Ther 2003; 2:1113–1120.

90. Sato S, Kajiyama Y, Sugano M, et al. Monoclonal antibody to HER-2/neu receptor enhances radiosensitivity of esophageal cancer cell lines expressing HER-2/*neu* oncoprotein. Int J Radiat Oncol Biol Phys 2005; 61:203–211.

91. Gong SJ, Jin CJ, Rha SY, Chung HC. Growth inhibitory effects of trastuzumab and chemotherapeutic drugs in gastric cancer cell lines. Cancer Lett 2004; 214:215–224.

92. Ciardiello F, Caputo R, Borriello G, et al. ZD1839 (IRESSA), an EGFR-selective tyrosine kinase inhibitor, enhances taxane activity in bcl-2 overexpressing, multidrug-resistant MCF-7 ADR human breast cancer cells. Int J Cancer 2002; 98:463–469.

93. Herbst RS. Review of epidermal growth factor receptor biology. Int J Radiat Oncol Biol Phys 2004; 59:21–26.

94. Mamane Y, Petroulakis E, Rong L, Yoshida K, Ler LW, Sonenberg N. eIF4E—from translation to transformation. Oncogene 2004; 23:3172–3179.

95. Hapke G, Yin MB, Rustum YM. Targeting molecular signals in chk1 pathways as a new approach for overcoming drug resistance. Cancer Metastasis Rev 2001; 20:109–115.

96. Sethi T, Rintoul RC, Moore SM, et al. Extracellular matrix proteins protect small cell lung cancer cells against apoptosis: a mechanism for small cell lung cancer growth and drug resistance in vivo. Nat Med 1999; 5:662–668.

97. St.Croix B, Kerbel RS. Cell adhesion and drug resistance in cancer. Current Opin Cell Biol 1997; 9:549–556.

98. Dimanche-Boitrel MT, Genne P, Duchamp O, Chauffert B. Confluence dependent resistance (CDR) to doxorubicin and E- cadherin expression in murine mammary cells. Canc Letts 1994; 85:171–176.

99. Zhang Y, Gonzalez V, Xu MJ. Expression and regulation of glutathione *S*-transferase P1-1 in cultured human epidermal cells. J Dermatol Sci 2002; 30:205–214.

100. Arber N, Han EK, Sgambato A, et al. A K-ras oncogene increases resistance to sulindac-induced apoptosis in rat enterocytes. Gastroenterology 1997; 113:1892–1900.

101. Ling CC, Endlich B. Radioresistance induced by oncogenic transformation. Radiat Res 1989; 120:267–279.

102. Riva C, el Khyari S, Rustum Y, Barra Y. Resistance to cytosine arabinoside in cells transfected with activated Ha-ras oncogene. Anticancer Res 1995; 15:1297–1302.

103. Sklar MD. Increased resistance to *cis*-diamminedichloroplatinum(II) in NIH 3T3 cells transformed by *ras* oncogenes. Cancer Res 1988; 48:793–497.

104. Koo HM, Monks A, Mikheev A, et al. Enhanced sensitivity to 1-β-D-arabinofuranosylcytosine and topoisomerase II inhibitors in tumor cell lines harboring activated ras oncogenes. Cancer Res 1996; 56:5211–5216.

105. Koo HM, McWilliams MJ, Alvord WG, Vande Woude GF. *Ras* oncogene-induced sensitization to 1-β-D-arabinofuranosylcytosine. Cancer Res 1999; 59:6057–6062.

106. Koo HM, Gray-Goodrich M, Kohlhagen G, et al. The ras oncogene-mediated sensitization of human cells to topoisomerase II inhibitor-induced apoptosis. J Natl Cancer Inst 1999; 91:236–244.
107. Blagosklonny MV. Targeting cancer cells by exploiting their resistance. Trends Mol Med 2003; 9:307–312.
108. Brown JM, Wilson G. Apoptosis genes and resistance to cancer therapy: what does the experimental and clinical data tell us? Cancer Biol Ther 2003; 2:477–490.
109. Dempke W, Voigt W, Grothey A, Hill BT, Schmoll HJ. Cisplatin resistance and oncogenes—a review. Anticancer Drugs 2000; 11:225–236.
110. Perez-Soler R. HER1/EGFR targeting: refining the strategy. Oncologist 2004; 9:58–67.
111. Amato RJ. Renal cell carcinoma: review of novel single-agent therapeutics and combination regimens. Ann Oncol 2005; 16:7–15.
112. Cowan-Jacob SW, Guez V, Fendrich G, et al. Imatinib (STI571) resistance in chronic myelogenous leukemia: molecular basis of the underlying mechanisms and potential strategies for treatment. Mini Rev Med Chem 2004; 4:285–299.
113. McCormick F. New-age drug meets resistance. Nature 2001; 412:281–282.
114. Ebos JM, Tran J, Master Z, et al. Imatinib mesylate (STI-571) reduces Bcr-Abl-mediated vascular endothelial growth factor secretion in chronic myelogenous leukemia. Mol Cancer Res 2002; 1:89–95.
115. Mayerhofer M, Valent P, Sperr WR, Griffin JD, Sillaber C. BCR/ABL induces expression of vascular endothelial growth factor and its transcriptional activator, hypoxia inducible factor-1α, through a pathway involving phosphoinositide 3-kinase and the mammalian target of rapamycin. Blood 2002; 100:3767–3775.
116. Deininger MW, Druker BJ. SRCircumventing imatinib resistance. Cancer Cell 2004; 6:108–110.
117. Shah NP, Tran C, Lee FY, Chen P, Norris D, Sawyers CL. Overriding imatinib resistance with a novel ABL kinase inhibitor. Science 2004; 305:399–401.
118. Hingorani SR, Tuveson DA. Targeting oncogene dependence and resistance. Cancer Cell 2003; 3:414–417.
119. Eisenberg BL, von Mehren M. Pharmacotherapy of gastrointestinal stromal tumours. Expert Opin Pharmacother 2003; 4:869–874.
120. Lynch TJ, Bell DW, Sordella R, et al. Activating mutations in the epidermal growth factor receptor underlying responsiveness of non-small-cell lung cancer to gefitinib. N Engl J Med 2004; 350:2129–2139.
121. Sordella R, Bell DW, Haber DA, Settleman J. Gefitinib-sensitizing EGFR mutations in lung cancer activate anti-apoptotic pathways. Science 2004; 305:1163–1167.
122. Pao W, Miller V, Zakowski M, et al. EGF receptor gene mutations are common in lung cancers from "never smokers" and are associated with sensitivity of tumors to gefitinib and erlotinib. Proc Natl Acad Sci U S A 2004; 101:13,306–13,311.
123. Blagosklonny MV. Gefitinib (iressa) in oncogene-addictive cancers and therapy for common cancers. Cancer Biol Ther 2004; 3:436–440.
124. Paez JG, Janne PA, Lee JC, et al. EGFR mutations in lung cancer: correlation with clinical response to gefitinib therapy. Science 2004; 304:1497–1500.
125. Pinkas-Kramarski R, Soussan L, Waterman H, et al. Diversification of Neu differentiation factor and epidermal growth factor signaling by combinatorial receptor interactions. EMBO J 1996; 15:2452–2467.
126. Kirschbaum MH, Marmor MD, Yarden Y. Oncogenic receptor tyrosine kinases. In: Rak J, ed. Oncogene-directed therapies. Totowa: Humana Press, 2003:47–76.
127. Viloria-Petit AM, Rak J, Hung M-C, Rockwell P, Goldstein N, Kerbel RS. Neutralizing antibodies against EGF and ErbB-2/*neu* receptor tyrosine kinases down-regulate VEGF production by tumor cells in vitro and in vivo: angiogenic implications for signal transduction therapy of solid tumors. Am J Pathol 1997; 151:1523–1530.
128. Yu JL, May L, Klement P, Weitz JI, Rak J. Oncogenes as regulators of tissue factor expression in cancer: implications for tumor angiogenesis and anti-cancer therapy. Semin Thromb Hemost 2004; 30:21–30.
129. Crombet-Ramos T, Rak J, Perez R, Viloria-Petit A. Antiproliferative, antiangiogenic and proapoptotic activity of h-R3: A humanized anti-EGFR antibody. Int J Cancer 2002; 101:567–575.
130. Viloria-Petit A, Crombet T, Jothy S, et al. Acquired resistance to the antitumor effect of epidermal growth factor receptor-blocking antibodies in vivo: a role for altered tumor angiogenesis. Cancer Res 2001; 61:5090–5101.
131. Rak J, Mitsuhashi Y, Sheehan C, et al. Oncogenes and tumor angiogenesis: differential modes of vascular endothelial growth factor up-regulation in ras-transformed epithelial cells and fibroblasts. Cancer Res 2000; 60:490–498.

132. Gatzemeier U. Targeting the HER1/EGFR receptor to improve outcomes in non-small-cell lung cancer. Oncology 2003; 17:7–10.
133. Mellinghoff IK, Sawyers CL. The emergence of resistance to targeted cancer therapeutics. Pharmacogenomics 2002; 3:603–623.
134. Chen CD, Welsbie DS, Tran C, et al. Molecular determinants of resistance to antiandrogen therapy. Nat Med 2004; 10:33–39.
135. Craft N, Shostak Y, Carey M, Sawyers CL. A mechanism for hormone-independent prostate cancer through modulation of androgen receptor signaling by the HER-2/neu tyrosine kinase. Nat Med 1999; 5:280–285.
136. Foley R, Hollywood D, Lawler M. Molecular pathology of prostate cancer: the key to identifying new biomarkers of disease. Endocr Relat Cancer 2004; 11:477–488.
137. Isaacs JT, Isaacs WB. Androgen receptor outwits prostate cancer drugs. Nat Med 2004; 10:26–27.
138. Folkman J. Tumor angiogenesis: therapeutic implications. N Engl J Med 1971; 285:1182–1186.
139. Rak J, Filmus J, Kerbel RS. Reciprocal paracrine interactions between tumor cells and endothelial cells. The "angiogenesis progression" hypothesis. Eur J Cancer 1996; 32A:2438–2450.
140. Hamada J, Cavanaugh PG, Miki K, Nicolson GL. A paracrine migration-stimulating factor for metastatic tumor cells secreted by mouse hepatic sinusoidal endothelial cells: identification as complement component C3b. Cancer Res 1993; 53:4418–4423.
141. Skobe M, Rockwell P, Goldstein N, Vosseler S, Fusenig NE. Halting angiogenesis suppresses carcinoma cell invasion. Nature Med 1997; 3:1222–1227.
142. Nicosia RF, Tchao R, Leighton J. Angiogenesis-dependent tumor spread in reinforced fibrin clot culture. Cancer Res 1983; 43:2159–2166.
143. Shan S, Robson ND, Cao Y, et al. Responses of vascular endothelial cells to angiogenic signaling are important for tumor cell survival. FASEB J 2004; 18:326–328.
144. Holash J, Maisonpierre PC, Compton D, et al. Vessel cooption, regression, and growth in tumors mediated by angiopoietins and VEGF. Science 1999; 284:1994–1998.
145. Folkman J. Tumor angiogenesis. Adv Cancer Res 1985; 43:175–203.
146. Hendrix MJ, Seftor EA, Hess AR, Seftor RE. Vasculogenic mimicry and tumour-cell plasticity: lessons from melanoma. Nat Rev Cancer 2003; 3:411–421.
147. Folkman J, Browder T, Palmblad J. Angiogenesis research: guidelines for translation to clinical application. Thromb Haemost 2001; 86:23–33.
148. Carmeliet P, Jain RK. Angiogenesis in cancer and other diseases. Nature 2000; 407:249–257.
149. Scholz D, Cai WJ, Schaper W. Arteriogenesis, a new concept of vascular adaptation in occlusive disease. Angiogenesis 2001; 4:247–257.
150. Yu JL, Rak JW. Host microenvironment in breast cancer development: inflammatory and immune cells in tumour angiogenesis and arteriogenesis. Breast Cancer Res 2003; 5:83–88.
151. Skobe M, Hawighorst T, Jackson DG, et al. Induction of tumor lymphangiogenesis by VEGF-C promotes breast cancer metastasis. Nat Med 2001; 7:192–198.
152. Stacker SA, Caesar C, Baldwin ME, et al. VEGF-D promotes the metastatic spread of tumor cells via the lymphatics. Nat Med 2001; 7:186–191.
153. Jain RK, Padera TP. Prevention and treatment of lymphatic metastasis by antilymphangiogenic therapy. J Natl Cancer Inst 2002; 94:785–787.
154. Alitalo K, Carmeliet P. Molecular mechanisms of lymphangiogenesis in health and disease. Cancer Cell 2002; 1:219–227.
155. Carmeliet P. Mechanisms of angiogenesis and arteriogenesis. Nat Med 2000; 6:389–395.
156. Scappaticci FA. Mechanisms and future directions for angiogenesis-based cancer therapies. J Clin Oncol 2002; 20:3906–3927.
157. St.Croix B, Rago C, Velculescu V, et al. Genes expressed in human tumor endothelium. Science 2000; 289:1197–1202.
158. Duarte A, Hirashima M, Benedito R, et al. Dosage-sensitive requirement for mouse Dll4 in artery development. Genes Dev 2004; 18:2474–2478.
159. Tang N, Wang L, Esko J, et al. Loss of HIF-1α in endothelial cells disrupts a hypoxia-driven VEGF autocrine loop necessary for tumorigenesis. Cancer Cell 2004; 6:485–495.
160. Bergers G, Song S, Meyer-Morse N, Bergsland E, Hanahan D. Benefits of targeting both pericytes and endothelial cells in the tumor vasculature with kinase inhibitors. J Clin Invest 2003; 111:1287–1295.
161. Folkman J. Clinical applications of research on angiogenesis. N Engl J Med 1995; 333:1757–1763.
162. Thorpe PE, Burrows FJ. Antibody-directed targeting of the vasculature of solid tumors. Breast Cancer Res Treat 1995; 36:237–251.

163. Hanahan D, Folkman J. Patterns and emerging mechanisms of the angiogenic switch during tumorigenesis. Cell 1996; 86:353–364.
164. Relf M, LeJeune S, Scott PA, et al. Expression of the angiogenic factors vascular endothelial cell growth factor, acidic and basic fibroblast growth factor, tumor growth factor β-1, platelet-derived endothelial cell growth factor, placenta growth factor, and pleiotrophin in human primary breast cancer and its relation to angiogenesis. Cancer Res 1997; 57:963–969.
165. Volpert OV, Dameron KM, Bouck N. Sequential development of an angiogenic phenotype by human fibroblasts progressing to tumorigenicity. Oncogene 1997; 14:1495–1502.
166. Holmgren L, O'Reilly MS, Folkman J. Dormancy of micrometastases: balanced proliferation and apoptosis in the presence of angiogenesis suppression. Nature Med 1995; 1:149–153.
167. Reiher FK, Volpert OV, Jimenez B, et al. Inhibition of tumor growth by systemic treatment with thrombospondin-1 peptide mimetics. Int J Cancer 2002; 98:682–689.
168. Hlatky L, Hahnfeldt P, Folkman J. Clinical application of antiangiogenic therapy: microvessel density, what it does and doesn't tell us. J Natl Cancer Inst 2002; 94:883–893.
169. Ferrara N. VEGF and the quest for tumour angiogenesis factors. Nat Rev Cancer 2002; 2:795–803.
170. Kerbel RS. A cancer therapy resistant to resistance. Nature 1997; 390:335–336.
171. Lengauer C, Kinzler KW, Vogelstein B. Genetic instabilities in human cancers. Nature 1998; 396:643–649.
172. Rak J, Kerbel RS. Treating cancer by inhibiting angiogenesis: New hopes and potential pitfalls. Cancer Metastasis Rev 1996; 15:231–236.
173. Kerbel RS, Yu J, Tran J, et al. Possible mechanisms of acquired resistance to anti-angiogenic drugs: implications for the use of combination therapy approaches. Cancer Metastasis Rev 2001; 20:79–86.
174. Yoshiji H, Harris SR, Thorgeirsson UP. Vascular endothelial growth factor is essential for initial but not continued in vivo growth of human breast carcinoma cells. Cancer Res 1997; 57:3924–3928.
175. Bergers G, Javaherian K, Lo KM, Folkman J, Hanahan D. Effects of angiogenesis inhibitors on multistage carcinogenesis in mice. Science 1999; 284:808–812.
176. Viloria-Petit A, Miquerol L, Yu JL, et al. Contrasting effects of VEGF gene disruption in embryonic stem cell-derived versus oncogene-induced tumors. EMBO J 2003; 22:4091–4102.
177. Kranenburg O, Gebbink MF, Voest EE. Stimulation of angiogenesis by Ras proteins. Biochim Biophys Acta 2004; 1654:23–37.
178. Dong J, Grunstein J, Tejada M, et al. VEGF-null cells require PDGFR α signaling-mediated stromal fibroblast recruitment for tumorigenesis. EMBO J 2004; 23:2800–2810.
179. Gunsilius E, Duba HC, Petzer AL, et al. Evidence from a leukaemia model for maintenance of vascular endothelium by bone-marrow-derived endothelial cells. Lancet 2000; 355:1688–1691.
180. Takahashi K, Mulliken JB, Kozakewich HPW, Rogers RA, Folkman J, Ezekowitz RAB. Cellular markers that distinguish the phases of hemangioma during infancy and childhood. J Clin Invest 1994; 93:2357–2364.
181. Holmgren L, Szeles A, Rajnavolgyi E, et al. Horizontal transfer of DNA by the uptake of apoptotic bodies. Blood 1999; 93:3956–3963.
182. Graeber TG, Osmanian C, Jacks T, et al. Hypoxia-mediated selection of cells with diminished apoptotic potential in solid tumours. Nature 1996; 379:88–91.
183. Malkin D. The role of p53 in human cancer. J Neurooncol 2001; 51:231–243.
184. Bunz F, Hwang PM, Torrance C, et al. Disruption of p53 in human cancer cells alters the responses to therapeutic agents. J Clin Invest 1999; 104:263–269.
185. Gudkov AV, Komarova EA. The role of p53 in determining sensitivity to radiotherapy. Nat Rev Cancer 2003; 3:117–129.
186. Chang BD, Xuan Y, Broude EV, et al. Role of p53 and p21[waf1/cip1] in senescence-like terminal proliferation arrest induced in human tumor cells by chemotherapeutic drugs. Oncogene 1999; 18:4808–4818.
187. Dameron KM, Volpert OV, Tainsky MA, Bouck N. Control of angiogenesis in fibroblasts by p53 regulation of thrombospondin-1. Science 1994; 265:1582–1584.
188. Yu JL, Rak JW, Carmeliet P, Nagy A, Kerbel RS, Coomber BL. Heterogeneous vascular dependence of tumor cell populations. Am J Pathol 2001; 158:1325–1334.
189. Yu JL, Rak JW, Coomber BL, Hicklin DJ, Kerbel RS. Effect of p53 status on tumor response to antiangiogenic therapy. Science 2002; 295:1526–1528.
190. Tamada H, Kitazawa R, Gohji K, Kitazawa S. Epigenetic regulation of human bone morphogenetic protein 6 gene expression in prostate cancer. J Bone Miner Res 2001; 16:487–496.

191. Brown EB, Campbell RB, Tsuzuki Y, et al. In vivo measurement of gene expression, angiogenesis and physiological function in tumors using multiphoton laser scanning microscopy. Nat Med 2001; 7:864–868.

192. Carmeliet P, Dor Y, Herbert JM, et al. Role of HIF-1α in hypoxia-mediated apoptosis, cell proliferation and tumour angiogenesis. Nature 1998; 394:485–490.

193. Akakura N, Kobayashi M, Horiuchi I, et al. Constitutive expression of hypoxia-inducible factor-1α renders pancreatic cancer cells resistant to apoptosis induced by hypoxia and nutrient deprivation. Cancer Res 2001; 61:6548–6554.

194. Abdalla SA, Behzad F, Bsharah S, et al. Prognostic relevance of microvessel density in colorectal tumours. Oncol Rep 1999; 6:839–842.

195. Rak J, Yu JL. Oncogenes and tumor angiogenesis: the question of vascular "supply" and vascular "demand." Semin Cancer Biol 2004; 14:93–104.

196. Bouck N, Stellmach V, Hsu SC. How tumors become angiogenic. Adv Cancer Res 1996; 69:135–174.

197. Rastinejad F, Polverini PJ, Bouck N. Regulation of the activity of a new inhibitor by angiogenesis by a cancer suppressor gene. Cell 1989; 56:345–355.

198. Grugel S, Finkenzeller G, Weindel K, Barleon B, Marme D. Both v-Ha-ras and v-raf stimulate expression of the vascular endothelial growth factor in NIH 3T3 cells. J Biol Chem 1995; 270:25,915–25,919.

199. Watnick RS, Cheng Y-N, Rangarajan A, Ince TA, Weinberg RA. Ras modulates Myc activity to repress thrombospondin-1 expression and increase tumor angiogenesis. Cancer Cell 2003; 3:219–231.

200. Zabrenetzky V, Harris CC, Steeg PS, Roberts DD. Expression of the extracellular matrix molecule thrombospondin inversely correlates with malignant progression in melanoma, lung and breast carcinoma cell lines. Int J Cancer 1994; 59:191–195.

201. Sparmann A, Bar-Sagi D. Ras-induced interleukin-8 expression plays a critical role in tumor growth and angiogenesis. Cancer Cell 2004; 6:447–458.

202. Yu JL, May L, Lhotak V, et al. Oncogenic events regulate tissue factor expression in colorectal cancer cells: implications for tumor progression and angiogenesis. Blood 2004; 104:1734–1741.

203. Mazure NM, Chen EY, Laderoute KR, Giaccia AJ. Induction of vascular endothelial growth factor by hypoxia is modulated by a phosphatidylinositol 3-kinase/Akt signaling pathway in Ha-ras-transformed cells through a hypoxia inducible factor-1 transcriptional element. Blood 1997; 90:3322–3331.

204. Laderoute KR, Alarcon RM, Brody MD, et al. Opposing effects of hypoxia on expression of the angiogenic inhibitor thrombospondin 1 and the angiogenic inducer vascular endothelial growth factor. Clin Cancer Res 2000; 6:2941–2950.

205. Filleur S, Volpert OV, Degeorges A, et al. In vivo mechanisms by which tumors producing thrombospondin 1 bypass its inhibitory effects. Genes Dev 2001; 15:1373–1382.

206. Filleur S, Courtin A, Ait-Si-Ali S, et al. SiRNA-mediated inhibition of vascular endothelial growth factor severely limits tumor resistance to antiangiogenic thrombospondin-1 and slows tumor vascularization and growth. Cancer Res 2003; 63:3919–3922.

207. Volpert OV, Zaichuk T, Zhou W, et al. Inducer-stimulated Fas targets activated endothelium for destruction by anti-angiogenic thrombospondin-1 and pigment epithelium-derived factor. Nat Med 2002; 8:349–357.

208. Denekamp J. Endothelial cell proliferation as a novel approach to targeting tumor therapy. Br J Cancer 1982; 45:136–139.

209. Tran J, Rak J, Sheehan C, et al. Marked induction of the IAP family anti-apoptotic proteins survivin and XIAP by VEGF in vascular endothelial cells. Biochem Biophys Res Commun 1999; 264:781–788.

210. Tran J, Master Z, Yu JL, Rak J, Dumont DJ, Kerbel RS. Induction of endothelial cell resistance to chemotherapy by VEGF mediated up-regulation of survivin. Proc Natl Acad Sci USA 2002; 99:4349–4354.

211. Klement G, Baruchel S, Rak J, et al. Continuous low-dose therapy with vinblastine and VEGF receptor-2 antibody induces sustained tumor regression without overt toxicity. J Clin Invest 2000; 105:R15–R24.

212. Browder T, Butterfield CE, Kraling BM, et al. Antiangiogenic scheduling of chemotherapy improves efficacy against experimental drug-resistant cancer. Cancer Res 2000; 60:1878–1886.

213. Bocci G, Francia G, Man S, Lawler J, Kerbel RS. Thrombospondin 1, a mediator of the antiangiogenic effects of low-dose metronomic chemotherapy. Proc Natl Acad Sci USA 2003; 100:12,917–12,922.

214. Garcia-Barros M, Paris F, Cordon-Cardo C, et al. Tumor response to radiotherapy regulated by endothelial cell apoptosis. Science 2003; 300:1155–1159.

215. Paris F, Fuks Z, Kang A, et al. Endothelial apoptosis as the primary lesion initiating intestinal radiation damage in mice. Science 2001; 293:293–297.

216. Lin X, Fuks Z, Kolesnick R. Ceramide mediates radiation-induced death of endothelium. Crit Care Med 2000; 28:N87–N93.

217. Garcia-Barros M, Lacorazza D, Petrie H, et al. Host acid sphingomyelinase regulates microvascular function not tumor immunity. Cancer Res 2004; 64:8285–8291.

218. Kim KJ, Li B, Winer J, et al. Inhibition of vascular endothelial growth factor-induced angiogenesis suppresses tumour growth in vivo. Nature 1993; 362:841–844.

219. Warren RS, Yuan H, Mati MR, Gillett NA, Ferrara N. Regulation by vascular endothelial growth factor of human colon cancer tumorigenesis in a mouse model of experimental liver metastasis. J Clin Invest 1995; 95:1789–1797.

220. Prewett M, Huber J, Li Y, et al. Antivascular endothelial growth factor receptor (fetal liver kinase 1) monoclonal antibody inhibits tumor angiogenesis and growth of several mouse and human tumors. Cancer Res 1999; 59:5209–5218.

221. Holash J, Davis S, Papadopoulos N, et al. VEGF-Trap: a VEGF blocker with potent antitumor effects. Proc Natl Acad Sci U S A 2002; 99:11,393–11,398.

222. Ferrara N. Role of vascular endothelial growth factor in physiologic and pathologic angiogenesis: therapeutic implications. Semin Oncol 2002; 29:10–14.

223. Shalaby F, Rossant J, Yamaguchi TP, et al. Failure of blood-island formation and vasculogenesis in Flk-1-deficient mice. Nature 1995; 376:62–66.

224. Fong GH, Rossant J, Gertsenstein M, Breitman ML. Role of the Flt-1 receptor tyrosine kinase in regulating the assembly of vascular endothelium. Nature 1995; 376:66–70.

225. Carmeliet P, Ferreira V, Breier G, et al. Abnormal blood vessel development and lethality in embryos lacking a single VEGF allele. Nature 1996; 380:435–439.

226. Ferrara N, Carver-Moore K, Chen H, et al. Heterozygous embryonic lethality induced by targeted inactivation of the VEGF gene. Nature 1996; 380:439–442.

227. Shi YP, Ferrara N. Oncogenic *ras* fails to restore an in vivo tumorigenic phenotype in embryonic stem cells lacking vascular endothelial growth factor (VEGF). Biochem Biophys Res Commun 1999; 254:480–483.

228. Grunstein J, Masbad JJ, Hickey R, Giordano F, Johnson RS. Isoforms of vascular endothelial growth factor act in a coordinate fashion to recruit and expand tumor vasculature. Mol Cell Biol 2000; 20:7282–7291.

229. Grunstein J, Roberts WG, Mathieu-Costello O, Hanahan D, Johnson RS. Tumor-derived expression of vascular endothelial growth factor is a critical factor in tumor expansion and vascular function. Cancer Res 1999; 59:1592–1598.

230. Inoue M, Hager JH, Ferrara N, Gerber HP, Hanahan D. VEGF-A has a critical, nonredundant role in angiogenic switching and pancreatic β cell carcinogenesis. Cancer Cell 2002; 1:193–202.

231. Hurwitz H, Fehrenbacher L, Novotny W, et al. Bevacizumab plus irinotecan, fluorouracil, and leucovorin for metastatic colorectal cancer. N Engl J Med 2004; 350:2335–2342.

232. Yang JC, Haworth L, Sherry RM, et al. A randomized trial of bevacizumab, an anti-vascular endothelial growth factor antibody, for metastatic renal cancer. N Engl J Med 2003; 349:427–434.

233. Malik AK, Gerber HP. Targeting VEGF ligands and receptors in cancer. Targets 2003; 2:48–57.

234. Miller KD. Recent translational research: antiangiogenic therapy for breast cancer—where do we stand? Breast Cancer Res 2004; 6:128–132.

235. Brown LF, Detmar M, Claffey KP, et al. Vascular permeability factor/vascular endothelial growth factor: A multifunctional angiogenic cytokine. In: Goldberg ID, Rosen EM, eds. Regulation of angiogenesis. Basel, Switzerland: Birkhauser, 1997:233–269.

236. Shweiki D, Neeman M, Itin A, Keshet E. Induction of vascular endothelial growth factor expression by hypoxia and by glucose deficiency in multicell spheroids: implications for tumor angiogenesis. Proc Natl Acad Sci U S A 1995; 92:768–772.

237. Yu J, Rak JW, Klement G, Kerbel RS. VEGF isoform expression as a determinant of blood vessel patterning in human melanoma xenografts. Cancer Res 2002; 62:1838–1846.

238. Gee MS, Procopio WN, Makonnen S, Feldman MD, Yeilding NM, Lee WM. Tumor vessel development and maturation impose limits on the effectiveness of anti-vascular therapy. Am J Pathol 2003; 162:183–193.

239. Inai T, Mancuso M, Hashizume H, et al. Inhibition of vascular endothelial growth factor (VEGF) signaling in cancer causes loss of endothelial fenestrations, regression of tumor vessels, and appearance of basement membrane ghosts. Am J Pathol 2004; 165:35–52.

240. Baffert F, Thurston G, Rochon-Duck M, Le T, Brekken R, McDonald DM. Age-related changes in vascular endothelial growth factor dependency and angiopoietin-1-induced plasticity of adult blood vessels. Circ Res 2004; 94:984–992.

241. Streubel B, Chott A, Huber D, et al. Lymphoma-specific genetic aberrations in microvascular endothelial cells in B-cell lymphomas. N Engl J Med 2004; 351:250–259.
242. Ebos JM, Tran J, Master Z, et al. Imatinib mesylate (STI-571) reduces Bcr-Abl-mediated vascular endothelial growth factor secretion in chronic myelogenous leukemia. Mol Cancer Res 2002; 1:89–95.
243. van der Schaft DW, Seftor RE, Seftor EA, et al. Effects of angiogenesis inhibitors on vascular network formation by human endothelial and melanoma cells. J Natl Cancer Inst 2004; 96:1473–1477.
244. Miller KD, Rugo H, Cobleigh M, et al. Phase III trial of capecitabine plus bevacizumab versus capecitabine alone in women with previously treated metastatic breast cancer. Breast Cancer Res Treat 2002; 76:S37.
245. Hurwitz H, Fehrenbacher L, Cartwright T, et al. Bevacizumab (a monoclonal antibody to vascular endothelial growth factor) prolongs survival in first-line colorectal cancer (CRC): results of a phase III trial of bevacizumbab in combination with bolus IFL (irinotecan, 5-fluorouracil, leucovorin) as first-line therapy in subjects with metastatic CRC. Proc Am Soc Clin Oncol 2003; 22:Abstract 3646.

5 PET Imaging of Response and Resistance to Cancer Therapy

David A. Mankoff, MD, PhD
and Kenneth A. Krohn, PhD

CONTENTS

SUMMARY

As cancer treatment moves towards more targeted therapy, there is an increasing need for tools to guide therapy selection and to evaluate response. Biochemical and molecular imaging can complement existing in vitro assay methods and is likely to play a key role in early drug testing and development, as well as future clinical practice. Imaging is ideally suited to assessing the spatial and temporal heterogeneity of cancer and to measure in vivo drug effects. This chapter highlights imaging approaches to guide cancer therapy, focusing on positron emission tomography and on those approaches that have undergone preliminary testing in patients. Examples showing how positron emission tomography imaging can be used to (1) assess the therapeutic target, (2) identify resistance factors, and (3) measure early response are described.

Key Words: Cancer imaging; PET; response; resistance; molecular imaging.

1. INTRODUCTION

As cancer treatment moves towards more-targeted therapy *(1)*, individualized to match the particular biologic features of a patient and his/her tumor, there is an increasing need for tools to guide therapy selection and to evaluate response. The current approach to patient management relies on in vitro assay of biopsy material to determine tumor biologic features; however, relying entirely on tissue sampling has two important limitations: (1) Tumors are heterogeneous; therefore, in vitro assay is prone to sampling error,

From: *Cancer Drug Discovery and Development: Cancer Drug Resistance*
Edited by: B. Teicher © Humana Press Inc., Totowa, NJ

especially with the increasing use of minimally invasive tumor sampling by needle biopsy. (2) In vitro assay does not adequately represent the complex interactions between the tumor, the host tissue, and the selected therapy in vivo. Emerging approaches to biochemical and molecular imaging offer the ability to make sophisticated and quantitative measurements of in vivo tumor biology and are therefore ideal for guiding targeted cancer treatment in conjunction with tissue sampling and in vitro assay. Radioisotope imaging using positron-emission tomography (PET) is particularly well suited for probing molecular pathways. In this chapter, we review the use of PET imaging to guide and monitor cancer therapy, with particular emphasis on approaches that are being translated into patient studies.

2. THE APPROACH TO CANCER IMAGING

Most of cancer imaging thus far, including the increasing use of ^{18}F-fluorodeoxyglucose (FDG) PET in clinical cancer care *(2)*, has been directed towards cancer detection and staging. This has been the principle guiding most clinical cancer imaging to date—find the cancer and determine where it has spread. To be able to localize tumor sites by radiopharmaceutical imaging requires imaging probes that have higher uptake in tumors than in normal background tissues. An illustrative set of targets for tumor detection is depicted in Fig. 1A. However, as imaging moves beyond cancer detection to address the need to characterize cancer as a tool to guide treatment, the paradigm for tumor imaging must expand. For guiding therapy, the absence of a particular tumor feature, for example, an oncogene product, may be as important as its presence. In this regard, cancer imaging must expand to include quantitative assays of tumor biology in addition to simply finding cancer sites. This implies a broader set of imaging targets, depicted in Fig. 1B. It also implies the need to simultaneously localize tumors (i.e., the existing paradigm) and measure their biology (i.e., the expanded cancer imaging paradigm). This need increases the importance of recent advances in multimodality imaging such as combined PET/computer tomography (CT) tomographs and the ability to coregister different images taken at different times (e.g., sequential images of two different PET radiopharmaceuticals) *(3)*.

In this chapter, we first review the basic principles of PET imaging and then address three tasks of importance in using imaging to guide cancer treatment: (1) measuring the expression of the therapeutic target, (2) identifying resistance factors, and (3) measuring early response. These are essential steps in choosing the cancer therapy that is most likely to be effective and in assuring that the chosen therapy is working.

3. BACKGROUND: PET IMAGING

3.1. Basic PET Principles

PET relies on the use of positron-emitting radiopharmaceuticals. Positron-electron annihilation after positron emission leads to two opposing 511 kev photons. PET tomographs are designed to detect "coincident" photon pairs along all possible projection lines through the body to reconstruct quantitative maps of tracer concentration. Tomographs primarily collect annihilation photon counts from the patient (emission scans); however, they also use transmission or attenuation scanning to correct for the body's absorption of photon pairs (*see* Fig. 2). Commercially available, dedicated PET tomographs achieve high sensitivity to annihilation photon pairs using a ring of detectors, either blocks of small crystals or larger continuous arrays of crystals, surrounding the patient. The practical

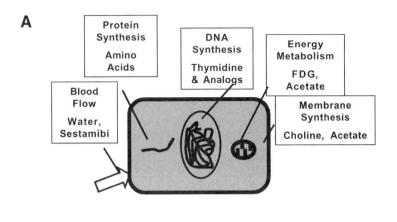

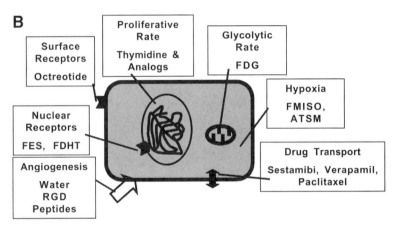

Fig. 1. Diagram of targets for positron-emission tomography imaging probes. The top of each box indicates the biologic process being targeted and the lower text refers to types of positron-emission tomography imaging probes. (Abbreviations are discussed in the text.) **(A)** In the standard approach to cancer imaging, probes are designed to detect and localize cancer, and must have higher uptake in tumor than normal tissue. **(B)** In the emerging approach using imaging to help guide therapy, probes are designed to measure specific cellular processes that will affect response to therapy, implying a different and broader set of targets.

PET Scanning Modes

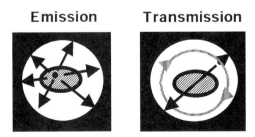

Fig. 2. Principles of positron-emission tomography (PET). Emission scanning captures annihilation photons from positron-emitting tracers in the patient. Transmission scanning uses a source external to the patient to measure photon attenuation. In PET/computer tomography devices, the transmission scan is typically performed by the computer tomography device.

spatial resolution for whole-body imaging using current instrumentation is 5–10 mm *(4)*. High-quality imaging of the torso can be achieved in approx 30 min, or conversely, dynamic images with fine time resolution (down to 10- to 15-s time resolution) can be obtained for kinetic analysis. More recently, PET and CT tomographs have been combined in the same gantry (PET/CT devices) to allow direct, mechanical coregistration of anatomy obtained from CT to functional characteristics obtained from PET *(3)*.

The use of radiation-emitting probes is driven by the need to detect very small amounts of the radiopharmaceutical, which is administered in such sufficiently small molar quantities that it does not perturb the system under study. There are two significant advantages of positron-emitting probes and PET over conventional radioisotope (single-photon or SPECT) imaging: (1) The detection of annihilation photon pairs avoids the need for physical collimation of the imaging detectors and results in higher resolution and the ability to measure absolute trace concentration. (2) Positron-emitters suitable for imaging include "biologic" nuclei such as ^{11}C and ^{18}F, offering a great deal of flexibility in designing radiopharmaceuticals to measure specific biologic processes.

3.2. Radioisotope Considerations

The use of a ^{11}C label offers the greatest flexibility in radiopharmaceutical design, given the ubiquity of carbon in biologic molecules. This makes [11]C a key radionuclide for investigational studies in a research setting. However, its short half-life (~20 min) makes it less feasible for routine clinical practice, and ^{11}C requires an on-site cyclotron and a new synthesis of radiopharmaceutical for each patient studied. [18]F has a more practical half-life (110 min), allowing regional distribution and multiple doses from a single "batch" of radiopharmaceutical. However, fluorine radiochemistry can pose a challenge, and fluorinated analogs of native biologic molecules require validation to show that they adequately match the biochemical properties of the native, nonfluorine-containing molecule.

Some biologic processes take longer than 2–4 h to study and therefore require longer-lived radioisotopes such as [124]I (4.2 d) or [64]C (12.7 h); however, the long half-life also carries a greater radiation burden to the patient relative to shorter-lived isotopes.

3.3. Imaging Protocols

Early studies of a particular imaging agent, where the imaging approaches are undergoing validation, require detailed imaging protocols that include dynamic imaging for one or more hours, often with blood sampling and metabolite analysis *(5–7)*. These studies are appropriate for pilot or early phase I/II studies, but impractical for larger clinical trials. Larger clinical trials (phase III) require radiopharmaceuticals that can be regionally distributed and, by necessity, need simplified and shorter imaging protocols with limited blood sampling. Whereas clinical feasibility is an important goal, it is a mistake, *a priori*, to limit the study of a new imaging probe to protocols simple enough for routine clinical imaging. The goal should be to study imaging agents in sufficient detail in early studies to be able to make intelligent choices about how to simplify subsequent protocols designed for routine use, while maintaining the validity of the procedure.

3.4. Image Analysis

There are several different approaches to image interpretation. The standard approach to image interpretation in clinical practice is purely qualitative, i.e., what is the pattern

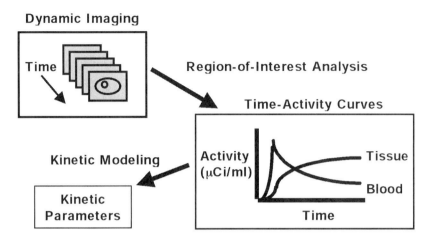

Fig. 3. Illustration of quantitative image analysis in positron-emission tomography. The tomograph captures dynamic tissue uptake profiles following radiopharmaceutical injection. The blood clearance curve, which serves as the input function for kinetic modeling, is obtained by blood sampling or from blood pool structures in the image. The blood and tissue curves are used, together with a model of radiopharmaceutical kinetics, to estimate parameters relevant to a particular tumor and its treatment.

of uptake? Largely qualitative image interpretation may be appropriate for tumor detection, but is unlikely to yield insights into quantitative in vivo tumor biology. The most detailed approach involves kinetic analysis (Fig. 3). Here, the blood clearance curve, obtained from dynamic images of a blood pool structure or from blood sampling, serves as the input to a compartmental model, from which relevant kinetic parameters can be estimated *(8)*. The most elegant, but computationally demanding application of kinetic analysis is to generate an image of kinetic parameters *(9)*, depicting quantitatively the regional behavior of the tracer and thus the regional biochemistry of the tumor or normal tissue.

In clinical practice, a more simplified and practical alternative to kinetic analysis, termed the standard uptake value (SUV), is often used. This is defined as the radiopharmaceutical tissue uptake (kBq/mL) divided by the injected dose per unit patient weight (MBq/kg). SUV has a value of 1 for a uniformly distributed tracer and a value greater than 1 in tissues where the compound accumulates. In some cases, SUV averaged over a designated period after injection is a reasonable approximation to tracer kinetics. However, in many instances, simple static uptake measures such as SUV are inadequate to describe the information on system dynamics that can be gleaned from PET imaging *(10)*. Here again, analysis of a new radiopharmaceutical should start with a detailed approach; subsequent simplification in the quantitative analysis should be based on rigorous initial tests with full knowledge of the potential inaccuracies of the simpler measures.

4. MEASURING THE THERAPEUTIC TARGET

4.1. Why Imaging?

In the approach to targeted, individualized therapy, the first step is to assess what targets are expressed in the tumor. An example would be measurement of the estrogen receptor in breast cancer before choosing hormonal therapy *(11)*. In current clinical practice, choices are based on in vitro assay of biopsy material. One might ask, "Why consider imaging rather than simply sample the tumor?" This is a reasonable but misleading question; it is not an either–or scenario. Imaging and tissue sampling are highly complementary. In vitro analysis can assay many features at once, whereas, because of practical limitations, imaging can measure only a few aspects of tumor biology for any one patient. However, it is difficult to measure changes in tumor biology and nearly impossible to measure in vivo drug effects through serial tissue sampling. Noninvasive imaging is ideally suited to both of these tasks. Furthermore, imaging can assess the regional heterogeneity of target expression and can guide sampling to those portions of the tumor most likely to yield the parameters relevant to clinical management. For example, in highly heterogeneous tumors such as soft-tissue sarcoma, PET imaging has been used to direct the biopsy towards the most active, phenotypically aggressive portion of the tumor for biopsy *(12)*. Furthermore, once tumors spread to multiple tumor sites, it is impractical to sample all tumor sites; however, there may be considerable site-to-site variability. This has been seen, for example, in studies of estrogen receptor (ER) expression in breast cancer, where ER-positive and ER-negative sites of disease arising from the same tumor may coexist *(13,14)*.

We discuss the example of ER imaging in breast cancer in some detail and then highlight briefly other approaches.

4.2. Example: PET Imaging of ER in Breast Cancer

PET imaging of ER in breast cancer provides a good example of issues related to PET imaging to identify a target. The majority of breast cancers express ER. ER expression is an indicator of prognosis and predicts the likelihood of responding to antiestrogen therapy *(11,15)*. A variety of agents has been tested for PET ER imaging *(16)* and new compounds continue to be evaluated *(16,17)*. A close analog of estradiol, the fluorinated estrogen, 16 α-[^{18}F]- fluoroestradiol-17β (FES) *(18)*, has shown the most promise in quantifying the functional ER status of breast cancer, either in the primary tumor or in metastatic lesions. Studies have shown that the quantitative level of FES uptake in primary tumors correlates with the level of ER expression measured by in vitro assay *(19)*. FES-PET provides sufficient image quality to image metastatic lesions with high sensitivity in patients with ER-positive tumors *(14)* at an acceptable radiation dose to the patient *(20)*.

FES-PET provides and important tool to characterize the entire volume of disease in an individual patient, especially in patients with recurrent or metastatic breast cancer, where tissue sampling at all sites is not feasible. FES-PET has shown heterogeneous uptake within the same tumor and between metastatic lesions, both qualitatively and quantitatively *(14,21)*. This comprehensive evaluation of functional ER status of the entire disease burden in patients will likely give important information about prognosis and help guide treatment selection (Fig. 4).

PET ER imaging can be used, in analogy to assay of ER in biopsy specimens, to predict the likelihood of response to hormonal therapy and thereby guide appropriate selection of patients for this type of treatment. Paralleling results showing that the level of ER expression predicts response to hormonal therapy *(22)*, studies by Mortimer, Dehdashti and colleagues *(23)* have shown that a higher level of FES uptake in advanced tumors predicts a greater chance of response to tamoxifen. Preliminary results in our center show similar results for patients with metastatic breast cancer treated with a variety of hormonal agents *(24)*. Serial FES-PET studies can also assess the functional response to

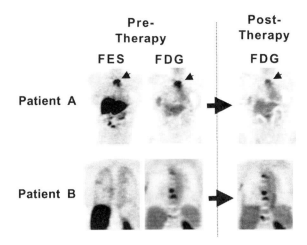

Fig. 4. Heterogeneous estrogen receptor expression in breast cancer and response to hormonal therapy. Images illustrate the correlation between 16 α-[^{18}F]- fluoroestradiol-17β (FES) uptake and subsequent response to hormonal therapy. Coronal images of FES uptake (left column) and ^{18}F-fluorodeoxyglucose (FDG) (middle column) uptake pretherapy, along with FDG uptake posthormonal therapy (left column) are shown for two patients (Patients A and B: top and bottom rows). Patient A had been previously treated with adjuvant tamoxifen and had a sternal recurrence of breast cancer 4 yr after primary tumor treatment. Her lesion had high pretherapy FES uptake in the lesion (arrows; image also shows liver and bowel uptake, both normal findings). FDG images taken before and after 6 wk of letrozole treatment show a significant decline in FDG uptake, with subsequent excellent clinical response. Patient B (bottom row) had newly diagnosed, but metastatic breast cancer that had not previously been treated. Her primary tumor was estrogen receptor-postive by immunohistochemistry and showed FES uptake (not shown). However, her pretherapy FES-positron-emission tomography (PET) showed absent uptake at bone metastases documented by multiple imaging modalities, including FDG PET. The patient received multiple hormonal treatments with no response of the bone metastases, indicated by the posttherapy FDG PET, despite response by the primary tumor. The patient ultimately had progression of bony metastases and succumbed to her disease.

hormonal therapy, or ER blockade in the case of tamoxifen, in the primary tumor or metastasis *(25)*. In the Mortimer study, substantial ER blockade in the primary tumor (about a 50% decrease in SUV from baseline) portended a good response to therapy *(23)*. In our laboratory, preliminary studies using FES in patients treated with the pure antiestrogen, fulvestrant, have shown incomplete blockade in some instances, predicting treatment failure and subsequent disease progression (Fig. 5). These exciting preliminary results show the potential of PET ER imaging to help guide appropriate, individualized breast cancer treatment and point the way for one future clinical use.

Other tracers for ER imaging may also play a role in breast cancer. Labeled analogs of commonly used hormonal agents such as tamoxifen and fulvestrant have been developed *(26,27)*, and may indicate the likelihood of response to specific agents. Conjugated estrogens have also been tested as a way to explore estrogen metabolism at the tumor site *(28)*. Other steroid receptor imaging agents such as progesterone receptor agents *(29)* and androgen receptor agents for prostate cancer *(30)* have undergone preliminary testing. In developing and testing these new agents, preclinical studies using appropriate animal models and animal imaging will be an important part of translating new compounds into clinical studies *(17)*.

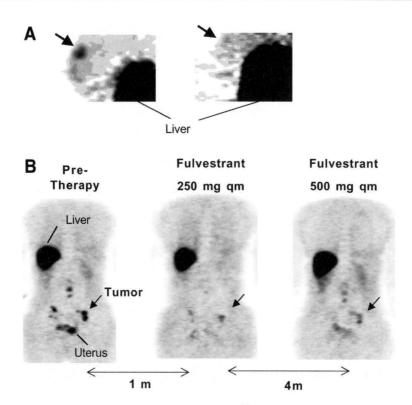

Fig. 5. Demonstration of in vivo drug effect by 16 α-[^{18}F]- fluoroestradiol-17β (FES)-positron-emission tomography (PET). Serial FES-PET images are shown for two women undergoing hormonal therapy (Patients **A** [top row] and **B**[bottom rows]. Patient A had a small primary breast tumor strongly expressing estrogen receptor (ER) (arrows). Thick sagittal images show high FES uptake pretherapy (left). After 2 mo of tamoxifen, the tumor size had reduced only slightly, but FES uptake was nearly eliminated, indicating complete blockade of the ER. The patient went on to have a partial response to treatment. Patient B had bony metastases in her lower spine and pelvis, which were recurrent from an ER+ primary tumor. She had an initial response to aromatase inhibitors, but subsequently progressed (not shown). Coronal FES-PET images at the time of disease progression (pretherapy, left) showed high uptake at multiple sites, one of which is indicated by the arrow. Uterine uptake is also seen. The patient was placed on fulvestrant, an antiestrogen. Images postfulvestrant (middle) show blockade of uterine uptake, but persistence of tumor uptake at some sites. Because of a lack of response by conventional imaging, the patient's oncologist increased her fulvestrant dose. Follow-up images on the higher dose (right) showed persistent FES uptake and reemergence of uptake at other sites seen pretherapy. Conventional imaging confirmed disease progression. These examples illustrate how PET can measure in vivo drug effects on the therapeutic target.

4.3. Other Examples of Imaging Therapeutic Targets

Other examples of targets measured by PET in preliminary studies include HER-2 *(31)*; angiogenesis, both nonspecifically by measuring blood flow *(32–34)* or by measuring specific components expressed in neovessels *(35)*; and other novel targets such as matrix metalloproteins *(36)*. In the future, it may also be possible to measure target expression in conjunction with gene therapy through imaging of transgenic reporters *(37)*. This approach has been demonstrated in animal models; however, the extent to which transgenes will play a role in patient imaging is less clear.

5. IDENTIFYING RESISTANCE MECHANISMS

5.1. Precedents for Therapy Resistance From In Vitro Studies

Even when a tumor expresses appropriate levels of the molecular target, therapy may fail if the tumor also has characteristics that will render it resistant to the chosen treatment. Examples of resistance factors identified by in vitro assay include the expression of HE-R2 as a resistance factor for hormone therapy *(24,38)*; the expression of P-glycoprotein (P-gp) as a resistance factor for doxorubicin, taxanes, and other chemotherapy agents that are P-gp substrates *(39)*; altered DNA repair mechanisms that provide resistance to alkylating agents *(40)*; and tumor hypoxia as a broad resistance factor for radiotherapy and cytotoxic chemotherapy *(41,42)*. Preliminary studies of PET agents targeted to each of these mechanisms have been undertaken in animal models and some human studies *(31,43–46)*. The ability to measure both the therapeutic target and specific resistance factors underlies the emerging role of PET in early drug testing *(47)*.

5.2. Imaging Hypoxia as a Resistance Factor

Tumor hypoxia has been established as a resistance factor for radiotherapy, and evolving evidence indicates it promotes tumor aggressiveness and resistance to a variety of systemic treatment modalities (41,42). Hypoxia also promotes genomic instability that favors survival of affected cells and leads to increased tumor heterogeneity. Imaging is ideally suited to determine the extent and heterogeneity of tumor hypoxia. Tumor hypoxia imaging by PET has received considerable attention and has undergone human testing for a number of tumors (reviewed in ref. *48*). Although hypoxia likely contributes to increased rates of glycolysis, supported by in vitro studies of FDG uptake *(49)*, a recent study in patients with a variety of tumor types showed that hypoxia was not predicted by FDG uptake *(50)*. Several PET agents specifically designed to image tumor hypoxia have been tested *(48)*. Of these, ^{18}F-fluoromisonidazole has the largest current body of preclinical validation studies and clinical experience *(43,48)* (Fig. 6). Other PET hypoxia tracers have also been studied in patients. Dehdashti et al. showed that high uptake of ^{62}Cu-ATSM predicted early progression in cervical cancer *(51)*. PET imaging holds great promise for identifying the subset of cancers with significant hypoxia, and will be important in selecting patients for alternate therapeutic strategies that overcome the resistance associated with hypoxia *(52)*.

5.2. Imaging the Drug Transporter P-gp

Drug efflux proteins, in particular P-gp, have been the topic of active investigations in cancer resistance. P-gp is a membrane transport protein for which a number of xenobiotics are substrates *(39)*. P-gp may mediate resistance by enhanced efflux of a number of chemotherapeutic agents, including agents like doxorubicin and taxol that are important in cancer treatment. Based on observations by Pinwica-Worms and others *(45)*, Ciarmello observed that enhanced washout of the SPECT agent, [^{99m}Tc]-sestamibi (MIBI), predicted resistance to epirubicin-based therapy of locally advanced breast cancer *(53)*. Other studies have observed low MIBI uptake, presumably caused by P-gp expression, as a predictor of response to P-gp-susceptible chemotherapy *(54,55)*. However, interpretation of MIBI images is confounded by the influence of blood flow, which is an important factor in its uptake and washout *(56)*. Alternative PET radiotracers such as ^{11}C-verapamil have been developed for imaging P-gp transport. Hendrickse *(44)* showed that verapamil could image P-gp transport in the brain in animal models. P-gp at

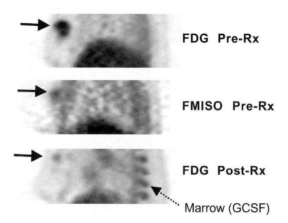

FDG Pre-Rx

FMISO Pre-Rx

FDG Post-Rx

Marrow (GCSF)

Fig. 6. Breast tumor hypoxia as a predictor of drug resistance. A patient with a large, locally advanced right breast tumor underwent ^{18}F-fluorodeoxyglucose (FDG) (top) and ^{18}F-fluoromi-sonidazole (FMISO)-positron-emission tomography (middle) pretherapy and after approx 10 wk of doxorubicin-based chemotherapy (bottom). Images are thick sagittal slices, similar to standard mammographic views. The pretherapy FDG study showed uniformly high FDG uptake throughout the tumor. FMISO-positron-emission tomography showed uptake suggestive of tumor hypoxia, but only close to the center of the tumor (arrow). Posttherapy images show a dramatic reduction in the extent and intensity of FDG uptake with residual activity in the part of the tumor that had FMISO uptake pretherapy, suggesting that the hypoxic core of the tumor was more resistant than the rest of the tumor. Residual viable tumor was found at surgery. Marrow uptake of FDG was also seen posttherapy (dashed arrow) because of granulocyte colony-stimulating factor (GCSF) administered for marrow support as part of the treatment.

the blood–brain barrier limits access of P-gp substrates to the brain parenchyma. Accordingly, Hendrickse showed that wild-type mice had low brain uptake of verapamil but high uptake in P-gp knockouts or with P-gp inhibition by cyclosporine-A. Early studies of this radiopharmaceutical applied to drug transport in the human brain are ongoing in our center *(57)*. Other tracers for P-gp transport, such as ^{18}F-paclitaxel have also been tested *(58)*. Probes to image other drug transporters that may affect cancer agent delivery and retention are being tested.

5.3. Is Altered Glycolysis a Resistance Factor?

Is altered glyocolysis a marker of tumor cell resistance to apoptosis, a key process in tumor response to therapy *(59)*? This intriguing (but untested) hypothesis arises, in part, from studies of glucose metabolism in cancer using FDG-PET. Circumstantial data supporting this hypothesis include the fact that high-FDG uptake is predictive of poor outcome for tumors treated with a variety of different treatments *(33,60–65)*. Our own studies in locally advanced breast cancer treated by neoadjuvant chemotherapy have suggested that an imbalance between glucose consumption, measured as the FDG flux, and delivery, measured as blood flow or as FDG transport (K_1) predicts poor response *(33,66)*. Several investigators have suggested that aberrant glycolysis, triggered either by intrinsic tumor properties or by local environmental stress factors, is part of a coordinated tumor response to avoid apoptosis *(67,68)*. More-recent in vitro data suggest that intermediates in the glycolytic pathway are key in initiating apoptosis and that alterations limit apoptosis *(69)*. Some gene products whose overexpression is associated with resistance to apoptosis, for example products of the PI3K/Akt pathway, are also associated with high glycolytic rates *(70)*. Thus, through a variety of mechanisms, altered glucose metabolism may be associated with broad drug resistance and may be manifested not simply as elevated FDG uptake, but as altered FDG kinetics *(66,71)*. We continue to investigate this intriguing hypothesis in ongoing studies in our laboratory.

6. MEASURING EARLY RESPONSE

6.1. Underlying Principles

As the choice of cancer treatments expands, there will be an increasing need to measure the efficacy of treatments early in the course of treatment. With many potentially effective treatments to choose from, it will be important to identify ineffective treatments early after initiation. This poses several challenges. A decrease in tumor size, the current standard in therapeutic monitoring, is a late event in response to treatment *(72)*. It is therefore desirable to be able to measure response well before any significant changes in tumor size would be expected. Additionally, some new therapies may be cytostatic instead of cytoreductive, in which case successful treatment may not lead to a decrease in tumor size at all. Studies of glucose metabolism using FDG-PET after a single dose of chemotherapy have supported the ability of in vivo biochemical imaging to measure early response *(73–76)*. However, imaging agents other than FDG that more directly measure cell growth and death will likely be even more effective at measuring early response.

In this context, it is important to distinguish tumor growth from cellular proliferation. A tumor may grow in size by generating more cells, but it can also increase in size if the cells grow larger (cellular hyperplasia) or generate more extracellular material. These two types of growth have different implications. Rapidly dividing (i.e., proliferating) tumors often carry poorer prognoses, but respond better to cytotoxic agents *(72)*. Enlarging, but nondividing tumors may not respond to cytotoxic agents and may dictate a different, possibly more localized, approach to treatment. Distinguishing between nonproliferative tumor growth and tumor proliferation is a task that benefits from a series of radiopharmaceuticals to image multiple facets of tumor biology at once. For example, images of cellular proliferation and tumor metabolism in the same imaging session may be very helpful.

6.2. Cellular Proliferation Imaging With ^{11}C-Thymidine

Decreased tumor proliferation is an early event in response to successful treatment *(72)*. This principle underlies the use of labeled thymidine and analogs to image cellular proliferation and early response to treatment (77). ^{11}C-thymidine (TdR) is incorporated into DNA but not RNA; therefore, thymidine uptake and retention in the tumor serves as a specific marker of cell division *(78–80)*.

Early clinical studies examined TdR-PET in a variety of tumors, including lymphomas *(81)*, head and neck tumors *(5,82,83)*, lung cancers *(84)*, sarcomas *(84)*, and a variety of intra-abdominal malignancies *(85)*. Some common features emerged. Images were often of lower contrast than FDG-PET, in part owing to image background from labeled TdR metabolites, both for the methyl compound *(5)* and the ring-2 compound *(7,86)*. Most patient series showed variability in tumor TdR uptake for different patients, and in many cases, uptake correlated with tumor grade or other pathologic features indicative of tumor growth. In general, these studies were pilot/feasibility studies, limited by the difficulty of synthesizing TdR and the need to analyze blood samples for metabolites or the requirement for a second scan with the major metabolite, $^{11}CO_2$.

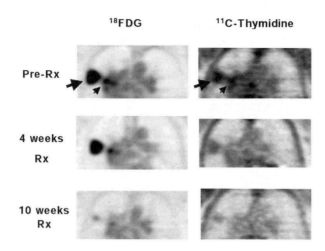

Fig. 7. Positron-emission tomography cellular proliferation imaging to measure response to treatment. Serial coronal images of a patient undergoing combined radiation therapy and chemotherapy for non-small cell lung cancer. Both ^{18}F-fluorodeoxyglucose (FDG) (left) and ^{11}C-thymidine (right) images show a decline in uptake in the primary tumor (large arrow) and a hilar metastasis (small arrow) over the course of treatment. Thymidine imaging shows evidence of a response earlier in the course of therapy, indicating the ability of cell proliferation imaging to measure early response to treatment.

Some more recent studies of TdR focused on early measurement of response, the application of cellular proliferation imaging that is most likely to find clinical use. Shields *(84)* studied a series of five patients with small cell lung cancer or high-grade sarcoma before and after a single cycle of chemotherapy with scans separated by 7–10 d. TdR-PET in these studies showed an early response to successful treatment, with a 100% decline in thymidine flux in the three patients who ultimately achieved a complete response, a 40% decline in a patient with a partial response, and no change in the patient with no response and ultimate disease progression. Changes in TdR flux were larger than changes in FDG metabolism assessed at the same times and differentiated responders from nonresponders better. This seminal study demonstrated the advantage of imaging cellular proliferation to assess early response, and sets forth a paradigm for future clinical applications. Whereas glucose metabolism fuels the growth process, it supports much more than proliferation, and so FDG images are much less specific than proliferation images. Thymidine is either catabolized or it is phosphorylated and eventually incorporated into DNA; therefore, thymidine imaging provides a uniquely specific measure of proliferation (Fig. 7).

A novel use of proliferation imaging to detect treatment effect has been described by Wells and colleagues *(87)*. In this elegant study, Wells showed that inhibition of the *de novo* thymidine synthesis pathway by an investigational thymidylate synthase inhibitor transiently increased thymidine flux through the alternative salvage pathway, quantified by TdR-PET. This approach demonstrated the ability of PET to measure an in vivo drug defect, and may be of clinical importance with the increasing use of capecitabine, a thymidylate synthase inhibitor *(88)*.

6.3. Cellular Proliferation Imaging Using Thymidine Analogs

Because of the short half-life of ^{11}C and the extensive metabolism of thymidine, TdR is not practical for routine clinical use outside of academic centers. This spurred the development of ^{18}F-labeled, nonmetabolized thymidine analogs to image tumor proliferation. The most promising thus far is ^{18}F fluoro-L-thymidine (FLT) *(89)*. The first human studies using FLT PET involved an international collaboration between our laboratory, Tuebingen University (Germany), and Wayne State University *(90)*. The studies involved a patient with lung cancer and demonstrated the high-image quality and low background afforded by FLT. Exquisite images can be obtained from injection of 3 mCi of FLT, and tumors are visualized at 45–60 min after injection. Recently, the radiation dosimetry has been published for FLT *(91)*, showing that repeat patient imaging is feasible with clinically acceptable radiation exposure for the subject. This is a critical issue for FLT, because it is likely to be used in clinical applications that require repeated studies to measure response to therapy. These studies paved the way for a series of pilot studies examining FLT-PET imaging for a variety of tumors.

Most early series focused on testing the feasibility of FLT-PET imaging and comparing FLT uptake to in vitro measures of tumor proliferation, typically the Ki-67 (MIB-1) index *(92)*. Some studies also compared FLT-PET to FDG-PET, given the established clinical role of FDG for staging in the tumor types studied. Studies have shown good correlation between FLT uptake and the Ki-67 index for a variety of tumors, including lung cancer *(93–95)*, lymphoma *(96)*, and colorectal cancer *(97)*. In cases where FDG-PET was also performed, the correlation for FLT uptake vs Ki-67 index was much better than the correlation for FDG uptake vs Ki-67. In some cases, the correlation between FDG uptake and Ki-67 was not statistically significant, confirming the earlier comment that FDG is used to fuel much more than cellular growth. These results have been summarized in a recent review *(77)*.

Most studies evaluated FLT uptake by a simple uptake measure (i.e., SUV) or by model-independent calculation of the flux of FLT trapping using graphical analysis. One exception was the study by Visvikis *(98)*, which applied a compartmental model to dynamic FLT data obtained in patients with colorectal cancer and found that the data were fit well by a three-parameter model. Estimates of flux by compartmental analysis agreed with estimates from graphical analysis. This result was distinct from experience at the University of Washington *(99,100)*; preliminary studies suggested that many tumors exhibited release of label from the trapped compartment for tumors, necessitating a k_4 parameter. A late downward curvature to the graphical analysis function indicated a finite k_4, causing discrepancies between compartmental and graphical estimates of flux. This was also reported in other preliminary studies *(101)*. These early studies support the hypothesis that FLT uptake reflects tumor proliferation; however, more work is needed to understand the kinetics of FLT in a variety of tumors and clinical settings in order to choose the optimal approach to image analysis. At this time, the approximation of a simple uptake parameter, such as SUV, or simple graphical analysis, as an index of response to treatment has not been validated.

Although preclinical models demonstrate the potential utility of FLT PET for measuring therapeutic response, limited data are available for this use in humans. Preliminary studies used FLT to monitor neoadjuvant breast cancer treatment *(101,102)* and showed that FLT could measure changes early in the course of treatment. Studies assessing FLT-PET to measure therapeutic response are underway in many centers and may give rise to multicenter trials in the near future.

More limited data are available for PET cellular proliferation imaging using thymidine analogs other than FLT. Tjuvajev *(103)* studied brain tumor patients using SPECT and ^{131}I-IUdR and found that early uptake of IUdR reflected blood–brain barrier breakdown around the brain tumor, but 24-h uptake reflected IUdR incorporation and tumor clinical and pathologic features. Similar results have been demonstrated for a positron-emitting version, [124]I-IUdR (104). This report supported the potential value of longer-lived thymidine analogs for measuring cellular proliferation, but the long half-life of [124]I and low-positron fraction lead to a high radiation burden that may limit its value for serial imaging. Boni (105) conducted a pilot study of [76]Br-BrUdR in melanoma patients and found that uptake by PET correlated with in vitro measures of proliferation by BrUdR uptake and Ki-67 immunohistochemistry. The limited clinical use of IUdR and BrUdR as PET imaging agents thus far reflects the currently limited availability of [124]I and [76]Br, and is confounded by the effect of their dehalogenation by in vivo metabolism.

6.4. Apoptosis Imaging

Besides an early decline in cell growth, effective treatments often lead to an early increase in cell death, typically by apoptosis (59). The SPECT agent ^{99m}Tc-annexin V has undergone preliminary validation as a way to image apoptosis in vivo (106) and a way to image early response to treatment (107). Annexin tracers labeled for use in PET offer better image quality and quantification, and are under development in many centers, including ours (108–110). The ability to image both changes in cell proliferation and cell death in response to treatment will be an effective means of characterizing how tumors respond to targeted therapy.

7. SUMMARY AND FUTURE DIRECTIONS

As cancer therapy becomes more targeted and individualized, new approaches to characterize tumor features and to guide therapy will be needed. PET imaging is uniquely suited to this task, and preliminary studies in patients have highlighted how imaging and tissue assay can work together to more effectively guide cancer treatment. To guide therapy, imaging must expand beyond its current role of tumor detection and staging, with an emphasis on imaging probes designed to measure particular aspects of tumor biology and on quantitative image analysis. Early studies provide examples of how imaging can be used to help guide early trials of new therapeutic agents and ultimately, to help make appropriate choices in clinical treatment. In vivo imaging is not intended to replace in vitro assay, but rather to expand the oncologist's ability to characterize the clinical biology of cancer in individual patients to make intelligent, individualized therapy choices.

REFERENCES

1. Kaklamani V, O'Regan RM. New targeted therapies in breast cancer. Semin Oncol 2004; 31:20–25.
2. Mankoff D, Bellon J. PET imaging of cancer: FDG and beyond. Semin Rad Oncol 2001; 11:16–27.
3. Alessio AM, Kinahan PE, Cheng PM, Vesselle H, Karp JS. PET/CT scanner instrumentation, challenges, and solutions. Radiol Clin North Am 2004; 42:1017–1032.
4. Surti S, Karp JS, Kinahan PE. PET instrumentation. Radiol Clin North Am 2004; 42:1003–1016.
5. Goethals P, van Eijkeren M, Lodewyck W, Dams R. Measurement of [methyl-carbon-11]thymidine and its metabolites in head and neck tumors. J Nucl Med 1995; 36:880–882.
6. Gunn RN, Yap JT, Wells P, et al. A general method to correct PET data for tissue metabolites using a dual-scan approach. J Nucl Med 2000; 41:706–711.
7. Shields AF, Mankoff D, Graham MM, et al. Analysis of 2-carbon-11-thymidine blood metabolites in PET imaging. J Nucl Med 1996; 37:290–296.
8. Mankoff DA, Muzi M, Zabib H. Quantitative analysis of nuclear oncologic images. In: Zabib H, ed. Qunatitative analysis of nuclear medicine images. Hingham: Springer, 2004.
9. Price JC. Principles of tracer kinetic analysis. Neuroimaging Clin N Am 2003; 13:689–704.
10. Mankoff DA, Muzi M, Krohn KA. Quantitative positron emission tomography imaging to measure tumor response to therapy: what is the best method? Mol Imaging Biol 2003; 5:281–285.

11. Sledge GJ, McGuire W. Steroid hormone receptors in human breast cancer. Adv Cancer Res 1983; 38:61–75.

12. Folpe AL, Lyles RH, Sprouse JT, Conrad EU, 3rd, Eary JF. (F-18) fluorodeoxyglucose positron emission tomography as a predictor of pathologic grade and other prognostic variables in bone and soft tissue sarcoma. Clin Cancer Res 2000; 6:1279–1287.

13. Hull DF, Clark GM, Osborne CK, Chamness GC, Knight WA, McGuire WL. Multiple estrogen receptor assays in human breast cancer. Cancer Res 1983; 43:413–416.

14. Dehdashti F, Mortimer JE, Siegel BA, et al. Positron tomographic assessment of estrogen receptors in breast cancer: a comparison with FDG-PET and in vitro receptor assays. J Nucl Med 1995; 36:1766–1774.

15. Reiner A, Neumeister B, Spona J, Reiner G, Schemper M, Jakesz R. Immunocytochemical localization of estrogen and progesterone receptor and prognosis in human primary breast cancer. Cancer Res 1990; 50:7057–7061.

16. Katzenellenbogen JA, Welch MJ, Dehdashti F. The development of estrogen and progestin radiopharmaceuticals for imaging breast cancer. Anticancer Res 1997; 17:1573–1576.

17. Aliaga A, Rousseau JA, Ouellette R, et al. Breast cancer models to study the expression of estrogen receptors with small animal PET imaging. Nucl Med Biol 2004; 31:761–770.

18. Kiesewetter DO, Kilbourn MR, Landvatter SW, et al. Preparation of four fluorine-18-labeled estrogens and their selective uptakes in target tissue of immature rats. J Nucl Med 1984; 25:1212–1221.

19. Mintun MA, Welch MJ, Siegel BA, et al. Breast cancer: PET imaging of estrogen receptors. Radiology 1988; 169:45–48.

20. Mankoff DA, Peterson LM, Tewson TJ, et al. [18F]fluoroestradiol radiation dosimetry in human PET studies. J Nucl Med 2001; 42:679–684.

21. Mankoff DA, Dehdashti F, Shields AF. Characterizing tumors using metabolic imaging: PET imaging of cellular proliferation and steroid receptors. Neoplasia 2000; 2:71–88.

22. Campbell FC, Elston CW, Blamey RW, et al. Quantitative oestradiol receptor values in primary breast cancer and response of metastases to endocrine therapy. Lancet 1981; 1:1317–1319.

23. Mortimer JE, Dehdashti F, Siegel BA, Trinkaus K, Katzenellenbogen JA, Welch MJ. Metabolic flare: indicator of hormone responsiveness in advanced breast cancer. J Clin Oncol 2001; 19:2797–803.

24. Linden HM, Link JM, Stekhova S, et al. HER2 Expression and uptake of [F-18]-fluoroestradiol (FES) predict response of breast cancer to hormonal therapy. J Nucl Med 2004; 45:85P.

25. McGuire A, Dehdashti F, Siegel B, et al. Positron tomographic assessment of 16α-[18F]fluro-17β-estradiol uptake in metastatic breast carcinoma. J Nucl Med 1991; 32:1526–1531.

26. Inoue T, Kim EE, Wallace S, et al. Positron emission tomography using [18F]fluorotamoxifen to evaluate therapeutic responses in patients with breast cancer: preliminary study. Cancer Biother Radiopharm 1996; 11:235–245.

27. Seimbille Y, Benard F, Rousseau J, et al. Impact on estrogen receptor binding and target tissue uptake of [18F]fluorine substitution at the 16α-position of fulvestrant (faslodex; ICI 182,780). Nucl Med Biol 2004; 31:691–698.

28. Brust P, Rodig H, Romer J, et al. Distribution of 16α-[18F]fluoro-estradiol-3,17β-disulfamate in rats, tumour-bearing mice and piglets. Appl Radiat Isot 2002; 57:687–695.

29. Dehdashti F, McGuire AH, VanBrocklin HF, et al. Assessment of 21-[18F]fluoro-16 α-ethyl-19-nonprogesterone as a positron-emitting radiopharmaceutical for the detection of progestin receptors in human breast carcinomas. J Nucl Med 1991; 32:1532–1537.

30. Larson SM, Morris M, Gunther H, et al. Tumor localization of 16β-18F-fluoro-5α-dihydrotestosterone versus 18F-FDG in patients with progressive, metastatic prostate cancer. J Nucl Med 2004; 45:366–373.

31. Gonzalez Trotter DE, Manjeshwar RM, Doss M, et al. Quantitation of small-animal 124I activity distributions using a clinical PET/CT scanner. J Nucl Med 2004; 45:1237–1244.

32. Wilson CBJH, Lammertsma AA, McKenzie CG, Sikora K, Jones T. Measurements of blood flow and exchanging water space in breast tumors using positron emission tomography: A rapid and non-invasive dynamic method. Cancer Res 1992; 52:1592–1597.

33. Mankoff DA, Dunnwald LK, Gralow JR, et al. Blood flow and metabolism in locally advanced breast cancer: relationship to response to therapy. J Nucl Med 2002; 43:500–509.

34. Zasadny KR, Tatsumi M, Wahl RL. FDG metabolism and uptake versus blood flow in women with untreated primary breast cancers. Eur J Nucl Med Mol Imaging 2003; 30:274–280.

35. Haubner R, Wester HJ, Burkhart F, et al. Glycosylated RGD-containing peptides: tracer for tumor F5targeting and angiogenesis imaging with improved biokinetics. J Nucl Med 2001; 42:326–336.

36. Zheng QH, Fei X, Liu X, et al. Synthesis and preliminary biological evaluation of MMP inhibitor radiotracers [11C]methyl-halo-CGS 27023A analogs, new potential PET breast cancer imaging agents. Nucl Med Biol 2002; 29:761–770.

37. Berger F, Gambhir SS. Recent advances in imaging endogenous or transferred gene expression utilizing radionuclide technologies in living subjects: applications to breast cancer. Breast Cancer Res 2001; 3:28–35.

38. Dowsett M, Harper-Wynne C, Boeddinghaus I, et al. HER-2 amplification impedes the antiproliferative effects of hormone therapy in estrogen receptor-positive primary breast cancer. Cancer Res 2001; 61:8452–8458.

39. Kaye SB. Multidrug resistance: clinical relevance in solid tumours and strategies for circumvention. Curr Opin Oncol 1998; 10(Suppl 1):S15–S19.

40. Dolan ME, Pegg AE. O-6-benzylguanine and its role in chemotherapy. Clin Cancer Res 1997; 3:837–847.

41. Teicher BA. Hypoxia and drug resistance. Cancer Metastasis Rev 1994; 13:139–168.

42. Sutherland R. Tumor hypoxia and gene expression. Acta Oncol 1998; 37:567–574.

43. Rasey JS, Koh W, Grierson JR, Grunbaum Z, Krohn KA. Radiolabeled fluoromisonidazole as an imaging agent for tumor hypoxia. Int J Radiation Oncol Biol Phys 1989; 17:985–992.

44. Hendrikse NH, de Vries EG, Eriks-Fluks L, et al. A new in vivo method to study P-glycoprotein transport in tumors and the blood-brain barrier. Cancer Res 1999; 59:2411–2416.

45. Piwnica-Worms D, Chiu ML, Budding M, Kronauge JF, Kramer RA, Croop JM. Functional imaging of multidrug-resistant P-glycoprotein with an organotechnetium complex. Cancer Research 1993; 53:977–984.

46. Zheng QH, Liu X, Fei X, et al. Synthesis and preliminary biological evaluation of radiolabeled O^6-benzylguanine derivatives, new potential PET imaging agents for the DNA repair protein O^6-alkylguanine-DNA alkyltransferase in breast cancer. Nucl Med Biol 2003; 30:405–415.

47. Aboagye EO, Price PM. Use of positron emission tomography in anticancer drug development. Invest New Drugs 2003; 21:169–181.

48. Rajendran JG, Krohn KA. Imaging tumor hypoxia. In: Bailey DL, Townsend dW, Valk PE, Maisey MN, eds. Positron emission tomography: principles and practice. London: Springer, 2002.

49. Clavo AC, Brown RS, Wahl RL. Fluorodeoxyglucose uptake in human cancer cell lines is increased by hypoxia. J Nucl Med 1995; 36:1625–1632.

50. Rajendran JG, Mankoff DA, O'Sullivan F, et al. Hypoxia and glucose metabolism in malignant tumors: evaluation by [18F]fluoromisonidazole and [18F]fluorodeoxyglucose positron emission tomography imaging. Clin Cancer Res 2004; 10:2245–2252.

51. Dehdashti F, Grigsby PW, Mintun MA, Lewis JS, Siegel BA, Welch MJ. Assessing tumor hypoxia in cervical cancer by positron emission tomography with 60Cu-ATSM: relationship to therapeutic response-a preliminary report. Int J Radiat Oncol Biol Phys 2003; 55:1233–1238.

52. Rischin D, Peters l, Hicks R, et al. Phase I trial of concurrent tirapazamine, cisplatin, and radiotherapy in patients with advanced head and neck cancer. J Clin Oncol 2001; 19:535–542.

53. Ciarmiello A, Vecchio SD, Silvestro P, et al. Tumor clearance of technetium 99m-sestamibi as a predictor of response to neoadjuvant chemotherapy for locally advanced breast cancer. J Clin Oncol 1998; 16:1677–1683.

54. Ceriani L, Giovanella L, Bandera M, Beghe B, Ortelli M, Roncari G. Semi-quantitative assessment of 99mTc-sestamibi uptake in lung cancer: relationship with clinical response to chemotherapy. Nucl Med Comm 1997; 18:1087–1097.

55. Kostakoglu L, Guc D, Canpinar H, et al. P-glycoprotein expression by technetium-99m-MIBI scintigraphy in hematologic malignancy. J Nucl Med 1998; 39:191–197.

56. Mankoff DA, Dunnwald LK, Gralow JR, et al. [Tc-99m]-sestamibi uptake and washout in locally advanced breast cancer are correlated with tumor blood flow. Nucl Med Biol 2002; 29:719–727.

57. Muzi M, Link JM, Mankoff DA, Collier AC, Yang X, Unadkat JD. Quantitative estimation of P-glycoprotein transport using [C-11]-verapamil. J Nucl Med 2003; 44:365P.

58. Kurziel KA, Kieswetter do, Carson RE, Eckelman WC, Herscovitch P. Biodistribution, radiation dose estimates, and in vivo P-gp modulation studies of 18F-paclitaxel in nonhuman primates. J Nucl Med 2003; 44:1330–1339.

59. Hockenbery D. Defining apoptosis. Am J Pathol 1995; 146:16–19.

60. Patronas NJ, Di Chiro G, Kufta C, et al. Prediction of survival in glioma patients by means of positron emission tomography. J Neurosurg 1985; 62:816–822.

61. Oshida M, Uno K, Suzuki M, et al. Predicting the prognoses of breast carcinoma patients with positron emission tomography using 2-deoxy-2-fluoro[18F]-D-glucose. Cancer 1998:2227–2234.

62. Tralins KS, Douglas JG, Stelzer KJ, et al. Volumetric analysis of 18F-FDG PET in glioblastoma multiforme: prognostic information and possible role in definition of target volumes in radiation dose escalation. J Nucl Med 2002; 43:1667–1673.

63. Vansteenkiste J, Fischer BM, Dooms C, Mortensen J. Positron-emission tomography in prognostic and therapeutic assessment of lung cancer: systematic review. Lancet Oncol 2004; 5:531–540.
64. Eary JF, O'Sullivan F, Powitan Y, et al. Sarcoma tumor FDG uptake measured by PET and patient outcome: a retrospective analysis. Eur J Nucl Med Mol Imaging 2002; 29:1149–1154.
65. Downey RJ, Akhurst T, Gonen M, et al. Preoperative F-18 fluorodeoxyglucose-positron emission tomography maximal standardized uptake value predicts survival after lung cancer resection. J Clin Oncol 2004; 22:3255–3260.
66. Tseng J, Dunnwald LK, Schubert EK, et al. [F-18]-FDG kinetics in locally advanced breast cancer: correlation with tumor blood flow and changes in response to neo-adjuvant chemotherapy. J Nucl Med 2004; 45:1829–1837.
67. Mathapala S, Rempel A, Pederson P. Aberrant glycolytic metabolism of cancer cells: a remarkable coordination of genetic, transcriptional, post-translational, and mutational events that lead to a critical role for type II hexokinase. J Biogenet Biomembr 1997; 29:339–343.
68. Brand K. Aerobic glycosis by proliferating cells: protection against oxidative stress at the expense of energy yield. J Bioenergetics and biomembranes 1997; 29:335–364.
69. Gottleib E, Heiden MV, Thompson C. Bcl-x_L prevents the initial disease in mitochondrial membrane potential and subsequent reactive oxygen species production during tumor necrosis factor alpha-induced apoptosis. Mol Cell Biol 2000; 20:5680–5689.
70. West KA, Castillo SS, Dennis PA. Activation of the PI3K/Akt pathway and chemotherapeutic resistance. Drug Resist Updat 2002; 6:234–248.
71. Spence A, Muzi M, Graham M, et al. Glucose metabolism in human malignant gliomas measured quantitatively with PET, 1-[C-11]glucose and FDG: analysis of the FDG lumped constant. J Nucl Med 1998; 39:440–448.
72. Tannock IF. Cell proliferation. In: Tannock IF, Hill RP, eds. The basic science of oncology. New York: McGraw-Hill, 1992:154–177.
73. Smith I, Welch A, Hutcheon A, et al. Positron emission tomography using [^{18}F]-fluorodeoxy-D-glucose to predict the pathologic response of breast cancer to primary chemotherapy. J Clin Oncol 2000; 18:1676–1688.
74. Schelling M, Avril N, Nahrig J, et al. Positron emission tomography using [^{18}F] fluorodeoxyglucose for monitoring primary chemotherapy in breast cancer. J Clin Oncol 2000; 18:1689–1695.
75. Romer W, Hanauske AR, Ziegler S, et al. Positron emission tomography in non-Hodgkin's lymphoma: assessment of chemotherapy with fluorodeoxyglucose. Blood 1998; 91:4464–4471.
76. Wieder HA, Brucher BL, Zimmermann F, et al. Time course of tumor metabolic activity during chemoradiotherapy of esophageal squamous cell carcinoma and response to treatment. J Clin Oncol 2004; 22:900–908.
77. Mankoff DA, Shields AF, Krohn KA. PET imaging of cellular proliferation (review). Radiol Clin North Am 2004; 43:153–167.
78. Cleaver JE. Thymidine metabolism and cell kinetics. Frontiers Biol 1967; 6:43–100.
79. Livingston RB, Ambus U, George SL, Freireich EJ, Hart JS. In vitro determination of thymidine-[H-3] labeling index in human solid tumors. Cancer Res 1974; 34:1376–1380.
80. Livingston RB, Hart JS. The clinical applications of cell kinetics in cancer therapy. Ann Rev Toxicol 1977; 17:529–543.
81. Martiat P, Ferrant A, Labar D, et al. In vivo measurement of carbon-11 thymidine uptake in non-Hodgkin's lymphoma using positron emission tomography. J Nucl Med 1988; 29:1633–1637.
82. van Eijkeren ME, De Schryver A, Goethals P, et al. Measurement of short-term ^{11}C-thymidine activity in human head and neck tumours using positron emission tomography (PET). Acta Oncol 1992; 31:539–543.
83. van Eijkeren ME, Thierens H, Seuntjens J, Goethals P, Lemahieu I, Strijckmans K. Kinetics of [methyl-^{11}C]thymidine in patients with squamous cell carcinoma of the head and neck. Acta Oncol 1996; 35:737–741.
84. Shields AF, Mankoff DA, Link JM, et al. Carbon-11-thymidine and FDG to measure therapy response. J Nucl Med 1998; 39:1757–1762.
85. Wells P, Gunn RN, Alison M, et al. Assessment of proliferation in vivo using 2-[^{11}C]thymidine positron emission tomography in advanced intra-abdominal malignancies. Cancer Res 2002; 62:5698–5702.
86. Shields AF, Graham MM, Kozawa SM, et al. Contribution of labeled carbon dioxide to PET imaging of carbon-11-labeled compounds. J Nucl Med 1992; 33:581–584.
87. Wells P, Aboagye E, Gunn RN, et al. 2-[^{11}C]thymidine positron emission tomography as an indicator of thymidylate synthase inhibition in patients treated with AG337. J Natl Cancer Inst 2003; 95:675–682.

88. Kaklamani VG, Gradishar WJ. Role of capecitabine (Xeloda) in breast cancer. Expert Rev Anticancer Ther 2003; 3:137–144.

89. Grierson JR, Shields AF. Radiosynthesis of 3'-deoxy-3'-[^{18}F]fluorothymidine: [^{18}F]FLT for imaging of cellular proliferation in vivo. Nucl Med Biol 2000; 27:143–156.

90. Shields AF, Grierson JR, Dohmen BM, et al. Imaging proliferation in vivo with [F-18]FLT and positron emission tomography. Nat Med 1998; 4:1334–1336.

91. Vesselle H, Grierson J, Peterson LM, Muzi M, Mankoff DA, Krohn KA. ^{18}F-Fluorothymidine radiation dosimetry in human PET imaging studies. J Nucl Med 2003; 44:1482–1488.

92. Pinder SE, Wencyk P, Sibbering DM, et al. Assessment of the new proliferation marker MIB1 in breast carcinoma using image analysis: associations with other prognostic factors and survival. Br J Cancer 1995; 71:146–149.

93. Vesselle H, Grierson J, Muzi M, et al. In vivo validation of 3'deoxy-3'-[(18)F]fluorothymidine ([(18)F]FLT) as a proliferation imaging tracer in humans: correlation of [(18)F]FLT uptake by positron emission tomography with Ki-67 immunohistochemistry and flow cytometry in human lung tumors. Clin Cancer Res 2002; 8:3315–3323.

94. Buck AK, Schirrmeister H, Hetzel M, et al. 3-deoxy-3-(^{18}F)fluorothymidine-positron emission tomography for noninvasive assessment of proliferation in pulmonary nodules. Cancer Res 2002; 62:3331–3334.

95. Buck AK, Halter G, Schirrmeister H, et al. Imaging proliferation in lung tumors with PET: ^{18}F-FLT versus ^{18}F-FDG. J Nucl Med 2003; 44:1426–1431.

96. Wagner M, Seitz U, Buck A, et al. 3'-[^{18}F]fluoro-3'-deoxythymidine ([^{18}F]-FLT) as positron emission tomography tracer for imaging proliferation in a murine B-cell lymphoma model and in the human disease. Cancer Res 2003; 63:2681–2687.

97. Francis DL, Freeman A, Visvikis D, et al. In vivo imaging of cellular proliferation in colorectal cancer using positron emission tomography. Gut 2003; 52:1602–1606.

98. Visvikis D, Francis D, Mulligan R, et al. Comparison of methodologies for the in vivo assessment of (18)FLT utilisation in colorectal cancer. Eur J Nucl Med Mol Imaging 2004; 31:169–178.

99. Muzi M, Mankoff DA, Grierson JR, Wells JM, Vesselle H, Krohn KA. The kinetic modeling of 3'-deoxy-3'-fluorothymidine in somatic tumors: mathematical studies. J Nucl Med 2005; 46:371–380.

100. Muzi M, Vesselle H, Grierson JR, et al. The kinetic analysis of FLT (3'-deoxy-3'-fluorothymidine) PET studies: validation studies in patients with lung cancer. J Nucl Med 2005; 46:274–282.

101. Pio BS, Park CK, Satyamurthy N, Czernin J, Phelps ME, Silverman DH. PET with fluoro-L-thmyidine allows early prediction of breast cancer response to chemotherapy. J Nucl Med 2003; 44:76P.

102. Dohmen BM, Shields AF, Dittman H, et al. Use of [^{18}F]FLT for breast cancer imaging. J Nucl Med 2001; 42:29P.

103. Tjuvajev JG, Macapinlac HA, Daghighian F, et al. Imaging of brain tumor proliferative activity with iodine-131-iododeoxyuridine. J Nucl Med 1994; 35:1407–1417.

104. Blasberg RG, Roelcke U, Weinreich R, et al. Imaging brain tumor proliferative activity with [^{124}I]iododeoxyuridine. Cancer Res 2000; 60:624–635.

105. Boni R, Blauenstein P, Dummer R, von Schulthess GK, Schubiger PA, Steinert HC. Non-invasive assessment of tumour cell proliferation with positron emission tomography and [^{76}Br]bromodeoxyuridine. Melanoma Res 1999; 9:569–573.

106. Blankenberg F, Ohtsuki K, Strauss HW. Dying a thousand deaths. Radionuclide imaging of apoptosis. Q J Nucl Med 1999; 43:170–176.

107. Belhocine T, Steinmetz N, Hustinx R, et al. Increased uptake of the apoptosis-imaging agent, [Tc-99m] recombinant human annexin V, in human tumor in human tumors after one course of chemotherapy, as a predictor of response and patient prognosis. Clin Cancer Res 2002; 8:2766–2774.

108. Grierson JR, Yagle KJ, Eary JF, et al. Production of ^{18}F-fluoroannexin for imaging apoptosis with PET. Bioconjug Chem 2004; 15:373–379.

109. Zijlstra S, Gunawan J, Burchert W. Synthesis and evaluation of a ^{18}F-labelled recombinant annexin-V derivative, for identification and quantification of apoptotic cells with PET. Appl Radiat Isot 2003; 58:201–207.

110. Yagle KJ, Eary JF, Tait JF, et al. Evaluation of ^{18}F-annexin V as a PET imaging agent in an animal model of apoptosis. J Nucl Med 2005; 46:658–666.

II | BIOLOGICAL RESISTANCE

6

Cancer Stem Cells

Implications for Development of More Effective Therapies

Ilia Mantle, PhD, Gabriela Dontu, PhD, Suling Liu, PhD, and Max S. Wicha, MD

CONTENTS

SUMMARY

Despite advances in the development of cytotoxic chemotherapies, the fact remains that for most common malignancies, metastatic disease remains incurable. Recent work has suggested that most, if not all, malignancies are driven by a small subpopulation of cells that have stem cell characteristics. These "tumor stem cells" are thought to arise either from normal tissue stem cells or from early progenitor cells through dysregulation of self-renewal pathways. The partial differentiation of cancer stem cells may result in tumor heterogeneity. One of the characteristics of this heterogeneity may be reflected in the resistance of cancer stem cells to cytotoxic chemotherapy. Evidence is presented that current chemotherapeutic regimens selectively target more differentiated cells in tumors, while sparing the tumor stem cell component. This may account for relapse following tumor regression. The mechanisms contributing to the resistance of tumor stem cells to cytotoxic agents may involve increased efficiency of DNA replication and repair mechanisms in stem cells, changes in cell cycle parameters, and the overexpression of antiapoptotic and transporter proteins in these cell populations.

From: *Cancer Drug Discovery and Development: Cancer Drug Resistance*
Edited by: B. Teicher © Humana Press Inc., Totowa, NJ

The tumor stem cell model of carcinogenesis has fundamental implications for the development of new cancer therapeutic agents, as well as for the design of clinical trials utilizing these agents. Strategies aimed at the targeting of cancer stem cell populations may lead to more effective therapies for the treatment of advanced malignancies.

Key Words: Cytotoxic chemotherapy; dysregulation; tumor heterogeneity; tumor stem cells; tumor stem cell model.

1. INTRODUCTION

Despite numerous advances in the development of antineoplastic agents, the fact remains that for most common malignancies, advanced disease remains incurable. Cytotoxic chemotherapies are often able to induce regression of cancer in patients, relieving symptoms, and improving quality of life. However, for most common malignancies, the tumors ultimately recur and become resistant to these agents. Recent work has suggested that most, if not all, malignancies, may contain a small subpopulation of cells that have stem cell characteristics. These "tumor stem cells" may drive tumorigenesis, and may display resistance to agents in our current pharmacologic armamentarium. In this chapter, we review recent evidence suggesting that cancers may arise from normal stem cells or their immediate progenitors, producing tumor heterogeneity and are driven by a "cancer stem cell" population. We explore potential molecular mechanisms accounting for resistance of these cancer stem cells to cytotoxic chemotherapy. Finally, based on an understanding of the biology of basic stem cell processes, we propose new strategies for therapeutic development that specifically target the cancer stem cell population. Targeting of this critical cell population may result in more effective treatments for advanced cancers.

2. TISSUE-SPECIFIC STEM CELLS AND THE ORIGIN OF CANCER

All tissues in the body are derived from the differentiation of organ-specific stem cells. These stem cells are defined by their capacity to undergo self-renewal, as well as to differentiate into the cell types that compose each organ. These tissue-specific stem cells are distinguished from embryonic stem cells in that their differentiation is largely restricted to cell types within a particular organ. Stem cells, by their long-lived nature, are subject to the accumulation of multiple mutations required for carcinogenesis. Over 40 yr ago, it was postulated that these tissue-specific stem cells may be the cell of origin of cancer *(1)*. Normal stem cells and their transformed counterparts share many characteristics, including the capacity for self-renewal, differentiation (although this is dysregulated in tumors), immortality as evidenced by telomerase expression, resistance to apoptosis, and ability to migrate and home to distant organ sites. Several recent reviews have explored the concept of the stem cell origin of tumors *(2–6)*. Recent studies of chronic myelogenous leukemia suggest that progenitor cells may also acquire mutations that allow them to self-renew *(6–8)*. A separate but related issue concerns the generation of tumor heterogeneity and the presence within tumors of tumor stem cells. If tumors arise through the transformation of stem or early progenitor cells and display various levels of differentiation, then tumor heterogeneity may be created, at least in part, by the aberrant differentiation of tumor stem cells and progenitor cells. Indeed, strong evidence has accumulated over the past decade that there exists within most, if not all tumors, a "stem cell population" that drives tumorigenesis. This was first demonstrated in human leukemia by John Dick's group *(9)*. They demonstrated that only a rare population of cells within leukemias, which expressed cell-surface markers similar to normal stem cells (CD34+CD38−), were able to transfer the leukemic phenotype to immunosuppressed nonobese, severe combined immunodeficient (NOD-SCID) mice. Furthermore, the tumors that developed in these mice recapitulated the characteristics of the leukemia from which the samples were derived. These studies, and subsequent ones *(10,11)*, have demonstrated that leukemias may contain a cellular hierarchy, with transformed tumor stem cells and other cells in various stages of differentiation. A similar model for stem cells in solid tumors was first demonstrated by our group in collaboration with Michael F. Clarke's laboratory *(12)*. We showed that human breast tumors contain a subpopulation of tumor stem cells that bear the cell-surface phenotype ESA+CD44+CD24−/lowLineage−. As few as 100 of these cells could form tumors in NOD-SCID mice, whereas 20,000 cells that did not bear this phenotype failed to form tumors. Furthermore, fitting a stem cell model, the tumors that were generated by the tumorigenic stem cells recapitulated the phenotypic heterogeneity found in the initial tumors.

More recently, several groups have provided evidence for the existence of tumor stem cells in human brain tumors. Dirks' group first demonstrated that human brain tumors contained a subpopulation of cells bearing the neural stem cell marker CD133 (2,13). These tumor stem cells were able to form tumor neurospheres in vitro, as well as to differentiate into tumors resembling those from the initial samples. Furthermore, they demonstrated that these sphere-forming cells are able to produce tumors when injected intracranially into NOD-SCID mice *(2)*. These tumors recapitulated the phenotypic heterogeneity found in the initial tumors. Cancer stem cells have also been isolated from human glioblastomas *(14,15)*. The existence of a tumor stem cell population has recently been described in human multiple myeloma. Richard Jones group *(16)* has found that human myelomas are generated from cells that lack the expression of syndecan (CD138), which is present on mature plasma cells. These "myeloma stem cells" are pre-B cells expressing CD20. All of the above studies point to the existence of a stem cell component within human tumors capable of transferring the malignant phenotype, as well as the more differentiated "nontumorigenic" cells that compose the bulk of the tumor. The percent of tumor stem cells within tumors may vary between different tumor types, as well as within each tumor type. Leukemic and myeloma stem cells may comprise as few as 1 out of 5 × 10^4 cells, whereas in solid tumors such as breast cancer and brain tumors, cells bearing the stem cell phenotype appear to be more abundant, comprising between 1 and 20% of the tumor cell population. Furthermore, there is evidence in brain tumors that the percent of stem cells within a tumor may be predictive of its clinical aggressiveness *(13)*.

3. BIOLOGICAL IMPLICATIONS OF CANCER STEM CELLS

As indicated above, the stem cell model of carcinogenesis suggests that tumor heterogeneity is generated through partial differentiation of tumor stem cells. In a sense then, tumorigenesis represents a form of abnormal organ development. This contrasts to earlier models that attribute the development of tumor heterogeneity to stochastic processes that result from random mutation and subsequent clonal selection. The development of cellular heterogeneity through differentiation of malignant stem and/or progenitor cells has implications for understanding the process of tumor metastasis, as well as for providing an explanation for the resistance of tumors to therapeutic agents. It has been hypothesized that metastasis results from random mutation and selection and is therefore a late event in tumor evolution. However, recent studies utilizing molecular profiling have cast doubt on this model. These studies have shown that the propensity of tumors to metastasize can be predicted by the molecular profile of the initial tumor, suggesting that the ability of tumor cells to metastasize is "hard-wired" into the genotype of the tumor. These results are more consistent with a stem cell model, which suggests that the metastatic propensity of a tumor is determined by its cell of origin as well as initial mutation profile, rather than being a late event in tumor evolution.

Another important issue in carcinogenesis is the interaction between transformed stem cells and their surrounding microenvironment. Normal stem cell behavior is tightly regulated by interactions between the stem cells and the surrounding environment. This environment, composed of neighboring cells, extracellular matrix, and soluble factors, has been termed the "stem cell niche." Evidence has accumulated that developing tumors also have important interactions with the surrounding environment. Indeed, the reciprocal interaction between tumor stem cells and their surrounding niche may play a fundamental role in tumor development. Recent studies have indicated that the stroma surrounding tumors has an altered gene expression profile compared to stroma surrounding normal tissue. This profile resembles that found in inflammatory tissue, suggesting similarities between wound healing and tumorigenesis (17). Interestingly, these studies provide a potential explanation for the role of inflammation in carcinogenesis in tumors such as gastric tumors. Interaction between tumor cells and their environment undoubtedly also plays a role in the sensitivity of these tumor cells to therapeutic agents. In this regard, it has been demonstrated that attachment of tumor cells to the extracellular matrix mediated by integrins, regulates their sensitivity to chemotherapy (18).

4. STEM CELLS AND CELL SURVIVAL

The generation of phenotypic heterogeneity through differentiation of tumor stem cells also has profound implications for understanding the sensitivity of these cells to chemotherapeutic agents, and for the development of new agents that target this tumor stem cell population.

By virtue of their fundamental importance in organogenesis, normal stem cells have evolved mechanisms that promote their survival and enhance their resistance to apoptosis. Examples of this can be found in organs where tissues undergo rapid turnover. In the mammary gland during pregnancy, there is marked proliferation and accumulation of mammary epithelial cells. These cells then undergo differentiation and produce milk proteins during lactation. The process of mammary involution that occurs following lactation is accompanied by massive apoptosis of differentiated cells. However, the stem cell component of the mammary gland is resistant to these apoptotic signals. These cells survive the involution process and regenerate the gland during subsequent pregnancies (19,20).

Resistance of stem cells to apoptosis can also be seen in colonic epithelial stem cells. These stem cells give rise to the rapidly proliferating cells, termed transient amplifying cells, which then differentiate and are shed into the intestine after they undergo apoptosis (21). Colonic stem cells are inherently resistant to this apoptotic process.

The inherent resistance of normal stem cells to apoptosis is also observed in patients undergoing cytotoxic chemotherapy treatments. When patients are given nonmyeloablative doses of cytotoxic chemotherapy, they experience transient decreases in their white blood cell counts. This is caused by apoptosis of differentiated neutrophil and myeloid precursors. The stem cells in the bone marrow are not ablated by these doses of chemotherapy and are able to regenerate a normal hematopoietic system after several weeks. Similarly, many of the gastrointestinal side effects of chemotherapy are caused by the induction of apoptosis in differentiating colonic epithelial cells. These injured cells are regenerated by stem cells that are able to survive these chemotherapeutic insults.

5. TUMOR STEM CELLS AND RESISTANCE TO CYTOTOXIC AGENTS

Just as normal stem cells may be more resistant to the induction of apoptosis by cytotoxic agents and radiation therapy than are more differentiated cells, so too, tumor stem cells may display increased resistance to these agents compared to the more differentiated cells that compose the bulk of the tumor. Supporting this concept, Craig Jordan's group has demonstrated that leukemic stem cells are more resistant to chemotherapy than are the more differentiated myeloblastic cells that constitute the vast majority of cells in leukemia (22). Similarly, Matsui et al. (16) have shown that myeloma stem cells are resistant to current therapies being used to treat myeloma, including chemotherapy and proteosome inhibitors. Previous observations regarding the in vitro behavior of "tumor spheroids" may also be related to the enrichment of stem cells in these structures. A number of groups, including Robert Kerbel's (23), have found that when tumor cells are cultured on nonadherent surfaces, they form floating colonies termed tumor spheroids. Cells in these tumor spheroids are considerably more resistant to both chemotherapy and radiation therapy, than are the same cells cultured as monolayers. These effects were not merely because of drug penetration or uptake. Interestingly, a number of laboratories, including our own, have recently shown that both normal and tumor cells growing in spheroids are highly enriched for "stem and early progenitor cells" (24). This raises the intriguing possibility that the relative resistance of tumor spheroids to chemotherapy and radiation therapy is because of enrichment of stem cells in these structures.

6. MECHANISMS OF STEM CELL RESISTANCE TO APOPTOSIS

As described, there is evidence that both normal stem cells and their malignant counterparts are more resistant to apoptosis than are the differentiated cells comprising the bulk of normal organs or tumors. Work in a number of laboratories has begun to elucidate the molecular mechanisms that may account for this resistance, which are described in the following four subheadings.

6.1. Cell Cycle Kinetics

Both normal stem cells and their malignant counterparts are slowly cycling cells that may contain a large fraction of cells that are in G_0 (25). In turn, these cells may give rise to "transit-amplifying cells" that have a substantially higher growth fraction. Chemotherapeutic agents, particularly those with cell cycle specificity, will thus have substantially more effects on transit amplifying, rapidly dividing cells, than relatively quiescent stem cells.

6.2. DNA Replication and Repair Mechanisms

Stem cells are defined by their ability to undergo self-renewal as well as differentiation. Self-renewal divisions are inherently different from divisions that occur in differentiating cells. Stem cell self-renewal may occur by either asynchronous or synchronous division. Asynchronous self-renewal results in a daughter cell with identical phenotype to the parent stem cell, as well as a second daughter cell that then undergoes differentiation. Because only a single stem cell is produced from this division, it can account for stem cell replenishment but not stem cell expansion. In contrast, a symmetric division resulting in two identical stem cells from a single stem cell can result in expansion of stem cell pools. The latter may occur during expansion of tumor stem cells in early tumor development. As first suggested by Cairns (26) and more recently confirmed by Potten et al. (27), symmetric cell division of stem cells involves an unusual DNA segregation event in which the parental strand of DNA is retained in the daughter stem cell, whereas the newly replicated strand is passed on to another daughter cell that undergoes differentiation. If this is the case, then DNA damaging agents may have less effect on tumor stem cells undergoing asymmetric cell division, because the DNA replication errors would be passed on to the more differentiated cells, rather than be maintained in the tumor stem cell. In addition, it has also been found that stem cells have increased levels of DNA repair enzymes (27–29). These mechanisms may have evolved to prevent accumulation of detrimental mutations and tumor formation. However, these same repair mechanisms may make tumor stem cells more resistant to DNA damaging therapeutic agents.

6.3. Antiapoptotic Proteins

Normal stem cells express higher levels of antiapoptotic proteins such as members of the Bcl-2 family, than do their more differentiated progeny. These cells also express inhibitors of apoptosis proteins. These proteins contribute to the resistance of stem cells to apoptotic insults. The expression of Bcl2 and or Bcl-X_L antiapoptotic proteins in cancer, has been associated with resistance to different drugs (30).

6.4. Transporter Proteins

One of the properties that has been used to isolate normal stem cells from a variety of organs is their ability to exclude Hoechst dyes. As first described by Goodell et al. (31), it was found that hematopoietic stem cells, are able to exclude Hoechst and rhodamine fluorescent dyes, a process that can be assessed by flow cytometry. These cells, termed the side or "SP population," show lower levels of staining because of the pumping action of ATP-binding cassette (ABC) transporters. The first transporter to be identified for its ability to efflux rhodamine and Hoechst in stem cells was ABCB1 or P-glycoprotein. More recently, the SP population has been redefined by the expression of a particular type of ABC transporter protein known as ABCG2 or breast cancer resistance protein (BCRP) that accounts for most of the Hoechst dye efflux in stem cells (32). SP populations have now been described also in neuronal stem cells and both human and rodent mammary stem cells (4,33). In addition to normal tissue stem cells, the existence of an SP population in tumorigenic stem cells has been demonstrated by recent studies showing that tumor SP cells are capable of generating tumors in mice to a much greater extent than tumor cells that do not exclude Hoechst dye. The specificity of this effect has been demonstrated by blocking these cellular pumps with agents such as verapamil (34). The presence of transporter proteins in both tumorigenic, as well as normal stem cells, may be one of the factors conferring on this stem cell population resistance to chemotherapy-induced apoptosis.

Failures in chemotherapy have been linked to the development of a multidrug resistance. In many cases, the initial shrinkage of a tumor is followed by the development of resistance to drugs to which the tumor was initially exposed, as well as to other drugs to which there was no prior exposure. Multidrug resistance is caused in part by the decrease in the accumulation of drugs inside the cells because of activity of ABC protein transporters *(34–37)*. BCRP, first described in breast cancers that were resistant to chemotherapy, has been found to be overexpressed in normal hematopoietic stem cells. Expression of BCRP may also protect stem cells against hypoxia. In stem cells, hypoxic environments induce the expression of BCRP that in turn prevents the detrimental accumulation of porphyrins (including heme) that can generate reactive oxygen species and damage the mitochondria *(38)*.

In addition to serving a protective mechanism in these cells, it has been suggested that these transporter proteins may play a direct role in stem cell biology by pumping out agents that induce cellular differentiation, thus keeping the stem cells in an undifferentiated state *(35,39)*. For example, ABC transporters have been shown to play a significant role in cell fate determination by exporting differentiation factors in *Dictyostelium (40,41)*.

7. SELF-RENEWAL AND SURVIVAL: ARE THESE PROCESSES LINKED?

As noted previously, stem cells are the only cells capable of undergoing self-renewal. Recent work has shed light on pathways that may regulate this process. A number of pathways that play in important role during development have been implicated in stem cell self-renewal. These pathways include Wnt, Hedgehog, Notch, as well as the transcription factor Bmi-1. Interestingly, each of these pathways when dysregulated has been found to promote carcinogenesis in murine models. Furthermore, there is accumulating evidence for dysregulation of these pathways in a variety of human malignancies. (For review of the role of these pathways in carcinogenesis, *see* refs. *42–45*.) In addition to their role in carcinogenesis, each of these pathways has also been linked to self-renewal of stem cells. For instance, Wnt signaling has been found to be involved in the self-renewal of hematopoietic stem cells. Dysregulation of this pathway has recently been demonstrated to play a role in the generation of chronic myelogenous leukemia. In this case, the activation of the Wnt pathway in myeloid progenitor cells may be responsible for expansion of leukemic clones. Hedgehog signaling has been implicated in a variety of human malignancies, including basal carcinoma of the skin *(46)* small cell lung cancer *(47)* as well as a number of gastrointestinal malignancies *(48)* including gastric cancer *(49)* and pancreatic cancer *(50)*.

Recently, evidence has been provided that this pathway is also dysregulated in human prostate *(51,52)* and breast *(53)* cancer. In addition to their role in self-renewal of stem cells, it now appears that each of these pathways is also linked to cell survival. For example, activation of Wnt signaling increases the generation of insulin-like growth factors, which in turn stimulate Akt, promoting cell survival *(54)*. These pathways may have evolved as important antineoplastic mechanisms, preventing stem cells from forming tumors. Simultaneous activation of self-renewal and survival pathways may be required for stem cell self-renewal and expansion. If this is the case, then specific targeting of the self-renewal pathways may provide an important approach to the induction of cell death in tumor stem cells.

8. CLINICAL IMPLICATIONS

The tumor stem cell model of carcinogenesis has fundamental implications for the development of new cancer therapeutic agents. In the past, antineoplastic agents have largely been developed through testing in animal models, as well as in phase II human clinical trials. In both of these, the end point has been shrinkage of tumors. Tumor response is usually defined in the clinic as the shrinkage of a tumor by at least 50%. However, if tumor stem cells are inherently resistant to chemotherapeutic agents and if these cells comprise only a minority of the tumor, then the shrinkage of tumors may merely reflect effects of chemotherapy on differentiated cells in a tumor rather than the tumor stem cell population. This may explain why induction of tumor regression often does not translate into clinically significant increases in patient survival. This has been illustrated for many tumor types including solid tumors and well as multiple myeloma, where patient survival does not correlate with changes in the M-protein levels (55). If the tumor stem cell model of carcinogenesis is correct, then we may need to devise new experimental paradigms for evaluation of antineoplastic agents that can target stem cell populations. It will be important to find and validate intermediate end points that accurately predict ultimate patient survival. In this regard, future clinical trial designs may involve such intermediate end points such as time to tumor progression following delivery of an agent that can target tumor stem cells.

The tumor stem cell model also has implications for interpreting molecular profiling studies. These studies have shown that tumor gene expression profiles have important prognostic and predictive value. Molecular profiling of tumors reflects gene expression patterns of a tumor stem cell component, as well as the bulk of the tumor that is derived from these stem cells. The fact that the initial gene expression patterns are predictive of subsequent behavior is consistent with a model in which tumor stem cells and their particular mutation spectrum determine the expression profile of the entire tumor. We have recently described the implications of gene profiling in directing the hormonal therapy of breast cancer (56). Most recently, a 21-gene expression profile of primary breast tumors has been shown to be useful in selecting patients for chemotherapy (57). These genes may reflect the profile of a particular group of breast tumors derived from a common progenitor or stem cell and the mutation subset that share clinical characteristics.

The tumor stem cell model of carcinogenesis also has important implications for understanding metastasis and tumor dormancy. Micrometastasis of tumor stem cells may carry a different prognosis from micrometastasis of more differentiated cells. This may explain why up to 50% of breast cancer and prostate cancer patients with micrometastasis to their bone marrow do not develop overt metastasis over a 10-yr period (58,59). One may postulate that some of these patients have metastasis of more differentiated cells, and only the metastasis of tumor stem cells will carry a poor prognosis. The elucidation of markers that define these stem cell populations will be necessary to confirm this hypothesis.

If the ultimate cure of various cancers depends on the elimination of tumor stem cells, one can question why several malignancies such as testicular carcinoma and choreocarcinoma are curable even in the metastatic setting with chemotherapy, whereas the vast majority of common malignancies are not. One might speculate that the stem cell component of testicular and choreocarcinoma are inherently different from other tissue stem cells because these involve germ cells (60). Indeed, chemotherapy treatment of these tumors also often results in residual masses that are found to be benign teratomas composed of differentiated cells. An understanding of the inherent differences between the stem cells of testicular cancer and choreocarinoma compared to those from other tumors may provide new clues for the development of therapies against these common tumor types.

9. OPPORTUNITIES FOR THERAPEUTIC DEVELOPMENT

The tumor stem cell model suggests that it may be necessary to modify the current paradigm in cancer drug development. If the eradication of cancers requires the targeting and elimination of tumor stem cells, then one must devise therapies that can selectively kill these tumor stem cells while sparing normal stem cells. Because many pathways such as those involved in self-renewal are shared between tumor stem cells and their normal counterparts, this may seem a formidable task. However, recent studies in animal models that have utilized agents that target these pathways indicate the feasibility of this approach. For instance, Notch signaling requires processing by the enzyme γ-secretase. γ-secretase inhibitors have recently been shown to have activity against breast cancers that overexpresses Notch 1 (61). Furthermore, in a murine model, these treatments appear to have little toxicity. Agents targeting Hedgehog signaling have recently been described to have antineoplastic activity. A Hedgehog inhibitor, cyclopamine, that specifically inhibits Hedgehog signaling by binding to the protein smoothend, was utilized to treat animals bearing a variety of tumor xenografts. Administration of cyclopamine to animals bearing prostatic cancer xenografts resulted in a dramatic regression of these tumors (51). Although the specific targeting of tumor stem cells by these agents has not yet been demonstrated, the fact that remissions obtained by this treatment were long lasting is consistent with the potential elimination of tumor stem cells (62). Furthermore, at least over brief periods, the administration of cyclopamine appeared to be nontoxic. A cyclopamine analog with 10 times the activity of the native compound has recently been shown to block medulloblastoma formation in a transgenic murine model (63), and this therapy also appears to be nontoxic. Elements of the Wnt pathway represent other potential tumor stem cell targets. Toward this end, small molecule inhibitors of Wnt signaling have recently been produced that specifically interfere with the binding of β-catenin to ternary complex factor transcription factors (64). It remains to be determined whether these small-molecule Wnt inhibitors have antitumor activity or toxicity.

In addition to targeting self-renewal pathways, it may be possible to target specific molecules present on tumor stem cells utilizing antibodies or antibody conjugated toxins. For example, Jones et al. have found that myeloma stem cells are pre-B cells that express CD20. This suggests that antibodies against CD20, such as the clinically available rituxamib, may have value in the treatment of myeloma by targeting its stem cell population. Furthermore, these studies suggest that the molecular profiling of tumor stem cells may identify new targets for therapeutic development.

10. CONCLUSIONS

In this chapter, we have reviewed evidence for the existence of tumor stem cells in a variety of human malignancies. These tumor stem cells that drive tumorigenesis may be resistant to currently available chemotherapeutic agents. These cells may therefore contribute to resistance of tumors to these agents as well as to relapse following treatment. If this is the case, then the development of more effective cancer therapies will require the targeting of the tumor stem cell population. A paradigm shift in cancer therapeutics may be required to develop agents that selectively target tumor stem cells while sparing their normal stem cell counterparts. Evaluation of these agents may require alterations in current clinical trial designs. Nevertheless, the recent elucidation of mechanisms that govern key events in both normal and tumor stem cells suggests the feasibility of selectively targeting these pathways to develop more effective cancer therapeutics.

REFERENCES

1. Till JE, McCullouch EA. A direct measurement of the radiation sensitivity of normal mouse bone marrow cells. Radiat Res 1961; 14:213–222.
2. Singh SK, Clarke ID, Hide T, et al. Cancer stem cells in nervous system tumors. Oncogene 2004; 23:7267–7273.
3. Al-Hajj M, Clarke M. Self-renewal and solid tumor stem cells. Oncogene 2004; 23:7274–7282.
4. Dontu G, Al-Hajj M, Abdallah WM, et al. Stem cells in normal breast development and breast cancer. Cell Prolif 2003; 36(Suppl 1):59–72.
5. Owens DM, Watt FM. Contribution of stem cells and differentiated cells to epidermal tumours. Nat Rev Cancer 2003; 3:444–451.
6. Reya T, Morrison SJ, Clarke MF, et al. Stem cells, cancer, and cancer stem cells. Nature 2001; 414:105–111.
7. Jamieson CH, Ailles LE, Dylla SJ, et al. Granulocyte-macrophage progenitors as candidate leukemic stem cells in blast-crisis CML. N Engl J Med 2004; 351:657–667.
8. Passeguâe E, Jamieson CH, Ailles LE, et al. Normal and leukemic hematopoiesis: are leukemias a stem cell disorder or a reacquisition of stem cell characteristics? Proc Natl Acad Sci U S A 2003; 100(Suppl 1):11,842–11,849.
9. Bonnet D, Dick JE, Department of Genetics RIHfSCUoTOC. Human acute myeloid leukemia is organized as a hierarchy that originates from a primitive hematopoietic cell. Nat Med 1997; 3:730–737.
10. Hope KJ, Jin L, Dick JE. Acute myeloid leukemia originates from a hierarchy of leukemic stem cell classes that differ in self-renewal capacity. Nat Immunol 2004; 5:738–743.
11. Dorrell C, Takenaka K, Minden MD, et al. Hematopoietic cell fate and the initiation of leukemic properties in primitive primary human cells are influenced by Ras activity and farnesyltransferase inhibition. Mol Cell Biol 2004; 24:6993–7002.
12. Al-Hajj M, Wicha M, Benito-Hernandez A, et al. Prospective identification of tumorigenic breast cancer cells. Proc Natl Acad Sci U S A 2003; 100:3983–3988.
13. Singh SK, Clarke ID, Terasaki M, et al. Identification of a cancer stem cell in human brain tumors. Cancer Res 2003; 63:5821–5828.
14. Yuan X, Curtin J, Xiong Y, et al. Isolation of cancer stem cells from adult glioblastoma multiforme. Oncogene 2004; 23:9392–9400.
15. Galli R, Binda E, Orfanelli U, et al. Isolation and characterization of tumorigenic, stem-like neural precursors from human glioblastoma. Cancer Res 2004; 64:7011–7021.
16. Matsui W, Huff CA, Wang Q, et al. Characterization of clonogenic multiple myeloma cells. Blood 2004; 103:2332–2336.
17. Mueller MM, Fusenig NE, Group T, et al. Friends or foes—bipolar effects of the tumour stroma in cancer. Nature reviews. Cancer 2004; 4:839–849.
18. Wang F, Hansen RK, Radisky D, et al. Phenotypic reversion or death of cancer cells by altering signaling pathways in three-dimensional contexts. J Natl Cancer Inst 2002; 94:1494–1503.
19. Hennighausen L, Robinson GW. Signaling pathways in mammary gland development. Dev Cell 2001; 1:467–475.
20. Strange R, Metcalfe T, Thackray L, et al. Apoptosis in normal and neoplastic mammary gland development. Microsc Res Tech 2001; 52:171–181.
21. Marshman E, Booth C, Potten CS. The intestinal epithelial stem cell. Bioessays 2002; 24:91–98.
22. Jordan CT, Guzman ML. Mechanisms controlling pathogenesis and survival of leukemic stem cells. Oncogene 2004; 23:7178–7187.
23. Mayer B, Klement G, Kaneko M, et al. Multicellular gastric cancer spheroids recapitulate growth pattern and differentiation phenotype of human gastric carcinomas. Gastroenterology 2001; 121:839–852.
24. Dontu G, Wicha MS. Survival of mammary stem cells in suspension culture: implications for stem cell biology and neoplasia. J Mammary Gland Biol Neoplasia 2005; 10:75–86.
25. Venezia TA, Merchant AA, Ramos CA, et al. Molecular signatures of proliferation and quiescence in hematopoietic stem cells. PLoS Biol 2004; 2:e301.
26. Cairns J. The cancer problem. Sci Am 1975; 233:64–72, 77–68.

27. Potten CS, Owen G, Booth D. Intestinal stem cells protect their genome by selective segregation of template DNA strands. J Cell Sci 2002; 115:2381–2388.
28. Park Y, Gerson SL. DNA repair defects in stem cell function and aging. Annu Rev Med 2004; 56:495–508.
29. Cai J, Weiss ML, Rao MS. In search of "stemness." Exp Hematol 2004; 32:585–598.
30. Wang S, Yang D, Lippman ME. Targeting Bcl-2 and Bcl-XL with nonpeptidic small-molecule antagonists. Semin Oncol 2003; 30:133–142.
31. Goodell MA, Brose K, Paradis G, et al. Isolation and functional properties of murine hematopoietic stem cells that are replicating in vivo. J Exp Med 1996; 183:1797–1806.
32. Doyle LA, Yang W, Abruzzo LV, et al. A multidrug resistance transporter from human MCF-7 breast cancer cells. Proc Natl Acad Sci U S A 1998; 95:15,665–15,670.
33. Alvi A, Clayton H, Joshi C, et al. Functional and molecular characterisation of mammary side population cells. Breast Cancer Res 2002; 5:E1.
34. Ross DD, Doyle LA. Mining our ABCs: pharmacogenomic approach for evaluating transporter function in cancer drug resistance. Cancer Cell 2004; 6:105–107.
35. Bunting KD. ABC transporters as phenotypic markers and functional regulators of stem cells. Stem Cells 2002; 20:11–20.
36. Gottesman MM, Fojo T, Bates SE. Multidrug resistance in cancer: role of ATP-dependent transporters. Nat Rev Cancer 2002; 2:48–58.
37. Dean M, Allikmets R. Complete characterization of the human ABC gene family. J Bioenerg Biomembr 2001; 33:475–479.
38. Krishnamurthy P, Ross DD, Nakanishi T, et al. The stem cell marker Bcrp/ABCG2 enhances hypoxic cell survival through interactions with heme. J Biol Chem 2004; 279:24,218–24,225.
39. Zhou S, Schuetz JD, Bunting KD, et al. The ABC transporter Bcrp1/ABCG2 is expressed in a wide variety of stem cells and is a molecular determinant of the side-population phenotype. Nat Med 2001; 7:1028–1034.
40. Good JR, Cabral M, Sharma S, et al. TagA, a putative serine protease/ABC transporter of Dictyostelium that is required for cell fate determination at the onset of development. Development 2003; 130:2953–2965.
41. Good JR, Kuspa A. Evidence that a cell-type-specific efflux pump regulates cell differentiation in *Dictyostelium*. Dev Biol 2000; 220:53–61.
42. Liu S, Dontu G, Wicha MS. Mammary stem cells, self-renewal pathways, and carcinogenesis. Breast Cancer Res 2005; 7:86–95.
43. Beachy PA, Karhadkar SS, Berman DM. Tissue repair and stem cell renewal in carcinogenesis. Nature 2004; 432:324–331.
44. Kopper L, Hajdu M. Tumor stem cells. Pathol Oncol Res 2004; 10:69–73.
45. Pardal R, Clarke MF, Morrison SJ. Applying the principles of stem cell biology to cancer. Nat Rev Cancer 2003; 3:895–902.
46. Wetmore C, Division of Pediatric Hematology Oncology DoP, Adolescent M, et al. Sonic hedgehog in normal and neoplastic proliferation: insight gained from human tumors and animal models. Current Opin Genet Dev 2003; 13:34–42.
47. Watkins DN, Berman DM, Burkholder SG, et al. Hedgehog signalling within airway epithelial progenitors and in small-cell lung cancer. Nature 2003; 422:313–317.
48. Oniscu A, James RM, Morris RG, et al. Expression of Sonic hedgehog pathway genes is altered in colonic neoplasia. J Pathol 2004; 203:909–917.
49. Xie K, Abbruzzese JL. Developmental biology informs cancer: the emerging role of the hedgehog signaling pathway in upper gastrointestinal cancers. Cancer Cell 2003; 4:245–247.
50. Thayer SP, di Magliano MP, Heiser PW, et al. Hedgehog is an early and late mediator of pancreatic cancer tumorigenesis. Nature 2003; 425:851–856.
51. Karhadkar SS, Bova GS, Abdallah N, et al. Hedgehog signalling in prostate regeneration, neoplasia and metastasis. Nature 2004; 431:707–712.
52. Fan L, Pepicelli CV, Dibble CC, et al. Hedgehog signaling promotes prostate xenograft tumor growth. Endocrinology 2004; 145:3961–3970.
53. Lewis MT. Hedgehog signaling in mouse mammary gland development and neoplasia. J Mammary Gland Biol Neoplasia 2001; 6:53–66.
54. Sinha D, Wang Z, Ruchalski KL, et al. Lithium activates the Wnt and phosphatidylinositol 3-kinase Akt signaling pathways to promote cell survival in the absence of soluble survival factors. Am J Physiol 2004; 288:F703–F713.
55. Kyle RA, Rajkumar SV, Division of H, et al. Multiple myeloma. New Engl J Med 2004; 351:1860–1873.

56. Dontu G, El-Ashry D, Wicha MS. Breast cancer, stem/progenitor cells and the estrogen receptor. Trends Endocrinol Metab 2004; 15:193–197.
57. Paik S, Shak S, Tang G, et al. A multigene assay to predict recurrence of tamoxifen-treated, node-negative breast cancer. N Engl J Med 2004; 351:2817–2826.
58. Braun S, Vogl FD, Janni W, et al. Evaluation of bone marrow in breast cancer patients: prediction of clinical outcome and response to therapy. Breast 2003; 12:397–404.
59. Braun S, Pantel K. Prognostic significance of micrometastatic bone marrow involvement. Breast Cancer Res Treat 1998; 52:201–216.
60. Masters JR, Koberle B. Curing metastatic cancer: lessons from testicular germ-cell tumours. Nat Rev Cancer 2003; 3:517–525.
61. Weijzen S, Rizzo P, Braid M, et al. Activation of Notch-1 signaling maintains the neoplastic phenotype in human Ras-transformed cells. Nat Med 2002; 8:979–986.
62. Sanchez P, Hernandez AM, Stecca B, et al. Inhibition of prostate cancer proliferation by interference with SONIC HEDGEHOG-GLI1 signaling. Proc Natl Acad Sci U S A 2004; 101:12,561–12,566.
63. Romer JT, Kimura H, Magdaleno S, et al. Suppression of the Shh pathway using a small molecule inhibitor eliminates medulloblastoma in Ptc1$^{+/-}$p53$^{-/-}$ mice. Cancer Cell 2004; 6:229–240.
64. Lepourcelet M, Chen YN, France DS, et al. Small-molecule antagonists of the oncogenic Tcf/β-catenin protein complex. Cancer Cell 2004; 5:91–102.

7 Therapeutic Resistance in Leukemia

William R. Waud, PhD

Contents

INTRODUCTION
DRUG-RESISTANT P388 LEUKEMIAS
CROSSRESISTANCE PROFILES
CONCLUSIONS
ACKNOWLEDGMENTS
REFERENCES

Summary

At Southern Research Institute, a series of in vivo drug-resistant murine P388 leukemias were developed for use in the evaluation of crossresistance and collateral sensitivity. These in vivo models have been used for the evaluation of new compounds of potential clinical interest. Crossresistance data coupled with knowledge of the mechanisms of resistance operative in the drug-resistant leukemias may identify useful guides for patient selection for clinical trials of new antitumor drugs and noncrossresistant drug combinations.

Key Words: P388 leukemia; drug-resistant tumor lines; drug resistance; therapeutic resistance.

1. INTRODUCTION

There have been major advances in the treatment of human leukemia *(1–4)*. Patients with acute lymphoblastic leukemia afford the best example. In children, the event-free survival rate for the standard-risk patient is approximately 80% at 4 yr and approx 65% for the high-risk patient. In adults, complete remissions occur in approximately 65–85% of the patients; however, the majority of these patients subsequently relapse, and overall, only 20–30% are cured. For acute myelogenous leukemia, less dramatic results have been achieved. In children, the complete remission rate is approximately 85%, but only 30–50% of the patients are long-term survivors. In adults, the majority of patients relapses, and ultimately dies from the consequences of resistant disease. Unlike acute leukemias, chronic leukemias are usually refractory to treatment. In adults, survival rates are 60–70% and 30–40% for 5 and 10 yr, respectively.

From: *Cancer Drug Discovery and Development: Cancer Drug Resistance*
Edited by: B. Teicher © Humana Press Inc., Totowa, NJ

Despite the successes in the management of human leukemias, certain obstacles remain. Among the most important is the development of resistance to the agents used for treatment. Understanding the resistance to various agents will facilitate the development of strategies to overcome the resistance.

At Southern Research Institute, a series of in vivo drug-resistant murine P388 leukemias has been developed for use in the evaluation of crossresistance and collateral sensitivity. These in vivo models have been used for the evaluation of new drugs of potential clinical interest. Crossresistance data, coupled with knowledge of the mechanisms of resistance operative in the drug-resistant leukemias, may yield insights into the mechanisms of action of the agents being tested. Similarly, crossresistance data, coupled with the mechanisms of action of various agents, may yield insights into the mechanisms of resistance operative in the drug-resistant leukemias. Furthermore, crossresistance data may identify potentially useful guides for patient selection for clinical trials of new antitumor drugs and possible noncrossresistant drug combinations.

Schabel and coworkers have published the most extensive summary of in vivo drug resistance and crossresistance data available (5). Their initial report included results of in vivo crossresistance studies of 74 antitumor drugs in 12 drug-resistant P388 leukemias. Previously, we expanded this crossresistance database for the drug-resistant P388 leukemias to include more clinically useful drugs, and we updated the database to include new candidate antitumor agents entering clinical trials (6). In this chapter, we have expanded this crossresistance database for the drug-resistant P388 leukemias to include four additional drug-resistant leukemias and have focused on clinically useful drugs. Furthermore, we have used the crossresistance data to gain insights into the mechanisms of resistance operative in these drug-resistant leukemias.

2. DRUG-RESISTANT P388 LEUKEMIAS

2.1. Selection Procedures

Eleven of the 16 drug-resistant P388 leukemias were developed at Southern Research Institute. B6D2F$_1$ mice (CD2F$_1$ mice for N,N'-bis(2-chloroethyl)-N-nitrosourea [BCNU], melphalan [L-PAM], etoposide [VP-16], and paclitaxel [PTX]) bearing intraperitoneal (ip) implants of 10^7 P388/0 cells were treated intraperitoneally with the drug of interest. When half the mice had died, tumor cells were harvested from a survivor that showed frank accumulation of ascites fluid. Transplantation of 10^7 cells intraperitoneally to healthy mice and ip treatment with the drug of interest was repeated until there was no further increase in resistance to the drug of interest.

The dosages and treatment schedules for the eleven drugs were as follows:

1. Actinomycin D (ACT-D): first treatment, 0.05 mg/kg/dose, days 4–12 postimplant; second treatment, 0.5 mg/kg, day 5; third treatment, 0.3 mg/kg, day 7; and subsequent treatments, 0.3 mg/kg, day 4.
2. 1-β-D-Arabinofuranosylcytosine (ara-C): 20 mg/kg/dose, days 1–9.
3. BCNU: first treatment, 20 mg/kg, day 3; and subsequent treatments, 25 mg/kg, day 2.
4. Cyclophosphamide (CPA): first treatment, 25 mg/kg/dose, days 1–24; second to fourth treatments, 25 mg/kg/dose, days 1–9; and subsequent treatments, 100 mg/kg, day 4.
5. Doxorubicin (ADR): first treatment, 1.5 mg/kg/dose, days 4–12; second treatment, 12.5 mg/kg, day 5; third treatment, 6 mg/kg, day 7; and subsequent treatments, 6 mg/kg, day 4.
6. 5-Fluorouracil (5-FU): 20 mg/kg/dose, days 1–9.

7. L-PAM: 2 mg/kg/dose, days 1–5.
8. Methotrexate (MTX): first and second treatments, 1.6 mg/kg/dose, days 1–9; third treatment, 2.4 mg/kg/dose, days 1–9; fourth to sixth treatments, 1.6 mg/kg/dose, days 1–9; and subsequent treatments, 0.75 mg/kg/dose, subcutaneously, days 1–9.
9. PTX: 15 mg/kg/dose, days 1–5.
10. Vincristine (VCR): 1 mg/kg/dose, days 1, 5, and 9.
11. VP-16: first and second treatments, 40 mg/kg/dose, days 3, 7, and 11; third treatment, 40 mg/kg/dose, days 3 and 7; fourth treatment, 40 mg/kg, day 3; fifth treatment, 40 mg/kg/dose, days 3 and 7; and sixth treatment, 40 mg/kg/dose, days 3, 7, and 11.

P388/amsacrine (AMSA), P388/dihydroxyanthracenedione (DIOHA), and P388/camptothecin (CPT) were obtained from Dr. Randall Johnson (GlaxoSmithKline, King of Prussia, PA), P388/cisplatin (DDPt) was received from Dr. Joseph Burchenal (Memorial Sloan-Kettering Cancer Center, New York, NY), and P388/mitomycin C (MMC) was obtained from Dr. William Rose (Bristol-Myers Squibb, Wallingford, CT). P388/0 was obtained from the Developmental Therapeutics Program Tumor Repository, Division of Cancer Treatment and Diagnosis, National Cancer Institute, Frederick, Maryland. P388/AMSA was developed by serial ip passage of P388/0 cells in CD2F$_1$ mice that were treated intraperitoneally with AMSA at a dosage of 4 mg/kg/dose on days 4–10 postimplant. After nine transplant generations, the treatment schedule was changed to days 1–7 (7). P388/DIOHA was developed by serial ip passage of P388/0 cells in CD2F$_1$ mice that were treated intraperitoneally with DIOHA (NSC 299195) at a dosage of 10 mg/kg on day 2. After 40 transplant generations, treatment was changed to 0.5 mg/kg/dose on days 1–7 (8). P388/CPT was developed by serial ip passage of P388/0 cells in B6D2F$_1$ mice that were treated intraperitoneally with CPT at a dosage of 3 mg/kg on day 2 for four transplant generations, 3 mg/kg on day 1 for the next three transplant generations, 6 mg/kg on day 1 for the next 29 transplant generations, and 9 mg/kg on day 1 for subsequent transplant generations (9). P388/DDPt was developed by serial ip passage of P388/0 cells in B6D2F$_1$ mice that were treated with DDPt at a dosage of 8 mg/kg on day 1 over successive generations until no increase in survival time was seen with any tolerated dose of DDPt (10). P388/MMC was developed by serial ip passage of P388/0 cells in CD2F$_1$ mice that were treated intraperitoneally with MMC at a dosage of 0.8 mg/kg/dose on days 1–4 over successive generations until no increase in survival was seen at an optimal dose of MMC (11).

Six of the drug-resistant P388 lines are passaged in the presence of drug. The treatments are as follows:

1. Actinomycin D: 0.2 mg/kg, intraperitoneally, day 4.
2. CPA: 100 mg/kg, intraperitoneally, day 1.
3. ADR: 4 mg/kg, intraperitoneally, day 4.
4. 5-FU: 15 mg/kg/dose, subcutaneously, days 1, 3, and 5.
5. L-PAM: 2.5 mg/kg, intraperitoneally, day 1.
6. MTX: 0.75 mg/kg/dose, subcutaneously, days 1–6.

2.2. Mechanisms of Resistance

Increased NAD-dependent aldehyde dehydrogenase activity has been demonstrated to be a mechanism of in vivo resistance to CPA in both P388 (12) and L1210 (13) leukemia.

There has been only one report concerning the mechanism(s) of resistance for P388/
L-PAM. Harrison et al. *(14)* reported an elevated intracellular glutathione (GSH) concentration for our P388/L-PAM in comparison to P388/0. Studies conducted with L1210/L-
PAM have shown the cells to have defective drug transport and increased intracellular
levels of GSH and GSH disulfide *(15,16)*.

Resistance to DDPt in P388/DDPt leukemia (selected for resistance in vivo before
chronic in vitro exposure to DDPt) is multifactorial *(17,18)*. P388/DDPt cells exhibit
decreased drug accumulation, elevated GSH, and increased DNA polymerase-β activity.
We have found that our in vivo P388/DDPt contains elevated DNA topoisomerase II
activity in comparison to P388/0 (unpublished results).

Whereas there appears to have been no published reports concerning the mechanisms(s)
of BCNU resistance in P388 leukemia, studies have shown that in vivo L1210/BCNU,
which has an elevated O^6-alkylguanine-DNA alkyltransferase content in comparison to
the parental L1210/0, exhibits a faster rate of repair of BCNU-induced damage to DNA
(19). Furthermore, L1210/BCNU exhibits an increased activation of DNA polymerase-
β *(20)*.

There has been only one report concerning the mechanism(s) of resistance for P388/
MMC. Kobayashi et al. reported that the accumulation of MMC in P388/MMC cells was
lower than that in the parental P388 cells *(21)*.

For P388/MTX, there have been reports of elevated dihydrofolate reductase activity
in cells selected for resistance in vitro *(22)* and increased expression of the *mdr1* gene
with little change in the energy-dependent drug efflux pump (as determined by
rhodamine efflux) in cells selected for resistance in vivo *(23)*. Even though the mechanisms of MTX resistance operative in P388/MTX have not been investigated extensively, studies have been conducted in both animal and human cells, especially with
other murine leukemias (e.g., L1210 and L5178Y). Resistance to MTX has been attributed to altered drug transport *(24)*, altered dihydrofolate reductase *(25)*, increased level
of dihydrofolate reductase resulting from gene amplification *(26)*, and defective metabolism to polyglutamate species *(27)*.

Resistance to 5-FU in P388/5-FU has been attributed to reduced initial uptake of drug,
decreased levels of uridine kinase and uracil phosphoribosyltransferase, and reduced
levels of 5-FU nucleotides *(28,29)*.

For P388/ARA-C, there appear to have been no published data concerning the
mechanisms(s) of resistance. Studies conducted with human and other murine (L1210,
L5178Y, and P815) leukemia cells resistant to ara-C have revealed several mechanisms
of resistance: decreased membrane nucleoside-binding sites, decreased deoxycytidine
kinase activity, increased cytidine deaminase activity, and increased intracellular cytidine triphosphate and deoxycytidine triphosphate pools *(30,31)*.

For P388/ACT-D (or L1210/ACT-D), there appear to have been no published reports
concerning mechanisms of resistance. Resistance to actinomycin D in Chinese hamster
cells has been attributed to differences in cell membrane in comparison to parental cells,
resulting in decreased drug permeability *(32)*.

Resistance to ADR in P388/ADR leukemia (selected for resistance in vivo) is multifactorial *(33,34)*. P388/ADR cells exhibit decreased drug accumulation, decreased formation of DNA single- and double-strand breaks, increased GSH transferase activity,
earlier onset of DNA repair, reduced DNA topoisomerase II activity and protein levels
(due to a fusion of the genes for topoisomerase II alpha and the retinoic acid receptor
[35]), and elevated P-glycoprotein.

Resistance to AMSA in P388/AMSA (selected for resistance in vivo) has been attributed in part to a decrease in DNA topoisomerase II activity *(36)* due to a rearrangement of the DNA topoisomerase II gene *(37)* and does not appear to be due to alterations in the cellular uptake or efflux of AMSA *(38)*. Studies in our laboratories have shown that P388/AMSA does not overexpress the *mdr1* gene in comparison to the parental P388/0 (unpublished results).

There have been no reported studies on the mechanisms of resistance of P388/DIOHA. Studies in our laboratories have shown that P388/DIOHA does not overexpress the *mdr1* gene in comparison to the parental P388/0 (unpublished results). Mitoxantrone-resistant HL-60 cells (selected for resistance in vitro) exhibit multidrug resistance but do not have altered drug transport or overexpression of P-glycoprotein *(39)*; however, P388 cells selected for resistance to mitoxantrone in vivo exhibit overexpression of P-glycoprotein and reduced DNA topoisomerase II activity and protein levels *(40)*.

Concerning the mechanisms of resistance of P388/VP-16, Higashigawa et al. reported that the pyrimidine triphosphate pools were significantly decreased in comparison to the parental P388/0 line *(41)*. Studies in our laboratories have shown that P388/VP-16 does not overexpress the *mdr1* gene but does exhibit decreased DNA topoisomerase II activity in comparison to the parental line *(42)*.

Resistance to CPT in P388/CPT (selected for resistance in vivo) has been attributed to a decrease in DNA topoisomerase I activity due to a rearrangement of the topoisomerase I gene *(37)*. Concomitant with this change has been an increase in DNA topoisomerase II activity.

P388/VCR (chronic selection in vivo) exhibits reduced intracellular accumulation and enhanced efflux of VCR in comparison to parental P388/0 *(43)*. The selection procedure apparently affects the observed crossresistance profile. P388/VCR (Japanese Foundation for Cancer Research), selected at 0.25 mg/kg/dose on days 2–10, is crossresistant to ADR and mitoxantrone, whereas our P388/VCR, selected at 1 mg/kg/dose on days 1, 5, and 9, is not crossresistant to ADR or mitoxantrone (Table 1) *(44)*. Studies in our laboratories have shown that our P388/VCR does not overexpress the *mdr1* gene in comparison to the parental P388/0 (unpublished results). HL-60/VCR (selected for resistant in vitro) exhibits reduced intracellular accumulation of VCR and increased levels of three surface glycoproteins, two of which are highly reactive with a monoclonal antibody against P-glycoprotein *(45)*. Various K562/VCR in vitro clones have been shown to have reduced intracellular accumulation and enhanced efflux of VCR; one clone was found to possess diminished amounts of β-tubulin *(46)*.

Even though the mechanisms of PTX resistance operative in P388/PTX have not been investigated, studies conducted with other tumor cell lines have revealed the resistance to be multifactorial—overexpression of the *mdr1* gene, molecular changes in the target molecule (β-tubulin), changes in apoptotic regulatory and mitosis checkpoint proteins, and more recently changes in lipid composition and potentially the overexpression of interleukin 6 *(47)*.

2.3. Experimental Design

CD2F$_1$ mice were implanted intraperitoneally with 10^6 cells of either P388/0 or a drug-resistant P388. Tumor implantation day was designated day 0. Drugs were administered intraperitoneally according to the schedules listed in the tables. Each drug was evaluated at several dosage levels (ranging from toxic to nontoxic), with each dosage level administered to 6–10 mice. Tumor-bearing control mice (12–20 per experiment) were untreated.

Table 1
Crossresistance of P388 Sublines Resistant to Various DNA
and Tubulin Binders to Clinically Useful Agents

Drug	NSC No.	$R_x{}^a$	ACT-D	ADR	AMSA	DIOHA	VP-16	CPT^b	VCR	PTX
Alkylating Agents										
Melphalan	8806	A	–	–	–		–		–	
Cyclophosphamide	26271	A	–	–	–	–			–	
Mitomycin C	26980	A	±	–				–^{e}	+	
Procarbazine	77213	D	–	–					–	
Cisplatin	119875	C	–	–	–^{c}		–^{c}	–^{e}	±	
BCNU	409962	A	–	–				–	–	
Antimetabolites										
Methotrexate	740	D	–	–	±		–		–	
6-Thioguanine	752	D	–	–					–	
6-Mercaptopurine	755	D	–	–					–	
5-Fluorouracil	19893	D	–	–^{d}	–^{d}		–		–	
PalmO-ara-C	135962	A	–	–	–				–	
Trimetrexate	249008	D		–					–	
Fludarabine	312887	D		=					–	
Gemcitabine	613327	E		–			–		–	
DNA Binders										
Actinomycin D	3053	A	+	+	+	–	+	–^{e}	–	
Doxorubicin	123127	A	±	+	+	–	+	–^{e}	–	+
Etoposide	141540	B	+	+	+	–	+		–	+
Amsacrine	249992	B	–	+	+	+	+	–^{e}	–	
Mitoxantrone	301739	B	+	+	+	+	+	–^{e}	–	
Tubulin Binders										
Vinblastine	49842	B	+	+	+		+		+	
Vincristine	67574	B	+	+	+	+	+		+	+
Paclitaxel	125973	C	±	±	+	–		–^{e}	–	+

CD2F$_1$ mice were implanted ip with 10^6 P388/0 or drug-resistant P388 cells on day 0. Data presented are for ip drug treatment at an optimal ($\leq$LD$_{10}$) dosage.

Resistance/crossresistance, +; marginal crossresistance, ±; no crossresistance, –; and collateral sensitivity, =.
^{a}Treatment schedule (R_x): A, day 1; B, days 1, 5, 9; C, days 1–5; D, days 1–9; E, days 1, 4, 7, 10.
^{b}Data from *Mol Pharmacol* 1990; 38:471–480.
^{c}Treatment schedule was days 1, 5, 9.
^{d}Treatment schedule was days 1–5.
^{e}Treatment schedule was days 1 and 5.

Mice were observed for lifespan. In each experiment, tumored groups were treated with a range of dosages of the appropriate drug to confirm the resistance of a drug-resistant P388 leukemia. Moreover, a drug-resistant P388 leukemia was compared directly in each experiment to P388/0, and the parallel groups of mice were treated identically with a single drug preparation. Experiments were typically repeated for confirmation.

Antitumor activity was assessed on the basis of percent median increase in lifespan (% ILS) and net $\log_{10}$ cell kill. Calculations of net $\log_{10}$ cell kill were made from the tumor doubling time that was determined from an internal tumor titration consisting of implants from serial 10-fold dilutions *(48)*. Long-term (45 to 60 d) survivors were excluded from calculations of % ILS and tumor cell kill. To assess tumor cell kill at the end of treatment, the survival time difference between treated and control groups was adjusted to account for regrowth of tumor cell populations that may occur between individual treatments *(49)*. The net $\log_{10}$ cell kill was calculated as follows:

$$\text{Net } \log_{10} \text{ cell kill} = [(T - C) - (\text{duration of treatment in days})] / 3.32 \times T_d$$

where $(T - C)$ is the difference in the median day of death between the treated (T) and control (C) groups, 3.32 is the number of doublings required for a population to increase

Table 2
Crossresistance of P388 Sublines Resistant to Various Alkylating Agents
and Antimetabolites to Clinically Useful Agents

Drug	NSC No.	R_x^a	CPA	L-PAM	DDPt	BCNU	MMC[b]	MTX	5-FU	ARA-C
Alkylating Agents										
Melphalan	8806	A	–	+	–	–				±
Cyclophosphamide	26271	A	+	–	–	–	–			+
Mitomycin C	26980	A	±	+	–	–	+	–		+
Procarbazine	77213	D	–							
Cisplatin	119875	B	–	+	+	–	±[c]	–		+
BCNU	409962	A	–	–	–	+	–			–
Antimetabolites										
Methotrexate	740	D			–		–[d]	+	+	+
6-Thioguanine	752	A					–[d]	–		
6-Mercaptopurine	755	D					–			
5-Fluorouracil	19893	D	–		–		–[d]		+	=
PalmO-ara-C	135962	A	–	–	–		–[d]	–	–	+
Trimetrexate	249008	D		±	–			–		–
Fludarabine	312887	D	=	=	=			–	=	+
Gemcitabine	613327	E	–	–	–			–		+
DNA Binders										
Actinomycin D	3053	A	–	±	–		±			
Doxorubicin	123127	A	–	–	–		+	–		–
Etoposide	141540	B	–	–	–		+[c]	–		–
Amsacrine	249992	B	–	+	=		–[c]	–		–
Mitoxantrone	301739	B		+	=			–		–
Tubulin Binders										
Vinblastine	49842	A					+			
Vincristine	67574	B	–	+	–		+[c]	–		+
Paclitaxel	125973	C		–	–			–		–

CD2F$_1$ mice were implanted ip with 10^6 P388/0 or drug-resistant P388 cells on day 0. Data presented are for ip drug treatment at an optimal ($\leq LD_{10}$) dosage.

Resistance/crossresistance, +; marginal crossresistance, ±; no crossresistance, –; and collateral sensitivity, =.

[a]Treatment schedule (R_x): A, day 1; B, days 1, 5, 9; C, days 1–5; D, days 1–9; E, days 1, 4, 7, 10.

[b]Data from *InVivo* 1987; 1:47–52.

[c]Treatment schedule was day 1.

[d]Treatment schedule was days 1 and 5.

$1 - \log_{10}$ U, and T_d is the mean tumor doubling time (days) calculated from a log-linear least-squares fit of the implant sizes and the median days of death of the titration groups.

Crossresistance was defined as decreased sensitivity (by $>2 - \log_{10}$ U of cell kill) of a drug-resistant P388 leukemia to a drug compared to that observed concurrently in P388/ 0 leukemia. Similarly, marginal crossresistance was defined as a decrease in sensitivity of approximately $2 - \log_{10}$ U. Collateral sensitivity was defined as increased sensitivity (by $>2 - \log_{10}$ U of cell kill) of a drug-resistant P388 leukemia to a drug over that observed concurrently in P388/0 leukemia.

3. CROSSRESISTANCE PROFILES

3.1. Resistance to Alkylating Agents

The crossresistance profile of P388/CPA to 14 different clinical agents is shown in Table 2. The P388/CPA line was crossresistant to one (MMC) of the five alkylating agents, no antimetabolites, no DNA-binding agents, and no tubulin-binding agents. Crossresistance of P388/CPA has also been observed for two other alkylating agents (chlorambucil and ifosfamide) *(50)*. Interestingly, there are differences among these three agents. Chlorambucil and ifosfamide, like CPA, each have two chloroethylating moieties, whereas MMC is from a different chemical class. Ifosfamide, CPA, and MMC require metabolic activation, and chlorambucil does not. Although P388/CPA is crossresistant to two chloroethylating agents, the line is not crossresistant to other chloroethylating agents (L-PAM and BCNU). Therefore, P388/CPA appears to be crossresistant only to a select group of alkylating agents with differing characteristics. P388/CPA appears to be collaterally sensitive to fludarabine.

The effect of 15 different clinical agents on P388/L-PAM is shown in Table 2. The P388/L-PAM line was crossresistant to approximately one half of the agents—two of four alkylating agents, one of four antimetabolites, three of five DNA-binding agents, and one of two tubulin-binding agents. The alkylating agents involved in crossresistance represent different chemical classes. Similarly, the DNA-interacting agents involved in crossre-sistance include agents with different mechanisms of action—inhibitors of DNA topoisomerase II (AMSA and mitoxantrone) and a DNA-binding agent (actinomycin D). However, the L-PAM-resistant line did not exhibit crossresistance to other inhibitors of DNA topoisomerase II (e.g., ADR and VP-16) or another DNA-binding agent (e.g., ADR).

The sensitivity of P388/DDPt to 17 different clinical agents is shown in Table 2. The P388/DDPt line was not crossresistant to any of these agents. Interestingly, the DDPt-resistant line was collaterally sensitive to three agents (fludarabine, AMSA, and mitoxantrone). Of these three agents, the latter two have been reported to interact with DNA topoisomerase II (51,52).

The crossresistance data for P388/BCNU have been limited to the evaluation of alkylating agents. The crossresistance profile of P388/BCNU to four different clinical agents is shown in Table 2. The BCNU-resistant line was not crossresistant to L-PAM, CPA, MMC, or DDPt.

The crossresistance profile of P388/MMC to 13 different clinical agents is shown in Table 2 (11). The P388/MMC line was crossresistant to approximately one half of the agents—one of three alkylating agents, zero of four antimetabolites, three of four DNA-binding agents, and two of two tubulin-binding agents. The pattern was similar to that observed for P388/L-PAM.

3.2. Resistance to Antimetabolites

The effect of 14 different clinical agents on P388/MTX is shown in Table 2. The P388/MTX line was not crossresistant to any of these agents.

The crossresistance data for P388/5-FU have been limited to antimetabolites. The sensitivity of the P388/5-FU line to three different agents is shown in Table 1. The P388/5-FU line was not crossresistant to palmO-ara-C (a slow-releasing form of ara-C) or fludarabine (possible collateral sensitivity). Crossresistance was observed for MTX.

The crossresistance profile of P388/ARA-C to 16 different clinical agents is shown in Table 2. The P388/ARA-C line was crossresistant to members of several functionally different classes of antitumor agents—four of five alkylating agents, three of five antimetabolites, none of four DNA-binding agents, and one of two tubulin-binding agents. Interestingly, the line was collaterally sensitive to 5-FU.

3.3. Resistance to DNA- and Tubulin-Binding Agents

The effect of 17 different clinical agents on P388/ACT-D is shown in Table 2. P388/ACT-D was not crossresistant to any alkylating agents or antimetabolites. It was, however, crossresistant to all of the drugs tested that are involved in multidrug resistance except for AMSA.

The crossresistance profile of P388/ADR to 21 different clinical agents is shown in Table 2. The P388/ADR line was not crossresistant to any of the antimetabolites and was marginally crossresistant to only one alkylating agent (MMC). Resistance was observed for all of the drugs tested that are reported to be involved in multidrug resistance (actinomycin D, ADR, VP-16, AMSA, mitoxantrone, vinblastine, VCR, and PTX). P388/ADR was collaterally sensitive to fludarabine.

The sensitivity of P388/AMSA to 14 different clinical agents is shown in Table 2. P388/AMSA was not crossresistant to any of the alkylating agents and was marginally crossresistant to only one antimetabolite. Crossresistance was observed for all of the drugs tested that are involved in multidrug resistance.

The crossresistance data for P388/DIOHA have been limited mainly to agents involved in multidrug resistance. The sensitivity of P388/DIOHA to seven different clinical agents is shown in Table 2. The P388/DIOHA line exhibited mixed multidrug resistance—crossresistance to AMSA and VCR but no crossresistance to actinomycin D, ADR, VP-16, or PTX.

The crossresistance profile of P388/VP-16 to 13 different clinical agents is shown in Table 2. The P388/VP-16 line was not crossresistant to any of the alkylating agents or antimetabolites; however, it was crossresistant to all of the drugs tested that are reported to be involved in multidrug resistance.

The sensitivity of P388/CPT to seven different clinical agents is shown in Table 2 (9). P388/CPT was not crossresistant to any of these agents.

The effect of 21 different clinical agents on P388/VCR is shown in Table 2. The P388/VCR line was crossresistant to three of the agents—MMC, DDPt (marginal), and vinblastine. Unexpectedly, P388/VCR was not crossresistant to many of the drugs tested that are involved in multidrug resistance (e.g., actinomycin D, ADR, VP-16, AMSA, mitoxantrone, and PTX).

The crossresistance data for P388/PTX have been limited to agents involved in multidrug resistance. The sensitivity of P388/PTX to three different clinical agents is shown in Table 2. The P388/PTX line was crossresistant to drugs that are involved in multidrug resistance (ADR, VP-16, and VCR).

4. CONCLUSIONS

Southern Research Institute has evaluated over 100 clinically useful antitumor drugs or new candidate antitumor agents in vivo against 24 drug-resistant P388 leukemias. We have presented here a portion of the results from those studies. Analysis of these data has revealed (1) possible noncrossresistant drug combinations and (2) possible mechanisms of drug resistance.

Schabel and coworkers (5) observed that except for crossresistance to other drugs with a similar chemical structure and/or biological function, resistance to one drug usually did not result in resistance to other drugs, particularly those of other functional classes. The additional data presented here confirm that original observation. P388/CPA, P388/DDPt, and P388/BCNU were not crossresistant to the alkylating agents tested (except for the marginal crossresistance of P388/CPA to MMC); P388/CPA and P388/DDPt were not crossresistant to antimetabolites, DNA-binding agents, or tubulin-binding agents. In contrast, P388/L-PAM was crossresistant to several of the alkylating agents and to representatives of the other functional classes; P388/MMC was crossresistant to most of the DNA- and tubulin-binding agents. The spectrum of crossresistance of an alkylating agent will depend on the individual agent.

P388/MTX was not crossresistant to the other clinical agents tested, whereas P388/5-FU was crossresistant to MTX. Similar to that observed for P388/L-PAM, P388/ARA-C was crossresistant to other antimetabolites and to representatives of two other functional classes. The spectrum of crossresistance of an antimetabolite will also depend on the individual agent.

Schabel and coworkers *(5)* also noted that crossresistance profiles were variable for the leukemia lines selected for resistance to large polycyclic anticancer drugs. P388/ACT-D, P388/ADR, P388/AMSA, P388/DIOHA, P388/VP-16, P388/CPT, and P388/VCR were not generally crossresistant to alkylating agents or antimetabolites. However, the crossresistance profiles to DNA- and tubulin-binding agents were quite variable. P388/ADR was crossresistant to all the listed agents, whereas P388/VCR was crossresistant only to vinblastine, and P388/CPT was not crossresistant to any of the tested agents. Generally, P388/ACT-D, P388/AMSA, P388/VP-16, and P388/PTX were crossresistant to DNA- and tubulin-binding agents, whereas P388/DIOHA exhibited a mixed multidrug resistance.

The crossresistance profile for P388/ADR was almost identical to that for another P388/ADR line selected for resistance in vivo *(53)*. The crossresistance profiles for P388/AMSA and P388/DIOHA were similar to those reported earlier by Johnson and coworkers for the same lines *(7,8)*. Notable differences with respect to agents involved in multidrug resistance were the appearance of crossresistance for our P388/AMSA to actinomycin D and VCR and the appearance and disappearance of crossresistance for our P388/DIOHA to VCR and ADR, respectively.

Six of the 16 drug-resistant leukemias exhibited collateral sensitivity to one or more drugs. These observations of collateral sensitivity suggest that a combination of one of the six drugs plus one of the corresponding agents for which collateral sensitivity was observed might exhibit therapeutic synergism. We have evaluated six such combinations and have observed therapeutic synergism for five of the combinations: ara-C + 5-FU, DDPt + fludarabine, DDPt + AMSA (unpublished results), CPA + DDPt *(54)*, and DDPt + mitoxantrone *(54)*. As always, none of the above approaches may be applied clinically without caution and concern for the recognized gap between preclinical prediction and clinical validation.

Examination of the crossresistance profiles has provided some insights into the mechanisms of resistance that are operative in some of these 16 drug-resistant P388 leukemias. The crossresistance of P388/CPA to alkylating agents of different chemical classes suggests that a mechanism of resistance other than aldehyde dehydrogenase is operative. Furthermore, the lack of crossresistance of P388/CPA to DDPt or L-PAM argues against the involvement of GSH or other thiols in the resistance. The crossresistance of P388/L-PAM to agents of different chemical classes and with different mechanisms of action suggests that another mechanism of resistance besides elevated GSH levels is operative. Whereas elevated GSH levels could explain the crossresistance to alkylating agents, it is not clear how elevated GSH levels would account for resistance to agents of the other functional classes. The observation of collateral sensitivity for P388/DDPt to two agents that have been reported to interact with DNA topoisomerase II suggests the possible involvement of the latter in DDPt resistance. Studies in our laboratories have shown that

P388/DDPt cells have more DNA topoisomerase II activity and protein than parental P388/0 cells (unpublished results). Increased DNA topoisomerase II activity has been reported for a DDPt-resistant human small cell lung carcinoma cell line *(55)*. The reported elevations in GSH are not apparently sufficient to result in crossresistance of P388/DDPt to L-PAM.

The reported mechanisms of resistance to ara-C have involved the uptake and metabolism of ara-C. However, the crossresistance of P388/ARA-C to several alkylating agents and one tubulin-binding agent suggests that another mechanism of resistance is involved.

The variability of the crossresistance profiles for P388/ACT-D, P388/ADR, P388/AMSA, P388/DIOHA, P388/VP-16, and P388/VCR to large polycyclic anticancer drugs prompted us to characterize biochemically these drug-resistant leukemias with respect to amplification of the *mdr1* gene, level of the 4.5-kb transcript, and level of P-glycoprotein. Preliminary studies have shown that our P388/ADR, which exhibits multidrug resistance, has increased expression of the *mdr1* gene, confirming the results reported for another in vivo selected P388/ADR leukemia *(33)*. However, P388/VP-16, which exhibits comparable multidrug resistance, did not overexpress the *mdr1* gene. P388/ACT-D and P388/AMSA, which exhibit multidrug resistance (although not as complete as P388/ADR), did not overexpress the *mdr1* gene. P388/DIOHA, which exhibits a mixed multidrug resistance, also did not overexpress the *mdr1* gene. Finally, P388/VCR, which does not exhibit multidrug resistance, did not overexpress the *mdr1* gene. Therefore, in vivo multidrug resistance does not require increased expression of the *mdr1* gene. Similar conclusions have been made for in vitro multidrug resistance, which has been called "atypical" multidrug resistance *(56)*.

In conclusion, the in vivo crossresistance profiles of 16 drug-resistant P388 leukemias to 22 clinically useful antitumor drugs have enabled the identification of possible noncrossresistant drug combinations and of insights into the mechanisms of resistance operative in some of the drug-resistant leukemias.

ACKNOWLEDGMENTS

The majority of this work was supported by contracts with the Developmental Therapeutics Program, Division of Cancer Treatment and Diagnosis, National Cancer Institute. The studies of gemcitabine and P388/VP-P388/VP-16 leukemia were supported by Eli Lilly and Company and by Burroughs Wellcome Company, respectively. The author gratefully acknowledges the technical assistance of the staff of the Cancer Therapeutics and Immunology Department. J. Tubbs assisted with data management, and K. Cornelius prepared the manuscript.

REFERENCES

1. Weinstein HJ, Tarbell NJ. Leukemias and lymphomas of childhood. In: DeVita VT Jr, Hellman S, Rosenberg SA, eds. Cancer: principles & practice of oncology, 6th edition. Philadelphia: Lippincott Williams & Wilkins, 2001:2235–2256.
2. Bloomfield CD, Caligiuri MA. Molecular biology of leukemias. In: DeVita VT Jr, Hellman S, Rosenberg SA, eds. Cancer: principles & practice of oncology, 6th edition. Philadelphia: Lippincott Williams & Wilkins, 2001:2389–2404.
3. Scheinberg DA, Maslak P, Weiss M. Acute leukemias. In: DeVita VT Jr, Hellman S, Rosenberg SA, eds. Cancer: principles & practice of oncology, 6th edition. Philadelphia: Lippincott Williams & Wilkins, 2001:2404–2433.
4. Kantarjian HM, Faderl S, Talpaz M. In: DeVita VT Jr, Hellman S, Rosenberg SA, eds. Cancer: principles & practice of oncology, 6th edition. Philadelphia: Lippincott Williams & Wilkins, 2001:2433–2447.

5. Schabel FM Jr, Skipper HE, Trader MW, Laster WR Jr, Griswold DP Jr, Corbett TH. Establishment of cross-resistance profiles for new agents. Cancer Treat Rep 1983; 67:905–922 (*see* correction, Cancer Treat Rep 1984; 68:453–459).

6. Waud WR, Griswold DP Jr. Therapeutic resistance in leukemia. In: Teicher BA, ed., Drug resistance in oncology. New York: Marcel Dekker, 1993:227–250.

7. Johnson RK, Howard WS. Development and cross-resistance characteristics of a subline of P388 leukemia resistant to 4'-(9-acridinylamino)methanesulfon-*m*-anisidide. Eur J Cancer Clin Oncol 1982; 18:479–487.

8. Johnson RK, Broome MG, Howard WS, Evans SF, Pritchard DF. Experimental therapeutic and biochemical studies of anthracenedione derivatives. In: Rozencweig M, Von Hoff DD, Staquet MJ, eds. New anticancer drugs: mitoxantrone and bisantrene. New York: Raven, 1983:1–28.

9. Eng WK, McCabe FL, Tan KB, et al. Development of a stable camptothecin-resistant subline of P388 leukemia with reduced topoisomerase I content. Mol Pharmacol 1990; 38:471–480.

10. Burchenal JH, Kalaher K, Dew K, Lokys L, Gale G. Studies of cross-resistance, synergistic combinations and blocking activity of platinum derivatives. Biochimie 1978; 60:961–965.

11. Rose WC, Huftalen JB, Bradner WT, Schurig JE. In vivo characterization of P388 leukemia resistant to mitomycin C. In Vivo 1987; 1:47–52.

12. Sladek NE, Landkamer GJ. Restoration of sensitivity to oxazaphosphorines by inhibitors of aldehyde dehydrogenase activity in cultured oxazaphosphorine-resistant L1210 and cross-linking agent-resistant P388 cell lines. Cancer Res 1985; 45:1549–1555.

13. Hilton J. Role of aldehyde dehydrogenase in cyclophosphamide-resistant L1210 leukemia. Cancer Res 1984; 44:5156–5160.

14. Harrison SD Jr, Brockman RW, Trader MW, Laster WR Jr, Griswold DP Jr. Cross-resistance of drug-resistant murine leukemias to deoxyspergualin (NSC 356894) in vivo. Invest New Drugs 1987; 5:345–351.

15. Redwood WR, Colvin M. Transport of melphalan by sensitive and resistant L1210 cells. Cancer Res 1980; 40:1144–1149.

16. Suzukake K, Petro BJ, Vistica DT. Reduction in glutathione content of L-PAM resistant L1210 cells confers drug sensitivity. Biochem Pharmacol 1982; 31:121–124.

17. Kraker AJ, Moore CW. Accumulation of *cis*-diamminedichloroplatinum(II) and platinum analogues by platinum-resistant murine leukemia cells in vitro. Cancer Res 1988; 48:9–13.

18. Kraker AJ, Moore CW. Elevated DNA polymerase beta activity in a *cis*-diamminedichloroplatinum(II) resistant P388 murine leukemia cell line. Cancer Lett 1988; 38:307–314.

19. Catapano CV, Broggini M, Erba E, et al. In vitro and in vivo methazolastone-induced DNA damage and repair in L-1210 leukemia sensitive and resistant to chloroethylnitrosoureas. Cancer Res 1987; 47:4884–4889.

20. Gorbacheva LB, Kukushkina GV, Durdeva AD, Ponomarenko NA. In vivo DNA damage and resistance to 1-methyl-1-nitrosourea and 1,3-*bis*(2-chloroethyl)-1-nitrosourea in L1210 leukemia cells. Neoplasma 1988; 35:3–14.

21. Kobayashi E, Okabe M, Kono M, et al. Comparison of uptake of mitomycin C and KW-2149 by murine P388 leukemia cells sensitive or resistant to mitomycin C. Cancer Chemother Pharmacol 1993; 32:20–24.

22. Mandelbaum-Shavit F, Ramu A. Dihydrofolate reductase activity in adriamycin and methotrexate sensitive and resistant P388 leukemia cells. Cell Biol Int Rep 1987; 11:389–396.

23. Fichtner I, Stein U, Hoffmann J, Winterfeld G, Pfeil D, Hentschel M. Characterization of four drug-resistant P388 sublines: resistance/sensitivity *in vivo*, resistance- and proliferation-markers, immunogenicity. Anticancer Res 1994; 14:1995–2004.

24. Sirotnak FM, Moccio DM, Kelleher LE, Goutas LJ. Relative frequency and kinetic properties of transport-defective phenotypes among methotrexate-resistant L1210 clonal cell lines derived in vivo. Cancer Res 1981; 41:4447–4452.

25. Goldie JH, Krystal G, Hartley D, Gudauskas G, Dedhar S. A methotrexate insensitive variant of folate reductase present in two lines of methotrexate-resistant L5178Y cells. Eur J Cancer 1980; 16:1539–1546.

26. Dolnick BJ, Berenson RJ, Bertino JR, Kaufman RJ, Nunberg JH, Schimke RT. Correlation of dihydrofolate reductase elevation with gene amplification in a homogeneously staining chromosomal region in L5178Y cells. J Cell Biol 1979; 83:394–402.

27. Cowan KH, Jolivet J. A novel mechanism of resistance to methotrexate in human breast cancer cells: lack of methotrexate polyglutamate formation. Clin Res 1983; 31:508A.

28. Tezuka M, Sugiyama H, Tamemasa O, Inaba M. Biochemical characteristics of a 5-fluorouracil-resistant subline of P388 leukemia. Gann 1982; 73:70–76.

29. Mulkins MA, Heidelberger C. Biochemical characterization of fluoropyrimidine-resistant murine leukemic cell lines. Cancer Res 1982; 42:965–973.

30. Brockman RW. Mechanisms of resistance. In: Sartorelli AC, Johns DG, eds. Handbook of experimental pharmacology. New series. Vol 38/1. New York: Springer, 1974:352–410.
31. Curt GA, Clendeninn NJ, Chabner BA. Drug resistance in cancer. Cancer Treat Rep 1984; 68:87–99.
32. Biedler JL, Riehm H. Cellular resistance to actinomycin D in Chinese hamster cells in vitro: cross-resistance, radioautographic, and cytogenetic studies. Cancer Res 1970; 30:1174–1184.
33. Deffie AM, Alam T, Seneviratne C, et al. Multifactorial resistance to adriamycin: relationship of DNA repair, glutathione transferase activity, drug efflux, and p-glycoprotein in cloned cell lines of adriamycin-sensitive and -resistant P388 leukemia. Cancer Res 1988; 48:3595–3602.
34. Deffie AM, Batra JK, Goldenberg GJ. Direct correlation between DNA topoisomerase II activity and cytotoxicity in adriamycin-sensitive and -resistant P388 leukemia cell lines. Cancer Res 1989; 49:58–62.
35. McPherson JP, Brown GA, Goldenberg GJ. Characterization of a DNA topoisomerase II alpha gene rearrangement in adriamycin-resistant P388 leukemia: expression of a fusion messenger RNA transcript encoding topoisomerase II alpha and the retinoic acid receptor alpha locus. Cancer Res 1993; 15:5885–5889.
36. Per SR, Mattern MR, Mirabelli CK, Drake FH, Johnson RK, Crooke ST. Characterization of a subline of P388 leukemia resistant to amsacrine: evidence of altered topoisomerase II function. Mol Pharmacol 1987; 32:17–25.
37. Tan KB, Mattern MR, Eng WK, McCabe FL, Johnson RK. Nonproductive rearrangement of DNA topoisomerase I and II genes: correlation with resistance to topoisomerase inhibitors. J Natl Cancer Inst 1989; 81:1732–1735.
38. Kessel D, Wheeler C, Chou T-H, Howard WS, Johnson RK. Studies on a mode of resistance to m-AMSA. Biochem Pharmacol 1982; 31:3008–3010.
39. Harker WG, Slade DL, Dalton WS, Meltzer PS, Trent JM. Multidrug resistance in mitoxantrone-selected HL-60 leukemia cells in the absence of P-glycoprotein over-expression. Cancer Res 1989; 49:4542–4549.
40. Kamath N, Grabowski D, Ford J, Kerrigan D, Pommier Y, Ganapathi R. Overexpression of P-glycoprotein and alterations in topoisomerase II in P388 mouse leukemia cells selected in vivo for resistance to mitoxantrone. Biochem Pharmacol 1992; 44:937–945.
41. Higashigawa M, Ido M, Ohkubo T, et al. Increased sensitivity to 1-β-D-arabinofuranosylcytosine in P388 murine leukemic cells resistant to etoposide. Leuk Res 1989; 13:39–42.
42. Waud WR, Vasanthakumar G, Schmid SM, et al. Characterization of an in vivo murine P388 leukemia resistant to etoposide. Proc Am Assoc Cancer Res 1992; 33:453.
43. Tsuruo T, Iida H, Tsukagoshi S, Sakurai Y. Overcoming of vincristine resistance in P388 leukemia in vivo and in vitro through enhanced cytotoxicity of vincristine and vinblastine by verapamil. Cancer Res 1981; 41:1967–1972.
44. Inaba M, Nagashima K, Sakurai Y. Cross-resistance of vincristine-resistant sublines of P388 leukemia to mitoxantrone with special emphasis on the relationship between in vitro and in vivo cross-resistance. Gann 1984; 75:625–630.
45. McGrath T, Center MS. Mechanisms of multidrug resistance in HL60 cells: evidence that a surface membrane protein distinct from P-glycoprotein contributes to reduced cellular accumulation of drug. Cancer Res 1988; 48:3959–3963.
46. Tsuruo T, Oh-Hara T, Saito H. Characteristics of vincristine resistance in vincristine resistant human myelogenous leukemia K562. Anticancer Res 1986; 6:637–641.
47. Yusuf RZ, Duan Z, Lamendola DE, Penson RT, Seiden MV. Paclitaxel resistance: molecular mechanisms and pharmacologic manipulation. Curr Cancer Drug Targets 2003; 3:1–19.
48. Schabel FM Jr, Griswold DP Jr, Laster WR Jr, Corbett TH, Lloyd HH. Quantitative evaluation of anticancer agent activity in experimental animals. Pharmacol Ther 1977; 1:411–435.
49. Lloyd HH. Application of tumor models toward the design of treatment schedules for cancer chemotherapy. In: Drewinko B, Humphrey RM, eds. Growth kinetics and biochemical regulation of normal and malignant cells. Baltimore: Williams & Wilkins, 1977:455–469.
50. Dykes DJ, Waud WR. Murine L1210 and P388 leukemias. In: Teicher B, ed., Tumor models in cancer research. Totowa: Humana Press, 2002:23–40.
51. Ho AD, Seither E, Ma DDF, Prentice G. Mitoxantrone-induced toxicity and DNA strand breaks in leukemic cells. Br J Haematol 1987; 65:51–55.
52. Nelson EM, Tewey KM, Liu LF. Mechanisms of antitimor drug action: poisoning of mammalian DNA topoisomerase II on DNA by 4′-(9-acridinylamino)methanesulfon-m-anisidide. Proc Natl Acad Sci U S A 1984; 81:1361–1365.
53. Johnson RK, Chitnis MP, Embrey WM, Gregory EB. In vivo characteristics of resistance and cross-resistance of an adriamycin-resistant subline of P388 leukemia. Cancer Treat Rep 1978; 62:1535–1547.

54. Schabel FM Jr, Trader MW, Laster WR Jr, Corbett TH, Griswold DP Jr. *cis*-Dichlorodiammine-platinum(II): combination chemotherapy and cross-resistance studies with tumors of mice. Cancer Treat Rep 1979; 63:1459–1473.

55. Jong S de, Timmer-Bosscha H, Vries EGE de, Mulder NH. Increased topoisomerase II activity in a cisplatin resistant cell line. Proc Am Assoc Cancer Res 1990; 31:337.

56. Danks MK, Yalowich JC, Beck WT. Atypical multiple drug resistance in a human leukemic cell line selected for resistance to teniposide (VM-26). Cancer Res 1987; 47:1297–1301.

8 Tumor Site Implantation and Animal Model Selection in Oncology

Anibal A. Arjona, PhD, and Enrique Alvarez, DVM, MA

SUMMARY

The goal of this chapter is to present several lines of evidence as to the importance of tumor site selection in oncology drug development. Tumor–host interactions differ according to the anatomical location of the tumor and can alter the pharmacodynamic effects of a drug candidate. In some instances, failure of a promising new drug to exhibit efficacy is attributed to drug resistance when instead, the lack of efficacy is a consequence of poor model characterization and selection. Orthotopic models are now presenting us with more-complex models to evaluate the activity of novel drug candidates. We present examples that demonstrate how implant site influences tumor growth kinetics and behavior; as a consequence of these influences, our interpretation of result with early stage drug candidates must be carefully considered.

In this chapter, we review a number of studies that support the notion that tumor implantation site represents a critical determinant for the successful and meaningful efficacy evaluation of chemotherapeutic agents.

Key Words: Tumor site; subcutaneous implantation; intradermal tumors; angiogenesis; hypoxia.

1. INTRODUCTION

The vast majority of *in vivo* drug development programs in oncology relies on transplantable tumor models. Recently, the broad screening of agents using syngeneic rodent tumors has been mostly replaced by the use of human tumor xenografts. Within the spectrum of models currently in use, orthotopic tumor models are adding to our under-

From: *Cancer Drug Discovery and Development: Cancer Drug Resistance*
Edited by: B. Teicher © Humana Press Inc., Totowa, NJ

standing of tumor–host interactions and drug response. Although relatively specialized and costly, orthotopic tumor models represent an important tool in drug development.

A number of issues particular to cancer drug development have the potential to create challenges to the successful testing of a drug candidate. Some of these early scientific decisions include the selection of tumor lines as well as validated *in vivo* models. The former defines drug activity *in vivo*. Tumor–host interactions differ according to the anatomical location of the tumor and can alter the pharmacodynamic effects of a drug candidate. In some instances, failure of a promising new drug to exhibit efficacy is attributed to drug resistance when instead, the lack of efficacy is a consequence of poor model characterization and selection. The application of novel technologies has led to the development and characterization of animal models to a fine resolution. This increases resolution can be used to guide the selection of tumor models that best reflect the drug target under evaluation. This particular concept applies well to the current development of targeted drug therapies in cancer.

The goal of this chapter is to present several lines of evidence as to the importance of tumor site selection in oncology drug development. Moreover, it presents a brief discussion on the background and supporting evidence found in the field of orthotopic models, a tool increasingly used to characterize new targeted therapies in oncology.

2. ORTHOTOPIC MODELS BACKGROUND AND CURRENT CHALLENGES

Currently, the cost of bringing drugs to market reaches in to the hundreds of millions of dollars *(1,2)*. The primary goal of drug development programs is to advance compounds that have the greatest potential to ameliorate or to cure human disease. Therefore, there is a great need to establish screening programs that select efficacious from nonefficacious compounds early in the development process. To date, a number of chemotherapeutic agents shown to be highly effective in preclinical animal models either lack or display reduced efficacy in clinical trials. These results can be attributed to the inherent limitations of today's pharmaceutical screening pathways *(3,4)*.

Tumor modeling has a long history in cancer research. It is a rapidly evolving field where many areas of research and efforts to "synthesize" the applicability of models continue. Killion and coworkers *(5)* outlined the characteristics of a successful preclinical animal tumor model. They stated that the model must reproduce the biology of human cancer; it should allow the study of relevant cellular and molecular events associated with growth and metastasis of tumors. Moreover, it must adequately reproduce the problems associated with a specific type and location of primary and metastatic cancer; it must also possess objective and quantitative end points of therapeutic responses. Finally, it must be reliable, reproducible, available, and affordable.

A perceived limitation of current models of transplantable tumors is that they do not possess a high degree of predictive value in identifying clinically active compounds *(6)*. One potential reason for this relative lack of predictive ability is the tendency to use concentrations of chemotherapeutic agents that represent maximum tolerated doses for mice rather than humans. As it has been suggested, the predictive value of some of the current preclinical tumor models increases and is reflective of the clinical response once the doses used are equivalent to the "clinically equivalent dose" *(7)*.

Another major limitation of current preclinical tumor models is that they often do not accurately replicate the stage of tumor development during which the chemotherapeutic agent is administered in clinical situations. In humans, most administration of a chemo-therapeutic agent occurs in situations where there is advanced, high-volume metastatic disease, whereas in mice a compound is generally given to animals exhibiting primary tumors with minimal metastatic disease.

In cancer research today, the subcutaneous xenograft tumor models represent the workhorse for testing the efficacy of new chemotherapeutic agents. This animal model possesses a number of advantages, namely it is rapid and reproducible (when compared to other models), it requires relatively minimal labor, and it is relatively inexpensive. In addition, tumor kinetics can be easily quantified (tumor size), and it is relatively easy to alter schedule conditions relative to tumor burden. Although useful, this model also generates an abundance of false-positive responses to drugs, probably a reflection of the dosages (maximum tolerated dose) and schedules that may not reflect the conditions use in the clinic. Another major disadvantage of subcutaneous xenograft tumor models is the general lack of metastasis. Studies have shown that subcutaneous implantation of cul-tured tumor cells or tumor fragments rarely leads to metastatic disease, a response that is in contrast to the natural course of human neoplastic disease *(8,9)*.

Since Paget postulated the "seed and soil" hypothesis *(10)*, cancer researchers have strived to generate animal models that resemble the course of human disease. Orthotopic implantation of tumors can generate tumors that growth and metastasize as their human counterparts. A response attributed to the effect that the environment exerts on the tumor cell's ability to express a particular set of genes. Keyes and coworkers *(11)* showed that, depending on the site of implantation (subcutaneous vs intraperitoneal), tumors produced substantially higher levels of angiogenic cytokines (vascular endothelial growth factor [VEGF] and basic fibroblast growth factor [bFGF]) when implanted intraperitoneally than subcutaneously.

In addition, numerous studies using orthotopic models show the site-specific depen-dence of therapy. For example, Onn and coworkers *(12)* reported significant differences in the response of various human lung cell lines to chemotherapeutic agents when im-planted orthotopically vs subcutaneously. They showed that in lung cancer cell lines implanted subcutaneously, paclitaxel induced tumor regression, whereas only a limited therapeutic response to paclitaxel occurred in tumors implanted orthotopically in the lung. These differences are probably the result of tissue–tumor interactions inducing the expression of specific genes. Farre and coworkers *(13)* assessed the influence of implan-tation site (orthotopic vs subcutaneous) on cell cycle and apoptotic gene regulation. In addition, they compared the effect of implantation site on influencing the metastatic process by comparing the behavior of tumor aliquots of two human pancreatic xenografts (NP18 and NP-9) implanted orthotopically, at the site of metastasis (liver) or in a nonmetastatic site (subcutaneous). They observed that implantation site changes tumor growth by altering apoptotic or cell cycle regulation in a tumor-specific manner. Whereas the NP18 tumor exhibited changes in Bcl2-antagonist of cell death /Bcl-X_L/caspase3 pathway, the NP9 tumor exhibited changes in proteins that regulate the cell cycle (extra-cellular signal-related kinase, proliferating cell nuclear antigen, and cyclin B1). Further-more, the site of tumor implantation influenced the location of the resulting metastasis.

These advantages of orthotopic-tumor xenograft models make them highly useful in preclinical development programs, as they are generally reflective of the clinical situa-tions. Orthotopic implantation of cells or tumor fragments is effective in inducing pri-mary tumor growth as well as metastasis. It has been suggested that surgical orthotopic implantation of tumor fragments may result in greater success rate regarding tumor take and metastasis than implantation of cell suspensions *(14,15)*.

One of the major drawbacks for the large-scale use of orthotopic models in preclinical screening programs remains the high level of technical skill required for successful implantation *(15)*. Another disadvantage of orthotopic-tumor xenograft models results from their ability to replicate the course of human disease, as this makes monitoring the kinetics of tumor growth and chemotherapeutic activity more complex. However, a number of groups continue to develop novel methodologies aimed at monitoring tumor kinetics in response to the chemotherapeutic agents' action. Katz and coworkers *(16)* demonstrated the feasibility of using a red fluorescent protein orthotopic pancreatic cancer cell model for the preclinical evaluation of chemotherapeutics. These authors use the MIA-PaCa-2 human pancreatic cancer cell line transduced with red fluorescent protein and grown subcutaneously. Tissue fragments from the subcutaneous implants were then implanted into the pancreas of nude mice. The authors then compare the effects of gemcitabine (intraperitoneally) and irinotecan (intravenously) on tumor growth with that of control mice by imaging the tumors sequentially. In this tumor mouse model, control animals exhibited a mean survival time of 21 d, whereas gemcitabine- and irinotecan-treated animals had mean survival times of 32.5 and 72 d, respectively. The authors concluded that this tumor is a highly metastatic model that reliably simulated the aggressive course of human pancreatic cancer.

Another approach used to monitor tumor kinetics is to measure tumor-specific markers or to engineer tumors to secrete a number of cytokines, which are then use to assess tumor growth and drug efficacy. Pesce and coworkers *(17)* suggested lactic dehydrogenase (LDH) isoenzymes as a useful indicator for detecting the presence and assessing the growth of human tumors in athymic mice. Circulating LDH cleared rapidly following an intravenous or intraperitoneal administration, decreasing to about 10% of the initial value by 12 hr. Solid tumors of HEp-2, T24, and SW733 cells implanted subcutaneously continuously released amounts of LDH that correlated with tumor mass.

More recently, Shih and coworkers *(18)* engineered tumors to express β-human chorionic gonadotropin hormone. Expression of this protein by the tumor and its secretion in the mouse urine served as a surrogate marker for tumor-growth kinetics and chemotherapeutic agent efficacy. Engineered cells were injected subcutaneously, intraperitoneally, intravenously and intrasplenic. β-Human chorionic gonadotropin levels were detected in the mice urine following 2, 1, 7 and 4 d after subcutaneous, intraperitoneal, intravenous, and intrasplenic injections, respectively. Furthermore, the levels continued to increase until the mice became moribund. Although useful in enabling researchers to monitor the progression and effect of chemotherapeutic agents, this tumor model does not provided the ability to assess the extent and location of tumor cells.

3. IMPLANT SITE SELECTION AND TUMOR MODEL KINETICS

Since Paget's postulated seed and soil hypothesis *(10)*, a number of studies have shown that tumor kinetics and responses to therapeutic agents differ according to their site of implantation. Cancer researchers continue to streamline screening pathways and to develop preclinical animal models aim at enhancing the model's ability to predict a compounds efficacy in the clinic. This volume clearly outlines our current knowledge and views regarding mechanisms of drug resistance. These mechanisms are various; however, it is possible to group them into several general categories such as pharmacodynamic, cellular, and molecular mechanisms. Whereas a tumor model might be intrinsically resistant—from a cellular or molecular perspective—to an experimental agent, the combined effect of the tumor–host interaction and anatomical implant site also affect the overall drug response. Improperly conducted studies or studies performed using a poorly characterize model could lead to the conclusion that the experimental agent is less active than otherwise predicted. A difference in response can result from changes in the pharmacodynamic profile of the experimental agent as the result of the tumor–host response. For example, Teicher and coworkers *(19)* reported a pharmacokinetic alteration of alkylating agents by a tumor–host response. In this study, in vivo selective pressures placed on a tumor by in vivo exposure to alkylating agents, and development of drug resistance, directly affected the pharmacokinetic profile of alkylating agents. They showed that tumor resistance in vivo resulted from broad pharmacodynamic alterations. They hypothesized that resistance arose from cytokine release from the resistant tumor and a concurrent host response. It is doubtful that these pronounced pharmacokinetic changes could have been anticipated *a priori*. The pharmacokinetic alterations observed in this study raise questions whether other model factors in addition to direct cellular resistance in vivo can alter the response to a drug in more subtle ways, thus altering the overall profile of a drug.

Before one considers how to select a particular tumor model and its implant site to develop our understanding on drug resistance, one must reflect on the model's fundamental role in research. As outlined by Harrison *(20)*, one finds a context with which to frame the use of the models in oncology research: "Models have provided a means to study not only the therapy of cancer but the biology of cancer as well." According to Harrison, tumor models allow for the description of four fundamental research areas: discovery, biology, mechanism, and development. Briefly, discovery refers to general drug screening, biology to cellular characteristics, mechanism to pharmacodynamics and finally development to prediction of clinical drug activity. We can frame the consideration of tumor implantation site and drug resistance within these four areas and evaluate how tumor site selection can affect each particular area.

Even though not a widely used in vivo model today, the VX2 rabbit carcinoma line represents an excellent example of how tumor implant site is an important factor to consider when studying drug effects. The VX2 rabbit model was initially described by Kidd and Rous in 1940 *(21)* and has been extensively used as a model of hypercalcemia of malignancy *(22,23)*. A paraneoplastic syndrome associated with alterations of calcium homeostasis. Clinical management of hypercalcemia is an important consideration as it adversely affects clinical outcome in cancer patients.

Hubbard and coworkers *(24)* described how the implantation site for the VX2 rabbit tumor directly affected the development of hypercalcemia in vivo. They evaluated endocrine changes and calcium levels associated with intramuscular vs intra-abdominal tumor implantation in rabbits. In this animal model, clinical hypercalcemia results from tumor implantation intramuscularly but not intra-abdominally. To characterize fully the model, the authors performed a direct comparison between animals implanted intra-abdominally and intramuscularly. The animal's serum calcium levels measured to establish the presence and degree of hypercalcemia. In addition, serum levels of 15-keto-13, 14-dihydro-prostaglandin E2 levels were determined using gas chromatography/mass spectrometry. The studies took place over a 5-wk period but did not directly measure tumor burden in the rabbits. The results showed that only animals with intramuscular tumor implants were significantly hypercalcemic when compared to animals with intra-abdominal tumor implants. Furthermore, calcium levels in naive animals did not differ significantly from intra-abdominally tumor implanted rabbits. Interestingly, plasma levels of 15-keto-13,

14-dihydro-prostaglandin E2 were equivalent for both tumor-implanted groups (but 10- to 20-fold higher than naive rabbits).

The authors hypothesized that the observed hypercalcemia in rabbits resulted from the general metabolism of prostaglandin E2 in the lungs. They suggested that intramuscular tumor implantation could promote venous drainage directing the tumor outflow to the lungs, whereas venous drainage from the intra-abdominal tumor implantation could allow for the metabolism of effluent through the liver before reaching the lungs, thereby explaining the overall differences in calcium homeostasis in this model. Whereas the authors did not attempt to alter the levels of hypercalcemia in the intramuscular or the abdominally implanted tumors, one can assume that the mechanisms involved in the resulting hypercalcemia would be specific to the implant site, and that they can exert a significant effect on potential therapeutics modalities.

Another example of the importance of tumor implantation site to the outcome of host response is the study of Malave and coworkers *(25)*, who evaluated the Lewis lung carcinoma model. They assessed the immune response of B6 male mice to the tumor as a function of the tumors' implantation site (the flank or the footpad [fp]). The authors stated:

> *The incidence of 3LL carcinoma was lower in B6 mice inoculated with small number of tumor cells in the flank than in those receiving a similar number of tumor cells in the fp. Lung metastases appeared earlier, and the number of metastatic nodules was significantly higher in mice bearing tumors in the flank than those in the fp.*

These observations could be the result of tumor implant efficacy, as the histological properties of both sites are different. The authors also compared and evaluated the host lymphatic organ weight of both implant sites. Again the authors described their findings:

> *. . . the flank 3LL carcinoma implant was followed by early and marked enlargement of the spleen, whereas the increase in spleen weight was delayed after fp 3LL implant. Thymus weight decreased gradually in either group, though thymus involution was faster in mice bearing flank tumors.*

The study does not contain a detailed explanation for the differences in tumor growth. These differences may result from immunogenicity, circulatory effects, and/or paracrine factor release. From a drug development standpoint, it is noteworthy how an *a priori* assumption regarding tumor implant site can adversely affect the outcome of a study. The VX2 rabbit and the Lewis lung carcinoma models lead us to conclude that a therapeutic agent applied to either model without a full understanding of the differential drug responses resulting from tumor site implantation can result in drawing erroneous conclusions regarding a novel agent's efficacy on a tumor.

It is clear from both examples that implant site influences tumor growth kinetics and behavior. These two studies represent broad scientific efforts to described tumor–host interactions. A specific example of how tumor implant site results in a differential response to antitumor interventions can found in the work of Hill and Denekamp *(26)*. The authors used the sarcoma F syngeneic tumor of the CBA mouse to evaluate the response of the tumor to hyperthermia, misonidazole and radiation therapy when implanted at various anatomical areas (ventral wall of thorax, distal tail, dorsal foot, and intramuscularly). As part of the initial characterization effort, the investigators measured latent time, tumor-doubling time, and tumor temperatures of the tumor at all implant sites. The results of this study indicate that the tumor implant site alters tumor growth kinetics. For tumors implanted in the chest, tail, foot and leg the doubling times were 1.2, 1.7, 1.6, and 0.6 d respectively. Basal tumor temperature was also influence by site of implantation. Again, for tumors implanted in the chest, tail, foot, and leg the recorded tumor temperatures were 34.9, 22.1, 27.5, and 35.8°C respectively. The authors noted that:

> *Tumors on the tail were consistently different from all other sites; they appeared later, grew slower, had the poorest blood flow, the lowest natural temperature, low drug concentration, and highest thermal enhancement ratio. Some of these features, but not all, were shared by tumors on the foot, which was also thought to be a constricted site. The growth rate and normal tumor temperature of the foot and tail tumors were similar, but in most other respects, the foot tumors matched the chest and leg tumors more closely. These data serve as a warning that the choice of an implant site for experimental hyperthermia studies should not be made lightly. That choice will carry with it many changes in the biological characteristics of the tumor; these should be considered alongside the obviously greater ease of experimentation and the reduced risk of whole body warming if tumors in the extremities are used.*

This study also demonstrated that the degree blood perfusion to the tumor resulting from the selection of implant site alters the tumor's temperature, and its response to radiation therapy with or without a radiosensitizer. Although these differences are not intuitively difficult to establish, the work of characterizing these differences is essential for the description of the model and its future application in the area of hyperthermia and radiation therapy research.

As discussed earlier, the application of modern technologies to the overall characterization of established models has increased our understanding of the available animal models. Preclinical model selection and knowledge of its limitations are crucial determinants for the establishment of a successful drug development program. The recent work of Keyes and coworkers *(27)* best exemplifies model characterization. They monitor the angiogenic cytokine profile of several well-established cell lines grown subcutaneously in vivo using Luminex technology. This system enabled them to simultaneously quantified circulating levels of basic fibroblast growth factor, vascular endothelial growth factor and transforming growth factor beta in nude mice bearing several human tumors. This effort generated an "angiogenic agent in vivo profile" for said models. In addition, the authors attempted to evaluate the correlation between tumor volume and cytokine levels. Several of the tumors tested show a positive correlation between VEGF levels and tumor volume (e.g., Calu-6 NSCLC, SW2 SCLC, HCT116 colorectal carcinoma, Caki-1 renal cell carcinoma, and HS746T gastric carcinoma). Interestingly, there was little evidence of VEGF production in animals bearing tumors <800 mm^3. Additionally, the levels of tumor growth factor-β also correlated with tumor volume in animals bearing GC3 colorectal carcinoma, HS746T gastric carcinoma, and the MX-1 breast carcinoma line. Whereas the work helps define the in vivo cytokine profile for several cell lines in vivo, of importance is the understanding of the cytokine levels in relation to a potential antiangiogenic agent. A well-characterized model enables researchers to select objectively a model to suit the molecular pathway targeted by a drug candidate. Subcutaneously implanted Caki-1 renal cell carcinoma tumors can serve as an example of the complexity of model selection and its impact on establishing agent efficacy. Keyes and coworkers *(25)* showed that maximal VEGF plasma level for this tumor type reach approximately 200 pg/mL. This result presents us with some important questions regarding the development of targeted therapies. For example, how would the knowledge of a circulating angiogenic factor profile in the model, guide the selection of a specific antiangiogenic factor inhibitor? Would it be more (or less) reasonable to test a specific VEGF neutralizing agent against a tumor model of high or low VEGF expression? How does the presence/absence of such an angiogenic profile influences one's interpretation of the overall agent efficacy?

A logical progression of the above referenced study was to evaluate the effect of implant site on the angiogenic cytokine profile of a number of tumors cell lines. Keyes and coworkers *(28)* measured VEGF, bFGF, and tumor necrosis factor-α circulating levels as well as tumor volumes of mice implanted with various human ovarian (A2780, OVCAR-3, and SKOV-3) or human pancreatic (BxPC-3, Panc-1, and AsPC3-3) carcinomas using Luminex technology. The tumors were implanted either subcutaneously or intraperitoneally. The data show that intraperitoneal implantation resulted in significantly elevated VEGF levels when compared to subcutaneously implanted tumors. For example, subcutaneously implanted A2780 and the SKOV-3 lines produced VEGF plasma levels of 350 pg/mL and 1500 pg/mL, respectively, whereas intraperitoneal implantation of these cell lines resulted in plasma levels of 1500 pg/mL and 3000 pg/mL, respectively. In contrast, one of the pancreatic tumor lines, BxPC-3, produced low levels of VEGF when implanted at either site. Another pancreatic tumor line, AsPC-1, responded similarly to the ovarian cell lines as subcutaneously implanted tumors produced plasma VEGF levels of 500 pg/mL, whereas intraperitoneal implantation resulted in a threefold increase in the overall VEGF levels. Of particular interest was the observation that when ascites production was evident, VEGF, and bFGF levels this fluid was many-fold higher than plasma levels. The researchers concluded that:

> *Different sites of tumor implantation will result in differences in levels of angiogenic cytokines secreted into the plasma of tumor bearing animals. These findings may be valuable for determining the model of choice for the in vivo evaluation of antiangiogenic agents.*

4. CONCLUSIONS

One of the major goals of an animal model in all indications is that it should display a similar course and involvement as that seen in humans. This has been, in most cases, very difficult to achieve. Historically, gross pathology has solely described differences in the natural course of a tumor model. The elucidation of the various cellular and biochemical differences associated with the various sites of tumor implantation presents a more challenging yet attainable goal.

In this chapter, we reviewed a number of studies that support the notion that tumor implantation site represents a critical determinant for the successful and meaningful efficacy evaluation of chemotherapeutic agents. Some key points include that it is of the utmost importance to recognize that the therapy of cancer is the therapy of metastatic disease and that it is essential to use or develop animal models to address specific questions with a clear understanding of an animal model's limitation.

As new technologies become available, rational tumor model selection should become the norm in drug developing/screening programs. Cancer researchers will continue to streamline screening pathways and to develop preclinical animal models capable of enhancing the model's ability to predict a compounds efficacy in the clinic.

REFERENCES

1. Dimasi JA, Hansen RW, Grabowski HG. The price of innovation: new estimates of drug development costs. J Health Econ 2003; 835:1–35.
2. Rawlins, M D. Cutting the cost of drug development. Nat Rev Drug Disc 2004; 3:360–364.
3. Schuh JCL. Trials, tribulations, and trends in tumor modeling in mice. Toxicol Pathol 2004; 32:53–66.
4. Bibby MC. Orthotopic models of cancer for preclinical evaluation: advantages and disadvantages. Eur J Cancer 2004; 40:852–857.
5. Killion JJ, Radinsky R, Fiddler IJ. Orthotopic models are necessary to predict therapy of transplantable tumors in mice. Cancer Metastasis Rev 1999; 17:279–284.
6. Kelland LR. "Of mice and men": values and liabilities of the athymic nude mouse model in anticancer drug development. Eur J Cancer 2004; 40:827–836.
7. Kerbel RS. What is the optimal rodent model for anti-tumor drug testing. Cancer Metastasis Rev 1999; 17:301–304.
8. Naito S, von Eschenbach AC, Fidler IJ. Different growth pattern and biologic behavior of human renal cell carcinoma implanted into different organs in nude mice. J Natl Cancer Inst 1987; 78:377–385.
9. Kozlowski JM, Fidler IJ, Campbell D, Xu ZL, Kaighn ME, Hart IR. Metastatic behavior of human tumor cell lines grown in the nude mouse. Cancer Res 1984; 44:3522–3529.
10. Paget S. The distribution of secondary growths in cancer of the breast. Lancet 1889; 1:571–573.
11. Keyes KA, Mann L, Teicher B, Alvarez E. Site-dependent angiogenic cytokine production in human tumor xenografts. Cytokine 2003; 21:98–104.
12. Onn A. Isobe T, Itasaka S, et al. Development of an orthotopic model to study the biology and therapy of primary human lung cancer in mice. Clin Cancer Res 2003; 9:5532–5539.
13. Farre L, Casanova I, Guerrero S, Trias M, Capella G, Mangues R. Heterotopic implantation alters the regulation of apoptosis and the cell cycle and generates a new metastatic site in a human pancreatic tumor xenograft model. FASEB J 2002; 16:975–982.
14. Fu X., Guadagni F, Hoffman RM. A metastatic nude-mouse model of human pancreatic cancer constructed orthotopically from histologically intact patient specimens. Proc Natl Acad Sci U S A 1992; 89:5645–5649.
15. Hoffman RM. Orthotopic metastatic models for anticancer drug discovery and evaluation: a bridge to the clinic. Invest New Drugs 1999; 17:343–359.
16. Katz MH, Takimoto S, Spivack D, Moossa AR, Hoffman RM, Bouvet M. A novel red fluorescent protein orthotopic pancreatic model for the preclinical evaluation of chemotherapeutics. J Surg Res 2003; 113:151–160.
17. Pesce A, Blubel HC, DiPersio L, Michael JG. Human lactic dehydrogenase as a marker for human tumor cells grown in athymic mice. Cancer Res 1977; 37:1998–2003.
18. Shih I-M, Torrance C, Sokoll LJ, Chan DW, Kinzler KW. Vogelstein B. Assessing tumors in living animals through measurement of urinary b-human chorionic gonadotropin. Nat Med 2000; 6:711–714.
19. Teicher BA, Herman TS, Holden SA, et al. Tumor resistance to alkylating agents conferred by mechanisms operative only in vivo. Science 1990; 247(4949 Pt 1):1457–1461.
20. Harrison S. Perspective on the history of tumor models. In: Teicher BA, ed. Tumor models in cancer research. Totowa: Humana Press, 2002:3–22.
21. Kidd JW, Rous P. A transplantable rabbit carcinoma originating in a virus-induced papilloma and containing the virus is masked or altered form. J Exp Med 1940; 71:813–837.
22. Doppelt SH, Slovik DM, Neer RM, Nolan J, Zusman RM, Potts JT. Gut-mediated hypercalcemia in rabbits bearing VX2 carcinoma: new mechanism for tumor-induced hypercalcemia. Proc Natl Acad Sci U S A 1982; 79:640–644.
23. Shilling T. In vivo models of hypercalcemia of malignancy. Recent Results Cancer Res 1994; 137:4475.
24. Hubbard WC, Hough AJ, Johnson RM, Oates JA. The site of VX2 tumor transplantation affects the development of hypercalcemia in rabbits. Prostaglandins 1980; 19:881–889.
25. Malave I, Blanca I, Fuji H. Influence of inoculation site on development of the Lewis lung carcinoma and suppressor cell activity in syngeneic mice. J Natl Cancer Inst 1979; 62:83–88.
26. Hill SA, Denekamp J. Site dependent response of tumours to combined heat and radiation. British J Radiol 1982; 55:905–912.
27. Keyes KA, Mann L, Cox K, Treadway P, Iversen P, Chen Y, Teicher BA. Circulating angiogenic growth factor levels in mice bearing human tumors using Luminex multiplex technology. Cancer Chemother Pharmacol 2003; 51:321–327.
28. Keyes KA, MannL, Teicher BA, Alvarez E. Site-dependent angiogenic cytokine production in human tumor xenografts. Cytokine 2003; 21: 98–104.

9 In Vivo Resistance

Beverly A. Teicher, PhD

Summary

The EMT6 mammary carcinoma sublines resistant to antitumor alkylating agents were produced by repeated exposure of fresh tumor-bearing hosts to each drug. These tumor lines have been used to extend understanding of drug resistance in a host organism. It is becoming clear as our knowledge of growth factors and cytokines has increased that the proliferation and metabolism of tumor cells, like those of normal cells, are influenced by these naturally occurring growth regulators. Our findings and those of others support the notion that the metabolism of tumor cells can be altered to enhance their survival via mechanisms that involve the autocrine and paracrine functions of growth factors and cytokines. Therapeutic resistance of a tumor in a host organism can evolve by a phenotypic change in the tumor cells that does not confer drug resistance on the isolated tumor cells but, which, through alterations in the handling of the drug by host.

Key Words: Cisplatin resistance; cyclophosphamide resistance; EMT-6 mammary carcinoma; in vivo resistance; transforming growth factor-β.

1. INTRODUCTION

The clinical problem of drug resistance was recognized when in the 1940s, Dr. Alfred Gilman's lymphoma patient failed to respond to a third course of nitrogen mustard after responding to the drug twice. Since then, elucidation of the mechanisms by which malignant cells develop a tolerance toward exposure to cytotoxic anticancer drugs has been a major area of investigation. Much of the research into drug resistance has been carried out in cells culture, most often using sublines cloned after repeated and/or chronic exposure of malignant cells to a specific agent. Although changes in cells developed in this manner were clear and often very well characterized, it has been more difficult to confirm that these changes correspond to the clinical problem *(1)*.

From: *Cancer Drug Discovery and Development: Cancer Drug Resistance*
Edited by: B. Teicher © Humana Press Inc., Totowa, NJ

The second most commonly used model is the transplantable tumor. This system has added knowledge beyond that which can be learned from cell culture, especially in the area of solid tumor physiology. Recognition of the physiological differences between solid tumors and normal tissues has permitted researchers to understand that a high degree of heterogeneity exists in the environmental conditions in which tumor cells survive in vivo. However, much of the work done with transplantable tumors has also focused on characteristics of singular tumor cells rather than on the tumor as a tissue interacting with the normal host tissues. The largest exception to this may be the study of interactions between the immune system and the tumor *(2)*.

One school of thought for overcoming drug resistance in the clinic is that drug resistance simply represents "under treatment" of the disease *(3)*. From this notion, treatment regimens consisting of high-dose combination chemotherapy with hematopoietic stem cell transplantation were developed and have been under clinical investigation for more than 10 yr *(4–13)*. Clinical protocols involving sequential high-dose regimens have also been reported *(14)*. The efficacy of this treatment approach, however, remains an open question. Preclinical in vivo modeling allows rigorous examination of many aspects of treatment, treatment combinations, sequences, and so on, that would be impossible to approach by clinical trial, because trial (because the number of variables involved) would require a prohibitively large number of patients. The scientific study of cancer therapy relevant to the high-dose setting has required the development of preclinical models that go beyond the conventional dose end points of increase in life span and tumor regression/ growth delay. High-dose therapy can be modeled using the tumor cell survival assay that allows tumor-bearing animals to be treated with "supralethal" doses of anticancer treatments with a quantitative measure of tumor cell killing *(15,16)* and using a tumor growth delay assay with transplant of hematopoietic stem cells from syngeneic donors *(17)*.

2. ACUTE IN VIVO RESISTANCE IN HIGH-DOSE THERAPY

The high-dose setting is the most informative situation in which to examine the effect of drug sequence and drug combination, because it is in the high-dose setting where the greatest potential cell killing effects can be obtained. In the design of sequential high-dose chemotherapy regimens, the selection of antitumor alkylating agents to be included in each intensification, and the interval between the intensifications are critical to the design of the therapy. The tumor cell survival assay and tumor growth delay assay using the murine EMT-6 mammary carcinoma were used as a solid tumor model in which to address these issues *(1)*. Tumor-bearing mice were treated with high-dose melphalan or cyclophosphamide (CTX) followed 7 or 12 d later by melphalan, CTX, thiotepa (THIO), or carboplatin (CARBO). After treatment with melphalan, both 7 and 12 d later, the tumor was resistant to each of the four drugs studied (Fig. 1). Treatment of the tumor-bearing animals with melphalan (30 mg/kg) on day 5 after tumor cell implantation followed by various doses of melphalan (20, 30, and 40 mg/kg) on day 12 or on day 17 resulted in marked resistance of the tumor to the second melphalan treatment, so that the first exposure to melphalan killed 2.5 logs of cells, but the second dose given 7 d later killed <1 log of EMT-6 tumor cells, and a dose given 12 d later killed about 1.5 logs of EMT-6 tumor cells. A similar pattern was seen if a dose of CTX was followed by a dose of melphalan (Fig. 1). The findings for the killing of bone marrow granulocyte-macrophage colony-forming units (GM-CFU) paralleled the findings in the tumor cells.

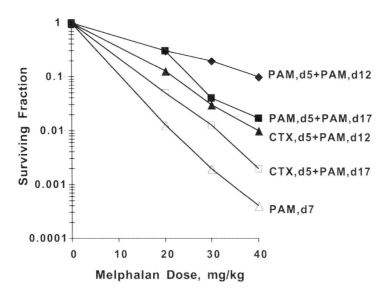

Fig. 1. Survival of EMT-6 tumor cells from animals treated with various doses of melphalan (PAM) on day (d)7 (△); with melphalan (30 mg/kg) on day 5, followed by various doses of melphalan on day 12 (◆) or day 17 (■); or with cyclophosphamide (CTX) (400 mg/kg) on day 5, followed by various doses of melphalan on day 12 (▲) or day 17 (□) after tumor implantation. Points are the means of three independent determinations *(1)*.

After treatment with CTX, both 7 and 12 d later, the tumor was resistant to melphalan and THIO but was not resistant to CTX or CARBO. When administered to the animals, a dose of CTX (400 mg/kg) killed about 2.5 logs of EMT-6 tumor cells (Fig. 2). Treatment of the tumor-bearing animals with melphalan (30 mg/kg) either 7 or 12 d before treatment with CTX resulted in <0.5 log and 1 log of tumor cell killing by CTX (400 mg/kg). On the other hand, treatment of the tumor-bearing animals with CTX (400 mg/kg) either 7 or 12 d before treatment with a second dose of CTX resulted in 3 logs and 2.5 logs of EMT-6 tumor cell killing by CTX (400 mg/kg). Again, parallel effects were seen with the response of bone marrow GM-CFU to these treatments. Administration of melphalan (30 mg/kg) to the tumor-bearing animals either 7 or 12 d before treatment with THIO or CARBO resulted in markedly decreased killing of EMT-6 tumor cells by THIO (Fig. 3) or CARBO (Fig. 4). Administration of CTX (400 mg/kg) either 7 or 12 d before THIO resulted in 1.5–2 logs of EMT-6 tumor cell killing by THIO (30 mg/kg), respectively (Fig. 3). Treatment with either melphalan or CTX decreased the killing of bone marrow GM-CFU by a subsequent dose of THIO. Administration of CTX (400 mg/kg) either 7 or 12 d before CARBO decreased EMT-6 by the drug to about 1.5 logs (Fig. 4). Neither prior treatment with melphalan nor prior treatment with CTX altered toxicity of CARBO toward bone marrow GM-CFU *(1)*.

To extend the interval between high-dose treatments to 14 and 21 d, after the first intensification, the tumor was transferred to second hosts that were either drug-treated or not drug-treated. When high-dose melphalan-treated tumors were treated with a second high dose of melphalan, the tumors were very resistant with the 14-d interval and less resistant with the 21-d interval. This small effect was evident in the bone marrow GM-CFU, except in the hosts pretreated with melphalan. When high-dose CTX-treated tumors

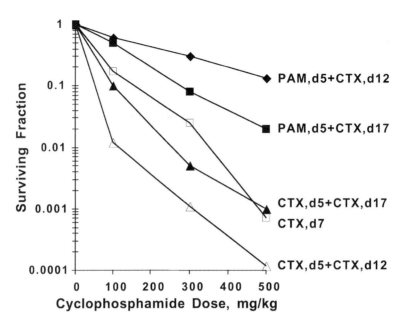

Fig. 2. Survival of EMT-6 tumor cells from animals treated with various doses of cyclophospha-mide (CTX) on day (d)7 (□); with melphalan (PAM) (30 mg/kg) on day 5, followed by various doses of cyclophosphamide on day 12 (◆) or day 17 (■); or with cyclophosphamide (CTX) (400 mg/kg) on day 5, followed by various doses of cyclophosphamide on day 12 (△) or day 17 (▲) after tumor implantation. Points are the means of three independent determinations *(1)*.

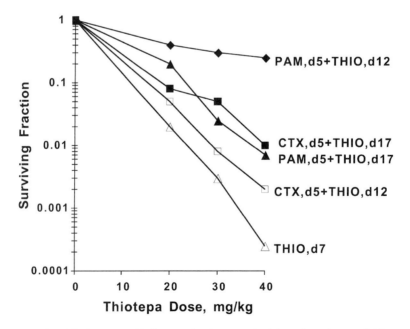

Fig. 3. Survival of EMT-6 tumor cells from animals treated with various doses of thiotepa (THIO) on day (d)7 (△); with melphalan (PAM) (30 mg/kg) on day 5, followed by various doses of thiotepa on day 12 (◆) or day 17 (▲); or with cyclophosphamide (CTX) (400 mg/kg) on day 5, followed by various doses of cyclophosphamide on day 12 (■) or day 17 (□) after tumor implantation. Points are the means of three independent determinations *(1)*.

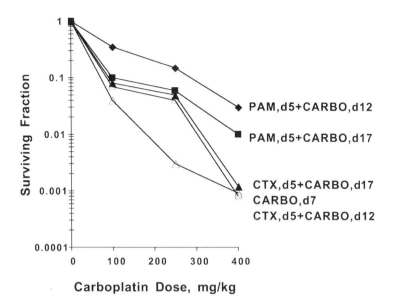

Fig. 4. Survival of EMT-6 tumor cells from animals treated with various doses of carboplatin (CARBO) on day (d)7 (□); with melphalan (PAM) (30 mg/kg) on day 5, followed by various doses of carboplatin on day 12 (◆) or day 17 (■); or with cyclophosphamide (CTX) (400 mg/kg) on day 5, followed by various doses of carboplatin on day 12 (△) or day 17 (▲) after tumor implantation. Points are the means of three independent determinations *(1)*.

were treated with a second high dose of CTX, drug resistance was observed both with the 14- and 21-d interval if the host was nonpretreated or was pretreated with melphalan, but not if the host was pretreated with CTX. The same was true in the bone marrow GM-CFU.

Tumor growth delay studies that allow the assessment of tumor response while the tumor remains in the host supported these findings the with high-dose CTX, melphalan, THIO, or CARBO resulted in additivity to greater-than-additive tumor growth delay. High-dose combination regimens required dose reduction of the drugs, which resulted in decreased tumor growth delays. Mice bearing the EMT-6 tumor received high-dose melphalan (30 mg/kg) or high-dose CTX (400 mg/kg) on day 5 and a second high-dose treatment on day 12 (Table 1). These animals received hematopoietic support consisting of peripheral blood cells from mobilized syngeneic donors on days 6 and 13 and recombinant GM-CFU on days 6 through 22. Tumor response to therapy was determined by tumor volume measurements. When animals bearing EMT-6 tumor were treated with melphalan on day 5, a tumor growth delay of 5.1 d was produced. Followed this dose of melphalan 7 d later with a second dose of melphalan or with high-dose cyclophsophamide, THIO, or CARBO resulted in tumor growth delays between 6.9 and 11.3 d that were greater than for melphalan but less than expected for independent additive effects of the drugs. A single high-dose treatment with CTX (400 mg/kg) on day 5 produced a tumor growth delay of 19.6 d. Treatment of these animals 7 d later with high-dose melphalan, CTX, THIO, or CARBO resulted in tumor resulted in tumor growth delays of 42.8, 46.4, 29.8, and 30.8 d, respectively, which were additive to greater than additive for independent effects of the drugs *(18–20)*.

The effect of two drug combinations in the high-dose setting was assessed by tumor growth delay (Table 2). The combination of high-dose CTX and high-dose THIO was

Table 1

Growth Delay of the EMT-6 Murine Mammary Carcinoma After Two High-Dose
Chemotherapy Treatments With Stem Cell Support

Treatment group	Tumor growth delay[a] (days)
Melphalan (30 mg/kg), day (d)5[b]	5.1 ± 0.4
Melphalan (30 mg/kg), d5 → melphalan (30 mg/kg), d12	7.2 ± 0.7
Melphalan (30 mg/kg), d5 → cyclophosphamide(400 mg/kg), d12	11.3 ± 1.4
Melphalan (30 mg/kg), d5 → thiotepa (30 mg/kg), d12	7.6 ± 0.5
Melphalan (30 mg/kg), d5 → carboplatin (250 mg/kg), d12	6.9 ± 0.8
Cyclophosphamide (400 mg/kg), d5	19.6 ± 1.4
Cyclophosphamide (400 mg/kg), d5 → melphalan (30 mg/kg), d12	42.8 ± 2.3
Cyclophosphamide (400 mg/kg), d5 → cyclophosphamide (400 mg/kg), d12	46.4 ± 2.0
Cyclophosphamide (400 mg/kg), d5 → thiotepa (30 mg/kg), d12	29.8 ± 1.5
Cyclophosphamide (400 mg/kg), d5 → carboplatin (250 mg/kg), d12	30.8 ± 1.3

[a]Tumor growth delay is the difference in days for treated vs control tumors to reach 500 mm^3. Control tumors reach 500 mm^3 in 12.2 ± 0.7 d after subcutaneous implant of 10^6 EMT-6 tumor cells.

[b]The tumor growth delays for the single drug treatments were melphalan (30 mg/kg), 5.1 ± 0.4 d; cyclophosphamide (400 mg/kg), 19.6 ± 1.4 d; thiotepa (30 mg/kg), 4.2 ± 0.5 d; and carboplatin (250 mg/kg), 9.0 ± 1.1 d.

Table 2

Growth Delay of the EMT-6 Mammary Carcinoma and Dose Intensity After High-Dose
Chemotherapy With Stem Cell Support

Treatment group	Dose intensity[a]	Tumor growth delay[b]
Cyclophosphamide (400 mg/kg), (d)7	1	19.2 ± 1.2
Thiotepa (30 mg/kg), d7	1	4.2 ± 0.5
Carboplatin (250 mg/kg), d7	1	9.0 ± 1.1
Cyclophosphamide (400 mg/kg), d7 + thiotepa (30 mg/kg), d7	2	6.3 ± 0.6/toxic
Cyclophosphamide (400 mg/kg), d7 + carboplatin (250 mg/kg), d7	2	Toxic
Cyclophosphamide (225 mg/kg), d7 + thiotepa (20 mg/kg), d7	1.2	5.8 ± 0.4
Cyclophosphamide (225 mg/kg), d7 + carboplatin (125 mg/kg), d7	1.1	8.8 ± 0.7
Thiotepa (30 mg/kg), d7 + carboplatin (250 mg/kg), d7	2	5.0 ± 0.4
Thiotepa (20 mg/kg), d7 + carboplatin (125 mg/kg), d7	1.2	4.4 ± 0.4

[a]Dose intensity indicates the relative summation of the dose of each regimen in which the dose intensity of each single high-dose drug is equal to 1.

[b]Tumor growth delay is the difference in days for treated versus control tumors to reach 500 mm^3. Control tumors reach 500 mm^3 in 12.2 ± 0.7 d after subcutaneous implant of 10^6 EMT-6 tumor cells.

toxic, in that more than 50% of the animals died within 2 wk after treatment. The tumor growth delay for the remaining animals was 6.3 d, much less than expected for additivity of the drug treatments. Treatment with high-dose CTX and high-dose CARBO was toxic. When the doses of the drugs were deduced to allow survival of the treated animals, the resulting tumor growth delays were less than those obtained with a full dose of the most effective single agent in each combination regimen. The reason for this finding at in part may be the severely depleted condition of these animals.

It can be concluded from the studies described above that the first administration of melphalan induced a metabolic condition in the host and in the tumor, which resulted in drug resistance that was slowly dissipating over a period of weeks. This finding is supported by a body of data from previous studies in cell culture (21–26) and in vivo (27,28) that show that exposure to melphalan resulted in decreased sensitivity to subsequent drug treatment, at least with antitumor alkylating agents. The sequential high-dose therapy tumor growth delay studies clearly show the diminished response of the EMT-6 tumor to treatment with high-dose melphalan, CTX, THIO, or CARBO 1 wk after a prior dose of melphalan. The exception to this was the bone marrow GM-CFU of animals treated with melphalan, in which the sensitivity of this tissue to melphalan was increased when exposed to the drug again on day 21 but not on days 12, 14, or 17.

Second, prior exposure to CTX results in much less or no drug resistance to administration of a second drug. In fact, administration of a second dose of CTX to animals that had already been treated with the drug can result in increased tumor cell killing compared with the initial treatment. This effect appears to be primarily an effect on the host, because when an untreated host or a host treated with melphalan bearing the CTX tumor was exposed to CTX, diminished sensitivity of the tumor to the drug was observed. Only when the host was treated with CTX was enhanced sensitivity to a second dose of CTX observed. Although a much smaller effect, the melphalan-treated tumors in the hosts treated with CTX were the most sensitive to the second dose of melphalan.

Exposure to cytotoxic therapy and especially to high-dose cytotoxic chemotherapy produces major metabolic responses in the host and in the tumor (19,27–29). Some of these responses are acute and short-lived, but other may last weeks or longer. These metabolic changes, although not permanent genetic alterations, clearly affect the response of the host and the tumor to subsequent exposures to cytotoxic anticancer agents. On the design of sequential and combination normal dose and high-dose treatment regimens, the response of the host and the tumor to prior therapy should be taken into account.

3. TRANSFORMING GROWTH FACTOR-β IN IN VIVO RESISTANCE

The EMT-6 mammary carcinoma sublines resistant to antitumor alkylating agents, CTX, THIO, cisplatin (CDDP), and CARBO were produced by repeated exposure of fresh tumor-bearing hosts to each drug (19). After 10 treatments, metastable, resistant tumors were produced. Although the tumors were resistant to drug treatment, the tumor cells in monolayer culture were not (19,20). As determined by the tumor cell survival assay from tumors treated in vivo at a level of 1 log (90%) of cell killing, the EMT-6/CDDP tumor is fourfold resistant to CDDP, and the EMT-6/CTX tumor is threefold resistant to CTX as compared with the EMT-6/Parent tumor (19). When the survival of bone marrow GM-CFU—an alkylating agent sensitive normal tissue—was assessed in mice bearing the EMT-6 parental tumor or the in vivo resistant EMT-6/CDDP, EMT-6/CTX, EMT-6/THIO, and EMT-6/CARBO tumors, the survival pattern of the bone marrow GM-CFU recapitulated the survival of the tumor cells, mimicking the development of resistance and reversion to sensitivity on removal of the selection pressure for each of the four alkylating agents (19,20). When the EMT-6 parental tumor was implanted in the opposite hind limb of the animals bearing the EMT-6/CDDP or EMT-6/CTX tumor, the survival of the parental tumor cells after treatment of the animals with the appropriate antitumor alkylating agent was enhanced. The EMT-6/CDDP tumor was crossresistant to CTX and melphalan, whereas the EMT-6/CTX tumor was somewhat resistant to CDDP and markedly sensitive to etoposide. In each case, the survival pattern of the bone marrow GM-CFU reflected the survival of the tumor cells. Thus, the presence of an alkylating agent-resistant tumor in an animal altered the drug response of the tissues distal to the resistant tumor *(19,20)*.

When the expression of several early response genes and genes associated with malignant disease was assessed in the EMT-6/Parent tumor and the EMT-6/CTX and EMT-6/CDDP in vivo resistant lines growing as tumors, it was found that, in the absence of treatment, the levels of mRNA for the genes c-*jun*, c-*fos*, c-*myc*, Ha-*ras* and *p53* were increased in the EMT-6/CTX and EMT-6/CDDP tumors as compared with the EMT-6/Parent tumor, whereas the expression of *erb-2* was similar in all three tumors *(19,30)*. There was increased expression of both c-*jun* and *erb-2* in the livers of tumor-bearing animals. The highest expression of both c-*jun* and *erb-2* occurred in the livers of animals bearing the EMT-6/CDDP tumor. Treatment of the animals with CDDP or CTX, in general, resulted in increased expression of both genes at 6 h posttreatment. The increased expression of these genes may impart metabolic changes in the tumors and/or hosts that contribute to the resistance of these tumors to specific antitumor alkylating agents *(30)*.

Several observations, including the fibrous nature of the resistant tumors, the increased metastatic potential of the resistant tumors, and the altered pharmacokinetics of the drugs in the resistant tumor-bearing hosts, led to the hypothesis that transforming growth factor-β (TGF-β) might be integrally involved in in vivo antitumor alkylating agent resistant in the EMT-6 tumor lines. Because it is difficult to maintain increased systemic levels of TGF-β by administering the protein to mimic the resistance phenotype, administration of TGF-β-neutralizing antibodies to animals bearing the resistant tumors in an attempt to reverse the resistance was chosen as the experimental design to address the hypothesis.

The potential role of transforming growth factor-β in in vivo resistance was examined by administration of transforming growth factor-β-neutralizing antibodies to animals bearing the EMT-6/Parent tumor or the antitumor alkylating resistant tumors, EMT-6/CTX or EMT-6/CDDP *(31)*. Treatment of tumor-bearing animals with anti-TGF-β antibodies by intraperitoneal injection daily on days 0–8 post-tumor cell implantation increased the sensitivity of the EMT-6/Parent tumor to CTX and CDDP and markedly increased the sensitivity of the EMT-6/CTX tumor to CTX and the EMT-6/CDDP tumor to CDDP, as determined by tumor cell survival assay. When animals bearing the EMT-6/Parent tumor or the EMT-6/CTX tumor were treated with a single dose of CTX, the tumor cell killing was obtained (Fig. 5). CTX (300 mg/kg) killed 2 logs of EMT-6/Parent tumor cells and less than 1 log of EMT-6/CTX tumor cells. CTX (500 mg/kg) killed 3.5 logs of EMT-6/Parent tumor cells but only 1.5 logs of EMT-6/CTX tumor cells. To assess the possibility the TGF-β might have a role in in vivo alkylating agent-resistance, animals bearing the EMT-6/Parent or EMT-6/CTX tumor were treated with anti-TGF-β 2G7, anti-TGF-β 4A11, or anti-TGF-β 2G7, and anti-TGF-β 4A11 daily by intraperitoneal injection on days 4–8 or daily on days 0–8 post-tumor cell implantation. No significant difference was observed in tumor growth rate by administration of these antibody treatments. There was no significant effect of the administration of anti-TGF-β 2G7 or anti-TGF-β 4A11 on days 4–8 on tumor cell killing by cyclophosphamide (300 mg/kg) in animals bearing either

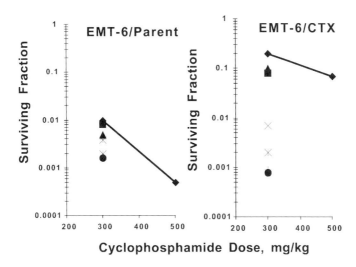

Fig. 5. Survival of EMT-6/Parent tumor cells and EMT-6/CTX tumor cells from tumors treated in vivo with cyclophosphamide (CTX) alone on day 8 (◆), antitransforming growth factor-β (TGF-β) 2G7 (1 mg/kg, intraperitoneally) for days 4–8; then, CTX on day 8 (■), anti-TGF-β 4A11 (1 mg/kg, intraperitoneally) for days 4–8; then, CTX on day 8 (▲), anti-TGF-β 2G7 (1 mg/kg, intraperitoneally) + anti-TGF-β 4A11 (1 mg/kg, intraperitoneally) for days 4–8; then, CTX on day 8 (X), anti-TGF-β 2G7 (1 mg/kg, intraperitoneally) for days 0–8; then, CTX on day 8 (*), anti-TGF-β 4A11 (1 mg/kg, intraperitoneally) for days 0–8; then, CTX on day 8 (◆), anti-TGF-β 2G7 (1 mg/kg, intraperitoneally) + anti-TGF-β 4A11 (1 mg/kg, intraperitoneally) for days 0–8; then, CTX on day 8 (+). Points are the means of three independent experiments *(31)*.

the EMT-6/Parent or EMT-/CTX tumor; however, treatment with the combination of anti-TGF-β 2G7 and anti-TGF-β 4A11 on days 4–8 post-tumor cell implantation resulted in increased tumor cell killing of both EMT-6/Parent tumor and EMT-6/CTX tumors by CTX (300 mg/kg). When treatment with antibodies to TGF-β was extended to the full period of tumor growth, days 0–8, a significant increase in the tumor cell killing of the EMT-6/Parent tumor by cyclophosphamide (300 mg/kg) was observed with each of the three antibody regimens ($p < 0.01$). A much greater effect on tumor cell killing by cyclophosphamide tumor was treated with any of the anti-TGF-β regimens on days 0–8. The effect of anti-TGF-β treatment on EMT-6/CTX tumor cell killing was not only highly significant ($p < 0.001$), but also resulted in the restoration of drug sensitivity to the level of the parent tumor in the EMT-6/CTX tumor cells (Fig. 5) *(31)*.

A similar study was carried out with animals bearing the EMT-6/Parent tumor and animals bearing the EMT-6/CDDP tumor treated with CDDP (Fig. 6). Treatment of animals bearing the EMT-6/Parent tumor or the EMT-6/CDDP tumor with a dose of CDDP (20 mg/kg) resulted in 1 log less killing of the EMT-6/CDDP tumor cells than of the EMT-6/Parent tumor cells. Treatment of animals bearing the EMT-6/Parent tumor or the EMT-6/CDDP tumor with 50 mg/kg of CDDP produced 4 logs less killing of the EMT-6/CDDP tumor cells than of the EMT-6/Parent tumor cells. The anti-TGF-β treatment regimens were the same as those described above. Administration of the antibodies to TGF-β on days 4–8 did not alter the response of the EMT-6/Parent tumor to treatment with CDDP (20 mg/kg), but significantly increased the killing of the EMT-6/CDDP tumor cells by CDDP (20 mg/kg) ($p < 0.01$). Administration of the antibodies to TGF-

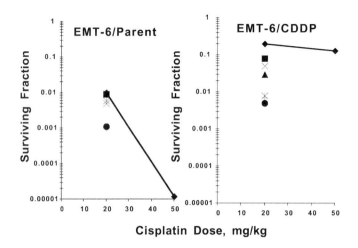

Fig. 6. Survival of EMT-6/Parent tumor cells and EMT-6/CDDP tumor cells from tumors treated in vivo with cisplatin (CDDP) alone on day 8 (♦); anti-transforming growth factor-β (TGF-β) 2G7 (1 mg/kg, intraperitoneally) for days 4–8; then, CDDP on day 8 (✳), anti-TGF-β 4A11 (1 mg/kg, intraperitoneally) for days 4–8; then, CDDP on day 8 (■), anti-TGF-β 2G7 (1 mg/kg, intraperitoneally) + anti-TGF-β 4A11 (1 mg/kg, intraperitoneally) for days 4–8; then, CDDP on day 8 (▲), anti-TGF-β 2G7 (1 mg/kg, intraperitoneally) for days 0–8; then, CDDP on day 8 (X), anti-TGF-β 4A11 (1 mg/kg, intraperitoneally) for days 0–8; then, CDDP on day 8 (♦), anti-TGF-β 2G7 (1 mg/kg, intraperitoneally) + anti-TGF-β 4A11 (1 mg/kg, intraperitoneally) for days 0–8; then, CDDP on day 8 (+). Points are the means of three independent experiments *(31)*.

β on days 0–8 increased the tumor cell killing of the EMT-6/Parent tumor cells by CDDP, but increased the tumor cell killing of the EMT-6/CDDP tumor cells by CDDP to a much greater degree ($p < 0.001$). The increase in the tumor cell killing in the EMT-6/CDDP tumor by treatment with anti-TGF-β on days 0–8 in addition to CDDP (20 mg/kg) was sufficient to produce cell killing of the EMT-6/CDDP tumor cells that was equivalent to

GM-CFU survival was determined from these same animals. The increase in the sensitivity in the tumors on treatment with the anti-TFG-β antibodies was also observed in increased sensitivity of the bone marrow GM-CFU to CTX and CDDP. Treatment of nontumor-bearing animals with the anti-TGF-β regimen did not alter blood ATP or serum glucose level but did decrease serum lactate levels. This treatment also decreased hepatic glutathione, glutathione *S*-transferase, glutathione reductase, and glutathione peroxidase in nontumor-bearing animals by 40–60%, but increased hepatic cytochrome P450 reductase in these normal animals. Animals bearing the EMT-6/CTX and EMT-6/CDDP tumors had higher serum lactate levels than normal or EMT-6/Parent tumor-bearing animals; these were decreased by the anti-TGF-β regimen. Treatment of animals bearing any of the three tumors with the anti-TGF-β regimen decreased by 30–50% the activity of hepatic glutathione *S*-transferase and glutathione peroxidase, and increased by 35–80% the activity of hepatic cytochrome P450 reductase. In conclusion, treatment with TGF-β-neutralizing antibodies restored drug sensitivity in the alkylating agent-resistant tumors, altering both the tumor and host metabolic status *(31)*.

Affecting in a therapeutically meaningful way on the resistance of EMT-6/CTX and EMT-6/CDDP tumors has been very difficult. Traditional approaches to antitumor alkylating agent resistance such as administration of thiol-depleting agents or administration of "chemosenstizer" such as etanidazole were not effective in restoring drug sensitivity to these tumors. The fibrous nature of the resistant tumors and the increased metastatic potential of the resistant tumors compared with the EMT-6/Parent tumor led to the hypothesis that TGF-β might be important in the genesis and maintenance of the in vivo resistant phenotype *(19,20,30,31)*.

The key to understanding mechanisms of therapeutic resistance in vivo lies in understanding the response of the tumor and host to exposure to cytotoxic therapy and how specific factors of that response after repeated fractions or courses of therapy result in a tumor that is no loner responsive to cytotoxic therapy. The initiation of a cytokine cascade or storm by repeated exposure to cytotoxic therapy has been recognized for several years in radiation therapy *(32–36)* and other disease areas *(37–39)*. The connection between this early burst of cytokine production and a perpetual production of TGF-β leading to postirradiation pulmonary fibrosis has also been established *(36)*. In the EMT-6 in vivo alkylating agent-resistant tumor lines, a connection has been established between increased levels of TGF-β and drug resistance *(20,31)*. The repeated induction of a cytokine cascade by sequential fractions of radiation or courses of chemotherapy may result in a metastable increase in TGF-β levels and to therapeutic resistance. Animals bearing EMT-6/CDDP tumors have higher circulating levels of TGF-β than do animals bearing the EMT-6/Parent tumor; however, when exposed to a cytotoxic insult (CTX or CDDP), a rapid and sustained induction of TGF-β occurred in animals bearing the EMT-6/Parent tumor, whereas in animals bearing the resistant tumors, a lesser and more short-lived induction of TGF-β occurred. In the tumor tissue, transcription of TGF-β was induced by the cytotoxic therapies. A marked increase in TGF-β protein occurred in the EMT-6/Parent tumors paralleling the changes seen in the circulating blood.

4. TARGETING THE VASCULATURE FOR DRUG RESISTANCE

The most clear-cut, direct-acting, most frequently found angiogenic factor in cancer patients is vascular endothelial growth factor (VEGF) *(40)*. The signal transduction pathways of the KDR/Flk-1 and Flt-1 receptors include tyrosine phosphorylation, downstream activation of protein kinase C and activation of the mitogen-activated protein kinase pathway *(41–46)*. Protein kinase C isoforms are centrally involved in signaling transduction pathways related to regulation of the cell cycle, apoptosis, angiogenesis, differentiation, invasiveness, senescence, and drug efflux *(47–53)*. When protein kinase C pathways were activated in human glioblastoma U973 cells by phorbol 12-myristate 13-acetate, VEGF mRNA expression was upregulated via a posttranscriptional mRNA stabilization mechanism *(54)*. Recent results provide evidence for the involvement of protein kinase C in the invasiveness of breast cancer cells through regulation of urokinase plasminogen activator *(55–57)*. Several studies have associated specific isoforms of protein kinase C with metabolic pathways in prostate cancer cells *(58–61)*. Protein kinase C has also been identified as an interesting therapeutic target for the treatment of malignant gliomas *(40,62)*.

To assess the contribution of protein kinase C activation to VEGF signal transduction, the effects of a protein kinase Cβ selective inhibitor, LY333531, which blocks the kinase activity of conventional and novel protein kinase C isoforms was studied *(63–67)*. LY333531 demonstrated antitumor activity alone and in combination with standard cancer therapies in the murine Lewis lung carcinoma and in several human tumor xenografts *(68)*. The National Cancer Institute 60-cell line identified the protein kinase C inhibitor UCN-01, 7-hydroxy-staurosporine. UCN-01 has undergone phase I clinical

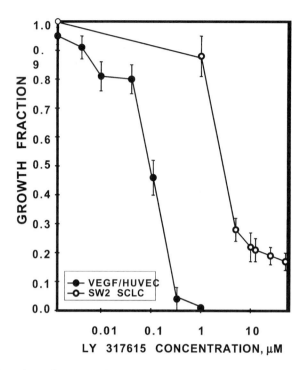

Fig. 7. Concentration-dependent growth inhibition of human umbilical vein endothelial cells and human SW2 small cell lung carcinoma cells after 72 h of exposure to various concentrations of LY317615 as determined by WST-1 assay. Points are the means of three determinations; bars represent standard errors of measurement.

trial *(69–71)*. UCN-01 has been shown to the in vitro and in vivo growth of many types of tumor cells including breast, lung, and colon cancer *(72–81)*.

The compound LY317615 (enzastaurin) is a potent and selective inhibitor of protein kinase Cβ *(82)*. When various concentrations of LY317615 were added to the cultures for 72 h, the proliferation of the VEGF (20 ng/mL)-stimulated human umbilical vein endothelial cells was profoundly inhibited by 600 n*M* of the compound (Fig. 7). In a similar experiment, when human SW2 small cell lung carcinoma cells were exposed to various concentrations of LY317615 for 72 h, a potency differential in the effect of the compound on the malignant cells versus the human umbilical vein endothelial cells was apparent.

Administration of LY317615 orally twice per day on days 1–10 postsurgical implant of VEGF impregnated filters resulted in markedly decreased vascular growth in the cornea of Fisher 344 female rats. A dose of 10 mg/kg of LY317615 or decreased vascular growth to about one half of the VEGF stimulated controls; whereas a dose of 30 mg/kg of LY317615 decreased vascular growth to the level of the unstimulated surgical control (Fig. 8) *(82)*. Administration of LY317615 (30 mg/kg) orally twice per day on days 1–10 postsurgical implantation of bFGF resulted in decreased vascular growth to a level of 26% of that of the bFGF control (Fig. 8).

Nude mice bearing human tumor sc xenografts were treated with LY317615 orally twice daily on days 4–14 or 14–30 post-tumor cell implantation. Tumors were collected and immunohistochemically stained for expression of endothelial specific markers, ei-

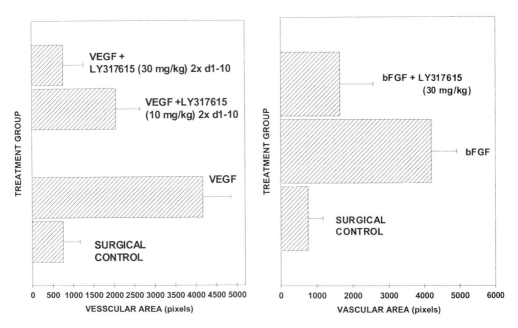

Fig. 8. Vascular area determined by image analysis and described in pixel number for Fisher 344 female rats implanted with a small filter disc (inside diameter of a 20-g needle) impregnated with vascular endothelial growth factor (VEGF) or basic fibroblast growth factor (bFGF) (except the surgical control). Animals were untreated or treated with LY317615 (10 or 30 mg/kg) administered orally twice per on days 1–10. Data are the means of four to six determinations from photographs on day 14; bars represent standard error measurements.

ther CD105 or CD31. The number of intratumoral vessels in the samples was quantified by counting stained regions in 10 high power microscope fields (×200). The number of intratumoral vessels was decreased from one half to one quarter of the controls in animals treated with LY317615 (30 mg/kg) (*see* Table 3) *(82–86)*. Although some of the tumors responded to LY317615 as an antiangiogenic agent, in no case was angiogenesis completely blocked as in the corneal micropocket neoangiogenesis model. The tumor growth delay in the tested tumors did not correlate with intratumoral vessel decrease (*see* Table 3). The plasma levels of VEGF in mice bearing the human SW2 SCLC and Caki-1 renal cell carcinomas treated or untreated with LY317615 were measured by the Luminex assay *(87–89)*. Plasma samples were obtained every 3 d starting on day 7 postimplantation and carried through treatment, as well as after the termination of treatment. Plasma VEGF levels were undetectable until tumor volumes were 500–600 mm^3 (Fig. 9). Plasma VEGF levels were similar between the treated and untreated groups through day 20, when plasma VEGF levels reached 75 pg/mL. Plasma VEGF levels in the SW2 control group continued to increase throughout the study reaching values of 400 pg/mL on day 40 postimplantation. On termination of treatment, plasma VEGF levels slightly increased to 100 ng/mL, which were still significantly decreased compared to the untreated control group. The VEGF levels in the control Caki-1 group continued to increase through the study and peaked at 225 pg/mL on day 49 post-tumor implantation. In the treatment group, the plasma levels remained suppressed compared to controls throughout the treatment period (days 21–39). The plasma VEGF levels, reaching a maximum of 37 pg/mL, remained suppressed out to day 53, which was 14 d after terminating treatment *(87–89)*.

Table 3
Intratumoral Vessel Counts and Tumor Growth Delay of Human Tumor Xenografts
Subcutaneously Implanted in Nude Mice Without Treatment or After Treatment
With LY317615 (30 mg/kg)

| | Intratumoral vessels | | | | Mean | Tumor growth |
| | Control | | LY317615 | | | |
Tumor	CD31	CD105	CD31	CD105	% normal	Delay (d)
SW2 small cell lung	80	50	24	28	43	9.7
MX-1 breast	26	7	17	4	61	21
HS746T gastric	19	11	15	7	71	15
Calu-6 NSCLC	17	20	8	10	48	9
T98G glioma	12	7.5	4.5	4	45	8.7
CaKi1 renal	10.5	11	1.5	2	16	15
HT29 colon	9.5	11	3	4.5	36	14
Hep3B HCC	7	4	3	1.5	40	20
SKOV-3 ovarian	5	4	2	1	33	—

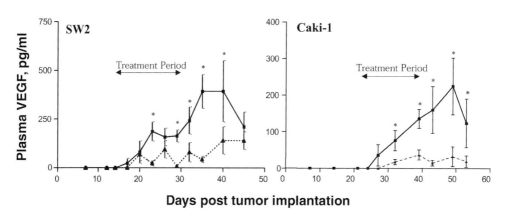

Days post tumor implantation

Fig. 9. Plasma vascular endothelial growth factor (VEGF) levels in nude mice bearing human SW2 SCLC, Caki-1 renal cell carcinoma or HCT116 colon carcinoma xenograft tumors, either untreated controls or treated with LY317615 orally twice daily on days 14–30 (21–39 for Caki-1 bearing mice). The data represent the average results for three trials, with each point being the average of nine individual tumors. Bars represent standard error measurements. Asterisks indicate statically significant differences ($p < 0.05$).

A sequential treatment regimen was used to examine the efficacy of LY317615 in the SW2 small cell lung cancer xenograft. Administration of LY317615 alone on days 14–30 post-tumor implantation over a dosage range from 3 to 30 mg/kg produced tumor growth delays between 7.4 and 9.7 d in the SW2 small cell lung cancer. The SW2 tumor is responsive to paclitaxel, and treatment with that drug alone produced a 25-d tumor growth delay. Treatment with paclitaxel followed by LY317615 (30 mg/kg) resulted in over 60 d of tumor growth delay, a 2.5-fold increased in the duration of tumor response. The SW2 small cell lung cancer was less responsive to carboplatin, which produced a tumor growth delay of 4.5 d in that tumor. Sequential treatment with carboplatin followed by LY317615 resulted in 13.1 d of tumor growth delay *(86)*. The antitumor activity of LY317615 alone and in combination with cytotoxic antitumor agents has been explored in several human tumor xenografts growing subcutaneously in nude mice *(86–89)*. Whereas in most of the tumor models the tumor growth delay produced by treatment with LY317615 as a single agent was not sufficient to predict single agent activity in the clinic, in combination regimens LY317615 was a useful addition to the therapeutic regimen. LY317615 is currently in phase I clinical trial *(90)*.

5. CONCLUSIONS

The reason why most patients with cancer are not cured by cytotoxic anticancer therapies is that their disease becomes less responsive to the therapy and/or their normal tissues reach a limit of tolerance to the therapy. It appears that malignant cells can become tolerant to the cytotoxic therapies. Many mechanisms for the development of this "drug tolerance" or "drug resistance" have been elucidated in cell culture; however, the translation of these observations in isolated malignant cells to drug resistance in tumors has been problematic *(19,20)*. In vivo survival advantage to repeated cytotoxic insults may be achieved by the induction of factors that are operative in complex tissues and require normal cells.

It is becoming clear, as our knowledge of growth factors and cytokines increases, that the proliferation and metabolism of tumor cells, like those of normal cells, are influenced by these naturally occurring growth regulators. Our findings and those of others support the notion that the metabolism of tumor cells can be altered to enhance their survival via mechanisms that involve the autocrine and paracrine functions of growth factors and cytokines. Therapeutic resistance of a tumor in a host organism can evolve by a phenotypic change in the tumor cells that does not confer drug resistance on the isolated tumor cells but which, through alterations in the handling of the drug by host tissues, leads to therapeutic resistance.

The implications of this type of resistance to the treatment of clinical disease are vast. The signal transduction pathways that control cellular responses to these proteins and peptides provide new targets for the medicinal chemist. Therapeutic strategies that focus on enhanced drug activation (such as cyclophosphamide in the liver) or decreased drug catabolism may provide new ways of improving the efficacy of chemotherapeutic agents.

REFERENCES

1. Teicher BA, Ara G, Keyes SR, Herbst RS, Frei E III. Acute in vivo resistance in high-dose therapy. Clin Cancer Res 1998; 4:483–491.
2. Teicher BA. In vivo resistance to antitumor alkylating agents. In: Teicher BA, ed. Drug resistance in oncology. New York: Marcel Dekker, 1993:263–290.
3. Schabel FM, Griswold DP, Corbett TH, Laster WR. Increasing therapeutic response rates to anticancer drugs by applying the basic principles of pharmacology. Pharmacol Therap 1983; 20:282–305.
4. Corringham R, Gilmore M, Prentice HG. High-dose melphalan with autologous bone marrow transplant: treatment of poor prognosis tumors. Cancer 1983; 52:1783–1787.
5. Fay JW, Levine MN, Phillips GL. Treatment of metastatic melanoma with intensive 1,3-*bis*(2-chloroethyl)-1-nitrosourea (BCNU) and autologous marrow transplantation (AMTX). Proc Amer Soc Clin Oncol 1981; 17:532.
6. Frei E III. Curative cancer chemotherapy. Cancer Res 1985; 45:6523–6537.
7. Frei E III, Antman K, Teicher BA. Bone marrow autotransplantation for solid tumors: prospects. J Clin Oncol 1989; 7:515–526.
8. Glode LM. Dose limiting extramedullary toxicity of high dose chemotherapy. Exp Hematol 1979; 7:265–278.

9. Knight WA III, Page CP, Kuhn JG. High-dose L-PAM and autologous marrow infusion for refractory solid tumors. Proc Amer Soc Clin Oncol 1984; 3:150.

10. McElwain TJ, Hedley DW, Burton G. Marrow autotransplantation accelerates hematological recovery in patients with malignant melanoma treated with high-dose melphalan. Brit J Cancer 1979; 40:72–80.

11. Peters WP, Eder JP, Henner WD, et al. High-dose combination alkylating agents with autologous bone marrow support: a Phase I trial. J Clin Oncol 1986; 4:646–654.

12. Phillips GL, Fay JW, Herzig GP, et al. Intensive 1,3-*bis*(2-chloroethyl)-1-nitrosourea (BCNU), NSC4366650 and cyropreserved autologous marrow transplantation for refractory cancer. Cancer 1983; 10:1892–1802.

13. Thomas ED. The role of marrow transplantation in the eradication of malignant disease. Cancer 1982; 49:1963–1969.

14. Ayash L, Elias A, Schwartz G, et al. Double dose-intensive chemotherapy with autologous stem cell support for metastatic breast cancer: no improvement in progression free survival by the sequence of high-dose melphalan followed by cyclophosphamide, thiotepa and carboplatin. J Clin Oncol 1996; 14:2984–2992.

15. Hill RP. Excision assays. In: RF Kallman, ed. Rodent tumor models in experimental cancer therapy. New York: Pergamon, 1987:67–75.

16. Teicher BA. Preclinical models for high dose therapy. In: Armitage JO, Antman KH, eds. High-dose cancer therapy: pharmacology, hematopoietins, stem cells, 3rd edition. Baltimore: Lippincott Williams & Wilkins, 2000:15–48.

17. Teicher BA, Northey D, Yuan J, Frei E III. High-dose therapy/stem cell support: comparison of mice and humans. Int J Cancer 1996; 65:695–699.

18. Teicher BA, Holden SA, Jacobs JL. Approaches to defining the mechanism of enhancement by Fluosol-DA 20% with carbogen of melphalan antitumor activity. Cancer Res 1987; 47:513–518.

19. Teicher BA, Herman TS, Holden SA, et al. Tumor resistance to alkylating agents conferred by mechanisms operative only in vivo. Science 1990; 247:1457–1461.

20. Teicher BA, Chatterjee D, Liu J, Holden SA, Ara G. Protection of bone marrow granulocyte macrophage colony-forming units in mice bearing in vivo alkylating agent resistant EMT-6 tumors. Cancer Chemother Pharmacol 1993; 32:315–319.

21. Frei E III, Teicher BA, Holden SA, Cathcart KNS, Wand Y. Preclinical studies and clinical correlation of the effect of alkylating agent dose. Cancer Res 1988; 48:6417–6423.

22. Frei E III, Teicher BA, Cucchi CA, et al. Resistance to alkylating agents: basic studies and therapeutic implications. In: Wooley PVI, Tew TD, eds. Mechanisms of drug resistance in neoplastic cells. New York: Academic, 1988:69–87.

23. Teicher BA Frei E III. Development of alkylating agent-resistant human tumor cell lines. Cancer Chemother Pharmacol 1988; 21:292–298.

24. Teicher BA, Frei E III. Alkylating agents. In: Gupta RS, ed. Drug resistance in mammalian cells: anticancer and other drugs. Boca Raton: CRC Press, 1989:1–31.

25. Teicher BA, Holden SA, Herman TS, et al. Characteristics of five human tumor cell lines and sublines resistant to *cis*-diamminedichloroplatinum II. Int J Cancer 1991; 47:252–260.

26. Holden SA Teicher BA, Frei E III. Long-term persistence and cytokinetics of human tumor cells in vitro following high-dose alkylating agent exposure. Cancer Lett 1994; 87:211–222.

27. Holden SA, Teicher BA, Ayash L, Frei E III. A preclinical model for sequential high dose chemotherapy. Cancer Chemother Pharmacol 1995; 36:61–64.

28. Holden SA, Emi Y, Kakeji Y, Northey D, Teicher BA. Host distribution and response to antitumor alkylating agents of EMT-6 tumor cells from subcutaneous tumor implants. Cancer Chemother Pharmacol 1997; 40:87–93.

29. Elias A. Dose-intensive therapy in lung cancer. Cancer Chemother Pharmacol 1997; 40(Suppl):S64–S69.

30. Chatterjee D, Liu CJ, Northey D, Teicher BA. Molecular characterization of the in vivo alkylating agent resistant murine EMT-6 mammary carcinoma tumors. Cancer Chemother Phamacol 1995; 35:423–431.

31. Teicher BA, Holden SA, Ara G, Chen G. Transforming growth factor-β in in vivo resistance. Cancer Chemother Pharmacol 1996; 37:601–609.

32. Anscher MS, Jirtle RL. Role of transforming growth factor-b abd hepatocyte growth factor in late normal tissue effects of radiation. Radiat Oncol Invest 1994; 1:305–313.

33. McBride WH. Cytokine cascades in late normal tissue radiation responses. Int J Radiat Oncol Biol Phys 1996; 33:232–234.

34. Randall K, Coggle JE. Expression of transforming growth factor-b1 in mouse skin during the acute phase of radiation damage. Int J Radiat Biol 1995; 68:301–309.

35. Rodemann HP, Bamberg M. Cellular basis of radiation-induced fibrosis. Radiotherap Oncol 1995; 35:83–90.
36. Rubin P, Johnston CJ, Williams JP, McDonald S, Finkelstein JN. A perpetual cascade of cytokines postirradiation leads to pulmonary fibrosis. Int J Radiat Oncol Biol Phys 1995; 33:99–109.
37. Zhan Y, Purton JF, Godfrey DJ, Cole TJ, Heath WR, Lew AM. Without peripheral interference, thymic deletion is mediated in a cohort of double-positive cells without classical activation. Proc Natl Acad Sci U S A 2003; 100:1197–1202.
38. Hatada T, Miki C. Nutritional status and postoperative cytokine response in colorectal cancer patients. Cytokine 2000; 12:1331–1336.
39. Hill GR, Ferrara JL. The primacy of the gastrointestinal tract as a target organ of acute graft-versus-host disease: rationale for the use of cytokine shields in allogeneic bone marrow transplantation. Blood 2000; 95:2754–2759.
40. Andratschke N, Grosu AL, Molls M, Nieder C. Perspectives in the treatment of malignant gliomas in adults. Anticancer Res 2001; 21:3541–3550.
41. Ellis LM, Takahashi Y, Liu W, Shaheen RM. Vascular endothelial growth factor in human colon cancer: biology and therapeutic implications. Oncologist 2000; 5(Suppl 1):S11–S15.
42. Xia P, Aiello LP, Ishii H, et al. Characterization of vascular endothelial growth factor's effect on the activation of protein kinase C, its isoforms, and endothelial cell growth. J Clinical Invest 1996; 98:2018–2026.
43. Guo D, Jia Q, Song HY, Warren RS, Donner DB. Vascular endothelial cell growth factor promotes tyrosine phosphorylation of mediators of signal transduction that contain SH2 domains. Association with endothelial cell proliferation. J Biol Chem 1995; 270:6729–6733.
44. Sawano A, Takahashi T, Yamaguchi S, Shibuya M. The phosphorylated 1169-tyrosine containing region of flt-1 kinase (VEGFR-1) is a major binding site for PLCγ. Biochem Biophys Res Commun 1997; 238:487–491.
45. McMahon G. VEGF receptor signaling in tumor angiogenesis. Oncologist 5(Suppl 1):3–11.
46. Buchner K. The role of protein kinase C in the regulation of cell growth and in signaling to the cell nucleus. J Cancer Res Clin Oncol 2000; 126:1–11.
47. Goekjian PG, Jirousek MR. Protein kinase C inhibitors as novel anticancer drugs. Exp Opin Invest Drugs 2001; 10:2117–2140.
48. O'Brian CA, Ward NE, Stewart JR, Chu F. Prospects for targeting protein kinase C isozymes in the therapy of drug-resistant cancer- an evolving story. Cancer Mets Rev 2001; 20:95–100.
49. Swannie HC, Kaye SB. Protein kinase C inhibitors. Curr Oncol Rep 2002; 4:37–46.
50. Way KJ, Chou E, King GL. Identification of PKC-isoform-specific biological actions using pharmacological approaches. Trends Pharmacol Sci 2000; 21:181–187.
51. Nishizuka Y, Intracellular signaling by hydrolysis of phospholipids and activation of protein kinase C. Science 1992; 8:607–614.
52. Blumberg PM, Acs P, Bhattacharyya DK, Lorenzo PS. Inhibitors of protein kinase C and related receptors for the lipophilic second-messenger sn-1,2-diacylglycerol. In: Gutkind JS, ed. Cell cycle control: the molecular basis of cancer and other diseases. Totowa: Humana Press, 2000:349–366.
53. Shen B-Q, Lee DY, Zioncheck TF. Vascular endothelial growth factor governs endothelial nitric-oxide synthase expression via a KDR/flk-1 receptor and protein kinase C signaling pathway. J Biol Chem 1999; 274:33,057–33,063.
54. Shih S-C, Mullen A, Abrams K, Mukhopadhyay M, Claffey KP. Role of protein kinase C isoforms in phorbol ester-induced vascular endothelial growth factor expression in human glioblastoma cells. J Biol Chem 1999; 274:15,407–15,414.
55. Silva D, English D, Lyons D, Lloyd FP. Protein kinase C induces motility of breast cancers by upregulating secretion of urokinase-type plsaminogen activator through activation of AP-1 and NF-κB. Biochem Biophys Res Commun 2002; 290:552–557.
56. Bhat-Nakshatri P, Sweeney CJ, Nakshatri H. Identification of signal transduction pathways involved in constitutive NF-κB activation in breast cancer cells. Oncogene 2002; 21:2066–2078.
57. Kim YW, Hur SY, Kim TE, et al. Protein kinase C modulates telomerase activity in human cervical cancer cells. Exp Mol Med 2001; 33:156–163.
58. Flescher E, Rotem R. Protein kinase C epsilon mediates the induction of P-glycoprotein in LNCaP prostate carcinoma cells. Cell Signal 2002; 14:37–43.
59. Sumitomo M, Ohba M, Asakuma J, et al. Protein kinase C delta amplifies ceramide formation via mitochondrial signaling in prostate cancer cells. J Clin Invest 2002; 109:827–836.
60. Ghosh PM, Bedolla R, Mikhailova M, Kreisberg JI. RhoA-dependent murine prostate cancer cell proliferation and apoptosis: role of protein kinase C zeta. Cancer Res 2002; 62:2630–2636.

61. Lin MF, Zhang XQ, Dean J, Lin FF. Protein kinase C pathway is involved in regulating the secretion of prostatic phosphatase in human prostate cancer cells. Cell Biol Int 2001; 25:1139–1148.
62. Da Rocha AB, Mans DR, Regner A, Schwartsmann G. Targeting protein kinase C: new therapeutic opportunity against high-grade malignant glioma? Oncologist 2002; 7:17–33.
63. Martelli AM, Sang N, Borgatti P, Capitani S, Neri LM. Multiple biological responses activated by nuclear protein kinase C. J Cellular Biochem 1999; 74:499–521.
64. Jirousek MR, Gillig JR, Gonzalez CM, et al. (*S*)-13-[(dimethylamino)methyl]-10,11,14,15-tetrahydro-4,9:16,21-dimetheno-1*H*,13*H*-dibenzo[*e*,*k*]pyrrolo[3,4-*h*][1,4,13]oxadiazacyclohexadecene-1,3(2*H*)-dione (LY333531) and related analogues: isozyme selective inhibitors of protein kinase C-β. J Med Chem 1996; 39:2664–2671.
65. Danis RP, Bingaman DP, Jirousek M, Yang Y. Inhibition of intraocular neovascularization caused by retinal ischemia in pigs by PKCβ inhibition with LY333531. Invest Ophthalmol Vis Sci 1998; 39:171–179.
66. Aiello LP, Bursell SE, Clermont A, et al. Vascular endothelial growth factor-induced retinal permeability is mediated by protein kinase C in vivo and suppressed by an orally effective β-isoform-selective inhibitor. Diabetes 1997; 46:1473–1480.
67. Ishii H, Jirousek MR, Koya D, et al. Amelioration of vascular dysfunctions in diabetic rats by an oral PKC β inhibitor [*see* comments], Science 1996; 272:728–731.
68. Yoshiji H, Kuriyama S, Ways DK, et al. Protein kinase C lies on the signaling pathway for vascular endothelial growth factor-mediated tumor development and angiogenesis. Cancer Res 1999; 59:4413–4418.
69. Teicher BA, Alvarez E, Mendelsohn LG, Ara G, Menon K, Ways DK. Enzymatic rationale and preclinical support for a potent protein kinase Cb inhibitor in cancer therapy. Adv Enzyme Regul 1999; 39:313–327.
70. Sausville EA, Arbuck SG, Messmann R, et al. Phase I trial of 72-hour continuous infusion UCN-01 in patients with refractory neoplasms. J Clin Oncol 2001; 19:2319–2333.
71. Dees E, O'Reilly S, Figg W, et al. A phase I and pharmacologic study of UCN-01, a protein kinase C inhibitor. Proc Am Soc Clin Oncol 2000; 19:797a.
72. Grosios K. UCN-01 Kyowa Hakko Kogyo Co. Curr Opin Invest Drugs 2001; 2:287–297.
73. Abe S, Kubota T, Otani Y, et al. UCN-01 (7-hydroxystaurosporine) inhibits in vivo growth of human cancer cells through selective perturbation of G1 phase checkpoint machinery. Jpn J Cancer Res 2001; 92:537–545.
74. Akinaga S, Gomi K, Morimoto M, Tamaoki T, Okabe M. Antitumor activity of UCN-01, a selective inhibitor of protein kinase C, in murine and human models. Cancer Res 1991; 51:4888–4892.
75. Senderowicz AM, Sausville EA. Preclinical and clinical development of cyclin-dependent kinase modulators. J Natl Cancer Inst 2000; 92:376–387.
76. Akiyama T, Yoshida T, Tsujita T, et al. G1 phase accumulation induced by UCN-01 is associated with dephosphorylation of Rb and CDK2 proteins as well as induction of CDK inhibitor p21/Cip1/WAF1/Sdi1 in p53-mutated human epidermoid carcinoma A431 cells. Cancer Res 1997; 57:1495–1501.
77. Sugiyama K, Akiyama T, Shimizu M, et al. Decrease in susceptibility toward induction of apoptosis and alteration in G1 checkpoint function as determinants of resistance of human lung cancer cells against the antisignaling drug UCN-01 (7-hydroxystaurosporine). Cancer Res 1999; 59:4406–4412.
78. Sarkaria JN, Busby EC, Tibbetts RS, et al. Inhibition of ATM and ATR kinase activities by the radiosensitizing agent, caffeine. Cancer Res 1999; 59:4375–4382.
79. Busby EC, Leistritz DF, Abraham RT, Karnitz LM, Sarkaria JN. The radiosensitizing agent 7-hydroxystaurosporine (UCN-01) inhibits the DNA damage checkpoint kinase hChk1. Cancer Res 2000; 60:2108–2112.
80. Graves PR, Yu L, Schwarz JK, et al. The Chk1 protein kinase and the Cdc25C regulatory pathways are targets of the anticancer agent UCN-01. J Biol Chem 2000; 275:5600–5605.
81. Chen X, Lowe M, Keyomarsi K. UCN-01-mediated G1 arrest in normal but not tumor breast cells is Rb-dependent and p53-independent. Oncogene 1999; 18:5691–5702.
82. Kruger EA, Blagosklonny MV, Dixon SC, Figg WD. UCN-01, a protein kinase C inhibitor, inhibits endothelial cell proliferation and angiogenic hypoxic response. Invasion Metastasis 1999; 18:209–218.
83. Teicher BA, Alvarez E, Menon K, et al. Antiangiogenic effects of a protein kinase C β-selective small molecule. Cancer Chemother Pharmacol 2002; 49:69–77.
84. Teicher BA, Menon K, Alvarez E, Galbreath E, Shih C, Faul MM. Antiangiogenic and antitumor effects of a protein kinase C β inhibitor in human HT-29 colon carcinoma and human Caki-1 renal cell carcinoma xenografts. Anticancer Res 2001; 21:3175–3184.

85. Teicher BA, Menon K, Alvarrez E, Galbreath E, Shih C, Faul MM. Antiangiogenic and antitumor effects of a protein kinase C β inhibitor in murine Lewis lung carcinoma and human Calu-6 non-small cell lung carcinoma xenografts. Cancer Chemother Pharmacol 2001; 48:473–480.

86. Teicher BA, Menon K, Alvarez E, Liu P, Shih C, Faul MM. Antiangiogenic and antitumor effects of a protein kinase C β inhibitor in human hepatocellular and gastric cancer xenografts. In Vivo 2001; 15:185–193.

87. Teicher BA, Menon K, Alvarez E, Galbreath E, Shih C, Faul MM. Antiangiogenic and antitumor effects of a protein kinase C Beta inhibitor in human T98G glioblastoma multiform xenografts. Clin Cancer Res 2001; 7:634–640.

88. Thornton DE, Keyes K, Mann L, et al. Determination of cancer growth factor biomarkers in plasma from mice bearing subcutaneous human tumor xenografts using Luminex Multiplex technology. Proc Am Assoc Cancer Res 2002; 43:897.

89. Keyes K, Cox K, Treadway P, et al. An in vitro tumor model: analysis of angiogenic factor expression after chemotherapy. Cancer Res 2002; 62:5597–5602.

90. Keyes K, Mann L, Cox K, et al. Circulating angiogenic growth factor levels in mice bearing human tumors using Luminex multiplex technology. Cancer Chemother Pharmacol 51:321–327.

10 Characteristics of the Metastatic Phenotype

The Melanoma Experience

Vladislava O. Melnikova, PhD
and Menashe Bar-Eli, PhD

Contents

Summary

Malignant progression and tumor metastasis is a complex process enabled by various molecular changes occurring in a subpopulation of tumor cells. The metastatic phenotype is associated with the cellular capacity for uncontrolled growth, resistance to apoptosis, high invasive potential, and effective neoangiogenesis. Whereas the contribution of genetic alterations to the metastatic dissemination is not yet clear, because both primary and metastatic tumors often have similar patterns of genetic mutations, the majority of the changes contributing to the metastatic phenotype are controlled epigenetically. In melanoma, the progression toward malignant disease and acquisition of the metastatic phenotype involves loss of activator protein 2 and gain in expression of activating transcription factor 1/cyclic adenosine monophosphate-responsive element-binding protein family transcription factors. Together with upregulation of activating transcription factor 2, Snail, nuclear factor-κB and other transcription factors, this results in deregulation of the expression of cellular adhesion molecules, matrix-degrading enzymes, as well as other factors that enable a complex interaction of tumor cells with extracellular milieu and other cells during malignant progression and metastatic dissemination. Furthermore, because of the need to survive mechanical and immuno-

From: *Cancer Drug Discovery and Development: Cancer Drug Resistance*
Edited by: B. Teicher © Humana Press Inc., Totowa, NJ

logical challenges, and changing nutritional environment during the dissemination process, metastatic cells are permanently selected for the superior survival capacity. As a result, metastatic cells are commonly characterized by their increased resistance to the chemotherapeutic treatment when compared to primary tumors. Here, we discuss some of the potential mechanisms contributing to drug resistance in melanoma.

Key Words: Melanoma; metastasis; angiogenesis; transcriptional regulation; AP-2, CREB.

1. INTRODUCTION

The development of tumor metastasis is a complex cascade of events. Potentially, metastatic cells have to exit the primary tumor site by loosening cell-to-cell contact, adhering to and degrading extracellular matrix, migrating through the subendothelial basement membrane of local postcapillary veins and lymphatic vessels and intravasate. Once in circulation, tumor cells face severe mechanical and immunosurveillance challenges. Surviving cells can arrest in the peripheral capillary bed of a distant organ, adhere to the subendothelial basement membrane, extravasate, adhere, and migrate through the extracellular matrix, and form a colony at the new metastatic site. Further induction of neoangiogenesis must occur to assure continuous growth. A selective pressure accompanying the process of development of metastasis results in a progressive loss of cells that actually left the primary tumor and an emergence of a metastatic "supercell." A recognized fundamental feature of solid malignancies is their genetic instability, which enables for random cell-to-cell genomic variation (genomic heterogeneity) to arise among cells of individual tumors. Genetically unstable cells may produce clones of cells with the mutations necessary for malignant behavior. Recent data also suggest that cells with higher metastatic potential may respond to the stimuli from the microenvironment with greater incidence of changes in gene expression, therefore emphasizing the role of dynamic epigenetic alterations in tumor progression *(1,2)*. Overall, the biological characteristics selected for during metastatic progression comprise of uncontrolled growth, resistance to apoptosis, and invasive properties including adhesion, motility, and proteolytic capacity.

Malignant melanoma has served as an excellent model for studying the molecular changes associated with the metastatic phenotype. This is partly because of the well-described sequential steps in the progression of the disease and successful identification of a number of accompanying molecular changes. Malignant melanoma arises from transformation and proliferation of melanocytes that are normally found in basal cell layer of the epidermis. Tumor growth can be biphasic or monophasic *(3)*. The biphasic pattern consists of a horizontal or radial initial growth phase followed by a subsequent vertical growth phase corresponding to the infiltration of the dermis and hypodermis. The monophasic growth pattern of melanoma consists of pure vertical growth mode. When the lesion enters the vertical growth phase, the repertoire of adhesion molecules changes as the tumor enters the dermis and acquires the capacity to metastasize (Fig. 1). As such, the single most important prognostic factor in malignant melanoma remains the vertical thickness of the primary tumor (i.e., the Breslow thickness).

In this chapter, we analyze our present knowledge about genetic and epigenetic changes associated with the progression of human melanoma. A special emphasis is made on recent developments in identification of the mechanisms of melanoma drug resistance.

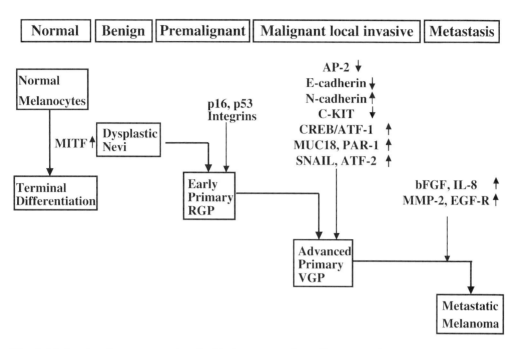

Fig. 1. Molecular changes associated with the progression of human melanoma. Abnormalities in the *p16/CDKN2* gene are usually an early event. Mutations in the *p53* gene are infrequent, but are observed in early stages. Abnormal functions of wild-type p53 were also observed. Transcription factor Snail normally functions in neural crest formation, but it also inhibits E-cadherin expression in melanoma cells. Alterations in c-KIT, melanoma cellular adhesion molecule (MCAM)/mucin (MUC)18 and N-cadherin, and integrins occur in the transition from radial initial growth phase (RGP) to vertical growth phase (VGP). The activator protein (AP)-2 transcription factor is not expressed in metastatic cells, whereas the transcription factors cyclic adenosine monophosphate response element-binding protein (CREB)/activating transcription factor (ATF)-1and ATF-2 are upregulated in these cells. The expression of genes involved in angiogenesis, invasion and apoptosis such as basic fibroblast growth factor (bFGF), interleukin (IL)-8, epidermal growth factor receptor (EGF-R), and protease-activated receptor (PAR)-1 correlates with higher metastatic potential of human melanoma cells.

2. GENETIC ALTERATIONS AND METASTATIC PROGRESSION

2.1. p16^INK4a/p14^ARF (CDKN2A) and p53 Tumor Suppressor Genes

Genetic mutations associated with initiation stage of cancers have been extensively described. Alterations in two major groups of genes are associated with cellular transformation process: tumor suppressors, mainly *p53, p16INK4a/p14ARF (CDKN2A)* or phosphatase and tensin (phosphatase and tensin homologue deleted in chromosome ten [*PTEN*]), and proto-oncogenes, mainly *K-, N-,* and *H-ras* or *BRAF* small tyrosine kinase protein-encoding genes. Inactivation of the *INK4a/Arf* melanoma susceptibility locus has been identified in approximately 20–30% of familial melanoma and 15–30% of sporadic melanomas *(4–10)*. The *INK4a/Arf* locus encodes two independent bona fide tumor suppressor proteins, which function as growth inhibitors and effectors of cellular senescence: the cyclin dependent kinase inhibitor p16^INK4a and the p53 activator p14^ARF (mouse p19^Arf). With respect to melanoma progression, several studies have shown near-similar frequencies of deletions and loss of heterozygosity alterations in matched primary melanomas and metastatic lesions (11–19). Recently, analysis of a large number of cases for p16^{INK4a} protein expression by immunohistochemistry demonstrated that p16^{INK4a} is lost in melanoma but not in nevi, and that metastatic lesions have a higher frequency of protein loss than primary tumors (11,17). In addition, the thickness of primary melanoma tumors has been correlated to higher occurrence of allelic loss or protein loss (14).

The tumor suppressor protein p53 functions as a latent, short-lived transcription factor (20) that induces expression of proteins involved in the cell cycle arrest, DNA repair, and/ or apoptosis, and represses transcriptional activation of growth-promoting genes (21,22). The p53 gene has been found to be mutated in 10–30% of cultured human melanoma cell lines (23–25), and at 0 or 20–25% frequency in melanoma tumor tissues (25–29). Although low frequency of mutations in p53 gene argues against its role in melanoma progression, a complex genetic profile including p16$^{INK4a(ARF)}$ + Ras(Braf) + p53 mutations shows greater correlation with aggressive disease/poor survival than, for example, the p16$^{INK4a(ARF)}$ + Ras(Braf) profile (30).

2.2. Activation of Ras-Braf-Mitogen-Activated Protein Kinase Pathway

The use of high-throughput genomic technologies aimed at global molecular profiling of cancer has recently led to the identification of oncogenic somatic mutations in the BRAF gene in 66% of primary sporadic human melanomas, as compared with lower rate in other cancers (31–39). All mutations were within the kinase domain, and 80% of them were a V600E (formerly recognized as V599E) (exon 15) substitution. The BRAF gene encodes for a serine/threonine kinase that is regulated by the binding with RAS protein (40). Mutations at V600 renders Braf protein constitutively active, resulting in increased phosphorylation and activation of downstream mitogen-activated protein kinase (MAPK) extracellular signal-regulated kinase (MEK)1/2 and extracellular signal-regulated kinase (ERK)1/2 mitogen-activated protein kinases (31). Activated ERK1/2 MAPK move into the nucleus where they phosphorylate and activate a number of transcription factors such as c-Fos and Elk-1 (41,42). ERK MAPK signaling plays a pivotal role in regulation of cell growth and proliferation. Sustained activation of ERKs is required to pass the G_1-restriction point of the cell cycle, and to induce expression of Cyclin D1 during mid-G_1 phase (43,44). A large number of growth factors necessary for the survival of normal melanocytes and involved in autocrine regulation of melanoma cell proliferation signal through the Ras/Raf/MAPK pathway. These factors include basic fibroblast growth factor (bFGF), hepatocyte growth factor (HGF), insulin-like growth factor, α-melanocyte stimulating hormone, epidermal growth factor, stem cell factor, and nerve growth factor (45–48).

An inverse correlation exists between the occurrence of mutations in the BRAF gene and in the RAS oncogene, which is activated in approximately 10–30% of human melanomas (49–52). Analysis of primary melanomas and corresponding metastases from 71 patients for BRAF mutations in exon 11 and exon 15 and N-RAS mutations in codon 61 showed that the vast majority of melanomas carried mutations in either one of the genes (53). Mutations in these genes appear to arise early during melanoma pathogenesis and are retained throughout tumor progression (53). Although some studies report an association between complex mutational profiles, including BRAF mutations and alterations at multiple tumor suppressor genes, and aggressive melanoma disease with poor survival (30,54), clearly more data are needed in order to link mutated BRAF to the disease progression and outcome.

2.3. PTEN *Tumor Suppressor Gene*

The *PTEN* tumor suppressor gene encodes for a lipid/protein phosphatase with dual specificity: by the lipid phosphatase activity, PTEN signals down the phosphatidylinositol-3-OH kinase/Akt pathway and regulates G_1 progression and apoptosis, whereas by protein phosphatase activity PTEN inhibits MAPK signaling *(55)*. PTEN is mutated in approximately 10% of primary and metastatic melanoma tumors (reviewed in ref. 56). Loss of heterozygosity occurs at higher frequency of approximately 40% in both primary and metastatic lesions, suggesting that alterations in PTEN occur early in melanoma development *(56)*. Loss of PTEN in melanoma results in the activation of Akt, which is detected in severely dysplastic nevi and most melanoma lesions but not in slightly dysplastic nevi *(57)*. Constitutive activation of Akt protein kinase in melanoma leads to upregulation of nuclear factor (NF)-κB, which is involved in regulating cell cycle, cell survival, and inflammatory cytokine signaling, and plays a pivotal role in malignant progression. This suggests that Akt activity may be an early marker for the malignant disease *(57)*.

3. REGULATION OF ADHESION, MOTILITY, AND INVASIVENESS DURING TUMOR PROGRESSION

The genetic alterations described above are generally associated with cellular transformation, uncontrolled proliferation, and, to some extent, participate in the control of neoangiogenesis required to support tumor growth. These characteristics are equally required for the growth of the primary as well as metastatic tumor. However, the analysis of melanoma-derived experimental cell lines with different metastatic potential reveals clear distinction in their invasive properties. As mentioned earlier, potentially metastatic cells have to be able to perform a complex task of dissemination. Several classes of molecules are involved in regulation of this multistep process. Their list includes, but is not limited to, adhesion molecules, matrix-degrading enzymes, motility factors and cytokines, and survival and growth factors and their receptors. In particular, malignant local invasive and metastatic melanoma phenotypes have been linked to downregulation of E-cadherin and upregulation of N-cadherin adhesion proteins, upregulation of the melanoma cellular adhesion molecule (MCAM) and protease-activated receptor (PAR)-1, activation of matrix metalloproteinases (MMPs) such as MMP-2, as well as overexpression of bFGF, interleukin (IL)-8, and epidermal growth factor receptor (*see* Fig. 1).

3.1. Cadherins

The cadherins are a family of Ca^{2+}-dependent cell adhesion molecules that function in promoting intracellular communications and heterotypic/homotypic adhesion and that play an integral part in cell–cell adherence junctions. Classic cadherins are divided into three subtypes: N (neural), E (epithelial), and P (placental). Changes in the subtype expression play an important role in segregation of cells into distinct tissues and in maintaining tissue architecture during early development *(58)*. Further, the cadherin family molecules have been shown to play a central role in maintaining homeostasis in the skin by regulating the interactions between melanocytes and epidermal keratinocytes, dermal fibroblasts, and endothelial cells. Loss of E-cadherin, which is now considered a natural metastasis suppressor, characterizes the majority of carcinomas. Inactivating germline mutations in the *CDH1* (E-cadherin-1) gene have been identified in diffuse gastric cancer, sporadic gastric cancer, and breast tumors *(59,60)*. Several paracrine and autocrine growth factors have been shown to induce tyrosine phosphorylation of the E-cadherin/β-catenin complex, resulting in downregulation of E-cadherin, and cell–cell adhesion *(60)*. During melanoma development, a progressive loss of E-cadherin expression is directly correlated with a loss of keratinocyte-mediated regulation of melanoma cell growth and expression of invasion-associated adhesion receptors such as MCAM/mucin (Muc)-18 *(61–65)*. Using skin reconstruction models, Hsu and colleagues demonstrated that restoration of E-cadherin expression in melanoma cells inhibited their invasion into dermis, restored keratinocyte-mediated growth control and downregulated expression of MCAM/Muc-18 and $\alpha_v\beta_3$ integrin molecules *(65)*. Loss of E-cadherin during melanoma progression appears to be associated with epigenetic silencing *(66)*. Two transcription factors, Snail and SIP1, have recently been shown to be important in the transcriptional silencing of the E-cadherin gene *(67,68)*. We have also previously demonstrated that loss of expression of a third transcription factor, activator protein (AP)-2, during progression of melanoma results in deregulation of E-cadherin expression *(69–71)*. It is presumed that loss of cell adhesion molecules such as E-cadherin produces a rich pool of tumor cells with loosen cell–cell contact, which can than leave the primary tumor site, eventually producing metastasis. Furthermore, during melanoma progression, the loss of functional E-cadherin is inversely correlated with a gain in expression of N-cadherin on melanoma cells *(64,65,72)*. N-cadherin expression in melanoma cells mediates homophilic adhesion between melanoma cells, facilitates gap-junctional formation with other N-cadherin-expressing cells in the stroma, including fibroblasts and endothelial cells. N-cadherin has been shown to promote the migration of melanoma cells over dermal fibroblasts *(73)*, whereas anti-N-cadherin antibodies can delay the transendothelial migration of melanoma cells and induce apoptosis of melanoma cells *(73–75)*.

3.2. Integrins

Integrins are a family of adhesion receptors that mediate adhesion to cell surface and matrix molecules. They play an important role in recognition and adherence of an invasive tumor cell to a new extracellular matrix. This process is accomplished by downregulation of original matrix receptors, such as $\alpha_5\beta_1$ fibronectin receptor and/or various laminin/collagen IV receptors such as $\alpha_6\beta_1$ or $\alpha_6\beta_4$ *(76)*, concomitant with overexpression of other integrins that promote rapid changes in adhesion/detachment cycles. Although many integrins have been implicated in mediating melanoma cell growth and metastasis, perhaps the most studied one is the vitronectin receptor $\alpha_v\beta_3$ *(77,78)*. Interaction between $\alpha_v\beta_3$ and extracellular matrix proteins serves to promote cell attachment, spreading, and migration. Expression of β_3 subunit correlates with vertical growth phase of melanomas *(81–84)*. In addition to mediating matrix adhesion, integrins like $\alpha_v\beta_3$ are involved in regulation of other important aspects of metastatic spreading: $\alpha_v\beta_3$ can bind and activate soluble proteolytic enzymes such as urokinase-type plasminogen activator (uPA) and MMP *(85)*, and facilitate transendothelial migration through interaction with L1 ligand on endothelial cells *(86)*.

3.3. MCAM/Muc-18

MCAM, also known as Muc-18, Mel-CAM, CD146, A32 antigen, and S-Endo-1 is a transmembrane glycoprotein that belongs to the immunoglobulin superfamily and functions as a Ca^{2+}-independent adhesion molecule. MCAM is strongly expressed by advanced primary and metastatic melanomas but is weaker and less frequent in nevus cells *(87)*. MCAM expression is also consistently present on other tumors such as angiosarcomas, Kaposi's sarcomas, leiomyosarcomas, placental site trophoblastic tumors, and choriocarcinomas *(88)*. When expressed on melanoma cells, MCAM mediates homotypic adhesion through interaction with a heterophilic ligand that remains to be identified *(89,90)*. Heterotypic adhesion between melanoma cells and endothelial cells has also been demonstrated via a heterophilic MCAM/ligand adhesion *(91)*. The level of expression of MCAM/Muc-18 by human melanoma cells has been shown to correlate directly with tumor progression and the acquisition of metastatic potential *(91–95)*. We showed that enforced expression of MCAM in MCAM-negative primary cutaneous melanoma SB-2 cells rendered them highly tumorigenic and increased their metastatic potential in nude mice as compared with parental and control transfected cells *(96)*. The transfected cells displayed increased homotypic adhesion, increased attachment to human endothelial cells, decreased ability to adhere to laminin, and increased invasiveness through Matrigel-coated filters *(96)*. Fully humanized anti-MCAM monoclonal antibody (ABX-MA1, obtained from Abgenix) inhibited tumor growth of MCAM-positive A375SM and WM2664 melanoma cells after subcutaneous injection in nude mice, and also greatly inhibited development of lung metastasis after intravenous injection *(97)*. This suggests that targeting inhibition of MCAM may prove to be a potent therapeutic modality.

3.4. Thrombin Receptor PAR-1

The thrombin receptor PAR-1 is a unique G-protein-coupled receptor that belongs to the protease-activated receptor family. PAR-1 has been implicated to play a central role in tumorigenesis and metastasis *(98–100)*. Overexpression of PAR-1 has been detected in metastatic melanoma cell lines *(101)*; human carcinoma cell lines including colon adenocarcinoma, laryngeal, breast, pancreatic; and oral squamous cell carcinoma *(98,100,102–105)*. Activation of PAR-1 receptor by serine protease thrombin (which is present in the circulation as well as local tumor sites) *(102,106–108)*, results in variety of cellular responses including activation of RAS, phosphoinositide 3 kinase (PI3K), and MAP kinases, which are all involved in cell growth, tumor promotion and carcinogenesis *(109,110)*. Furthermore, PAR-1 activation induces expression of genes required for cell adhesion, invasion and tumor angiogenesis, including $\alpha_{IIb}\beta_3$, $\alpha_v\beta_3$, and $\alpha_v\beta_5$ integrins, MMP-2, uPA, platelet-derived growth factor, IL-8, vascular endothelial growth factor (VEGF) and bFGF *(102,111–118)*.

3.5. Matrix-Degrading Enzymes

Invasion requires increased activity of matrix-degrading enzymes such as serine-protease family (uPA, elastase, plasmin, and cathepsin G), the matrix metalloproteinases (gelatinases, stromelysins, matrilysins) and the cysteine proteinases (cathepsin B, L) *(119)*. In tumor cells, regulation of the activity of one or several of these enzymes is often distorted because of either inappropriate trafficking, for example in case of cathepsins, or downregulation of their inhibitors *(120,121)*. Transcriptional upregulation of MMP2 expression has also been documented in malignant melanoma, and involves increased activity of cAMP response element-binding (CREB) protein and downregulation of AP-2 transcription factors *(122)*. A combined action of the matrix-degrading enzymes results in fragmentation of the matrix proteins, allowing easy migration of tumor cells, and release of some matrix-bound growth factors and cytokines and chemokines.

3.6. Motility Factors

Migration of tumor cells through the extracellular matrix, local basement membrane, and subendothelial basement membrane may be regulated by both autocrine and paracrine motility factors. In many cancer types, tumor cells are characterized by production of an autocrine motility factor and expression of autocrine motility factor receptor *(123)*, as well as high constitutive production of another cytokine, autotaxin (reviewed in ref. *60*). In addition, practically all paracrine cytokines are capable of inducing motility response in tumor cells *(60)*. One of the most prominent paracrine motility cytokines is HGF/scatter factor, which is frequently produced by mesenchymal cells, and tumor cells often express its receptor, the c-met oncoprotein *(124)*.

3.7. Melanoma Angiogenesis

The growth of the primary and metastatic tumors is controlled by the rate of angiogenesis and hence, by the angiogenic factors promoting it. Melanomas are considered to be highly angiogenic. Melanoma cells produce large amounts of multiple angiogenic factors including VEGF *(125–128)*, IL-8 *(129–131)*, platelet-derived endothelial cell growth factor *(132,133)*, and bFGF *(134,136)*. VEGF, also known as vascular permeability factor, is a strong specific mitogen for endothelial cells and may also stimulate endothelial cell migration and reorganization *(137,138)*. Platelet-derived endothelial cell growth factor, also known as thymidine phosphorylase and gliostatin, stimulates endothelial cell mitogenesis and chemotaxis in vitro and is strongly angiogenic in vivo, possibly through modulation of nucleotide metabolism *(139)*, bFGF, which belongs to the family of heparin-binding growth factors, is a multifunctional protein having a well-established key role in tumor angiogenesis *(140–142)*. IL-8, which belongs to the superfamily of CXC chemokines, is a multifunctional cytokine that exhibits potent angiogenic activities both in vitro and in vivo, and also acts as an autocrine growth factor for melanoma cells *(143–145)*.

The angiogenic activity of IL-8 produced by monocytes and macrophages was first demonstrated by Koch and colleagues *(143)*. They found that human recombinant IL-8 was potently angiogenic when implanted in a rat cornea and induced proliferation and chemotaxis of human umbilical vein endothelial cells. The involvement of IL-8 in tumor angiogenesis was first demonstrated in human bronchogenic carcinoma *(146)*. Tumor cell-derived IL-8 induces endothelial cell chemotaxis in vitro and corneal neovascularization in vivo. These observations have been confirmed in many other types of human tumors including melanomas *(147)*. Now, IL-8 is considered to be one of the most potent angiogenic factors secreted by melanoma cells. The question of how IL-8 exerts its angiogenic activity, however, remains unknown. We have recently demonstrated that metastatic melanoma cells producing IL-8 or primary cutaneous melanoma (IL-8-negative) transfected with the IL-8 gene displayed upregulation of MMP-2 expression and activity and increased invasiveness through Matrigel-coated filters *(148)*. Activation of MMP-2 by IL-8 can enhance the invasion of host stroma by tumor cells and increase angiogenesis and, hence, metastasis. In addition, IL-8 has been shown recently to act directly on vascular endothelial cells and to serve as a survival factor *(149)*. Thus, multiple mechanisms seem to be involved in IL-8 action, including direct effects on tumor and vascular endothelial cell proliferation, angiogenesis, and migration. These observations suggested that IL-8 could be a crucial mediator of angiogenesis, tumor growth, and metastasis in melanoma and offered a potential target for immunotherapies against human melanomas.

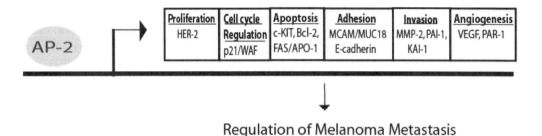

Proliferation	Cell cycle	Apoptosis	Adhesion	Invasion	Angiogenesis
HER-2	Regulation	c-KIT, Bcl-2,	MCAM/MUC18	MMP-2, PAI-1,	VEGF, PAR-1
	p21/WAF	FAS/APO-1	E-cadherin	KAI-1	

Regulation of Melanoma Metastasis

Fig. 2. A model for the role of loss of activator protein (AP)-2 transcription factor in the progression of human melanoma. AP-2 may act as a tumor suppressor by regulating a number of genes involved in tumor growth and metastasis of melanoma.

Recently, we used a fully human anti-IL-8 antibody (ABX-IL8, obtained from Abgenix) to neutralize the IL-8 secreted by melanoma cells and examine its effect on tumor growth. ABX-IL8 did not inhibit the proliferation of melanoma cells in vitro *(150)*. However, ABX-IL8 suppressed the tumorigenicity and metastatic potential of metastatic human melanoma A375SM and TXM-13 cells in vivo. ABX-IL8 displayed potent inhibition of MMP-2 activity in melanoma cells, and inhibited the invasion of tumor cells through basement membrane in vitro. Inhibition of tumor growth and metastasis by ABX-IL8 *in vivo* correlated with decreased vascularization of melanomas in nude mice that was at least partially because of decreased MMP-2 expression *(150)*. These results suggest that blocking of IL-8 by ABX-IL8 suppresses angiogenesis and metastasis of human melanoma. Thus, the human IL-8 neutralizing antibody ABX-IL8 may be beneficial for melanoma therapy either alone or in combination with other chemotherapeutic or antiangiogenic agents *(150)*.

4. TRANSCRIPTIONAL REGULATION OF METASTASIS-RELATED GENES IN MELANOMA

Loss or gain of transcription factor gene function plays a major role in tumor progression *(69,70,92,151–155)*. In melanomas, advancement toward malignant local invasive and metastatic phenotypes is associated with loss of expression of the transcription factor AP-2, and overexpression of CREB, activating transcription factor (ATF)-1, ATF-2, Snail, and nuclear factor (NF)-κB *(see* Fig. 1) *(69,70,152–155)*.

4.1. Activator Protein 2

The progression of human melanoma is associated with loss of expression of the transcription factor AP-2 *(69,70)*. Inactivation of AP-2 in SB-2 nonmetastatic primary cutaneous melanoma cells by using a dominant-negative AP-2, the *AP-2B* gene has been shown to augment cell tumorigenicity in nude mice *(71)*. Enforced overexpression of AP-2 in metastatic melanoma cells inhibited greatly tumor cell growth at subcutaneous sites and abrogated formation of lung metastasis after intravenous injection *(152)*. In metastatic melanoma cells, loss of AP-2 is directly linked to overexpression of MCAM/Muc-18, PAR-1, and MMP-2, and loss of expression of tyrosine-kinase receptor c-KIT (Fig. 2) *(69,70,101)*. Other studies have shown that AP-2 regulates additional genes involved in melanoma development and progression, including E-cadherin, *p21/WAF-1, c-erbB-*

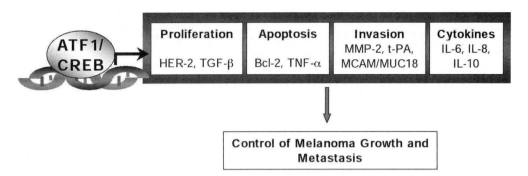

Fig. 3. A model for the role of cyclic adenosine monophosphate response element-binding protein (CREB)/ activated transcription factor (ATF)-1 overexpression in the progression of human melanoma. CREB/ATF-1 regulate several genes involved in tumor growth and metastasis of human melanoma.

2/HER-2/neu, plasminogen activator inhibitor type I *(PAI-1)*; insulin-like growth factor-binding protein-5 *(IGFBP-5)*, transforming growth factor-α *(TGF-α)*, *HGF*, vascular endothelial growth factor/vascular permeability factor *(VEGF/VPF)*, and c-*Myc (156–163)*.

4.2. Activating Transcription Factor 1/cAMP-Responsive Element-Binding Protein

The transition of melanoma cells from radial to vertical growth phase is associated with overexpression of ATF-1 and CREB *(152)*. Both transcriptional factors have been implicated in cAMP and Ca^{2+}-induced signaling. Quenching of CREB activity in metastatic melanoma cells by means of a dominant-negative form of CREB (KCREB) led to a decrease in their tumorigenicity and metastatic potential in nude mice *(164)*. We identified two mechanisms that explain how overexpression of CREB/ATF-1 contributes to the metastatic phenotype. The first is one in which CREB/ATF-1 play an essential role in invasion by regulating the CRE-dependent expression of the metalloproteinase MMP-2 and the adhesion molecule MCAM/Muc-18 genes (Fig. 3) *(164)*. In the second mechanism, CREB and ATF-1 act as survival factors for human melanoma cells. Expression of dominant-negative form of CREB (KCREB) in metastatic melanoma cells sensitized them to thapsigargin-induced apoptosis *(165)*. Analogously, intracellular expression of an inhibitory anti-ATF-1 single chain antibody fragment (ScFv) in MeWo melanoma cells suppressed their tumorigenicity and metastatic potential in nude mice *(166)*. ScFv anti-ATF-1 rendered the melanoma cells susceptible to thapsigargin-induced apoptosis in vitro and caused massive apoptosis in tumors transplanted subcutaneously into nude mice, confirming that AFT-1/CREB act as survival factors for human melanoma cells *(166)*.

4.3. Activating Transcription Factor 2

Another member of the CREB/ATF family of transcription factors that has been implicated in melanoma progression is ATF-2. It has been demonstrated that the nevi stage of melanoma can be induced in vitro by chronic stimulation of melanocytes with inflammatory mediators of HGF/scatter factor *(167,168)*. Activated ATF-2 affects expression of multiple genes, including c-*Jun*, E-selectin, cyclin A, *TNF-α*, and transforming growth factor-β *(169–173)*. Many of these genes regulate cell growth, differentiation, immune response and cell death. ATF-2 has been implicated in the resistance of late stage melanoma to UV-induced apoptosis through upregulation of the NF-κB pathway *(174)*.

Notably, it has been shown that tumorigenic and metastatic potential of melanoma cells could be reduced by blocking ATF-2 protein function with a synthetic ATF-2-derived peptide *(175,176)*.

4.4. Snail

Snail is a transcription factor that plays an important role in human embryonic development. One of the major mechanisms by which activation of Snail contributes to metastatic progression is associated with its regulation of E-cadherin expression. In melanoma cells, overexpression of Snail has been shown to suppress expression of E-cadherin *(177)*. Additionally, in bladder, colorectal, and pancreatic carcinoma, the downregulation of E-cadherin was observed to correlate with an overexpression of Snail *(178,179)*. It appears that Snail and AP-2 regulate E-cadherin gene in an inverse manner; the former suppresses and the latter promotes its expression.

4.5. Nuclear Factor-κB

NF-κB, a member of the RelA/NF-κB family of transcription factors, is involved in multiple cellular processes, including inflammation, cell cycle regulation, apoptosis, and oncogenesis. Constitutive activation of NF-κB has been described in a great number of solid tumors, and this activation appears to support cancer cell survival and to reduce the sensitivity against chemotherapeutic drugs. Normal melanocytes and nonmetastatic melanoma cells express no or low levels of NF-κB, whereas metastatic melanoma cells constitutively exhibit a high level of NF-κB activity *(180–182)*. Transfection of highly metastatic human melanoma variant cells with a dominant-negative mutant inhibitor of NF-κB, I-κBα expression vector (I-κBαM), decreased the level of constitutive NF-κB activity, inhibited subcutaneous tumor growth, and prevented lung metastasis in nude mice. Notably, the slow-growing subcutaneous tumors formed by the I-κBαM-transfected cells exhibited a decrease in microvessel density (angiogenesis), which correlated with a decrease in the level of IL-8 and VEGF expression *(155,183)*. Furthermore, inactivation of NF-κB by means of the ringer-finger-deleted TRAF-2 mutant has been shown to sensitize melanoma cells to apoptosis *(184)*.

5. DRUG RESISTANCE IN METASTATIC MELANOMA

Chemotherapy for metastatic melanoma is disappointing, there being anecdotal cases of complete remission. As described above, drug resistance in melanoma cells can be associated with overexpression of CREB/ATF-1 and NF-κB transcription factors. A growing number of evidence also suggest that activation of mitogen-activated protein kinase cascade is directly involved in chemoresistance.

Dacarbazine (DTIC) is considered the gold standard for treatment, having a response rate of 15–20%, but most responses are not sustained. Recently, we showed that DTIC induced IL-8 and VEGF protein overexpression and secretion via transcriptional upregulation in several melanoma cell lines *(185)*. The MAPK signal transduction pathway seemed to regulate at least partially the activation of IL-8, whereas it was not involved in VEGF promoter regulation. Metastatic melanoma cell lines secreting high levels of IL-8 and VEGF were more resistant to DTIC than early primary melanomas secreting low levels of the cytokines *(185)*. Accordingly, transfection of the primary nonmetastatic cutaneous melanoma SB-2 cells with the *IL-8* gene rendered them resistant to the cytotoxic effect of the drug, whereas the addition of IL-8-neutralizing antibody to metastatic melanoma MeWo cells lowered their sensitivity to DTIC *(185)*. Furthermore, to analyze the long-term effect of DTIC and its role in tumor growth and metastasis in vivo, we have generated DTIC-resistant cell lines by repeatedly exposing two of the primary cutaneous melanoma cell lines SB2 and MeWo to increasing concentrations of DTIC *(186)*. The selected DTIC-resistant cell lines, SB2-D and MeWo-D, exhibited increased tumor growth and metastatic behavior in nude mice. Higher levels of phosphorylation of RAF, MEK, and ERK protein kinases, as well as more IL-8, VEGF, MMP-2, and microvessel density (CD31) were found in tumors produced by SB2-D and MeWo-D in vivo as compared with those produced by their parental counterparts *(186)*. These results imply that treatment of melanoma patients with DTIC may produce a considerable hazard by selecting cells with a more aggressive melanoma phenotype. Reasonably, combination treatment with anti-VEGF/IL-8 or MEK inhibitors may potentiate the therapeutic effects of DTIC.

Similar to DTIC, treatment of melanoma cells with cisplatin has also been shown to induce ERK activation *(187)*. Furthermore, activation of MAPKs, when achieved by overexpression of mutant N-ras, increased cisplatin resistance in human melanoma cells by inducing overexpression of the antiapoptotic protein bcl-2 and inhibiting cell death *(188,189)*. Nevertheless, in studies using ERK inhibitor PD 98059, sensitization of melanoma cells to treatment with cisplatin was proven successful only in a limited number of cell lines *(187)*. Perhaps, one of the factors to consider when attempting to sensitize cells to chemotherapeutic drugs using MAPK inhibitors, is a frequent loss of apoptosis effectors proteins such as Apaf-1 in metastatic melanomas *(190)*, which may render cells chemoresistant even when survival signals are abrogated.

6. CONCLUDING REMARKS

In melanoma, genetic mutations in proto-oncogenes such as *BRAF* or *RAS* may be detected as early as in benign dysplastic nevi. Premalignant lesions characterized by radial growth frequently contain additional mutations in tumor suppressors genes *p16INK4a or/and p14ARF*, and, less frequently, *PTEN*, or *p53*. The progression to malignant local invasive disease, and metastatic dissemination is controlled molecularly through differential expression of transcription factors such as AP-2, CREB/ATF-1, ATF-2, Snail, microphthalmia-associated transcription factor, and NF-κB, resulting in the acquisition of the metastatic phenotype. Crucial step in melanoma progression is a loss of AP-2 and overexpression of ATF-1/CREB family transcription factors. The balance between these two effectors appears to be critical for regulating the repertoire of cell surface adhesion molecules such as MCAM/Muc-18, production of matrix degrading enzymes and angiogenic factors and receptors such as MMP-2 and PAR-1, expression of survival and apoptosis-related proteins such as fatty acid synthase/APO-1 and Bcl-2, and proliferation (HER-2).

The therapeutic modalities to control tumor growth and metastasis of human melanoma are very limited. Recent studies show that practical chemotherapeutic drugs such as DTIC or cisplatin, whereas being toxic, induce a stress response in melanoma cells that results in activation of MAPK cascade and stimulation of IL-8 and VEGF production. These are potent survival, angiogenic, and invasion-associated factors. Their overexpression may promote the invasion of host stroma by tumor cells and hence, the metastatic disease. In vitro, long-term cell treatment with DTIC selects for the resistant cells with very high levels of IL-8 and VEGF production, implying that treatment of melanoma patients with DTIC may produce a considerable hazard by selecting cells with a more aggressive melanoma phenotype. Reasonably, combination treatment of DTIC with anti-VEGF/IL-8 or MEK inhibitors may potentiate the therapeutic effects of the cytotoxic drug. Furthermore, based on our observations that MCAM/Muc-18 and IL-8 play a major role in the acquisition of the metastatic phenotype in human melanoma, we have developed two fully human antibodies targeting these molecules. In this chapter, we have presented evidence that these antibodies inhibited tumor growth, invasion, angiogenesis, and metastasis of melanoma in animal models. Currently, both of these antibodies are being evaluated in clinical trials.

REFERENCES

1. Hendrix MJ, Seftor RE, et al. Transendothelial function of human metastatic melanoma cells: role of the microenvironment in cell-fate determination. Cancer Res 2002; 62:6658.
2. Eshel R, Neumark E, Sagi-Assif O, Witz IP. Receptors involved in microenvironment-driven molecular evolution of cancer cells. Semin Cancer Biol 2002; 12:139–147.
3. de Braud F, Khayat D, Kroon BB, Valdagni R, Bruzzi P, Cascinelli N. Malignant melanoma. Crit Rev Oncol Hematol 2003; 47:35–63.
4. Fountain JW, Bale SJ, Housman DE and Dracopoli NC. Genetics of melanoma. Cancer Surv 1990; 9:645–671.
5. Flores JF, Walker GJ, Glendening JM, et al. Loss of the p16INK4a and p15INK4b genes, as well as neighboring 9p21 markers, in sporadic melanoma. Cancer Res 1996; 56:5023–5032.
6. Piccinin S, Doglioni C, Maestro R, et al. p16/CDKN2 and CDK4 gene mutations in sporadic melanoma development and progression. Clin Lab Med 1997; 20:667–690.
7. Halushka FG and Hodi FS. Molecular genetics of familial cutaneous melanoma. J Clin Oncol 1998; 16:670–682.
8. Monzon J, Liu L, Brill H, Goldstein AM, et al. CDKN2A mutations in multiple primary melanomas. N Engl J Med 1998; 338:879–887.
9. Gruis NA, van der Velden PA, Bergman W and Frants RR. Familial melanoma; CDKN2A and beyond. J Investig Dermatol Symp Proc 1999; 4:50–54.
10. Bishop DT, Demenais F, Goldstein AM, Bergman W, et al. Geographical variation in the penetrance of CDKN2A mutations for melanoma. J Natl Cancer Inst 2002; 94:894–903.
11. Ghiorzo P, Villaggio B, Sementa AR, et al. Expression and localization of mutant p16 proteins in melanocytic lesions from familial melanoma patients. Hum Pathol 2004; 35:25–33.
12. Talve L, Sauroja I, Collan Y, Punnonen K, Ekfors T. Loss of expression of the p16INK4/CDKN2 gene in cutaneous malignant melanoma correlates with tumor cell proliferation and invasive stage. Int J Cancer 1997; 74:255–259.
13. Pollock PM, Welch J, Hayward NK. Evidence for three tumor suppressor loci on chromosome 9p involved in melanoma development. Cancer Res 2001; 61:1154–1161.
14. Cachia AR, Indsto JO, McLaren KM, Mann GJ, Arends MJ. CDKN2A mutation and deletion status in thin and thick primary melanoma. Clin Cancer Res 2000; 6:3511–3515.
15. Straume O, Sviland L and Akslen LA. Loss of nuclear p16 protein expression correlates with increased tumor cell proliferation (Ki-67) and poor prognosis in patients with vertical growth phase melanoma. Clin Cancer Res 2000; 6:1845–1853.
16. Vuhahula E, Straume O and Akslen LA Frequent loss of p16 protein expression and high-proliferative activity (Ki-67) in malignant melanoma from black Africans. Anticancer Res 2000; 20:4857–4862.
17. Pavey SJ, Cummings MC, Whiteman DC, et al. Loss of p16 expression is associated with histological features of melanoma invasion. Melanoma Res 2000; 12:539–547.
18. Chang TG, Wang J, Chen LW, et al. Loss of expression of the p16 gene is frequent in malignant skin tumors. Biochem Biophys Res Commun 1997; 230:85–88.
19. Palmieri G, Cossu A, Ascierto PA, et al. Melanoma Cooperative Group. Definition of the role of chromosome 9p21 in sporadic melanoma through genetic analysis of primary tumours and their metastases, Br. J. Cancer 2000; 83:1707–1714.
20. Harris CC. p53: at the crossroads of molecular carcinogenesis and risk assessment. Science 1993; 262:1980–1981.
21. Ko LJ, Prives C. p53: puzzle and paradigm. Genes Dev 1996; 10:1054–1072.

22. Levine AJ. p53, the cellular gatekeeper for growth and division. Cell 1997; 88:323–31.
23. Volkenandt M, Schlegel U, Nanus DM and Albino AP. Mutational analysis of the human p53 gene in malignant melanoma. Pigment Cell Res 1991; 4:35–40.
24. Weiss J, Schwechheimer K, Cavenee WK, Herlyn M and Arden KC. Mutation and expression of the p53 gene in malignant melanoma cell lines. Int J Cancer 1993; 54(4):693–699.
25. Albino AP, Vidal MJ, McNutt NS, et a. Mutation and expression of the p53 gene in human malignant melanoma. Melanoma Res 1994; 4:35–45.
26. Lubbe J, Reichel M, Burg G, Kleihues P. Absence of p53 gene mutations in cutaneous melanoma. J Invest Dermatol 1994; 102:819–821.
27. Papp T, Jafari M, Schiffmann D. Lack of p53 mutations and loss of heterozygosity in non-cultured human melanocytic lesions. J Cancer Res Clin Oncol 1996; 122:541–548.
28. Sparrow LE, Soong R, Dawkins HJ, Iacopetta BJ, Heenan PJ. p53 gene mutation and expression in naevi and melanomas. Melanoma Res 1995; 5:93–100.
29. Hartmann A, Blaszyk H, Cunningham JS, et al. Overexpression and mutations of p53 in metastatic malignant melanomas. Int J Cancer 1996; 67:313–317.
30. M. Daniotti M, Oggionni T, Ranzani V, et al. BRAF alterations are associated with complex mutational profiles in malignant melanoma. Oncogene 2004; 23:5968–5977.
31. Davies H, Bignell GR, Cox C, Stephens P, et al. Mutations of the BRAF gene in human cancer. Nature 2002; 417:949–954.
32. Brose MS, Volpe P, Feldman M, et al. BRAF and RAS mutations in human lung cancer and melanoma. Cancer Res 2002; 62:6997–7000.
33. Cohen Y, Xing M, Mambo E, et al. BRAF mutation in papillary thyroid carcinoma. J Natl Cancer Inst 2003; 95:625–627.
34. Dong J, Phelps RG, Qiao R, et al. BRAF oncogenic mutations correlate with progression rather than initiation of human melanoma. Cancer Res 2003; 63:3883–3885.
35. Gorden A, Osman I, Gai W, et al. Analysis of BRAF and N-RAS mutations in metastatic melanoma tissues. Cancer Res 2003; 63:3955–3957.
36. Pollock PM, Pearson JV, Hayward NK. Compilation of somatic mutations of the CDKN2 gene in human cancers: non-random distribution of base substitutions. Genes Chromosomes Cancer 1996; 15:77–88.
37. Rajagopalan H, Bardelli A, Lengauer C, Kinzler KW, Vogelstein B, Velculescu VE. Tumorigenesis: RAF/RAS oncogenes and mismatch-repair status. Nature 2002; 418:934.
38. Weber A, Langhanki L, Sommerer F, Markwarth A, Wittekind C, Tannapfel A. Mutations of the BRAF gene in squamous cell carcinoma of the head and neck. Oncogene 2003; 22:4757–4759.
39. Xu X, Quiros RM, Gattuso P, Ain KB, Prinz RA. High prevalence of BRAF gene mutation in papillary thyroid carcinomas and thyroid tumor cell lines. Cancer Res 2003; 63:4561–4567.
40. Mercer KE, Pritchard CA. Raf proteins and cancer: B-Raf is identified as a mutational target. Biochim Biophys Acta 2000; 1653:25–40.
41. Lenormand P, Sardet C, Pages G, L'allemain G, Brunet A, Pouyssegur J. Growth factors induce nuclear translocation of MAP kinase (p42MAPK and p44MAPK) but not their activator MAP kinase kinase (p45MAPKK) in fibroblasts. J Cell Biol 1993; 122:1079–1088.
42. Treisman R. Ternary complex factors: growth factor regulated transcriptional activators. Curr Opin Genet Dev 1994; 4:96–101.
43. Pages G, Lenormand P, L'Allemain G, Chambard JC, Meloche S, Pouyssegur J. Mitogen-activated protein kinases p42mapk and p44mapk are required for fibroblast proliferation. Proc Natl Acad Sci USA 1993; 90:8319–8323.
44. Welsh CF, Roovers K, Villanueva J, Liu Y, Schwartz MA, Assoian RK. Timing of cyclin D1 expression within G1 phase is controlled by Rho. Nat Cell Biol 2001; 3:950–957.
45. Mattei S, Colombo MP, Melani C, Silvani A, Parmiani G, Herlyn M. Expression of cytokine/growth factors and their receptors in human melanoma and melanocytes. Int J Cancer 1994; 56:853–857.
46. Lazar-Molnar E, Hegyesi H, Toth S, Falus A. Autocrine and paracrine regulation by cytokines and growth factors in melanoma. Cytokine 2000; 12:547–54.
47. Nesbit M, Nesbit HKE, Bennett J, et al. Basic fibroblast growth factor induces a transformed phenotype in normal human melanocytes. Oncogene 1999; 18:6469–6476.
48. Satyamoorthy K, Li G, Vaidya B, Patel D, Herlyn M. Insulin-like growth factor-1 induces survival and growth of biologically early melanoma cells through both the mitogen-activated protein kinase and β-catenin pathways. Cancer Res 2001; 61:7318–7324.

49. Albino AP, Nanus DM, Mentle IR, et al. Analysis of ras oncogenes in malignant melanoma and precursor lesions: correlation of point mutations with differentiation phenotype. Oncogene 1989; 4:1363–1374.

50. van't Veer LJ, Burgering BM, Versteeg R, et al. N-*ras* mutations in human cutaneous melanoma from sun-exposed body sites. Mol Cell Biol 1989; 9:3114–3116.

51. Jafari M, Papp T, Kirchner S, et al. Analysis of ras mutations in human melanocytic lesions: activation of the ras gene seems to be associated with the nodular type of human malignant melanoma. J Cancer Res Clin Oncol 1995;121:23–30.

52. Omholt K, Karsberg S, Platz A, Kanter L, Ringborg U, Hanson J. Screening of N-*ras* codon 61 mutations in paired primary and metastatic cutaneous melanomas: mutations occur early and persist throughout tumor progression. Clin Cancer Res 2002; 8:3468–3474.

53. Omholt K, Platz A, Kanter L, Ringborg U, Hansson J. *NRAS* and *BRAF* mutations arise early during melanoma pathogenesis and are preserved throughout tumor progression. Clin Cancer Res 2003; 9:6483–6488.

54. Houben R, Becker JC, Kappel A, et al. Constitutive activation of the Ras–Raf signaling pathway in metastatic melanoma is associated with poor prognosis. J Carcinog 2000; 3:6.

55. Wu H, Goel V and Haluska FG. PTEN signaling pathways in melanoma. Oncogene 2003; 20:3113–3122.

56. Rodolfo M, Daniotti M, Vallacchi V. Genetic progression of metastatic melanoma. Cancer Lett 2004; 214:133–147.

57. Dhawan P, Singh AB, Ellis DL, Richmond A. Constitutive activation of Akt/protein kinase B in melanoma leads to up-regulation of nuclear factor-κB and tumor progression. Cancer Res 2002; 62:7335–7342.

58. Vleminckx K, Kemler R. Cadherins and tissue formation: integrating adhesion and signaling. Bioessays 1999; 21:211–220.

59. Guilford P. E-cadherin downregulation in cancer: fuel on the fire? Mol Med Today 1999; 5:172–177.

60. Timar J, Csuka O, Orosz Z, Jeney A, Kopper L. Molecular pathology of tumor metastasis. I. Predictive pathology. Pathol Oncol Res 2001; 7:217–230.

61. Shih IM, Elder DE, Hsu MY, Herlyn M. Regulation of Mel-CAM/MUC18 expression on melanocytes of different stages of tumor progression by normal keratinocytes. Am J Pathol 1994; 145:837–845.

62. Valyi-Nagy IT, Hirka G, Jensen PJ, Shih IM, Juhasz I, Herlyn M. Undifferentiated keratinocytes control growth, morphology, and antigen expression of normal melanocytes through cell-cell contact. Lab Invest. 1993; 69:152–159.

63. Danen EH, de Vries TJ, Morandini R, Ghanem GG, Ruiter DJ, van Muijen GN. E-cadherin expression in human melanoma. Melanoma Res 1996; 6:127–131.

64. Hsu MY, Wheelock MJ, Johnson KR, Herlyn M. Shifts in cadherin profiles between human normal melanocytes and melanomas. J Investig Dermatol Symp Proc 1996; 1:188–194.

65. Hsu MY, Meier FE, Nesbit M, et al. E-cadherin expression in melanoma cells restores keratinocyte-mediated growth control and down-regulates expression of invasion-related adhesion receptors. Am J Pathol 2000; 156:1515–1525.

66. Mortarini R, Anichini A. From adhesion to signalling: roles of integrins in the biology of human melanoma. Melanoma Res 1993; 3:87–97.

67. Poser I, Dominguez D, de Herreros AG, Varnai A, Buettner R, Bosserhoff AK. Loss of E-cadherin expression in melanoma cells involves up-regulation of the transcriptional repressor Snail. J Biol Chem 2001; 276:24,661–24,666.

68. Comijn J, Berx G, Vermassen P, et al. The two-handed E box binding zinc finger protein SIP1 downregulates E-cadherin and induces invasion. Mol Cell 2001; 7:1267–1278.

69. Jean D, Gershenwald JE, Huang S, et al. Loss of AP-2 results in up-regulation of MCAM/MUC18 and an increase in tumor growth and metastasis of human melanoma cells. J Biol Chem 1998; 273:16,501–16,508.

70. Huang S, Jean D, Luca M, Tainsky MA, Bar-Eli M. Loss of AP-2 results in downregulation of c-KIT and enhancement of melanoma tumorigenicity and metastasis. EMBO J 1998; 17:4358–4369.

71. Gershenwald JE, Sumner W, Calderone T, Wang Z, Huang S, Bar-Eli M. Dominant-negative transcription factor AP-2 augments SB-2 melanoma tumor growth in vivo. Oncogene 2001; 20:3363–3375.

72. Tang A, Eller MS, Hara M, Yaar M, Hirohashi S, Gilchrest BA. E-cadherin is the major mediator of human melanocyte adhesion to keratinocytes in vitro. J Cell Sci 1994; 107:983–992.

73. Li G, Satyamoorthy K, Herlyn M. N-cadherin-mediated intercellular interactions promote survival and migration of melanoma cells. Cancer Res 2001; 61:3819–3825.
74. Sandig M, Voura EB, Kalnins VI, Siu CH. Role of cadherins in the transendothelial migration of melanoma cells in culture. Cell Motil Cytoskeleton 1997; 38:351–364.
75. Voura EB, Sandig M, Siu CH. Cell-cell interactions during transendothelial migration of tumor cells. Microsc Res Tech 1998; 43:265–275.
76. Juliano RL, Varner JA. Adhesion molecules in cancer: the role of integrins. Curr Opin Cell Biol 1993; 5:812–818.
77. Danen EH, Van Muijen GN, Ruiter DJ. Role of integrins as signal transducing cell adhesion molecules in human cutaneous melanoma. Cancer Surv 1995; 24:43–65.
78. Mortarini R, Anichini A. From adhesion to signalling: roles of integrins in the biology of human melanoma. Melanoma Res 1993; 3:87–97.
79. Seftor RE, Seftor EA, Hendrix MJ. Molecular role(s) for integrins in human melanoma invasion. Cancer Metastasis Rev 1999; 18:359–375.
80. Johnson JP. Cell adhesion molecules in the development and progression of malignant melanoma. Cancer Metastasis Rev 1999; 18:345–357.
81. Albelda SM, Mette SA, Elder DE, Stewart R, Damjanovich L, Herlyn M, et al. Integrin distribution in malignant melanoma: association of the β 3 subunit with tumor progression. Cancer Res 1990; 50:6757–6764.
82. Danen EH, Jansen KF, Van Kraats AA, Cornelissen IM, Ruiter DJ, Van Muijen GN. Alpha v-integrins in human melanoma: gain of α v β 3 and loss of α v β 5 are related to tumor progression in situ but not to metastatic capacity of cell lines in nude mice. Int J Cancer 1995; 61:491–496.
83. Natali PG, Hamby CV, Felding-Habermann B, et al. Clinical significance of α(v)β3 integrin and intercellular adhesion molecule-1 expression in cutaneous malignant melanoma lesions. Cancer Res 1997; 57:1554–1160.
84. Schadendorf D, Gawlik C, Haney U, Ostmeier H, Suter L, Czarnetzki BM. Tumour progression and metastatic behaviour in vivo correlates with integrin expression on melanocytic tumours. J Pathol 1993; 170:429–434.
85. Brooks PC, Stromblad S, Sanders LC, et al. Localization of matrix metalloproteinase MMP-2 to the surface of invasive cells by interaction with integrin alpha v β 3. Cell 1996; 85:683–693.
86. Voura EB, Ramjeesingh RA, Montgomery AM, Siu CH. Involvement of integrin alpha(v)β(3) and cell adhesion molecule L1 in transendothelial migration of melanoma cells. Mol Biol Cell 2001; 12:2699–2710.
87. Lehmann JM, Holzmann B, Breitbart EW, Schmiegelow P, Riethmuller G, Johnson JP. Discrimination between benign and malignant cells of melanocytic lineage by two novel antigens, a glycoprotein with a molecular weight of 113,000 and a protein with a molecular weight of 76,000. Cancer Res 1987; 47:841–845.
88. Shih IM, Wang TL, Westra WH. Diagnostic and biological implications of mel-CAM expression in mesenchymal neoplasms. Clin Cancer Res 1996; 2:569–75.
89. Shih IM, Elder DE, Speicher D, Johnson JP, Herlyn M. Isolation and functional characterization of the A32 melanoma-associated antigen. Cancer Res 1994; 54:2514–20.
90. Johnson JP, Bar-Eli M, Jansen B, Markhof E. Melanoma progression-associated glycoprotein MUC18/MCAM mediates homotypic cell adhesion through interaction with a heterophilic ligand. Int J Cancer 1997; 73:769–774.
91. Shih LM, Hsu MY, Palazzo JP, Herlyn M. The cell-cell adhesion receptor Mel-CAM acts as a tumor suppressor in breast carcinoma. Am J Pathol 1997; 151:745–751.
92. Luca M, Hunt B, Bucana CD, Johnson JP, Fidler IJ, Bar-Eli M. Direct correlation between MUC18 expression and metastatic potential of human melanoma cells. Melanoma Res 1993; 3:35–41.
93. Holzmann B, Brocker EB, Lehmann JM, et al. Tumor progression in human malignant melanoma: five stages defined by their antigenic phenotypes. Int J Cancer 1987; 39:466–471.
94. Kraus A, Masat L, Johnson JP. Analysis of the expression of intercellular adhesion molecule-1 and MUC18 on benign and malignant melanocytic lesions using monoclonal antibodies directed against distinct epitopes and recognizing denatured, non-glycosylated antigen. Melanoma Res 1997; 7(Suppl 2):S75–S81.
95. Shih IM, Elder DE, Hsu MY, Herlyn M. Regulation of Mel-CAM/MUC18 expression on melanocytes of different stages of tumor progression by normal keratinocytes. Am J Pathol 1994; 145:837–845.
96. Xie S, Luca M, Huang S, Gutman M, Reich R, Johnson JP, Bar-Eli M. Expression of MCAM/MUC18 by human melanoma cells leads to increased tumor growth and metastasis. Cancer Res 1997; 57:2295–2303.

97. Mills L, Tellez C, Huang S, et al. Fully human antibodies to MCAM/MUC18 inhibit tumor growth and metastasis of human melanoma. Cancer Res 2002; 62:5106–5114.
98. Even-Ram S, Uziely B, Cohen P, et al. Thrombin receptor overexpression in malignant and physiological invasion processes. Nat Med 1998; 4:909–914.
99. Nierodzik ML, Chen K, Takeshita K, et al. Protease-activated receptor 1 (PAR-1) is required and rate-limiting for thrombin-enhanced experimental pulmonary metastasis. Blood, 1998; 92:3694–3700.
100. Henrikson KP, Salazar SL, Fenton JW II, Pentecost BT. Role of thrombin receptor in breast cancer invasiveness. Br J Cancer 1998; 79:401–416.
101. Telez C, Bar-Eli M. Role and regulation of the thrombin receptor (PAR-1) in human melanoma. Oncogene 2003; 22:3130–3137.
102. Wojtukiewicz MZ, Tang DG, Ben-Josef E, Renaud C, Walz DA, Honn KV. Solid tumor cells express functional "tethered ligand" thrombin receptor. Cancer Res 1995; 55:698–704.
103. Kaufmann R, Schafberg H, Rudroff C, Nowak G. Thrombin receptor activation results in calcium signaling and protein kinase C-dependent stimulation of DNA synthesis in HEp-2g laryngeal carcinoma cells. Cancer 1997; 80:2068–2074.
104. Rudroff C, Schafberg H, Nowak G, Weinel R, Scheele J, Kaufmann R. Characterization of functional thrombin receptors in human pancreatic tumor cells (MIA PACA-2). Pancreas 1998; 16:189–194.
105. Liu Y, Gilcrease MZ, Henderson Y, Yuan XH, Clayman GL, Chen Z. Expression of protease-activated receptor 1 in oral squamous cell carcinoma. Cancer Lett 2001; 169:173–180.
106. Zacharski LR, Memoli VA, Morain WD, Schlaeppi JM, Rousseau SM. Cellular localization of enzymatically active thrombin in intact human tissues by hirudin binding. Thromb. Haemost 1995; 73:793–797.
107. Ornstein DL and Zacharski LR. Treatment of cancer with anticoagulants: rationale in the treatment of melanoma. Int J Hematol 2001; 73:157–161.
108. Nierodzik ML, Chen K, Takeshita K, et al. Protease-activated receptor 1 (PAR-1) is required and rate-limiting for thrombin-enhanced experimental pulmonary metastasis. Blood 1998; 92:3694–3700.
109. Grand RJ, Turnell AS, Grabham PW. Cellular consequences of thrombin-receptor activation. Biochem J 1996; 313:353–368.
110. Macfarlane SR, Seatter MJ, Kanke T, Hunter GD, Plevin R. Proteinase-activated receptors. Pharmacol Rev 2001; 53:245–282.
111. Senger DR, Ledbetter SR, Claffey KP, Papadopoulos-Sergiou A, Peruzzi CA, Detmar M. Stimulation of endothelial cell migration by vascular permeability factor/vascular endothelial growth factor through cooperative mechanisms involving the $\alpha v \beta 3$ integrin, osteopontin, and thrombin. Am J Pathol 1996; 149:293–305.
112. Even-Ram SC, Maoz M, Pokroy E, et al. Tumor cell invasion is promoted by activation of protease activated receptor-1 in cooperation with the $\alpha v \beta 5$ integrin. J Biol Chem 2001; 276:10,952–10,962.
113. Zucker S, Conner C, DiMassmo BI, et al. Thrombin induces the activation of progelatinase A in vascular endothelial cells. Physiologic regulation of angiogenesis. J Biol Chem 1995; 270:23,730–23,738.
114. Yoshida E, Verrusio EN, Mihara H, Oh D, Kwaan HC. Enhancement of the expression of urokinase-type plasminogen activator from PC-3 human prostate cancer cells by thrombin. Cancer Res 1994; 54:3300–3304.
115. Shimizu S, Gabazza EC, Hayashi T, Ido M, Adachi Y, Suzuki K. Thrombin stimulates the expression of PDGF in lung epithelial cells. Am J Physiol 2000; 279:L503–L510.
116. Ueno A, Murakami K, Yamanouchi K, Watanabe M, Kondo T. Thrombin stimulates production of interleukin-8 in human umbilical vein endothelial cells. Immunology 1996; 88:76–81.
117. Huang YQ, Li JJ, Hu L, Lee M, Karpatkin S. Thrombin induces increased expression and secretion of VEGF from human FS4 fibroblasts, DU145 prostate cells and CHRF megakaryocytes. Thromb Haemost 2001; 86:1094–1098.
118. Cucina A, Borrelli V, Di Carlo A, et al. Thrombin induces production of growth factors from aortic smooth muscle cells. J Surg Res 1999: 82;61–66.
119. Duffy MJ: Proteases as prognostic markers in cancer. Clin Cancer Res 1996; 2:613–618.
120. Meyer T, Hart IR: Mechanisms of tumour metastasis. Eur J Cancer 1998; 34:214–221.
121. Sloane BF, Moin K, Krepela E, et al. Cathepsin B and its endogenous inhibitors: the role in tumor malignancy. Cancer Metastasis Rev 1990; 9:333–352.
122. Gershenwald JE, Sumner W, Calderone T, Wang Z, Huang S, Bar-Eli M. Dominant-negative transcription factor AP-2 augments SB-2 melanoma tumor growth in vivo. Oncogene 2001; 20:3363–3375.
123. Silletti S, Paku S, Raz A. Tumor cell motility and metastasis. Autocrine motility factor as an example of ecto/exoenzyme cytokines. Pathol Oncol Res 1997 ;3:230–254.

124. Ma PC, Maulik G, Christensen J, Salgia R. c-Met: structure, functions and potential for therapeutic inhibition. Cancer Metastasis Rev 2003; 22:309–325.

125. P'tgens AJG, Lubsen NH, van Altena MC, Schoenmakers JGG, Ruiter DJ, de Waal RMW. Vascular permeability factor expression influences tumor angiogenesis in human melanoma lines xenografted to nude mice. Am J Pathol 1995; 146:197–209.

126. Oku T, Tjuvajev JG, Miyagawa T, et al. Tumor growth modulation by sense and antisense vascular endothelial growth factor gene expression: effects on angiogenesis, vascular permeability, blood volume, blood flow, fluorodeoxyglucose uptake, and proliferation of human melanoma intracerebral xenografts. Cancer Res 1998; 58:4185–4192.

127. Claffey KP, Brown LF, del Aguila LF, et al. Expression of vascular permeability factor/vascular endothelial growth factor by melanoma cells increases tumor growth, angiogenesis, and experimental metastases. Cancer Res 1996; 56:172–181.

128. Rofstad EK, Danielsen T. Hypoxia-induced angiogenesis and vascular endothelial growth factor secretion in human melanoma. Br J Cancer 1998; 77:897–902.

129. Singh RK, Gutman M, Radinsky R, Bucana CD, Fidler IJ. Expression of interleukin 8 correlates with the metastatic potential of human melanoma cells in nude mice. Cancer Res, 1994; 54:3242–3247.

130. Luca M, Huang S, Gershenwald JE, Sing RK, Reich R, Bar-Eli M. Expression of interleukin-8 by human melanoma cells up-regulates MMP-2 activity and increases tumor growth and metastases. Am J Pathol 1997; 151:1105–1113.

131. Kunz M, Hartmann A, Flory E, et al. Anoxia-induced up-regulation of interleukin-8 in human malignant melanoma. Am J Pathol 1999; 155:753–763.

132. Leyva A, Appel H, Kraal I, Pinedo HM. Differential metabolism of thymidine in human lymphoid and melanoma cells in vitro. Anticancer Res 1984; 4:173–178.

133. Asgari MM, Haggerty JG, McNiff JM, Milstone LM, Schwartz PM. Expression and localization of thymidine phosphorylase/platelet-derived endothelial cell growth factor in skin and cutaneous tumors. J Cutan Pathol 1999; 26:287–294.

134. Halaban R, Kwon BS, Ghosh S, Delli Bovi P, Baird A. bFGF as an autocrine growth factor for human melanoma. Oncogene Res 1988; 3:177–186.

135. Becker D, Meier CB, Herlyn M. Proliferation of human malignant melanomas is inhibited by antisense oligodeoxynucleotides targeted against basic fibroblast growth factor. EMBO J 1989; 8:3685–3691.

136. Wang Y, Becker D. Antisense targeting of basic fibroblast growth factor and fibroblast growth factor receptor-1 in human melanomas blocks intratumoral angiogenesis and tumor growth. Nat Med 1997; 3:887–893.

137. Dvorak HF, Brown LF, Detmar M, Dvorak AM. Vascular permeability factor/vascular endothelial growth factor, microvascular hyperpermeability, and angiogenesis. Am J Pathol 1995; 146:1029–1039.

138. Ferrara N. Vascular endothelial growth factor. Eur J Cancer 1996; 32A:2413–2422.

139. Griffiths L, Stratford IJ. Platelet-derived endothelial cell growth factor thymidine phosphorylase in tumour growth and response to therapy. Br J Cancer 1997; 76:689–693.

140. Slavin J. Fibroblast growth factors: at the heart of angiogenesis. Cell Biol Int 1995; 19:431–444.

141. Ellis LM, Fidler IJ. Angiogenesis and metastasis. Eur J Cancer 1996; 32:2451–2460.

142. Bikfalvi A, Klein S, Pintucci G, Rifkin DB. Biological roles of fibroblast growth factor-2. Endocr Rev 1997; 18:26–45.

143. Koch AE, Polverini PJ, Kunkel SL, et al. Interleukin-8 as a macrophage derived mediator of angiogenesis. Science 1992; 258:1798–1801.

144. Bar-Eli M. Role of interleukin-8 in tumor growth and metastasis of human melanoma. Pathobiology 1999; 67:12–18.

145. Schadendorf D, Moller A, Algermissen B, Worm M, Sticherling M, Czarnetzki BM. 1993. IL-8 produced by human malignant melanoma cells in vitro is an essential autocrine growth factor. J Immunol 1993; 151:2667–2675.

146. Smith DR, Polverini PJ, Kunkel SL, et al. Inhibition of interleukin 8 attenuates angiogenesis in bronchogenic carcinoma. J Exp Med 1994; 179:1409–1415.

147. Westphal JR, Van't Hullenaar R, Peek R, et al. Angiogenic balance in human melanoma: Expression of VEGF, bFGF, IL-8, PDGF, and angiostatin in relation to vascular density of xenografts in vivo. Int J Cancer 2000; 86:768–776.

148. Luca M, Huang S, Gershenwald JE, Singh RK, Reich R, Bar-Eli M. Expression of interleukin-8 by human melanoma cells up-regulates MMP-2 activity and increases tumor growth and metastasis. Am J Pathol 1997; 151:1105–1113.

149. Yoshida S, Ono M, Shono T, et al. Involvement of interleukin-8, vascular endothelial growth factor, and basic fibroblast growth factor in tumor necrosis factor α-dependent angiogenesis. Mol Cell Biol 1997; 17:4015–4023.

150. Huang S, Mills L, Mian B, et al. Fully humanized neutralizing antibodies to interleukin-8 (ABX-IL8) inhibit angiogenesis, tumor growth, and metastasis of human melanoma. Am J Pathol 2002; 161:125–134.

151. Jean D, Bar-Eli M. Regulation of tumor growth and metastasis of human melanoma by the CREB transcription factor family. Mol Cell Biochem 2000; 212:19–28.

152. Nyormoi O, Bar-Eli M. Transcriptional regulation of metastasis-related genes in human melanoma. Clin Exp Metastasis 2003; 20:251–263.

153. Ronai Z, Yang YM, Fuchs SY, Adler V, Sardana M, Herlyn M. ATF2 confers radiation resistance to human melanoma cells. Oncogene 1998; 16:523–531.

154. Batlle E, Sancho E, Franci C, et al. The transcription factor snail is a repressor of E-cadherin gene expression in epithelial tumour cells. Nat Cell Biol 2000; 2:84–89.

155. Huang S, DeGuzman A, Bucana CD, Fidler IJ. Level of interleukin-8 expression by metastatic human melanoma cells directly correlates with constitutive NF-κB activity. Cytokines Cell Mol Ther 2000; 6:9–17.

156. Cowley GP, Smith ME. Cadherin expression in melanocytic naevi and malignant melanomas. J Pathol 1996; 179:183–187.

157. Jiang H, Su ZZ, Lin JJ, Goldstein NI, Young CS, Fisher PB. The melanoma differentiation associated gene mda-7 suppresses cancer cell growth. Proc Natl Acad Sci USA 1996; 93:9160–9165.

158. Natali PG, Nicotra MR, Digiesi G, et al. Expression of gp185HER-2 in human cutaneous melanoma: implications for experimental immunotherapeutics. Int J Cancer 1994; 56:341–346.

159. Descheemaeker KA, Wyns S, Nelles L, Auwerx J, Ny T, Collen D. Interaction of AP-1-, AP-2-, and Sp1-like proteins with two distinct sites in the upstream regulatory region of the plasminogen activator inhibitor-1 gene mediates the phorbol 12-myristate 13-acetate response. J Biol Chem 1992; 267:15,086–15,091.

160. van den Oord JJ, Vandeghinste N, De Ley M, De Wolf-Peeters C. Bcl-2 expression in human melanocytes and melanocytic tumors. Am J Pathol 1994; 145:294–300.

161. Gille J, Swerlick RA, Caughman SW. Transforming growth factor-α-induced transcriptional activation of the vascular permeability factor (VPF/VEGF) gene requires AP-2-dependent DNA binding and transactivation. EMBO J 1997; 16:750–759.

162. Silins G, Grimmond S, Egerton M, Hayward N. Analysis of the promoter region of the human VEGF-related factor gene. Biochem Biophys Res Commun 1997; 230:413–418.

163. Werner H, Stannard B, Bach MA, LeRoith D, Roberts CT Jr. Cloning and characterization of the proximal promoter region of the rat insulin-like growth factor I (IGF-I) receptor gene. Biochem Biophys Res Commun 1990; 169:1021–1027.

164. Xie S, Price JE, Luca M, Jean D, Ronai Z, Bar-Eli M. Dominant-negative CREB inhibits tumor growth and metastasis of human melanoma cells. Oncogene 1997; 15:2069–2075.

165. Jean D, Harbison M, McConkey DJ, Ronai Z, Bar-Eli M. CREB and its associated proteins act as survival factors for human melanoma cells. J Biol Chem 1998; 273:24884–90.

166. Jean D, Tellez C, Huang S, et al. Inhibition of tumor growth and metastasis of human melanoma by intracellular anti-ATF-1 single chain Fv fragment. Oncogene 2000; 19:2721–2730.

167. Medrano EE, Farooqui JZ, Boissy RE, Boissy YL, Akadiri B, Nordlund JJ. Chronic growth stimulation of human adult melanocytes by inflammatory mediators in vitro: implications for nevus formation and initial steps in melanocyte oncogenesis. Proc Natl Acad Sci USA 1993; 90:1790–1794.

168. Recio JA, Merlino G. Hepatocyte growth factor/scatter factor induces feedback up-regulation of CD44v6 in melanoma cells through Egr-1. Cancer Res 2003; 63:1576–1582.

169. Kim SJ, Wagner S, Liu F, O'Reilly MA, Robbins PD, Green MR. Retinoblastoma gene product activates expression of the human TGF-β 2 gene through transcription factor ATF-2. Nature 1992; 358:331–334.

170. Gupta S, Campbell D, Derijard B, Davis RJ. Transcription factor ATF2 regulation by the JNK signal transduction pathway. Science 1995; 267:389–393.

171. Kaszubska W, Hooft van Huijsduijnen R, Ghersa P, et al. Cyclic AMP-independent ATF family members interact with NF-κ B and function in the activation of the E-selectin promoter in response to cytokines. Mol Cell Biol 1993; 13:7180–7190.

172. Shimizu M, Nomura Y, Suzuki H, et al. Activation of the rat cyclin A promoter by ATF2 and Jun family members and its suppression by ATF4. Exp Cell Res 1998; 239:93–103.

173. Tsai EY, Jain J, Pesavento PA, Rao A, Goldfeld AE. Tumor necrosis factor α gene regulation in activated T cells involves ATF-2/Jun and NFATp. Mol Cell Biol 1996; 16:459–467.
174. Ivanov VN, Ronai Z. Down-regulation of tumor necrosis factor α expression by activating transcription factor 2 increases UVC-induced apoptosis of late-stage melanoma cells. J Biol Chem 1999; 274:14,079–14,089.
175. Bhoumik A, Ivanov V, Ronai Z. Activating transcription factor 2-derived peptides alter resistance of human tumor cell lines to ultraviolet irradiation and chemical treatment. Clin Cancer Res 2001; 7:331–342.
176. Ivanov VN, Ronai Z. p38 protects human melanoma cells from UV-induced apoptosis through down-regulation of NF-κB activity and Fas expression. Oncogene 2000; 19:3003–3012.
177. Poser I, Dominguez D, de Herreros AG, Varnai A, Buettner R, Bosserhoff AK. Loss of E-cadherin expression in melanoma cells involves up-regulation of the transcriptional repressor Snail. J Biol Chem 2001; 276:24,661–24,666.
178. Batlle E, Sancho E, Franci C, et al. The transcription factor snail is a repressor of E-cadherin gene expression in epithelial tumour cells. Nat Cell Biol 2000; 2:84–89.
179. Cano A, Perez-Moreno MA, Rodrigo I, et al. The transcription factor snail controls epithelial-mesenchymal transitions by repressing E-cadherin expression. Nat Cell Biol 2000; 2:76–83.
180. Arlt A, Schafer H. NFκB-dependent chemoresistance in solid tumors. Int J Clin Pharmacol Ther 2002; 40:336–47.
181. Duffey DC, Chen Z, Dong G, et al. Expression of a dominant-negative mutant inhibitor-κBα of nuclear factor-κB in human head and neck squamous cell carcinoma inhibits survival, proinflammatory cytokine expression, and tumor growth in vivo. Cancer Res 1999; 59:3468–3874.
182. McNulty SE, Tohidian NB, Meyskens FL Jr. RelA, p50 and inhibitor of κ B α are elevated in human metastatic melanoma cells and respond aberrantly to ultraviolet light B. Pigment Cell Res 2001; 14:456–465.
183. Huang S, DeGuzman A, Bucana CD, Fidler IJ. Nuclear factor-κB activity correlates with growth, angiogenesis, and metastasis of human melanoma cells in nude mice. Clin Cancer Res 2000; 6:2573–2581.
184. Ivanov VN, Fodstad O, Ronai Z. Expression of ring finger-deleted TRAF2 sensitizes metastatic melanoma cells to apoptosis via up-regulation of p38, TNFα and suppression of NF-κB activities. Oncogene 2001; 20:2243–2253.
185. Lev DC, Ruiz M, Mills L, McGary EC, Price JE, Bar-Eli M. Dacarbazine causes transcriptional up-regulation of interleukin 8 and vascular endothelial growth factor in melanoma cells: a possible escape mechanism from chemotherapy. Mol Cancer Ther 2003; 8:753–763.
186. Lev DC, Onn A, Melinkova VO, et al. Exposure of melanoma cells to dacarbazine results in enhanced tumor growth and metastasis in vivo. J Clin Oncol 2004; 22:2092–2100.
187. Mandic A, Viktorsson K, Heiden T, Hansson J, Shoshan MC. The MEK1 inhibitor PD98059 sensitizes C8161 melanoma cells to cisplatin-induced apoptosis. Melanoma Res 2001; 11:11–19.
188. Jansen B, Schlagbauer-Wadl H, Eichler HG, et al. Activated N-ras contributes to the chemoresistance of human melanoma in severe combined immunodeficiency (SCID) mice by blocking apoptosis. Cancer Res 1997; 57:362–365.
189. Borner C, Schlagbauer Wadl H, et al. Mutated N-ras upregulates Bcl-2 in human melanoma in vitro and in SCID mice. Melanoma Res 1999; 9:530.
190. Soengas MS, Capodieci P, Polsky D, et al. Inactivation of the apoptosis effector Apaf-1 in malignant melanoma. Nature 2001; 409:207–211.

11 The Microenvironment and Drug Resistance

Patrice J. Morin, PhD

CONTENTS

SUMMARY

Although much of the research into cancer drug resistance has focused on the cancer cells themselves, it is becoming increasingly clear that the tumor microenvironment can significantly affect the success of chemotherapy. The interactions between the tumor cells and their environment can be classified into three main categories: (1) cell–cell contacts, (2) interactions with the extracellular matrix, and (3) interactions with soluble factors/cytokines. Each of these interactions can influence the sensitivity of the tumor cells to treatment-induced apoptosis and can therefore affect the outcome of therapy. The pathways responsible for these effects are just beginning to be elucidated.

Key Words: Microenvironment; extracellular matrix; cytokines; growth factors; drug resistance; chemoresistance; apoptosis; anoikis.

1. INTRODUCTION

Much of the research into cancer drug resistance has focused on the cancer cells, but it is becoming increasingly clear that host factors can significantly affect the success of chemotherapy. For example, immune modulation, the pharmacological clearance of drug, and poor tolerance to the side effects can all affect the outcome of therapy *(1)*. Normal cells require cell contacts and growth factors for their survival. Moreover, it is now accepted that the tumor microenvironment, including the contacts between the tumor cells, can also influence the survival of cancer cells during treatment. This effect is clearly related to the ability of the environment to affect signaling pathways important for cell survival, cell cycle checkpoints, and other processes relevant to the response of cells to cytotoxic drugs. The apoptotic response of cancer cells in response to chemotherapeutic agents can therefore be affected by pathways controlled, at least in part, by the microen-

From: *Cancer Drug Discovery and Development: Cancer Drug Resistance*
Edited by: B. Teicher © Humana Press Inc., Totowa, NJ

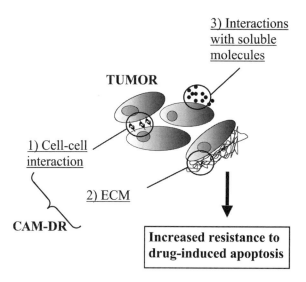

Fig. 1. Mechanisms of environment-mediated drug resistance. Cancer cells can develop drug resistance through three main types of interactions with the microenvironment: (1) direct cell-cell contacts, (2) extracellular matrix (ECM) interactions, both of which constitute cell-adhesion-mediated drug resistance (CAM-DR), and (3) binding of soluble molecules.

vironment. The importance of these noncell autonomous mechanisms of drug resistance has attracted an increasing amount of attention and will be discussed in this chapter

1.1. The Tumor Microenvironment

The cancer cell occupies an abnormal environment with altered extracellular matrix (ECM), increased amount of proteases, growth factors, as well as abnormal hypoxic conditions and altered stroma *(2)*. The first clue that the environment could affect tumor cell survival in the presence of cytotoxic agents was noted over 30 yr ago, when it was observed that multicellular spheroids of tumor cells were more resistant to anticancer agents than the corresponding monolayer cultures, and that these differences were not because of a compromised ability of the drug to penetrate the spheroids *(3)*. In addition to direct cell–cell contacts, the interactions of cancer cells with various soluble factors and with components of the ECM can drastically affect the apoptotic sensitivity of these cells and their response to chemotherapeutic drugs (Fig. 1). The multidrug resistance phenotype that results from direct cell contact with the ECM or other cells has been coined "cell-adhesion-mediated drug resistance," or CAM-DR *(4)*, and appears to be related to an adhesion-dependent suppression of apoptosis. In the next subheading, each type of tumor cell–microenvironment interaction is described.

2. DRUG RESISTANCE

As mentioned above, the interactions between tumor cells and the environment can be divided into two main categories: the cell-adhesion-type interactions and the soluble factor interactions (*see* Fig. 1). The cell adhesion interactions can further be divided into direct cell–cell contact interactions and cell–ECM interactions. Drug resistance that stems from these last two types of interactions has been termed CAM-DR *(4)*.

2.1. Cell-Adhesion-Mediated Drug Resistance

2.1.1. Cell–Cell Contacts (Multicellular Resistance)

The first indications that cell–cell interactions may influence survival to cytotoxic drugs came to light when it was observed that multicellular spheroids were more resistant to radiation exposure than cells grown in monolayers *(5)*. This particular type of drug resistance, observed when cells are grown as three-dimensional (3-D) masses, as been coined multicellular resistance (MR) *(6)* and can be considered a subtype of CAM-DR. Indeed, it appears that cells grown as 3-D cultures more closely recapitulate the drug resistance properties of in vivo cells compared to the more typical 2-D (monolayers) cultures used in most laboratories *(7)*. MR has been shown to encompass a wide variety of cytotoxic agents, including alkylating agents *(8,9)*, taxol *(10)*, and multidrug resistance *(11)*. In addition, since the initial study *(5)*, many reports have confirmed that MR can protect cells from ionizing radiation *(9,12,13)*. Similar findings of MR have been reported in many different experimental systems (Table 1) *(7,11,14,15)*. Interestingly, it has also been shown that cell–cell interaction disruption (using an anticadherin antibody) can sensitize cancer cells to a host immune response *(16)*.

Although the exact mechanisms of MR are still being elucidated, cadherin molecules have been shown to play an important role. E-cadherin, an epithelial homophilic cell–cell adhesion molecule, was shown to play role in the MR exhibited by human Lovo and MCF-7 cancer cells *(17)*. Indeed, the presence of a neutralizing E-cadherin antibody could decreases p27 levels and drug resistance in 3-D cultures, but did not affect drug resistance in 2-D cultures of cells that did not express E-cadherin. Similar findings were reported in HT-29 cells where treatment of cells with neutralizing E-cadherin antibodies was found to decrease resistance to a variety of agents such as 5-fluorouracil, paclitaxel, vinblastine, and etoposide but not cisplatin *(18)*. This is consistent with findings that p27 plays a major role in chemoresistance and that E-cadherin can upregulate p27 *(19,20)*. Interestingly, it was shown that forced overexpression of p27 in cells expressing E-cadherin, abolished the effects of neutralizing E-cadherin antibodies on the proliferation of these cells *(19)*, clearly implicating p27 downstream of E-cadherin. Consistent with this hypothesis downregulation of p27 has been associated with drug resistance in many experimental systems *(21,22)*. In addition, it was recently reported that the *PMS2* gene and the overall mismatch repair gene activity was downregulated in spheroids of EMT-6 cells compared to monolayer cultures, suggesting a new mechanisms as a determinant of MR *(23)*.

2.1.2. Extracellular Matrix

The ECM, a complex assembly of collagen, proteoglycans and other molecules, is an important constituent of normal tissues and provides essential cues for cell development, migration, adhesion, proliferation, survival, and other metabolic functions *(24)*. ECM components typically interact with integrins, a family of α- and β-transmembrane proteins, which associate to form heterodimeric receptors *(25)*. The roles of integrins in cell survival have been studied extensively, and it is now known that the loss of ECM–integrin interactions can lead to anoikis, a specialized form of apoptosis *(26)*. For example, early studies showed that fibronectin can promote anchorage-independent growth of eosinophils and Chinese hamster ovary cells through mechanisms that involve inhibition of anoikis *(27,28)*. There are certainly reasons to believe that the same types of mechanisms may also promote resistance to drug-mediated apoptosis *(29)*. Indeed, tumor cells are

Table 1

Select Studies on the Effect of the Microenvironment on Cancer Drug Resistance

Type of resistance	Cell line/cancer	Culture system	Drug(s)	Reference
Multicellular	MCF7 and MCF7-MDR	Spheroids	MDR	11
Multicellular	EMT-6 murine mammary sublines	Spheroids	Cisplatin, Phosphoramide	8
Multicellular	4 Human ovarian carcinoma cell lines	Spheroids	Taxol	10
Multicellular	V79 Chinese hamster cells	Spheroids	Radiation	5
Multicellular	HT29 colon carcinoma cell line	Xenograft	Immune response	16
Multicellular	EMT-6 murine mammary, MCF-7	Spheroids, xeno	Alkylating (4HC)	20
Multicellular	OVCAR 3	Spheroids	Radiation	13
Multicellular	Human squamous carcinoma cell lines (A431 and CaSki)	Spheroids	Radiation	12
Multicellular	Human Lovo and MCF-7	Spheroids	?	17
Multicellular	EMT-6 murine mammary sublines	Spheroids	5-FU, Taxol, vinblastine, etoposide	18
Multicellular	EMT-6 murine mammary sublines	Spheroids	alkylating agents, cisplatin	23
ECM-mediated	Tumor endothelium	Monolayers	Etoposide	30
ECM-mediated	Small cell lung cancer lines	Monolayers	Etoposide, cyclophosphamide, and γ-radiation	31
ECM-mediated	LS174T and LiM6 colon cancer lines	Monolayers	5-FU, Camptothecin, etoposide	32
ECM-mediated	Ovarian cancer cell line	Monolayers	Cisplatin	33
ECM-mediated	Small cell lung cancer	Monolayers	Doxorubicin, etoposide	34
ECM-mediated	HMT-3522 murine epithelial cell cancer model	3-D cultures	Fas, etoposide	35
ECM-mediated	RPMI 8226 myeloma cell line	Suspension	Doxorubicin, melphalan	39
ECM-mediated	RPMI 8226 myeloma cell line	Suspension	Etoposide	40
ECM-mediated	PC3 prostate cancer cell line	Monolayers	TNF-α	41
Soluble factor (IL-6)	Multiple myeloma primary tumors and cell lines	Suspension, patients	Dexamethasone	63
Soluble factor (IL-6)	Prostate cancer cell lines PC-3 and DU145	Monolayers	Cisplatin, etoposide, adriamycin	64
Soluble factor (IL-6)	MCF-7 cell line derivatives	Monolayers	Doxorubicin, vincristine, taxol	65
Soluble factor (HGF)	Rhabdomyosarcomas cell lines	Suspension/mono layers	Ionizing radiations, vincristine, etoposide,	70
Soluble factor (IGF-1)	Murine colon cancer cell line	Monolayers	Actinomycin, lovastatin, doxorubicin	71
Soluble factor (FGF-2)	HT1376 bladder cancer cell line line	Monolayers, xenografts	Cisplatin	72
Soluble factor (IGF)	HepG2 and Huh-7	Monolayers	Anthracycline	74

ECM, extracellular matrix; 5-FU, Fluorouracil; 3-D, three-dimensional; TNF-α, tumor necrosis factor-α; IL-6, interleukin 6; HGF, hepatocyte growth factor; IGF-1, insulin-like growth factor I; FGF-2, fibroblast growth factor 2.

surrounded by ECM produced by neighboring stromal cells, the cancer cells themselves, or other cells in the tumor microenvironment. These ECM components can interact with tumor cell integrins and affect their behavior, including their sensitivity to apoptosis. For example, adhesion to fibronectin or other ECM components such as various collagens and laminins has been shown to prevent drug-induced apoptosis *(30–35)*. In many systems, integrins were shown to be the mediator of these effects. Other studies have demonstrated the involvement of other ECM proteins such as collagen IV, fibronectin, and tenascin, which are elevated in small cell lung cancer *(34)*. These ECM proteins were found to protect small cell lung cancer cells from chemotherapy-induced apoptosis using various chemotherapeutic drugs, and there was evidence that the signaling was through the integrin $\beta 1$ receptor.

Interestingly, some evidence suggest that integrin-mediated changes in polarity and tissue architecture may be key in drug resistance as opposed to simple activation of the integrin receptors. Weaver and collaborators recently showed that in breast cancer cells, reconstituted basement membrane, a specialized ECM for epithelial cells, can lead to the formation of polarized structures, which are essential in protecting these cells from chemotherapy-induced apoptosis *(35,36)*. As a clue to possible downstream signals that may result from these interactions, chemoresistance was accompanied by nuclear factor (NF)-κB activation, a transcription factor that has been involved in mediating survival signals *(37)*. Similarly, myeloma cells strongly induce NF-κB when adhered to fibronectin *(38)*.

The effects of ECM on myeloma cell survival has been studied extensively. It has been demonstrated that fibronectin interactions with the β-1 integrins may be important in inhibiting drug-induced apoptosis and therefore promoting cell survival *(39)*. Again, similar to what was observed with MR, p27 appeared to play an important role *(40)*, suggesting that these different mechanisms of drug resistance may converge at the molecular level. In addition, up-regulation of Bcl-2 *(28)* and, as mentioned above, activation of NF-κB *(38)* may also play a role in fibronectin-mediated cell survival. Fibronectin has also been shown to promote survival in many solid tumors such as prostate cancer *(41)*, breast cancer *(42)*, and colon cancer *(32)*.

In addition to integrins, other receptors are known to interact with the ECM. For example, CD44 has been shown to bind hyaluronate *(43)*, collagen *(44)*, and fibronectin *(45)*. In a fashion similar to the integrins, the CD44 receptor is involved in a wide range of physiological processes, including invasion and survival. In addition, many tumors have been shown to overexpress abnormal CD44 variant, especially colon cancer cells *(46)*, where it has been suggested to contribute to drug resistance *(47)*. Again, the increased drug resistance was attributable to a decrease in sensitivity to drug-induced apoptosis *(47,48)*. Similar findings have been reported in other cancers, including lymphoid malignancies *(49)*.

In the past several years, the tumor vasculature has emerged as a prime target for cancer therapy using specific antiangiogenic compounds *(50–52)*. The tumor vasculature is also a target of conventional chemotherapy and the efficacy of cancer drugs may, at least in part, be because of their ability to destroy the tumor vasculature *(53)*. It has been reported that fibronectin can inhibit drug-mediated apoptosis in tumor-derived endothelial cells *(30)*, making this interaction an attractive new target for tumor therapy *(54)*, and providing evidence that ECM interactions can also protect tumors through their ability to provide survival signals to endothelial cells during chemotherapy.

Because tumor cells are known to produce ECM components, there is a possibility that they may produce their own favorable ECM, thereby increasing their resistance to chemotherapy. Indeed, a study of ovarian cancer gene expression recently found that collagen VI is one of the genes most highly upregulated in a model of acquired cisplatin resistance in vitro *(55)*. In addition, collagen VI is expressed in many ovarian tumors in vivo but absent from normal ovarian epithelial cells. It has been hypothesized that the tumor cells may produce collagen VI and other ECM components to reorganize the ECM and increase their resistance to apoptosis *(56)*. Indeed, ovarian cells adhered to collagen VI exhibit an increased survival when exposed to a variety of anticancer drugs *(55)*. In addition, it has been suggested that the tumor cells may secrete various cytokines and growth factors that may lead the neighboring stroma to produce protective ECM proteins *(57)*.

An important point that will need to be clarified is whether the ECM interactions necessary for tumor survival in the presence of drug are dependent on tumor type. It appears likely that different cancers will have different optimal requirements for ECM-mediated protection. For example, collagen IV and laminin have been shown to increase resistance of lung cancer cells to various agents *(34)*. Our own work shows that collagen VI, but not collagen I, may be crucial in establishing interactions leading to cisplatin resistance in ovarian cancer *(55)*. A reconstituted basement membrane (Matrigel) is necessary for decreasing drug-induced apoptosis in breast cancer cells *(35)*. Whereas these interactions are likely to be extremely complex and tumor specific, it is possible that they will lead to the activation of similar intracellular pathways that may in turn represent an attractive target for therapy aimed at reversing chemoresistance (*see* Section 3.).

2.2. Soluble Factors: Growth Factors, Cytokines

The tumor microenvironment is also rich in soluble factors, cytokines, growth factors, secreted by the stroma or by the tumor cells themselves. Interleukin (IL)-6, a cytokine secreted by bone marrow stromal cells, has been observed to be a survival factor in various normal, leukemic, and myeloma cells *(58–62)*. IL-6 can protect against chemo-therapy-induced apoptosis and therefore induce drug resistance in myeloma cells *(63)*. Interestingly, IL-6 has also been shown to promote drug resistance in prostate cancer cells *(64)*, and autocrine production of IL-6 has been shown to cause drug resistance in breast cancer *(65)*. Activation of the IL-6 receptor is believed to lead to downstream signaling through the Janus kinase/signal transducer and activator of transcription pathway *(66)*, the mitogen-activated protein kinase cascade *(67)*, the phosphoinositide 3 kinase/Akt pathway *(68)*, and X-linked mammalian inhibitor of apoptosis protein *(69)*, all of which are believed to be important in controlling survival and apoptosis. Growth factors also influence drug response in solid tumors. For example, pathways involving insulin-like growth factor I, epidermal growth factor, hepatocyte growth factor, and basic fibroblast growth factor have all been shown to influence the survival of various cancers in the presence of chemotherapeutic drugs *(70–74)*.

2.3. Alterations of the Physical Properties of the Environment Affecting Drug Delivery

In addition to its effects on tumor cell signaling, the environment may also affect the ability of therapeutic agents to effectively reach the tumor cells *(75)*. For example, the ECM can influence physical properties such as mechanical stiffness in the tumor, affecting diffusion of drugs *(76)*. Overall, the limited ability of drugs to reach tumor cells, especially cells that are distant from blood vessels, may be an important component of the effect of the environment on drug resistance *(77)*.

3. REVERSAL STRATEGIES

Drug resistance is a major problem that has attracted significant attention from researchers in the field of cancer research. However, from a clinical standpoint, most efforts have focused on the identification of alternative therapies against resistant tumors as opposed to the identification of targets that may reverse the resistance to conventional, proven therapy. Whereas, in principle, this represents a sound strategy, in practice it has been observed that tumor cells often exhibit crossresistance to many antitumor agents. This may be due, at least in part, to the fact that these cells tend to be generally more resistant to apoptosis *(78)*, and that this phenomenon may not be compound dependent. Importantly, the identification of specific pathways responsible for drug resistance may provide targets for combination therapy aimed at circumventing or decreasing resistance *(79)*. Therefore, intervention aimed at reducing the interactions between the environment and the tumor cells may increase the efficiency of cytotoxic therapy. For example, inhibition of the interactions between the ECM and the integrins or blocking of downstream signaling pathways represent promising avenues *(80)*. In addition, inhibition of various growth factors receptors such as epidermal growth factor receptor may also sensitize tumor cells to conventional chemotherapy *(73,81)*. This area of research is crucial, as it is becoming increasingly evident that even treatment with new generation of mechanism-based targeted drugs such as Gleevec®, a highly specific Bcr-Abl kinase inhibitor, can lead to the development of resistance in the treated cells.

4. CONCLUSIONS/PERSPECTIVES

Whereas it is clear that conventional mechanisms such as altered expression or mutations of genes involved in DNA repair, growth, and apoptosis are crucial in the development of drug resistance, there is a broad range of evidence for a role of the microenvironment (*see* Table 1). The resistant tumors arising from strong selection during chemotherapy will be a sum of the genetic changes that favor tumor growth in the presence of the drug, including those affecting the interactions of the cells with their environment. Although much energy has been devoted to identifying the cell-autonomous mechanisms leading to drug resistance, increasing efforts are being devoted to understanding the effects of the microenvironment on resistance. These efforts will likely lead to a more global understanding of the mechanisms involved in drug resistance and may provide novel specific targets for drugs aimed at reversing drug resistance.

REFERENCES

1. Gottesman MM. Mechanisms of cancer drug resistance. Annu Rev Med 2002; 53:615–627.
2. Liotta LA, Kohn E. Anoikis: cancer and the homeless cell. Nature 2004; 430:973–974.
3. Durand RE, Sutherland RM. Effects of intercellular contact on repair of radiation damage. Exp Cell Res 1972; 71:75–80.
4. Dalton WS. The tumor microenvironment as a determinant of drug response and resistance. Drug Resist Updat 1999; 2:285–258.
5. Sutherland RM, Durand RE. Cell contact as a possible contribution to radiation resistance of some tumours. Br J Radiol 1972; 45:788–789.
6. Green SK, Frankel A, Kerbel RS. Adhesion-dependent multicellular drug resistance. Anticancer Drug Des 1999; 14:153–168.
7. St. Croix B, Kerbel RS. Cell adhesion and drug resistance in cancer. Curr Opin Oncol 1997; 9:549–556.
8. Kobayashi H, Man S, Graham CH, Kapitain SJ, Teicher BA, Kerbel RS. Acquired multicellular-mediated resistance to alkylating agents in cancer. Proc Natl Acad Sci U S A 1993; 90:3294–3298.

9. St. Croix BS, Rak JW, Kapitain S, Sheehan C, Graham CH, Kerbel RS. Reversal by hyaluronidase of adhesion-dependent multicellular drug resistance in mammary carcinoma cells. J Natl Cancer Inst 1996; 88:1285–1296.

10. Frankel A, Buckman R, Kerbel RS. Abrogation of taxol-induced G2-M arrest and apoptosis in human ovarian cancer cells grown as multicellular tumor spheroids. Cancer Res 1997; 57:2388–2393.

11. dit Faute MA, Laurent L, Ploton D, Poupon MF, Jardillier JC, Bobichon H. Distinctive alterations of invasiveness, drug resistance and cell-cell organization in 3D-cultures of MCF-7, a human breast cancer cell line, and its multidrug resistant variant. Clin Exp Metastasis 2002; 19:161–168.

12. Kwok TT, Sutherland RM. The influence of cell-cell contact on radiosensitivity of human squamous carcinoma cells. Radiat Res 1991; 126:52–57.

13. Filippovich IV, Sorokina NI, Robillard N, Chatal JF. Radiation-induced apoptosis in human ovarian carcinoma cells growing as a monolayer and as multicell spheroids. Int J Cancer 1997; 72:851–859.

14. Teicher BA, Herman TS, Holden SA, et al. Tumor resistance to alkylating agents conferred by mechanisms operative only in vivo. Science 1990; 247(Pt 1):1457–1461.

15. Desoize B, Jardillier J. Multicellular resistance: a paradigm for clinical resistance? Crit Rev Oncol Hematol 2000; 36:193–207.

16. Green SK, Karlsson MC, Ravetch JV, Kerbel RS. Disruption of cell-cell adhesion enhances antibody-dependent cellular cytotoxicity: implications for antibody-based therapeutics of cancer. Cancer Res 2002; 62:6891–68900.

17. Nakamura T, Kato Y, Fuji H, Horiuchi T, Chiba Y, Tanaka K. E-cadherin-dependent intercellular adhesion enhances chemoresistance. Int J Mol Med 2003; 12:693–700.

18. Green SK, Francia G, Isidoro C, Kerbel RS. Antiadhesive antibodies targeting E-cadherin sensitize multicellular tumor spheroids to chemotherapy in vitro. Mol Cancer Ther 2004; 3:149–159.

19. St Croix B, Sheehan C, Rak JW, Florenes VA, Slingerland JM, Kerbel RS. E-Cadherin-dependent growth suppression is mediated by the cyclin-dependent kinase inhibitor p27[KIP1]. J Cell Biol 1998; 142:557–571.

20. St. Croix B, Florenes VA, Rak JW, et al. Impact of the cyclin-dependent kinase inhibitor p27[Kip1] on resistance of tumor cells to anticancer agents. Nat Med 1996; 2:1204–1210.

21. Brown I, Shalli K, McDonald SL, et al. Reduced expression of p27 is a novel mechanism of docetaxel resistance in breast cancer cells. Breast Cancer Res 2004; 6:R601–R107.

22. Nahta R, Takahashi T, Ueno NT, Hung MC, Esteva FJ. P27[kip1] down-regulation is associated with trastuzumab resistance in breast cancer cells. Cancer Res 2004; 64:3981–3986.

23. Francia G, Man S, Teicher B, Grasso L, Kerbel RS. Gene expression analysis of tumor spheroids reveals a role for suppressed DNA mismatch repair in multicellular resistance to alkylating agents. Mol Cell Biol 2004; 24:6837–6849.

24. survival. J Cell Sci 2002; 115(Pt 19):3729–3738.

25. Jin H, Varner J. Integrins: roles in cancer development and as treatment targets. Br J Cancer 2004; 90:561–565.

26. Frisch SM, Screaton RA. Anoikis mechanisms. Curr Opin Cell Biol 2001; 13:555–562.

27. Anwar AR, Moqbel R, Walsh GM, Kay AB, Wardlaw AJ. Adhesion to fibronectin prolongs eosinophil survival. J Exp Med 1993; 177:839–843.

28. Zhang Z, Vuori K, Reed JC, Ruoslahti E. The α 5 β 1 integrin supports survival of cells on fibronectin and up-regulates Bcl-2 expression. Proc Natl Acad Sci U S A 1995; 92:6161–6165.

29. Shain KH, Dalton WS. Cell adhesion is a key determinant in de novo multidrug resistance (MDR): new targets for the prevention of acquired MDR. Mol Cancer Ther 2001; 1:69–78.

30. Hoyt DG, Rusnak JM, Mannix RJ, Modzelewski RA, Johnson CS, Lazo JS. Integrin activation suppresses etoposide-induced DNA strand breakage in cultured murine tumor-derived endothelial cells. Cancer Res 1996; 56:4146–4149.

31. Kraus AC, Ferber I, Bachmann SO, et al. In vitro chemo- and radio-resistance in small cell lung cancer correlates with cell adhesion and constitutive activation of AKT and MAP kinase pathways. Oncogene 2002; 21:8683–8695.

32. Kouniavsky G, Khaikin M, Zvibel I, et al. Stromal extracellular matrix reduces chemotherapy-induced apoptosis in colon cancer cell lines. Clin Exp Metastasis 2002; 19:55–60.

33. Maubant S, Cruet-Hennequart S, Poulain L, et al. Altered adhesion properties and alphav integrin expression in a cisplatin-resistant human ovarian carcinoma cell line. Int J Cancer 2002; 97:186–194.

34. Sethi T, Rintoul RC, Moore SM, et al. Extracellular matrix proteins protect small cell lung cancer cells against apoptosis: a mechanism for small cell lung cancer growth and drug resistance in vivo. Nat Med 1999; 5:662–668.

35. Weaver VM, Lelievre S, Lakins JN, et al. β4 integrin-dependent formation of polarized three-dimensional architecture confers resistance to apoptosis in normal and malignant mammary epithelium. Cancer Cell 2002; 2:205–216.

36. Zahir N, Weaver VM. Death in the third dimension: apoptosis regulation and tissue architecture. Curr Opin Genet Dev 2004; 14:71–80.

37. Wang CY, Mayo MW, Baldwin AS Jr. TNF- and cancer therapy-induced apoptosis: potentiation by inhibition of NF-κB. Science 1996; 274(5288):784–787.

38. Landowski TH, Olashaw NE, Agrawal D, Dalton WS. Cell adhesion-mediated drug resistance (CAM-DR) is associated with activation of NF-κB (RelB/p50) in myeloma cells. Oncogene 2003; 22:2417–2421.

39. Damiano JS, Cress AE, Hazlehurst LA, Shtil AA, Dalton WS. Cell adhesion mediated drug resistance (CAM-DR): role of integrins and resistance to apoptosis in human myeloma cell lines. Blood 1999; 93:1658–1667.

40. Hazlehurst LA, Damiano JS, Buyuksal I, Pledger WJ, Dalton WS. Adhesion to fibronectin via β1 integrins regulates p27[kip1] levels and contributes to cell adhesion mediated drug resistance (CAM-DR). Oncogene 2000; 19:4319–4327.

41. Fornaro M, Plescia J, Chheang S, et al. Fibronectin protects prostate cancer cells from tumor necrosis factor-alpha-induced apoptosis via the AKT/survivin pathway. J Biol Chem 2003; 278:50,402–50,411.

42. Noti JD, Johnson AK. Integrin α 5 β 1 suppresses apoptosis triggered by serum starvation but not phorbol ester in MCF-7 breast cancer cells that overexpress protein kinase C-alpha. Int J Oncol 2001; 18:195–201.

43. Aruffo A, Stamenkovic I, Melnick M, Underhill CB, Seed B. CD44 is the principal cell surface receptor for hyaluronate. Cell 1990; 61:1303–1313.

44. Carter WG, Wayner EA. Characterization of the class III collagen receptor, a phosphorylated, transmembrane glycoprotein expressed in nucleated human cells. J Biol Chem 1988; 263:4193–4201.

45. Jalkanen S, Jalkanen M. Lymphocyte CD44 binds the COOH-terminal heparin-binding domain of fibronectin. J Cell Biol 1992; 116:817–825.

46. Matsumura Y, Tarin D. Significance of CD44 gene products for cancer diagnosis and disease evaluation. Lancet 1992; 340:1053–1058.

47. Bates RC, Edwards NS, Burns GF, Fisher DE. A CD44 survival pathway triggers chemoresistance via lyn kinase and phosphoinositide 3-kinase/Akt in colon carcinoma cells. Cancer Res 2001; 61:5275–5283.

48. Lakshman M, Subramaniam V, Rubenthiran U, Jothy S. CD44 promotes resistance to apoptosis in human colon cancer cells. Exp Mol Pathol 2004; 77:18–25.

49. Allouche M, Charrad RS, Bettaieb A, Greenland C, Grignon C, Smadja-Joffe F. Ligation of the CD44 adhesion molecule inhibits drug-induced apoptosis in human myeloid leukemia cells. Blood 2000; 96:1187–1190.

50. Boehm T, Folkman J, Browder T, O'Reilly MS. Antiangiogenic therapy of experimental cancer does not induce acquired drug resistance. Nature 1997; 390:404–407.

51. O'Reilly MS, Boehm T, Shing Y, et al. Endostatin: an endogenous inhibitor of angiogenesis and tumor growth. Cell 1997; 88:277–285.

52. Folkman J. Angiogenesis inhibitors: a new class of drugs. Cancer Biol Ther 2003; 2(Suppl 1):S127–S133.

53. Miller KD, Sweeney CJ, Sledge GW Jr. Redefining the target: chemotherapeutics as antiangiogenics. J Clin Oncol 2001; 19:1195–1206.

54. Kalluri R. Basement membranes: structure, assembly and role in tumour angiogenesis. Nat Rev Cancer 2003; 3:422–433.

55. Sherman-Baust CA, Weeraratna AT, Rangel LBA, et al. Remodeling of the extracellular matrix through overexpression of collagen VI contributes to cisplatin resistance in ovarian cancer cells. Cancer Cell 2003; 3:377–86.

56. Morin PJ. Drug resistance and the microenvironment: nature and nurture. Drug Resist Updat 2003; 6:169–172.

57. Rintoul RC, Sethi T. Extracellular matrix regulation of drug resistance in small-cell lung cancer. Clin Sci (Lond) 2002; 102:417–424.

58. Lotem J, Sachs L. Selective regulation of the activity of different hematopoietic regulatory proteins by transforming growth factor β 1 in normal and leukemic myeloid cells. Blood 1990; 76:1315–1322.

59. Lotem J, Cragoe EJ Jr, Sachs L. Rescue from programmed cell death in leukemic and normal myeloid cells. Blood 1991; 78:953–960.

60. Klein B, Zhang XG, Lu ZY, Bataille R. Interleukin-6 in human multiple myeloma. Blood 1995; 85:863–872.

61. Chauhan D, Kharbanda S, Ogata A, et al. Interleukin-6 inhibits Fas-induced apoptosis and stress-activated protein kinase activation in multiple myeloma cells. Blood 1997; 89:227–234.
62. Lichtenstein A, Tu Y, Fady C, Vescio R, Berenson J. Interleukin-6 inhibits apoptosis of malignant plasma cells. Cell Immunol 1995; 162:248–255.
63. Frassanito MA, Cusmai A, Iodice G, Dammacco F. Autocrine interleukin-6 production and highly malignant multiple myeloma: relation with resistance to drug-induced apoptosis. Blood 2001; 97:483–489.
64. Borsellino N, Belldegrun A, Bonavida B. Endogenous interleukin 6 is a resistance factor for *cis*-diamminedichloroplatinum and etoposide-mediated cytotoxicity of human prostate carcinoma cell lines. Cancer Res 1995; 55:4633–4639.
65. Conze D, Weiss L, Regen PS, et al. Autocrine production of interleukin 6 causes multidrug resistance in breast cancer cells. Cancer Res 2001; 61:8851–8858.
66. Catlett-Falcone R, Landowski TH, Oshiro MM, et al. Constitutive activation of Stat3 signaling confers resistance to apoptosis in human U266 myeloma cells. Immunity 1999; 10:105–115.
67. Ogata A, Chauhan D, Teoh G, et al. IL-6 triggers cell growth via the Ras-dependent mitogen-activated protein kinase cascade. J Immunol 1997; 159:2212–2221.
68. Hideshima T, Nakamura N, Chauhan D, Anderson KC. Biologic sequelae of interleukin-6 induced PI3-K/Akt signaling in multiple myeloma. Oncogene 2001; 20:5991–6000.
69. Yamagiwa Y, Marienfeld C, Meng F, Holcik M, Patel T. Translational regulation of x-linked inhibitor of apoptosis protein by interleukin-6: a novel mechanism of tumor cell survival. Cancer Res 2004; 64:1293–1298.
70. Jankowski K, Kucia M, Wysoczynski M, et al. Both hepatocyte growth factor (HGF) and stromal-derived factor-1 regulate the metastatic behavior of human rhabdomyosarcoma cells, but only HGF enhances their resistance to radiochemotherapy. Cancer Res 2003; 63:7926–7935.
71. Guo YS, Jin GF, Houston CW, Thompson JC, Townsend CM Jr. Insulin-like growth factor-I promotes multidrug resistance in MCLM colon cancer cells. J Cell Physiol 1998; 175:141–148.
72. Miyake H, Hara I, Gohji K, Yoshimura K, Arakawa S, Kamidono S. Expression of basic fibroblast growth factor is associated with resistance to cisplatin in a human bladder cancer cell line. Cancer Lett 1998; 123:121–126.
73. Navolanic PM, Steelman LS, McCubrey JA. EGFR family signaling and its association with breast cancer development and resistance to chemotherapy (review). Int J Oncol 2003; 22:237–252.
74. Alexia C, Fallot G, Lasfer M, Schweizer-Groyer G, Groyer A. An evaluation of the role of insulin-like growth factors (IGF) and of type-I IGF receptor signalling in hepatocarcinogenesis and in the resistance of hepatocarcinoma cells against drug-induced apoptosis. Biochem Pharmacol 2004; 68:1003–1015.
75. Jain RK. Vascular and interstitial barriers to delivery of therapeutic agents in tumors. Cancer Metastasis Rev 1990; 9:253–266.
76. Jain RK. The next frontier of molecular medicine: delivery of therapeutics. Nat Med 1998; 4:655–657.
77. Tannock IF, Lee CM, Tunggal JK, Cowan DS, Egorin MJ. Limited penetration of anticancer drugs through tumor tissue: a potential cause of resistance of solid tumors to chemotherapy. Clin Cancer Res 2002; 8:878–884.
78. Bunz F. Cell death and cancer therapy. Curr Opin Pharmacol 2001; 1:337–341.
79. Baird RD, Kaye SB. Drug resistance reversal—are we getting closer? Eur J Cancer 2003; 39:2450–2461.
80. Damiano JS. Integrins as novel drug targets for overcoming innate drug resistance. Curr Cancer Drug Targets 2002; 2:37–43.
81. Ciardiello F, De Vita F, Orditura M, Tortora G. The role of EGFR inhibitors in nonsmall cell lung cancer. Curr Opin Oncol 2004; 16:130–135.

III BIOCHEMICAL RESISTANCE

12 Glutathione and Glutathione *S*-Transferases in Drug Resistance

Victoria J. Findlay, PhD,
Danyelle M. Townsend, PhD,
and Kenneth D. Tew, PhD

Contents

Summary

The major roles of glutathione (GSH) and glutathione S-transferases (GSTs) in the detoxification of xenobiotics predicts their important role in drug resistance. As such, both GSH and GSTs have been manipulated as targets in the design of novel chemotherapeutic drugs. The discovery that GSTs have additional roles in the cell as regulatory molecules in the mitogen-activated protein kinase pathways together with the more recent discovery of GSH as a regulatory posttranslational modification lend further weight to their already important roles in the anticancer drug resistance response. These findings highlight the importance of these targets in the creation of future novel anticancer drugs. This chapter gives a brief overview of the importance of both GSH and GST in the response to anticancer drug resistance, and highlights some of the anticancer drugs currently being investigated at various stages in the process from lab to clinic.

Key Words: Glutathione; glutathione S-transferase; drug resistance; cancer; MAPK pathway.

1. GENERAL INTRODUCTION

Reactive oxygen species (ROS) are generated as a result of normal cellular metabolism, which is critical for the generation of energy in biological systems. Although low amounts of ROS are easily tolerated by the cell, abnormally high levels of ROS induce

From: *Cancer Drug Discovery and Development: Cancer Drug Resistance*
Edited by: B. Teicher © Humana Press Inc., Totowa, NJ

oxidative stress (OS), leading to cellular damage. In fact, ROS are implicated in a wide variety of diseases including Parkinson's, Alzheimer's, and cancer *(1)*. ROS are also produced after exposure to ionizing radiation, selected chemotherapeutic agents, hyperthermia, inhibition of antioxidant enzymes, or depletion of cellular reductants such as NADPH and glutathione (GSH). Consequently, cells have evolved protective mechanisms including antioxidants that detoxify ROS, and tolerable levels are maintained because of a complex redox buffering system.

The sensitivity of cells to OS depends on their intrinsic antioxidant systems, in particular, the levels of GSH within the cell. When GSH levels are low, the cellular environment will be oxidizing and the functioning of enzymes, particularly those with thiol groups, will be altered. A caveat to this complex defense system is the fact that the production of ROS is a mechanism shared by many chemotherapeutic agents. The ability of cells to detoxify exogenous substrates means that components of the cellular redox system may be targeted to enhance cell killing in the case of tumors.

2. GLUTATHIONE

GSH homeostasis is maintained in cells by a complex series of balanced pathways. *De novo* synthesis can occur through the γ-glutamyl cycle, where the three constituent amino acids (Glu-Cys-Gly) are combined with rate-limiting catalysis through γ-glutamylcysteine synthetase. Salvage of GSH can occur through the cleavage activity of the membrane associated γ-glutamyl transpeptidase, which can recycle constituents of the molecule. Whereas intracellular concentrations of GSH may vary considerably, 0.1–10 mM are not uncommonly found in mammalian cells (10–30 μM in plasma). Glutathione can occur in reduced (GSH), oxidized (GSSG), or in mixed disulfide forms, and its ubiquitous abundance is testament to its biological importance. The GSH:GSSG ratio is the major cellular redox sensor and determines the antioxidative capacity of the cell, although it can be affected by other redox sensors within the cell. As such, intracellular GSH contributes toward redox balance, and the variety of pathways that synthesize or use GSH influence this homeostasis. Owing to its reactivity and high intracellular concentrations, GSH has been implicated in resistance to several chemotherapeutic agents. Included among these are platinum-containing compounds, alkylating agents such as melphalan, anthracyclines including doxorubicin, as well as arsenic.

GSH participates in many cellular reactions directly as a free radical and ROS scavenger and indirectly as a cofactor in enzymatic reactions. During these processes, GSH is oxidized to GSSG. To restore homeostasis, GSSG is subsequently reduced by the NADPH-dependent glutathione reductase. GSH also reacts with exogenous substrates such as the aforementioned drugs that are subsequently removed from the cellular milieu via efflux through the multidrug resistance-associated protein, a member of the ATP-binding cassette transporter superfamily. In this capacity, GSH has a major role in the cell's survival to commonly used chemotherapeutic agents.

3. GSH IN SIGNALING

One of the more interesting conundrums to emerge from the completion of the genome project is the realization that humans are a composite of <30,000 genes, and yet complexity of protein structure/function seems distinctly more layered. In the burgeoning era of proteomics, it becomes clear that the central dogma of genetic determinism can be influ-

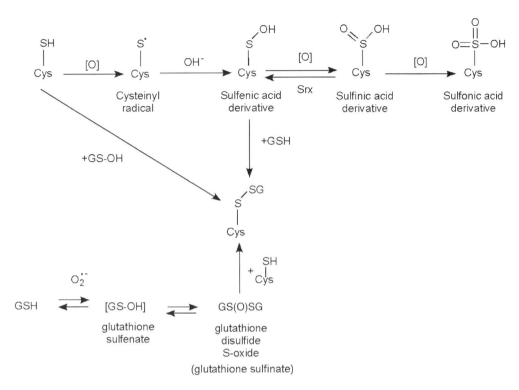

Fig. 1. Possible mechanisms of reactive oxygen species-induced protein glutathionylation. Reactive oxygen species may induce glutathionylation of protein thiols by many different routes. Those highlighted here include the direct oxidation of protein cysteines to generate a reactive protein thiol intermediate such as the reactive cysteinyl radical or sulfenic acid which further reacts with glutathione (GSH) to form a mixed disulfide. Alternatively, a mixed disulfide is formed through reaction with oxidized forms of GSH, i.e., GS-OH or GS(O)SG.

enced by a number of processes that include, polymorphic variants, gene splicing events, exon shuffling, protein domain rearrangements, and the large number of posttranslational modifications that contribute to alterations in tertiary and quaternary protein structure. Amongst these, phosphorylation, glycosylation, methylation, and acetylation can account for a large proportion of modifications. More recently, however, addition of GSH to available Cys residues (glutathionylation) has been shown to be of consequence (Fig. 1). The importance of modifying Cys residues is not necessarily restricted to redox regulation, but now seems to be a plausible event that can lead to changes in protein function and thereby signaling processes, particularly in response to a divergent number of stresses *(2)*. By adding GSH to a target protein, an additional negative charge is introduced (as a consequence of the Glu residue), and a change in protein conformation is made likely. The implication from this somewhat terse analysis is that cells actively participate in the stochastic production of multiple protein building blocks with the intent of realizing functional nonredundancy. Adding a further layer of complexity is the understanding that proteins do not act in isolation in a cellular milieu. Rather, essential protein:protein interactions govern how cellular events unfold. This process has proved to be significant to the regulation of JNK (c-Jun N-terminal kinase) signaling by GST-π *(3,4)*. This same paradigm seems to hold for thioredoxin and GST-μ with respect to the apoptosis signal-regulating kinase, ASK1 *(5)*, implying the possible existence of a general regulatory mechanism for kinases that may involve GSH and associated pathways *(6)*.

Emergent literature suggests that direct glutathionylation of critical signaling molecules may serve as a trigger for cellular events that are influenced by oxidative stress *(7,8)*. More specifically, Cross and Templeton *(8)* identified that site-specific glutathionylation of the ATP-binding domain of mitogen-activated protein kinase (MAPK) kinase kinase (MEKK1) functions as an inhibitory regulator of the MAPK pathway in response to oxidative stress. In this capacity it serves to distinguish between ASK1, which promotes an apoptotic signal, and MEKK1 which promotes a cell survival signal, toward MAPK kinase 4 and stress-activated protein kinase/JNK1 *(8)*. In addition, this inhibitory modification appears to be "dominant" over activation of the kinase by phosphorylation.

The small GTPase Ras modulates diverse signaling pathways and modification, by nitrosation, of its critical Cys-118 in the GTP-binding region has been shown to lead to an increase in Ras activity and to downstream signaling. However, more recent studies show glutathionylation of Ras at Cys-118 is a critical step in the redox-sensitive signaling leading to the activation of p38 and Akt, events that contribute to hypertrophic signaling induced by angiotensin II (AII) *(7)*. AII increases production of ROS from NAD(P)H oxidase that activates downstream kinases p38 and Akt, a response that contributes to vascular dystrophy.

NE-F2 related factor (Nrf2) is a redox-sensitive transcription factor that has been implicated in cellular responses to OS. Nrf2 regulates numerous genes through the antioxidant response element, such as GSH synthesis enzymes *(9,10)*. Generation of ROS leads to the dissociation of Nrf2 from its cytoplasmic anchor Kelch-like ECH-associating protein 1, which allows Nrf2 to relocate to the nucleus where antioxidant response element responsive genes become actively transcribed *(11)*. This dissociation is largely because of modification of key cysteine residues in Kelch-like ECH-associating protein 1. Recent studies now implicate GSH in the dissociation/nuclear translocation of Nrf2, through a type I (thiylation) redox switch, which is distinct from the transcription factor binding to DNA regulated by thioredoxin *(12)*.

Glutathionylation is emerging as a significant posttranslational modification that affects protein function and cellular response. The relevance of glutathionylation with respect to disease state, and the question of whether or not it is protective or detrimental in nature is an ongoing "hot spot" in research. The future promises to hold many potentially interesting insights into the significance of this modification and the importance of GSH within the cell will continue to grow.

4. GLUTATHIONE *S*-TRANSFERASE

GSTs (EC 2.5.1.18) are a family of phase II detoxification enzymes that promote the conjugation of GSH to an electrophilic center of endogenous and exogenous compounds, resulting in the formation of the corresponding GSS conjugates *(13)*. The mechanism by which GSTs increase the rate of GSH conjugation involves deprotonation of GSH to GS by a tyrosine residue, which functions as a base catalyst. GST isoenzymes have been divided into at least seven classes based on amino acid sequence similarity, five of which are cytosolic (designated α, μ, π, θ, and κ), and two are membrane-bound. Several isoenzymes, including those from μ, π, and θ, have been shown to be polymorphic in humans (for a review, *see* ref. *14*).

Development of drug resistance is a key element in the failure of chemotherapy treatment. Exposure to anticancer agents leads to the induction and expression of gene products that protect the cell. GSTs have been implicated in the development of resistance toward chemotherapy agents *(15)*. It is plausible that GSTs serve two distinct roles in the development of drug resistance via direct detoxification as well as acting as an inhibitor of the MAPK pathway. Hence, it is not surprising that high levels of GSTs have been reported in a large number of tumors types *(15)*.

The connection between GST and their role in the regulation of MAPK pathways is relatively recent. GST-π plays a key role in the regulation of the MAPK pathway through a protein:protein interaction with JNK, a kinase involved in stress response *(3,16)*. In nonstressed cells, JNK activity is low and is located in the cytoplasm bound to GST-π. Under conditions of OS, more specifically UV irradiation and H_2O_2 treatment, oligomerization of GST-π occurs together with the release and phosphorylation of JNK. Phosphorylated JNK is the active form, which then translocates to the nucleus, activating downstream transcription factors involved in gene expression and/or the induction of apoptosis. The precise mechanism of the disruption of the complex is unknown; however, oligomerization of the GST monomers implicates intermolecular disulfide bridge formation between available Cys residues. Furthermore, the lack of catalytic activity for the regulation of the JNK pathway, shown by the mutation of the essential Tyr (Tyr-7) residue in the active site of the enzyme, suggests a novel nonenzymatic role for this enzyme *(3)*. Upstream regulation of the MAPK pathways by GST is also observed, as demonstrated by the GST-μ:ASK1 complex. ASK1 is a MAP kinase kinase kinase (MAPKKK) that activates JNK and p38 pathways leading to cytokine- and stress-induced apoptosis *(17)*. ASK1 is activated in response to OS and heat shock. Like JNK, the activity of ASK1 is low in nonstressed cells because of its sequestration via protein:protein interactions with GST-μ and or thioredoxin *(5,18)*. The mechanism by which ASK1 is released from and activated by either of these proteins is distinct. GST-μ is responsive to heat shock, whereas thioredoxin responds to OS. The discovery of the involvement of GSTs in the regulation of these MAPK pathways, together with the known involvement of other small redox-regulated proteins adds an extra layer of complexity to these MAPK pathways with respect to signaling towards cell survival or cell death.

Other recent studies have broadened the role of GSTs. Small redox active protein families such as peroxiredoxin (Prx) have the potential to heterodimerize with GST-π. Studies have shown that full activation of PrxVI requires heterodimerization of the oxidized protein with GST-π, followed by glutathionylation of its conserved Cys (Cys-47) in a sterically protected region *(19)*. Dissociation from GST-π, followed by spontaneous reduction of glutathionylated protein by GSH, results in catalytically active protein. Whereas PrxVI contains a single Cys residue, six other mammalian Prxs have been identified that all contain two conserved cysteine residues *(20)*. This observation broadens the functional importance of GST-π into yet another arena.

5. GSH AND GSTs AS THERAPEUTIC AGENTS

GSTs are upregulated in a number of human tumors and as such, are promising therapeutic targets in research. A number of potential anticancer agents have been designed with this in mind using several different approaches. The first approach was to design inhibitors of GST exploiting its role as a detoxifying enzyme. Another approach was to find inhibitors of the protein:protein interaction of GST with kinases from the stress-activated protein kinase pathways. A third strategy involved the exploitation of the elevation of GSTs in tumors, with particular emphasis of the π isoform, through design of GST-activated prodrugs.

In the past, modulation of GSH and GST has been attempted as a means to improve response to cancer drugs. Lowering GSH levels in order to increase drug response being the ultimate goal. Use of, for example, buthionine sulfoximine and ethacrynic acid, whereas effective in their experimental effects on each system, was not successful enough in the clinic to merit continued development (21,22). One consequence of these approaches was the conceptual design of a peptidomimetic inhibitor of GST-π, γ-glutamyl-S-(benzyl)cysteinyl-R-‾phenyl glycine diethyl ester (TLK199). It was shown to potentiate the toxicity of numerous anticancer agents in different tumor cell lines. In addition, TLK199 was shown to be an inhibitor of multidrug resistance-associated protein, which is a known multidrug efflux transporter (23). Preclinical and mechanism of action studies with this agent revealed an unexpected effect in animals, namely that the drug possessed myeloproliferative activity through disruption of the GST-π:JNK complex (24,25). As an extension of these data, the company has sponsored a phase I/II trial of TLK199 (now named Telintra™) in patients with myelodysplastic syndrome.

Another novel GSH peptidomimetic anticancer agent, NOV-002, is a platinum coordination complex of oxidized glutathione. This drug has undergone significant clinical testing in Russia, and evidence of efficacy has been reported in 340 patients with diseases such as non-small cell lung cancer, colorectal, pancreatic, and breast cancer (26). These trials are now being repeated in the United States. Of interest, the drug also acted on the bone marrow, with increases in circulating lymphocyte, monocytes, T-cell, and NK cell counts.

Examples of GSH-activated prodrugs, which ultimately takes advantage of the elevated levels of GSH, include the novel thiopurine prodrugs cis-6-(2-acetylvinylthio) purine (cis-AVTP) and trans-6-(2-acetylvinylthio)guanine (trans-AVTG), which are α,β-unsaturated conjugates of the thiopurines 6-mercaptopurine and 6-thioguanine, respectively. These prodrugs have been shown to react rapidly with cellular thiols (like GSH) to yield the respective thiopurines as the major metabolites (27). As already mentioned, these drugs take advantage of the elevated levels of GSH observed in tumor cells, and the upregulated levels of GSH associated with chemotherapeutic drug resistance. Indeed, less bone marrow and intestinal toxicity was observed in mice after multiple treatments with the prodrugs than after equivalent treatments with 6-thioguanine (28). More recently, cytotoxicity analysis using the National Cancer Institutes' anticancer screening program showed the prodrugs to have enhanced in vitro cytotoxicity when compared with the parent thiopurines (29).

Many efforts are focused on GST-targeted agents. The rationale for such efforts lies with accumulated observations about GST expression in tumor and normal tissues. In particular, the association between high levels of expression of GST isozymes and malignancy and drug resistance (30) provided an ideal rationale for the design of GST-π activated prodrugs. In many instances, the GST-π isozyme can accumulate to levels that make it one of the more prevalent cytosolic proteins. In addition, even when the selecting drug is not a substrate for GST-π, its expression is most readily enhanced in drug resistant cells. Such data complicated interpretation of the connection between GST-π and drug resistance in cell culture (31) and in clinical trials (26). Largely because of the connection between GST-π, JNK, and apoptosis pathways (16), there is now a clearer understanding of why increased GST-π is associated with so many divergent acquired drug resistant situations.

Exploitation of elevated levels of GSTs to preferentially activate drugs led to the development of γ-glutamyl-α-amino-β(2-ethyl-N,N,N',N'-tetrakis (2-chloroethyl) phosphorodiamidate)-sulfonyl)-propionyl-(R)-‾phenylglycine (TLK286) and O^2-[2,4-

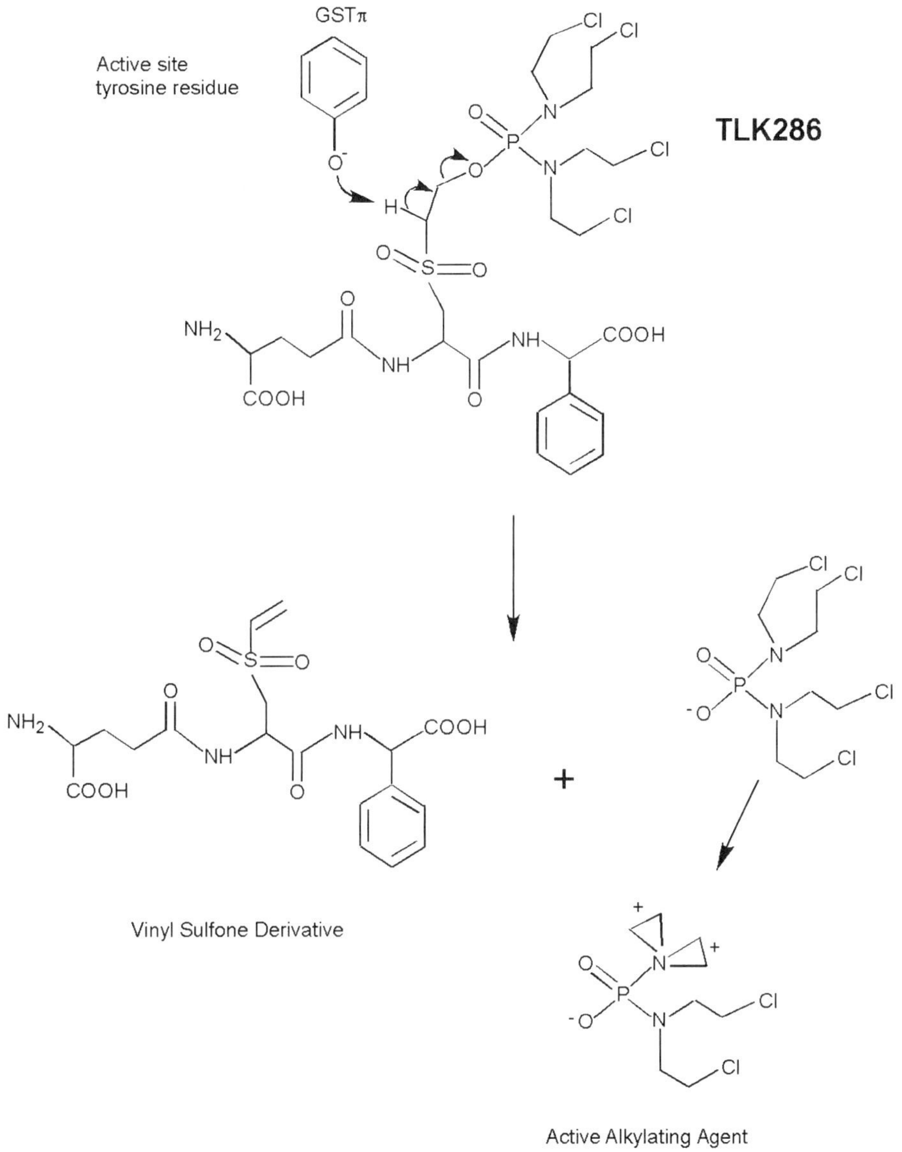

Fig. 2. Structure of γ-glutamyl-α-amino-β(2-ethyl-*N,N,N',N'*-tetrakis (2-chloroethyl) phosphoro-diamidate)-sulfonyl)-propionyl-(R)-⁻phenylglycine (TLK286) and its activation by glutathione *S*-transferase-π (GST-π).

dinitro-5-(*N*-methyl-*N*-4-carboxyphenylamino) phenyl] 1-*N,N*-dimethylamino)diazen-1-ium-1,2-diolate (PABA/NO). The early rationale for design, synthesis and testing of TLK286 incorporated the principle that enhanced tumor GST-π levels would preferentially activate more of the toxic phosphorodiamidate alkylating species (Fig. 2) with a commensurate advantage in therapeutic index *(32,33)*. Drug sensitivity is correlated with increased levels of GST-π both in vitro and in vivo. TLK286 is also under active testing in phase III settings for a number of disease states including non-small cell, ovarian, and colon cancers.

Another more recent example of a GST-activated prodrug is PABA/NO, a novel nitric oxide-releasing agent *(34)*. Studies show that cells lacking GST-π in vitro are less sensitive to the cytotoxic effects of PABA/NO. The activation of JNK and p38 also appears to be important for the cytotoxic effects of PABA/NO, as the inhibition of these pathways led to a reduction in cell death. In vivo antitumor data suggest PABA/NO as a good lead compound for further structure activity and drug discovery efforts.

6. CONCLUDING REMARKS

The traditional view of ROS is that they have a negative effect on cell function and viability, and therefore, substances that inhibit their reactivity (i.e., antioxidants) must be beneficial to cells. The increasing recognition of roles of ROS in cell signaling and modification of gene expression has forced a reevaluation of this simplistic view *(35)*. It has been demonstrated that GSH and GSTs have roles that extend much further than simple detoxification reactions. Indeed, it is not unreasonable to predict that glutathionylation may provide regulatory control complementary to other well-studied and established posttranslational modifications. Future studies will shed an advanced knowledge of the proteins involved in the cells response to "stress" and the interplay of proteins within the cell, with not only themselves in an enzymatic manner, but with other proteins in a regulatory fashion.

REFERENCES

1. Townsend DM, Tew KD, Tapeiro H. The importance of glutathione in human disease. Biomed Pharmacother 2003; 57:145–155.
2. Giustarini D, Rossi R, Milzani A, Colombo R, Dalle-Donne I. S-glutathionylation: from redox regulation of protein functions to human diseases. J Cell Mol Med 2004; 8:201–212.
3. Adler V, Yin Z, Fuchs SY, et al. Regulation of JNK signaling by GST-π.. EMBO J 1999; 18:1321–1334.
4. Wang T, Arifoglu P, Ronai Z, Tew KD. Glutathione S-transferase P1-1 (GSTP1-1) inhibits c-jun N-terminal kinase (JNK1) signaling through interaction with the C terminus. J Biol Chem 2001; 276:20,999–21,003.
5. Saitoh M, Nishitoh H, Fujii M, et al. Mammalian thioredoxin is a direct inhibitor of apoptosis signal-regulating kinase (ASK) 1. EMBO J 1998; 17:2596–2606.
6. Adler, Yin Z, Tew KD and Ronai Z. Role of redox potential and reactive oxygen species in stress signaling. Oncogene 1999; 18:6104–6111.
7. Adachi T, Pimentel DR, Heibeck T, et al. S-glutathiolation of Ras mediates redox-sensitive signaling by angiotensin II in vascular smooth muscle cells. J Biol Chem 2004; 279:29,857–29,862.
8. Cross JV, Templeton DJ. Oxidative stress inhibits MEKK1 by site-specific glutathionylation in the ATP binding domain. Biochem J 2004; 381:675–683.
9. Moinova HR, Mulcahy RT. Up-regulation of the human γ-glutamylcysteine synthetase regulatory subunit gene involves binding of Nrf-2 to an electrophile response element. Biochem Biophys Res Commun 1999; 261:661–668.
10. Kwak MK, Kensler TW, Casero RA. Induction of phase 2 enzymes by serum oxidized polyamines through activation of Nrf2: effect of the polyamine metabolite acrolein. Biochem Biophys Res Commun 2003; 305:662–670.
11. Nguyen T, Sherratt PJ, Pickett CB. Regulatory mechanisms controlling gene expression mediated by the antioxidant response element. Annu Rev Pharmacol Toxicol 2003; 43:233–260.
12. Hansen JM, Watson WH, Jones DP. Compartmentation of Nrf-2 redox control: Regulation of cytoplasmic activation by glutathione and DNA binding by thioredoxin-1. Toxicol Sci 2004; 82:308–317.
13. Armstrong RN. Structure, catalytic mechanism and evolution of the glutathione transferases. Chem Res Toxicol 1997; 10:2–18.
14. Townsend DM, Tew KD. The role of glutathione S-transferase in anti-cancer drug resistance. Oncogene 2003; 22:7369–7375.

15. Tew KD. Glutathione-associated enzymes in anticancer drug resistance. Cancer Res 1994; 54:4313–4320.

16. Yin Z, Ivanov V, Habelhah H, Tew KD, Ronai Z. Glutathione *S*-transferase p elicits protection against H_2O_2-induced cell death via coordinated regulation of stress kinases. Cancer Res 2000; 60:4053–4057.

17. Ichijo H, Nshida E, Irie K, et al. Induction of apoptosis by ASK1, a mammalian MAPKKK that activates SAPK/JNK and p38 signaling pathways. Science 1997; 275:90–94.

18. Cho SG, Lee YH, Park HS, et al. Glutathione *S*-transferase mu modulates the stress-activated signals by suppressing apoptosis signal-regulating kinase 1. J Biol Chem 2001; 276:12,749–12,755.

19. Manevich Y, Feinstein SI, Fisher AB. Activation of the antioxidant enzyme 1-CYS peroxiredoxin requires glutathionylation mediated by heterodimerization with πGST. Proc Natl Acad Sci U S A 2004; 101:3780–3785.

20. Kang SW, Baines IC, Rhee SG. Characterization of a mammalian peroxiredoxin that contains one conserved cysteine. J Biol Chem 1998; 273:6303–6311.

21. O'Dwyer PJ, LaCreta F, Nash S, et al. Phase I study of thiotepa in combination with the glutathione transferase inhibitor ethacrynic acid. Cancer Res 1991; 51:6059–6065.

22. Bailey HH, Ripple G, Tutsch KD, et al. Phase I study of continuous-infusion L-S,R-buthionine sulfoximine with intravenous melphalan. J Natl Cancer Inst 1997; 89:1789–1796.

23. O'Brien ML, Kruh GD, Tew KD. The influence of coordinate overexpression of glutathione phase II detoxification gene products on drug resistance. J Pharmacol Exp Ther 2000; 294:480–487.

24. Ruscoe JE, Rosario LA, Wang T, et al. Pharmacological or genetic manipulation of glutathione *S*-transferase P1-1 (GSTpi) influences cell proliferation pathways. J Pharmacol Exp Ther 2001; 298:339–345.

25. Gate L, Majumdar RS, Lunk A, Tew KD. Increased myeloproliferation in glutathione S-transferase pi-deficient mice is associated with a deregulation of JNK and Janus kinase/STAT pathways. J Biol Chem 2004; 279:8608–8616.

26. Tew KD, Monks A, Barone L, et al. Glutathione-associated enzymes in the human cell lines of the National Cancer Institute Drug Screening Program. Mol Pharmacol 1996; 50:149–159.

27. Gunnarsdottir S, Rucki M, Elfarra AA. Novel glutathione-dependent thiopurine prodrugs: evidence for enhanced cytotoxicity in tumor cells and for decreased bone marrow toxicity in mice. J Pharmacol Exp Ther 2002; 301:77–86.

28. Gunnarsdottir S, Rucki M, Phillips LA, Young KM, Elfarra AA. The glutathione-activated thiopurine prodrugs *trans*-6-(2-acetylvinylthio)guanine and *cis*-6-(2-acetylvinylthio)purine cause less in vivo toxicity than 6-thioguanine after single- and multiple-dose regimens. Mol Cancer Ther 2002; 1:1211–1220.

29. Gunnarsdottir S, Elfarra AA. Cytotoxicity of the novel glutathione-activated thiopurine prodrugs *cis*-AVTP [*cis*-6-(2-acetylvinylthio)purine] and *trans*-AVTG [*trans*-6-(2-acetylvinylthio)guanine] results from the national cancer institute's anticancer drug screen. Drug Metab Disp 2004; B32:321–327.

30. Townsend DM, Tew KD. Cancer drugs, genetic variation and the glutathione-*S*-transferase gene family. Am J Pharmacogenomics 2003; 3:157–172.

31. Schisselbauer JC, Silber R, Papadopoulos E, Abrams K, LaCreta FP, Tew KD. Characterization of glutathione S-transferase expression in lymphocytes from chronic lymphocytic leukemia patients. Cancer Res 1990; 50:3562–3568.

32. Morgan AS, Sanderson PE, Borch RF, et al. Tumor efficacy and bone marrow-sparing properties of TER286, a cytotoxin activated by glutathione *S*-transferase. Cancer Res 1998; 58:2568–2575.

33. Rosario LA, O'Brien ML, Henderson CJ, Wolf CR, Tew KD (2000) Cellular responses to a glutathione *S*-transferase P1-1 activated prodrug. Mol Pharmacol 2000; 58:167–174.

34. Findlay VJ, Townsend DM, Saavedra JE, et al. Tumor cell responses to a novel glutathione *S*-transferase-activated nitric oxide-releasing prodrug. Mol Pharmacol 2004; 65:1070–1079.

35. Forman HJ, Fukuto JM, Torres M. Redox signaling: thiol chemistry defines which reactive oxygen and nitrogen species can act as second messengers. Am J Physiol 2004; 287:C246–C256.

13 Metallothioneins in Drug Resistance

Faiyaz Notta, MSc *and D. James Koropatnick,* PhD

Contents

Summary

Metallothioneins (MTs) are a family of proteins that bind some, but not all, heavy metal ions essential for eukaryotic cell function (for example, zinc and copper), and some that are both toxic and not required for cell function (for example, cadmium and mercury). A role for MTs in metabolism and detoxication of heavy metals is strongly suggested by the sensitivity of many MT genes to induction by heavy metals and the ability of MT proteins to bind to many inducing metal ions. However, MT genes are also induced by nonmetal toxins and the expression of MTs varies during normal physiological events (proliferation, differentiation, and cell cycle), suggesting a role or roles not directly related to heavy metal stress. One such role may be the homeostatic regulation of zinc availability. Assessment of function of cells with abrogated MT expression (antisense downregulation of MT and MT gene knockout), increased MT expression by virtue of transient or stable transfection of heterologous MT expression vectors, and in vitro observation of direct and indirect interaction of MT protein with cellular zinc-requiring enzymes and transcription factors has implicated MTs in events modulating resistance to anticancer drug therapy, including zinc-dependent monocyte/macrophage activation, hormone responsiveness, and transcription factor activity. Evidence exists to suggest that MT (1) regulates immune cell functions by mediating the activity of signal transduction proteins and transcription factors involved in monocyte activation; (2) participates in resisting the effects of damage induced by toxins by

From: *Cancer Drug Discovery and Development: Cancer Drug Resistance*
Edited by: B. Teicher © Humana Press Inc., Totowa, NJ

regulating the function of the zinc-sensitive transcription factor metal transcription factor 1, the antiapoptotic protein nuclear factor-κB, and the tumor suppressor protein p53, and signaling through the glucocorticoid hormone receptor and other possibly other hormone receptors; and (3) mediates these events in whole or in part by regulating zinc. The importance of inflammation, hormone response, antiapoptotic and zinc-dependent transcription factor function, and zinc regulation in cellular resistance to toxins, coupled with understanding of how MT influences them, sets the stage for rational therapeutic targeting of MT to enhance cancer treatment while sparing normal tissues.

Key Words: Metallothioneins; glutathione; cisplatin; free radical scavengers; protein sulfhydryls.

1. METALLOTHIONEINS AND METAL HOMEOSTASIS
1.1. Metallothionein Proteins

Metallothioneins (MTs) are a family of small (less than 10 kDa), metal-inducible, metal-binding proteins found in a wide variety of organisms including bacteria, fungi, and eukaryotic plants and animals. They are typically composed of 61 or 62 amino acids (depending on the organism and MT isotype) organized into two globular domains (α and β). Both domains contain a high proportion of cysteine residues—eleven in the α-domain and nine in the β-domain—that are responsible for noncovalent, high-affinity metal ion binding by digonal, trigonal, and tetrahedral associations (1). In mammals, zinc (and, to a minor degree, copper) are the predominant metals bound to MT in the absence of appreciable levels of other metal ions with higher affinity (for example, silver, mercury, copper, and cadmium). Notably, MTs are the single most abundant group of intracellular zinc-binding proteins in eukaryotic cells (2). Five to 10% of zinc in human hepatocytes is bound to MTs (3). An essential biological function for MTs has not been identified, although the remarkable homology among MT protein isotypes and across species (4) implies that such a function or functions exists.

Although MTs have long been associated with resistance to toxicity resulting from exposure to toxic metals and generators of reactive oxygen, their capacity to interact directly with metal ions and oxygen radicals has been taken as evidence that they protect by acting simply as "sacrificial scavengers" to intercept and directly inactivate toxic molecules (5). More recently, it has been suggested that MTs play an indirect role by controlling zinc bioavailability to zinc-requiring proteins that act in a broad range of physiological events, including proteins that themselves directly mediate resistance to toxic events and those that act indirectly by receiving and transducing extracellular signals that alter cellular resistance to toxicity (transcription factors, hormone receptors, metalloproteinases, superoxide dismutase and catalase, among others [6]). In this chapter, we review the evidence surrounding this concept. Understanding the role(s) of MTs in events mediated by these molecules can, potentially, lead to targeting MT expression and/or function as a therapeutic anticancer drug therapy.

1.2. MT Genes

Humans possess 16 MT genes clustered on the q13 region of chromosome 16, including at least 11 that encode MT-1 (*MT-1A, -1B, -1E, -1F, -1G, -1H, -1I, -1J, -1K, -1L,* and *-1X,* some of which appear to be incompetent in directing production of MT protein), and single copies of MT-2 (also referred to as MT-2A), MT-3, and MT-4. Related genes (metallothionein-like 5 [*MTL-5*], encoding tesmin protein; and *MT-M* and *MT-E*) have also been reported (reviewed in ref. *7*). Rodents have only four MT genes, clustered on chromosome 8 (*MT-1*, *MT-2*, *MT-3*, and *MT-4*) *(2–4)*, although additional MT-related mouse genes (mouse *MTL-5* and "MT-1 activator") have been reported (reviewed in ref. *7*). MT-1 and MT-2 are expressed at basal and inducible levels in virtually all tissues, with highest capacity for expression in liver. MT-3 and MT-4 are restricted to certain tissues, with MT-3 produced predominantly in brain in glutaminergic neurons, and at very low levels in pancreas and intestine *(8–11)*. MT-4 is limited to squamous epithelial cells of the skin and tongue *(8)*. A role for MTs in detoxication of metals is supported by the ability of MT to bind to, and be induced by, heavy metals. However, MT-1 and MT-2 are expressed in virtually all tissues and are correlated with a wide variety of physiological events not directly associated with toxic metal insult. Increased expression of both are associated with proliferation, without metal induction, in a human prostate stem cell line *(12)*, in rat kidney undergoing compensatory hypertrophy *(13)*, in proliferating human cancer cells *(9,12,14,15)*, and in human monocytes undergoing respiratory burst *(16,17)*. The level and intracellular location of MT-1 and MT-2 is developmentally regulated in some cells and tissues *(7,18–24)*. MTs may protect against carcinogenesis *(25–28)*, and nuclear MT has been proposed to regulate and/or protect against nuclear oxidant events during cell cycle progression *(29,30)*, including oxidant-induced nuclear zinc release *(31)*—MTs are capable of binding and inactivating reactive oxygen intermediates and may also protect against these toxic species *(29,32,33)*. MTs are, therefore, associated with proliferation, hypertrophy, differentiation, immune cell activation, and resistance to toxins of multiple types in addition to toxic heavy metals.

2. METALLOTHIONEINS AND ZINC

The multiple circumstances under which MTs are expressed has fuelled speculation about their function(s). Notably, MTs are bound primarily to zinc in mammalian cells, suggesting a role in homeostasis of this multifunctional metal ion. A broad range of proteins important in the processes described above require zinc for activity and zinc-associated MTs could supply zinc to (or, depending on relative affinity, sequester zinc away from) mammalian metalloproteins, including transcription factors and hormone receptors *(34,35)*. Unlike strongly redox-active ionic copper and iron, the participation of zinc ions in oxidation-reduction reactions does not readily lead to the formation of damaging free radicals as side products. In addition, zinc can act as an antioxidant to inhibit oxidation by other redox-active metal ions. Zinc competes with redox-active metal ions (including those of iron and copper) for binding to cellular macromolecules, decreasing their capacity to generate toxic hydroxyl radicals (HO•) through Fenton-like reactions *(36)*, and association of zinc with sulfhydryl groups also protects proteins (including δ-aminolevulinate dehydratase, alanyl tRNA synthetase, farnesyltransferase, tubulin, dihydroorotase, and zinc finger proteins) against oxidative denaturation *(37)*. Zinc, therefore, contributes to the structure and activity of enzymes and DNA-binding proteins with less danger of oxidative damage to DNA and other molecules required for cell viability and normal function: a quality that may explain the fact that zinc is an essential cofactor in over 3000 signal transduction proteins and transcription factors, and more than 300 enzymes, including copper/zinc superoxide dismutase with activity in preventing superoxide radical damage, and DNA repair proteins responsible for maintaining the restoring DNA integrity after damage *(32,38)*.

Zinc is a dietary micronutrient that is absorbed by the intestine, associated primarily with albumin in blood, and transported into and within cells by the ZRT-, IRT-like protein, and cation diffusion facilitator families of zinc transporters *(39)*. Albumin has a relatively low affinity for zinc and zinc-albumin constitutes a small, readily available zinc pool that can be rapidly exhausted to produce mild to severe deficiency *(40–42)*. Zinc deficiency is, in fact, a reality in a significant portion of the North American population, with 10% of individuals consuming less than half the recommended level *(43)*. Deficiency is associated with a broad range of clinical disorders (including sickle cell anemia, renal disease, chronic gastrointestinal disorders and acrodermatitis enteropoathica, and HIV infection) and is common in children with diarrhea and among the elderly. Zinc status is tightly linked to antibody and cell-mediated immune integrity in humans and animals *(42,44,45)*. Furthermore, zinc deficient cell culture *(46)* and rodent models *(47)* have increased susceptibility to oxidative damage to DNA and proteins, and zinc supplementation offers protection against progression of pathologies associated with free radical-induced damage, including age-related macular degeneration in humans *(48,49)*, chemically induced diabetes in mice *(44)*, and UV-induced DNA damage and death in human fibroblasts in culture. The antioxidant capacity of zinc, coupled with the requirement of multiple proteins regulating cellular responses to redox damage for zinc, suggest that zinc deficiency can contribute to the development and progression of diseases (including cancer) by enhancing damage to genes and proteins, and by altering or impairing zinc-dependent responses to that damage *(50)*.

The urgent mammalian requirement for zinc, coupled with the ease with which it is depleted, suggest that multiple mechanisms exist to maintain and regulate the cellular supply of zinc ions. Evidence exists to support the concept that MTs are homeostatic molecules, and alteration of MT levels in cells will affect the activities of zinc-requiring proteins that mediate cell functions including signal reception and transduction, gene transcription, and immune cell activation *(51,52)*.

3. METALLOTHIONEIN, ZINC, AND ZINC-REQUIRING PROTEIN FUNCTION

DNA metabolizing and signal transduction proteins require zinc *(52–54)*. For example, glucocorticoid receptor (GR) and estrogen receptor, among other members of a multigene hormone receptor family, require association with zinc for stability and activity *(55)*. Removal of zinc from GR by chelation produces an apoprotein that does not bind to glucocorticoid response elements in DNA. DNA binding is restored by zinc addition *(34,53)*. Although in vivo requirement of MTs for hormone receptor function has not been demonstrated, MT genes are classically inducible by glucocorticoid hormones and hormone analogues *(56,57)*, the cellular level of zinc-associated MT is positively correlated with glucocorticoid receptor activity in rodent cells *(58)*, and MTs have been demonstrated in vitro to donate or remove zinc from hormone receptors (reversible zinc exchange in vitro between MT-2 and the estrogen receptor zinc finger has been reported in vitro *[7]*). Although a role for MT in regulating the zinc status of hormone receptors is an intriguing possibility, there is no direct evidence MTs suppress or enhance receptor activity by modulating zinc availability—under normal conditions, zinc might be directly available to zinc-requiring proteins, without association with "zinc gatekeepers" or "zinc chaperones." A critical question arises: Is zinc association with zinc-requiring proteins regulated to control the activity of those proteins? For this to be possible, the availability of zinc within cells must necessarily be limited. A readily available pool of zinc for all proteins requiring them would frustrate strategies to control access to zinc ions. However, virtually all cellular zinc is associated with macromolecules and "free" zinc is extremely limited *(53)*. Storage of zinc ions by association with high-affinity molecules, coupled with direct or indirect transfer from that binding species to zinc-requiring (and possibly zinc-regulated) molecules would constitute a point of potential control, especially where zinc levels are limited. Furthermore, chaperone-mediated regulation of essential metals has been observed and described. Copper, for example, is regulated by specific transporters and intracellular chaperones elucidated in yeast, but which imply analogous metal ion regulation in higher eukaryotes, including humans *(59)*. Evidence now suggests that MTs may act as intracellular zinc chaperones, regulating zinc availability to proteins that mediate resistance to damage and cellular responses to damage events.

4. REGULATION OF MT GENE EXPRESSION

MT-1 and *MT-2* genes are widely expressed in many tissues and cell types. Expression is maintained at basal levels in the absence of administration of exogenous agents, and in response to an exceptionally broad range of signaling events mediated by multiple transcription factors including AP1, AP2, SP1, steroid hormone receptors, cytokines, and others *(7)*. Transcription factors that mediate both basal and induced MT gene expression interact with multiple promoter/enhancer elements, often involving transcription factor interactions that are poorly understood. However, it is clear that metal response elements ([MREs] present in multiple copies in *MT-1* and *MT-2* genes), antioxidant response elements (overlapping with an upstream stimulatory factor-binding site in *MT-1* genes), and glucocorticoid response elements, and signal transducer and activator of transcription response elements are of high importance, in addition to others. Variations in chromatin structure, DNA methylation, and poorly understood posttranscriptional events also appear to modulate MT expression *(7)*. Stress from heat, cold, physical trauma and other conditions—including oxidative stress induced by administrative of exogenous chemicals that generate hydroxyl radicals (hydrogen peroxide) and superoxide radicals (*tert*-butyl hydroquinone and menadione), and mitochondria-specific reactive oxygen generators (antimycin A and 2,4-dinitrophenol *[60]*)—induce MTs in many organs in whole animals *(61)*. MTs are classically induced by soluble metal ions to which they bind (zinc, cadmium, mercury, copper, and Bi), and by some metals that do not bind to MTs (nickel and cobalt) *(62)*. These metal ions enter cells by multiple processes *(2)* including specific eukaryotic metal ion transporters *(39,63)*. MREs embedded in the promoters of MT and other genes bind the transcription factor metal transcription factor (MTF)-1 *(64,65)*, which is essential for basal, metal-induced, and oxidant stress-induced MT induction *(66)*.

5. METAL TRANSCRIPTION FACTOR 1

MTF-1 is an MRE-binding protein that is ubiquitously expressed in mammalian cells *(67)*. Homozygous knockout of MTF-1 genes in mice is lethal to embryonic mice because of the essential nature of the protein for liver development and stress responses *(68,69)*. On the other hand, MTF-1 can be eliminated in adult mice without compromising viability, although MTF-1 conditional knockout mice have increased susceptibility to heavy metal stress *(70)*. MTF-1 appears to play dual roles—one in liver development that is essential for viability, and the other in response to cell stress that is required only under those stress conditions.

MTF-1 contains, in the N-terminal region, six Cys2-His2 "zinc fingers" that mediate noncovalent interaction of the protein with DNA. MTF-1 protein is maintained by constitutive MTF-1 gene transcription and mRNA translation in human and rodent cell lines *(71)*, although the MTF-1 protein is prevented from mediating high basal MT gene activity, limiting its access into the nucleus. Stress or metal ion exposure induces MTF-1 translocation from the cytoplasm to the nucleus where MTF-1 binds to MREs in the promoter region of *MT-1* and *MT-2* genes, including direct or indirect interactions with components of the RNA polymerase II transcriptional complex *(72,73)*. Although MTF-1 binding to DNA is reversibly activated by a variety of metal ions that induce MTs, zinc (and only zinc) directly binds to MTF-1 *(74,75)*. Of the six zinc fingers, four or five are normally bound to zinc under physiological conditions. On the other hand, one (and possibly two) is a "zinc-sensing" finger that is not occupied by metal in the absence of excess added zinc, even when zinc levels are adequate to maintain viability *(76)*. MTF-1 is, therefore, both zinc dependent (i.e., requiring zinc for activity) and zinc sensitive (i.e., has variable activity within the range of physiological variation in intracellular zinc concentrations), and variations in zinc availability regulate MTF-1 activity. However, the mechanism(s) by which MTF-1 is regulated appear to be more complex than simple zinc association. MTF-1 can be phosphorylated on metal induction through activation of a kinase signaling cascade including protein kinase C (PKC), phosphoinositiol-3 kinase, c-jun N-terminal kinase, and a tyrosine-specific kinase *(77)*, suggesting that metal ions can activate MTF-1 by stimulating kinase activity. Release of MTF-1 from inhibitory regulatory molecules has also been proposed as process to regulate activity *(78)*. Although it is clear that zinc is a critical component of MTF-1 activation, its association with MTF-1 does not appear to be the sole activating event.

MTF-1 activates, not only MT genes, but also other genes important in response to stress and resistance to toxicity. γ-Glutamyl-cysteine synthetase heavy chain (γ-GSChc) is a key enzyme for synthesis of the radical scavenger glutathione (GSH), and has been suggested to be MTF-1-regulated *(79)*. GSH has been implicated in resistance to several chemotherapeutic agents, including platinum-containing compounds, alkylating agents (for example, melphalan), anthracyclines (including doxorubicin), and arsenic. A requirement for GSH in multidrug resistance protein-mediated anthracycline resistance (and possibly arsenic resistance) through efflux of these toxic agents has suggested by demonstration of impaired multidrug resistance protein activity following GSH depletion. On the other hand, GSH levels in embryonic livers in MTF-1 knockout mice have been observed to be at least as high as in wild-type littermates. This suggests that MTF-1 direction of γ-GCShc expression may not be critical, at least under these developmental circumstances *(80)*.

In addition to γ-GCShc, the genes encoding the transcription factor C/EBP-α, embryonic α-fetoprotein, the zinc transporter ZnT-1, and placental growth factor are also likely targets of MTF-1 *(81)*. C/EBP-α participates in maintaining the differentiated, nonproliferative state in hepatocytes *(82)*, and is induced during acute phase response *(83,84)*, indicating a role in response to stress. α-Fetoprotein, in addition to other functions, is a scavenger of heavy metal ions and reactive oxygen *(85)*. ZnT-1 plays an important role in regulating intracellular zinc levels and metabolism *(86)*, and placental growth factor is a member of the vascular endothelial growth factor family of angiogenic factors and is induced in an MTF-1-dependent manner in fibroblasts *(87)*. Furthermore, MTF-1 appears to be directly involved in tumor development. Loss of MTF-1 results in

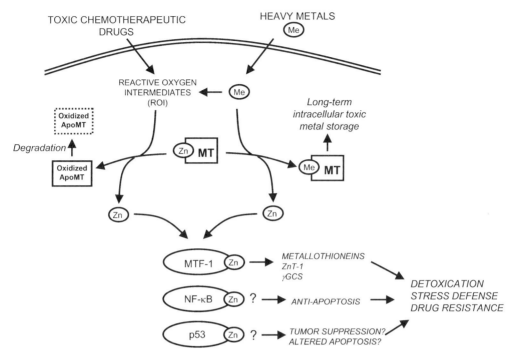

Fig. 1. Model of proposed "metal sensor" and "zinc regulatory" roles for metallothionein. Metal ions or reactive oxygen (exogenous or endogenous) leads to release of zinc from metallothioneins. Released zinc activates zinc-sensitive, zinc-dependent transcription factors mediating drug resistance (*see* text for details). Me, heavy metal ions; MT, metallothioneins; ApoMT, metallothioneins partially or completely depleted of zinc; Zn, zinc ions; MTF-1, metal transcription factor 1; NF-κB, nuclear factor κB; p53, tumor suppressor protein 53; ZnT-1, zinc transporter 1; γ-GCS, γ-glutamyl cysteine synthetase, a key enzyme in the production of glutathione.

increased activity of transforming growth factor β1 and tissue transglutaminase (both of which are involved in extracellular matrix production), and delayed tumor growth and reduced vasculature density in *ras*-transformed mouse embryonic fibroblasts *(88)*. Overall, MTF-1 appears to be a critical transcription factor, not only in mediating cellular responses to stresses induced by a variety of toxins including chemotherapeutic agents, but also in physiological events contributing to tumor growth and malignancy.

The activity of MTF-1 and other zinc-binding transcription factors depends on a metalloregulatory protein or proteins that do not, themselves, have DNA-binding or transactivation capacity *(35)*. Such a metalloregulatory protein would respond to an array of disparate signals by adding or removing zinc, and only zinc, from zinc-requiring transcription factors. Metallothioneins are candidates for this role (Fig. 1). They bind different metals with different avidity—zinc associates with MT with a stability constant (~1011) that is ~100-fold less than that of copper, mercury, silver, or cadmium *(18)*. Zinc displaced by binding to higher-avidity metals *(125)* or by redox conditions present during stress *(45)* would be available to zinc-dependent proteins. Such a high affinity, metal- and stress-responsive zinc carrier, capable of supplying zinc to both high avidity proteins (by direct transfer) or to low-avidity proteins (by release of zinc after reactive oxygen interaction with MTs) would conceivably be important in maintaining an intracellular store of zinc when dietary sources are limited. In support of this, *MT-1/MT-2* knockout mice *(89,90)* have heightened sensitivity to zinc deficiency leading to retarded kidney development and *in utero* mortality *(91)*. In addition, in vitro transcriptional activation of MRE-driven genes by MTF-1 requires zinc-saturated MT—free zinc alone, or zinc-deprived MT, are not sufficient *(65,78)*. MT appears, therefore, to be a necessary factor in regulating zinc availability to zinc-dependent MTF-1. Similarly, in rodent cells transfected with a reporter gene driven by an MTF-1-responsive promoter, increased MT-1 levels enhanced zinc-induced gene expression, an observation that correlates MT with MTF-1-mediated transcription in a concentration-dependent manner *(92)*. Furthermore, mouse fibroblasts adapted to growth in severely zinc-depleted medium have amplified MT genes and elevated MT gene expression, suggesting that MT confers an advantage in coping with scarce zinc, possibly by acting as a high affinity storage depot to conserve zinc for selected physiological processes necessary for survival under conditions when dietary zinc is not readily available, is in high demand because of stress, or both *(93)*. Thus, MTs can mediate zinc-responsive gene expression and may regulate zinc availability, especially under low environmental zinc conditions where increased zinc transport would have diminished capacity to increase intracellular zinc levels.

6. METALLOTHIONEIN AND NUCLEAR FACTOR-κB AND p53 ACTIVITY

The Rel family nuclear factor (NF)-κB transcription factors are candidates for regulation by MT. They are dimers, with the p50/p65 complex the most abundant form in mammals *(94)*. NF-κB interacts with an inhibitory protein (an inhibitor of NF-κB [IκB] family member) in cytoplasm *(95)* or the nucleus *(96)* to block nuclear localization and transcriptional activity. IκBs are degraded in response to diverse stimuli to allow NF-κB to enter the nucleus, bind target DNA elements, and regulate genes involved in immune response, growth, and apoptosis *(94)*. NF-κB is required to protect cells from apoptosis induced by tumor necrosis factor (TNF) and other stimuli through activation of antiapoptotic genes *(97)*. Like NF-κB, MTs are antiapoptotic—antisense downregulation of MT expression stimulates apoptotic death *(98,99)*. Contradictory reports either support *(99–101)* or do not support *(102–104)* a role for MT in regulating NF-κB *(105)*. To resolve the controversy, we examined NF-κB protein levels and NF-κB-dependent reporter gene activity in clonal fibroblastic cell lines from normal (MT-WT) and *MT-1/MT-2* knockout (MT-KO) embryonic mouse kidneys. Using a time-resolved dissociation-enhanced lanthanide fluoroimmunoassay immunoassay developed in our laboratory to improve measurement of MT *(106)*, we confirmed lower basal levels of MT and lack of metal-induced MT in MT-KO cells. MT-KO cell lines had dramatically reduced levels of NF-κB subunit p65 (but not of the NF-κB p50 subunit, or of IκBα), had less than half the expression of a transfected NF-κB-dependent reporter, and were more sensitive to apoptosis induced by *tert*-butylhydroperoxide. Decreased nuclear localization of p65 in MT-KO clones was not responsible for differences in NF-κB activity. In fact, MT-KO cells had higher nuclear levels of p65 than MT-WT cells in spite of lower overall cellular levels, suggesting that MT regulates the specific activity of NF-κB. Reconstitution of MT by stable incorporation of mouse MT-1 expression in multiple clonal populations of MT-KO cells (MT-KO$_2^{+mt}$) increased NF-κB p65 (but not IκBα or NF-κB p50), and increased NF-κB-dependent reporter activity and resistance to apoptosis. These observations strongly support a role for MT in regulating NF-κB subunit levels and NF-κB function.

The mechanism by which MTs mediate NF-κB is not known, but there is a wealth of evidence to suggest that they regulate zinc *(6,58)*. However, in vitro evidence reveals that MTs can both donate and sequester zinc depending on relative affinity, overall zinc status, and cellular location of MTs and zinc-dependent proteins *(6)*. MT-1 and MT-2 bind 7 zinc atoms, but only one or two are readily available for transfer *(107)*. The remaining zincs require disruption of zinc-thiol coordinate covalent bonds for release. It is possible that MTs with an incomplete complement of zinc (apo-MT) could sequester zinc when it is scarce, lowering zinc availability to other proteins. For example, moderate overexpression of MT-2 in a human breast cancer-derived cell line (MCF-7) enhanced the transcriptional activity of the zinc-dependent transcription factor and tumor suppressor protein p53, but high-level overexpression suppressed p53 activity *(106)*. Zinc-depleted MT has also been reported to selectively activate enzymes in which zinc is bound at an inhibitory site, without removing zinc from the catalytic site of metalloenzymes—an effect suggested by the authors to be because of selective sequestration of zinc by MT *(108)*. Finally, cells selected for survival under low zinc conditions had high MT expression, but transcription of a transfected MTF-1-responsive reporter construct was suppressed, consistent with the interpretation that, in low zinc, MT sequestered scarce zinc ions away from zinc-sensing MTF-1. These observations are consistent with the hypothesis that, in low zinc, zinc-dependent transcription factor activity (including transcription factors such as p53 and NF-κB that have important roles in modulating apoptosis and sensitivity to toxins) may be (1) more dependent on MT than in the presence of sufficient zinc (if MT has a full complement of seven zinc ions, with one or two available for transfer to zinc-requiring proteins), or (2) inversely dependent on MT (if MT binds less than seven zinc ions, bound in the molecule's interior and unavailable for ready transfer). If either of these hypotheses is correct, then the case for zinc regulation by MT to mediate NF-κB and/or will be strengthened. If not, then the alternative hypothesis that MTs regulate NF-κB activity independent of zinc will grow in importance. These possibilities have implications for NF-κB function in the face of variable zinc levels in humans. Investigation of the role of MT in regulating NF-κB activity through zinc regulation, by assessing NF-κB function in cells with altered MT and depleted or supplemented zinc levels, is an important area for further investigation.

7. METALLOTHIONEIN AND GLUCOCORTICOID HORMONE RESPONSIVENESS

A mouse mammary tumor cell line (2305) with a stable, mouse mammary tumor virus-driven vector containing a chloramphenicol acetyltransferase (*CAT*) reporter gene has been used to test the role of MT in GR activity. This vector responds to the artificial glucocorticoid dexamethasone (DEX), which stimulates GR translocation to the nucleus and GR-mediated transcription. An antisense MT-1 expression vector (capable of down-regulating both MT-1 and MT-2) reduced MT-1 mRNA to only 40% of the amount in control cells *(109)*. This resulted in a small (approximately 10%) but significant decrease in DEX-induced CAT activity. Considering that zinc in fetal bovine serum medium (~4 μM) could be an alternative source and diminish the putative role of MT as a zinc regulator, the serum was chelated to reduce zinc to less than 0.3 μM. Under these conditions, DEX responsiveness was reduced by 25% in MT-expressing cells—a nearly threefold enhancement of suppression *(109)*. Furthermore, zinc, mercury, and heat shock treatment of 2305 cells (but not copper or cadmium induction) enhanced response of a DEX-inducible CAT reporter construct *(58,110)*. The significant factor that correlated with enhancement of hormone response was not the absolute MT protein level, but the level of zinc-associated MT. For example, treatment with cadmium or copper increased MT, but the resulting cadmium- and copper-bound MT had no effect on DEX-induced CAT expression. Heat shock did not increase MT protein, but increased both the amount of MT associated with zinc and DEX-responsiveness. Collectively, these data strengthen the concept that MT mediates GR activity by regulating zinc. The importance of MT in GR activity is accentuated under conditions of low zinc availability, consistent with the susceptibility of MT knockout mice to adverse effects associated with zinc deprivation.

The multiple functions of GR in events related to cancer (growth, development, and death), and the potential of the stress- and metal-inducible protein MT to mediate GR activity, suggests that modulating MT expression may alter tumor cell growth and development, potentially for therapeutic benefit.

8. METALLOTHIONEIN, INFLAMMATION, AND CANCER

Cell-mediated immune responses, including infiltration of macrophages into tumors during inflammation, have profound impact on tumor progression. The implications of inflammation for tumor behavior are complex and can be neutral, lead to tumor rejection, or lead to enhanced tumor growth depending on tumor characteristics and the nature of the inflammatory response *(111)*. However, suppression of cell-mediated immune responses is associated with many tumors, including melanoma, colorectal, and prostate cancer *(112,113)*. Modulation of inflammatory responses, particularly suppression, may be of value in inhibiting human tumor growth.

Zinc is essential for proteins mediating activation of monocyte/macrophages *(114,115)*. Activation proceeds through a G-protein-linked pathway, including phosphorylation of protein kinases leading to a cascade of events resulting in cytokine production and arachidonate release. PKC and inositol 1,4,5-triphosphate are activated, and active PKC releases NF-κB from IκBα. Released NF-κB is translocated to the nucleus to control transcription of multiple genes mediating activation, including IL-1α, IL-1β, and TNF-α *(116,117)*. There is circumstantial evidence that MTs may mediate innate immunity (which includes monocyte/macrophage action among the action of other cell types)—MT-KO mice are protected against TNF-induced systemic inflammatory response syndrome, and MT-1-overexpressing transgenic mice are more sensitized to the lethal effects of TNF, compared to wild-type mice *(118)*, consistent with the hypothesis that MT influences the activity of zinc-requiring monocyte activation proteins.

MT expression is elevated in primary human monocytes, and a human monocytic cell line (THP-1), after activation *(16)*. Although it was initially hypothesized that increased MT was not involved in the activation process and only provided protection against damaging reactive oxygen generated during activated monocytes undergoing respiratory burst, antisense RNA to suppress basal, cadmium, and lipopolysaccharide (LPS)- and cadmium-induced MT in human THP-1 monocytes completely abolished subsequent LPS and granulocyte-colony stimulating factor activation, without reducing viability *(17)*. Therefore, MT induction concomitant with activation did not appear to mediate resistance to resistance to reactive oxygen. Loss of activation potential as a result of MT downregulation indicated a role for MT in monocyte activation.

MT-KO mice provide a model to study the effect of MT loss on primary monocyte/ macrophages. These animals are phenotypically normal but sensitive to cadmium and oxidant activity, and have reduced zinc uptake suggesting that zinc homeostasis in these animals is disturbed *(119)*. Innate immune function (monocyte/macrophage activation) is compromised in MT-KO mouse monocytes, consistent with reduced sensitivity to systemic inflammatory response syndrome in MT-KO mice *(120)*. Characterization of the effects of MT loss and gain on monocyte/macrophage action, and assessment of the putative zinc homeostatic role of MT as the mechanism by which it mediates monocyte/ macrophage function, will be important future areas of investigation with implications for strategies for cancer treatment through modulation of inflammation.

8.1. Metal Salts Inhibit LPS-Induced Activation Without Decreasing Cell Viability

Metal salts can inhibit cell activity through direct toxicity to critical cellular molecules and structures. On the other hand, they can also change cell behavior by inducing specific genes (including MT). Therefore, metals may affect cell function by directly damaging cell components, or by transmitting or influencing signals controlling gene expression. To explore this, the ability of low-level metal salt pretreatment to alter monocyte behavior without decreasing viability has been measured. Treatment of THP-1 cells with low levels of zinc, cadmium, or mercury had no effect on viability or proliferation, but significantly induced MT mRNA and dramatically reduced LPS activation potential *(120)*. Zinc chloride pretreatment of primary human peripheral blood monocytes similarly inhibited activation potential *(16)*. Interestingly, LPS induction after zinc pretreatment dramatically decreased MT mRNA and protein expression (opposite to the effect of LPS activation of cells not pretreated with metal salts), suggesting a novel zinc-induced alteration in MT gene response to LPS in monocytes *(16)*. Zinc levels used were similar to those found in normal human serum *(121)*, and had no toxic effect as assessed by dye exclusion and radiolabel incorporation during run-on transcription in isolated nuclei.

These data indicate that nontoxic pretreatment of monocytes with metal salts induces MT and diminishes human monocyte activation potential. Given the apparent importance of MT in mediating activation revealed by antisense MT and in MT-KO mice, this was unexpected, but of potential therapeutic interest (particularly with respect to zinc) to treat pathological conditions involving chronic upregulation of innate immune functions (such as rheumatoid arthritis, infectious disease, and inflammatory bowel disease *[122]* and cancer *[111–113]*). There are at least three possible explanations. First, MT levels might need to be in a relatively narrow range to mediate induction of activation: either increasing or decreasing those levels would have a negative effect. Second, metal treatment might affect activity of signaling proteins mediating activation, without decreasing cell viability and without involvement of MT. Third, metal treatment can affect expression of other genes in addition to those encoding MT. Non-MT factors induced by metals might act independently, or in conjunction with MT, to inhibit activation potential. Exploration of these possibilities using cells with genetically altered MT expression, and monocytes isolated from transgenic MT-overexpressing *(123)* and MT-KO mice *(89,90)* with elevated and abolished MT expression (respectively) will be important. The activation potential of these cells, with or without metal pretreatment, will assess the involvement of MT in monocyte activation, and in metal-induced suppression of activation.

9. THE CONNECTION BETWEEN GR, NF-κB, AND INFLAMMATION

There is an important connection between immune function, NF-κB and GR activity, and the potential influence of MT. Both NF-κB and GR control the expression of many inflammatory and immune genes, including those regulating monocyte/macrophage activity (both IL-1β and TNF-α activate/are activated by NF-κB in a proinflammatory regulatory loop, and glucocorticoids induce anti-inflammatory genes and inhibit pro-inflammatory gene expression) *(124)*. NF-κB engages in crosstalk with other transcription factors important in innate immune function, including GR *(125)*. GR transrepresses NF-κB (and vice versa) through a direct protein:protein interaction with the p65 subunit of NF-κB, the component revealed to be regulated by MT in studies of MT-KO and MT-WT cells *(105)*. Close examination of the role of MT in regulating these factors and functions separately, and their influence on each other, has important implications for enhancing therapy (combining drugs to target both transcription factors and signaling pathways, and MTs) of pathological conditions involving innate immune action, including cancer.

10. CONCLUSION

Metallothioneins can act as sacrificial scavengers to directly intercept toxins (including metal ions and reactive oxygen species) that can damage cells and/or transmit signals regulating multiple physiological events, including resistance and sensitivity to toxic agents. In addition, a new role for metallothioneins as regulators of zinc-requiring and zinc-sensing transcription factors is emerging. Those transcription factors, including NF-κB, p53, GR, and MTF-1 have important roles in regulating cellular events important in inflammation and apoptosis, proliferation, and tumor development and progression. Critical questions that require further investigation include evaluation of the putative role of MT in regulating the zinc status of transcription factors to modulate their activity, and assessment of the potential to alter MT in tumors or normal cells to enhance the effectiveness of chemotherapeutic drugs designed to induce apoptosis, or to alter signaling events in human tumors for therapeutic benefit.

ACKNOWLEDGMENTS

Some of the work described in this review was supported by grants to J.K. from the Canadian Institutes of Health Research (CIHR). F.N. is supported by a CIHR Strategic Training Program Scholarship.

REFERENCES

1. Stillman MJ, Presta A. Characterizing metal ion interactions with biological molecules—the spectroscopy of metallothionein. In: Zalups RK and Koropatnick J, eds. Molecular biology and toxicology of metals. New York: Taylor and Francis, 2000:1–33.
2. Andrews GK. Regulation of metallothionein gene expression. Prog Food Nutr Sci 1990; 14:193–258.
3. Kagi JHR. Overview of metallothionein. Methods Enzymol 1991; 205:613–626.
4. Miles AT, Hawksworth GM, Beattie JH, Rodilla V. Induction, regulation, degradation, and biological significance of mammalian metallothioneins. Crit Rev Biochem Mol Biol 2000; 35:35–70.
5. Thornalley PH, Vasak M. Possible role for metallothionein in protection against radiation-induced oxidative stress. Kinetics and mechanism of its reaction with superoxide and hydroxyl radicals. Biochim Biophys Acta 1985; 827:36–44.
6. Koropatnick J, Zalups RK. Toxic and essential metals in the cellular response to signals, In: Zalups RK and Koropatnick J, eds. Molecular biology and toxicology of metals. New York: Taylor and Francis, 2000:551–576.

7. Haq F, Mahoney M, Koropatnick J. Signaling events for metallothionein induction. Mut Res 2003; 533:211–226 (review).

8. Quaife CJ, Findley SD, Erickson JC, et al. Induction of a new metallothionein isoform (MT-4) occurs during differentiation of stratified squamous epithelia. Biochemistry 1994; 33:7250–7259.

9. Kontozoglou TE, Banerjee D, Cherian MG. Immunohistochemical localization of metallothionein in human testicular embryonal carcinoma cells. Virchows Archiv A Pathol Anat 1989; 415:545–549.

10. Moffat P, Seguin C. Expression of the gene encoding MT-3 in organs of the reproductive system. DNA Cell Biol 1998; 17:501–510.

11. Somji S, Garrett SH, Sens MA, Gurel V, Sens DA. Expression of metallothionein isoform 3 (MT-3) determines the choice between apoptotic or necrotic cell death in Cd^{+2}-exposed human proximal tubule cells. Toxicol Sci 2004; 80:358–366.

12. Koropatnick J, Kloth DM, Kadhim S, Chin JL, Cherian MG. Metallothionein expression and resistance to cisplatin in a human germ cell tumor cell line. J Pharmaceut Exp Ther 1995; 275:1681–1687.

13. Zalups RK, Fraser J, Koropatnick J. Enhanced transcription of metallothionein genes in rat kidney: effect of uninephrectomy and compensatory renal growth. Am J Physiol 1995; 37:F643–F650.

14. Nagel WW, Vallee BL. Cell cycle regulation of metallothionein in human colonic cancer cells. PNAS 1995; 92:579–583.

15. Meskel HH, Cherian MG, Martinez VJ, Veinot LA, Frei JV. Metallothionein as an epithelial proliferative compartment marker for DNA flow cytometry. Mod Pathol 1993; 6:756–760.

16. Leibbrandt MEI, Koropatnick J. Activation of human monocytes with lipopolysaccharide induces metallothionein expression and is diminished by zinc. Toxicol Appl Pharmacol 1994; 124:72–81.

17. Leibbrandt MEI, Khokha R, Koropatnick J. Antisense down-regulation of metallothionein in a human monocytic cell line alters adherence, invasion, and the respiratory burst. Cell Growth and Differ 1994; 5:17–25.

18. Hamer DH. Metallothionein. Ann Rev Biochem 1986; 55:913–951.

19. Ouellette AJ. Metallothionein mRNA expression in fetal mouse organs. Dev Biol 1982; 92:240–246.

20. Koropatnick J, Duerksen JD. Nuclease sensitivity of alpha-feprotein, metallothionein-1, and immunoglobulin gene sequences in mouse during development. Dev Biol 1987; 122:1–10.

21. Slotkin SH, Cherian MG. Elevated metallothionein expression in human fetal liver. Paed Res 1989; 24:326–329.

22. Panemangalore M, Banerjee D, Onosaka S, Cherian MG. Changes in the intracellular accumulation and distribution of metallothionein in rat liver and kidney during postnatal development. Dev Biol 1983; 97:95–102.

23. Nartey NO, Banerjee D, Cherian MG. Immunohistochemical localization of metallothionein in cell nucleus and cytoplasm of fetal human liver and kidney and its changes during development. Pathology 1987; 19:233–238.

24. Cherian MG. The significance of the nuclear and cytoplasmic localization of metallothionein in human liver and tumour cells. Env Health Persp 1994; 102:131–135.

25. Zhang B, Satoh M, Nishimura N, et al. Metallothionein deficiency promotes mouse skin carcinogenesis induced by 7,12-dimethylbenz[a]anthracene. Cancer Res 1998; 58:1–12.

26. Suzuki JS, Nishimura N, Zhang B, et al. Metallothionein deficiency enhances skin carcinogenesis induced by 7,12-dimethylbenz(a)anthracene and 12-O-tetradecanoylphorbol-13-acetate in metallothionein-null mice. Carcinogenesis 2003; 24:1123–1132.

27. Cherian MG, Jayasurya A, Bay BH. Metallothioneins in human tumors and potential roles in carcinogenesis. Mutat Res 2003; 533:201–209.

28. Theocharis SE, Margeli AP, Klijanienko JT, Kouraklis GP. Metallothionein expression human neoplasia. Histopathology 2004; 45:103–118.

29. Takahashi Y, Ogra Y, Suzuki KT. Nuclear trafficking of metallothionein requires oxidation of a cytosolic partner. J Cell Physiol 2005; 202:563–569.

30. Takahashi Y, Ogra Y, Suzuki KT. Synchronized generation of reactive oxygen species with the cell cycle. Life Sci 2004; 75:301–311.

31. Spahl DU, Berendji-Grun D, Suschek CV, Kolb-Bachofen V, Kroncke KD. Regulation of zinc homeostasis by inducible NO synthase-derived NO: nuclear metallothionein translocation and intranuclear Zn^{2+} release. PNAS 2003; 100:13952–13957.

32. Tamai KT, Gralla EB, Ellerby LM, Valentine JS, Thiele DJ. Yeast and mammalian metallothioneins functionally substitute for yeast copper-zinc superoxide dismutase. PNAS 1993; 90:131–135.

33. Schwarz MA, Lazo JS, Yalowich JC, et al. Cytoplasmic metallothionein overexpression protects NIH 373 cells from tert-butyl hydroperoxide toxicity. J Biol Chem 1994; 269:15,238–15,243.

34. Vallee BL, Coleman JE, Auld DS. Zinc fingers, zinc clusters, and zinc twists in DNA-binding protein domains. PNAS 1991; 88:999–1003.

35. Koropatnick J, Leibbrandt MEI. Effects of metals on gene expression. In: Goyer RA, Cherian MG, eds. Handbook of experimental pharmacology, toxicology of metals—biochemical aspects. Berlin: Springer, 1995:93–113.

36. Conte E, Narindrasorasak S, Sarkar B. In vivo and in vitro iron-replaced zinc finger generates free radicals and causes DNA damage. J Biol Chem 1996; 271:5125–5130.

37. Powell SR. The antioxidant properties of zinc. J Nutr 2000; 130:1447S–1454S.

38. Prasad AS. Zinc Deficiency. BMJ 2003; 326:409–410.

39. Gaither LA, Eide DJ. Eukaryotic zinc transporters and their regulation. Biometals 2001; 14:251–270.

40. Davis SR, Cousins RJ. MT expression in animals: a physiological perspective on function. J Nutr 2000; 130:1085–1088.

41. Chan S, Gerson B, Subramaniam S. The role of copper, molybdenum, selenium, and zinc in nutrition and health. Clin Lab Med 1998; 18:673–685.

42. Tapiero H, Tew, KD. Trace elements in human physiology and pathology: zinc and metallothioneins. Biomed Pharmacother 2003; 57:399–411.

43. Wakimoto P, Block G. Dietary intake, dietary patterns, and changes with age: an epidemiological perspective. J Gerontol A Biol Sci Med Sci 2001; 56:65–80.

44. Fraker PJ, King LE, Laakko T, Vollmer TL. The dynamic link between the integrity of the immune system and zinc status. J Nutr 2000; 130:1399S–1406S.

45. Mocchegiani E, Muzzioli M, Giacconi R. Zinc, metallothioneins, immune responses, survival and ageing. Biogerontology 2000; 1:133–143.

46. Ho E, Ames BN. Low intracellular zinc induces oxidative DNA damage, disrupts p53, NFκB and AP1 binding and affects DNA repair in a rat glioma cell line. Proc Natl Acad Sci U S A 2002; 99:16,770–16,775.

47. Oteiza PL, Olin KL, Fraga CG, Keen CL. Oxidant defense systems in testes from zinc-deficient rats. Proc Soc Exp Biol Med 1996; 213:85–91.

48. Mittra RA. New treatments for age-related macular degeneration. Minn Med 2003; 86:40–46.

49. Age-Related Eye Disease Study Research Group. A rondomized, placebo-controlled, clinical trial of high-dose supplementation with vitamins C and E, beta carotene, and zinc for age-related macular degeneration and vision loss. AREDS report 8. Arch Ophthalmol 2001; 119:1417–1436.

50. Datta K, Sinha S, Chattopadhyay P. Reactive oxygen species in health and disease. Natl Med J India 2000; 13:304–310.

51. Czupryn M, Brown WE, Vallee BL. Zinc rapidly induces a metal response element-binding factor. PNAS 1992; 89:10,395–10,399.

52. O'Halloran TV. Transition metals in control of gene expression. Science 1993; 261:715–725.

53. Vallee BL, Falchuk, FH. The biochemical basis of zinc physiology. Physiol Rev 1993; 73:79–118.

54. Coleman JE. Zinc proteins: enzymes, storage proteins, transcription factors, and replication proteins. Ann Rev Biochem 1992; 61:897–946 (review).

55. Evans RM. The steroid and thyroid hormone receptor superfamily. Science 1998; 240:889–895 (review).

56. Hager LJ, Palmiter RD. Transcriptional regulation of mouse liver metallothionein-1 gene by glucocorticoids. Nature 1981; 291:340–342.

57. Karin M, Andersen RD, Slater E, Smith K, Herschman HR. Metallothionein mRNA induction in HeLa cells in response to zinc or dexamethasone is a primary induction response. Nature 1980; 286:295–297.

58. DeMoor JM, Kennette WA, Collins OM, Koropatnick J. Zinc-metallothionein levels are correlated with enhanced glucocorticoid responsiveness in mouse cells exposed to Zn Cl$_2$, HgCl$_2$, and heat shock. Toxicol Sci 2001; 64:67–76.

59. Ress EM, Thiele DJ. From aging to virulence: forging connections through the study of copper homeostasis in eukaryotic micro. Curr Opin Microbiol 2004; 7:175–184.

60. Kondoh M, Inoue Y, Atagi S, Futakawa N, Higashimoto M, Sato M. Specific induction of metallothhionein synthesis by mitochondrial oxidative stress. Life Sci 2001; 69:2137–2146.

61. Ghoshal K, Wang Y, Sheridan JF, Jacob ST. Metallothionein induction in response to restraint stress: transcriptional control, adaptation to stress, and role of glucocorticoid. J Biol Chem 1998; 273:27,904–27,910.

62. Palmiter RD. Regulation of metallothionein genes by heavy metal appears to be mediated by a zinc-sensitive inhibitor that interacts with a constitutively active transcription factor, MTF-1. Proc Natl Acad Sci U S A 1994; 91:1219–1223.

63. Nelson N. Metal ion transporters and homeostasis. EMBO J 1999; 18:4361–4371.
64. Lichtlen P, Wang Y, Belser T, et al. Target gene search for the metal-responsive transcription factor MTF-1. Nucleic Acids Res 2001; 29:1514–1523.
65. Zhang B, Georgiev O, Hagmann M, et al. Activity of metal-responsive transcription factor 1 by toxic heavy metals and H_2O_2 in vitro is modulated by metallothionein. Mol Cell Biol 2003; 23:8471–8485.
66. Heuchel R, Radtke F, Georgiev O, Stark G, Aguet M, Schaffner W. The transcription factor MTF-1 is essential for basal and heavy metal-induced metallothionein gene transcription. EMBO J 1994; 13:2870–2875.
67. Westin G, Schaffner W. A zinc-responsive factor interacts with a metal-regulated enhancer element (MBE) of the mouse metallothioinein-1 gene. EMBO J 1988; 7:3763–3770.
68. Heuchel R, Radtke F, Georgiev O, Stark G, Aguet M, Schaffner W. The transcription factor MTF-1 is essential for basal and heavy metal-induced metallothionein gene expression. EMBO J 1994; 13:2870–2875.
69. Radtke, Heuchel R, Georgiev O, et al. Cloned transcription factor MTF-1 activates the mouse metallothionein-1 promoter. EMBO J 1993; 12:1355–1362.
70. Wang Y, Wimmer U, Lichtlen P, et al. Metal-responsive transcription factor-1 (MTF-1) is essential for embryonic liver development and heavy metal detoxification in the adult liver. FASEB J 2004; 18:1071–1079.
71. Saydam N, Adams TK, Steiner F, Schaffner W, Freedman JH. Regulation of metallothionein transcription by the meta-responsive transcription factor MTF-1. J Biol Chem 2002; 277:20,438–20,445.
72. Smirnova IV, Bittel DC, Ravindra H, Jiang GK, Andrews GK. Zinc and cadmium can promote the rapid nuclear translocation of MTF-1. J Biol Chem 2000; 275:9377–9384.
73. Kelly EJ, Quaife CJ, Froelick GJ, Palmiter RD. Metallothionein 1 and 2 protect against zinc deficiency and zinc toxicity in mice. J Nutr 1996; 126:1782–1790.
74. Dalton TP, Bittel D, Andrews GK. Reversible activation of mouse metal response element-binding transcription factor-1 DNA binding involves zinc interaction with the zinc finger domain. Mol Cell Biol 1997; 17:2781–2789.
75. Andrews GK, Bittel D, Dalton T, et al. New insights into the mechanisms of cadmium regulation of mouse metallothionein-1 gene expression. In: Klaassen CD, ed. Metallothionein IV. Basel: Birkhauser, 1999:227–232.
76. Chen X, Agarwal A, Giedroc DP. Structural and functional heterogeneity among the zinc fingers of human MRE-binding transcription factor-1. Biochemistry 1998; 37:11,152–11,161.
77. LaRochelle O, Gane V, Charron J, Soh JW, Seguin C. Phosphorylation is involved in the activation of metal-regulatory transcription factor 1 in response to metal ions. J Biol Chem 2001; 276:41,879–41,888.
78. Bi Y, Palmiter RD, Wood KM, Qiang MA. Induction of metallothionein 1 by phenolic antioxidants requires metal-activated transcription factor 1 (MTF-1) and zinc. Biochem J 2004; 380:695–703.
79. Lichtlen P, Schaffner W. The "metal transcription factor" MTF-1: biological facts and medical implications. Swiss Med Wkly 2001; 131:647–652.
80. Benderra Z, Trussardi A, Morjani H, Villa AM, Doglia SM, Manfait M. Regulation of cellular glutathione modulates nuclear accumulation of daunorubicin in human MCF7 cells overexpressing multidrug resistance associated protein. Eur J Cancer 2000; 36:428–434.
81. Lichtlen P, Wang Y, Belser T, et al. Target gene search for the metal-responsive transcription factor MTF-1. Nucl Acids Res 2001; 29:1514–1523.
82. Timchenko NA, Harris TE, Wilde M, et al. CCAAT/enhancer binding protein alpha regulates p21 protein and hepatocyte proliferration in newborn mice. Mol Cell Biol 1997; 17:7353–7361.
83. Wang ND, Finegold MJ, Bradley A, Ou CN, Abdelsayed SV, Darlington GJ. Impaired energy homeostasis in C/EBP alpha knockout mice. Science 1995; 269:1108–1112.
84. Burgess-Beusse BL, Darlington GJ. C/EBP alpha is critical for the neonatal acute-phase response to inflammation. Mel. Cell Biol 1998; 28:7269–7277.
85. Mizejewski GJ. Alpha-fetoprotein as a biologic response modifier: relevance to domain and subdomain structure. Proc Soc Exp Biol Med 1997; 215:333–362.
86. Cuajungco MP, Lees GJ. Zinc metabolism in the brain: relevance to human neurodegenerative disorders. Neurobiol Dis 1997; 4:137–169.
87. Green CJ, Lichtlen P, Huynh NT, Yanovsky M, Schaffner W, Murphy BJ. Placenta growth cator gene expression is induced by hypoxia in fibroblasts: a central role for metal transcription factor MTF-1. Cancer Res 2001; 61:2696–2673.
88. Haroon ZA, Amin K, Lichtlen P, et al. Loss of metal transcription factor-1 suppresses tumor growth through enhanced matrix deposition. FASEB J 2004; 18:1176–1184.

89. Michalska AE, Choo KH. Targeting and germ-line transmission of a null mutation at the metallo-thionein-1 and -2 loci in mouse. PNAS 1993; 90:8088–8092.

90. Masters BA, Kelly EJ, Quaife CJ, Brinster RL, Palmiter RD. Targeted disruption of metallothionein 1 and 2 genes increases sensitivity to cadmium. PNAS 1994; 91:584–588.

91. Kelly EJ, Quaife CJ, Froelick GJ, Palmiter RD. Metallothionein-1 and -2 protect against zinc deficiency and zinc toxicity in mice. J Nutr 1996; 126:1782–1790.

92. Palmiter RD. Constitutive expression of metallothionein-3, but not MT-1, inhibits growth when cells become zinc deficient. Toxicol Appl Pharmacol 1995; 135:139–146.

93. Suhy DA, Simon KD, Linzer DI, O'Halloran TV. Metallothionein is part of a zinc-scavenging mecha-nism for cell survival under conditions of extreme zinc deprivation. J Biol Chem 1999; 274:9183–9192.

94. Siebenlist U, Franzoso G, Brown K. Structure, regulation and function of NF-κB. Annu Rev Cell Biol 1994; 10:405–455.

95. Karin M. The beginning of the end: IκB kinase (IKK) and NF-κB activation. J Biol Chem 1999; 27:27,339–27,342.

96. Nelson G, Paraoan L, Spiller DG, et al. Multi-parameter analysis of the kinetics of NF-κB signaling and transcription in single living cells. J Cell Sci 2002; 115:1137–1148.

97. Wang CY, Cusack JC Jr, Liu R, Baldwin AS Jr. Control of inducible chemoresistance: enhanced anti-tumour therapy through increased apoptosis by inhibition of NF-κB. Nature Med 1999; 5:412–417.

98. Tsangaris GT, Tzortzatou-Stathopoulou F. MT expression prevents apoptosis: a study with antisense phosphorothioate oligodeoxynucleotides in a human T cell line. Anticancer Res 1998; 18:2423–2433.

99. Abdel-Mageed AB, Agrawal KC. Activation of NF-κB: potential role in MT-mediated mitogenic response. Cancer Res 1998; 58:2335–2338.

100. Kanekiyo M, Itoh N, Kawasaki A, Tanaka J, Nakanishi T, Tanaka K. Zinc-induced activation of the human cytomegalovirus major immediate-early promoter is mediated by metallothionein and NF-κB. Toxicol Appl Pharmacol 2001; 173:146–153.

101. Kanekiyo M, Itoh N, Kawasaki A, et al. Metallothionein modulates LPS-stimulated tumour necrosis factor expression in mouse peritoneal macrophages. Biochem J 2002; 361:363–369.

102. Sakurai A, Hara S, Okano N, Kondo Y, Inoue J, Imura N. Regulatory role of MT in NF-κB activation. FEBS Lett 1999; 455:55–58.

103. Crowthers KC, Kline V, Giardina C, Lynes MA. Augmented humoral immune function in metallothionein-null mice. Toxicol Appl Pharmacol 2000; 166:161–172.

104. Papouli E, Defais M, Larminat F. Overexpression of MT-2 sensitizes rodent cells to apoptosis induced by DNA cross-linking agent through inhibition of NF-κB activation. J Biol Chem 2002; 277:4764–4769.

105. Butcher HL, Kennette WA, Collins O, Zalups RK, Koropatnick J. Metallothionein mediates the level and activity of NF-κB in murine fibroblasts. J Pharmacol Exp Ther 2004; 310:589–598.

106. Meplan C, Richard MJ, Hainaut P. Metalloregulation of the tumor suppressor protein p53: zinc medi-ates the renaturation of p53 after exposure to metal chelators in vitro and in intact cells. Oncogene 2000; 19:5227–5236.

107 Maret W. Cellular zinc and redox status converge in the metallothionein/thionein pair. J Nutr 2003; 133:1460S–1462S.

108. Maret W, Jacob C, Vallee BL, Fischer EH. Inhibitory sites in enzymes: zinc removal and reactivation by thionein. PNAS 1998; 96:1936–1940.

109. Koropatnick J, DeMoor JM, Collins OM. Metallothionein and glucocorticoid responsiveness. In: Klaassen CD ed., Metallothionein IV. Basel: Birkhäuser, 1999:261–266.

110. DeMoor JM, Koropatnick DJ. Metals and cellular signaling in mammalian cells. Cell Mol Biol 2000; 46:367–381.

111. Blankenstein T. The role of inflammation in tumour growth and tumour suppression. Novartis Found Symp 2004; 256:205–210.

112. Dalgleish AG, O'Byrne KJ. Chronic immune activation and inflammation in the pathogenesis of AIDS and cancer. Adv Cancer Res 2002; 84:231–276.

113. Nelson WG, De Marzo AM, DeWeese TL, Isaacs WB. The role of inflammation in the pathogenesis of prostate cancer. J Urol 2004; 172(Suppl):S6–S12.

114. Szallasi Z, Bogi K, Gohari S, Biro T, Acs P, Blumberg PM. Non-equivalent roles for the first and second zinc fingers of protein kinase Cδ. Effect of their mutation on phorbol ester-induced translocation in NIH 3T3 cells. J Biol Chem 1996; 27:18,299–18,301.

115. Otsuka M, Fujita M, Aoki T, et al. Novel zinc chelators with dual activity in the inhibition of the kappa B site-binding proteins HIV-IP1 and NF-κB. J Med Chem 1995; 38:3264–3270.

116. Hancock WW, Grey ST, Hau L, et al. Binding of activated protein C to a specific receptor on human mononuclear phagocytes inhibits intracellular calcium signaling and monocyte-dependent proliferative response. Transplantation 1995; 60:1525–1532.

117. Meier RW, Niklaus G, Dewald B, Fey MF, Tobler A. Inhibition of the arachidonic acid pathway prevents induction of IL-8 mRNA by phorbol ester and changes the release of IL-8 from HL-60 cells: differential inhibition of induced expression of IL-8, TNFα, and IL-1α. J Cell Physiol 1995; 165:62–70.

118. Waelput W, Broekaert D, Vandekerckhove J, Brouckaert P, Tavernier J, Libert C. A mediator role for metallothionein in tumor necrosis factor-induced lethal shock. J Exp Med 2001; 11:1617–1624.

119. Coyle P, Philcox JC, Rofe AM. Hepatic zinc in metallothionein-null mice following zinc challenge: in vivo and in vitro studies. Biochem J 1995; 309:25–31.

120. Koropatnick J, Zalups RK. Effect of non-toxic mercury, zinc or cadmium pretreatment on the capacity of human monocytes to undergo lipopolysaccharide-induced activation. J Pharmacol 1997; 120:797–806.

121. Goyer A. Toxicology of metals. In: Amdur MO, Doull J, Klaassen CD, eds. Toxicology—the basic science of poisons, 4th edition. New York: Pergamon, 1991.

122. Vassalli P. The pathophysiology of tumour necrosis factors. Ann Rev Immunol 1992; 10:411–452.

123. Palmiter RD, Sandgren EP, Koeller DM, Brinster RL. Distal regulatory elements from the mouse metallothionein locus stimulate gene expression in transgenic mice. Mol Cell Biol 1993; 13:5266–5275.

124. Adcock IM, Caramori G. Cross-talk between pro-inflammatory transcription factors and glucocorticoids. Immunol Cell Biol 2001; 79:376–384.

125. Karin M. New twists in gene regulation by glucocorticoid receptor: is DNA binding dispensable? Cell 1998; 93:487–490.

14 Molecular Determinants of Intrinsic Multidrug Resistance in Cancer Cells and Tumors

Elena Monti, *PhD*

CONTENTS

SUMMARY

Intrinsic drug or multidrug resistance in previously untreated tumors is often the major obstacle to the success of cancer chemotherapy. Understanding the molecular mechanisms underlying these conditions is a prerequisite to the design of novel strategies aimed at improving current clinical protocols. This chapter focuses on recent experimental evidence concerning two of the features most commonly encountered in multidrug resistant cancer cells: (over)expression of multidrug transporters and disabling of apoptotic pathways.

Key Words: Apoptosis; intrinsic resistance; LRP; MRP; P-glycoprotein.

1. INTRODUCTION

It is common knowledge that tumors derived from different tissues exhibit widely varying degrees of susceptibility to anticancer agents, from the exquisitely sensitive testicular germ cell tumors to the drug refractory pancreatic and glial cancers. Failure of tumors to respond to anticancer drugs can depend on host-related factors and/or on the genetic makeup of cancer cells (Table 1; for a recent review see ref. *1*). Some of these factors (e.g., alterations of drug targets, deficits in specific drug-metabolizing enzymes) result in resistance to a small number of structurally or functionally related drugs. All too often, though, tumors are found to be simultaneously resistant to several drugs differing in chemical structure and/or mechanism of action; that is to say, they exhibit the notorious multidrug resistant (MDR) phenotype. Host and cellular factors can both contribute to the MDR phenotype (Fig. 1), drastically restricting viable chemotherapeutic options.

From: *Cancer Drug Discovery and Development: Cancer Drug Resistance*
Edited by: B. Teicher © Humana Press Inc., Totowa, NJ

Table 1
Factors Involved in Anticancer Drug Resistance

Host factors	Immunomodulation
	Pharmacogenetic features:
	    failure to achieve optimal serum drug levels due
	    to altered ADME[a]
	    low tolerance to drug-induced side effects
	    (requiring use of suboptimal drug doses)
	Restricted drug access to tumor site
	Microenvironmental cues

Genetic/epigenetic features of cancer cells	Altered expression of drug transporters Quali-/quantitative alterations of drug target(s) Changes in intracellular drug handling/metabolism Changes in DNA repair activities Alterations in apoptotic pathways

[a]ADME, absorption, distribution, metabolism, excretion.

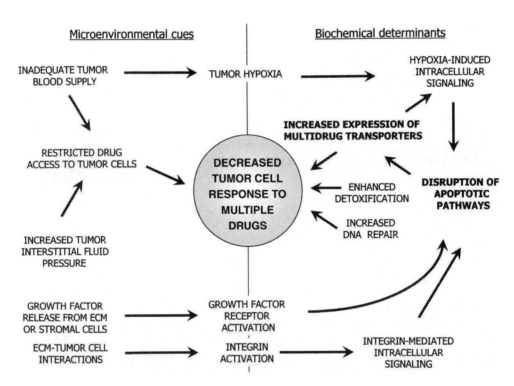

Fig. 1. Biological and bochemical mechanisms of drug resistance.

Our current understanding of the mechanisms underlying MDR was largely derived from studies based on selection and analysis of drug-resistant sublines in monolayer tissue culture systems. However, such studies completely overlook the importance of host-related factors and microenvironmental cues in tumor cell response, and generally fail address the problem of the inherent resistance encountered in the clinic in drug naive tumors. Yet, intrinsic or *de novo* resistance plays a critical role in the limited success of chemotherapy in some types of cancer, including colorectal and pancreatic carcinomas, non-small cell lung cancers and melanomas. Furthermore, intrinsic resistance, albeit usually present at low levels, may facilitate acquisition of additional cytoprotective features, leading to a full-blown resistant phenotype. Thus, understanding the genesis of intrinsic resistance may provide a rational basis for improvement of current therapeutic protocols, including those involving novel targeted agents.

The following paragraphs will review the state of the art concerning some aspects of intrinsic anticancer drug resistance, with an emphasis on mechanisms underlying the MDR phenotype. Factors related to tumor microenvironment have emerged as critical determinants of inherent chemoresistance in solid tumors; however, they will only briefly be dealt with, as they are specifically addressed by other authors in this book. The present chapter focuses on the role played by multispecific drug transporters and by disruption of apoptotic pathways in the response of unselected cancer cells to anticancer drugs; other biochemical determinants of resistance, such as glutathione-dependent detoxification processes and DNA repair enzyme activities, will be discussed elsewhere in this volume.

2. MICROENVIRONMENTAL CUES AND DRUG RESISTANCE

The notion that tumor cells respond very differently to therapy when they grow as a solid mass than when they grow as cell suspensions or monolayers can be traced back to the early 1970s *(2)*; Teicher and colleagues subsequently showed that very high levels of resistance to anticancer agents can be achieved under in vivo growth conditions that disappear in vitro *(3)*. Since then, the consequences of three-dimensional growth on tumor cell behavior has been extensively investigated using multicellular spheroids (MS) to reproduce some of the aspects encountered in solid tumors. As the tumor mass increases in size, increasingly severe limitations are imposed on the diffusion of oxygen and nutrients, eventually leading to heterogeneous cell behavior in different regions of the tumor, as regards both cell proliferation and response to cytotoxic agents (reviewed in ref. *4*). On oxygen deprivation, the cells initiate a pleiotropic adaptive response centered on activation of the transcription factor hypoxia-inducible factor (HIF)-1 *(5)*. Whereas this may lead to apoptotic death of a fair percentage of cells in a tumor population, survivors become tolerant to hypoxia-induced damage, likely by disabling one or more steps in apoptotic pathways. Such changes may also help tumor cells to overcome other insults, including chemotherapy-induced DNA damage, and thus may contribute to drug resistance *(6)*. Interestingly, tumor cells grown as MS have been found to express important biochemical determinants of drug resistance, such as high levels of the multidrug-specific transporter ATP-binding cassette ABCB1 (also known as P-glycoprotein) *(7)* and reduced activity of the mismatch repair system *(8)*, and many of these alterations can depend on HIF-1 activation *(9,10)*.

Also critical for solid tumor growth is the network of mutual interactions that the tumor cell establishes with neighboring tumor cells, with different types of normal cells present in the tumor stroma and with components of the extracellular matrix. Homotypic interactions among tumor cells are mediated by the E-cadherin family of surface proteins, and disruption of these interactions was found to restore sensitivity of MS to various drugs *(11)*. Other mechanisms depend instead on tumor cell interactions with components of the extracellular matrix, shifting the focus on the role of the integrin family of membrane glycoproteins as a likely source for cytoprotective signals that may ultimately lead to drug resistance (reviewed in ref. *12*). In summary, tumor chemoresistance, particularly in solid tumors, depends at least in part on survival signals developed under stressful conditions during tumor growth and/or on the ability of tumor cells to establish and maintain an efficient network of homo- and heterotypic interactions with other cells and with the tumor stroma. The design of novel approaches to overthrow these cellular strategies, e.g., by targeting the HIF-1 transcription factor *(5,13)*, is under way.

3. MULTISPECIFIC DRUG TRANSPORTERS AND INTRINSIC DRUG RESISTANCE

3.1. ABC Transporters

Most transporters involved in the MDR phenotype belong to the superfamily of the ABC (ATP-binding cassette) membrane transport proteins, which to date includes 48 members, grouped into seven subfamilies (A–G) *(14)*. The first to be identified, in 1976, was the 170 P-glycoprotein (now indicated as ABCB1), a surface glycoprotein decreasing drug accumulation in Chinese hamster ovary cells selected for resistance to the antimitotic agent colchicine *(15)*. This was followed in 1992 by the discovery of a second transporter, named multidrug resistance-associated protein (MRP, later changed into MRP-1 and, finally, into ABCC1) *(16)* in an MDR human lung cancer cell line, in which neither ABCB1 overxpression nor significant decreases in intracellular drug accumulation were apparent. ABCC1 was subsequently recognized as the prototype of a new subfamily of transporters, of which to date it remains the best-characterized member *(14,17)*. ABCB1 and ABCC1 substrate specificities show partial overlaps; however, important differences between the two transporters have been described, including a distinct preference for hydrophobic, weakly basic compounds for ABCB1, and for organic anions in the case of ABCC1. ABCC1 is the main transporter involved in elimination of drugs and endogenous compounds conjugated to glutathione (GSH), glucuronate or sulfate, which suggests an ubiquitous role in general detoxification mechanisms; interestingly, GSH seems to act as a cofactor for the transport of drugs that are not appreciably conjugated with GSH, such as vincristine and doxorubicin (DOX). In addition, ABCC1 was found to be insensitive to the action of ABCB1 inhibitors, such as verapamil (VP) or cyclosporin A (CsA). Finally, the levels of resistance imparted by ABCC1 are sensibly lower than those attained by ABCB1-expressing cells, and this has led to hypothesize that ABCC1 may be more relevant to the clinical intrinsic resistance. Among other studies, data obtained by our group in a monoclonal line (LoVo 7) derived from untreated human colon adenocarcinoma LoVo cells and exhibiting low-level spontaneous resistance to DOX support this hypothesis *(18)*. More recently, another ABC transporter, ABCG2 (also known as mitoxantrone resistance protein, MXR, or breast cancer resistance protein, BCRP) has also been involved in MDR in some tumors *(19)*. Although MDR ABC transporters were first identified in cancer cells selected in vitro for drug resistance, they were also subsequently identified in many normal tissues *(20,21)*, where they are believed to act as cytoprotectants against noxious xenobiotics and endogenous substances. An impressive body of experimental evidence has accumulated over the years, supporting a role for ABC transporters, and particularly ABCB1 and ABCC1, in acquired MDR, whereas studies on the mechanisms of intrinsic resistance have lagged considerably behind, mainly because of difficulties in obtaining experimental models reproducing the clinical situation. Drug-selected cells generally exhibit high levels of resistance (which is infrequent in clinical tumors), because of macroscopic alterations in the expression of drug efflux pumps and other critical determinants; the more subtle changes that lead to levels of resistance comparable to those observed in the clinic in untreated tumors are much more difficult to detect, and even when they *are* detected, it is hard to predict their impact on the overall outcome of drug treatment. To address this problem, Allen and colleagues tested the effects of eliminating basal ABCB1 and ABCC1 expression on drug response by comparing mouse cell lines carrying either functional or targeted null alleles of the gene encoding either or both transporters *(22)*. In this experimental model, expression of the two transporters, at levels that are more readily related to those detected in untreated tumors, was found to contribute to the basal resistance to substrate drugs, suggesting that even low levels of expression of ABCB1 and ABCC1, such as those that can be found in unselected cells, can substantially affect innate drug sensitivity of clinical tumors.

Recent studies used oligonucleotide arrays *(23)* or quantitative real-time RT–PCR (reverse transcriptase-polymerase chain reaction) *(24)* to analyze correlations between expression of ABC transporters and sensitivity to libraries of anticancer agents in the panel of 60 human cancer cell lines (the NCI-60) used by the National Cancer Institute to screen for anticancer activity. The cell lines in the panel were derived from a wide variety of tumors with different tissue origins, and as most of them have not been selected in the laboratory they may be more representative of drug resistance in the clinic than cells selected for resistance in vitro. Both studies underscored the prominent role played by ABC transporters in determining drug resistance in tumor cells and confirmed the negative correlation between ABCB1 expression and cytotoxicity of a broad spectrum of anticancer agents (whereas for ABCC1 and ABCG2 correlative evidence was found to be much weaker).

The role of ABC transporters in clinical resistance, and particularly in the resistant phenotypes encountered in drug naive patients with solid malignancies, is still the object of much debate. In general, a clear-cut correlation between protein levels and response to drug treatment is not easy to demonstrate, mainly because of technical difficulties in accurately measuring levels of ABC transporters in tumor samples and normal tissues. A relatively recent meta-analysis of studies examining ABCB1 expression in breast cancer indicates that a substantial fraction of tumors already expresses the protein at the time of clinical detection, and that this feature exhibits a significant positive correlation with a poor response to chemotherapy *(25)*. As overexpression of the *ABCB1* gene has been associated to other defects that *per se* are known to favor drug resistance, including *p53* mutations *(26)* and HIF-1 activation *(9)*, it is unclear whether increased ABCB1 levels can be considered as an independent prognostic factor. Increases in ABCB1 and ABCC1 (as well as lung resistance protein [LRP]; *see* Subheading 3.2.) expression were also reported early on during colorectal carcinogenesis *(27)*: MDR proteins appear to counteract colorectal carcinogenesis by protecting the epithelium against further environmentally induced genetic damage; however, as additional genetic changes take over on the way to malignant progression, the cytoprotective action of drug transporters is bypassed, and its overexpression becomes a negative feature by reducing response to drug treatment. In contrast, in acute lymphoblastic leukemia *de novo* resistance seems to depend only on ABCB1 expression, whereas ABCC1 (and LRP) expression is much less frequent *(28)*.

One issue that is particularly relevant to the role of ABC transporters in unselected tumor cells concerns their subcellular localization, which might affect intracellular drug distribution. One of the first hints that altered intracellular drug distribution may contribute to the MDR phenotype came from the work of Schuurhuis and colleagues *(29)*, who showed that resistance modifiers, such as VP, caused a redistribution of the cytotoxic agent DOX from the cytoplasm to the nucleus, thus facilitating its access to the target.

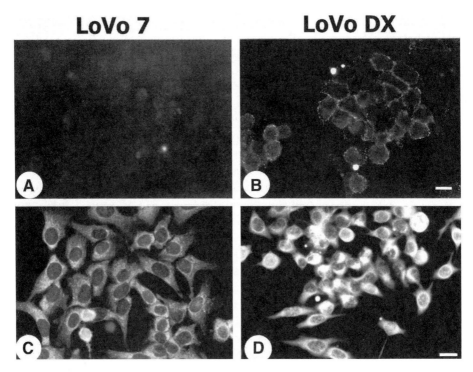

LoVo 7   LoVo DX

Fig. 2. Surface **(A,B)** and intracytoplasmic **(C,D)** expression of ABCB1 in human colon adenocardinoma cells LoVo 7 (intrinsically resistant to doxorubicin) and LoVo DX (selected in vitro for resistance to doxorubicin). *See* text and ref. *33*.

Although in tumor cells with an acquired MDR ABCB1 is mainly located at the plasma membrane, several other cellular compartments have been indicated as potential sites for ABCB1 functional activity, including the nucleus and nuclear envelope and intracyto-plasmic vesicles, generally related to the Golgi apparatus (reviewed in ref. *30*); this strategic localization might have profound bearings on drug resistance, as it might prevent drug access to its primary targets (DNA and/or DNA-related enzymes) by active extrusion from the nucleus and/or sequestration into intracytoplasmic compartments. To date, a role for intracellular ABCB1 in drug resistance remains to be firmly established; Larsen et al., after an extensive review of resistance mechanisms associated with changes in intracellular distribution of anticancer drugs, conclude that intracellular expression of ABCB1 is irrelevant to the MDR phenotype *(31)*. However, studies performed in unselected human melanoma cell lines as well as in a primary culture from a human metastatic melanoma lesion showed that ABCB1 is not expressed at the plasma membrane, but only at intracellular sites (mainly the Golgi apparatus). Treatment with the ABCB1 inhibitors VP and CsA was found to inhibit drug transit from the nucleus to the Golgi apparatus and its subsequent efflux from the cell, thereby increasing drug sensitivity *(32)*. These results are supported by our data in LoVo 7 cells *(33)*. In this cell line, evidence of the presence of intracellular ABCB1 was obtained by flow cytometry, immunofluorescence, immunoelectronmicroscopy, and immunoprecipitation, whereas surface expression was virtually absent (Fig. 2). This expression was accompanied by a slower time course in both DOX accumulation and efflux in LoVo 7 cells as compared to the parental cell line; ABCB1 inhibition by CsA was able to restore cell kinetics to the parental pattern. Thus, ABCB1 inhibitors may be useful not only to reverse or prevent acquired drug resistance, but also to sensitize drug naive, untreated tumors to substrate drugs. Intracytoplasmic localization has also been reported for ABCC1 *(32,34)*, and is believed to contribute significantly to drug resistance in some contexts *(31)*.

3.2. Lung Resistance Protein

LRP is not an ABC transporter; it was first identified by Scheper and colleagues *(35)* in a non-small cell lung cancer (NSCLC) selected for resistance to doxorubicin and is expressed at high levels in many tumors, as well as in normal tissues *(36)*. LRP was subsequently found to be identical to the major vault protein, concurring to the formation of multisubunit ribonucleoprotein particles ("vaults") that are present in the cytoplasm and at (or near) the nuclear membrane of all eukaryotic cells, where they are believed to be involved in nucleocytoplasmic transport. The resistance phenotype mediated by LRP, therefore, may be explained by transport of anticancer drugs *away* from their nuclear targets (reviewed in ref. *37*). An extensive study measuring ABCB1, ABCC1, and LRP mRNA and protein levels in the NCI-60 panel showed that, among the three MDR proteins, LRP expression correlated best with in vitro drug resistance to both classic MDR-related drugs (i.e., ABCB1 substrates) and non-MDR drugs *(38)*. The importance of LRP as a determinant of intrinsic resistance versus diverse anticancer agents has been subsequently confirmed in a number of different cell lines *(39)*. Studies by our group have demonstrated that LRP is expressed in LoVo 7 cells *(18,33)*, and that it is also associated to intrinsic resistance to DOX in the NSCLC cell line A549 *(40,41)*. Besides the evidence obtained in tumor cell lines, several groups demonstrated that LRP is also overexpressed in human tumors, including acute myeloid leukemia, childhood acute lymphoblastic leukemia, multiple myeloma, soft tissue sarcoma, ovarian cancer, breast and colorectal carcinoma, and this is generally associated to poor response to chemotherapy and/or shorter overall survival *(37)*. In contrast, Harada et al. *(42)* have demonstrated an inverse correlation between LRP expression and response to chemotherapy in NSCLC, whereas LRP overexpression seems to be a rare event in *de novo* adult acute lymphoblastic leukemia *(28)*. In addition, expression of LRP stably transfected into the ovarian carcinoma cell line A2780 was found to lead to increased number of vault particles, but does not confer a drug resistant phenotype *(43)*. These results, together with the observation that embryonic stem cells from *LRP–/–* mice were no more sensitive to a wide array of cytotoxic agents than cells obtained from *LRP+/+ mice (44)*, suggest that whereas LRP overexpression may contribute significantly to drug resistance in some tumors (and in the cell lines derived therein), the role of LRP seems to depend largely on the context.

4. APOPTOSIS AND DRUG RESISTANCE

Cell death by apoptosis can occur through at least two distinct but interconnected pathways, converging on activation of several members of a family of cysteine proteases called caspases. The extrinsic (or death receptor-dependent) pathway is triggered by interaction of death-inducing cytokines, such as Fas ligand, tumor necrosis factor (TNF)-α or TNF-related apoptosis-inducing ligand (TRAIL), with their respective membrane receptors (Fas/CD95, TNF-R1 and DR4/DR5), resulting in formation of an intracellular complex (the death-inducing signaling complex) whose ultimate effect is activation of the initiator caspase 8. In some cell types (type I), the extrinsic pathway is sufficient to induce cell death, whereas in others (type II), the intervention of the intrinsic pathway must also be engaged through caspase 8-mediated cleavage of the cytoplasmic protein Bid, a member of the Bcl-2 family of apoptosis regulators (45,46). The intrinsic (or mitochondrial) pathway is initiated by various cellular stresses, resulting in the release of proapoptotic factors from the mitochondrial intermembrane space, including cytochrome-c, the caspase-independent AIF (apoptosis-inducing factor) and Smac/Diablo (second mitochondrial activator of caspases/direct inhibitor of apoptosis protein [IAP]-binding protein with low pI); in the presence of dATP, a complex (the apoptosome) is formed from cytochrome-c, Apaf-1 (adaptor protein apoptosis activating factor) and inactive procaspase 9, leading to activation of initiator caspase 9. From this point on, both pathways proceed identically with activation of effector caspases (mainly caspases 3, 6, and 7), cleavage of key intracellular components and, ultimately, cell death. The intrinsic pathway is regulated by the tumor suppressor p53 through transcriptional activation or repression of a number of target genes and can be modulated positively or negatively at the mitochondrial level by members of the Bcl-2 family of proteins. A further level of control is exerted trough the activity of IAPs, a family of polypeptides inhibiting caspase activity (reviewed in ref. 47 and references therein).

It has been said that the ability of cells to evade apoptosis is an essential hallmark of cancer, and that disabling apoptosis represents an obligatory step on the way to a full-blown malignant phenotype (48). A number of excellent reviews have addressed this aspect in the past few years (e.g., refs. 49–53), underscoring the fact that cancer cells, and particularly those from solid tumors, are subject to strong selective pressure during tumor development and metastasis formation and that, in order to eventually "make it," they must be able to survive a number of diverse insults, from immune attack to nutrient and oxygen deprivation. Thus, disabling cell death programs has emerged as a winning strategy, allowing tumor cells to overcome the many hurdles threatening to block their progression. Unfortunately, it has also become clear that there are striking similarities in the way in which tumor cells respond to physiologic and pharmacologic insults. Studies performed nearly 25 yr ago showed that apoptosis accompanies tumor regression during chemotherapy with such diverse agents as actinomycin D, mitomycin C, and cytosine arabinoside (54). Since then, the hypothesis that the majority of cytotoxic drugs used in cancer chemotherapy act by triggering apoptosis, at least at therapeutic concentrations, has gained wide acceptance, even though evidence for drug-induced apoptosis is admittedly hard to obtain in the clinic (53) and other modalities of cell death have been recognized as contributing to the final outcome of therapy (55). Thus, apoptosis provides a link between tumor development and tumor response to treatment: alterations in the apoptotic machinery are built-in features in most cancer cells, and this makes them inherently resistant to agents requiring intact apoptotic pathways. As advanced and metastatic cancers have necessarily proven themselves most efficient in evading apoptotic cell death during their history, it is not surprising that they are also intrinsically most efficient in resisting therapeutic interventions (56). Notably, as anticancer drugs with widely differing intracellular targets impinge on the same intracellular death pathways, such inherently resistant phenotype encompasses different classes of compounds and, therefore, can be considered as the ultimate form of multidrug resistance.

So, the past decade of drug resistance research has witnessed a distinct shift in focus from mechanisms upstream of drug-target interactions responsible for "classic" MDR (such as overexpression of drug efflux pumps and/or detoxification enzymes) to events related to the cell's ability to detect and respond to the damage resulting from drug-target interactions. Whereas mutations in cancer cells most often target upstream regulators in the intrinsic pathway, such as *p53* and/or *Bcl-2*-related genes, alterations that disrupt apoptosis downstream of the mitochondrion can also occur, albeit less frequently. A case in point is represented by Apaf-1 (the adaptor protein involved in apoptosome formation), the expression of which is lost in metastatic melanoma through deletion of one allele of the corresponding gene, and methylation-induced silencing of the other, possibly contributing to the well-known inherent chemoresistance of these tumors *(57,58)*. Drug-induced apoptosis has been shown to depend mainly on activation of the intrinsic pathway *(59)*, even though the death receptor pathway has also been proposed to contribute to drug resistance in a cell-specific fashion *(46)*. The following paragraphs will briefly review the role played by key components of apoptotic pathways in *de novo* drug resistance of cancer cells and human tumors.

4.1. Death Receptors

The death receptor pathway can be recruited by anticancer agents (mainly through p53 activation) and contribute to the overall response to chemotherapy in some settings *(60,61)*. Blocking antibodies against Fas, or Fas mutations were found to abolish 5-fluorouracil-induced cytotoxicity in mouse thymocytes and in some human colon cancer cell lines; however, neither anti-Fas antibodies nor Fas mutations were able to interfere with etoposide- or DOX-induced apoptosis in acute lymphoblastic leukemia or multiple myeloma cells (reviewed in ref. *62*). In addition, experiments using cells from mice with functional mutations in the death receptor pathway indicated that it is dispensable for the cytotoxic action of chemotherapeutic agents *(63)*. Disabling of the extrinsic pathway can be observed in a subset of melanomas, through death receptor downregulation or expression of decoy receptors, or, again, through upregulation of FLIP (Fas-associated death domain-like interleukin-1β-converting enzyme inhibitor protein), which inhibits caspase 8 activation *(58)*; however, whereas these defect may help explain how melanoma cells evade immune surveillance, the specific contribution of the extrinsic pathway to clinical drug resistance remains to be defined.

4.2. p53

The p53 tumor suppressor is activated in response to several stress signals, including those deriving from DNA damage, hypoxia, or aberrant oncogene expression, to promote cell cycle arrest, DNA repair, senescence, and apoptosis (reviewed in refs. *64* and *65*). p53 controls and directs such diverse cellular responses mainly through transcriptional activation of an ever-increasing number of target genes *(66)*. Among the earliest to be identified were genes encoding the cyclin-dependent kinase inhibitor p21^{WAF1}, which is the main responsible for cell cycle arrest, and GADD45, participating in DNA repair processes. Several target genes whose products are involved in apoptosis control have also been identified, starting from the proapoptotic Bcl-2 family member Bax and the death receptor Fas/CD95, to the more recently discovered DR5 (acting as membrane receptor for the death-inducing ligand TRAIL) and the BH3-only proteins PUMA and Noxa. Whereas upregulation of these effectors alone is sufficient to initiate apoptosis, other proteins encoded by p53 target genes require that the cells be subjected to additional proapoptotic stimuli, including exposure to cytotoxic drugs, whereby they could exert a chemosensitizing effect *(66)*. This class of targets includes Apaf-1, the BH3-only protein Bid, and the effector caspase 6. Besides inducing expression of proapoptotic factors, p53 was also found to repress that of a number of antiapoptotic regulators, including Bcl-2 and the IAP family member survivin *(67)*.

Given the role played by p53 in apoptosis, it is not surprising that p53 should be selected strongly against during tumorigenesis: p53 is in fact the most commonly mutated gene in human cancers *(68)*. In addition, p53 function can be lost through a number of other mechanisms, including binding and/or degradation by virally encoded oncoproteins; overexpression of the murine double minute (Mdm)2 protein, which also binds p53 blocking its transcriptional activity and targeting it for proteolytic degradation; loss of p19ARF, that binds and neutralizes Mdm2; defects in posttranslational modifications (phosphorylation, acetylation) of p53; altered subcellular localization of p53; and defects in the effector pathways downstream of p53 activation *(64)*.

In addition to its role in suppressing tumorigenesis, p53-dependent apoptosis contributes to chemotherapy-induced cell death *(50)*. Studies performed over a decade ago by comparing oncogenically transformed fibroblasts from wild-type and p53-deficient mice demonstrated that p53 plays a critical role in promoting apoptosis on treatment with ionizing radiation and several genotoxic chemotherapeutic drugs, that is, p53-deficient cells displayed a multi-drug-resistant phenotype *(69)*. A broader analysis on the NCI-60 panel found that cell lines with *p53* mutations were generally more resistant to treatment that cell lines with wild-type *p53 (70)*. Possibly contributing to chemoresistance in the absence of functional p53 is also the ability of the wild-type form of the protein to downregulate some ABC transporters, including ABCB1 and ABCC1, as well as the fact that some mutated forms of p53 actually increase ABCB1 levels *(26)*. Thus, several aspects of p53 function would favor cell sensitivity to cytotoxic agents. However, some notable exceptions *(71)* indicate that p53 status is not a universal predictor of treatment response, in part because not all drugs absolutely require p53 for their apoptosis-inducing effects *(51)*. In the clinic, loss of p53 has been linked to chemoresistance in a wide spectrum of tumor types *(50,72)*. In lymphoid malignancies, patients with *p53* mutations are remarkably resistant to therapy and display very short survival times; however, in this type of malignancy loss of p53 tends to be very rare in primary tumors, and becomes more frequent in relapsed tumors, suggesting it occurs as part of an acquired MDR phenotype, rather than as an inherent feature of this type of malignancies. Among solid tumors, p53 status was indicated as a strong predictor of therapeutic failure, relapse, and death in breast carcinomas *(73)* and in gastric and colon cancer *(74)*. However, other studies failed to establish a significant correlation between p53 levels and response to chemotherapy (e.g., *see* ref. *75*); in bladder cancer, *p53* mutations were actually found to correlate with *increased* drug sensitivity *(76)*. In summary, clinical as well as experimental data have emerged to support both positive and negative correlations between *p53* mutations and drug sensitivity. One possible explanation for this apparent paradox lies in the very pleiotropic nature of p53 target genes, which would lead to opposing cell responses following exposure to cytotoxic drugs: on one hand, loss of the p53-dependent apoptotic program might promote drug resistance by making tumors less responsive to therapy, whereas loss of p53-dependent damage-induced checkpoints might enhance sensitivity by making tumor cells more vulnerable to DNA-damaging agents. Thus, the actual impact of p53 status on treatment outcome might be related to the mode of drug action, tissue of tumor origin or the precise genetic makeup of individual tumors. In addition, it has recently become clear that p53 is a member of an emerging protein family *(77)* and that other members, such as p73, may compensate for p53 loss in some settings: a recent study showed that the induction of apoptosis by p53 requires the presence of p73 *(78)*; however, p73 can induce apoptosis in tumor cells lacking functional p53; whereas mutant p53 can block p73 function *(79)*. The picture is further complicated by the existence of different isoforms for p73, (as well as for the other member of the family, p63), some of which (TA) can substitute for p53 and transactivate proapoptotic genes, whereas others (ΔN) act in a dominant negative fashion and can block chemotherapy-induced apoptosis in tumor cells that retain wild-type p53 *(80)*. Finally, at least some of the difficulties in relating *p53* mutations to clinical parameters depend on technical problems inherent in the methodologies employed to assess p53 status in clinical specimens. Immunohistochemistry (IHC) is still the most widely employed method to detect p53, but a number of drawbacks make this method less than optimal: (1) as wild-type p53 protein has a very short half-life, it is assumed that all of the detected p53 corresponds to the mutated protein, but, depending on the context, this can lead to gross over- or underestimation of the actual incidence of mutations; (2) not all p53 mutations are functionally equivalent; (3) p53 function can be lost in spite of the presence of wild-type protein because of defects in regulatory pathways; and (4) IHC relies on subjective data evaluation. Direct sequence analysis and yeast functional assays represent distinct improvements in accuracy over IHC, but they suffer from the same inability to identify mutations in modifiers of p53 activity (such as Mdm2 or p19ARF) or downstream effectors (e.g., Bax). Consequently, to establish a correlation between p53 function and tumor chemosensitivity/resistance, a complete analysis of the p53 pathway is required, which has only recently been made feasible by the advent of DNA and protein "array" technologies.

4.3. The Bcl-2 Family

To date, the mammalian Bcl-2 family of proteins includes ~20 different polypeptides sharing a variable number of conserved regions, named Bcl-2 homology (BH) domains, that are involved in both homo- and heterotypic protein–protein interactions *(81)*. Members of the family are grouped according to the number of BH regions, which also confers different functional properties: proteins containing BH1-4, such as Bcl-2 itself and Bcl-X_L, are antiapoptotic, whereas multidomain proteins lacking BH4, such as Bax and Bak, promote apoptosis. Following appropriate stimuli, proapoptotic proteins in this latter group translocate from the cytoplasm to the outer mitochondrial membrane, oligomerize to form pore-like structures, and promote release of proapoptotic factors from the mitochondrial intermembrane space. Translocation to mitochondria is aided by yet another subfamily of Bcl-2 proteins, the so-called BH3-only proteins, including Bad, the p53 targets Noxa and PUMA, and the already-mentioned Bid. Antiapoptotic members of the family exert their function, at least in part, by sequestering BH3-only proteins in stable complexes, thereby preventing Bax and Bak activation; in addition, they exert direct effects on mitochondrial channels, blocking mitochondrial release of proapoptotic factors *(82)*. Mutations or altered expression of Bcl-2 family proteins can drastically alter drug response in experimental systems, and the evidence is strongest for Bcl-2 itself. Expression of exogenous Bcl-2 has been found early on to protect cultured cells against the majority of agents used for cancer chemotherapy *(83)*, whereas downregulation of Bcl-2 increases chemsensitivity in tumor cell lines and animal models (reviewed in ref. *84*). Studies in clinical samples have demonstrated a correlation between high expression of Bcl-2 and poor prognosis in a number of human cancers, including acute myeloid and lymphoblastic leukemias, non-Hodgkin's lymphomas, and prostate cancer (reviewed in ref. *85*). Similar observations support the involvement of Bcl-X_L in drug resistance, as high Bcl-X_L levels, whether intrinsic or induced by transfection, inhibit chemotherapy-induced apoptosis in experimental models *(86,87)*, and high Bcl-X_L levels correlate high with poorer prognosis in patients with such diverse tumors as intermediate grade lymphomas *(88)*, squamous cell carcinoma of the oropharynx *(89)*, and soft tissue sarcomas *(90)*.

Among proapoptotic multidomain members of the Bcl-2 family, Bax is probably the most extensively investigated: in HCT116 human adenocarcinoma cells, as well as in other in vitro models, *BAX* deletion has been reported to inhibit drug-induced apoptosis *(91,92)*; similar considerations apply to Bak *(93)*. Interestingly, mismatch repair-deficient tumors of the colon-rectum have been reported to harbor inactivating frameshift mutations in a single *BAX* allele *(94)*, probably leading to reduced Bax protein levels; this alteration could very well contribute to the well-known inherent resistance of this tumor type. However, the effects of Bax and Bak alterations on drug sensitivity in vivo remain to be established; evidence obtained in both in vitro models and in vivo suggests that it is the ratio of pro- to antiapoptotics members of the Bcl-2 family rather than absolute levels of any given protein that will ultimately tip the balance towards chemosensitivity or chemoresistance (e.g. ref. *95*).

Very little information is available regarding the role of BH3-only proteins in tumor response to chemotherapy. A recent report indicates that the level of Bid expression is closely associated with sensitivity of hepatocellular carcinoma cells to chemotherapeutic drugs *(96)*; moreover, a synthetic peptide corresponding to the minimal sequence of the BH3 domain has been shown to enhance anthracycline-induced cell death in a human ovarian carcinoma cell line *(97)*. Finally, recent evidence indicates that the BH3-only proteins Noxa and PUMA mediate drug-induced cytotoxicity both in cancer cells and in mice *(98)*. However, to date there is not sufficient evidence to support a role for this subfamily in clinical intrinsic chemoresistance.

4.4. Caspases

Caspases are a family of twelve (currently identified) aspartate-specific cysteine proteases, six of which (caspases 3, 6, 7, 8, 9, and 10) have been definitely implicated in apoptosis in various model systems and classified as "initiator" or "upstream" caspases, such as caspases 8 and 9, and "effector" or "downstream" caspases, according to their respective functions along the apoptotic cascades *(99)*. The ability of anticancer drugs to trigger caspase activation appears to be a critical determinant of drug sensitivity/resistance. In spite of the key role played by caspases in death execution, caspase mutations have been observed infrequently in cancer cells *(100)*; however, inactivation by epigenetic mechanisms has also been reported *(101)*, and reexpression of caspase 8, through demethylation by 5-aza-2'-deoxycytidine or direct gene transfer, has been shown to sensitize a variety of tumor cell lines towards death receptor- as well as drug-induced apoptosis *(102)*. In addition, caspase 9 function can be lost in some melanomas through upregulation of heat shock protein 70, which blocks caspase 9 activation by the apoptosome *(103)*. On the other hand, evidence suggesting that individual caspases may be dispensable for apoptosis, at least in some systems, has also been reported: for example, MCF-7 breast carcinoma cells, which lack caspase 3 owing to a deletion in the *CASP-3* gene, are still able to undergo apoptosis following treatment with TNF or staurosporine *(104)*, and are exquisitely sensitive to the cytotoxic action of most agents currently used in breast cancer therapy. These data suggest the existence of a degree of functional redundancy in caspase-mediated proteolytic cascades, especially among effector caspases, as well as the possibility of context-dependence in the overall effects of caspase activation.

4.5. Inhibitor of Apoptosis Proteins

Members of this family of polypeptides were originally identified in baculoviruses as part of viral strategies aimed at suppressing apoptotic programs in infected cells. Multiple members of the family, such as cIAP-1 and -2, X-linked mammalian inhibitor of apoptosis protein (XIAP), melanoma-IAP/livin and survivin, have been identified in human cells, and most have been found to block the activity and/or activation of both up- and downstream caspases. This is achieved by binding the enzymes and facilitating their ubiquitylation and subsequent degradation. Activity of IAPs can be upregulated by activation of the antiapoptotic transcription factor NF-κB, as well as by binding to mitochondrially released Smac/Diablo, which causes displacement of IAPs from their caspase-binding partners (reviewed in ref. *105*). Evidence obtained in both in vitro and in vivo settings suggests that IAPs may play a role in the inherent chemoresistance of some tumor types: high expression of different IAPs is associated with poor prognosis in prostate cancer *(106)* and acute childhood myeloid leukemia *(107)*; XIAP was found to inhibit cisplatin-induced cell death in a number of human ovarian cancer cell lines *(108)* and in DU145 prostate cancer cells *(109)*, whereas antisense downregulation of XIAP was found to restore cisplatin sensitivity in both experimental models, as well as to sensitize NIH-H460 human non-small cell lung cancer in vitro and in vivo to the cyotoxic action of DOX, paclitaxel, vinorelbine, and etoposide *(110)*; ML-IAP/livin is upregulated in melanoma cell lines *(111)*, and its inhibition by Smac/Diablo was found to restore sensitivity to doxorubicin-induced apoptosis in MCF-7 breast carcinoma cells *(112)*. However, a recent attempt to correlate expression of these polypeptides with drug sensitivity NCI-60 panel failed to demonstrate the postulated negative correlation *(113)*. Survivin was also identified as a member of the IAP family whose expression is extremely common in embryos and in fetal tissues, drastically downregulated in the adult and upregulated in most human cancers (for a review, *see* ref. *114*), suggesting that survivin reactivation is important during tumorigenesis. However, a number of features set survivin apart from the rest of the family, including its cell cycle-dependent expression and its subcellular localization on spindle microtubules, leading to a dual role in apoptosis suppression and regulation of cell division *(115)*. In addition, whereas the mechanism of caspase inhibition by other IAPs has been characterized (*see* above), in the case of survivin it is not yet clear, whether the effect depends on direct or indirect interactions. Growing evidence indicates a correlation between elevated survivin levels and poor prognosis, e.g., in acute myelogenous leukemia, neuroblastoma, and malignant glioma, as well as cancers of the colon, prostate, ovary, breast, pancreas, and esophagus *(62)*. Zaffaroni and Daidone recently reviewed substantial in vitro and clinical evidence correlating survivin levels and poor response to paclitaxel *(116)*. Ribozyme-mediated downregulation of survivin was shown to sensitize melanoma cells to both topotecan and cisplatin *(117,118)*. Interestingly, the naturally occurring dietary compound resveratrol was also found to sensitize a number of established and primary cancer cell lines to the action of cytotoxic agents including DOX, cisplatin, cytosine arabinoside, and etoposide by downregulating survivin through transcriptional and posttranscriptional mechanisms *(119)*.

4.6. Cell Survival Pathways

Although signaling pathways involved in cell survival may not directly act downstream of anticancer drugs, recent studies indicate that they can synergize with antiapoptotic mutations to reduce chemosensitivity. Activation of the phosphoinositol-3-kinase (PI3K)/Akt/phosphatase and tensin homologue deleted in chromosome ten (PTEN) pathway (reviewed in ref. *120*) occurs downstream of a number of oncogenic products, such as Ras and the HER receptors, and suppresses cell death programs by direct or indirect disabling of proapoptotic signals. Dysregulation of this pathway in cancer can be because of a variety of mechanisms, including *Akt* amplification, loss of the negative regulator PTEN, and constitutive activation of upstream positive regulators. Evidence in support of a role for this pathway in response to chemotherapeutic agents can be summarized as follows: (1) Constitutively active Akt was found to reduce topotecan-induced apoptosis in A549 NSCLC cells *(121)*. (2) Inactivation of Akt by overexpression of PTEN enhances the response of SHIN-3 ovarian cancer cells to irinotecan *(122)* and of LNCaP prostate cells to DOX and vincristine *(123)*. (3) Inhibition of PI3K/Akt by the PI3K inhibitor LY294002 accelerated and enhanced DOX-induced cell death in human lung adenocarcinoma NCI-H522 cells *(124)*. (4) A new selective pharmacologic Akt inhibitor has recently been shown to sensitize HL60 human acute promyelocytic leukemia cells to anticancer drugs, including cytosine arabinoside and etoposide, as well as to the proapoptotic ligand TRAIL and to ionizing radiation *(125)*.

The NF-κB pathway depends on activation of a transcription factor modulating several components of the mitochondrial and death receptor pathways, thereby suppressing apoptosis and possibly contributing to chemoresistance *(126,127)*. Treatment with cytotoxic agents induces NF-κB functional activation as part of a cellular response to genotoxic stress; thus, NF-κB is implicated in a form of short-term inducible chemoresistance. However, constitutive activation through chromosomal amplification, overexpression, and rearrangement of genes coding for Rel/NF-κB factors has been noted in many human hematopoietic and solid tumors *(128)*. Persistent nuclear NF-κB activity was also described in several human cancer cell types, as a result of constitutive activation of upstream signaling kinases or mutations inactivating IκB (inhibitory κB) subunits. Thus, NF-κB may also be involved in inherent drug resistance, that could be overcome by forced expression of its inhibitor IκB or by the proteasome inhibitor bortezomib (PS-341), that blocks IκB degradation; both types of interventions were in fact found to restore sensitivity of multiple myeloma cells to melphalan and DOX *(129)* and of pancreatic cancer cells to paclitaxel *(130)*.

5. CONCLUSIONS AND PERSPECTIVES

Enhanced understanding of the mechanisms of drug resistance, even though derived largely from in vitro models of acquired resistance, has suggested ways to improve the clinical management of tumors inherently refractory to chemotherapy. Early attempts at circumventing ABCB1-mediated MDR by using inhibitors like VP and CsA have met with disappointing outcomes, possibly because the inhibitors were too weak, or because of their unpredictable pharmacokinetic interactions. Novel ABCB1 inhibitors, such as XR9576 (tariquidar), are currently in clinical trials, but it is still too early to predict their efficacy as clinical tools. Other strategies (such as use of hammerhead ribozymes) directed at inhibiting ABCB1 as well as other MDR transporters are currently being developed *(131)*. Similarly, several different approaches have been devised to target apoptotic defects in order to restore sensitivity to cytotoxic agents, and these include, among others, blocking of Bcl-2 (or Bcl-X$_L$) by antisense agents or by BH3-like small molecules disrupting interactions between pro- and antiapoptotic Bcl2 family members; use of ribozymes to downregulate survivin and possibly other IAP family members; direct stimulation of the death receptor pathway by treatment with recombinant TRAIL; restoring p53 function by direct gene transfer, by blocking negative p53 regulators, such as Mdm-2 or the E6 protein from human papilloma viruses, or by using small molecules that promote correct folding of mutant forms of p53 *(84,116,131)*. None of these strategies has been clinically validated as yet, and the whole concept has suffered a severe blow from the rejection by the Food and Drug Administration of the anti-Bcl2 antisense agent oblimersen sodium (Genasense®) in combination with the cytotoxic drug dacarbazine for the treatment of malignant melanoma, because of its failure to improve overall survival over dacarbazine alone. Several issues will have to be considered if chemosensitizers are to be successfully incorporated into chemotherapeutic regimens (possibly including the choice of alternative endpoints). Perhaps it is most important to emphasize that drug resistance, especially when inherent to untreated tumors, results from one of innumerable possible combinations of cellular mechanisms, often organized as networks that have only just begun to be unraveled; thus, it is unlikely that targeting a single mechanism may go a long way in restoring chemosensitivity. A better strategy could be trying to target multiple mechanisms at the same time, as suggested by a recent experimental study of the combined effects of antisense oligonucleotides directed at Bcl-2 and ABCC1 on DOX cytotoxicity in SCLC cells *(132)*. Resolving the intricate interactions among proteins within the integrated systems responsible for chemosensitivity/ resistance, using approaches such as DNA, tissue and protein microarrays and proteomics and with the aid of novel mathematical models, will hopefully provide a framework that will accelerate both drug discovery and its translation to the clinical management of chemoresistant disease.

REFERENCES

1. Gottesman MM. Mechanisms of cancer drug resistance. Annu Rev Med 2002; 53:516–527.
2. Durand RE, Sutherland RM. Effects of intercellular contact on repair of radiation damage. Exp Cell Res 1972; 71:75–80.
3. Teicher BA, Herman TS, Holden SA, et al. Tumor resistance to alkylating agents conferred by mechanisms operative only in vivo. Science 1990; 247:1457–1461.
4. Desoize B, Jardillier J-C. Multicellular resistance: a paradigm for clinical resistance? Crit Rev Oncol Hematol 2000; 36:193–207.
5. Semenza GL. Targeting HIF-1 for cancer therapy. Nat Rev Cancer 2003; 3:721–732.
6. Harris AL. Hypoxia—a key regulatory factor in tumor growth. Nature Rev Cancer 2002; 3:712–732.
7. Wartenberg M, Frey C, Diedershagen H, et al. Development of an intrinsic P-glycoprotein-mediated doxorubicin resistance in quiescent cell layers of large, multicellular prostate tumor spheroids. Int J Cancer 1998; 75:855–863.
8. Francia G, Man S, Teicher B, et al. Gene expression analysis of tumor spheroids reveals a role for suppressed DNA mismatch repair in multicellular resistance to alkylating agents. Mol Cell Biol 2004; 24:6837–6849.

9. Wartenberg M, Ling FC, Müschen M, et al. Regulation of the multidrug resistance transporter P-glycoprotein in multicellular tumor spheroids by hypoxia-inducible factor (HIF-1) and reactive oxygen species. FASEB J 2003; 17:503–505.

10. Mihaylova VT, Bindra RS, Yuan J, et al. Decreased expression of the DNA mismatch repair gene *Mlh1* under hypoxic stress in mammalian cells. Mol Cell Biol 2003; 23:3265–3273.

11. Green SK, Francia G, Isidoro C, Kerbel RS. Antiadhesive antibodies targeting E-cadherin sensitize multicellular tumor spheroids to chemotherapy in vitro. Mol Cancer Ther 2004; 3:149–159.

12. Damiano JS. Integrins as novel drug targets for overcoming innate drug resistance. Curr Cancer Drug Targets 2002; 2:37–43.

13. Giaccia A, Siim BG, Johnson RS. HIF-1 as a target for drug development. Nat Rev Drug Discov 2003; 2:803–811.

14. Gottesman MM, Fojo T, Bates SE. Multidrug resistance in cancer: role of ATP-dependent transporters. Nat Rev Cancer 2002; 2:48–58.

15. Juliano RL, Ling V. A surface glycoprotein modulating drug permeability in Chinese hamster ovary cell mutants. Biochim Biophys Acta 1976; 455:162–152.

16. Cole SP, Bhardwaj G, Gerlach JH, et al. Overexpression of a transporter gene in a multidrug-resistant human lung cancer cell line. Science 1992; 258:1650–1654.

17. Borst P, Evers R, Kool M, Wijnholds J. A family of drug transporters: the multidrug resistance-associated proteins. J Natl Cancer Inst 2000; 92:1295–1302.

18. Dolfini E, Dasdia T, Arancia G, et al. Characterization of a clonal human colon adenocarcinoma line intrinsically resistant to doxorubicin. Br J Cancer 1997; 76:67–76.

19. Miyake K, Mickley L, Litman T, et al. Molecular cloning of cDNAs which are highly overexpressed in mitoxantrone-resistant cells. Demonstration of homology to ABC transport genes. Cancer Res 1999; 59:8–13.

20. Fojo AT, Ueda K, Slamon DJ, et al. Expression of multidrug-resistance gene in human tumors and tissues. Proc Natl Acad Sci U S A 1987; 84:265–269.

21. Flens MJ, Zaman GJ, van der Valk P, et al. Tissue distribution of the multidrug resistance protein. Am J Pathol 1996; 148:1237–1247.

22. Allen JD, Brinkhuis RF, van Deemter L, et al. Extensive contribution of the multidrug transporters P-glycoprotein and Mrp1 to basal drug resistance. Cancer Res 2000; 60:5761–5766.

23. Huang Y, Anderle P, Bussey KJ, et al. Membrane transporters and channels: role of the transportome in cancer chemosensitivity and chemoresistance. Cancer Res 2004; 64:4294–4301.

24. Szakács G, Annereau JP, Lababidi S, et al. Predicting drug sensitivity and resistance: profiling ABC transporter genes in cancer cells. Cancer Cell 2004; 6:129–137.

25. Trock BJ, Leonessa F, Clarke R. Multidrug resistance in breast cancer: a meta-analysis of Mdr1/gp170 expression and its possible functional significance. J Natl Cancer Inst 1997; 89:917–931.

26. Bush JA, Li G. Cancer chemoresistance: the relationship between p53 and multidrug transporters. Int J Cancer 2002; 98:323–330.

27. Meijer GA, Schroeijers AB, Flens MJ, et al. Increased expression of multidrug resistance related proteins Pgp, MRP1, and LRP/MVP occurs early in colorectal carcinogenesis. J Clin Pathol 1999; 52:450–454.

28. Damiani D, Michelutti A, Michieli M, et al. P-glycoprotein, lung resistance-related protein and multidrug resistance-associated protein in de novo adult acute lymphoblastic leukaemia. Br J Haematol 2002; 116:519–527.

29. Schuurhuis GJ, Broxterman HJ, Cervantes A, et al. Quantitative determination of factors contributing to doxorubicin resistance in multidrug-resistant cells. J Natl Cancer Inst 1989; 81:1887–1892.

30. Molinari A, Calcabrini A, Meschini S, et al. Subcellular detection and localization of the drug transporter P-glycoprotein in cultured tumor cells. Curr Protein Pept Sci 2002; 3:653–670.

31. Larsen AK, Escargueil AE, Skladanowski A. Resistance mechanisms associated with altered intracellular distribution of anticancer agents. Pharmacol Ther 2000; 85:217–229.

32. Molinari A, Calcabrini A, Meschini S, et al. Detection of P-glycoprotein in the Golgi apparatus of drug-untreated human melanoma cells. Int J Cancer 1998; 75:885–893.

33. Meschini S, Marra M, Calcabrini A, et al. Role of the lung resistance-related protein (LRP) in the drug sensitivity of cultured tumor cells. Toxicol In Vitro 2002; 16:389–398.

34. Krishnamachary N, Center MS. The MRP gene associated with a non-P-glycoprotein multidrug resistance encodes a 190-kDa membrane bound glycoprotein. Cancer Res 1993; 53:3658–3661.

35. Scheper RJ, Broxterman HJ, Scheffer GL, et al. Overexpression of an M_r 110,000 vesicular protein in non-P-glycoprotein-mediated multidrug resistance. Cancer Res. 1993; 53:1475–1479.

36. Izquierdo MA, Scheffer GL, Flens MJ, et al. Broad distribution of the multidrug resistance-related vault lung resistance protein in normal human tissues and tumors. Am J Pathol 1996; 148:877–887.
37. Scheffer GL, Schroeijers AB, Izquierdo MA, et al. Lung resistance-related protein/major vault protein and vaults in multidrug-resistant cancer. Curr Opin Oncol 2000; 12:550–556.
38. Izquierdo MA, Shoemaker RH, Flens MJ, et al. Overlapping phenotypes of multidrug resistance among panels of human cancer-cell lines. Int J Cancer 1996; 65:230–237.
39. Laurencot CM, Scheffer GL, Scheper RJ, Shoemaker RH. Increased LRP mRNA expression is associated with the MDR phenotype in intrinsically resistant human cancer cell lines. Int J Cancer 1997; 72:1021–1026.
40. Meschini S, Calcabrini A, Monti E, et al. Intracellular P-glycoprotein expression is associated with the intrinsic multidrug resistance phenotype in human colon adenocarcinoma cells. Int J Cancer 2000; 87:615–628.
41. Gariboldi MB, Ravizza R, Riganti L, et al. Molecular determinants of intrinsic resistance to doxorubicin in human cancer cell lines. Int J Oncol. 2003; 22:1057–1064.
42. Harada T, Ogura S, Yamazaki K, et al. Predictive value of expression of P53, Bcl-2 and lung resistance-related protein for response to chemotherapy in non-small cell lung cancers. Cancer Sci 2003; 94:394–399.
43. Siva AC, Raval-Fernandes S, Stephen AG, et al. Up-regulation of vaults may be necessary but not sufficient for multidrug resistance. Int J Cancer 2001; 92:195–202.
44. Mossink MH, van Zon A, Franzel-Luiten E, et al. Disruption of the murine major vault protein (MVP/LRP) gene does not induce hypersensitivity to cytostatics. Cancer Res 2002; 62:7298–7304.
45. Scaffidi C, Fulda S, Srinivasan A, et al. Two CD95 (APO-1/Fas) signaling pathways. EMBO J 1998; 17:1675–1687.
46. Fulda S, Meyer E, Friesen C, et al. Cell type specific involvement of death receptor and mitochondrial pathways in drug-induced apoptosis. Oncogene 2001; 20:1063–1075.
47. Igney FH, Krammer PH. Death and anti-death: tumour resistance to apoptosis. Nature Rev Cancer 2002; 2:277–288.
48. Hanahan D, Weinberg RA. The hallmarks of cancer. Cell 2000; 100:57–70.
49. Schmitt CA, Lowe SW. Apoptosis and therapy. J Pathol 1999; 187:127–137.
50. Johnstone RW, Ruefli AA, Lowe SW. Apoptosis: a link between cancer genetics and chemotherapy. Cell 2002; 108:153–164.
51. Herr I and Debatin KM. Cellular stress response in apoptosis and cancer therapy. Blood 2001; 98:2603–2614.
52. Debatin KM. Apoptosis pathways in cancer and cancer therapy. Cancer Immunol Immunother 2004; 53:153–159.
53. Kaufmann SH, Vaux DL. Alterations in the apoptotic machinery and their potential role in anticancer drug resistance. Oncogene 2003; 22:7414–7430.
54. Searle J, Lawson TA, Abbott PJ, et al. An electron-microscope study of the mode of cell death induced by cancer-chemotherapeutic agents in populations of proliferating normal and neoplastic cells. J Pathol 1975; 116:129–38.
55. Wyllie AH, Golstein P. More than one way to go. Proc Natl Acad Sci U S A 2000; 93:11–13.
56. Stein WD, Bates SE, Fojo T. Intractable cancers: the many faces of multidrug resistance and the many targets it presents for therapeutic attack. Curr Drug Targets 2004; 5:333–346.
57. Soengas MS, Capodieci P, Polsky D, et al. Inactivation of the apoptosis effector Apaf-1 in malignant melanoma. Nature 2001; 409:207–211.
58. Soengas MS, Lowe SW. Apoptosis and melanoma chemoresistance. Oncogene 2003; 22:3138–3151.
59. Debatin KM, Poncet D, Kroemer G. Chemotherapy: targeting the mitochondrial cell death pathway. Oncogene 2002; 21:8786–8803.
60. Fulda S, Los M, Friesen C, Debatin KM. Chemosensitivity of solid tumor cells in vitro is related to activation of the CD95 system. Int J Cancer 1998; 76:105–114.
61. Fulda S, Debatin KM. Signaling through death receptors in cancer therapy. Curr Opin Pharmacol 2004; 4:327–332.
62. Mow BM, Blajeski AL, Chandra J, Kaufmann SH. Apoptosis and the response to anticancer therapy. Curr Opin Oncol 2001; 13:453–462.
63. Los M, Wesselborg S, Schulze-Osthoff K. The role of caspases in development, immunity, and apoptotic signal transduction: lessons from knockout mice. Immunity 1999; 10:629–639.
64. Vousden KH, Lu X. Live or let die: the cell's response to p53. Nature Rev Cancer 2002; 2:594–604.

65. Hofseth LJ, Hussain SP, Harris CC. p53: 25 years after its discovery. Trends Pharmacol Sci 2004; 25:177–181.
66. Sax JK, el-Deiry W. p53 downstream targets and chemosensitivity, Cell Death Differ 2003; 10:413–417.
67. Friedman JS, Lowe SW. Control of apoptosis by p53. Oncogene 2003; 22:9030–9040.
68. Hussain SP, Harris CC. Molecular epidemiology of human cancer: contribution of mutation spectra studies of tumor suppressor genes. Cancer Res 1998; 58:4023–4037.
69. Lowe SW, Ruley HE, Jacks T, Housman DE. p53-dependent apoptosis modulates the cytotoxicity of anticancer agents. Cell 1993; 74:957–967.
70. Weinstein JN, Myers TG, O'Connor PM, et al. An information-intensive approach to the molecular pharmacology of cancer. Science 1997; 275:343–349.
71. Bunz F, Hwang PM, Torrance C, et al. Disruption of p53 in human cancer cells alters the responses to therapeutic agents. J Clin Invest. 1999; 104:263–269.
72. Wallace-Brodeur RR, Lowe SW. Clinical implications of p53 mutations. Cell Mol Life Sci 1999; 55:64–75.
73. Degeorges A, de Roquancourt A, Extra JM, et al. Is p53 a protein that predicts the response to chemotherapy in node negative breast cancer? Breast Cancer Res Treat 1998; 47:47–55.
74. Hosaka N, Ichikawa Y, Ishikawa T, et al. Correlation of immunohistochemical p53 labeling index with inhibition rate in chemosensitivity test in gastric and colon cancer. Anticancer Res 2001; 21:229–235.
75. Rozan S, Vincent-Salomon A, Zafrani B, et al. No significant predictive value of c-erbB-2 or p53 expression regarding sensitivity to primary chemotherapy or radiotherapy in breast cancer. Int J Cancer 1998; 79:27–33.
76. Cote RJ, Esrig D, Groshen S, Jones PA, Skinner DG. p53 and treatment of bladder cancer. Nature 1997; 385:123–125.
77. Jost CA, Marin MC, Kaelin WJ. p73 is a human p53-related protein that can induce apoptosis. Nature 1997; 389:191–194.
78. Flores ER, Tsai KY, Crowley D, et al. p63 and p73 are required for p53-dependent apoptosis in response to DNA damage. Nature 2002; 416:560–564.
79. Irwin MS, Kondo K, Marin MC, et al. Chemosensitivity linked to p73 function. Cancer Cell 2003; 3:403–410.
80. Zaika AI, Slade N, Erster SH, et al. DeltaNp73, a dominant-negative inhibitor expression interferes with p53-independent apoptotic pathways. J. Exp. Med 2002; 196:765–780.
81. Cory S, Huang DC, Adams JM. The Bcl-2 family: roles in cell survival and oncogenesis. Oncogene 2003; 22:8590–8607.
82. Martinou JC, Green DR. Breaking the mitochondrial barrier. Nature Rev Mol Cell Biol 2001; 2:63–67.
83. Miyashita T, Reed JC. bcl-2 gene transfer increases relative resistance of S49.1 and WEHI7.2 lymphoid cells to cell death and DNA fragmentation induced by glucocorticoids and multiple chemotherapeutic drugs. Cancer Res 1992; 52:5407–5411.
84. Bettaieb A, Dubrez-Daloz L, Launay S, et al. Bcl-2 proteins: targets and tools for chemosensitisation of tumor cells. Curr Med Chem Anti-Canc Agents 2003; 3:307–318.
85. Reed JC. Dysregulation of apoptosis in cancer. J Clin Oncol 1999; 17:2941–2953.
86. Violette S, Poulain L, Dussaulx E, et al. Resistance of colon cancer cells to long-term 5-fluorouracil exposure is correlated to the relative level of Bcl-2 and Bcl-X_L in addition to Bax and p53 status. Int J Cancer 2002; 98:498–504.
87. Liu R, Page C, Beidler DR, et al. Overexpression of Bcl-x_L promotes chemotherapy resistance of mammary tumors in a syngeneic mouse model. Am J Pathol 1999; 155:1861–1867.
88. Bairey O, Zimra Y, Shaklai M, et al. Bcl-2, Bcl-X, Bax, and Bak expression in short- and long-lived patients with diffuse large B-cell lymphomas. Clin Cancer Res 1999; 5:2860–2866.
89. Aebersold DM, Kollar A, Beer KT, et al. Involvement of the hepatocyte growth factor/scatter factor receptor c-met and of Bcl-x_L in the resistance of oropharyngeal cancer to ionizing radiation. Int J Cancer 2001; 96:41–54.
90. Kohler T, Wurl P, Meye A, et al. High bad and bcl-x_L gene expression and combined bad, bcl-xL, bax and bcl-2 mRNA levels: molecular predictors for survival of stage 2 soft tissue sarcoma patients. Anticancer Res 2002; 22:1553–1559.
91. Theodorakis P, Lomonosova E, Chinnadurai G. Critical requirement of BAX for manifestation of apoptosis induced by multiple stimuli in human epithelial cancer cells. Cancer Res 2002; 62:3373–3376.
92. Zhang L, Yu J, Park BH, Kinzler KW, Vogelstein B. Role of BAX in the apoptotic response to anticancer agents. Science 2000; 290:989–992.
93. Wei MC, Zong WX, Cheng EH, et al. Proapoptotic BAX and BAK: a requisite gateway to mitochondrial dysfunction and death. Science 2001; 292:727–730.

94. Rampino N, Yamamoto H, Ionov Y, et al. Somatic frameshift mutations in the BAX gene in colon cancers of the microsatellite mutator phenotype. Science 1997; 275:967–969.

95. Pepper C, Hoy T, Bentley P. Elevated Bcl-2/Bax are a consistent feature of apoptosis resistance in B-cell chronic lymphocytic leukaemia and are correlated with in vivo chemoresistance. Leuk Lymphoma 1998; 28:355–361.

96. Miao J, Chen GG, Chun SY, et al. Bid sensitizes apoptosis induced by chemotherapeutic drugs in hepatocellular carcinoma. Int J Oncol 2004; 25:651–659.

97. Minko T, Dharap SS, Fabbricatore AT. Enhancing the efficacy of chemotherapeutic drugs by the suppression of antiapoptotic cellular defense. Cancer Detect Prev 2003; 27:193–202.

98. Villunger A, Michalak EM, Coultas L, et al. p53- and drug-induced apoptotic responses mediated by BH3-only proteins puma and noxa. Science 2003; 302:1036–1038.

99. Degterev A, Boyce M, Yuan J. A decade of caspases. Oncogene 2003; 22:8543–8567.

100. Kim H, Lee J, Soung Y, Park W, et al. Inactivating mutations of caspase-8 gene in colorectal carcinomas. Gastroenterology 2003; 125:708–715.

101. Hopkins-Donaldson S, Ziegler A, Kurtz S, et al. Silencing of death receptor and caspase-8 expression in small cell lung carcinoma cell lines and tumors by DNA methylation. Cell Death Differ 2003; 10:356–364.

102. Fulda S, Kufer MU, Meyer E, et al. Sensitization for death receptor- or drug-induced apoptosis by re-expression of caspase-8 through demethylation or gene transfer. Oncogene 2001; 20:5865–5877.

103. Beere HM, Green DR. Stress management—heat shock protein-70 and the regulation of apoptosis. Trends Cell Biol 2001; 11:6–10.

104. Janicke RU, Sprengart ML, Wati MR, Porter AG. Caspase-3 is required for DNA fragmentation and morphological changes associated with apoptosis. J Biol Chem 1998; 273:9357–9360.

105. Salvesen GS, Duckett CS. IAP proteins: blocking the road to death's door. Nat Rev Mol Cell Biol 2002; 3:401–410.

106. Krajewska M, Krajewski S, Banares S, et al. Elevated expression of inhibitor of apoptosis proteins in prostate cancer. Clin Cancer Res 2003; 9:4914–4925.

107. Tamm I, Richter S, Oltersdorf D, et al. High expression levels of X-linked inhibitor of apoptosis protein and survivin correlate with poor overall survival in childhood de novo acute myeloid leukemia. Clin Cancer Res 2004; 10:3737–3744.

108. Li J, Feng Q, Kim JM, et al. Human ovarian cancer and cisplatin resistance: possible role of inhibitor of apoptosis proteins. Endocrinology 2001; 142:370–380.

109. Amantana A, London CA, Iversen PL, Devi GR. X-linked inhibitor of apoptosis protein inhibition induces apoptosis and enhances chemotherapy sensitivity in human prostate cancer cells. Mol Cancer Ther 2004; 3:699–707.

110. Hu Y, Cherton-Horvat G, Dragowska V, et al. Antisense oligonucleotides targeting XIAP induce apoptosis and enhance chemotherapeutic activity against human lung cancer cells in vitro and in vivo. Clin Cancer Res 2003; 9:2826–2836.

111. Vucic D, Stennicke HR, Pisabarro MT, et al. ML-IAP, a novel inhibitor of apoptosis that is preferentially expressed in human melanomas. Curr Biol 2000; 10:1359–1366.

112. Vucic D, Deshayes K, Ackerly H, et al. SMAC negatively regulates the anti-apoptotic activity of melanoma inhibitor of apoptosis (ML-IAP). J Biol Chem 2002; 277:12,275–12,279.

113. Tamm I, Kornblau SM, Segall H, et al. Expression and prognostic significance of IAP-family genes in human cancers and myeloid leukemias. Clin Cancer Res 2000; 6:1796–1803.

114. Altieri D. The molecular basis and potential role of survivin in cancer diagnosis and therapy. Trends Mol Med 2001; 7:542–547.

115. Reed JC, Bischoff JR. BIRinging chromosomes through cell division - and survivin the experience. Cell 2000; 102:545–548.

116. Zaffaroni N, Daidone MG. Survivin expression and resistance to anticancer treatments: perspectives for new therapeutic interventions. Drug Resist Updat 2002; 5:65–72.

117. Pennati M, Binda M, De Cesare M, et al. Ribozyme-mediated down-regulation of survivin expression sensitizes human melanoma cells to topotecan in vitro and in vivo. Carcinogenesis 2004; 25:1129–1136.

118. Pennati M, Colella G, Folini M, et al. Ribozyme-mediated attenuation of survivin expression sensitizes human melanoma cells to cisplatin-induced apoptosis. J Clin Invest 2002; 109:285–286.

119. Fulda S, Debatin KM. Sensitization for anticancer drug-induced apoptosis by the chemopreventive agent resveratrol. Oncogene 2004; 23:6702–6711.

120. Vivanco I, Sawyers CL. The phosphatidylinositol 3-kinase–AKT pathway in human cancer. Nature Rev Cancer 2002; 2:489–501.

121. Nakashio A, Fujita N, Rokudai S, et al. Prevention of phosphatidylinositol 3'-kinase-Akt survival signaling pathway during topotecan-induced apoptosis. Cancer Res 2000; 60:5303–5309.

122. Saga Y, Mizukami H, Suzuki M, et al. Overexpression of PTEN increases sensitivity to SN-38, an active metabolite of the topoisomerase I inhibitor irinotecan, in ovarian cancer cells. Clin Cancer Res 2002; 8:1248–1252.

123. Huang H, Cheville JC, Pan Y, et al. PTEN induces chemosensitivity in PTEN-mutated prostate cancer cells by suppression of Bcl-2 expression. J Biol Chem 2001; 276:38830–38836.

124. Zhao Y, You H, Yang Y, et al. Distinctive regulation and function of PI3K/Akt and MAPKs in doxorubicin-induced apoptosis of human lung adenocarcinoma cells. J Cell Biochem 2004; 91:621–632.

125. Martelli AM, Tazzari PL, Tabellini G, et al. A new selective AKT pharmacological inhibitor reduces resistance to chemotherapeutic drugs, TRAIL, all-*trans*-retinoic acid, and ionizing radiation of human leukemia cells. Leukemia 2003; 17:1794–1805.

126. Mayo MW, Baldwin AS. The transcription factor NF-κB: control of oncogenesis and cancer therapy resistance. Biochim Biophys Acta 2000; 1470:M55–M62.

127. Wang CY, Mayo MW, Baldwin AS Jr. TNF-a and cancer therapy-induced apoptosis: potentiation by inhibition of NF-κB. Science 1996; 274:784–787.

128. Panwalkar A, Verstovsek S, Giles F. Nuclear factor-κB modulation as a therapeutic approach in hematologic malignancies. Cancer 2004; 100:1578–1589.

129. Mitsiades N, Mitsiades CS, Richardson PG, et al. The proteasome inhibitor PS-341 potentiates sensitivity of multiple myeloma cells to conventional chemotherapeutic agents: therapeutic applications. Blood 2003; 101:2377–2380.

130. Dong QG, Sclabas GM, Fujioka S, et al. The function of multiple IκB : NF-κB complexes in the resistance of cancer cells to Taxol-induced apoptosis. Oncogene 2002; 21:6510–6509.

131. Fojo T, Bates S. Strategies for reversing drug resistance. Oncogene 2003; 22:7512–7523.

132. Pakunlu RI, Wang Y, Tsao W, et al. Enhancement of the efficacy of chemotherapy for lung cancer by simultaneous suppression of multidrug resistance and antiapoptotic cellular defense: novel multicomponent delivery system. Cancer Res 2004; 64:6214–6224.

15 New and Revised Concepts in Multidrug Resistance

Sestamibi, SNPs, Substrates, and Stem Cells

Susan E. Bates, MD, John Deeken, MD, Chaohong Fan, MD, PhD, and Robert W. Robey, BChE

CONTENTS

SUMMARY

Drug resistance resulting from the outward efflux of anticancer agents by ATP binding cassette (ABC) transporters such as P-glycoprotein (P-gp) has been well described in vitro in laboratory models. The extent to which multidrug transporters are responsible for clinical drug resistance has been more difficult to determine. In one sense, P-gp can be viewed as a molecular target that was tested in the clinic before there was an adequate understanding of the diseases that were best to study, and before the best inhibitors had been identified. We now recognize that several factors may have impeded the results of clinical trials testing P-gp modulators. First, inhibitors either were not sufficiently potent or required a reduction in anticancer drug dose. Alternatively, the presence of other ABC transporters, such as the multidrug resistance-associated protein (MRP1) and the ABC half-transporter ABCG2, may have confounded the results. A single-nucleotide polymorphism (SNP) that limits the expression of P-gp could prevent inhibitor therapy from benefiting patients, and increase toxicity as well. The goal of this chapter is to evaluate

From: *Cancer Drug Discovery and Development: Cancer Drug Resistance*
Edited by: B. Teicher © Humana Press Inc., Totowa, NJ

new directions in the study of ABC transporters in multidrug resistance, offering fresh approaches to the fundamental question that asks whether ABC transporters are important molecular targets for anticancer drug development.

Key Words: Multidrug resistance; SNPs; gP170; setamibi; multidrug resistance; stem cells.

1. INTRODUCTION

At a time when targeted therapies generate front-page news reports, it is tempting to dismiss P-glycoprotein (P-gp) and multidrug resistance (MDR)1 as a dated concept. Whereas P-gp modulators could be considered one of the earliest targeted therapies, none has entered the clinical armamentarium. Disappointing outcomes of clinical trials of P-gp inhibitors have led many to turn away from these studies. Yet, work in various laboratories and from various vantages continues to suggest the importance of this hypothesis. It can be argued that the discovery of verapamil as a modulator of multidrug resistance led to the translation of the hypothesis to clinical trials too early, before there was sufficient understanding of the best diseases to study and before there was development of the best agents for study.

Whereas admittedly simplistic, at the core of every cancer death lies a drug resistant cell. Were it not for the problem of drug resistance, our success in the treatment of cancer would be much greater, and the outcomes more favorable. Drug resistance, both intrinsic and acquired, remains the primary cause of the failure of cancer therapy. Intrinsic drug resistance is a vexing problem responsible for the refractory nature of cancers arising from the pancreas, liver, and kidney, among others. Acquired resistance, a frustrating outcome of initially successful chemotherapy, emerges at variable intervals after a successful chemotherapy outcome, conferring tolerance to previously effective therapies and often to untried but potentially effective chemotherapeutics. Acquired resistance in breast, ovarian, and refractory lymphomas, among others, derails an apparently successful outcome, and eventually leads to the emergence of a cancer indistinguishable in large part from those we regard as intrinsically resistant. The similarity between inherently resistant cancers and those with acquired tolerance has been regarded as sufficient evidence for the use of either as a model of the other.

Acquired drug resistance was first observed in a laboratory model in 1950, in mouse leukemic cells passaged in mice treated with 4-amino-N^{10}-methyl-pteroylglutamic acid *(1)*. Fifty years later, we have numerous laboratory models of drug resistance, but little real understanding of drug resistance in clinical tumors. In 1972, Dano described drug resistance because of the active outward transport of chemotherapeutic agents *(2)*. Daunorubicin- and vinblastine-resistant cells were found to have energy-dependent transport of daunorubicin that could be inhibited by vinblastine, vincristine, and other anthracyclines. The multidrug resistance phenotype was thus characterized by resistance to structurally unrelated anticancer agents, display of active outward transport, and overexpression of a 170-kDa cell membrane glycoprotein that became known as P170 or P-gp*(3,4)*. As critical as this discovery was, it was the observation that drug resistance could be reversed by the addition of several different compounds, including verapamil, that brought P-gp into prominence as a potential target for improving cancer therapy *(5)*.

P-gp is a member of the ATP-binding cassette (ABC) transporter family of proteins that includes several members that confer drug resistance by the extrusion of anticancer agents from the cell through ATP-dependent drug efflux. To date, 48 human ABC genes have been identified and classified into seven distinct subfamilies, ABCA through ABCG

(6). However, it is likely that only a subset of these 48 transporters will be shown to be drug efflux pumps. Those isolated from drug-resistant cell lines are the most promising candidates, and indeed, it is these for which the evidence is most convincing. By contrast, the evidence supporting a role in drug resistance for ABC transporters identified first either in a normal tissue context or *in silico* is less compelling.

2. ABC TRANSPORTER INVOLVEMENT IN DRUG RESISTANCE

P-gp, a member of the B subfamily of ABC genes encoded by the *MDR1* gene (*ABCB1*), was among the first ABC transporters to be identified, as described above. Data from mice in which the *mdr1* genes have been deleted, and increasingly, from clinical pharmacology, have proven that P-gp plays an important role in normal tissue protection and normal human pharmacology (reviewed in ref. *7*). As a corollary, despite convincing evidence that P-gp mediates resistance in cancer cell lines in the laboratory, proof that P-gp is important in clinical drug resistance has been difficult to obtain. Other transporter proteins include the multidrug resistance-related protein (MRP1, ABCC1) and related family members ABCC2 to -9 *(8)*, and the half-transporter ABCG2 (breast cancer resistance protein [BCRP], mitoxantrone resistance protein [MXR], ABCP) *(9)*. These transporters are also involved in normal physiologic functions. The substrates overlap somewhat, although MRP family members have an affinity for organic anion substrates, and ABCG2 is noteworthy for its transport of mitoxantrone, camptothecin analogues, methotrexate and methotrexate polyglutamates *(8,9)*. Several approaches have been used to evaluate a link between a given ABC transporter and clinical drug resistance. These approaches were most extensively carried out for P-gp and included assays of levels in drug resistant human cancers, assays of levels in tumor tissue before and after therapy, and clinical outcomes of patients treated with transport inhibitors. This latter strategy was widely adopted as an approach for understanding the role of P-gp in drug resistance, and multiple clinical trials were launched using inhibitors that had limited potency, or inhibitors that interfered with the cytochrome P450 system resulting in the need to reduce the dose of the anticancer agent. The first generation inhibitors such as verapamil and quinidine were never shown to inhibit P-gp—the molecular target—in patients. The second-generation inhibitors, such as VX710 and PSC 833, were shown to inhibit P-gp in patients, but the pharmacokinetic interaction delayed excretion of the anticancer agent, and resulted in toxicity requiring reduction of anticancer drug doses (reviewed in ref. *10*). In short, the results of the early trials were disappointing and suggested that P-gp inhibitors would offer, at best, modest improvements in response duration. Subsequently, several large randomized clinical trials testing valspodar (PSC 833), and even the third-generation inhibitor tariquidar (XR 9576), were either negative or closed early for excess toxicity in the experimental arm, offering further disappointment *([11,12]*; D. Norris, Xenova, personal communication). Glimmers of clinical benefit have been seen in a few trials, including two acute myeloid leukemia (AML) trials, one using cyclosporine as a modulator *(13)* and the other with valspodar in a subset of patients whose leukemic cells had detectable P-gp function *(12)*. Many of these clinical trials have been reviewed elsewhere and will not be the subject of this chapter (*see* refs. *10*, *14*, and *15*). Rather, this chapter evaluates new directions in the study of ABC transporters in multidrug resistance, which may offer fresh approaches to the fundamental question of whether ABC transporters are important molecular targets for anticancer drug development. First, we examine the question of transporter expression in cancer. Second, we turn to the imaging studies that support the development of ABC transporters as clinical targets in anticancer therapy. Third, the evidence that single-nucleotide polymorphisms (SNPs) may affect ABC transporter expression and function is reviewed. Finally, reports on new ABC transporter substrates and the new cancer stem cell hypothesis are summarized. Taken together, these approaches suggest that ABC transporters continue to be important molecular targets for anticancer drug development.

3. EXPRESSION OF ABC TRANSPORTERS IN HUMAN TUMORS

For many oncologists, one of the dreams for anticancer therapy of the future is that it will be individualized. The advent of molecularly targeted therapy provides substance for that imagination. Demonstration of the target in a tumor determines whether the targeted therapy will be selected. For some targets, demonstration of the target's expression in a cancer is sufficient. Thus, the demonstration of bcr-abl in chronic myeloid leukemia is sufficient, with the level of expression inconsequential. More recently, we have learned that for some targets, such as the epidermal growth factor receptor (EGFR) in lung cancer, the existence of an acquired mutation is more important than the level of its expression *(16)*. A clinical assay allowing the simple detection of EGFR mutations will allow the definition of a subgroup of patients in which that therapy has far greater potential to succeed. For others, such as ErbB2 detection in breast cancer, the degree of overexpression is critical *(17)*. In this setting, the impact of an accurate assay cannot be overstated. One example can be found in the ErbB2 detection assays used to define therapy for Herceptin. The response rate for patients with ErbB2 expression level 3+ was assessed at 35%, in contrast to a 0% response rate for expression level 2+ *(18)*. For P-gp, a standardized clinical assay was not developed before the launch of dozens of clinical trials. Studied before we understood how important it was to detect the molecular target in the tumor being treated, this single flaw may have been the most critical one in clinical trials of P-gp inhibitors.

Indeed, one must recognize that 25 yr after its first description a defined assay for this transporter has not been delineated. It is clearly not certain that an assay demonstrating activity of an ABC transporter would lead to clinical benefit. However, it is unlikely that P-gp can be developed as a clinical target without having the ability to detect its activity and select the patient population that would have potential benefit. Expression data for MRP1 and ABCG2 in cancer are more limited than those available for P-gp.

Studies in acute myelogenous leukemia have consistently demonstrated expression of a functional transporter in leukemic samples (reviewed in refs. *10* and *15*). These studies, spanning over a decade, have utilized immunohistochemical assays, RNA assays, and flow cytometric functional studies. The results have consistently demonstrated P-gp expression or activity in 30–60% of AML samples before treatment. These studies have reported that expression is associated with a greater likelihood of developing resistant disease, or poorer outcome, and have also shown increased expression in refractory samples. Because of this repeated detection of functional P-gp, AML has been the subject of multiple clinical trials testing P-gp inhibition. Recently, a large number of studies have reported the expression of ABCG2 (BCRP) in acute leukemia. The results of these latter studies have been confusing, with some reporting significant levels of expression; another, an impact on clinical outcome; and others reporting no correlation *(9)*. An explanation for this confusion may lie in the poor concordance of the assays for ABCG2 in AML as noted by Suvannasankha et al. *(19)*. One of the largest studies examined BCRP (ABCG2) expression by RT-PCR and P-gp function in 149 AML samples *(20)*. Achievement of complete remission and improved survival were significantly correlated with absence of both transporters in the leukemic samples.

P-gp expression in solid tumors has been more difficult to quantify. It is overexpressed at baseline in chemotherapy-resistant tumors such as colon and kidney cancer, and is upregulated after disease progression following chemotherapy in malignancies such as leukemia and breast cancer. As noted above, the assays for P-gp expression are not validated. Thus, the most reliable reports are those that include pre- and posttherapy sampling, although the possibility of a publication bias has to be recognized when generating an analysis of this type. Table 1 demonstrates a selected series of such studies. Many of the studies report an increase in P-gp expression, suggesting that resistance mediated by P-gp is being acquired during treatment with chemotherapy. Several specific disease types warrant mention. A meta-analysis estimated the incidence of P-gp expression in breast cancer at 40%. A recent study evaluating expression in breast cancer by immunohistochemistry, reported a 66% frequency of P-gp expression and a 61% frequency of MRP1 expression (21). There was no relationship between P-gp expression and relapse-free or overall survival. In ovarian cancer, the incidence appears to be lower. However, a recent report concluded that expression of P-gp in tumors at the time of second look surgery was associated with poorer survival (22). This result is consistent with another recent study that measured mRNA levels of *MDR1*, *MRP2*, and topoisomerase I in ovarian tumor samples (23). In this study, low *MDR1* expression was significantly associated with a prolonged overall survival time, although not with progression-free survival. Both of these studies thus demonstrate a concept that is relevant for clinical trials of P-gp inhibitors—response and relapse following initial therapy that features principally a potent non-P-gp substrate such as cisplatin is more likely to be related to that agent than to the expression of P-gp. Both of the studies contrast with a slightly older study in ovarian cancer that found no correlation with expression and survival (24).

Another tumor type in which classical multidrug resistance may play an important role is in sarcoma. Studies in soft tissue sarcoma have reproducibly reported expression of P-gp in a sizeable proportion of clinical samples (25). A meta-analysis concluded that whereas P-gp did not predict response to chemotherapy, expression was associated with a worse prognosis, as defined by disease progression within 2 yr (25). Both P-gp and MRP1 are expressed in a majority of chemotherapy-naive soft tissue sarcomas (26). A recent study examining 86 cases of surgically resected soft tissue sarcoma noted very high levels of MDR1 and MRP3 expression in the histologic subtype, malignant peripheral nerve sheath tumors (27). Posl et al. noted a 64.4% incidence before chemotherapy and an 82.9% incidence after chemotherapy (28). Although some studies have reported a correlation with clinical outcome, others have not, so that whereas the frequent detection of MDR1/P-gp in sarcoma is established, its interpretation is not.

The identification of multiple other ABC family members able to transport anticancer agents has complicated matters further, raising the possibility that clinical trial results were compromised by the presence of undetected, and uninhibited, ABC transporters. Thus, a number of studies have addressed the question of whether multiple ABC transporters could be responsible for drug resistance. Burger et al. analyzed mRNA levels of ABCG2, lung resistance protein, MRP1, MRP2, and MDR1 in 59 breast tumor specimens (29). Interestingly, MDR1 expression was the strongest predictor of a poor outcome. Diestra et al. evaluated expression of P-gp, MRP1, lung resistance protein, and BCRP in bladder cancer (30). Whereas P-gp was associated with reduced progression-free survival, the presence of MRP1 was associated with an improved response to chemotherapy.

Table 1

P-glycoprotein Expression in Paired Samples

Author, year	Histology	Method	n	Pretreatment	n	Posttreatment
Mechetner 1998 (91)	Breast cancer	JSB-1 IHC	359	11%		30%
Chevillard, 1996 (92)	Breast cancer	IHC	63	14%		43%
Linn 1997 (93)	Breast cancer	JSB-1 IHC	40	64%	40	57%
Chung 1997 (94)	Breast cancer	JSB-1 IHC	23	26%	23	57%
Lizard-Nacol 1999 (95)	Breast cancer	RT-PCR	75	92%		96%
Faneyte 2001 (96)	Breast cancer	JSB-1 IHC	80	0	88	0
Rudas 2003 (97)	Breast cancer	IHC	80	55%	68	100%
Han 2000 (98)	AML		109		36	
Grogan 1993 (99)	Myeloma	IHC	47	6%	49	43%
Zhou 1995 (100)	AML	RT-PCR	51	18%	40	33%
Nakagawa 1997 (129)	Bladder cancer	IHC	33	67%	28	86%
Tada 2002 (101)	Bladder cancer	RT-PCR	63	5.7-fold increase in residual tumors.		
				4.5-fold increase in recurrent tumors.		
Van der Zee 1995 (102)	Ovarian cancer	IHC	89	15%	38	48%
Penson 2004 (22)	Ovarian cancer	C219, C494	32	59%	32	59%
		IHC				
Posl, 1997 (28)	High-grade central osteosarcoma	JSB-1 IHC	58	64.4%		82.9%

IHC, immunohistochemistry, RT-PCR, reverse transcription-polymerase chain reaction; AML, acute myeloid leukemia.

It will be important to examine multiple ABC transporters in future clinical trials in order to make accurate assessments of the role of a single transporter in a given tumor type.

4. DETECTION OF ABC TRANSPORTER FUNCTION IN CANCER BY RADIONUCLIDE IMAGING

A critical step toward the understanding of the role of ABC transporters in clinical drug resistance is the development of an imaging tool that could be used to identify patients who have transporter-mediated resistance. Two radionuclide agents approved for use in cardiac imaging, ^{99m}Tc-sestamibi and ^{99m}Tc-tetrofosmin, have been evaluated in cancer by various investigators. The uptake and clearance of the agents have almost invariably been associated with response to chemotherapy, and the same parameters have often been significantly correlated with P-gp expression. Thus, the agents offer the possibility of a real-time diagnostic assay for detection of drug resistance mediated by P-gp. Potentially more significant is the demonstration that a P-gp inhibitor could increase accumulation of the agents in tumors. This has been confirmed, primarily for sestamibi, in combination with valspodar, biricodar, and tariquidar (31–35). Thus, these imaging tools offer the possibility of providing both a diagnostic assay and a surrogate assay for inhibition of the molecular target. Table 2 details the results of some 20 imaging studies evaluating ^{99m}Tc-sestamibi uptake or washout in diverse malignancies.

Although the sample size in each study presented in Table 2 is small and almost certainly underpowered, the geographic diversity of the studies and the similarity of the results speak to their validity. Impaired drug accumulation, as measured by the sestamibi surrogate, results in impaired chemotherapy response. Consistently, higher sestamibi uptake is correlated with a better response to chemotherapy. As an example, in 25 patients studied in Barcelona, the mean tumor uptake ratio of ^{99m}Tc-sestamibi was higher (7.70 ± 5.20) than the mean ratio in nonresponding patients (2.21 ± 1.0) (36). The results for most of the studies show similar differences in uptake. It could be considered that a two- to threefold change in drug accumulation is too modest to be of clinical significance, although few oncologists would advocate the converse (i.e., a 50% reduction in the dosage of anticancer therapies).

In multiple studies, there was also a difference in tumor uptake related to P-gp expression. Again, a roughly twofold decreased sestamibi uptake in tumors with detectable P-gp expression was noted by several investigators (37–39). This result is consistent with the increased tumor accumulation of sestamibi observed following administration of P-gp modulators. At least three studies have reported increases in sestamibi in tumors and P-gp-expressing normal tissues (32–35). With tariquidar, a third-generation P-gp modulator, the magnitude of the increase in the area under the curve (AUC) ranged from 0 to 278% in normal liver and from 36 to 263% in visible tumor masses in 13 of 17 patients (31). It is interesting that this increase in sestamibi accumulation is of the same order of magnitude as the difference between P-gp-expressing and nonexpressing tumors in the studies noted above.

It should be noted that the planar sestamibi imaging methodology is likely to underestimate actual differences. This can be ascribed to the detection of uptake in regions of interest that include all of the tissue between the tumor and the camera detector, as well as the tissue located behind the tumor in that plane. The inclusion of nontumor tissue in the overlapping areas will diminish differences between patients.

Table 2

Clinical Correlates in Sestamibi Imaging

Author, year	Country	Tumor type	n	Clinical correlate	p -Value
Moretti 1996 (103)	France	Breast cancer	13	Only P-gp$^+$ breast cancer was one of three that were MIBI negative.	NS
Del Vecchio 1997 (104)	Italy	Breast cancer	30	Higher retention of MIBI associated with low P-gp.	<0.001
Kostakoglu 1998 (105)	Turkey	Breast cancer	30	T/B ratios lower with strong P-gp expression.	<0.001
Ciarmiello 1998 (106)	Italy	Breast cancer	39	Rapid MIBI clearance with residual disease.	<0.01
Kao 2001 (107)	Taiwan	Breast cancer	24	T/B MIBI ratio lowest with both P-gp and MRP expression.	<0.05
Takamura 2001 (108)	Japan	Breast cancer	46	T/N$_d$ MIBI ratio higher in tumors responding to chemotherapy. P-gp but not MDR1 mRNA higher in tumors with low MIBI T/N$_d$ ratios.	<0.01
Del Vecchio 2002 (109)	Italy	Breast cancer	33	MIBI efflux with apoptotic pathway activation.	<0.001
Mubashar 2002 (37)	UK	Breast cancer	20	T/B ratio inversely correlated with P-gp expression.	<0.001
Alonso 2002 (110)	Uruguay	Breast cancer	33	Higher MIBI T/B ratio with response to chemotherapy.	<0.0001
Fuster 2002 (36)	Spain	Breast cancer	25	Higher RI with response to chemotherapy.	0.20
				Higher MIBI uptake with response to chemotherapy.	<0.0001
				Higher MIBI uptake with negative P-gp expression.	NS
Kim 2002 (111)	Japan	Breast cancer	13	Higher MIBI uptake in responding tumors.	NS
Cayre 2002 (112)	France	Breast cancer	45	Negative MIBI scan is associated with nonresponse to chemotherapy.	<0.05
				In IDC, MIBI uptake is inversely correlated with MDR1 expression.	0.0015
Cayre 2004 (113)	France	Breast cancer	98	Low tumor uptake with improved survival; low uptake with ILC histology.	<0.005
Kao 2001 (114)	Taiwan	Lymphoma	25	T/B ratio higher in patients with good response and negative P-gp expression.	<0.01
Ohta 2001 (115)	Japan	Lymphoma	45	Early-uptake ratio, no difference; 2-hr update correlates with response.	0.016

Study	Country	Cancer	N	Finding	p
Song 2003 (116)	Korea	Lymphoma	17	Retention index higher in patients with response to chemotherapy.	0.014
Yamamato 2001 (117)	Japan	SCLC	33	Higher early MIBI uptake ratio with response to chemotherapy.	<0.01
Lim 2000 (118)	Korea	SCLC	28	T/N ratio higher in those with complete or partial response.	
Nishiyama 2000 (119)	Japan	NSCLC	38	Higher T/N ratio and RI in responder group.	<0.05
Zhou 2001 (120)	Japan	Lung cancer	34	L/N_d higher in P-gp$^-$ tumors.	0.0324
				L/N_{wr} higher in P-gp$^-$ tumors.	0.0269
Hsu 2002 (121)	Taiwan	NSCLC	30	Higher T/L ratio with good clinical response and negative for P-gp expression.	<0.05
Pace 2000 (122)	Italy	Myeloma	30	Negative scan associated with best response.	<0.001
Fonti 2004 (123)	Italy	Myeloma	17	MIBI washout rate higher in bone marrow with highest P-gp.	<0.05
Burak 2003 (42)	Turkey	Osteosarcoma	24	Higher clearance with expression of MRP. Lower clearance with therapy response.	0.007 0.005
Burak 2001 (124)	Turkey	Bone and STS	25	Higher clearance with expression of P-gp.	<0.01
Kawata 2004 (39)	Japan	Gastric cancer	36	Lower 30- and 120-min uptake ratios with P-gp positivity.	<0.0001
Wang 2004 (38)	China	Hepatocellular	78	No MIBI uptake, and higher washout rates in tumors with P-gp expression.	0.035

MIBI, ^{99m}Tc-sestamibi; P-gp, P-glycoprotein; NS, not significant; T/B, tumor-to-background ratio; T/N_d, tumor-to-normal ratio; MDR1, multidrug resistance 1; RI, retention index; ILC, invasive lobular carcinoma; SCLC, small cell lung cancer; NSCLC, non-small cell lung cancer; L/N_d, delayed lesion-to-normal ratio; L/N_{wr}, lesion-to-normal washout ratio; T/L, tumor-to-normal lung tissue ratio; STS, soft tissue sarcoma.

It is unlikely, however, that P-gp is the sole determinant in sestamibi accumulation. The multidrug transporter MRP1 has also been shown to transport sestamibi *(40,41)*. In the studies noted above, there was a correlation of sestamibi uptake and MRP1 expression in some studies but not in others. These mixed results may be related to differences in methodology or in tumor type, for example, a statistically significant correlation was observed in osteosarcoma *(42)*, but no correlation in gastric cancer *(39)*. The general lack of uptake of sestamibi in the central nervous system—even in the presence of the P-gp inhibitor tariquidar—proves that factors other than P-gp control uptake. Indeed, disruption of the blood–brain barrier results in sestamibi visualization of primary and metastatic brain tumors against the normal negative background of the brain *(43)*.

One final note in the development of sestamibi imaging for multidrug resistance is the caveat that sestamibi provides a surrogate for chemotherapy accumulation, but it is not known how accurate that surrogate is. Other imaging agents have been evaluated including tetrofosmin, also a substrate for both P-gp and MRP1 *(41)*. Although fewer in number, studies with tetrofosmin have also shown that uptake and washout rates correlate with P-gp expression and chemotherapy responsiveness *(44–47)*. The development of imaging tools using actual antineoplastic agents has lagged. Positron-emission tomography imaging with ^{18}F-paclitaxel in combination with tariquidar in monkeys demonstrated increases in the tissue AUC normalized to plasma AUC of 54 and 97% in the liver and lung, respectively, with no change in kidney uptake *(48)*. These changes are somewhat lower than the normal tissue uptake in the sestamibi studies noted above; the factors responsible for this are unknown—both the different species and the different transport substrate are candidates.

Taken together, these results support the continued evaluation of imaging agents as diagnostic assays for the detection of P-gp and other ABC transporters, and support the continued study of therapies aimed at overcoming P-gp-mediated drug transport.

5. SNPs IN ABC TRANSPORTERS

Genetic variants in the *MDR1* gene and their phenotypic implications have been extensively studied over the past 5 yr. Since Hoffmeyer et al. reported in 2000 that a SNP in exon 26 correlated with reduced levels of expression of the P-gp transporter on the luminal surface of the small intestine *(49)*, research groups from around the world have studied the gene for further SNPs and their physiologic effects. Known SNPs in exon coding regions of the *MDR1* gene are reported in Table 3 *(50)*. It is worth noting that an additional seven SNPs located in noncoding introns have been described and have no known effect to date.

Researchers have tracked the ethnic distribution of these variants, as well as investigated the effects on disease risk, treatment response, and drug metabolism. Although there have been conflicting results, the T/T genotype related to the C3435T polymorphism has been associated with reduced gastrointestinal P-gp expression *(49,51)* and reduced drug excretion *(52–54)*. Further, linkage between the common SNPs in exons 12, 21, and 26 has been suggested in some studies *(7)*. The exact effect on drug metabolism from these SNPs has been controversial, with differing results reported by various researchers when examining different combinations of SNPs. The reader is referred to several excellent reviews of this subject *(7,55,56)*. Known racial and ethnic allelic variations in the three most studied SNPs are listed in Table 4. As noted in Table 3, the C3435T SNP found to affect P-gp expression in the duodenum is a synonymous polymorphism, meaning that it does not affect the amino acid sequence of the protein.

Table 3
Multidrug Resistance 1 Exon-Encoded
Single-Nucleotide Polymorphisms

SNP	Location	Translation impact
T-12C	Exon 1	Noncoding
G-1A	Exon 2	Translation
A61G	Exon 2	Asn21Asp
T307C	Exon 5	Phe103Leu
G1199A	Exon 11	Ser400Asn
C1236T	Exon 12	Gly412Gly
G2677T/A	Exon 21	Ala893Ser/Thr
G2995A	Exon 24	Ala999Thr
C3435T	Exon 26	Ile1145Ile
C3396T	Exon 26	Wobble

This raises the question of whether certain SNPs could be linked to regulatory sites up or downstream of the *MDR1* gene *(50,57–59)*.

SNPs of the *MDR1* gene have been reported to correlate with disease processes, including ulcerative colitis and Parkinson's disease *(60,61)*, presumably through enhanced susceptibility to environmental toxin exposure. A similar role in oncology has also been proposed. Jamroziak et al. compared children with acute lymphoblastic lymphoma with age-matched controls, and found that individuals with the T/T genotype at position 3435 had a higher risk of developing acute lymphoblastic lymphoma, with an odds ratio of 1.8 *(62)*. The authors postulate that lower levels of P-gp result in a long-term increased exposure of stem cells or other vulnerable cells to carcinogens, thereby allowing initiation and progression of malignancy. The same study also reported that those with the wild-type C/C genotype had a poorer response to therapy and a worse prognosis *(62)*.

These results and others highlight the possibility that *MDR1* SNPs may affect drug sensitivity. Kafka et al. found that patients with locally advanced breast cancer with the homozygous 3435T genotype had an improved response and a higher complete remission rate to preoperative chemotherapy than patients with the wild-type or heterozygous genotype *(63)*. Woodahl et al. investigated the G1199A SNP—an allelic variant not thought to be linked to other SNPs and found in more than 5% of Caucasians—and found that LLC-PK1 epithelial cells expressing this polymorphism were more resistant to vinblastine and vincristine *(64)*. As with the expression and pharmacokinetic correlations noted above, the association between drug sensitivity and SNPs has been controversial.

As mentioned, a sizable body of research has investigated the role of the *MDR1*-encoded P-gp in inducing drug resistance and the possible clinical benefit in inhibiting the efflux pump. Little recent research has investigated the effect of SNPs on P-gp inhibition. An exception was the work of Kuppens et al., who reported on the oral bioavailability of docetaxel when given with the P-gp blocking agent OC144-093 *(65)*. One of 12 patients had variant alleles, and the pharmacokinetic parameters in this single patient were not different from those in the other 11 patients. Larger trials will be needed to answer the question of whether the SNPs alter the effect of P-gp inhibitors.

Even without the certainty of whether the polymorphic variants would affect P-gp inhibition, it seems clear that genetic factors could control the inducibility or the level of expression of *MDR1*, thus confounding the results of clinical trials correlating *MDR1*

Table 4
Allelic Frequencies by Ethnicity and Nationality

SNP Location	C1236T Exon 12		G2677T/A Exon 21			C3435T Exon 26	
Allele Ethnicity/nationality	C	T	G	T	A	C	T
Korean	38	62	44	37	19	63	37
European Caucasians			56	42	2	46	54
Portuguese			52	48		35–43	57–65
British Caucasians						48	52
Spanish						48	52
European Americans						67	33
African Americans						84–86	14–16
Kenyan						83	17
Ghanaian						83	17
Sudanese						73	27
Chinese						53	47
Filipino						59	41
Saudi Arabian						55	45

SNP, single-nucleotide polymorphism.
Sources: refs. 57, 125, 126, and 127.

expression with resistance, with clinical course, or with the results of P-gp inhibition. A sizeable number of studies have evaluated *MDR1* expression in different patient populations, concluding in many cases that tumors in patients with relapse following therapy have higher levels of *MDR1* expression. If a SNP were associated with reduced expression of *MDR1*, or with limited inducibility, then exposure to the anticancer agent would not necessarily be associated with increased levels. A case in point is the clinical trial in acute leukemia that tested PSC 833 in combination with cytosine arabinoside, daunorubicin, and etoposide and closed early for toxicity in the treated group *(12)*. There was a suggestion of benefit in the subset of patients who had detectable activity of P-gp as measured by a flow cytometric assay *(12)*. One can speculate that the effect of a variant SNP preventing increased *MDR1* expression despite the selection pressure induced by prior chemotherapy would be a subset of patients who could not receive benefit. Treatment of patients with such a variant, even with P-gp substrates, would effectively push the cancer in the direction of other mechanisms of drug resistance, and obviate the utility of a P-gp inhibitor in that patient population. Patients whose *MDR1* expression could increase would have resistance mediated by P-gp, and so could benefit from the addition of an inhibitor. A further extension of that hypothesis is that those patients would have intrinsically higher P-gp levels in their normal stem cells and tissues, and that chemotherapy in the presence of a P-gp modulator would be less toxic for those patients. The observation in the Baer study that the subset of patients with P-gp-positive leukemic cells had no toxic deaths is certainly compatible with such a hypothesis. Indeed, the study closed early because of toxicity, but had the patients been selected for those with detectable efflux in their leukemic cells, there may have been both benefit and reduced toxicity.

Laboratory data with ABCG2 show that variations in amino acid sequence may indeed affect the success of a transport inhibitor. Whereas the natural product fumitremorgin C appears to behave equivalently in cells bearing a gain of function mutation in ABCG2 at amino acid 482, other inhibitors such as novobiocin and some taxane derivatives function less efficiently *(66,67)*. This mutation has not been found as a SNP but has been characterized as a hot spot, having been found in multiple cell lines selected for drug resistance *(68,69)*. It remains to be seen whether the mutation could occur in a particular clinical setting. Beyond the mutation at 482, several polymorphic variants have been described. One of these, 421C>A, results in a protein in which the glutamine at residue 141 has been substituted by lysine. This variant results in impaired transport activity and, some report, impaired expression at the cell surface *(70–72)*. As a result, cells expressing the variant ABCG2 have increased sensitivity to ABCG2 substrate drugs such as mitoxantrone, topotecan, and SN-38. It has been speculated that a group of patients carrying this variant would have enhanced sensitivity to the toxicities of substrates such as irinotecan and topotecan; however, proof of this has been difficult to obtain, potentially because of confounding effects of other polymorphic proteins *(73)*. Evaluation of this question is ongoing. As with the discussion for *MDR1*, the presence of a variant limiting expression could have an impact on the results of expression studies or clinical trials evaluating the role of ABCG2 in clinical drug resistance.

6. EXPANDING NUMBERS OF SUBSTRATES FOR ABC TRANSPORTERS

The focus of this chapter is delineation of the evidence arguing for the importance of multidrug transporters in cancer. The steadily expanding recognition of new substrates and inhibitors can be included in such an argument. One of the noteworthy features of

Table 5
ABCG2 Substrates

Mitoxantrone
Topotecan
Irinotecan
SN38
Methotrexate
Methotrexate (MTX) polyglutamates
STI571 (Gleevec®)
Flavopiridol
Photodynamic therapy agents
Indolocarbazole topo I inhibitors (rebeccamycin)
Novel camptothecins
Homocamptothecin
Anthelmintic benzimidazoles
Cimetidine
AZT
Sulfated estrogens
2-amino-1-methyl-6-phenylimidazo[4,5-b]pyridine (PhIP)
Hoechst 33342
Pheophorbide a
BODIPY-prazosin
[Lysotracker Green]
[Rhodamine 123]

The number of reported substrates for ABCG2 (breast cancer resistance protein) continues to grow. The top half of the table includes anticancer agents both approved and in development; the lower half includes compounds used in treatment of other diseases, a carcinogen, and fluorescent dyes. Compounds in square brackets are substrates only for ABCG2 with a mutation at amino acid 482.
ABCG2, ATP-binding cassette transporter G2.

P-gp is the diversity of substrates that are transported. Recent studies have focused on identification of orally absorbed nononcologic agents in widespread clinical use, including digoxin, HIV protease inhibitors, tricyclic antidepressants, and antibiotics (7,74). Work with the National Cancer Institute drug screen matching drug sensitivity profiles in the 60-cell line panel suggested that there were hundreds, if not thousands, of substrates for P-gp (75,76). The number of substrates for MRP1 discovered by this methodology was not as great, perhaps because of the need for some MRP1 substrates to be conjugated with glutathione, sulfate, or a glucuronide and the disparate ability of cancer cell lines to carry out this function (8). Data being gathered for ABCG2 suggest a degree of diversity in substrates akin to that of P-gp (9). The diversity of substrates for all three of the transporters suggests that new compounds in development should be screened for vulnerability to drug transport. Table 5 provides an updated list of ABCG2 substrates.

7. ABC TRANSPORTERS AND THE CANCER STEM CELL HYPOTHESIS

Another emerging line of evidence supporting the role of ABC transporters in oncologic drug resistance is that involving the cancer stem cell hypothesis. According to this hypothesis, a malignant tumor, whereas originating from a single malignant clone, is composed of several compartments of cells with differing capacities for self-renewal. The existence of a pluripotent, self-renewing stem cell in normal bone marrow has been firmly established for some time, and recent evidence has pointed toward the existence of such cells in normal tissues as well. In normal tissues, these cells are not thought to be as pluripotent as embryonic stem cells; rather there exists pluripotency within tissue specificity. These tissue-specific stem cells retain the self-renewing capacity that is the hallmark of the stem cell, and have been touted as potential therapeutic tools in several disease processes.

In bone marrow, the stem cell population has been identified phenotypically based on efflux of the fluorescent dye Hoechst 33342, known as the "side population" or SP phenotype (77). Because Goodell et al. demonstrated reversal of the SP phenotype by verapamil, it was believed the SP phenotype was determined by P-gp. However, Zhou and colleagues found side-population cells in Mdr1a/1b$^{-/-}$ cells and recognized that the SP phenotype in mice is determined by the presence of Abcg2, for which Hoechst 33342 is a substrate (78). This was later shown to be true in human hematopoietic stem cells as well (79,80). Whereas both P-gp and ABCG2 are expressed in SP cells, ABCG2 is believed to be primarily responsible for the SP phenotype because bone marrow from Abcg2$^{-/-}$ mice display a sharp reduction in the number of SP cells (81). SP cells have also been identified in an increasing number of normal tissues, including normal brain, kidney, heart, and breast tissues. Tissue-specific stem cells carry lineage-specific markers in addition to the SP phenotype.

Increasingly, it appears that cancers are also composed of pluripotent cells with self-renewing capabilities existing alongside other compartments of cells that are malignant and yet have lineage-specific markers without a long-term self-renewing capacity. Several investigators have reported evidence of distinct cell compartments within a tumor mass, including breast cancer, brain tumors, neuroblastomas, and gastrointestinal cancers (82–85). Hirschmann-Jax and colleagues found SP cells in primary tumors from patients with neuroblastoma, and noted high expression of ABCG2 and ABCA3 in the SP cells, promoting survival when the cells were exposed to cytotoxic drugs. If this hypothesis is correct, the logical conclusion is that anticancer therapy should be directed toward the population with self-renewal capacity. As an aside, it should be noted that the converse cannot be assumed—that is, the presence of an SP phenotype cannot be the sole defining feature of the stem cell. To be sure, drug-resistant cells and cancer cells derived from normal tissues that express ABCG2 in the mature, terminally differentiated state may exhibit ABCG2 expression as part of the cancer phenotype.

By definition, the long-term, self-renewing capacity of the stem cell implies enhanced repair capabilities and resistance mechanisms that allow survival and regeneration despite injury. How much overlap these mechanisms have with the cellular mechanisms characterized in cancer cells is not yet known. These mechanisms likely exist in cancer stem cells, too. ABCG2 expression offers a first line of defense for stem cells against toxins that are also substrates. For example, Abcg2 expression was found to confer hematopoietic protection from mitoxantrone in mice (81). It appears that in hematopoietic cells, both ABCG2 and MDR1 are preferentially expressed by the earliest progenitors, whereas MDR1 is expressed by more mature progenitors (81,86). One of the earlier phenotypic descriptions of the stem cell compartment was that it was rhodamine dull (87). This phenotype could not be ascribed to ABCG2, expression because rhodamine has been shown to be a substrate only for a mutated form of ABCG2 and not for the wild-type form (66). MDR1 expression in hematopoietic progenitors has also been reported to have a protective role (88).

In tissue-specific stem cells, the SP phenotype has been demonstrated, indicating ABCG2 expression. Whether MDR1 is expressed by more mature progenitors in this setting, whether some stem cells express both, or whether there are differences among different tissue-specific stem cell types remains to be determined (89,90). The extent to which cancers replicate the normal tissue stem cell and differentiation pathway is not clear. As therapies are directed toward the stem cell phenotype, it will be important either to identify agents that are not substrates, or to develop agents in combination with inhibitors of the transporters. Differences between stem cells among specific tumor types could allow anticancer therapies to be directed more specifically against these cells, sparing stem cells in noninvolved tissues.

8. CONCLUSION

In summary, in the 30 yr since the discovery of P-gp, the importance of the "multidrug" ABC transporters in normal physiology has emerged. It has become clear that these transporters play roles in normal stem cells, in the blood–brain barrier, in protection from toxic xenobiotics, in drug excretion, and it is very likely that they partially mediate interindividual differences in drug sensitivity. Our understanding of the role of multidrug transporters in drug resistance in cancer is still evolving. The disappointing results of clinical trials with P-gp inhibitors have led many investigators to take a wait-and-see attitude toward the further development of these agents. However, the development of imaging agents that are substrates for transporters offers the possibility of determining in the clinical setting whether drug accumulation can be modulated. This is perhaps the most logical and straightforward approach for future studies, and the ability to document ABC transporter activity in the clinical setting offers the potential of selecting patients most likely to benefit. Such a strategy could allow ABC transporters to join the growing group of molecular targets that are identified before therapy is offered. These agents soon will include, in addition to estrogen and progesterone receptors as time-honored examples, HER-2 in breast cancer; EGFR mutations in lung cancer; and cKit mutations in gastrointestinal stromal tumors. Detection of patients whose tumors have detectable ABC transporter activity offers not only the possibility of identifying patients who may benefit from inhibitor therapy, but also offers the possibility of avoiding patients who may suffer undue toxicity due to SNPs that confer a lower level of transporter expression in normal and malignant tissues. Whereas this latter point is entirely speculative, this possibility could explain the striking differences in toxicity in subsets of patients treated with P-gp inhibitors in randomized trials ([11,12]; D. Norris, Xenova, unpublished data). P-gp was a molecular target discovered before the era of targeted therapy and before we understood how targeted therapies needed to be developed. Perhaps this early molecular target can now become a "validated" target for anticancer therapy.

REFERENCES

1. Burchenal JH, Robinson E, Johnston SF, Kushida, MN. The induction of resistance to 4-amino-N[10]-methyl-pteroylglutamic acid in a strain of transmitted mouse leukemia. Science 1950; 111:116.
2. Dano K. Active outward transport of daunomycin in resistant Ehrlich ascites tumor cells. Biochim Biophys Acta 1973; 323:466–183.
3. Beck WT, Mueller TJ, Tanzer LR. Altered surface membrane glycoproteins in vinca alkaloid-resistant human leukemic lymphoblasts. Cancer Res 1979; 39:2070–2076.
4. Riordan JR, Ling V. Purification of P-glycoprotein from plasma membrane vesicles of chinese hamster ovary cell mutants with reduced colchicine permeability. J Biol Chem 1979; 254:12,701–12,705.
5. Tsuruo T, Iida H, Tsukagoshi S, et al. Overcoming of vincristine resistance in P388 leukemia in vivo and in vitro through enhancing cytotoxicity of vincristine and vinblastine by verapamil. Cancer Res 1981; 41:1967–1972.

6. Dean M, Rzhetsky A, Allikmets R. The human ATP-binding cassette (ABC) transporter superfamily. Genome Res 2001; 11:1156–1166.

7. Marzolini C, Paus E, Buclin T, Kim RB. Polymorphisms in human MDR1 (P-glycoprotein): recent advances and clinical relevance. Clin Pharmacol Ther 2004; 75:13–33.

8. Kruh GD, Zeng H, Rea PA, Liu G, Chen ZS, Lee K, Belinsky MG. MRP subfamily transporters and resistance to anticancer agents. J Bioenerg Biomembr 2001; 33:493–501.

9. Doyle LA, Ross DD. Multidrug resistance mediated by the breast cancer resistance protein BCRP (ABCG2). Oncogene 2003; 22:7340–7358.

10. Leonard GD, Polgar O, Bates SE. ABC transporters and inhibitors: new targets, new agents. Curr Opin Investig Drugs 2002; 3:1652–1659.

11. Joly F, Mangioni C, Nicoletto M, et al. A phase 3 study of PSC 833 in combination with paclitaxel and carboplatin (PC-PSC) versus paclitaxel and carboplatin (PC) alone in patients with stage IV or suboptimally debulked stage III epithelial ovarian cancer or primary cancer of the peritoneum. Proc Am Soc Clin Oncol 2002.

12. Baer MR, George SL, Dodge RK, O'Loughlin KL, et al. Phase 3 study of the multidrug resistance modulator PSC-833 in previously untreated patients 60 years of age and older with acute myeloid leukemia: Cancer and Leukemia Group B Study 9720. Blood 2002; 100, 1224–1232.

13. List AF, Spier C, Greer J, et al. Phase I/II trial of cyclosporine as a chemotherapy-resistance modifier in acute leukemia. J Clin Oncol 1993; 11:1652–1660.

14. Leonard GD, Fojo T, Bates SE. The role of ABC transporters in clinical practice. Oncologist 2003; 8:411–424.

15. Bates SE. Solving the problems of multidrug resistance: ABC transporters in clinical oncology, in ABC Proteins: From Bacteria to Man (Holland IB, Cole SPC, Kuchler K, Higgins CF, Eds), Elsevier Science, London, 2002:359–391.

16. Paez JG, Janne PA, Lee JC, et al. EGFR mutations in lung cancer: correlation with clinical response to gefitinib therapy. Science 2004; 304:1497–1500.

17. Ross JS, Fletcher JA, Bloom KJ, Linette GP, Stec J, Symmans WF, Pusztai L, Hortobagyi GN. Targeted therapy in breast cancer: the HER-2/neu gene and protein. Mol Cell Proteomics 2004; 3:379–398.

18. Vogel CL, Cobleigh MA, Tripathy D, et al. Efficacy and safety of trastuzumab as a single agent in first-line treatment of HER2-overexpressing metastatic breast cancer. J Clin Oncol 2002; 20:719–726.

19. Suvannasankha A, Minderman H, O'Loughlin KL, et al. Breast cancer resistance protein (BCRP/MXR/ABCG2) in acute myeloid leukemia: discordance between expression and function. Leukemia 2004; 18:1252–1257.

20. Benderra Z, Faussat AM, Sayada L, et al. Breast cancer resistance protein and P-glycoprotein in 149 adult acute myeloid leukemias. Clin Cancer Res 2004; 10:7896–7902.

21. Larkin A, O'Driscoll L, Kennedy S, et al. Investigation of MRP-1 protein and MDR-1 P-glycoprotein expression in invasive breast cancer: a prognostic study. Int J Cancer 2004; 112:286–294.

22. Penson RT, Oliva E, Skates SJ, et al. Expression of multidrug resistance-1 protein inversely correlates with paclitaxel response and survival in ovarian cancer patients: a study in serial samples. Gynecol Oncol 2004; 93:98–106.

23. Materna V, Pleger J, Hoffmann U, Lage H. RNA expression of MDR1/P-glycoprotein, DNA-topoisomerase I, and MRP2 in ovarian carcinoma patients: correlation with chemotherapeutic response. Gynecol Oncol 2004; 94:152–160.

24. Arts HJ, Katsaros D, de Vries EG, Massobrio M, et al. Drug resistance-associated markers P-glycoprotein, multidrug resistance-associated protein 1, multidrug resistance-associated protein 2, and lung resistance protein as prognostic factors in ovarian carcinoma. Clin Cancer Res 1999; 5:2798–2805.

25. Pakos EE, Ioannidis JP. The association of P-glycoprotein with response to chemotherapy and clinical outcome in patients with osteosarcoma. A meta-analysis. Cancer 2003; 98:581–589.

26. Komdeur R, Plaat BE, Hoekstra HJ, Molenaar et al. Expression of P-glycoprotein, multidrug resistance-associated protein 1, and lung resistance-related protein in human soft tissue sarcomas before and after hyperthermic isolated limb perfusion with tumor necrosis factor-α and melphalan. Cancer 2001; 91:1940–1948.

27. Oda Y, Saito T, Tateishi N, Ohishi Y, et al. ATP-binding cassette superfamily transporter gene expression in human soft tissue sarcomas. Int J Cancer 2005; 114(6):854–862.

28. Posl M, Amling M, Grahl K, et al. P-glycoprotein expression in high grade central osteosarcoma and normal bone cells. An immunohistochemical study. Gen Diagn Pathol 1997; 142:317–325.

29. Burger H, Foekens JA, Look MP, et al. RNA expression of breast cancer resistance protein, lung resistance-related protein, multidrug resistance-associated proteins 1 and 2, and multidrug resistance gene 1 in breast cancer: correlation with chemotherapeutic response. Clin Cancer Res 2003; 9:827–836.

30. Diestra JE, Condom E, Del Muro XG, et al. Expression of multidrug resistance proteins P-glycoprotein, multidrug resistance protein 1, breast cancer resistance protein and lung resistance related protein in locally advanced bladder cancer treated with neoadjuvant chemotherapy: biological and clinical implications. J Urol 2003; 170:1383–1387.

31. Agrawal M, Abraham J, Balis FM, et al. Increased 99mTc-sestamibi accumulation in normal liver and drug-resistant tumors after the administration of the glycoprotein inhibitor, XR9576. Clin Cancer Res 2003; 9:650–656.

32. Luker GD, Facasso PM, Dobkin J, Piwnica-Worms D. Modulation of the multidrug resistance P-glycoprotein: detection with technetium-99m-sestamibi in vivo. J Nucl Med 1997; 38:369–372.

33. Bakker M, van der Graaf WT, Piers DA, et al. 99mTc-Sestamibi scanning with SDZ PSC 833 as a functional detection method for resistance modulation in patients with solid tumours. Anticancer Res 1999; 19:2349–2353.

34. Chen CC, Meadows B, Regis J, Kalafsky G, Fojo T, Carrasquillo JA, Bates SE. Detection of in vivo p-glycoprotein inhibition by PSC 833 using Tc-99m sestamibi. Clin Cancer Res 1997; 4:545–552.

35. Peck RA, Hewett J, Harding MW, et al. Phase I and pharmacokinetic study of the novel MDR1 and MRP1 inhibitor biricodar administered alone and in combination with doxorubicin. J Clin Oncol 2001; 19:3130–3141.

36. Fuster D, Munoz M, Pavia J, et al. Quantified 99mTc-MIBI scintigraphy for predicting chemotherapy response in breast cancer patients: factors that influence the level of 99m Tc-MIBI uptake. Nucl Med Commun 2002; 23:31–38.

37. Mubashar M, Harrington KJ, Chaudhary KS, et al. 99mTc-sestamibi imaging in the assessment of toremifene as a modulator of multidrug resistance in patients with breast cancer. J Nucl Med 2002; 43:519–525.

38. Wang H, Chen XP, Qiu FZ. Correlation of expression of multidrug resistance protein and messenger RNA with 99mTc-methoxyisobutyl isonitrile (MIBI) imaging in patients with hepatocellular carcinoma. World J Gastroenterol 2004; 10:1281–1285.

39. Kawata K, Kanai M, Sasada T, Iwata S, Yamamoto N, Takabayashi A. Usefulness of 99mTc-sestamibi scintigraphy in suggesting the therapeutic effect of chemotherapy against gastric cancer. Clin Cancer Res 2004; 10:3788–3793.

40. Chen WS, Luker KE, Dahlheimer JL, Pica CM, Luker GD, Piwnica-Worms D. Effects of MDR1 and MDR3 P-glycoproteins, MRP1, and BCRP/MXR/ABCP on the transport of (99m)Tc-tetrofosmin. Biochem Pharmacol 2000; 60:413–426.

41. Hendrikse NH, Franssen EJ, van der Graaf WT, et al. 99mTc-sestamibi is a substrate for P-glycoprotein and the multidrug resistance-associated protein. Br J Cancer 1998; 77:353–358.

42. Burak Z, Moretti JL, Ersoy O, et al. 99mTc-MIBI imaging as a predictor of therapy response in osteosarcoma compared with multidrug resistance-associated protein and P-glycoprotein expression. J Nucl Med 2003; 44:1394–1401.

43. Baldari S, Restifo Pecorella G, Cosentino S, Minutoli F. Investigation of brain tumours with (99m)Tc-MIBI SPET. Q J Nucl Med 2002; 46:336–345.

44. Fuster D, Vinolas N, Mallafre C, Pavia J, Martin F, Pons F. Tetrofosmin as predictors of tumour response. Q J Nucl Med 2003; 47:58–62.

45. Liang JA, Shiau YC, Yang SN, et al. Using technetium-99m-tetrofosmin scan to predict chemotherapy response of malignant lymphomas, compared with P-glycoprotein and multidrug resistance related protein expression. Oncol Rep 2002; 9:307–312.

46. Yeh JJ, Hsu WH, Huang WT, Wang JJ, Ho ST, Kao A. Technetium-99m tetrofosmin SPECT predicts chemotherapy response in small cell lung cancer. Tumour Biol 2003; 24:151–155.

47. Liu TJ, Shiau YC, Tsai SC, Wang JJ, Ho ST, Kao A. Predicting multidrug resistance-related protein and P-glycoprotein expression with technetium-99m tetrofosmin mammoscintigraphy. Breast 2003; 12:58–62.

48. Kurdziel KA, Kiesewetter DO, Carson RE, Eckelman WC, Herscovitch, P. Biodistribution, radiation dose estimates, and in vivo P-gp modulation studies of 18F-paclitaxel in nonhuman primates. J Nucl Med 2003; 44:1330–1339.

49. Hoffmeyer S, Burk O, von Richter O, et al. Functional polymorphisms of the human multidrug-resistance gene: multiple sequence variations and correlation of one allele with P-glycoprotein expression and activity in vivo. Proc Natl Acad Sci U S A 2000; 97:3473–3478.

50. Cascorbi I, Gerloff T, Johne A, et al. Frequency of single nucleotide polymorphisms in the P-glycoprotein drug transporter MDR1 gene in white subjects. Clin Pharmacol Ther 2001; 69:169–174.

51. Nakamura T, Sakaeda T, Horinouchi M, et al. Effect of the mutation (C3435T) at exon 26 of the MDR1 gene on expression level of MDR1 messenger ribonucleic acid in duodenal enterocytes of healthy Japanese subjects. Clin Pharmacol Ther 2002; 71:297–303.

52. Kim RB, Leake BF, Choo EF, et al. Identification of functionally variant MDR1 alleles among European Americans and African Americans. Clin Pharmacol Ther 2001; 70:189–99.

53. Fellay J, Marzolini C, Meaden ER, et al. Response to antiretroviral treatment in HIV-1-infected individuals with allelic variants of the multidrug resistance transporter 1: a pharmacogenetics study. Lancet 2002; 359:30–36.

54. Hitzl M, Drescher S, van der Kuip H, et al. The C3435T mutation in the human MDR1 gene is associated with altered efflux of the P-glycoprotein substrate rhodamine 123 from CD56+ natural killer cells. Pharmacogenetics 2001; 11:293–298.

55. Sakaeda T, Nakamura T, Okumura K. Pharmacogenetics of MDR1 and its impact on the pharmacokinetics and pharmacodynamics of drugs. Pharmacogenomics 2003; 4:397–410.

56. Sparreboom A, Danesi R, Ando Y, Chan J, Figg WD. Pharmacogenomics of ABC transporters and its role in cancer chemotherapy. Drug Resist Updat 2003; 6:71–84.

57. Yi SY, Hong KS, Lim HS, et al. variant 2677A allele of the MDR1 gene affects fexofenadine disposition. Clin Pharmacol Ther 2004; 76:418–427.

58. Drescher S, Schaeffeler E, Hitzl M, et al. MDR1 gene polymorphisms and disposition of the P-glycoprotein substrate fexofenadine. Br J Clin Pharmacol 2002; 53:526–534.

59. Tang K, Ngoi SM, Gwee PC, et al. Distinct haplotype profiles and strong linkage disequilibrium at the MDR1 multidrug transporter gene locus in three ethnic Asian populations. Pharmacogenetics 2002; 12:437–450.

60. Schwab M, Schaeffeler E, Marx C, et al. Association between the C3435T MDR1 gene polymorphism and susceptibility for ulcerative colitis. Gastroenterology 2003; 124:26–33.

61. Drozdzik M, Bialecka M, Mysliwiec K, Honczarenko K, Stankiewicz J, Sych Z. Polymorphism in the P-glycoprotein drug transporter MDR1 gene: a possible link between environmental and genetic factors in Parkinson's disease. Pharmacogenetics 2003; 13:259–263.

62. Jamroziak K, Mlynarski W, Balcerczak E, et al. Functional C3435T polymorphism of MDR1 gene: an impact on genetic susceptibility and clinical outcome of childhood acute lymphoblastic leukemia. Eur J Haematol 2004; 72:314–321.

63. Kafka A, Sauer G, Jaeger C, et al. Polymorphism C3435T of the MDR-1 gene predicts response to preoperative chemotherapy in locally advanced breast cancer. Int J Oncol 2003; 22:1117–1121.

64. Woodahl EL, Yang Z, Bui T, Shen DD, Ho RJ. Multidrug resistance gene G1199A polymorphism alters efflux transport activity of P-glycoprotein. J Pharmacol Exp Ther 2004; 310:1199–1207.

65. Kuppens IE, Bosch TM, van Maanen MJ, et al. Oral bioavailability of docetaxel in combination with OC144-093 (ONT-093; Cancer Chemother Pharmacol 2005; 55:72–78.

66. Robey RW, Honjo Y, Morisaki K, et al. Mutations at amino acid 482 in the ABCG2 gene affect substrate and antagonist specificity. Br J Cancer 2003; 89:1971–1978.

67. Minderman H, Brooks TA, O'Loughlin KL, Ojima I, Bernacki RJ, Baer MR. Broad-spectrum modulation of ATP-binding cassette transport proteins by the taxane derivatives ortataxel (IDN-5109, BAY 59-8862; and tRA96023. Cancer Chemother Pharmacol 2004; 53:363–369.

68. Honjo Y, Hrycyna CA, Yan QW, et al. Acquired mutations in the MXR/BCRP/ABCP gene alter substrate specificity in MXR/BCRP/ABCP-overexpressing cells. Cancer Res 2001; 61:6635–6639.

69. Allen JD, Jackson SC, Schinkel AH. A mutation hot spot in the Bcrp1 (Abcg2) multidrug transporter in mouse cell lines selected for Doxorubicin resistance. Cancer Res 2002; 62:2294–2299.

70. Imai Y, Nakane M, Kage K, et al. C421A polymorphism in the human breast cancer resistance protein gene is associated with low expression of Q141K protein and low-level drug resistance. Mol Cancer Ther 2002; 1:611–616.

71. Mizuarai S, Aozasa N, Kotani H. Single nucleotide polymorphisms result in impaired membrane localization and reduced atpase activity in multidrug transporter ABCG2. Int J Cancer 2004; 109:238–246.

72. Morisaki K, Robey RW, Ozvegy-Laczka C, et al. Single nucleotide polymorphisms modify the transporter activity of ABCG2. Cancer Chemother Pharmacol 2005; 56(2):161–172.

73. de Jong FA, Marsh S, Mathijssen RH, et al. ABCG2 pharmacogenetics: ethnic differences in allele frequency and assessment of influence on irinotecan disposition. Clin Cancer Res 2004; 10:5889–5894.

74. Eichelbaum M, Fromm MF, Schwab M. Clinical aspects of the MDR1 (ABCB1) gene polymorphism. Ther Drug Monit 2004; 26:180–185.

75. Lee JS, Paull K, Alvarez M, et al. Rhodamine efflux patterns predict P-glycoprotein substrates in the National Cancer Institute Drug Screen. Mol Pharmacol 1994; 46:627–638.

76. Alvarez M, Paull K, Monks A, et al. Generation of a drug resistance profile by quantitation of mdr-1/P-glycoprotein in the cell lines of the NCI anticancer drug screen. J Clin Invest. 1995; 95:2205–2214.

77. Goodell MA, Brose K, Paradis G, Conner AS, Mulligan RC. Isolation and functional properties of murine hematopoietic stem cells that are replicating in vivo. J Exp Med 1996; 183:1797–1806.

78. Zhou S, Schuetz JD, Bunting KD, et al. The ABC transporter Bcrp1/ABCG2 is expressed in a wide variety of stem cells and is a molecular determinant of the side-population phenotype. Nat Med 2001; 7:1028–1034.

79. Scharenberg CW, Harkey MA, Torok-Storb B. The ABCG2 transporter is an efficient Hoechst 33342 efflux pump and is preferentially expressed by immature human hematopoietic progenitors. Blood 2002; 99:507–512.

80. Kim M, Turnquist H, Jackson J, et al. The multidrug resistance transporter ABCG2 (breast cancer resistance protein 1) effluxes Hoechst 33342 and is overexpressed in hematopoietic stem cells. Clin Cancer Res 2002; 8:22–28.

81. Zhou S, Morris JJ, Barnes Y, Lan L, Schuetz JD, Sorrentino BP. Bcrp1 gene expression is required for normal numbers of side population stem cells in mice, and confers relative protection to mitoxantrone in hematopoietic cells in vivo. Proc Natl Acad Sci U S A 2002; 99:12,339–12,344.

82. Al-Hajj M, Wicha MS, Benito-Hernandez A, Morrison SJ, Clarke MF. Prospective identification of tumorigenic breast cancer cells. Proc Natl Acad Sci U S A 2003; 100:3983–3988.

83. Hemmati HD, Nakano I, Lazareff JA, et al. Cancerous stem cells can arise from pediatric brain tumors. Proc Natl Acad Sci U S A 2003; 100:15,178–15,183.

84. Singh SK, Clarke ID, Terasaki M, et al. Identification of a cancer stem cell in human brain tumors. Cancer Res 2003; 63:5821–5828.

85. Hirschmann-Jax C, Foster AE, Wulf GG, et al. A distinct "side population" of cells with high drug efflux capacity in human tumor cells. Proc Natl Acad Sci U S A 2004; 101:14,228–14,233.

86. Bunting KD. ABC transporters as phenotypic markers and functional regulators of stem cells. Stem Cells 2002; 20:11–20.

87. Bertoncello I, Hodgson GS, Bradley TR. Multiparameter analysis of transplantable hemopoietic stem cells: I. The separation and enrichment of stem cells homing to marrow and spleen on the basis of rhodamine-123 fluorescence. Exp Hematol 1985; 13:999–1006.

88. Smeets M, Raymakers R, Vierwinden G, et al. A low but functionally significant MDR1 expression protects primitive haemopoietic progenitor cells from anthracycline toxicity. Br J Haematol 1997; 96:346–355.

89. Lechner A, Leech CA, Abraham EJ, Nolan AL, Habener JF. Nestin-positive progenitor cells derived from adult human pancreatic islets of Langerhans contain side population (SP) cells defined by expression of the ABCG2 (BCRP1) ATP-binding cassette transporter. Biochem Biophys Res Commun 2002; 293:670–674.

90. Terunuma A, Jackson KL, Kapoor V, Telford WG, Vogel JC. Side population keratinocytes resembling bone marrow side population stem cells are distinct from label-retaining keratinocyte stem cells. J Invest Dermatol 2003; 121:1095–1103.

91. Mechetner E, Kyshtoobayeva A, Zonis S, et al. Levels of multidrug resistance (MDR1) P-glycoprotein expression by human breast cancer correlate with in vitro resistance to taxol and doxorubicin. Clin Cancer Res 1998; 4:389–398.

92. Chevillard S, Pouillart P, Beldjord C, et al. Sequential assessment of multidrug resistance phenotype and measurement of S-phase fraction as predictive markers of breast cancer response to neoadjuvant chemotherapy. Cancer 1996; 77:292–300.

93. Linn SC, Pinedo HM, van Ark-Otte J, et al. Expression of drug resistance proteins in breast cancer, in relation to chemotherapy. Int J Cancer 1997; 71:787–795.

94. Chung HC, Rha SY, Kim JH, et al. P-glycoprotein: the intermediate end point of drug response to induction chemotherapy in locally advanced breast cancer. Breast Cancer Res Treat 1997; 42:65–72.

95. Lizard-Nacol S, Genne P, Coudert B, et al. MDR1 and thymidylate synthase (TS) gene expressions in advanced breast cancer: relationships to drug exposure, p53 mutations, and clinical outcome of the patients. Anticancer Res 1999; 19:3575–3581.

96. Faneyte IF, Kristel PM, van de Vijver MJ. Determining MDR1/P-glycoprotein expression in breast cancer. Int J Cancer 2001; 93:114–122.

97. Rudas M, Filipits M, Taucher S, et al. Expression of MRP1, LRP and P-gp in breast carcinoma patients treated with preoperative chemotherapy. Breast Cancer Res Treat 2003; 81:149–157.

98. Han K, Kahng J, Kim M, et al. Expression of functional markers in acute nonlymphoblastic leukemia. Acta Haematol 2000; 104:174–180.

99. Grogan TM, Spier CM, Salmon SE, et al. P-glycoprotein expression in human plasma cell myeloma: correlation with prior chemotherapy. Blood 1993; 81:490–495.

100. Zhou DC, Zittoun R, Marie JP. Expression of multidrug resistance-associated protein (MRP) and multidrug resistance (MDR1) genes in acute myeloid leukemia. Leukemia 1995; 9:1661–1666.

101. Tada Y, Wada M, Migita T, et al. Increased expression of multidrug resistance-associated proteins in bladder cancer during clinical course and drug resistance to doxorubicin. Int J Cancer 2002; 98:630–635.

102. van der Zee AG, Hollema H, et al. Value of P-glycoprotein, glutathione S-transferase pi, c-erbB-2, and p53 as prognostic factors in ovarian carcinomas. J Clin Oncol 1995; 13:70–78.

103. Moretti JL, Azaloux H, Boisseron D, Kouyoumdjian JC, Vilcoq J. Primary breast cancer imaging with technetium-99m sestamibi and its relation with P-glycoprotein overexpression. Eur J Nucl Med 1996; 23:980–986.

104. Del Vecchio, S, Ciarmiello, A, Pace, L, et al. Fractional retention of technetium-99m-sestamibi as an index of P-glycoprotein expression in untreated breast cancer patients. J Nucl Med 1997; 38:1348–1351.

105. Kostakoglu L, Ruacan S, Ergun EL, Sayek I, Elahi N, Bekdik CF. Influence of the heterogeneity of P-glycoprotein expression on technetium-99m-MIBI uptake in breast cancer. J Nucl Med 1998; 39:1021–1026.

106. Ciarmiello A, Del Vecchio S, Silvestro P, et al. Tumor clearance of technetium 99m-sestamibi as a predictor of response to neoadjuvant chemotherapy for locally advanced breast cancer. J Clin Oncol 1998; 16:1677–1683.

107. Kao CH, Tsai SC, Liu TJ, et al. P-Glycoprotein and multidrug resistance-related protein expressions in relation to technetium-99m methoxyisobutylisonitrile scintimammography findings. Cancer Res 2001; 61:1412–1414.

108. Takamura Y, Miyoshi Y, Taguchi T, Noguchi S. Prediction of chemotherapeutic response by Technetium 99m—MIBI scintigraphy in breast carcinoma patients. Cancer 2001; 92:232–239.

109. Del Vecchio S, Zannetti A, Ciarmiello A, et al. Dynamic coupling of 99mTc-MIBI efflux and apoptotic pathway activation in untreated breast cancer patients. Eur J Nucl Med Mol Imaging 2002; 29:809–814.

110. Alonso O, Delgado L, Nunez M, et al. Predictive value of (99m)Tc sestamibi scintigraphy in the evaluation of doxorubicin based chemotherapy response in patients with advanced breast cancer. Nucl Med Commun 2002; 23:765–771.

111. Kim R, Osaki A, Hirai T, Toge T. Utility of technetium-99m methoxyisobutyl isonitrile uptake analysis for prediction of the response to chemotherapy in advanced and relapsed breast cancer. Breast Cancer 2002; 9:240–247.

112. Cayre A, Cachin F, Maublant J, et al. Single static view 99mTc-sestamibi scintimammography predicts response to neoadjuvant chemotherapy and is related to MDR expression. Int J Oncol 2002; 20:1049–1055.

113. Cayre A, Cachin F, Maublant J, Mestas D, Penault-Llorca F. Does 99mTc-sestamibi uptake discriminate breast tumors? Cancer Invest 2004; 22:498–504.

114. Kao CH, Tsai SC, Wang JJ, et al. Technetium-99m-sestamethoxyisobutylisonitrile scan as a predictor of chemotherapy response in malignant lymphomas compared with P-glycoprotein expression, multidrug resistance-related protein expression and other prognosis factors. Br J Haematol 2001; 113:369–374.

115. Ohta M, Isobe K, Kuyama J, et al. Clinical role of Tc-99m-MIBI scintigraphy in non-Hodgkin's lymphoma. Oncol Rep 2001; 8:841–845.

116. Song HC, Lee JJ, Bom HS, et al. Double-phase Tc-99m MIBI scintigraphy as a therapeutic predictor in patients with non-Hodgkin's lymphoma. Clin Nucl Med 2003; 28:457–462.

117. Yamamoto Y, Nishiyama Y, Fukunaga K, Satoh K, Fujita J, Ohkawa M. 99mTc-MIBI SPECT in small cell lung cancer patients before chemotherapy and after unresponsive chemotherapy. Ann Nucl Med 2001; 15:329–335.

118. Lim SC, Park KO, Kim YC, Na KJ, Song H, Bom HS. Comparison of Tc-99m sestamibi, serum neuron-specific enolase and lactate dehydrogenase as predictors of response to chemotherapy in small cell lung cancer. Cancer Biother Radiopharm 2000; 15:381–386.

119. Nishiyama, Y, Yamamoto, Y, Satoh, K, et al. Comparative study of Tc-99m MIBI and TI-201 SPECT in predicting chemotherapeutic response in non-small-cell lung cancer. Clin Nucl Med 2000; 25, 364–369.

120. Zhou J, Higashi K, Ueda Y, et al. Expression of multidrug resistance protein and messenger RNA correlate with (99m)Tc-MIBI imaging in patients with lung cancer. J Nucl Med 2001; 42:1476–1483.
121. Hsu WH, Yen RF, Kao CH, et al. Predicting chemotherapy response to paclitaxel-based therapy in advanced non-small-cell lung cancer (stage IIIb or IV) with a higher T stage (> T2). Technetium-99m methoxyisobutylisonitrile chest single photon emission computed tomography and P-glycoprotein express ion. Oncology 2002; 63:173–179.
122. Christen RD, Isonishi S, Jones JA, et al. Signaling and drug sensitivity. Cancer Metastasis Rev 1994; 13:175–189.
123. Fonti R, Del Vecchio S, Zannetti A, et al. Functional imaging of multidrug resistant phenotype by 99mTc-MIBI scan in patients with multiple myeloma. Cancer Biother Radiopharm 2004; 19:165–170.
124. Burak Z, Ersoy O, Moretti JL, et al. The role of 99mTc-MIBI scintigraphy in the assessment of MDR1 overexpression in patients with musculoskeletal sarcomas: comparison with therapy response. Eur J Nucl Med 2001; 28:1341–1350.
125. Ameyaw MM, Regateiro F, Li T, et al. MDR1 pharmacogenetics: frequency of the C3435T mutation in exon 26 is significantly influenced by ethnicity. Pharmacogenetics 2001; 11:217–221.
126. Cascorbi I, Gerloff T, Johne A, et al. Frequency of single nucleotide polymorphisms in the P-glycoprotein drug transporter MDR1 gene in white subjects. Clin Pharmacol Ther 2004; 75:169–171.
127. Bernal ML, Sinues B, Fanlo A, Mayayo E. Frequency distribution of C3435T mutation in exon 26 of the MDR1 gene in a Spanish population. Ther Drug Monit 2003; 25:107–111.
128. Cavaco I, Gil J-P, Gil-Berglund E, Ribeiro V. CYP3A4 and MDR1 alleles in a Portuguese population. Clin Chem Lab Med 2003; 41:1345–1350.
129. Nakagawa M, Emoto A, Nasu N, et al. Clinical significance of multi-drug resistance associated protein and P-glycoprotein in patients with bladder cancer. J Urol 1997; 157(4):1260–1264; discussion 1264–1265.

16 Cisplatin Resistance

Molecular Basis of a Multifaceted Impediment

Zahid H. Siddik, PhD

CONTENTS

SUMMARY

cis-Diammine-dichloro-platinum^{II} (cisplatin) is an inorganic, square-planar coordination complex that has become one of the most important drugs in the clinical management of cancers over the last three decades. It is similar to classical alkylating agents, in that the central platinum atom interacts covalently with DNA to also form adducts, which are the cytotoxic lesions. When these adducts are detected by damage recognition proteins, signals are transduced that culminate in the activation of apoptosis. However, cisplatin resistance arises when dysregulation of genes reduces the level of adducts formed, reduces recognition of adducts, or inhibits the apoptotic process. Alternatively, prosurvival pathways may become upregulated to increase cell proliferation even when DNA damage is extensive. It is rare to find a single mechanism of resistance within a tumor; in general, several mechanisms coexist to create a complex multifaceted dilemma, which confounds cancer treatment strategies. However, additional platinum-based agents with different spectrums of antitumor activity are entering the clinic, but it is likely that more-potent leads may be identified from among the large reservoir of existing platinum-based agents, provided the multifaceted nature of cisplatin resistance is better appreciated. Although a number of mechanisms have become firmly established in the literature, it appears that several more will be added in time, based on the

From: *Cancer Drug Discovery and Development: Cancer Drug Resistance*
Edited by: B. Teicher © Humana Press Inc., Totowa, NJ

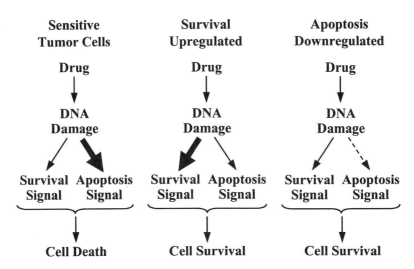

Fig. 1. DNA damage generates both survival and apoptotic signals. Cell fate will depend on the relative strength of the two sets of signals. Upregulation of survival pathways and/or downregulation of apoptotic pathways will induce drug resistance.

increasing number of resistance-inducing genes that have been identified from differential gene expression profiles.

Key Words: Cisplatin; resistance; molecular mechanism; DNA adducts; damage recognition; DNA damage tolerance; cell cycle; apoptosis.

1. CONCEPT OF CISPLATIN RESISTANCE AND ITS MULTIFACETED NATURE

Genetic changes are at the heart of cancer development. Although cancer may arise as a result of a key genetic defect, a number of compensatory molecular changes ensue to enable tumor cells to attenuate or override cell cycle regulatory controls and, thereby, proliferate unabated. Interestingly, no cancers from two individuals, even from the same tissue, are identical in their expression profile of genetic abnormalities. It is remarkable then that such cancers respond similarly to therapeutic interventions with a given regimen. This suggests that a favorable antitumor response depends predominantly on the proper functioning of a few critical genes involved in signal transduction pathways, which on activation by antitumor drugs, tip the balance in favor of apoptosis (Fig. 1). In this regard, *cis*-diammine-dichloro-platinum[II] (cisplatin) is considered a potent inducer of apoptosis, and, therefore, has played a clinically important role in the management of several cancers, including those of the ovary, testes, and the head and neck. This spectrum of antitumor activity also suggests that common apoptotic-inducing signal transduction pathways are activated by cisplatin in tumors of different tissue origin. The high potency of this drug is readily appreciated by considering that in 1970, before the advent of cisplatin, only about 5% of young men with metastatic testicular cancer survived, whereas now greater than 80% of such cases are cured *(1)*.

Cisplatin-induced cytotoxicity involves a complex process, ranging from initial drug entry into cells to the final stages of apoptosis (Fig. 2). For cisplatin, the therapeutic molecular event that initiates the cytotoxic process is DNA damage *(2)*, with the N7-

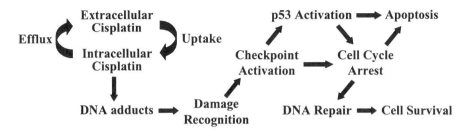

Fig. 2. The process involved in cisplatin-induced cytotoxicity. If any stage of the process toward apoptosis is disrupted, resistance will ensue.

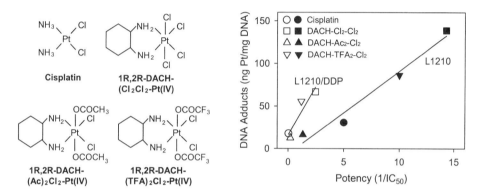

Fig. 3. Structure of cisplatin and analogs, and correlation between potency and the level of total DNA adducts. Data from isogenic sensitive (L1210) and cisplatin-resistant (L1210/DDP) murine leukemia cells are presented. The lines were generated by linear regression. (Adapted with permission from ref. *170*).

position of adenine and guanine providing prime nucleophilic sites for the platinum drug to form DNA–DNA interstrand and intrastrand crosslinks *(3)*. The major cytotoxic adducts, however, appear to be ApG and GpG (where "p" is a phosphate linking the two bases) intrastrand crosslinks, which account for 85–90% of total DNA lesions *(4,5)*. Although these adducts transduce signals to produce the characteristic inhibition of DNA synthesis and suppression of RNA transcription that are associated with cisplatin, such cellular responses to DNA damage do not necessarily correlate with cytotoxicity *(6,7)*. On the other hand, gross adduct levels do correlate directly with the level of cell killing *(2,8)*, and this indicates that adducts transduce additional signals that facilitate cell death. In this regard, apoptotic signals are the more critical event for antitumor responses that may translate into clinical cures, as with testicular cancers. Correlation between DNA damage and cellular drug sensitivity does not only apply to cisplatin, but also extends to platinum analogs. As indicated in Fig. 3, a linear relationship has been demonstrated in the sensitive murine L1210 leukemia model between adduct levels and potency (defined as the reciprocal of IC_{50} drug concentration) for cisplatin and the three analogs shown. Such a relationship is not as well correlated in the isogenic cisplatin-resistant L1210/DDP model. This suggests that different mechanisms of action are at play for each of the platinum drugs, and these transduce signals with good efficiency to the apoptotic machinery in sensitive cells, but with relatively lower efficiency in the resistant model where the main signal transduction pathways activated by cisplatin are disrupted. Such disruptions in signaling are the basis for acquired cisplatin resistance and crossresistance to other platinum and nonplatinum agents, and explain why antitumor responses to cisplatin do not always translate into cures. Indeed, in small cell lung and ovarian cancers, the significant initial cisplatin response rates of up to 70% lead to a 5-yr survival rate of only 5–10 and 25–30%, respectively *(9,10)*. Nevertheless, it is apparent that in model systems, cell death can still be accomplished in resistant cells, but with a relatively higher drug input. Clinical resistance, on the higher hand, is defined as a failure of tumor cells to undergo apoptosis at clinically relevant doses or at clinically achievable plasma drug concentrations. Therefore, the exact level of resistance in patients is difficult to define, but refractory tumors may be at least twofold resistant, because such tumors become responsive when the standard clinical dose of cisplatin is doubled *(11)*. Moreover, acquired resistance may not always be ascribed to the failure/attenuation of apoptotic signal transduction pathways, as resistance can arise through upregulation in other pathways that shift the delicate balance toward cell survival (*see* Fig. 1).

Cisplatin resistance does not necessarily have to be acquired. Intrinsic mechanisms in tumor cells also impede cisplatin-mediated cell death and are ascribed to preexisting signaling defects, which are presumed to be similar to those observed in acquired resistance. For instance, LNCaP prostate tumor cells selected for metastatic potential demonstrate intrinsic resistance to cisplatin, and this resistance, like acquired resistance, can be circumvented by the DACH-Ac$_2$-Cl$_2$-Pt^{IV} analog shown in Fig. 3 *(12–14)*. Although a single mechanism of resistance in a cell line is possible *(15)*, it is not unusual to find that the underlying cause of resistance is multifaceted, as indicated by the concurrent presence of several resistance mechanisms within a tumor cell *(16,17)*. Furthermore, the spectrum of resistance mechanisms varies between cell lines, and some mechanisms may be absent in certain resistant models *(5)* and expressed in others only when the tumor is grown in vivo *(18)*. Unfortunately, the several resistance mechanisms within a tumor are often unrelated and arise sequentially, so that final resistance acquired through cisplatin exposure can be high *(19)*. Irrespective of their specific characteristics, resistance mechanisms are an impediment to clinical management of the disease, and this is further compounded by the fact that tumors acquiring resistance to cisplatin are fully crossresistant to the platinum analog carboplatin *(20)* and also to diverse unrelated antitumor drugs *(21)*. This suggests that cisplatin, carboplatin, and the unrelated agents likely share common mechanisms of resistance. In such cases, the mechanistically distinct platinum analogs oxaliplatin *(22)* and DACH-Ac$_2$-Cl$_2$-Pt^{IV} *(14)* can be of particular clinical interest for their ability to circumvent cisplatin resistance.

In essence, cisplatin resistance occurs because of a failure of cells to induce apoptosis. This failure arises as a result of molecular alterations that either attenuate the level and persistence of DNA damage, reduce transduction of DNA damage signals reaching the apoptotic machinery, upregulate survival pathways, or a combination of these. The specific mechanisms are detailed in the following subheadings.

2. REDUCED ADDUCT LEVELS AS A CAUSATIVE FACTOR

Because the level of DNA–DNA adducts and their persistence correlates directly with cisplatin cytotoxicity *(2,8)*, changes in gene expression within the cell that reduce the level of these DNA lesions will induce resistance. The four main mechanisms that attenuate adduct levels are reduced drug uptake, enhanced drug efflux, increased inactivation of cisplatin, and enhanced adduct repair.

2.1. Reduced Drug Uptake

Although a few studies have demonstrated a lack of change in cisplatin uptake in cisplatin-resistant cells *(15)*, these appear to be isolated incidences. In fact, reduced drug uptake is prevalent and surfaces early in the genesis of drug resistant clones. Reduced drug accumulation of about 20–70% has been observed in a variety of cisplatin-resistant cell lines, and so it represents a significant factor *(5)*. In a few of these cell lines, reduced uptake can be the principal mechanism of resistance. Because reduced influx can be demonstrated over a wide range of extracellular cisplatin concentrations, it has been suggested that the defect is in the passive nonsaturable drug uptake process *(4,23)*. However, cisplatin uptake via an energy-dependent active transport involving Na^+/K^+ ATPase or a gated ion channel has been suggested *(24,25)*, and the possibility exists that defect in this system may also contribute to cisplatin resistance. Recently, cisplatin uptake via the high-affinity copper transport protein (Ctr)1 has been proposed in yeast and mammalian cells *(26–28)*. This is supported by evidence that deletion of the *Ctr1* gene was associated with reduced cisplatin uptake *(28)*, and, conversely, cells engineered for increased expression of this gene increased uptake of cisplatin by about 1.5-fold. Interestingly, exposure of cells to cisplatin results in decrease of Ctr1 within minutes, which is suggestive of degradation or poisoning of the transporter protein *(28)*. However, the significance of Ctr1 in cisplatin resistance is unclear. Although deletion of *Ctr1* resulted in the drug-resistant phenotype *(28)*, increased expression of this gene that enhanced drug uptake did not induce sensitivity to cisplatin *(27)*. In contrast to these studies, which manipulated *Ctr1* expression in sensitive cells to examine modulation of drug sensitivity, one report has identified significant (>50%) reduction in *Ctr1* mRNA, and corresponding reduction in cisplatin uptake, in a stable fivefold cisplatin-resistant human small cell lung cancer cell line derived through traditional chronic exposure of isogenic sensitive cells to cisplatin *(29)*. Moreover, in this study, increased expression of *Ctr1* by transfection increased cisplatin sensitivity of both sensitive and resistant cell line pair. Therefore, the preponderance of these early data does seem to implicate *Ctr1* gene in cisplatin resistance.

2.2. Enhanced Drug Efflux

As with reduced drug uptake, enhanced drug efflux in resistant cells can also affect a net decrease in intracellular cisplatin levels and contribute to the drug-resistant phenotype. Although cisplatin efflux as a mechanism has been discounted in some model systems *(17,24)*, several studies have demonstrated upregulation of exporter proteins in response to chronic cisplatin treatment. Of these, the multidrug resistance-associated (MRP) gene family is a major focus of investigations. The MRP family is composed of at least seven members (MRP1-7), which are ATP-dependent proteins and localized in the cell membrane. Several of these have been associated with cellular efflux of a variety of drugs and, more significantly, their presence has been demonstrated in tumor cells *(30)*. However, of the MRP members, only MRP1 and MRP2 may be of significance, and then only in some cisplatin-resistant tumor models *(31)*. The role of MRP2 (canalicular multispecific organic anion transporter; ATP-binding cassette transporter C2) appears to be of greater importance, and is supported by increased gene expression of this member in cisplatin-resistant cells *(32)*. Additional support has been provided through demonstration that cisplatin resistance can be induced following transfection of *MRP2* gene expression vector, or, conversely, through sensitization of cells to cisplatin following expression of *MRP2* antisense *(33,34)*.

In the past few years, an additional family of ATPase exporter genes has been linked to cisplatin resistance. Investigations on cisplatin efflux have centered around two family members, *ATP7A* and *ATP7B*, which are copper-transporting genes that are overexpressed in cisplatin-resistant tumor cells *(26,35,36)*. Studies indicate that human tumor cells transfected with *ATP7A* or *ATP7B* acquire significant resistance to both cisplatin and copper. However, it is not clear whether this acquisition of cisplatin resistance is because of enhanced cisplatin efflux, as intracellular levels of cisplatin do not decrease in such engineered cells *(37)*. It appears that ATP7A and ATP7B may initiate efflux of cisplatin directly into the vesicular compartment, which reduces nuclear access of cisplatin to affect DNA damage, and this in turn reduces cytotoxicity. Although the significance of the copper transporter in cancer has been highlighted by a recent proposal to use overexpression of *ATP7B* as a clinical marker of chemoresistance to cisplatin in ovarian cancer *(38)*, this contrasts with the reported lack of change in the expression of *ATP7A* and *ATP7B* in five nonovarian cisplatin-resistant cell lines when compared to their isogenic sensitive counterparts *(29)*. A remote possibility is that increased expression of these efflux transporters in cisplatin resistance is tissue-type specific, but it will require future studies to clarify this and amplify the clinical significance of these export proteins.

Other proteins implicated in cisplatin efflux include the multidrug resistance (MDR) P-glycoprotein or the major vault/lung resistance-related protein (MVP/LRP) transporter, but the supporting evidence is weak *(39)*. Indirect evidence, however, demonstrates that in advanced ovarian cancer, overexpression of P-glycoprotein is associated with a poor response to cisplatin-based regimen *(40)*. Similar poor response to the platinum regimen has also been demonstrated in this disease expressing increased levels of MVP/LRP *(41)*. It is apparent that further data are needed to draw definitive conclusions on the role of P-glycoprotein and MVP/LRP in cisplatin resistance.

2.3. Increased Inactivation of Cisplatin

Cisplatin is a neutral inorganic molecule, which undergoes aquation reactions to become activated before it can react with nucleophilic sites on the DNA. This interaction can also occur with other nucleophilic components, which include glutathione (GSH) and the cysteine-rich metallothionein in the cytoplasm. Thus, any increases in such thiols will enhance inactivation and sequestration of cisplatin in the cytoplasm, reduce the availability of the antitumor agent in the nucleus to form DNA adducts, and induce resistance.

Several preclinical and clinical studies have demonstrated that increases in GSH do indeed correlate with cisplatin resistance *(5,42)*. Such elevations have been ascribed to coordinate increases in the expression of the γ-glutamylcysteine synthetase (γ-*GCS*) gene (involved in GSH biosynthesis) and the transcription factor c-Jun *(43)*. Although the reaction between aquated cisplatin and GSH can occur spontaneously, this reaction in part may also be catalyzed by the xenobiotic detoxication enzyme GSH-*S*-transferase-π, the increased level of which is also implicated in cisplatin resistance *(44)*. This is supported by evidence that patients with head and neck cancer survive longer when their tumors have a low level of GSH-*S*-transferase-π than when their tumors have high levels *(45)*. The role of elevated GSH in cisplatin resistance may also be due in part to GSH-mediated increase in either the repair of DNA adducts *(5)* or the capacity to suppress apoptosis *(46,47)*. As with GSH, metallothioneins also interact with and inactivate cisplatin. Because metallothioneins are rich in thiol-containing cysteine residues, increases in this protein of up to fivefold in cisplatin-resistant murine and human tumor models can provide a substantially greater potential to inactivate cisplatin and enhance the resistance phenotype *(48,49)*.

2.4. Enhanced Adduct Repair

An increase in the rate of repair of drug-induced DNA adducts constitutes an important mechanism of cisplatin resistance. The resultant decrease in cisplatin-mediated cell killing has been demonstrated in several murine and human tumor cell lines *(8,19,50)*. The twofold increase in repair is probably the upper limit as further increases are not observed even when resistance to cisplatin continues to rise in chronic drug exposure protocols *(51,52)*.

Removal of platinum adducts from the DNA involves the nucleotide excision repair (NER) pathway. NER is a complex process involving some 17 different proteins *(53)*, but changes in only a few rate-limiting proteins is sufficient to enhance repair capacity *(54)*. It is not surprising then that cisplatin resistance arises with increases in the excision repair crosscomplementing (ERC)C1 or ERCC1/xeroderma pigmentosum group (XP)F proteins, but not ERCC3 *(55,56)*. Overexpression of ERCC1 and another NER protein, XPA, have also been demonstrated in patient's tumors that are refractory to cisplatin *(57)*. Based on these observations, one may predict that a defect in NER may hypersensitize tumor cells to cisplatin. This has indeed been demonstrated, together with restoration of normal drug sensitivity when NER integrity is reestablished *(51,58)*. Similarly, the high sensitivity of testicular tumor cells to cisplatin correlates with their reduced repair capacity as a result of low levels of XPA and ERCC1/XPF *(59,60)*. NER has broad specificity, such that increased repair from cisplatin exposure also increases repair of structurally diverse platinum-based drugs *(61,62)*. This may explain in part both the inability of specific platinum drugs, such as oxaliplatin, to fully circumvent cisplatin resistance and the crossresistance observed with structurally diverse nonplatinum drugs.

Although the NER complex can remove cisplatin-induced DNA adducts by both global genomic and transcription-coupled nucleotide excision repair (TC-NER), the significance of TC-NER in cisplatin resistance is considered by some as doubtful *(51,51,63)*. This emanates from the finding that several proteins, such as ERCC1 and XPA, play a key role in TC-NER, but demonstrate a preference for repairing interstrand platinum crosslinks rather than the lethal intrastrand adducts of cisplatin. This, however, is countered by the demonstration that cells deficient specifically in TC-NER, but not global genomic repair, are hypersensitive to cisplatin *(58)*. Moreover, breast cancer 1 (*BRCA1*) is involved in TC-NER (64), and overexpression or inhibition of this breast and ovarian cancer susceptibility gene leads to cisplatin resistance or sensitivity, respectively *(65)*. However, the role of BRCA in DNA repair is dependent on members of the Fanconi anemia family of proteins. In this regard, the Fanconi anemia F gene is downregulated by epigenetic silencing in sensitive 2008 cells, but expressed in cisplatin-resistant 2008/C13 cells to facilitate interaction with BRCA proteins and promote cisplatin adduct repair *(66)*. Irrespective of the specific mechanism involved, a general conclusion is that an increased rate of repair of DNA adducts by NER generally induces cisplatin resistance.

3. DEFECTIVE DNA DAMAGE RECOGNITION

Before signal transduction pathways can be activated to initiate specific cellular responses, such as repair, the damage to the DNA by cisplatin has to be recognized. This is done by specific proteins that do not necessarily recognize the specific DNA adduct, but rather the physical distortions or kinks created in the DNA helix by the damage *(67)*.

Such distortions can differ between interstrand and intrastrand adducts, and between one platinum agent and another. There are more than 20 DNA damage recognition proteins, including human mutS homolog-2 (hMSH2), high mobility group (HMG)1/2, human mRNA for upstream binding factor, and TATA box binding factor, with each recognizing one or more qualitatively distinct DNA distortion *(61,68)*. More recent data have demonstrated that the p53 molecule in its nascent form also has the capacity to recognize and bind to DNA–cisplatin adducts, but in addition, p53 can enhance the binding of the recognition protein HMG1 to the adduct *(69,70)*. Because several proteins may recognize the same distortion, multiple signaling pathways can be activated by a single type of DNA lesion. With cisplatin, several types of intrastrand adducts are formed (including GpG, ApG, GpXpG and ApXpG, where "X" is any base), which may require recognition by an array of proteins, and this is consistent with the observation that several cellular effects are observed when DNA is damaged by this agent. Interestingly, the spectrum of these effects may be different with structurally different platinum analogs, such as the clinically active oxaliplatin and satraplatin (JM216). This stems from the understanding that adducts of cisplatin and these agents may be differentially recognized, as has been reported with HMG1 or components of the mismatch repair (MMR) complex, which show greater preference for interacting with cisplatin adducts *(68,71)*. An alternative proposal to explain the variety of cellular response is that a single recognition protein transduces multiple signals following DNA damage by cisplatin. Support for this concept is provided by a recent study with XPC using gene microarrays. This recognition protein is involved in NER, but defect in the *XPC* gene not only affects other DNA repair genes, but also downstream genes involved in cell cycle, cell proliferation, and apoptotic response *(72)*. Thus, recognition of cisplatin-induced DNA adducts by a single protein is capable of inducing a cascade of cellular responses that, when integrated downstream, determine the final fate of the cell.

Because damage recognition proteins can affect cell death, the converse is also true that loss of damage recognition can render cells insensitive to cisplatin. This is well demonstrated by loss of the integrity of the MMR complex, which normally facilitates cisplatin-mediated apoptosis after attempting futile repair of DNA adducts *(73)*. The MMR complex consists of a number of proteins, including hMutL-α (heterodimer of hMLH1 and PMS2) and hMutS-α (a heterodimer of hMSH2 and hMSH6). Of these, hMSH2 (as a monomer or the hMutSα heterodimer) is involved directly in recognizing GpG intrastrand adduct of cisplatin *(68,71,73)*. Both hMLH1 or hMSH2 are reported to be downregulated or mutated in some cancers, and because these abnormalities attenuate apoptotic activity, response to cisplatin is significantly reduced *(71,73–75)*. Thus, loss of MMR integrity induces cisplatin resistance.

4. INCREASED DNA DAMAGE TOLERANCE

Molecular mechanisms of resistance involving transport, thiols, and DNA repair serve to reduce the formation and persistence of cytotoxic DNA adducts. However, the ability of cells to tolerate a greater level of cisplatin adducts is a significant factor in cisplatin resistance. Indeed, several reports have demonstrated an excellent correlation between DNA damage tolerance and resistance *(19,76,77)*. Such a correlation can be seen in Fig. 4, which demonstrates that this relationship applies to both murine L1210 and human A2780 tumor models.

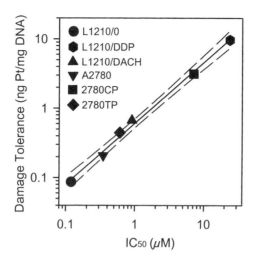

Fig. 4. Relationship between DNA damage tolerance and antitumor activity (IC_{50}) of cisplatin. Data were derived from murine (L1210) and human (A2780) isogenic tumor models, which are sensitive (L1210/0, A2780), cisplatin-resistant (L1210/DDP, 2780CP), or resistant to oxaliplatin or teraplatin (L1210/DACH, 2780TP). The line is a linear regression fit, and shown with 95% confidence limits. (Adapted with permission from ref. 77).

Tolerance to DNA adducts is a function of the individual resistance mechanism: a defect in the signal transduction pathway can only culminate in resistance if cells can tolerate an increased level of DNA damage. This can be reconciled by considering that cell death is a net result of both prosurvival and proapoptotic signals, and either an increase in intensity and/or duration of prosurvival signals or suppression of proapoptotic signals in resistant cells will inhibit apoptosis (*see* Fig. 1), even when DNA damage has reached or exceeded the normal cytotoxic threshold of sensitive tumor cells. The mechanisms contributing to DNA damage tolerance, including those involving p53 and HER-2/*neu*, are considered under Sections 6. and 7. However, the ability to tolerate high levels of DNA adducts and survive requires that DNA replication and cellular proliferation continue unabated. To facilitate this, resistant cells have acquired an enhanced capacity to replicate DNA past the adduct, and then initiate postreplication repair *(51)*. In this respect, defects in hMLH1 or hMSH6 appear to enhance replicative bypass by three- to sixfold *(73)*, but this increase may also occur independent of changes in such MMR proteins *(78)*. Moreover, increased tolerance to DNA adducts and replicative bypass in MMR-deficient cells can be exacerbated by coexistence of other cellular defects, such as loss of p53 *(74,79)*.

5. INHIBITION OF APOPTOSIS

As highlighted, cisplatin is a potent inducer of apoptosis. Loss of apoptotic signal allows tumor cells to raise the threshold of DNA damage that induces cell death. This is the basic concept of DNA damage tolerance, as discussed above. A major player in inducing apoptosis with cisplatin is the tumor suppressor p53, which is also a sequence-specific transcription activator *(80,81)*. Under normal circumstances, DNA damage signals to affect apoptosis are propagated via checkpoint kinases ataxia telangiectasia mutated protein (ATM) and ATM- and Rad3-related protein (ATR), with cisplatin showing preference for ATR *(82)*. Once activated, ATR induces p53 by phosphorylation, both directly at Ser-15 and via either Chk1 at Ser-20 or mitogen-activated protein kinase (MAPK) cascade at Thr-81 *(83,84)*. The functionally activated p53 has the capacity to transactivate several genes, with the *bax* gene being critical for executing the well-orchestrated process of cisplatin-mediated apoptosis *(85,86)*. The next step in this process involves the translocation of cytosolic Bax to the mitochondria, where a cascade of events affects the release of apoptogenic factors (such as cytochrome *c* and second mitochondria-derived activator of capsase/direct inhibitor of apoptosis protein [IAP]-binding protein with low pI), which activate the caspase 9/caspase 3 pathway to finally affect the apoptotic process of DNA fragmentation *(87)*. Apoptosis induced by cisplatin also occurs through the fatty acid synthase/fatty acid synthase ligand-activated caspase 8/caspase 3 pathway *(88)*, but this pathway for cisplatin appears to be of lower significance. Nevertheless, it serves to amplify the notion that several options are available to induce cisplatin-induced cell death, and when the most efficient pathway for apoptosis becomes defective, the cell can activate another pathway when the higher threshold for DNA damage is reached.

The apoptotic process is tightly regulated by the ratio between Bax and its closely related antiapoptotic partner, Bcl-2. When the Bax:Bcl-2 ratio is increased by cisplatin, either by elevation of Bax or down-regulation of *bcl-2*, mitochondrial levels of proapoptogenic Bax/Bax homodimers exceed levels of antiapoptotic Bcl-2/Bcl-2 homodimers, and, thereby, initiate the apoptotic process *(89)*. Based on this understanding, it is easy to appreciate that cisplatin resistance will be observed when tumor cells overexpress *bcl-2 (90)*. This resistance may not be due entirely to a failure to initiate directly the final steps in apoptosis, but may also occur via an indirect effect. This is best appreciated by considering that overexpression of *bcl-2* is reported to increase levels of GSH *(47)*, which, as discussed, could reduce cytotoxicity through several possible mechanisms.

In addition to Bcl-2, members of IAP, represented by the survivin and X-linked inhibitor of apoptosis protein (XIAP) molecules, also are known to induce resistance when overexpressed *(91,92)*. These inhibitors directly or indirectly inhibit the caspase cascade to prevent activation of apoptosis by cisplatin. This is also consistent with the finding that activation of caspases 3, 8, and 9 is attenuated in cisplatin-resistant cells *(91,93)*. Other mechanisms that inhibit the apoptotic process, such as those related to p53 and HER-2/*neu*, are discussed in Sections 6. and 7.

6. LOSS OF p53 TUMOR SUPPRESSOR FUNCTION

The significance of p53 in cancer is profound. From a therapeutic viewpoint, the p53 is not only involved in apoptosis, as discussed above, but also in response to checkpoint activation following the formation of DNA–platinum adducts. Loss of apoptosis and checkpoint response are two of several negative outcomes affected by defects in p53 function *(94)*.

6.1. p53 Gene Status and Defective Function

The p53 protein represents a critical player in activating apoptosis and affecting the cytotoxicity of cisplatin (*see* Fig. 2). Its close relative p73 provides a parallel pathway for cisplatin-induced cell death *(95)*, but very little is known of any defect in this homolog protein or its function that could mediate cisplatin resistance. On the other hand, defect

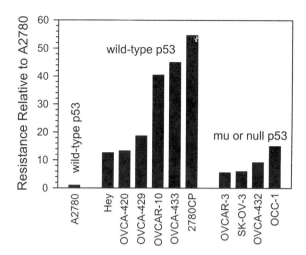

Fig. 5. The status of p53 and cisplatin resistance in an ovarian tumor panel. Cells having wild-type p53 tend to be sensitive to cisplatin, as exemplified by ovarian A2780 cells. However, among resistant models, those having wild-type p53 are generally more resistant to cisplatin than those with mutant or null p53.

in p53 functions are frequent and, therefore, it plays a significant role in cisplatin resistance. The major defect occurs when p53 becomes mutated, so that the three-dimensional structure of p53 is altered and it can no longer bind to DNA in a sequence-specific manner to transactivate genes, including the cyclin-dependent kinase (CDK) inhibitor *p21Waf1/ Cip1*, the p53 feedback inhibitor murine double minute 2 (*mdm2*), growth arrest and DNA damage-inducible *gadd45a* gene, and the proapoptotic *bax* gene. Approximately half of all cancers harbor mutant p53 *(96)*, and the therapeutic consequence of this is readily appreciated by considering the relationship between *p53* gene status and durable responses among cancers considered sensitive to cisplatin. In this regard, the greatest cure rate is observed in seminomatous germ cell tumors, which harbor predominantly wild-type p53, whereas a relatively lower cure rate is noted in ovarian, head and neck, and metastatic bladder cancers, which demonstrate a 40–60% p53 mutation frequency *(97–99)*. However, within a given disease type, such as ovarian cancer, the response and 5-yr survival rates after cisplatin-based treatment are significantly greater in patients with tumors expressing wild-type p53 than mutant p53 *(98,100)*. This differential response is confirmed in model systems where tumor cells expressing mutant p53 are defective in apoptotic response and, therefore, resistant to cisplatin *(80,85,90)*.

Although cisplatin resistance because of mutant p53 is understandable, the numerous reports of resistance in the presence of wild-type p53 present a conceptual challenge. In ovarian cancer, about a half of the patients with wild-type p53 tumors fail cisplatin therapy *(101)*. In testicular cancer, on the other hand, the incidence is more dramatic, with almost all of the small numbers of refractory tumors still harboring wild-type p53 *(102)*. In these cases, it is not uncommon to ascribe resistance to the likely presence of other molecular defects within the tumors, such as microsatellite instability *(103)*. However, it is interesting to note that in model systems, cisplatin resistance is actually associated with the presence of wild-type p53 *per se*, and this resistance can be substantially greater than in mutant or null p53 cells *(14,97,104)*. This is seen in Fig. 5, which demonstrates that the resistance of wild-type p53 models is generally greater in a cisplatin-resistant ovarian tumor panel composed predominantly of models established from clinical samples after patients became resistant to cisplatin (except 2780CP, which was made resistant by exposing drug-naive A2780 cells to cisplatin in tissue culture). The underlying basis for resistance in wild-type p53 models has been ascribed in some systems to a lack of p53 induction, whereas in others, a selective loss of p53 function appears to be the major cause *(12,13,19,104)*. The molecular explanation for this defect in the p53 pathway is not known, but these reports demonstrate that the defect and the resistance disappear when the mechanistically distinct platinum analog DACH-Ac$_2$-Cl$_2$-Pt^{IV} *(see* Fig. 3) is used as the cytotoxic agent. Because of this differential response, it is difficult to implicate involvement of the likely modifiers of p53, such as MDM2 *(105)*, p14^{ARF} *(106)*, or the human papillomavirus-16 E6 oncogene *(107)*, as possible explanations for defective p53 function, because these would also affect the cytotoxicity of the platinum analog. It is plausible that independent pathways exist for activation of p53, and that the pathway inhibited to affect cisplatin resistance is not required for the cytotoxicity of the analog. This is analogous to the dependency on MMR for transducing apoptotic signals of cisplatin, but not oxaliplatin *(108)*.

6.2. Checkpoint Response in Cisplatin Resistance

Considering that cisplatin resistance can be greater in wild-type p53 cells than in mutant or null cells implies that inactivation of the wild-type p53 in such resistant cells could actually reduce resistance to the level seen in p53-defective cells. Such a counterintuitive consideration may indeed provide a logical explanation for the unexpected observation that in wild-type p53 tumor cells with apoptotic defect, disruption of p53 function increases cisplatin sensitivity *(109,110)*. Surprisingly, a similar sensitization to cisplatin is also observed when the downstream p53-dependent *p21*$^{Waf1/Cip1}$ gene is deleted *(111)*. This places the p21$^{Waf1/Cip1}$ protein squarely in the position of inhibiting cisplatin-induced cell death. How the p53/p21$^{Waf1/Cip1}$ pathway mediates resistance in the select group of wild-type p53 tumor models is not precisely known. However, the current concept of p53 is that it activates both Bax, which is the downstream effector of apoptosis, and p21$^{Waf1/Cip1}$, an inhibitor of CDK and effector of cell cycle arrest that permits DNA repair and, therefore, promotes survival. Thus, one may speculate that a differentially greater induction of p21$^{Waf1/Cip1}$ than Bax, perhaps dictated by cell context, will tip the apoptosis-survival balance in favor of cell survival. An alternative mechanism suggests that the presence of p21$^{Waf1/Cip1}$ prevents uncoupling of S- and M-phases of the cell cycle, and this facilitates cell survival by affecting a normal checkpoint response at the G$_2$/M phase *(112)*.

Although the above explanations for sensitization of tumor cells lacking p21$^{Waf1/Cip1}$ appear valid, several contrasting reports indicate that cisplatin sensitivity in fact requires increased expression of p21$^{Waf1/Cip1}$ *(113–115)*. This is supported by recent evidence, which confirms that cisplatin resistance is associated with a defect in the p53/p21$^{Waf1/Cip1}$ pathway and, more specifically, with the lack of p21$^{Waf1/Cip1}$ induction *(12,13,19)*. Because the p53/p21$^{Waf1/Cip1}$ pathway is an integral component of the DNA damage checkpoint response machinery, it is likely that resistance is because of loss of this checkpoint response and failure of the cell cycle to arrest. An important question, therefore, to ask in this regard is from which phase of the cell cycle is the primary apoptotic signal normally generated, but attenuated in the absence of p21$^{Waf1/Cip1}$. With cisplatin, checkpoint response in tumor cells results in a transient S-phase arrest, which is followed by a durable G_2/M-phase arrest, but arrest in these phases is independent of p53 status *(104)*. This would seem to argue against S- and G_2/M-phase checkpoint responses as inducers of the p53/p21$^{Waf1/Cip1}$ pathway-dependent apoptotic signal. In support of this is the consensus that G_2/M-phase arrest is in fact inhibitory to the cytotoxic process, primarily because pharmacological abrogation of G_2/M arrest increases cellular sensitivity to cisplatin *(116,117)*. This raises the possibility that G_1-phase checkpoint response mediated through p21$^{Waf1/Cip1}$ is the transducer of the cell death signal. In this respect, the G_1-phase checkpoint response in tumor cells treated with cisplatin is reported to be quite robust, as judged by an almost complete inhibition of G_1-phase CDK4 and CDK2 kinase activities *(118)*. However, it needs to be acknowledged that cisplatin is not recognized for inducing significant G_1-phase arrest, but this is probably because G_1-phase CDK inhibition occurs late when cells are already stuck at the G_2/M interface. A recent study has provided an excellent direct correlation between the ability of tumor models in the NCI 60-cell line panel to demonstrate G_1 arrest by ionizing radiation and cisplatin sensitivity *(119)*. Moreover, the analog DACH-Ac$_2$-Cl$_2$-Pt^{IV} (*see* Fig. 3) only activates the G_1-phase checkpoint to affect cytotoxicity *(120)*. These considerations collectively provide good support for loss of G_1-phase checkpoint response as an effector of cisplatin resistance.

The ability of p21$^{Waf1/Cip1}$ to both inhibit and induce apoptosis has created much confusion, and has been the subject of several reviews *(121,122)*. In both of these opposing functions, cisplatin resistance by p21$^{Waf1/Cip1}$ is mediated by its affect on cell cycle checkpoint response: Resistance in one case is because of a positive G_2/M checkpoint response, whereas in the other, the loss of G_1-phase checkpoint response is implicated. The exact mechanisms are not known. However, defective regulations may involve any number of molecular pathways to alter (1) p21$^{Waf1/Cip1}$ expression by posttranscriptional modification that stabilize its mRNA, (2) expression of transcriptional activators that facilitate transactivation of the p21$^{Waf1/Cip1}$ promoter, and (3) posttranslational modification that stabilize the protein *(123)*. For instance, upregulation of posttranslational phosphorylation of p21$^{Waf1/Cip1}$ by the MAPK *(124)* or the phosphatidylinositol 3 kinase (PI3-K)/Akt pathway *(125,126)* could switch the function of p21$^{Waf1/Cip1}$ from an inducer of apoptosis to an inhibitor (*see* Section 7.1.). This is plausible, as phosphorylation by the upregulated PI3K/Akt pathway has been demonstrated to promote cyctoplasmic localization of p21$^{Waf1/Cip1}$ *(127)*, which then is prevented from interacting with the CDKs in the nucleus and participating in checkpoint response. Although, evidence exists to propose that preventing p21$^{Waf1/Cip1}$ from participating in checkpoint response mediates cisplatin resistance, the data is still not definitive at the present time. However, a plausible model is presented in Fig. 6 to indicate how p21$^{Waf1/Cip1}$ could determine cell fate.

7. UPREGULATION OF HER-2/*NEU* SURVIVAL SIGNALING

The *HER-2/neu* proto-oncogene, which has extensive homology to the epidermal growth factor receptor, encodes the p185 transmembrane receptor tyrosine kinase *(128)*. This oncogene is overexpressed in about 20–30% of breast and ovarian cancer patients, and its proliferative stimulus leads to a poor response of these cancers to cisplatin *(129,130)*. Although there are isolated reports that induction of p185 tyrosine phosphorylation activity increases sensitivity to cisplatin *(131)*, in general, this induction is associated with the onset of cisplatin resistance and confirmed in model systems engineered for *HER-2/neu* overexpression *(132)*. This has led to exploration of strategies to potentiate cisplatin cytotoxicity by either inhibiting the kinase activity with emodin or

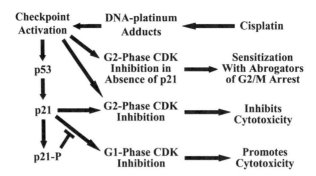

Fig. 6. A model depicting the role of p21 in checkpoint response and the fate of cells exposed to cisplatin. The presence of functional p21 inhibits G_1-phase cyclin-dependent kinases (CDKs), which transduces an apoptotic signal. The p21 can also contribute to inhibition of G_2-phase CDK, and this is depicted as inhibiting cytotoxicity. CDK inhibition in the G_2 phase is not dependent on p21, but without p21, the G_2 arrest is not as robust and can be abrogated to sensitize cells to cisplatin. Phosphorylation of p21 inhibits checkpoint response and, therefore, cell death.

with an HER-2/*neu* antibody *(133,134)*. The signaling from activation of the HER-2/*neu* receptor is propagated through either the PI3-K/Akt pathway or the Src-homology and collagen homology/growth factor receptor-binding protein 2/son of sevenless pathway, which in turn activates the downstream Ras/MAPK *(128)*. Both the PI3-K/Akt and the Ras/MAPK pathways are intimately involved in the onset of cisplatin resistance.

7.1. Enhanced Activity of the PI3-K/Akt Pathway

The PI3-K/Akt pathway regulates several cellular functions, such as cell growth and survival. In cisplatin-sensitive tumor cells, however, basal activity of the PI3-K/Akt is essential for the induction of p21[Waf1/Cip1] by cisplatin *(126)*. This allows cells to arrest the cell cycle and respond to the stress created by DNA damage, including repairing the DNA for survival and, conversely, activating apoptosis if the repair is incomplete. This regulatory function of Akt can be disrupted when its expression and its serine–threonine protein kinase activity are increased by upstream overexpression of *HER-2/neu (135)*. However, mechanisms other than HER-2/*neu* may also be responsible for increasing Akt activity, and this is deduced primarily from considering that overexpression of *HER-2/neu* is observed in 20–30% of ovarian cancers *(129)*, whereas elevated active Akt levels is found in almost 70% of this cancer *(136)*. One likely possibility involves the phosphatase and tensin homolog deleted on chromosome ten, which normally is a negative regulator of Akt, but mutation in the phosphatase and tensin homolog deleted on chromosome ten gene allows Akt to become constitutively active *(137)*. Irrespective of the mechanism involved, hyperactive Akt phosphorylates p21[Waf1/Cip1] at Thr-145, and thereby prevents nuclear localization of the CDK inhibitor to affect cell cycle arrest *(127)*. Thus, p21[Waf1/Cip1] function could be either promoted or attenuated by the PI3/Akt pathway, depending on the strength of the upstream signal. More importantly, inhibition of this p21[Waf1/Cip1] function provides a valid mechanism to explain the observation that upregulation of Akt induces cisplatin resistance *(135,138,139)*.

Because enhanced Akt activity disrupts multiple cellular functions *(137)*, it is reasonable to expect that cisplatin resistance from upregulation of Akt activity will not be because of a single dysfunction, but rather to several dysfunctions, as can be seen in Fig. 7.

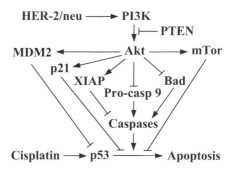

Fig. 7. Upregulated phosphatidylinositol 3 kinase/Akt pathway induces cisplatin resistance. Overexpression of HER-2/*neu* and/or loss of phosphatase and tensin homolog deleted on chromosome ten increase Akt activity, which negatively affects the function of multiple proteins, and these collectively inhibit cisplatin-mediated apoptotic process.

One downstream effector of Akt activation is mammalian target of rapamycin; it is elevated in 55% of ovarian cancers and, like Akt, reduces sensitivity of tumors to cisplatin *(136)*. Increased Akt activity has also been reported to induce phosphorylation of the MDM2 oncoprotein, which then translocates to the nucleus *(140,141)*. Increases in nuclear levels of this oncoprotein reduce p53 activity by ubiquitination, and induce cisplatin resistance by an enforced loss of p53-mediated apoptosis. Apoptosis can also be lost by inactivation of the proapoptotic protein Bad following its phosphorylation at Ser-136 by Akt, and this has been demonstrated as a significant factor in inhibiting cisplatin-mediated cell death *(139)*. Further inhibition of apoptosis has been observed as a result of Akt inducing inactivating-phosphorylation at Ser-196 of the procaspase 9 protease *(142)*.

An additional Akt-dependent mechanism that suppresses cisplatin cytotoxicity also involves disruption of the caspase cascade, and requires coordinated interaction between Akt and XIAP *(91)*. It appears that sensitivity of ovarian 2008 tumor cells to cisplatin is conferred by the drug's ability to decrease XIAP, but this ability is lost in cisplatin-resistant 2008/C13 cells *(143)*. Similarly, reinduction of cell death by cisplatin in resistant DU145 prostate tumor cells can be accomplished by decreases in XIAP and Akt levels, with a concomitant activation of the caspase cascade *(144)*. Thus, it becomes apparent that the inability of cisplatin to decrease XIAP levels via the ubiquitin pathway is a factor that mediates resistance. How this happens is now becoming clearer, with reports indicating that activated Akt phosphorylates XIAP and prevents cisplatin-mediated degradation of this inhibitor *(145,146)*.

Insofar as Akt is critical in inducing cisplatin resistance, it is useful to consider the role of Akt isoforms in this negative function. Three isoforms of Akt have been identified so far, and all can be activated through phosphorylation at two critical sites (for instance, Thr-308 and Ser-473 of Akt1) by phosphoinositide-dependent protein kinases 1 and 2, and, therefore, all have the potential to inhibit cisplatin cyotoxicity. However, studies appear to indicate that Akt2 and Akt3 are the more significant in inducing the cisplatin resistance phenotype *(138)*.

7.2. Enhanced Activity of the Ras/MAPK Pathway

MAPK subfamily members p38α, Janus kinase ([JNK] or stress-activated protein kinase) and extracellular signal-regulated kinase (ERK) participate in integrating extracellular signals to regulate cell proliferation, differentiation, and apoptosis *(147)*. Reports indicate that all three kinase members are activated in tumor cells exposed to cisplatin, with ERK activation being the most sensitive, and, therefore, the most critical for cisplatin-induced apoptosis at low clinically relevant concentrations *(87)*. The significant role of ERK is also borne out from the demonstration that its activation by cisplatin contributes to p53 stability via phosphorylation at Ser-15 *(148)*, and that its inhibition by PD98059 induces cisplatin resistance *(149)*. Similarly, JNK activation leads to induction of p53, whereas maintaining JNK in an inactive state decreases p53-dependent cell killing of tumor cells by cisplatin *(150,151)*.

Both ERK and JNK MAPK pathways are regulated by orderly signaling through upstream Ras, which is activated transiently in a stimulus-dependent fashion. The signaling for ERK is mediated downstream by the Ras/RAF/mitogen-activated or extracellular signal-regulated protein kinase (MEK) pathway, whereas JNK is activated via the Ras/MAPK ERK kinase kinase (MEKK)/MKK pathway *(128)*. Although regulated Ras-dependent activation of MAPK is essential for p53-dependent apoptosis by cisplatin, resistance appears when tumor cells overexpress *Ras* or harbor mutant Ras, which then transduce aberrant signaling to the MAPK subfamily members to promote cell proliferation *(152–155)*. This proliferation could be because of two possibilities: a direct stimulus of the cell cycle machinery or a net balance favoring cell survival from loss of apoptotic activity. The latter possibility is supported by the finding that ERK is capable of phosphorylating the proapoptotic Bad at Ser-112 to inhibit cisplatin-induced cytotoxicity *(139)*.

It is clear from consideration of the literature that Ras/MAPK, like PI3-K/Akt, provides another example of a pathway that activates both cell survival and cell death pathways, and the switch between survival and death is likely dependent on the relative intensity and duration of signals transduced along the pathways following DNA damage. In support of this is the finding that sensitive cells require an 8- to 12-h persistence of active JNK signaling after cisplatin exposure to induce apoptosis, whereas resistant cells maintain the activated JNK signaling for a significantly reduced time of only 1–3 h *(156)*. Thus, loss of downstream signaling by JNK may attenuate apoptosis. In the case of Ras/ MAPK, the likely components that could modulate survival-death decisions are the transcription factors, such as c-Myc and c-Jun, which are activated by ERK and JNK, respectively *(128,157,158)*. This is also consistent with the finding that c-Jun normally induces p73 to facilitate an alternative mode (to p53) of cell killing by cisplatin, whereas absence of this transcription factor leads to platinum resistance *(159)*. Details for the c-Jun-dependent induction of p73 are sketchy, but there are several pieces of evidence that may shed some light on the process: (1) cisplatin signaling through p73 requires the nonreceptor tyrosine kinase c-Abl and functional MMR complex *(95)*, (2) activation of c-Abl and JNK by cisplatin is MMR dependent *(108,160)*, (3) cisplatin fails to activate JNK in cells lacking c-Abl *(161)*, (4) cells lacking MMR are cisplatin resistant (*see* Subheading 3.), and (5) c-Abl phosphorylates MEKK in response to cisplatin-induced DNA damage *(162)*. Thus, recognition of cisplatin-induced DNA adducts, in part by MMR, may activate c-Abl and Ras, which independently or cooperatively regulate the same MEKK/ MKK/JNK pathway to activate c-Jun. This transcription factor then activates p73 to affect cisplatin-induced apoptosis. In contrast to this proapoptotic function of normal levels of active c-Jun, overexpression of c-Jun and other such transcriptional factors switches their function toward prosurvival, and in such cases downregulation of the

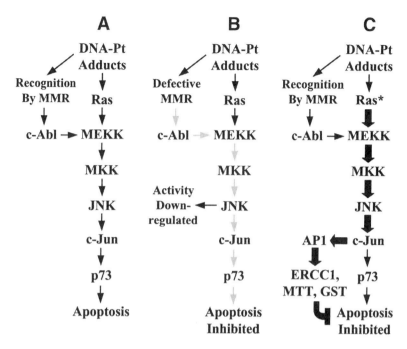

Fig. 8. A model for the modulatory role of Janus kinase (JNK) mitogen-activated protein kinase (MAPK) pathway on cisplatin cytotoxicity by p73. In (**A**), the pathway in sensitive cells is activated through mismatch repair (MMR) and c-Abl, and the downstream activation of c-Jun induces p73 to affect cell death. If MMR or c-Abl is defective, as in (**B**), the signal is weakened (shown by gray-shaded arrows) and incapable of maintaining JNK activity for a sufficient time period to induce c-Jun, and this leads to resistance. In (**C**), the mutant Ras* is constitutively active, and the greater intensity of signals (shown by wider arrows) induce excision repair crosscomplementing (ERC)C1, metallothionein (MTT), glutathione (not shown), and glutathione-*S*-transferase (GST), which collectively inhibit apoptosis to induce cisplatin resistance.

transcriptional factor is capable of reversing cisplatin resistance *(43,161)*. A mechanism that may explain how overexpression of c-Jun may induce resistance is by considering its involvement as a component within the AP1 transcription complex. This complex induces such genes as *ERCC1*, *metallothionein*, and *GST (154)*, so that increased levels of c-Jun could conceivably enhance expression of these genes, with a resultant effect that DNA-platinum adducts will be reduced. Furthermore, c-Jun overexpression is associated with an increase in GSH levels also *(43)*, and this has the potential of exacerbating the reduction in adduct levels to induce cisplatin resistance. A model to explain the possible role of JNK in p73-dependent apoptosis and in cell survival is depicted in Fig. 8.

8. GENE EXPRESSION PROFILES AND MISCELLANEOUS MECHANISMS

The multifaceted or multifactorial nature of cisplatin resistance was apparent two decades ago, and additional mechanisms in support of this have been since identified incrementally. The advent of gene expression profile technology, however, is now providing potential opportunities to examine mechanisms on a global scale. However, the utility of such a technology will depend on the accuracy and reproducibility of the data, which in turn will depend on the context of the cell lines used, the concentration of cisplatin that the cells are exposed to, and the time point at which the cells are harvested to determine the expression profile. For instance, in a well-defined system, cisplatin-induced gene expression in the presence of wild-type p53 is significantly different from cells with inactivated or mutant p53 *(163)*. This is understandable because p53-transactivated genes would be absent and p53-repressed genes would be present when p53 is inactive or mutant. Therefore, without knowledge of the status of normal genes (wild type vs mutant vs null), the power of gene expression profiling can be reduced. With appropriate design, however, some of the limitations could be overcome.

One approach to identify genes contributing to cisplatin resistance is to compare gene expression profiles from microarray analysis of sensitive and resistant cell lines. In this respect, it is worth mentioning three recent reports to highlight the interest and to assess the utility of the approach. In one report using head and neck tumor models, about 60 genes were identified that were differentially expressed in the cisplatin-resistant group *(164)*, but none of these genes could be associated with any of the resistance mechanisms discussed in this chapter. In the second study with two isogenic cisplatin sensitive-resistant pairs of bladder cancer cell lines, the disparity between the two resistant models was overtly apparent: 51 genes were downregulated and 11 upregulated in one resistant model, but in contrast, only nine were downregulated and four upregulated in the second *(165)*. Interestingly, five downregulated genes were common to both models, but none of the upregulated genes was common. Again, none of the differentially expressed genes was recognizable with the mechanisms firmly established for cisplatin resistance. In the third example, *in silico* exploration of gene expression profiles and functional response from a 60-cell line panel in the vast NCI database yielded five genes that correlated with resistance *(119)*, but none correlated with known mechanisms. These studies serve to demonstrate that gene expression profiles generate much data, but their failure to identify and confirm genes already known to be involved in mediating cisplatin resistance requires a degree of caution. However, gene expression profiles can provide opportunities to identify novel genes that have not been implicated previously in inducing resistance. Such genes include inositol 1,4,5-triphosphate receptor type 1, which is downregulated in resistance, and c-*met*, which is overexpressed *(164,165)*. How these genes modulate cisplatin-induced cell death is not known.

Changes in expression of other genes, identified recently using alternative techniques and demonstrated as decreasing cisplatin sensitivity, include downregulation of serine/arginine-rich protein-specific kinase 1 *(166)*, upregulation of transcription factor Ets-1 *(167)* and overexpression of dihydrodiol dehydrogenase *(168)*. Once again, their precise mechanism remains elusive at this time.

9. CONCLUSION

Cisplatin resistance is a net effect of multiple mechanisms that either inhibit apoptosis, promote cell survival, or both. The multifaceted nature of resistance continues to become more complex as more genes inducing cisplatin resistance are identified from gene expression profiles. Because many of these mechanisms coexist within a resistant tumor cell, the task of identifying therapeutic approaches that will be effective against cisplatin refractory disease become daunting. However, cell fate depends on net balance between prosurvival and prodeath signals induced by cisplatin, so the challenge for the future is to acquire specific knowledge that will aid in identifying and activating a dominant apoptotic pathway that will overcome the sum effects of prosurvival signaling pathways.

It is ironic that agents developed or in development to circumvent cisplatin resistance are also platinum-based, and these include oxaliplatin and the DACH-Ac$_2$-Cl$_2$-Pt^{IV} analog. This, however, may be reconciled from the understanding that platinum complexes fall into at least 12 mechanistically distinct groups *(169)*, with candidate agents from any 1 of the 11 groups providing the potential to circumvent resistance of cisplatin and cisplatin-like compounds clustered in the twelfth group. Undoubtedly, a rational, concerted approach will be needed to identify the ideal compound.

ACKNOWLEDGMENTS

Supported by NIH Grants CA77332 and CA82361.

REFERENCES

1. Masters JR, Koberle B. Curing metastatic cancer: lessons from testicular germ-cell tumours. Nat Rev Cancer 2003; 3:517–525.
2. Roberts JJ, Pera MF Jr. DNA as a target for anticancer coordination compounds. In: Lippard SJ, ed. Platinum, gold, and other metal chemotherapeutic agents: chemistry and biochemistry. Washington, DC: American Chemical Society, 1983:3–25.
3. Eastman A. The formation, isolation and characterization of DNA adducts produced by anticancer platinum complexes. Pharmacol Ther 1987; 34:155–166.
4. Kelland LR. Preclinical perspectives on platinum resistance. Drugs 2000; 59(Suppl 4):S1–S8.
5. Kelland LR. New platinum antitumor complexes. Crit Rev Oncol Hematol 1993; 15:191–219.
6. Sorenson CM, Eastman A. Influence of *cis*-diamminedichloroplatinum^{II} on DNA synthesis and cell cycle progression in excision repair proficient and deficient Chinese hamster ovary cells. Cancer Res 1988; 48:6703–6707.
7. Jordan P, Carmo-Fonseca M. Molecular mechanisms involved in cisplatin cytotoxicity. Cell Mol Life Sci 2000; 57:1229–1235.
8. Fraval HN, Roberts JJ. Excision repair of *cis*-diamminedichloroplatinum^{II}-induced damage to DNA of Chinese hamster cells. Cancer Res 1979; 39:1793–1797.
9. Giaccone G. Clinical perspectives on platinum resistance. Drugs 2000; 59:(Suppl 4):S9–S17; discussion 37–38 (review).
10. Ozols RF. Ovarian cancer: new clinical approaches. Cancer Treat Rev 1991; 18(Suppl A):S77–S83.
11. Ozols RF, Corden BJ, Jacob J, Wesley MN, Ostchega Y, Young RC. High-dose cisplatin in hypertonic saline. Ann Intern Med 1984; 100:19–24.
12. Mujoo K, Watanabe M, Khokhar AR, Siddik ZH. Increased sensitivity of a metastatic model of prostate cancer to a novel tetravalent platinum analog. Prostate 2005; 62:91–100.
13. Mujoo K, Watanabe M, Nakamura J, Khokhar AR, Siddik ZH. Status of p53 phosphorylation and function in sensitive and resistant human cancer models exposed to platinum-based DNA damaging agents. J Cancer Res Clin Oncol 2003; 129:709–718.
14. Siddik ZH, Hagopian GS, Thai G, Tomisaki S, Toyomasu T, Khokhar AR. Role of p53 in the ability of 1,2-diaminocyclohexane-diacetato-dichloro-*t*^{IV} to circumvent cisplatin resistance. J Inorg Biochem 1999; 77:65–70.
15. Kelland LR, Mistry P, Abel G, et al. Mechanism-related circumvention of acquired *cis*-diamminedichloroplatinum^{II} resistance using two pairs of human ovarian carcinoma cell lines by ammine/amine platinum(IV) dicarboxylates. Cancer Res 1992; 52:3857–3864.
16. Richon VM, Schulte N, Eastman A. Multiple mechanisms of resistance to *cis*-diamminedichloroplatinum^{II} in murine leukemia L1210 cells. Cancer Res 1987; 47:2056–2061.
17. Teicher BA, Holden SA, Kelley MJ, et al. Characterization of a human squamous carcinoma cell line resistant to *cis*-diamminedichloroplatinum^{II}. Cancer Res 1987; 47:388–393.
18. Teicher BA, Herman TS, Holden SA, et al. Tumor resistance to alkylating agents conferred by mechanisms operative only in vivo. Science 1990; 247(Pt 1):1457–1461.
19. Siddik ZH, Mims B, Lozano G, Thai G. Independent pathways of p53 induction by cisplatin and X-rays in a cisplatin-resistant ovarian tumor cell line. Cancer Res 1998; 58:698–703.
20. Gore M, Fryatt I, Wiltshaw E, Dawson T, Robinson B, Calvert A. Cisplatin/carboplatin cross-resistance in ovarian cancer. Br J Cancer 1989; 60:767–769.

21. Ozols RF. Chemotherapy for advanced epithelial ovarian cancer. Hematol Oncol Clin North Am 1992; 6:879–894.

22. Misset JL, Bleiberg H, Sutherland W, Bekradda M, Cvitkovic E. Oxaliplatin clinical activity: a review. Crit Rev Oncol Hematol 2000; 35:75–93.

23. Yoshida M, Khokhar AR, Siddik ZH. Biochemical pharmacology of homologous alicyclic mixed amine platinum^{II} complexes in sensitive and resistant tumor cell lines. Cancer Res 1994; 54:3468–3473.

24. Andrews PA, Velury S, Mann SC, Howell SB. cis-Diamminedichloroplatinum^{II} accumulation in sensitive and resistant human ovarian carcinoma cells. Cancer Res 1988; 48:68–73.

25. Gately DP, Howell SB. Cellular accumulation of the anticancer agent cisplatin: a review. Br J Cancer 1993; 67:1171–1176.

26. Safaei R, Howell SB. Copper transporters regulate the cellular pharmacology and sensitivity to Pt drugs. Crit Rev Oncol Hematol 2005; 53:13–23.

27. Holzer AK, Samimi G, Katano K, et al. The copper influx transporter human copper transport protein 1 regulates the uptake of cisplatin in human ovarian carcinoma cells. Mol Pharmacol 2004; 66:817–823.

28. Ishida S, Lee J, Thiele DJ, Herskowitz I. Uptake of the anticancer drug cisplatin mediated by the copper transporter Ctr1 in yeast and mammals. Proc Natl Acad Sci U S A 2002; 99:14,298–14,302.

29. Song I-S, Savaraj N, Siddik ZH, et al. Roles of Human copper transporter Ctr1 in the transport of platinum-based antitumor agents in cisplatin-sensitive and cisplatin-resistant cells. Mol Cancer Ther 2004; 3:1543–1549. Erratum in 4:864.

30. Borst P, Evers R, Kool M, Wijnholds J. A family of drug transporters: The multidrug resistance-associated proteins. J Natl Cancer Inst 2000; 92:1295–1302.

31. Shen DW, Goldenberg S, Pastan I, Gottesman MM. Decreased accumulation of ^{14C}carboplatin in human cisplatin-resistant cells results from reduced energy-dependent uptake. J Cell Physiol 2000; 183:108–116.

32. Kool M, de Haas M, Scheffer GL, Scheper RJ, et al. Analysis of expression of cMOAT (MRP2), MRP3, MRP4, and MRP5, homologues of the multidrug resistance-associated protein gene (MRP1), in human cancer cell lines. Cancer Res 1997; 57:3537–3547.

33. Cui Y, Konig J, Buchholz JK, Spring H, Leier I, Keppler D. Drug resistance and ATP-dependent conjugate transport mediated by the apical multidrug resistance protein, MRP2, permanently expressed in human and canine cells. Mol Pharmacol 1999; 55:929–937.

34. Koike K, Kawabe T, Tanaka T, et al. A canalicular multispecific organic anion transporter (cMOAT) antisense cDNA enhances drug sensitivity in human hepatic cancer cells. Cancer Res 1997; 57:5475–5479.

35. Komatsu M, Sumizawa T, Mutoh M, Chen ZS, Terada K, Furukawa T, et al. Copper-transporting P-type adenosine triphosphatase (ATP7B) is associated with cisplatin resistance. Cancer Res 2000; 60:1312–1316.

36. Katano K, Kondo A, Safaei R, et al. Acquisition of resistance to cisplatin is accompanied by changes in the cellular pharmacology of copper. Cancer Res 2002; 62:6559–6565.

37. Samimi G, Safaei R, Katano K, et al. Increased expression of the copper efflux transporter ATP7A mediates resistance to cisplatin, carboplatin, and oxaliplatin in ovarian cancer cells. Clin Cancer Res 2004; 10:4661–4669.

38. Nakayama K, Kanzaki A, Ogawa K, Miyazaki K, Neamati N, Takebayashi Y. Copper-transporting P-type adenosine triphosphatase (ATP7B) as a cisplatin based chemoresistance marker in ovarian carcinoma: comparative analysis with expression of MDR1, MRP1, MRP2, LRP and BCRP. Int J Cancer 2002; 101:488–495.

39. Mossink MH, Van Zon A, Franzel-Luiten E, et al. Disruption of the murine major vault protein (MVP/LRP) gene does not induce hypersensitivity to cytostatics. Cancer Res 2002; 62:7298–7304.

40. Baekelandt MM, Holm R, Nesland JM, Trope CG, Kristensen GB. P-glycoprotein expression is a marker for chemotherapy resistance and prognosis in advanced ovarian cancer. Anticancer Res 2000; 20:1061–1067.

41. Izquierdo MA, van der Zee AG, Vermorken JB, et al. Drug resistance-associated marker Lrp for prediction of response to chemotherapy and prognoses in advanced ovarian carcinoma. J Natl Cancer Inst 1995; 87:1230–1237.

42. Godwin AK, Meister A, O'Dwyer PJ, Huang CS, Hamilton TC, Anderson ME. High resistance to cisplatin in human ovarian cancer cell lines is associated with marked increase of glutathione synthesis. Proc Natl Acad Sci U S A 1992; 89:3070–3074.

43. Pan B, Yao KS, Monia BP, et al. Reversal of cisplatin resistance in human ovarian cancer cell lines by a c-jun antisense oligodeoxynucleotide (ISIS 10582): evidence for the role of transcription factor overexpression in determining resistant phenotype. Biochem Pharmacol 2002; 63:1699–1707.

44. Goto S, Iida T, Cho S, Oka M, Kohno S, Kondo T. Overexpression of glutathione *S*-transferase pi enhances the adduct formation of cisplatin with glutathione in human cancer cells. Free Radic Res 1999; 31:549–558.

45. Shiga H, Heath EI, Rasmussen AA, et al. Prognostic value of p53, glutathione S-transferase pi, and thymidylate synthase for neoadjuvant cisplatin-based chemotherapy in head and neck cancer. Clin Cancer Res 1999; 5:4097–4104.

46. Slater AF, Nobel CS, Maellaro E, Bustamante J, Kimland M, Orrenius S. Nitrone spin traps and a nitroxide antioxidant inhibit a common pathway of thymocyte apoptosis. Biochem J 1995; 306(Pt 3):771–778.

47. Rudin CM, Yang Z, Schumaker LM, et al. Inhibition of glutathione synthesis reverses Bcl-2-mediated cisplatin resistance. Cancer Res 2003; 63:312–318.

48. Kelley SL, Basu A, Teicher BA, Hacker MP, Hamer DH, Lazo JS. Overexpression of metallothionein confers resistance to anticancer drugs. Science 1988; 241:1813–1815.

49. Kasahara K, Fujiwara Y, Nishio K, et al. Metallothionein content correlates with the sensitivity of human small cell lung cancer cell lines to cisplatin. Cancer Res 1991; 51:3237–3242.

50. Lai GM, Ozols RF, Smyth JF, Young RC, Hamilton TC. Enhanced DNA repair and resistance to cisplatin in human ovarian cancer. Biochem Pharmacol 1988; 37:4597–4600.

51. Chaney SG, Sancar A. DNA repair: enzymatic mechanisms and relevance to drug response. J Natl Cancer Inst 1996; 88:1346–1360.

52. Eastman A, Schulte N. Enhanced DNA repair as a mechanism of resistance to *cis*-diamminedichloroplatinum^{II}. Biochemistry 1988; 27:4730–4734.

53. Friedberg EC. How nucleotide excision repair protects against cancer. Nat Rev Cancer 2001; 1:22–33.

54. Reed E. Platinum-DNA adduct, nucleotide excision repair and platinum based anti- cancer chemotherapy. Cancer Treat Rev 1998; 24:331–344.

55. Ferry KV, Hamilton TC, Johnson SW. Increased nucleotide excision repair in cisplatin-resistant ovarian cancer cells: role of ERCC1-XPF. Biochem Pharmacol 2000; 60:1305–1313.

56. Lee KB, Parker RJ, Bohr V, Cornelison T, Reed E. Cisplatin sensitivity/resistance in UV repair-deficient Chinese hamster ovary cells of complementation groups 1 and 3. Carcinogenesis 1993; 14:2177–2180.

57. Dabholkar M, Vionnet J, Bostick-Bruton F, Yu JJ, Reed E. Messenger RNA levels of XPAC and ERCC1 in ovarian cancer tissue correlate with response to platinum-based chemotherapy. J Clin Invest 1994; 94:703–708.

58. Furuta T, Ueda T, Aune G, Sarasin A, Kraemer KH, Pommier Y. Transcription-coupled nucleotide excision repair as a determinant of cisplatin sensitivity of human cells. Cancer Res 2002; 62:4899–4902.

59. Koberle B, Masters JR, Hartley JA, Wood RD. Defective repair of cisplatin-induced DNA damage caused by reduced XPA protein in testicular germ cell tumours. Curr Biol 1999; 9:273–276.

60. Welsh C, Day R, McGurk C, Masters JR, Wood RD, Koberle B. Reduced levels of XPA, ERCC1 and XPF DNA repair proteins in testis tumor cell lines. Int J Cancer 2004; 110:352–361.

61. Chaney SG, Vaisman A. Specificity of platinum-DNA adduct repair. J Inorg Biochem 1999; 77:71–81.

62. Jennerwein MM, Eastman A, Khokhar AR. The role of DNA repair in resistance of L1210 cells to isomeric 1,2- diaminocyclohexaneplatinum complexes and ultraviolet irradiation. Mutat Res 1991; 254:89–96.

63. Larminat F, Bohr VA. Role of the human *ERCC-1* gene in gene-specific repair of cisplatin- induced DNA damage. Nucleic Acids Res 1994; 22:3005–3010.

64. Gowen LC, Avrutskaya AV, Latour AM, Koller BH, Leadon SA. BRCA1 required for transcription-coupled repair of oxidative DNA damage. Science 1998; 281:1009–1012.

65. Husain A, He G, Venkatraman ES, Spriggs DR. BRCA1 up-regulation is associated with repair-mediated resistance to *cis*-diamminedichloroplatinum^{II}. Cancer Res 1998; 58:1120–1123.

66. Taniguchi T, Tischkowitz M, Ameziane N, et al. Disruption of the Fanconi anemia-BRCA pathway in cisplatin-sensitive ovarian tumors. Nat Med 2003; 9:568–574.

67. Bellon SF, Coleman JH, Lippard SJ. DNA unwinding produced by site-specific intrastrand cross-links of the antitumor drug cis-diamminedichloroplatinum^{II}. Biochemistry 1991; 30:8026–8035.

68. Chaney SG, Campbell SL, Bassett E, Wu Y. Recognition and processing of cisplatin- and oxaliplatin-DNA adducts. Crit Rev Oncol Hematol 2005; 53:3–11.

69. Fojta M, Pivonkova H, Brazdova M, et al. Recognition of DNA modified by antitumor cisplatin by "latent" and "active" protein p53. Biochem Pharmacol 2003; 65:1305–1316.

70. Imamura T, Izumi H, Nagatani G, et al. Interaction with p53 enhances binding of cisplatin-modified DNA by high mobility group 1 protein. J Biol Chem 2001; 276:7534–7540.

71. Fink D, Aebi S, Howell SB. The role of DNA mismatch repair in drug resistance. Clin Cancer Res 1998; 4:1–6.
72. Wang G, Dombkowski A, Chuang L, Xu XX. The involvement of XPC protein in the cisplatin DNA damaging treatment-mediated cellular response. Cell Res 2004; 14:303–314.
73. Vaisman A, Varchenko M, Umar A, et al. The role of hMLH1, hMSH3, and hMSH6 defects in cisplatin and oxaliplatin resistance: correlation with replicative bypass of platinum- DNA adducts. Cancer Res 1998; 58:3579–3585.
74. Anthoney DA, McIlwrath AJ, Gallagher WM, Edlin AR, Brown R. Microsatellite instability, apoptosis, and loss of p53 function in drug- resistant tumor cells. Cancer Res 1996; 56:1374–1381.
75. Brown R, Hirst GL, Gallagher WM, et al. hMLH1 expression and cellular responses of ovarian tumour cells to treatment with cytotoxic anticancer agents. Oncogene 1997; 15:45–52.
76. Johnson SW, Laub PB, Beesley JS, Ozols RF, Hamilton TC. Increased platinum-DNA damage tolerance is associated with cisplatin resistance and cross-resistance to various chemotherapeutic agents in unrelated human ovarian cancer cell lines. Cancer Res 1997; 57:850–856.
77. Yoshida M, Khokhar AR, Siddik ZH. Cytotoxicity and tolerance to DNA adducts of alicyclic mixed amine platinum[II] homologs in tumor models sensitive and resistant to cisplatin or tetraplatin. Oncol Rep 1998; 5:1281–1287.
78. Mamenta EL, Poma EE, Kaufmann WK, Delmastro DA, Grady HL, Chaney SG. Enhanced replicative bypass of platinum-DNA adducts in cisplatin- resistant human ovarian carcinoma cell lines. Cancer Res 1994; 54:3500–3505.
79. Lin X, Ramamurthi K, Mishima M, Kondo A, Christen RD, Howell SB. P53 modulates the effect of loss of DNA mismatch repair on the sensitivity of human colon cancer cells to the cytotoxic and mutagenic effects of cisplatin. Cancer Res 2001; 61:1508–1516.
80. Fan S, el Deiry WS, Bae I, Freeman J, Jondle D, Bhatia K, et al. p53 gene mutations are associated with decreased sensitivity of human lymphoma cells to DNA damaging agents. Cancer Res 1994; 54:5824–5830.
81. Segal-Bendirdjian E, Mannone L, Jacquemin-Sablon A. Alteration in p53 pathway and defect in apoptosis contribute independently to cisplatin-resistance. Cell Death Differ 1998; 5:390–400.
82. Zhao H, Piwnica-Worms H. ATR-mediated checkpoint pathways regulate phosphorylation and activation of human Chk1. Mol Cell Biol 2001; 21:4129–4139.
83. Appella E, Anderson CW. Post-translational modifications and activation of p53 by genotoxic stresses. Eur J Biochem 2001; 268:2764–2772.
84. Shieh SY, Ahn J, Tamai K, Taya Y, Prives C. The human homologs of checkpoint kinases Chk1 and Cds1 (Chk2) phosphorylate p53 at multiple DNA damage-inducible sites. Genes Dev 2000; 14:289–300.
85. Perego P, Giarola M, Righetti SC, et al. Association between cisplatin resistance and mutation of p53 gene and reduced bax expression in ovarian carcinoma cell systems. Cancer Res 1996; 56:556–562.
86. Sugimoto C, Fujieda S, Seki M, et al. Apoptosis-promoting gene (bax) transfer potentiates sensitivity of squamous cell carcinoma to cisplatin in vitro and in vivo. Int J Cancer 1999; 82:860–867.
87. Wang X, Martindale JL, Holbrook NJ. Requirement for ERK activation in cisplatin-induced apoptosis. J Biol Chem 2000; 275:39,435–39,443.
88. Muller M, Wilder S, Bannasch D, et al. p53 activates the CD95 (APO-1/Fas) gene in response to DNA damage by anticancer drugs. J Exp Med 1998; 188:2033–2045.
89. del Bello B, Valentini MA, Zunino F, Comporti M, Maellaro E. Cleavage of Bcl-2 in oxidant- and cisplatin-induced apoptosis of human melanoma cells. Oncogene 2001; 20:4591–4595.
90. Eliopoulos AG, Kerr DJ, Herod J, et al. The control of apoptosis and drug resistance in ovarian cancer: influence of p53 and Bcl-2. Oncogene 1995; 11:1217–1228.
91. Asselin E, Mills GB, Tsang BK. XIAP regulates Akt activity and caspase-3-dependent cleavage during cisplatin-induced apoptosis in human ovarian epithelial cancer cells. Cancer Res 2001; 61:1862–1868.
92. Ikeguchi M, Liu J, Kaibara N. Expression of survivin mRNA and protein in gastric cancer cell line (MKN-45) during cisplatin treatment. Apoptosis 2002; 7:23–29.
93. Ono Y, Nonomura N, Harada Y, et al. Loss of p73 induction in a cisplatin-resistant bladder cancer cell line. Mol Urol 2001; 5:25–30.
94. Sionov RV, Haupt Y. The cellular response to p53: the decision between life and death. Oncogene 1999; 18:6145–6157.
95. Gong JG, Costanzo A, Yang HQ, et al. The tyrosine kinase c-Abl regulates p73 in apoptotic response to cisplatin-induced DNA damage [see Comments]. Nature 1999; 399:806–809.
96. Soussi T. The p53 tumor suppressor gene: from molecular biology to clinical investigation. Ann N Y Acad Sci 2000; 910:121–137.

97. Bradford CR, Zhu S, Ogawa H, et al. P53 mutation correlates with cisplatin sensitivity in head and neck squamous cell carcinoma lines. Head Neck 2003; 25:654–661.

98. Reles A, Wen WH, Schmider A, et al. Correlation of p53 mutations with resistance to platinum-based chemotherapy and shortened survival in ovarian cancer. Clin Cancer Res 2001; 7:2984–2997.

99. Sarkis AS, Bajorin DF, Reuter VE, et al. Prognostic value of p53 nuclear overexpression in patients with invasive bladder cancer treated with neoadjuvant MVAC. J Clin Oncol 1995; 13:1384–1390.

100. van der Zee AG, Hollema H, Suurmeijer AJ, et al. Value of P-glycoprotein, glutathione S-transferase pi, c-erbB-2, and p53 as prognostic factors in ovarian carcinomas. J Clin Oncol 1995; 13:70–78.

101. Lavarino C, Pilotti S, Oggionni M, et al. *p53* gene status and response to platinum/paclitaxel-based chemotherapy in advanced ovarian carcinoma. J Clin Oncol 2000; 18:3936–3945.

102. Mayer F, Honecker F, Looijenga LH, Bokemeyer C. Towards an understanding of the biological basis of response to cisplatin-based chemotherapy in germ-cell tumors. Ann Oncol 2003; 14:825–832.

103. Mayer F, Gillis AJ, Dinjens W, et al. Microsatellite instability of germ cell tumors is associated with resistance to systemic treatment. Cancer Res 2002; 62:2758–2760.

104. Hagopian GS, Mills GB, Khokhar AR, Bast RC Jr., Siddik ZH. Expression of p53 in cisplatin-resistant ovarian cancer cell lines: modulation with the novel platinum analogue (1R, 2R- diaminocyclo-hexane)(trans-diacetato)(dichloro)-platinum(IV). Clin Cancer Res 1999; 5:655–663.

105. Meek DW. Mechanisms of switching on p53: a role for covalent modification? Oncogene 1999; 18:7666–7675.

106. Deng X, Kim M, Vandier D, et al. Recombinant adenovirus-mediated p14(ARF) overexpression sensitizes human breast cancer cells to cisplatin. Biochem Biophys Res Commun 2002; 296:792–798.

107. Kessis TD, Slebos RJ, Nelson WG, et al. Human papillomavirus 16 E6 expression disrupts the p53-mediated cellular response to DNA damage. Proc Natl Acad Sci U S A 1993; 90:3988–3992.

108. Nehme A, Baskaran R, Nebel S, et al. Induction of JNK and c-Abl signalling by cisplatin and oxaliplatin in mismatch repair-proficient and -deficient cells. Br J Cancer 1999; 79:1104–1110.

109. Fan S, Smith ML, Rivet DJ, et al. Disruption of p53 function sensitizes breast cancer MCF-7 cells to cisplatin and pentoxifylline. Cancer Res 1995; 55:1649–1654.

110. Hawkins DS, Demers GW, Galloway DA. Inactivation of p53 enhances sensitivity to multiple chemotherapeutic agents. Cancer Res 1996; 56:892–898.

111. Fan S, Chang JK, Smith ML, Duba D, Fornace AJ Jr, O'Connor PM. Cells lacking *CIP1/WAF1* genes exhibit preferential sensitivity to cisplatin and nitrogen mustard. Oncogene 1997; 14:2127–2136.

112. Waldman T, Lengauer C, Kinzler KW, Vogelstein B. Uncoupling of S phase and mitosis induced by anticancer agents in cells lacking p21. Nature 1996; 381:713–716.

113. Lincet H, Poulain L, Remy JS, et al. The p21(cip1/waf1) cyclin-dependent kinase inhibitor enhances the cytotoxic effect of cisplatin in human ovarian carcinoma cells. Cancer Lett 2000; 161:17–26.

114. Qin LF, Ng IO. Exogenous expression of p21(WAF1/CIP1) exerts cell growth inhibition and enhances sensitivity to cisplatin in hepatoma cells. Cancer Lett 2001; 172:7–15.

115. Kawasaki T, Tomita Y, Bilim V, Takeda M, Takahashi K, Kumanishi T. Abrogation of apoptosis induced by DNA-damaging agents in human bladder-cancer cell lines with p21/WAF1/CIP1 and/or p53 gene alterations. Int J Cancer 1996; 68:501–505.

116. Demarcq C, Bunch RT, Creswell D, Eastman A. The role of cell cycle progression in cisplatin-induced apoptosis in Chinese hamster ovary cells. Cell Growth Differ 1994; 5:983–993.

117. O'Connor PM, Fan S. DNA damage checkpoints: implications for cancer therapy. Prog Cell Cycle Res 1996; 2:165–173.

118 He G, Siddik ZH, Kuang J. Reevaluation of the effect of cisplatin on the cell cycle checkpoints. Proc Am Assoc Cancer Res 2001; 42:A4887, 4901.

119. Vekris A, Meynard D, Haaz MC, Bayssas M, Bonnet J, Robert J. Molecular determinants of the cytotoxicity of platinum compounds: the contribution of in silico research. Cancer Res 2004; 64:356–362.

120. Kuang J, He G, Huang Z, Khokhar AR, Siddik ZH. Bimodal effects of 1R,2R-diaminocyclo-hexane(trans-diacetato)(dichloro)platinum^{IV} on cell cycle checkpoints. Clin Cancer Res 2001; 7:3629–3639.

121. Gartel AL, Tyner AL. The role of the cyclin-dependent kinase inhibitor p21 in apoptosis. Mol Cancer Ther 2002; 1:639–649.

122. Liu S, Bishop WR, Liu M. Differential effects of cell cycle regulatory protein p21(WAF1/Cip1) on apoptosis and sensitivity to cancer chemotherapy. Drug Resist Updat 2003; 6:183–195.

123. Gartel AL, Tyner AL. Transcriptional regulation of the p21$^{WAF1/CIP1}$ gene. Exp Cell Res 1999; 246:280–289.

124. DeHaan RD, Yazlovitskaya EM, Persons DL. Regulation of p53 target gene expression by cisplatin-induced extracellular signal-regulated kinase. Cancer Chemother Pharmacol 2001; 48:383–388.

125. Li Y, Dowbenko D, Lasky LA. AKT/PKB phosphorylation of p21$^{Cip/WAF1}$ enhances protein stability of p21Cip/WAF1 and promotes cell survival. J Biol Chem 2002; 277:11,352–11,361.

126. Mitsuuchi Y, Johnson SW, Selvakumaran M, Williams SJ, Hamilton TC, Testa JR. The phosphatidylinositol 3-kinase/AKT signal transduction pathway plays a critical role in the expression of p21$^{WAF1/CIP1/SDI1}$ induced by cisplatin and paclitaxel. Cancer Res 2000; 60:5390–5394.

127. Zhou BP, Liao Y, Xia W, Spohn B, Lee MH, Hung MC. Cytoplasmic localization of p21$^{Cip1/WAF1}$ by Akt-induced phosphorylation in HER-2/neu-overexpressing cells. Nat Cell Biol 2001; 3:245–252.

128. Hung MC, Lau YK. Basic science of HER-2/neu: a review. Semin Oncol 1999; 26(Suppl 12):51–59.

129. Slamon DJ, Godolphin W, Jones LA, et al. Studies of the HER-2/neu proto-oncogene in human breast and ovarian cancer. Science 1989; 244:707–712.

130. Hengstler JG, Lange J, Kett A, et al. Contribution of c-erbB-2 and topoisomerase IIα to chemoresistance in ovarian cancer. Cancer Res 1999; 59:3206–3214.

131. Arteaga CL, Winnier AR, Poirier MC, et al. p185c-erbB-2 signal enhances cisplatin-induced cytotoxicity in human breast carcinoma cells: association between an oncogenic receptor tyrosine kinase and drug-induced DNA repair. Cancer Res 1994; 54:3758–3765.

132. Tsai CM, Yu D, Chang KT, Wu LH, Perng RP, Ibrahim NK, et al. Enhanced chemoresistance by elevation of p185neu levels in HER-2/neu-transfected human lung cancer cells. J Natl Cancer Inst 1995; 87:682–684.

133. Pietras RJ, Fendly BM, Chazin VR, Pegram MD, Howell SB, Slamon DJ. Antibody to HER-2/neu receptor blocks DNA repair after cisplatin in human breast and ovarian cancer cells. Oncogene 1994; 9:1829–1838.

134. Zhang L, Hung MC. Sensitization of HER-2/neu-overexpressing non-small cell lung cancer cells to chemotherapeutic drugs by tyrosine kinase inhibitor emodin. Oncogene 1996; 12:571–576.

135. Bacus SS, Altomare DA, Lyass L, et al. AKT2 is frequently upregulated in HER-2/neu-positive breast cancers and may contribute to tumor aggressiveness by enhancing cell survival. Oncogene 2002; 21:3532–3540.

136. Altomare DA, Wang HQ, Skele KL, et al. AKT and mTOR phosphorylation is frequently detected in ovarian cancer and can be targeted to disrupt ovarian tumor cell growth. Oncogene 2004; 23:5853–5857.

137. West KA, Castillo SS, Dennis PA. Activation of the PI3K/Akt pathway and chemotherapeutic resistance. Drug Resist Updat 2002; 5:234–248.

138. Gagnon V, Mathieu I, Sexton E, Leblanc K, Asselin E. AKT involvement in cisplatin chemoresistance of human uterine cancer cells. Gynecol Oncol 2004; 94:785–795.

139. Hayakawa J, Ohmichi M, Kurachi H, et al. Inhibition of BAD phosphorylation either at serine 112 via extracellular signal-regulated protein kinase cascade or at serine 136 via Akt cascade sensitizes human ovarian cancer cells to cisplatin. Cancer Res 2000; 60:5988–5994.

140. Zhou BP, Hung MC. Novel targets of Akt, p21$^{Cip1/WAF1}$, and MDM2. Semin Oncol 2002; 29(Suppl 11):62–70.

141. Mayo LD, Donner DB. The PTEN, Mdm2, p53 tumor suppressor-oncoprotein network. Trends Biochem Sci 2002; 27:462–467.

142. Cardone MH, Roy N, Stennicke HR, et al. Regulation of cell death protease caspase-9 by phosphorylation. Science 1998; 282:1318–1321.

143. Mansouri A, Zhang Q, Ridgway LD, Tian L, Claret FX. Cisplatin resistance in an ovarian carcinoma is associated with a defect in programmed cell death control through XIAP regulation. Oncol Res 2003; 13:399–404.

144. Amantana A, London CA, Iversen PL, Devi GR. X-linked inhibitor of apoptosis protein inhibition induces apoptosis and enhances chemotherapy sensitivity in human prostate cancer cells. Mol Cancer Ther 2004; 3:699–707.

145. Dan HC, Sun M, Kaneko S, et al. Akt phosphorylation and stabilization of X-linked inhibitor of apoptosis protein (XIAP). J Biol Chem 2004; 279:5405–5412.

146. Fraser M, Leung BM, Yan X, Dan HC, Cheng JQ, Tsang BK. p53 is a determinant of X-linked inhibitor of apoptosis protein/Akt-mediated chemoresistance in human ovarian cancer cells. Cancer Res 2003; 63:7081–7088.

147. Dent P, Grant S. Pharmacologic interruption of the mitogen-activated extracellular- regulated kinase/mitogen-activated protein kinase signal transduction pathway: potential role in promoting cytotoxic drug action. Clin Cancer Res 2001; 7:775–783.

148. Persons DL, Yazlovitskaya EM, Pelling JC. Effect of extracellular signal-regulated kinase on p53 accumulation in response to cisplatin. J Biol Chem 2000; 275:35,778–35,785.

149. Yeh PY, Chuang SE, Yeh KH, Song YC, Ea CK, Cheng AL. Increase of the resistance of human cervical carcinoma cells to cisplatin by inhibition of the MEK to ERK signaling pathway partly via enhancement of anticancer drug-induced NFκB activation. Biochem Pharmacol 2002; 63:1423–1430.

150. Fuchs SY, Adler V, Pincus MR, Ronai Z. MEKK1/JNK signaling stabilizes and activates p53. Proc Natl Acad Sci U S A 1998; 95:10,541–10,546.

151. Gebauer G, Mirakhur B, Nguyen Q, Shore SK, Simpkins H, Dhanasekaran N. Cisplatin-resistance involves the defective processing of MEKK1 in human ovarian adenocarcinoma 2008/C13 cells. Int J Oncol 2000; 16:321–325.

152. Woessmann W, Chen X, Borkhardt A. Ras-mediated activation of ERK by cisplatin induces cell death independently of p53 in osteosarcoma and neuroblastoma cell lines. Cancer Chemother Pharmacol 2002; 50:397–404.

153. Van't Veer LJ, Hermens R, van den Berg-Bakker LA, et al. The *ras* oncogene activation in human ovarian carcinoma. Oncogene 1988; 2:157–165.

154. Dempke W, Voigt W, Grothey A, Hill BT, Schmoll HJ. Cisplatin resistance and oncogenes—a review. Anticancer Drugs 2000; 11:225–236.

155. Fan J, Banerjee D, Stambrook PJ, Bertino JR. Modulation of cytotoxicity of chemotherapeutic drugs by activated H-ras. Biochem Pharmacol 1997; 53:1203–1209.

156. Mansouri A, Ridgway LD, Korapati AL, et al. Sustained activation of JNK/p38 MAPK pathways in response to cisplatin leads to Fas ligand induction and cell death in ovarian carcinoma cells. J Biol Chem 2003; 278:19,245–19,256.

157. Leppa S, Bohmann D. Diverse functions of JNK signaling and c-Jun in stress response and apoptosis. Oncogene 1999; 18:6158–6162.

158. Robinson MJ, Cobb MH. Mitogen-activated protein kinase pathways. Curr Opin Cell Biol 1997; 9:180–186.

159. Toh WH, Siddique MM, Boominathan L, Lin KW, Sabapathy K. c-Jun regulates the stability and activity of the p53 homologue, p73. J Biol Chem 2004; 279:44,713–44,722.

160. Stojic L, Brun R, Jiricny J. Mismatch repair and DNA damage signalling. DNA Repair (Amst) 2004; 3:1091–1101.

161. Kartalou M, Essigmann JM. Mechanisms of resistance to cisplatin. Mutat Res 2001; 478:23–43.

162. Kharbanda S, Pandey P, Yamauchi T, et al. Activation of MEK kinase 1 by the c-Abl protein tyrosine kinase in response to DNA damage. Mol Cell Biol 2000; 20:4979–4989.

163. Lapouge G, Millon R, Muller D, et al. Cisplatin-induced genes as potential markers for thyroid cancer. Cell Mol Life Sci 2005; 62:53–64.

164. Akervall J, Guo X, Qian CN, et al. Genetic and expression profiles of squamous cell carcinoma of the head and neck correlate with cisplatin sensitivity and resistance in cell lines and patients. Clin Cancer Res 2004; 10:8204–8213.

165. Tsunoda T, Koga H, Yokomizo A, et al. Inositol 1,4,5-trisphosphate (IP$_3$) receptor type1 (IP$_3$R1) modulates the acquisition of cisplatin resistance in bladder cancer cell lines. Oncogene 2005; 24:1396–1402.

166. Schenk PW, Stoop H, Bokemeyer C, et al. Resistance to platinum-containing chemotherapy in testicular germ cell tumors is associated with downregulation of the protein kinase SRPK1. Neoplasia 2004; 6:297–301.

167. Wilson LA, Yamamoto H, Singh G. Role of the transcription factor Ets-1 in cisplatin resistance. Mol Cancer Ther 2004; 3:823–832.

168. Deng HB, Adikari M, Parekh HK, Simpkins H. Ubiquitous induction of resistance to platinum drugs in human ovarian, cervical, germ-cell and lung carcinoma tumor cells overexpressing isoforms 1 and 2 of dihydrodiol dehydrogenase. Cancer Chemother Pharmacol 2004; 54:301–307.

169. Fojo T, Farrell N, Ortuzar W, Tanimura H, Weinstein J, Myers TG. Identification of non-cross-resistant platinum compounds with novel cytotoxicity profiles using the NCI anticancer drug screen and clustered image map visualizations. Crit Rev Oncol Hematol 2005; 53:25–34.

170. Kido Y, Khokhar AR, al Baker S, Siddik ZH. Modulation of cytotoxicity and cellular pharmacology of 1,2-diaminocyclohexane platinum (IV) complexes mediated by axial and equatorial ligands. Cancer Res 1993; 53:4567–4572.

17 Regulation of the Cellular Pharmacology and Cytotoxicity of Cisplatin by Copper Transporters

Roohangiz Safaei, PhD
and Stephen B. Howell, MD

CONTENTS

SUMMARY

There is now a large body of evidence to indicate that the copper (Cu) transporters copper transporter receptor (CTR)1, ATP7A, and ATP7B regulate the cellular pharmacology and cytotoxicity of cisplatin (DDP), and that these proteins can mediate acquired DDP resistance. Cells that have acquired resistance to cisplatin demonstrate crossresistance to Cu and vice versa. The crossresistance between DDP and Cu is characterized by parallel changes in Cu and DDP accumulation and altered expression of the Cu efflux transporters ATP7A and ATP7B. Yeast, mouse, and human cells engineered to alter the expression of CTR1, ATP7A or ATP7B exhibit altered sensitivity to both Cu and DDP. Detailed studies of uptake and efflux indicate that each protein can alter the cellular pharmacology of DDP and in some cases, DDP analogs. Immunohistochemical studies of human tumors have identified associations between increased expression of either ATP7A or ATP7B and poor response to treatment with

From: *Cancer Drug Discovery and Development: Cancer Drug Resistance*
Edited by: B. Teicher © Humana Press Inc., Totowa, NJ

one or another of the platinum drugs. Whereas other transporters may also participate in the influx and efflux of the platinum drugs, available evidence supports the concept that DDP enters the cell, is distributed within the cell, and is exported by mechanisms that have evolved to manage Cu homeostasis.

Key Words: Cisplatin; copper; copper transporters metal complexes metallotrans-porters.

1. INTRODUCTION

Cisplatin (DDP) is one of the most widely effective anticancer drugs currently available. It reacts with DNA, RNA, and proteins to form platinum (Pt) adducts that activate multiple signaling pathways that trigger apoptosis and other cell death mechanisms *(1–3)*. However, repeated exposure to DDP results in the emergence of resistance, and such resistance is often accompanied by cross-resistance to a variety of other metals and metalloids (Table 1). In the majority of cases (70–90%), acquisition of resistance to DDP is accompanied by reduced accumulation of the drug *(4)*. In many instances, there is a direct relationship between the extent of DDP accumulation, the degree of DNA damage *(5)* and sensitivity to the cytotoxic effect of this drug *(6)*. Because DDP is highly polar and does not diffuse readily across lipid membranes, defective accumulation in DDP-resistant cells suggest alterations in the expression or function of DDP transporters *(7)*.

The cellular accumulation of DDP is relatively slow compared to that of many other classes of chemotherapeutic agents. Uptake is modulated by metabolic factors *(7)*, temperature *(8)*, pH *(9–11)*, K$^+$ ions *(12)*, and reducing agents *(13–15)*, supporting the involvement of specific transporters in the influx process (reviewed in ref. *7*). Very few candidate DDP transporters have been identified. Rather than transporting DDP, several transporters known to modulate DDP accumulation. For example, the Na$^+$/K$^+$-ATPase *(12)*, the Ca^{2+}-ATPase *(16)*, and the vacuolar ATPase *(17)* are known to alter DDP uptake through secondary effects on the proteins that do directly transport DDP. Others, such as the organic cation transporters, that have been reported to regulate the cellular accumulation of DDP and exhibit altered expression levels in DDP-resistant cells (*see* ref. *11* and the references therein), also seem unlikely to play a direct role considering that DDP is an inorganic molecule and data on its ability to be transported as a conjugated compound is still lacking.

The influx of DDP in human tumor cells has been reported to increase linearly with extracellular DDP concentration and to exhibit no saturation *(7)*. However, because of the difficulty in measuring very small amounts of Pt, the majority of studies have used DDP concentrations well above the peak concentrations of free drug attained in the plasma of cancer patients, and the kinetic parameters of DDP influx at concentrations below 1 μM have not been well defined.

The efflux of DDP is energy dependent and requires Ca$^+$ ions; it is biphasic with a very rapid initial phase and a slow secondary phase *(18)*. Until recently, the search for proteins capable of effluxing DDP failed to yield a strong candidate. P-glycoprotein 1 (ATP-binding cassette transporter [ABC]B1) does not play a major role *(19)*. Thus far, no correlation has been found between the expression of this transporter and DDP resistance in tumor samples *(19)* or in cell lines (*see*, for example, ref. *20*). Nor is there a connection between DDP accumulation and the expression of this ABC transporter in tumor cells *(21)* or transgenic multidrug resistance gene (*mdr1a*)$^{-/-}$ mice *(22)*. Other members of the ABC transporter family, particularly ABCC2 (multidrug-related protein [MRP]2) have also been considered as potential exporters of DDP. However, although the ABCC2

Table 1
Crossresistance Between Platinum Drugs, Metals, and Metalloids

Metal	Pt drug	Cell type	Phenotype	Reference
	DDP;	Human KCP-4	↑ Efflux	(81)
	L-OHP	Human leukemia CCRF-	Low level crossresistance to gold	(82)
Au	DDP	CEM/CDDP		
Cd, Bi, Ca, K Mg, V, Se, Cu, Zn, Fe	DDP	Human ovarian cells A2780 and 2780/CP20	Various degrees of crossresistance	(83)
Cd, Zn, Cu, Hg, Ni, As	DDP	Cd-rA7 and Cd-rB5, Metallothionein null fibroblast	↓ Drug accumulation; ↑ Efflux	(84)
As, Sb, Cd	DDP	Human hepatoma and a cervical adenocarcinoma	↓ Drug accumulation	(85)
Cd	DDP	Human ovarian carcinoma A2780/CP70	↓ Drug accumulation; ↑ increased tolerance to higher levels of DNA damage	(86)
Cd, Zn, Sb	DDP	Human ovarian 2008/C13*5.25	↓ Drug accumulation; ↑ glutathione; ↑ metallothioneins	(87)
Cd	JM15; DDP	Human ovarian carcinoma 41M and CH1	↑ Glutathione; no change in drug accumulation; ↓ DNA adducts	(88)
Cd	DDP	Subline of human ovarian carcinoma A2780	No change in metallothionein mRNA; high resistance to DDP; low resistance to Cd	(89)
As, Sb, Cd, Ni	DDP	Rat liver cells exposed to arsenite	↓ Drug accumulation; no change in glutathione levels	(90)
Cd	DDP; CBDCA	Human bladder cancer cells J82/MMC	No change in drug accumulation; ↑ glutathione transferase	(91)

Pt, platinum; DDP, cisplatin; L-OHP, oxaliplatin; Au, gold; Cd, cadmium; Bi, bismuth; Ca, calcium; K, potassium; Mg, magnesium; V, vanadium; Se, selenium; Cu, copper; Zn, zinc; Fe, iron; Hg, mercury; Ni, nickel; As, arsenic; Sb, antimony; CBDCA, carboplatin.

protein seems to play a role in some cases of DDP resistance *(23)*, it is clearly not involved in other cases *(24)* (reviewed in ref. *25*). It is of interest that the expression of some ABC transporters, such as ABCB1 *(26)*, ABCC2, and ABCC3 (MRP3) *(27)*, is induced following exposure to DDP. This might explain the crossresistance between DDP and metalloids such as arsenite that are substrates of these transporters *(28)*.

A substantial body of evidence has emerged over just the past several years, indicating that the major influx and efflux transporters responsible for Cu homeostasis regulate the sensitivity of cells to the cytotoxic effects of DDP and several of the other clinically available Pt drugs, and that they do so by modulating influx and sequestration mechanisms so as to limit the amount of the drug reaching critical targets in the cell.

2. CU HOMEOSTASIS IN MAMMALIAN CELLS

The proteins that mediate Cu homeostasis accomplish two main functions: they distribute Cu to cuproenzymes involved in critical cellular functions such as electron transport, neurotransmission, and iron metabolism in various subcellular compartments, and they serve to protect the cell against the potential toxicity of Cu. Cu^{+1} is highly toxic, both by virtue of its ability to undergo oxidation with the generation of oxygen free radicals and its ability to interact directly with proteins, RNA, and DNA. Chelation of Cu^{+1} by the metal-binding sequences (MBS) of the Cu-homeostasis proteins keeps the free Cu^{+1} concentration below $10^{-18} M$/cell *(29)*, while at the same time transferring Cu^{+1} to Cu requiring enzymes in different subcellular compartments. The components of the Cu-homeostasis system include influx and efflux transporters, chelating and buffering molecules, and metallochaperones. Many of these elements have been conserved during evolution to the degree that they can complement function between different species. Figure 1 presents a schematic diagram of the major components that control Cu homeostasis.

Cysteine, methionine, and histidine-rich motifs, known as the MBS, are found in many of the proteins that play central roles in Cu homeostasis. The MBS contain core CXXC sequences that are also found in transport and regulatory proteins that control the cellular accumulation of other metals such as mercury (Hg), magnesium (Mg), and cadmium (Cd) *(30)*. Many of these proteins have several copies of this motif arranged in tandem. Several of these protein motifs have been studied by NMR and X-ray crystallography and have been shown to fold in a very similar way *(31)*. Interaction of MBS motifs of the Cu-homeostasis proteins with other metals such as Cd^{+2}, zinc (Zn^{+2}), Hg^{+2}, and gold (Au^{+1}) has been detected by circular dichroism *(32)* and immobilized metal ion affinity chromatography and metal blots *(33)*. These studies support the idea that some elements of the Cu-homeostasis system may function to detoxify other metalloids as well as protect the cell against the toxicity of Cu.

2.1. Cu Influx

The influx of Cu^{+1} through the plasma membrane of human cells is mediated mainly by the 190-amino acid Cu transporter hCtr1 *(34)*. Ctr1 is essential for mammalian development as indicated by the death *in utero* of Ctr1$^{-/-}$ transgenic mice *(35,36)*. Figure 2 presents a schematic drawing of Ctr1. Ctr1 is found in both the plasma and internal membranes *(36,37)*, and its extracellular region contains two MBSs that play a role in scavenging Cu under conditions of Cu starvation. When the extracellular Cu concentration is in a physiologic range, two methionines in the extracellular domain (residues 40 and 45) and two methionines in the second transmembrane region are necessary for Cu

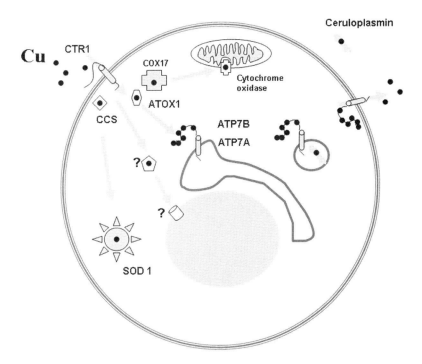

Fig. 1. Schematic drawing of the major copper (Cu)-homeostasis pathways in mammalian cells. Cu is taken up by hCTR1 and transferred to metallochaperones antioxidant ATOX1, copper chaperone for (superoxide dismutase [SOD]) (CCS), and cytochrome c oxidase COX17 which transfer it to ATP7A and ATP7B, Cu-Zn superoxide dismutase, and cytochrome c oxidase, respectively. ATP7A and ATP7B tranfer Cu into the trans-Golgi network, where it is loaded onto cuproenzymes such as tyrosinase and ceruloplasmin. Cu binding to ATP7A and ATP7B also induces subcellular trafficking of vesicles that contain the two proteins from the trans-Golgi network to more peripheral locations.

transport *(38)*. The details of the mechanism by which Ctr1 transports Cu across the plasma membrane remain to be determined. It has been suggested that Ctr1 binds Cu via the methionine and histidine-rich amino terminal domain and transports it across the membrane through pores that it forms by oligomeric association *(38)*. The hydrophilic C-terminal cytosolic domain of Ctr1 is capable of delivering Cu^{+1} directly to the chaperone antioxidant ATOX1 in vitro *(39)*. Ctr1 binds an average of 4 Cu^{+1} atoms/molecule with an average dissociation constant of $K_d = 10^{-19}$, a value similar to that estimated for the yeast chaperone Atx1 and an N-terminal domain of the yeast Ccc2 Cu export pump *(40)*.

hCtr1 is not the only Cu influx transporter in eukaryotic cells. Recent studies have identified two other transporters capable of moving Cu across a bilayer member. The first of these is the divalent metal transporter (also known as natural resistance associated macrophage protein 2). The second is the divalent cation transporter 1, which can transport both Cu and several other divalent metals such as Mg, cobalt, and Cd *(41)*. No information is available as to whether either of these proteins can transport DDP.

2.2. Intracellular Cu Sequestration and Subcellular Distribution

Several cysteine-rich proteins can bind Cu in the cytoplasm, mitochondria, and nucleus, and the roles of metallothioneins and glutathione have been extensively studied. Cu can

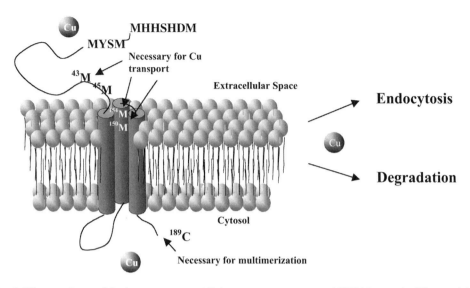

Fig. 2. The topology of the human copper (Cu) transporter receptor (CTR)1 protein. The methionine residues (M) involved in Cu import and multimerization of the protein are marked.

induce the expression of metallothioneins *(42)*, and these bind Cu, providing an intracellular reservoir *(43)*. Although glutathione can potentially bind Cu, this peptide may not function to protect the cell as free Cu catalyses glutathione oxidation, resulting in the production of H_2O_2 and hydroxyl radicals *(44)*. Some organisms, such as *Mycobacterium scrofulaceum*, sequester Cu^{+2} in the form of black $CuSO_4$ precipitates *(45)*, but this is not known to occur in human cells.

Although the sequestration of Cu into a solvent-shielded region within metallothionein is one mechanism by which cells can potentially limit exposure to Cu, metallothioneins cannot perform the critical function of delivering Cu to specific organelles and/or Cu-requiring proteins. This task is performed by metallochaperones that deliver Cu in a highly specific manner to intracellular Cu transporters and Cu-requiring proteins. These proteins are highly conserved in plants, bacteria, yeast, and animal cells. As shown in Fig. 1, the metallochaperones known to be involved in subcellular trafficking of Cu in mammalian cells include ATOX1 (HAH1) that delivers Cu to the P-type ATPases ATP7A and ATP7B at the *trans*-Golgi network *(46,47)*, cytochrome *c* oxidase COX17 that delivers Cu to COX in mitochondria *(48)*, and copper chaperone for superoxide dismutase (SOD) that loads Cu onto cytoplasmic SOD1 *(49)*. These metallochaperones act as both scavengers and carriers of Cu. The function of at least two of these metallochaperones is essential for embryonic development. Deletion of the *ATOX1* gene in mice causes prenatal mortality *(50)*, indicating that delivery of Cu to ATP7A and ATP7B by ATOX1 is critical to the loading of this metalloid onto essential Cu-requiring enzymes such as tyrosinase, lysyl oxidase, and ceruloplasmin *(51)*. Similarly, homozygous mutations of *COX17* in mice cause embryonic death between days E8.5 and E10 *(52)*. The mortality time course is similar to that of *CTR1–/–* mice *(35,36)*.

2.3. Cu Efflux

Efflux of Cu from cells is mediated largely by ATP7A and ATP7B *(53)*. These pumps are very similar to the P-type ATPases of bacteria and yeast in both structure and function

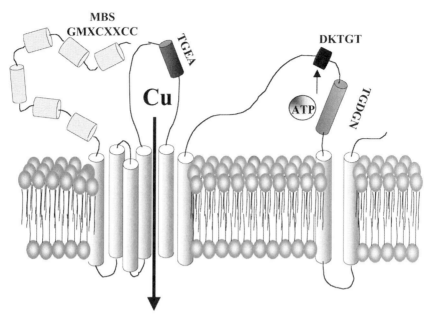

Fig. 3. Schematic diagram of the transmembrane organization of copper (Cu) export ATPases ATP7A and ATP7B. The metal/binding sites (MBS) structures with CXXC motifs at the N-terminal domain, the DKTG phosphorylation site, the TGDN AT- binding site, and the TGEA phosphatase domain are conserved in all P-type ATPases.

(reviewed in ref. *30*). The mammalian ATP7A and ATP7B proteins have eight transmembrane segments and two large cytosolic domains as shown schematically in Fig. 3. Like other P-type ATPases, human Cu ATPases have a single catalytic monomer of 165–170 kDa, which can be inhibited by vanadates *(54)*, and form an intermediate acylphosphate through the addition of γ-phosphate from ATP to an aspartic acid residue. ATP7A and ATP7B also have four signature motifs found in other P-type ATPases: the TGEA phosphatase motif, the DKTGT motif with an invariant aspartate residue, a conserved cysteine and proline (CPC) motif in the proposed cation transduction channel, and an ATP-binding sequence (GDGIND) at the carboxy terminal domain. Both proteins have six characteristic MBS motifs at their N-terminal domain, each containing a core MXCXXC sequence that coordinates Cu^{+1} via the two cysteine residues (reviewed in ref. *53*). The Cu-binding activities of the N-terminal MBS motifs and the intramembrane CPC motif appear to be needed for phosphorylation of the Cu ATPases *(55)*. MBS motifs 5 and 6 have a unique role in regulating catalytic activity, possibly through induction of conformational changes required for the transition between high- and low-affinity states *(53)*.

Mutations that disable the function of ATP7A and ATP7B cause Menkes and Wilson's diseases, respectively. Menkes disease is an X-linked Cu-deficiency disorder that is usually fatal in early childhood. Patients with this disease present with mental retardation and neurodegeneration, mostly as a result of a deficiency of Cu-dependent enzymes necessary for brain development *(56)*. Wilson's disease is an autosomal recessive disorder characterized by a marked increase of Cu in the liver and brain caused by a reduced capacity to excrete Cu through biliary and other pathways. Cu accumulates in hepatocytes and brain cells, leading to cirrhosis and neurodegeneration, and Cu is deposited in the cornea producing the characteristic Kaiser-Fleischer rings *(57)*. LEC rats, which spontaneously develop fulminant hepatitis and hepatocellular carcinoma and exhibit excessive hepatic Cu and Fe accumulation, are thought to be an animal model of Wilson's disease *(58)*.

3. ALTERATIONS IN Cu-HOMEOSTASIS PROTEINS IN Cu-RESISTANT CELLS

As it is the case for the Pt drugs, cells exposed repeatedly to high concentrations of Cu become resistant to the toxic effects of this metalloid. There is now strong evidence that ATP7A and ATP7B can function individually to protect the cell against toxic levels of Cu. Chinese hamster ovary cells selected for acquired resistance to Cu were shown to have amplified the *ATP7A* gene *(59)*. Similarly, repeated exposure of the hepatocarcinoma cell line HuH7 to Cu resulted in a resistant population in which the expression of ATP7B mRNA and protein was increased *(60)*. Forced expression of either ATP7A or ATP7B in human fibroblasts was found to render them Cu resistant *(59)*. However, these Cu ATPases are not the only proteins functioning in Cu homeostasis that can mediate Cu resistance through altered expression level. A variety of Cu-resistant cells has high concentrations of metallothioneins, and a specific role for the protection of nuclei has been proposed for these proteins *(61)*. Interestingly, high-level resistance to Cd-, Pt-, a Cu-containing compounds was noted in cell lines that have high nuclear/cytoplasmic metallothionein concentration ratios *(42)*. In many Cu-resistant cells, metallothionein genes become amplified in tandem arrays *(42)*. However, it is not clear whether metallothioneins alone can render a cell resistant to Cu without the participation of other Cu homeostatic proteins. The role of Cu-binding proteins other than ATP7A, ATP7B, and metallothioneins in the development of Cu resistance is less clear. For example, it is not yet known whether reduction of Ctr1 function is found in cells selected for Cu resistance.

Recent studies have identified a number of other proteins that regulate sensitivity to Cu. Loss of the mouse U2af1-rs1 region 1 protein causes Cu toxicosis in the Bedlington terriers *(62)*. This Cu-homeostasis protein lacks a Cu-binding site but modulates Cu homeostasis through interaction with ATP7B *(62)*. The amyloid precursor protein contains a Cu-binding site, and null mutations of the gene encoding this protein result in Cu accumulation in the brain of mice *(63)*. It has been suggested that amyloid precursor protein serves as a barrier to Cu import in the brain *(64)*. Whether the expression or function of these proteins is altered in cells selected for Cu resistance has not yet been determined.

4. CROSSRESISTANCE BETWEEN Cu AND DDP

It has been known for some time that cells selected for resistance to DDP share some phenotypic characteristics with cells selected for resistance to other metalloids *(28)*. As shown in Table 1, cells selected for resistance to DDP are often crossresistant to Cu *(65)*. Where they have been examined, cells selected for resistance to Cu have also been shown to be crossresistant to DDP. Analyses of two Cu-resistant hepatocarcinoma sublines, CuR23 and CuR27, selected from the parental HuH7 cell line by repeated exposure to $CuSO_4$, demonstrated crossresistance to DDP *(66)*. Interestingly, irrespective of the agent used for selection, in all cases examined to date, the level of resistance to DDP has always been higher than the level of resistance to Cu. For example, human ovarian carcinoma cells selected for resistance to DDP were found to be 2- to 30-fold more resistant to DDP but only two- to fourfold more resistant to Cu *(65)*. Whereas the

Cu-selected CuR23 and CuR27 sublines were, respectively, 2.0- and 1.8-fold more resistant to Cu, they were 8.3- and 8.6-fold more resistant to DDP *(66)*. Why such modest degrees of resistance to Cu are associated with much greater degrees of resistance to DDP is unknown.

Analyses of three human ovarian carcinoma cell lines, 2008/C13*5.25, A2780/CP, and IGROV-1/CP, selected for resistance to DDP and found to be crossresistant to Cu did not reveal consistent changes in the level of *CTR1* mRNA expression but did show increased expression of either ATP7A or ATP7B in each resistant subline. Higher expression of ATP7A mRNA and protein was found in both the 2008/C13*5.25 and A2760/CP cells, whereas the IGROV-1/CP cells exhibited increased expression of ATP7B *(65)*. A prostate cancer cell line selected for resistance to DDP has also been reported to overexpress ATP7B *(67)*.

Analyses of the Cu-resistant CuR23 and CuR27 cell lines revealed no alterations in expression of either glutathione or metallothioneins when compared to the HuH7 parental line *(60)*. However, these cells were found to express, respectively, 2.3- and 2.4-fold more ATP7B protein than the parental HuH7 cells *(66)*. In the absence of any change in the metallothioneins, glutathione, and ABC transporters, MRP2, MRP3, and MRP5 (R. Safaei, unpublished), enhanced export of DDP by ATP7B is most the likely to be responsible for the crossresistance of CuR23 and CuR27 to DDP.

The fact that Cu causes cell death primarily through the generation of oxidative damage, whereas DDP kills cells primarily through the formation of adducts in DNA, suggests that crossresistance between Cu and DDP can be attributed to components of the Cu-homeostasis pathways that affect both compounds rather than to a defect further downstream in the apoptotic pathway. Systematic analyses of the available Cu and DDP crossresistant cell lines have not yet been performed; however, such studies are likely to provide additional insight into which components of the Cu-homeostasis pathway are most strongly associated with the crossresistant phenotype.

5. PARALLEL CHANGES IN THE CELLULAR PHARMACOLOGY OF DDP AND Cu IN CROSSRESISTANT CELLS

Analyses of cells selected for resistance to either DDP or Cu have demonstrated defects in the accumulation of both Cu and DDP that are summarized in Table 2. The ovarian carcinoma cell lines 2008/C13*5.25, A2780/CP and IGROV-1/CP, each selected for resistance to DDP, had 1-min rates for DDP that were, respectively, 23, 30, and 55% of that in the parental cells *(65)*. The resistant sublines accumulated only 39, 25, and 44% as much Cu. Similar results were obtained from studies of the accumulation of Cu and DDP in CuR27 cells that were selected for resistance to Cu *(66)*. During the first minute of exposure, the accumulation of DDP and Cu in the CuR27 cells were, respectively, 74 and 64% of those in the parental HuH7 cells. Similar results were obtained when accumulation was measured after 1 h of exposure to DDP or Cu.

The time course of the efflux of DDP and Cu from drug-sensitive cells was found to be quite similar. The first phase of efflux is very rapid and results in the loss of a large fraction of the Cu and DDP present in the cells. In contrast, the second phase of efflux is very slow and accounts for a much smaller fraction of the total cellular DDP or Cu that is lost from the cells. Cells selected for resistance to DDP or Cu exhibited increased rates of efflux. In the case of human ovarian carcinoma 2008/C13*5.25 cells, the initial efflux rate of DDP was increased by 2.3 ± 0.2-fold and that of Cu was increased 2.4 ± 0.1-fold *(65)*. Similarly, the initial rate of efflux in CuR27 cells was 2.5-fold faster for DDP and

Table 2
Changes in the Cellular Pharmacokinetic Parameters Found in Cisplatin and Copper
Crossresistant Cells

	Cells selected for resistance to DDP		Cells selected for resistance to Cu	
	DDP	Cu	DDP	Cu
Resistance	↑(2- to 38-fold)	↑(1.9- to 2-fold)	↑(8- to 10-fold)	↑(1.5- to 18-fold)
Accumulation	↓(38–67%)	↓(26–56%)	↓	↓
Basal levels	–	↓ (22–56%)		↓
Initial efflux rate	↑(23–55%)	↑ (56–75%)	↑	↑
DNA–Pt adduct	↓(10–38%)			
Expression of Cu transporters	Altered		Altered	

DDP, cisplatin; Cu, copper; Pt, platinum.

6.5-fold faster for Cu *(66)*. These results demonstrate a parallelism between the changes that occurred in the cellular pharmacology of Cu and DDP in both DDP-resistant and Cu-resistant cells. A further indication that Cu-homeostasis mechanisms are involved in this phenomenon came from the observation that both Cu- and DDP-resistant cells contained much lower levels (22–56% of control) of Cu when grown in standard tissue culture medium, suggesting that Cu homeostasis was defective in DDP-resistant cells, a finding consistent with the observed higher levels of ATP7A or ATP7B found in these cells *(65,66)*. Table 3 summarizes the effects of forced expression of Cu transporters on the cellular pharmacology of Cu and DDP.

6. ROLE OF CTR1 IN DDP INFLUX

Analysis of yeast and mammalian genetic variants has demonstrated that the major Cu influx transporter Ctr1 can regulate both sensitivity to the cytotoxic effect of DDP and its cellular accumulation. The initial report that *ctr1–/– Saccharomyces cerevisiae* accumulated less DDP *(68)* was rapidly followed by a confirmatory report that also demonstrated defective accumulation of carboplatin (CBDCA) and oxaliplatin *(69)*. Further evidence of the importance of Ctr1 was provided by a study of mouse fibroblast cell lines established from *CTR1–/–* knockout mice that exhibited reduced DDP uptake and increased DDP resistance *(68)*. More recent work *(70,71)* using *hCTR1*-transfected A2780 human ovarian carcinoma cells showed that overexpression of *CTR1* enhanced the accumulation of both Cu and DDP, although the effect was much larger for the former than the latter. Interestingly, the increase in DDP whole-cell accumulation was not accompanied by a significant increase in delivery of Pt to DNA or an increase in sensitivity to the cytotoxic effect of DDP. This suggests that, when *CTR1* is forcibly overexpressed, the excess DDP entering the cell is sequestered in a compartment from which it does not have immediate access to the nucleus or other key cytotoxic targets.

Additional studies with human ovarian carcinoma A2780 cells have now shown that both Cu and DDP reduce the level of expression of Ctr1(Table 3). Using Western blot analysis and confocal digital deconvolution microscopy, it was found that exposure to DDP triggered the loss of hCtr1 from the cell in a concentration and time-dependent

Table 3
Parallel Changes in the Cellular Pharmacokinetic Parameters for Cisplatin and Copper in Cells Molecularly Engineered to Express Altered Levels of Copper Transporters

Gene	Overexpression/ knockout	DDP				CuSO$_4$			Basal
		Fold resistance	Pt content	Efflux rate	Pt–DNA adduct	Fold resistance	Cu content	Efflux rate	Cu content
ATP7B	Overexpression	↑	↓	↑	↑	↑	↓	↑	↓
ATP7A	Overexpression	↑	↓	–	No change	↑	↓	↑	↓
hCTR1	Overexpression	No change	↑	–	No change	No change	↑	–	↑
MCTR1[a]	Knockout	↑	↓		↓	↑	↓		
yCTR1[b]	Knockout	↑	↓			↑	↓		

DDP, cisplatin; CuSO$_4$, cupric sulfate; Pt, platinum; Cu copper.
[a]Mouse.
[b]Yeast.

manner *(70)*. Exposure to as little as 0.5 μ*M* DDP for 5 min reduced the hCtr1 level whereas exposure to DDP concentrations ≥2.0 μ*M* caused almost complete disappearance. The loss of hCtr1 was observed within 1 min of the start of exposure to 2 μ*M* DDP. Treatment of cells with 100 μ*M* Cu for 5 min produced a much smaller effect. Pretreatment of cells with 2 μ*M* DDP for 5 min resulted in a 50% decrease in Cu uptake, documenting that the DDP-induced loss of hCtr1 detected by Western blot analysis and digital confocal imaging was functionally significant. Thus, DDP downregulates the amount of its major influx transporter in human ovarian carcinoma cells in a concentration and time-dependent manner. This effect was observed at DDP concentrations within the range found in the plasma of patients being treated with DDP, and occurred very quickly relative to the half-life of the drug.

A large number of questions about the interaction of the Pt drugs with Ctr1 remain to be addressed. The ability of DDP to cause the disappearance of Ctr1 from the cell suggests that DDP binds to Ctr1, but the differences in potency between Cu and DDP hint at differences in the conformation of the N-terminal extracellular domain in the bound state. Whether DDP enters the cell through a true channel formed by Ctr1 or whether Ctr1 serves as a carrier to conduct DDP into an endocytotic entry route remains unknown, as does the mechanism by which DDP causes the disappearance of Ctr1 from the cell. The ability of DDP to trigger the disappearance of an influx transporter important to its own entry has interesting clinical implications. First, differential expression of Ctr1 in various normal tissues may explain the pattern of dose-limiting toxicity observed in man. Second, a pharmacological intervention directed at blocking Ctr1 degradation may improve drug uptake into tumor cells.

7. EFFECT OF ATP7A ON THE CELLULAR PHARMACOLOGY AND CYTOTOXICITY OF DDP

The effect of ATP7A on the cellular pharmacology and cytotoxicity of DDP and other Pt drugs has been investigated in several different systems (Table 3). In one set of studies, an ATP7A expression vector was transfected into Me32a fibroblasts, originally established from a patient with Menkes disease, that express neither ATP7A nor ATP7B. The ATP7A-transfected cells were found to accumulate less Cu and DDP and were less sensitive to the cytotoxic effect of both agents than the parental ATP7A-deficient Me32a cells *(72)*. In another study, human ovarian carcinoma 2008 cells were found to be more resistant to DDP when transfected with an ATP7A expression vector even when the increase in the ATP7A expression over the endogenous levels was quite small *(73)*.

Whereas increased expression of ATP7A produced parallel effects on sensitivity to the cytotoxic effect of Cu and DDP, there is evidence that these two compounds interact differently with this efflux transporter. Pt accumulates in vesicles expressing ATP7A in cells exposed to DDP, and a fluorescent analog of DDP was found in vesicles that express ATP7A by confocal analysis of ovarian carcinoma 2008 cells *(74)*, suggesting that ATP7A mediates the sequestration of DDP into vesicles of the secretory pathway. However, clear differences have been demonstrated in the ability of Cu and DDP to trigger intracellular movement of ATP7A. Whereas Cu efficiently triggered redistribution of ATP7A from the perinuclear region to more peripheral reaches of the cell, DDP did not *(72)*. Thus, whereas the available studies indicate that ATP7A can mediate resistance to DDP and modulate its cellular pharmacology, a mechanistic understanding of how the ATP7A-mediated vesicular export pathway handles Cu and DDP differently is not yet in hand.

The evidence that ATP7A controls sensitivity to the cytotoxic effect of DDP in experimental systems has raised the question of whether its expression in tumors is associated with response to treatment. An immunohistochemical study demonstrated substantial heterogeneity of ATP7A staining among 54 patients with ovarian carcinoma *(75)*. Whereas there was no clear association between ATP7A expression in the tumor prior to treatment and subsequent response, in some patients, treatment with a Pt drug-based regimen was associated with enrichment for ATP7A-expressing cells in the tumor obtained after treatment, and this subgroup of patients had also significantly poorer survival rates. Whereas ATP7A is a candidate marker of Pt drug resistance, the larger studies needed for validation must consider the expression of Ctr1, ATP7B, and possibly other Cu-homeostasis proteins as well.

8. EFFECT OF ATP7B ON THE CELLULAR PHARMACOLOGY AND CYTOTOXICITY OF DDP

The evidence that ATP7B can mediate resistance to DDP is now quite compelling, as this effect has been observed in multiple experimental models, and an association between expression and subsequent response has been reported for several different types of human malignancies. Transfection of epidermoid carcinoma KB-3-1 cells with an ATP7B expression vector was reported to render them 8.9-fold more resistant to DDP and two-fold more resistant to Cu *(67)*. Subsequent studies demonstrated that forced expression of ATP7B in human ovarian and head and neck carcinoma cells conferred resistance to Cu, DDP, and a variety of DDP analogs *(76)*.

Analyses of Cu and Pt accumulation levels in cells transfected with ATP7B expression vectors (Table 3) suggests that this protein has a direct role in the efflux of DDP as well as Cu. Cells engineered to overexpress ATP7B were found to have lower basal levels of Cu when compared to empty vector-transfected cells, similar to the situation found in ovarian carcinoma cells selected for resistance to DDP *(76)*. Forced overexpression of ATP7B resulted in reduced accumulation of DDP *(67)* and a detailed study of ^{64}Cu and ^{14}C-CBDCA kinetics in these cells demonstrated reduced accumulation of Pt in DNA and enhanced efflux of both compounds *(76)*.

Table 4 summarizes the results of a number of immunohistochemical and mRNA analyses of the association between ATP7B expression and clinical outcome of Pt drug-based therapy. In general, higher expression of ATP7B was correlated with an unfavorable response to treatment with Pt-containing agents (for examples, *see* refs. *77* and *78*). No such correlation was found between the expression of other efflux drug transporters such as MRP1, MRP2, MDR1, or LPR and response to Pt drug therapy *(77,78)*. An association was also found between the level of ATP7B expression and presence of poorly differentiated or undifferentiated cells in tumors *(77,78)*.

9. SUMMARY AND CONCLUSIONS

Current data are consistent with the concept that the transporters that control Cu homeostasis also regulate sensitivity to DDP by controlling its uptake, intracellular transport, and efflux. Based on the fact that DDP interacts with cysteine, methionine, and histidine residues in other proteins, it is possible that the CXXC and other motifs that chelate Cu in the Cu-binding proteins also bind DDP. The fact that all three of the major Cu transporters modulate DDP sensitivity has led to the hypothesis that following exposure to clinically relevant concentrations of DDP, the drug is not free in the cell but is

Table 4

Correlation Between Drug Resistance in Human Tumors and Expression of Gene Products for Copper Transporters ATP7A and ATP7B

Tumor type	Cu protein	Detection method	Pt drug	Outcome	Reference
Breast carcinoma	ATP7B	IHC; RT-PCR	DDP	No correlation between the outcome of therapy and the expression of MDR1, MRP1, LRP, and BCRP was found.	(77)
Ovarian carcinoma	ATP7B	RT-PCR	DDP	43.9% of samples were positive for ATP7B expression; ATP7B expression was significantly higher in undifferentiated cells; no correlation between the outcome of therapy and the expression of MDR1, MRP1, LRP, and BCRP was found.	(78)
Esophageal carcinoma	ATP7B	IHC	DDP	70.5% of samples were positive for ATP7B expression; ATP7B expression correlated with unfavorable outcome of therapy.	(92)
Oral squamouse carcinoma	ATP7B	IHC	DDP	ATP7B expression significantly correlated with unfavorable outcome of therapy.	(93)
Gastric carcinoma	ATP7B	IHC	DDP	41.2% of samples were positive for ATP7B expression; ATP7B expression was significantly higher in undifferentiated cells.	(94)
Hepatocellular carcinoma	ATP7B	IHC	DDP	Various degrees of staining were observed in 21.1% (4/19) of samples; study suggested correlation between high expression and unfavorable outcome of therapy.	(95)
Ovarian carcinoma	ATP7B	IHC	DDP	34.6% (36 of 104 cases) of samples were positive for ATP7B expression; significantly higher positivity in poorly/moderately differentiated carcinoma cells; ATP7B-positive tumors had a significantly inferior response to chemotherapy.	(96)
Prostate, breast, testes, kidney, pancreas, liver, thyroid, ovary, lung, endometrial, colon, and other tumors	ATP7A	IHC	Pt-based	All except liver and endometrial tumors expressed higher levels of ATP7A compared to normal issue; upregulation of ATP7A expression correlated negatively with survival.	(75)

Cu, copper; Pt, platinum; IHC, immunohistochemistry; RT-PCR, reverse transcription-polymerase chain reaction; DDP, cisplatin; MDR1, multidrug resistance 1; MRP1, multidrug-related protein 1; LRP, lung resistance-related protein; BCRP, breast cancer-related protein.

shuttled from a transporter to chaperones that deliver it to key intracellular targets including DNA. This hypothesis provides a framework for a set of experiments in which the level of each known Cu-binding protein is altered to map the importance of sequential steps in the passage of DDP into the cell and through the various subcellular compartments.

The hypothesis that DDP utilizes pathways that have evolved to manage Cu homeostasis provides an interesting explanation for a long-standing conundrum in the field. Whereas DDP is known to react readily with glutathione and a variety of other thiols whose cytoplasmic concentration is >1,000 times higher than that of DDP, this drug is still effective at killing cells even at very low concentrations. It has been difficult to understand how DDP ever wends its way through such a sea of thiols and arrives at DNA in a form that is still capable of forming adducts. The concept that, like Cu, DDP may be secured in redox-protected pockets formed by metallochaperones provides a mechanistically attractive explanation. However, the role of Cu chaperones in binding or delivering DDP has yet to be explored.

It is important to note that none of the Cu transporters has yet been formally shown to bind DDP or transport it across a lipid bilayer membrane. As ATP7A and ATP7B function as monomers (79), it should be possible to study their ability to transport DDP using vesicles from cells engineered to express high levels of these proteins, or by assembling recombinant proteins in artificial membranes. In view of the fact that Ctr1 shows high selectivity for Cu as opposed to other metals, and a preference for Cu^{+1} rather than Cu^{+2}, it is intriguing that this transporter mediates the uptake of DDP, and, at least in yeast, CBDCA and oxaliplatin as well. The finding that some of the Cu-binding proteins can bind other metals, and the fact that Cu and DDP can both interact with cysteine, methionine, and histidine-rich motifs, makes it likely that DDP can bind to a number of Cu transporters and chaperones but the differences in the coordination chemistry of Cu and DDP suggest that the structural features of the Cu and DDP-loaded proteins are probably different. Such structural differences may account for the fact that Cu can trigger trafficking of ATP7A but DDP cannot (73). Whereas the hypothesis that Cu transporters directly transport DDP is attractive, it remains possible that they regulate intracellular levels of DDP indirectly by affecting Cu-dependent activities such as ATP production or simply by acting as Pt drug traps. Secondary regulatory effects on Pt drug transport have been reported for other transporters such as the Na/K-ATPase (12), the Mg-ATPase (80), the Ca-ATPase (16), and the vacuolar ATPase (17).

If the transporters and chaperones that regulate Cu homeostasis do constitute the primary cellular conduits for DDP, then one would expect these to be altered in cells selected for acquired DDP resistance. Indeed, increased expression of either ATP7A or ATP7B has been observed in ovarian carcinoma cells selected for resistance to DDP (65), although it has not been proven that either protein is the actual cause of the resistant phenotype in these cells. Whether the higher ATP7A and ATP7B levels are because of changes in gene copy number, transcription, translation, or protein stability has not yet been determined, but because both the phenotype and the high levels of these proteins are stable over multiple generations, a mutational origin is likely.

Whereas there may be other transporters that mediate influx or efflux of the Pt drugs and whose alteration can contribute to the acquired DDP resistant phenotype, a careful dissection of the mechanism by which the Cu transporters modulate sensitivity to the cytotoxic effects of these drugs promises to provide novel insights into how to prevent the emergence of resistance or overcome it once it becomes apparent. Substantial work remains to be done in order to understand the mechanisms that control Pt drug influx and efflux and to map the subcellular pathways by which these drugs move inside the cells. Gaining insight into the manner of involvement of the Cu homeostasis mechanism in this process provides a starting point.

REFERENCES

1. Inoue K, Mukaiyama T, Mitsui I, Ogawa M. In vitro evaluation of anticancer drugs in relation to development of drug resistance in the human tumor clonogenic assay. Cancer Chemoth Pharm 1985; 15:208–213.
2. Wilson AP, Ford CH, Newman CE, Howell A. Cisplatin and ovarian carcinoma. In vitro chemosensitivity of cultured tumor cells from patients receiving high dose cisplatin as first line treatment. Brit J Cancer 1987; 56:763–773.
3. Andrews PA, Jones JA, Varki NM, Howell SB. Rapid emergence of acquired cis-diammine-dichloroplatinum[II] resistance in an in vivo model of human ovarian carcinoma. Cancer Commun 1990; 2:93–100.
4. Kelland LR. New platinum antitumor complexes. Crit Rev Oncol Hematol 1993; 15:191–219.
5. Jekunen AP, Hom DK, Alcaraz JE, Eastman A, Howell SB. Cellular pharmacology of dichloro(ethylene-diamine)platinum(II) in cisplatin-sensitive and resistant human ovarian carcinoma cells. Cancer Res 1994; 54:2680–2687.
6. Loh SY, Mistry P, Kelland LR, Abel G, Harrap KR. Reduced drug accumulation as a major mechanism of acquired resistance to cisplatin in a human ovarian carcinoma cell line: circumvention studies using novel platinum (II) and (IV) ammine/amine complexes. Br J Cancer 1992; 66:1109–1115.
7. Gately DP, Howell SB. Cellular accumulation of the anticancer agent cisplatin: a review. Br J Cancer 1993; 67:1171–1176.
8. Okuda M, Tsuda K, Masaki K, Hashimoto Y, Inui K. Cisplatin-induced toxicity in LLC-PK1 kidney epithelial cells: role of basolateral membrane transport. Toxicol Lett 1999; 106:229–235.
9. Amtmann E, Zoller M, Wesch H, Schilling G. Antitumoral activity of a sulphur-containing platinum complex with an acidic pH optimum. Cancer Chemother Pharmacol 2001; 47:461–466.
10. Atema A, Buurman KJ, Noteboom E, Smets LA. Potentiation of DNA-adduct formation and cytotoxicity of platinum-containing drugs by low pH. Int J Cancer 1993; 54:166–172.
11. Endo T, Kimura O, Sakata M. Carrier-mediated uptake of cisplatin by the OK renal epithelial cell line. Toxicology 2000; 146:187–195.
12. Andrews PA, Mann SC, Huynh HH, Albright KD. Role of the Na+-, K+-ATPase in the accumulation of cis-diammine- dichloroplatinum[II] in human ovarian carcinoma cells. Cancer Res 1991; 51:3677–3681.
13. Chiang CD, Song EJ, Yang VC, Chao CC. Ascorbic acid increases drug accumulation and reverses vincristine resistance of human non-small-cell lung-cancer cells. Biochem J 1994; 301:759–764.
14. Sarna S, Bhola RK. Chemo-immunotherapeutical studies on Dalton's lymphoma in mice using cisplatin and ascorbic acid: synergistic antitumor effect in vivo and in vitro. Arch Immunol Ther Exp 1993; 41:327–333.
15. Zhang JG, Zhong LF, Zhang M, et al. Amelioration of cisplatin toxicity in rat renal cortical slices by dithiothreitol in vitro. Hum Exp Toxicol 1994; 13:89–93.
16. Aggarwal SK, Niroomand-Rad I. Effect of cisplatin on the plasma membrane phosphatase activities in ascites sarcoma-180 cells: a cytochemical study. J Histochem Cytochem 1983; 31:307–317.
17. Torigoe T, Izumi H, Ishiguchi H, et al. Enhanced expression of the human vacuolar H+-ATPase c subunit gene (ATP6L) in response to anticancer agents. J Biol Chem 2002; 277:36,534–36,543.
18. Mann SC, Andrews PA, Howell SB. Short-term cis-diamminedichloroplatinum (II) accumulation in sensitive and resistant human ovarian carcinoma cells. Cancer Chemoth Pharm 1990; 25:236–240.
19. Schadendorf D, Herfordt R, Czarnetzki BM. P-glycoprotein expression in primary and metastatic malignant melanoma. Br J Dermatol 1995; 132:551–555.
20. Wada H, Saikawa Y, Niida Y, et al. Selectively induced high MRP gene expression in multidrug-resistant human HL60 leukemia cells. Exp Hematol 1999; 27:99–109.
21. Hiss D, Gabriels G, Jacobs P, Folb P. Tunicamycin potentiates drug cytotoxicity and vincristine retention in multidrug resistant cell lines. Eur J Cancer 1996; 32:2164–2172.
22. Saito T, Zhang ZJ, Ohtsubo T, et al. Homozygous disruption of the mdr1a P-glycoprotein gene affects blood–nerve barrier function in mice administered with neurotoxic drugs. Acta Otolaryngol 2001; 121:735–742.

23. Chen ZS, Kawabe T, Ono M, et al. Effect of multidrug resistance-reversing agents on transporting activity of human canalicular multispecific organic anion transporter. Mol Pharmacol 1999; 56:1219–1228.

24. Shen DW, Goldenberg S, Pastan I, Gottesman MM. Decreased accumulation of [14C] carboplatin in human cisplatin-resistant cells results from reduced energy-dependent uptake. J Cell Physiol 2000; 183:108–116.

25. Borst P, Evers R, Kool M, Wijnholds J. A family of drug transporters: the multidrug resistance-associated proteins. J Natl Cancer Inst 2000; 92:1295–1302.

26. Pu YS, Tsai TC, Cheng AL, et al. Expression of MDR-1 gene in transitional cell carcinoma and its correlation with chemotherapy response. J Urol 1996; 156:271–275.

27. Schrenk D, Baus PR, Ermel N, Klein C, Vorderstemann B, Kauffmann HM. Up-regulation of transporters of the MRP family by drugs and toxins. Toxicol Lett 2001; 120:51–57.

28. Naredi P, Heath DD, Enns RE, Howell SB. Cross-resistance between cisplatin, antimony potassium tartrate, and arsenite in human tumor cells. J Clin Invest 1995; 95:1193–1198.

29. Rae TD, Schmidt PJ, Pufahl RA, Culotta VC, O'Halloran TV. Undetectable intracellular free copper: the requirement of a copper chaperone for superoxide dismutase. Science 1999; 284:805–808.

30. Solioz M, Vulpe C. CPx-type ATPases: a class of p-type ATPases that pump heavy metals. Trends Biochem Sci 1996; 21:237–241.

31. Steele RA, Opella SJ. Structures of the reduced and mercury-bound forms of MerP, the periplasmic protein from the bacterial mercury detoxification system. Biochemistry 1997; 36:6885–6895.

32. Lutsenko S, Petrukhin K, Cooper MJ, Gilliam CT, Kaplan JH. N-terminal domains of human copper-transporting adenosine triphosphatases (the Wilson's and Menkes disease proteins) bind copper selectively in vivo and in vitro with stoichiometry of one copper per metal-binding repeat. J Biol Chem 1997; 272:18,939–18,944.

33. DiDonato M, Narindrasorasak S, Forbes JR, Cox DW, Sarkar B. Expression, purification, and metal binding properties of the N- terminal domain from the wilson disease putative copper-transporting ATPase (ATP7B). J Biol Chem 1997; 272:33,279–33,282.

34. Zhou B, Gitschier J. hCTR1: A human gene for copper uptake identified by complementation in yeast. Proc Natl Acad Sci U S A 1997; 94:7481–7486.

35. Kuo YM, Zhou B, Cosco D, Gitschier J. The copper transporter CTR1 provides an essential function in mammalian embryonic development. Proc Natl Acad Sci U S A 2001; 98:6836–6841.

36. Lee J, Prohaska JR, Thiele DJ. Essential role for mammalian copper transporter Ctr1 in copper homeostasis and embryonic development. Proc Natl Acad Sci U S A 2001; 98:6842–6847.

37. Klomp AE, Tops BB, Van Denberg IE, Berger R, Klomp LW. Biochemical characterization and subcellular localization of human copper transporter 1 (hCTR1). Biochem J 2002; 364:497–505.

38. Eisses JF, Kaplan JH. Molecular characterization of hCTR1, the human copper uptake protein. J Biol Chem 2002; 277:29,162–29,1671.

39. Xiao Z, Loughlin F, George GN, Howlett GJ, Wedd AG. C-terminal domain of the membrane copper transporter Ctr1 from Saccharomyces cerevisiae binds four Cu(I) ions as a cuprous-thiolate polynuclear cluster: sub-femtomolar Cu(I) affinity of three proteins involved in copper trafficking. J Am Chem Soc 2004; 126:3081–3090.

40. Ralle M, Lutsenko S, Blackburn NJ. X-ray absorption spectroscopy of the copper chaperone HAH1 reveals a linear two-coordinate Cu(I) center capable of adduct formation with exogenous thiols and phosphines. J Biol Chem 2003; 278:23,163–23,170.

41. Puig S, Thiele DJ. Molecular mechanisms of copper uptake and distribution. Curr Opin Chem Biol 2002; 6:171–180.

42. Coyle P, Philcox JC, Carey LC, Rofe AM. Metallothionein: the multipurpose protein. Cell Mol Life Sci 2002; 59:627–647.

43. Suzuki KT, Someya A, Komada Y, Ogra Y. Roles of metallothionein in copper homeostasis: responses to Cu-deficient diets in mice. J Inorg Biochem 2002; 88:173–182.

44. Kachur AV, Koch CJ, Biaglow JE. Mechanism of copper-catalyzed oxidation of glutathione. Free Radic Res 1998; 28:259–269.

45. Mergeay M. Towards an understanding of the genetics of bacterial metal resistance. Trends Biotechnol 1991; 9:17–24.

46. Harada M, Kumemura H, Sakisaka S, et al. Wilson disease protein ATP7B is localized in the late endosomes in a polarized human hepatocyte cell line. Int J Mol Med 2003; 11:293–298.

47. Petris MJ, Mercer JF, Culvenor JG, Lockhart P, Gleeson PA, Camakaris J. Ligand-regulated transport of the Menkes copper P-type ATPase efflux pump from the Golgi apparatus to the plasma membrane: a novel mechanism of regulated trafficking. EMBO J 1996; 15:6084–6095.

48. Amaravadi R, Glerum DM, Tzagoloff A. Isolation of a cDNA encoding the human homolog of COX17, a yeast gene essential for mitochondrial copper recruitment. Hum Genet 1997; 99:329–333.

49. Culotta VC, Klomp LW, Strain J, Casareno RL, Krems B, Gitlin JD. The copper chaperone for superoxide dismutase. J Biol Chem 1997; 272:23,469–23,472.

50. Hamza I, Faisst A, Prohaska J, Chen J, Gruss P, Gitlin JD. The metallochaperone Atox1 plays a critical role in perinatal copper homeostasis. Proc Natl Acad Sci U S A 2001; 98:6848–6852.

51. Hamza I, Prohaska J, Gitlin JD. Essential role for Atox1 in the copper-mediated intracellular trafficking of the Menkes ATPase. Proc Natl Acad Sci U S A 2003; 100:1215–1220.

52. Takahashi Y, Kako K, Kashiwabara S, et al. Mammalian copper chaperone Cox17p has an essential role in activation of cytochrome C oxidase and embryonic development. Mol Cell Biol 2002; 22:7614–7621.

53. Lutsenko S, Petris MJ. Function and regulation of the mammalian copper-transporting ATPases: insights from biochemical and cell biological approaches. J Membr Biol 2003; 191:1–12.

54. Dijkstra M, In't Veld G, van den Berg GJ, Muller M, Kuipers F, Vonk RJ. Adenosine triphosphate-dependent copper transport in isolated rat liver plasma membranes. J Clin Invest 1995; 95:412–416.

55. Bissig KD, Wunderli-Ye H, Duda PW, Solioz M. Structure-function analysis of purified Enterococcus hirae CopB copper ATPase: effect of Menkes/Wilson disease mutation homologues. Biochem J 2001; 357:217–223.

56. Mercer JF, Llanos RM. Molecular and cellular aspects of copper transport in developing mammals. J Nutr 2003; 133:1481S–1484S.

57. Brewer GJ. Wilson disease and canine copper toxicosis. Am J Clin Nutr 1998; 67:1087S–1090S.

58. Shim H, Harris ZL. Genetic defects in copper metabolism. J Nutr 2003; 133:1527S–1531S.

59. Camakaris J, Petris MJ, Bailey L, et al. Gene amplification of the Menkes (MNK; ATP7A) P-type ATPase gene of CHO cells is associated with copper resistance and enhanced copper efflux. Hum Mol Genet 1995; 4:2117–2123.

60. Schilsky ML, Stockert RJ, Kesner A, et al. Copper resistant human hepatoblastoma mutant cell lines without metallothionein induction overexpress ATP7B. Hepatology 1998; 28:1347–1356.

61. Cousins RJ. Metallothionein—aspects related to copper and zinc metabolism. J Inherit Metab Dis 1983; 6(Suppl 1):S15–S21.

62. Tao TY, Liu F, Klomp LW, Wijmenga C, Gitlin JD. The copper toxicosis gene product Murr1 directly interacts with the Wilson Disease protein. 2003; 278:41,593–41,596.

63. White AR, Reyes R, Mercer JF, et al. Copper levels are increased in the cerebral cortex and liver of APP and APLP2 knockout mice. Brain Res 1999; 842:439–444.

64. Bayer TA, Schafer S, Simons A, et al. Dietary Cu stabilizes brain superoxide dismutase 1 activity and reduces amyloid Aβ production in APP23 transgenic mice. Proc Natl Acad Sci U S A 2003; 100:14,187–14,192.

65. Katano K, Kondo A, Safaei R, et al. Acquisition of resistance to cisplatin is accompanied by changes in the cellular pharmacology of copper. Cancer Res 2002; 62:6559–6565.

66. Safaei R, Katano K, Samimi G, et al. Cross-resistance to cisplatin in cells with acquired resistance to copper. Cancer Chemother Pharmacol 2004; 53:239–246.

67. Komatsu M, Sumizawa T, Mutoh M, et al. Copper-transporting P-type adenosine triphosphatase (ATP7B) is associated with cisplatin resistance. Cancer Res 2000; 60:1312–1316.

68. Ishida S, Lee J, Thiele DJ, Herskowitz I. Uptake of the anticancer drug cisplatin mediated by the copper transporter Ctr1 in yeast and mammals. Proc Natl Acad Sci U S A 2002; 99:14,298–14,302.

69. Lin X, Okuda T, Holzer A, Howell SB. The copper transporter CTR1 regulates cisplatin uptake in saccharomyces cerevisiae. Mol Pharmacol 2002; 62:1154–1159.

70. Holzer AK, Katano K, Klomp LW, Howell SB. Cisplatin rapidly down-regulates its own influx transporter hCTR1 in cultured human ovarian carcinoma cells. Clin Cancer Res 2004; 10:6744–6749.

71. Holzer AK, Samimi G, Katano K, et al. The copper influx transporter human copper transport protein 1 regulates the uptake of cisplatin in human ovarian carcinoma cells. Mol Pharmacol 2004; 66:817–823.

72. Samimi G, Katano K, Holzer AK, Safaei R, Howell SB. Modulation of the cellular pharmacology of cisplatin and its analogs by the copper exporters ATP7A and ATP7B. Mol Pharmacol 2004; 66:25–32.

73. Samimi G, Safaei R, Katano K, et al. Increased expression of the copper efflux transporter ATP7A mediates resistance to cisplatin, carboplatin and oxaliplatin in ovarian cancer cells. Clin Cancer Res 2004; 10:4661–4669.

74. Safaei R, Samimi G, Holzer AK, et al. Intracellular localization and trafficking of fluorescein-labeled cisplatin in human ovarian carcinoma cells. Clin Cancer Res 2005; 11(Pt 1):756–767.

75. Samimi G, Varki NM, Wilczynski S, Safaei R, Alberts DS, Howell SB. Increase in expression of the copper transporter ATP7A during platinum drug-based treatment is associated with poor survival in ovarian cancer patients. Clin Cancer Res 2003; 9:5853–5859.

76. Katano K, Safaei R, Samimi G, Holzer A, Rochdi M, Howell SB. The copper export pump ATP7B modulates the cellular pharmacology of carboplatin in ovarian carcinoma cells. Mol Pharmacol 2003; 64:466–473.

77. Kanzaki A, Toi M, Neamati N, et al. Copper-transporting P-type adenosine triphosphatase (ATP7B) is expressed in human breast carcinoma. Jpn J Cancer Res 2002; 93:70–77.

78. Nakayama K, Kanzaki A, Ogawa K, Miyazaki K, Neamati N, Takebayashi Y. Copper-transporting P-type adenosine triphophatase (ATP7B) as a cisplatin-based chemoresistance marker in ovarian carcinoma: comparative analysis with expression of MDR1, MRP, LRP and BCRP. Int J Cancer 2002; 101:488–495.

79. Solioz M, Odermatt A, Krapf R. Copper pumping ATPases: common concepts in bacteria and man. FEBS Lett 1994; 346:44–47.

80. Nechay BR, Neldon SL. Characteristics of inhibition of human renal adenosine triphosphatases by cisplatin and chloroplatinic acid. Cancer Treat Rep 1984; 68:1135–1141.

81. Schilder RJ, Hall L, Monks A, et al. Metallothionein gene expression and resistance to cisplatin in human ovarian cancer. Int J Cancer 1990; 45:416–422.

82. Naredi P, Heath DD, Enns RE, Howell SB. Cross-resistance between cisplatin and antimony in a human ovarian carcinoma cell line. Cancer Res 1994; 54:6464–6468.

83. Mellish KJ, Kelland LR. Mechanisms of acquired resistance to the orally active platinum-based anticancer drug *bis*-acetato-ammine-dichloro-cyclohexylamine platinum (i.v.) (JM216) in two human ovarian carcinoma cell lines. Cancer Res 1994; 54:6194–6200.

84. Lee KB, Parker RJ, Reed E. Effect of cadmium on human ovarian cancer cells with acquired cisplatin resistance. Cancer Lett 1995; 88:57–66.

85. Singh SV, Xu BH, Jani JP, et al. Mechanism of cross-resistance to cisplatin in a mitomycin C-resistant human bladder cancer cell line. Int J Cancer 1995; 61:431–436.

86. Nicholson DL, Purser SM, Maier RH. Differential cytotoxicity of trace metals in cisplatin-sensitive and -resistant human ovarian cancer cells. Biometals 1998; 11:259–263.

87. Chen ZS, Mutoh M, Sumizawa T, et al. An active efflux system for heavy metals in cisplatin-resistant human KB carcinoma cells. Exp Cell Res 1998; 240:312–320.

88. Shen D-W, Pastan I, Gottesman MM. Cross-resistance to methotrexate and metals in human cisplatin-resistant cell lines results from a pleiotropic defect in accumulation of these compounds associated with reduced plasma membrane binding proteins. Cancer Res 1998; 58:268–275.

89. Yanagiya T, Imura N, Kondo Y, Himeno S. Reduced uptake and enhanced release of cadmium in cadmium-resistant metallothionein null fibroblasts. Life Sci 1999; 65:PL177–PL182.

90. Coronnello M, Marcon G, Carotti S, et al. Cytotoxicity, DNA damage, and cell cycle perturbations induced by two representative gold(III) complexes in human leukemic cells with different cisplatin sensitivity. Oncol Res 2000; 12:361–370.

91. Romach EH, Zhao CQ, Del Razo LM, Cebrian ME, Waalkes MP. Studies on the mechanisms of arsenic-induced self tolerance developed in liver epithelial cells through continuous low-level arsenite exposure. Toxicol Sci 2000; 54:500–508.

92. Higashimoto M, Kanzaki A, Shimakawa T, et al. Expression of copper-transporting P-type adenosine triphosphatase in human esophageal carcinoma. Int J Mol Med 2003; 11:337–341.

93. Miyashita H, Nitta Y, Mori S, et al. Expression of copper-transporting P-type adenosine triphosphatase (ATP7B) as a chemoresistance marker in human oral squamous cell carcinoma treated with cisplatin. Oral Oncol 2003; 39:157–162.

94. Ohbu M, Ogawa K, Konno S, et al. Copper-transporting P-type adenosine triphosphatase (ATP7B) is expressed in human gastric carcinoma. Cancer Lett 2003; 189:33–38.

95. Sugeno H, Takebayashi Y, Higashimoto M, et al. Expression of copper-transporting P-type adenosine triphosphatase (ATP7B) in human hepatocellular carcinoma. Anticancer Res 2004; 24:1045–1048.

96. Nakayama K, Kanzaki A, Terada K, et al. Prognostic value of the Cu-transporting ATPase in ovarian carcinoma patients receiving cisplatin-based chemotherapy. Clin Cancer Res 2004; 10:2804–2811.

18 Resistance To Taxanes

Lee M. Greenberger, PhD
and Deepak Sampath, PhD

CONTENTS

SUMMARY

Resistance to two taxanes, paclitaxel and docetaxel, is frequently observed in cancer patients and limits successful therapy. In experimental systems, resistance to paclitaxel and docetaxel are mediated by alterations in tubulin (the primary site of action of taxanes), proteins that interact with microtubules, energy-dependent efflux pumps, apoptotic proteins, and signal transduction pathways. Clinical correlations with some of these alterations exist, but have not been fully elucidated. Strategies to overcome or circumvent resistance to paclitaxel or docetaxel include inhibition of efflux pumps (which have largely proven to be unsuccessful), the use of novel taxanes or other chemically distinct classes of polymerizing agents that do not interact with drug efflux pumps (currently in clinical trials), and regulation of apoptotic or signal transduction pathways that would restore sensitivity to taxanes. Understanding the basis of resistance at the clinical level is likely to be difficult and complex, but holds the promise of providing a therapeutic opportunity specific to taxane-resistant cancer cells.

Key Words: Taxanes; resistance; microtubules; tubulin; transporters; P-glycoprotein; apoptosis; signal transduction.

From: *Cancer Drug Discovery and Development: Cancer Drug Resistance*
Edited by: B. Teicher © Humana Press Inc., Totowa, NJ

1. INTRODUCTION

Resistance is a relatively new chapter in the long history of taxanes and their use in oncology. Originally mentioned as toxic substances isolated from the leaves of the yew tree, such as *Taxus baccata* L. in 1856 *(1)*, as a component of clarified butter for use in treating cancer in 1912 *(2)*, and as a cytotoxic isolated from the bark of *T. brevifolia* in the National Cancer Institute's screening program in 1962 *(3)*, the first isolated taxane that had anticancer activity in tissue culture systems, designated taxol (Fig. 1), was reported in 1971 by Wall and coworkers *(4)*. A breakthrough came in 1979 when Susan Horwitz's laboratory found that taxol stabilized microtubules *(5)*, which was in contrast to the depolymerizing agents: vinca alkaloids and colchicine. It took an additional 13 years to develop a suitable formulation and source of taxol that ultimately led to its approval for use in cancer patients beginning in 1992 *(6)*. Taxol® is also known as paclitaxel; the latter name will be used in this chapter.

As early as 1978, and reaffirmed over the following decade, it was apparent that paclitaxel was not equally effective in human tumor xenograft model systems *(7)*. This was reemphasized in the early phase II trials that took place in the mid 1980s, where paclitaxel had good, weak, and poor activity when tested in patients with ovarian carcinoma, melanoma, and renal carcinoma, respectively *(8–10)*. Ultimately, paclitaxel was approved for use in patients with ovarian, lung, or breast cancers. Paclitaxel given as monotherapy to patients with these types of advanced cancers induces a 15–25% response rate and a 10- to 13-mo median survival time *(11)*. It is now apparent that patients with certain tumor types (i.e., colon and renal) have very low response rates to taxane-containing regimens and therefore, have inherent resistance. More insidious is the case where some patients initially respond to paclitaxel, but then fail to respond on repeated courses of therapy. These patients have acquired resistance. Therefore, resistance to taxanes is a major limiting factor in successful taxane therapy.

A second taxane, docetaxel (also known as Taxotere®) *(12)*, with good anticancer activity in preclinical models *(13)* was reported in 1991 and has also been used to treat lung and breast cancer since 1996 and 1999, respectively *(6)*. Paclitaxel and docetaxel are highly related molecules (*see* Fig. 1). Both contain a baccatin III core composed of four fused rings including a four-membered oxetane ring; the C-10 position is deacetylated in docetaxel. Both baccatin cores are esterified at the C-13 position of the A ring; paclitaxel and docetaxel have an *N*-benzoyl-β-phenylisoserine *(14)* and an *N-tert*-butoxycarbonyl-β-phenylisoserine *(12)* side chain, respectively.

It stands to reason that if the molecular basis for resistance to taxane were understood, then resistance to paclitaxel or docetaxel might be avoided. This chapter provides an overview of the mechanisms of resistance to taxanes. In the final analysis, one striking observation is clear. Resistance to taxanes is complex and can occur by multiple mechanisms including alteration in microtubules, transporters, proteins that regulate the cell cycle, apoptotic machinery, and signal transduction pathways (Fig. 2). The importance of these mechanisms regarding the treatment of human disease will require careful evaluation of qualitative and quantitative changes for each mechanism. Reassembling all the data, or perhaps finding key markers, will be necessary to identify those patients with tumors that will respond well to taxanes or require therapeutic strategies to circumvent resistance.

1.1. Microtubule Structure and Function

A working knowledge of how taxanes interact with its primary (but probably not only) target, the microtubule *(15)*, and how it induces cell death is needed before discussing

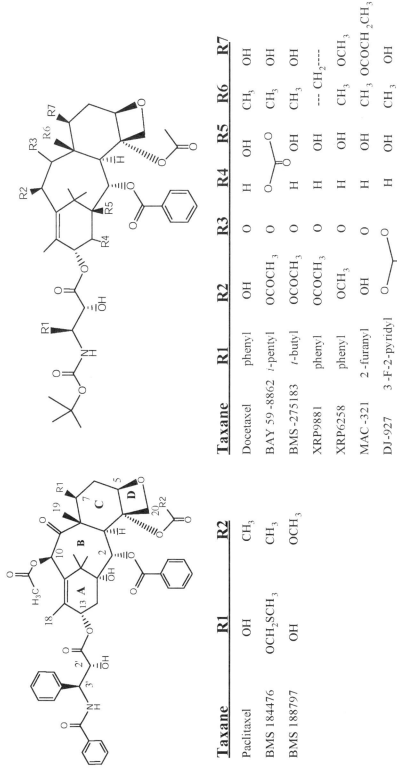

Fig. 1. Chemical structure of taxanes.

Taxane	R1	R2
Paclitaxel	OH	CH_3
BMS 184476	OCH_2SCH_3	CH_3
BMS 188797	OH	OCH_3

Taxane	R1	R2	R3	R4	R5	R6	R7
Docetaxel	phenyl	OH	O	H	OH	CH_3	OH
BAY 59-8862	i-pentyl	$OCOCH_3$	O	O–C(=O)–O	OH	CH_3	OH
BMS-275183	t-butyl	$OCOCH_3$	O	H	OH	CH_3	OH
XRP9881	phenyl	OCH_3	O	H	OH	--- CH_2---	
XRP6258	phenyl	OCH_3	O	H	OH	CH_3	OCH_3
MAC-321	2-furanyl	OH	O	H	OH	CH_3	$OCOCH_2CH_3$
DJ-927	3-F-2-pyridyl	O–CH_2–CH_2–N	O	H	OH	CH_3	OH

331

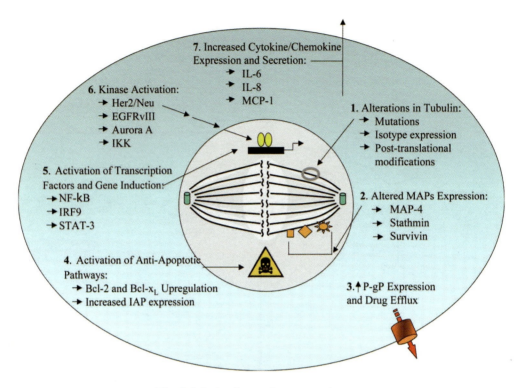

Fig. 2. Mechanisms of taxane resistance.

resistance mechanism. Microtubules are highly dynamic polymers whose essential element is the α/β-tubulin heterodimer (Fig. 3A). Each subunit binds GTP. One molecule is tightly bound to α-tubulin at a nonexchangeable site. The second molecule binds to a homologous site in β-tubulin at the exchangeable site; it undergoes hydrolysis and is required for normal tubulin polymerization. Under certain conditions, the dimer binds in a head to tail fashion to form linear protofilaments (Fig. 3A). About 13 protofilaments associate in parallel to a cylindrical axis to form the microtubule of 25 nm in diameter and up to micrometers in length. The polymer is initially formed from a short microtubule nucleus located at the so-called "–" end; in the case of the dividing cell this is found within the centrosome. Although the protofilament can grow from both ends, α-/β-tubulin dimers are added more quickly to the opposite or "+" end. The microtubule can elongate slowly or shorten rapidly by adding or removing tubulin dimers from the existing polymer, respectively. The conversion from growing to shrinking is called catastrophe, whereas the conversion from shrinking to growing is called rescue. The transition between these two behaviors is known as dynamic instability *(16)*.

How do microtubules participate in cell division? After chromosome replication during cell division, microtubules emanating from a centrosome undergo pronounced elongation and capture one of the sister chromatids at the kinetochore (central region of the chromosome). This can allow for rapid poleward movement of the bound chromosome. However, simultaneously or soon after this event, the sister kinetochore becomes attached to microtubules emanating from the opposite centrosome and the chromosomes align at the metaphase plate (*see* Fig. 3B). Then, during anaphase, the sister chromatids separate and move to the opposite poles; this is coordinated with widening of the distance

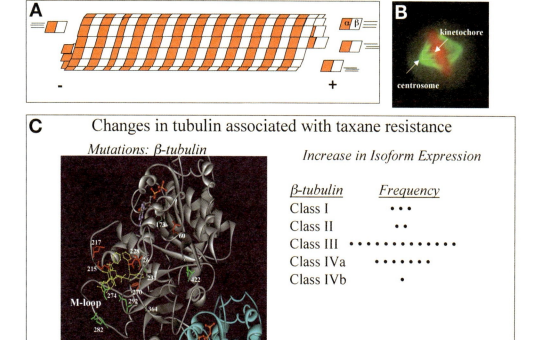

Fig. 3. Resistance to taxanes mediated by microtubules. (**A**) The α/β-tubulin heterodimer is the basic subunit of the protofilament. Net elongation of the protofilament can occur at both ends, but predominately by addition of the tubulin heterodimer to the "+" end. About 13 protofilaments associate to form the microtubule (boxed area in [**B**]). The +-end of the microtubule can switch from slow elongation (rescue) to rapid shrinking (catastrophe) resulting in dynamic instability. (B) Early in mitosis (prophase), the microtubules grow from the centrosome and capture the sister chromatids at the kinetochore. The microtubule (stained green using an antibody to tubulin) assist in assembling the chromatids (stained red using propidium iodide) at the metaphase plate. Once achieved, the sister chromatid separate during anaphase and move to the opposite poles. This is mediated, in part, by a shortening of the kinetochore microtubules. (**C**) Resistance to taxanes has been associated with point mutations in tubulin and overexpression of certain isoforms of tubulin. Point mutations found in paclitaxel (green)- or epothilone (red)-selected cell lines are shown with respect to the structure of β-tubulin cocrystallized with paclitaxel (indicated in yellow and located near the microtubule [M]-loop) (PDB accession code: 1JFF). The structure of GDP and GTP, within β- and α-tubulin, respectively, is indicated in the ball-and-stick model. A portion of α-tubulin is shown in the bottom right of the figure. The incidence of increased expression of isoforms of β-tubulin are tallied from Table 1 of ref. *20*.

between the poles. These events require rapid elongation and contraction of microtubules and are distinct compared with the relatively quiescent microtubules in the cytoplasm present during interphase. All antimicrotubule agents induce a blockage at the G_2/M phase of the cell cycle during the metaphase/anaphase transition by inhibiting the micro-tubule-dependent movement of sister chromatids to the opposite pole of the cell, as well as inhibiting the lengthening of the interpolar distance.

At substoichiometric ratios compared with tubulin, all antimitotics including taxanes act in a similar manner. They inhibit dynamic instability, causing improper tensioning of the mitotic apparatus and/or insufficient microtubule contraction required to move the chromosomes to the pole. At equal stoichiometric ratios, taxanes induce the polymerization of microtubules (in a GTP-independent manner) from purified tubulin *(5)* or in cells *(17)* and stabilize the microtubule against depolymerization. They do so by binding to the β-subunit *(18)* within polymerized tubulin *(19)*. A great deal of information on the molecular interaction of taxanes with tubulin have been obtained by: (1) mapping the sites of interaction of bovine brain tubulin with photoaffinity labeling analogs of paclitaxel *(20)*, (2) examining electron crystallographic interaction of taxanes with zinc-induced sheets of tubulin *(18,21)*, and (3) reevaluating the crystallographic data using fluorescence energy transfer spectroscopy and solid-state rotational echo double-resonance *(22)* or nuclear magnetic resonance studies *(23)*. The paclitaxel-binding site resides near the so-called microtubule (M)-loop within β-tubulin (*see* Fig. 3C). This region interacts with the H3 helix of the adjacent β-tubulin within the adjacent protofilament. It has been proposed that conformational changes in the M-loop that are induced by paclitaxel would stabilize the interaction between protofilaments *(18)*. Five other classes of structurally diverse natural products, epothilones, discodermolide, laulimalide, eleutherobin, sarcodictyins, also enhance tubulin polymerization *(15)*. The binding sites for epothilone A and paclitaxel overlap within tubulin but are distinct *(24)*.

1.2. Experimental Models of Taxane Resistance

Our understanding of the molecular basis of resistance to taxanes is founded largely on experimental work done using tumor cells grown in tissue culture or animals. Once established, the clinical correlation with the mechanism has been explored. This approach has some obvious limitations. In much of the work, when tumor cells in tissue culture are grown in the presence of continuous and multiple ascending concentrations of paclitaxel or docetaxel over a period of many weeks or months, they develop resistance to taxanes. It is clear that this type of exposure does not approximate the periodic exposure to taxanes in animals or humans (e.g., from every day for a short period up to once every 21 d), nor does it replicate the tumor environment. More-recent work has suggested relationships between taxane resistance and changes in the control of apoptosis, cell division, and signaling pathways. This work is also largely based on experiments in tissue culture where certain proteins have been manipulated or correlated with taxane resistance.

2. RESISTANCE TO TAXANES ASSOCIATED WITH CHANGES IN MICROTUBULES

At least four factors immediately related to tubulin can influence the polymerization state of microtubules and have been associated with taxane resistance. First, mutations in tubulin have been associated with taxane resistance. Second, changes in the expression of tubulin isomers can occur. In humans, six β-tubulin and at least five α-tubulin isoforms have been described *(25,26)*. The isomers are highly conserved with differences within a single species of 4–16% for β-tubulins and approximately 10% for α-tubulins *(26,27)*. The most variable regions are located in the last 15–20 amino acids of the carboxy terminal. The human (H)β-isoforms are grouped according to classes: class I, HM40; class II, Hβ9; class III, Hβ4, class IVa, Hβ5; class IVb, Hβ2; and class VI, HJβ1. The α-isoforms are classified as follows: group 1, bα-1 and kα-1; group 2, TUBA4; group 3, TUBA2; and group 4, TUBA8. Third, numerous other proteins that bind to tubulin, such as microtubule-associated proteins (MAPs) *(28)* and stathmins *(29)* stabilize and destabilize the microtubule, respectively. Fourth, posttranslational modifications of tubulin including glutamylation, glycylation, acetylation, tyrosination, and phosphorylation may alter polymerization of tubulin. All of these modifications, with the exception of acetylation, occur in the C-terminal 20 amino acids of tubulin. This region also is the same region that interacts with many MAPs. An excellent detailed review on the mechanisms of paclitaxel resistance related to microtubules is available *(20)*. An overview is provided here.

2.1. Mutations in Tubulin

Numerous point mutations in tubulin have been found in a variety of tumor cell lines selected for resistance to paclitaxel or have crossresistance to paclitaxel after cells are selected for resistance to epothilones. Cells selected for survival in the presence of paclitaxel are often coselected with a so-called P-glycoprotein-inhibitor, because P-glycoprotein frequently mediates resistance to paclitaxel by itself *(see* Section 3.). Most of the mutations are found in class I β-tubulin *(see* Fig. 3C), which is the predominate (and therefore, most easily assessed) isoform found in cancer cells *(30)*. Mutations are often found in a single tubulin allele and therefore, may be coexpressed with wild-type tubulin or if solely expressed, require that the wild-type gene be silenced. The mutations in β-tubulin associated with paclitaxel selection are: human $(h)26^{Asp \to Glu}$ *(31)*, hamster (ha) $26^{Asp \to Glu}$ *(32)*, ha $60^{Val \to Ala}$ *(32)*, ha $215^{Leu \to His}$ *(33)*, ha $215^{Leu \to Phe}$ *(33)*, ha $215^{Leu \to Arg}$ *(33)*, ha $217^{Leu \to Arg}$ *(33)*, ha $228^{Leu \to Phe}$ *(33)*, ha $228^{Leu \to His}$ *(33)*, and h $270^{Phe \to Val}$ *(34)*. The mutations in β-tubulin associated with epothilone A- or B-selection are: h $173^{Pro \to Ala}$ *(35)*, h $231^{Ala \to Thr}$ *(36)*, h $274^{Thr \to Ile}$ *(37)*, h $282^{Arg \to Gln}$ *(37)*, h $292^{Gln \to Glu}$ *(35,36)*, h $364^{Ala \to Thr}$ *(34)*, and h $422^{Tyr \to Cys}$ *(35)*. However, mutations are not limited to β-tubulin, because an A549 lung carcinoma selected for resistance to paclitaxel contains a mutation in kα-1 tubulin $(h$ $379^{Ser \to Arg})$ *(38)*. The differences between the mutations observed in paclitaxel- and epothilone-selected cells compared with the preferential resistance to selecting agent has been used, in conjunction with crystallographic data, to argue that paclitaxel and epothilone have similar binding domains in β-tubulin, but the binding pockets are unique *(24)*.

Mutations may reduce the affinity of paclitaxel to tubulin or alter the stability of tubulin. Consistent with the first possibility, residue 274^{Thr} makes contact with the oxetane ring of taxanes, residue 26^{Asp} makes contact with the C-3′ NHCO-phenyl group of paclitaxel, residue 270^{Phe} makes contact with paclitaxel's C3′ phenyl and C4-OAc groups, and residues 217^{Leu} and 219^{Leu} make hydrophobic contact with the two-phenyl ring of paclitaxel *(21)*. Consistent with the second possibility, mutations within the M-loop $(h$ $282^{Arg \to Gln})$ or residues that influence the orientation of the M-loop $(h$ $292^{Gln \to Glu})$ may influence lateral interaction between adjacent protofilaments. In addition, mutations near the C terminus $(\alpha\text{-}379^{Ser \to Arg}$, β$\text{-}364^{Ala \to Thr}$, and β$\text{-}422^{Tyr \to Cys})$ reside in regions that interact with MAPs, which by themselves alter microtubule stability. Finally, the Pro-to-Ala mutaton at β-173 occurs at a site that is involved with ribose binding at the exchangeable GTP site as well as longitudinal contacts between tubulin dimers *(35)*. GTP binding and hydrolysis is an essential regulatory mechansm of microtubule stability. The way that mutations would alter the stability is explained as follows *(39)*. Normally, cells control the ratio of polymerized microtubules to depolymerized tubulin. Any shift from a set point ratio could induce resistance. Therefore, paclitaxel-resistant cells may shift the equilibrium towards the depolymerized form of tubulin. This may explain why some paclitaxel-resistant cells with tubulin mutations actually become dependent on paclitaxel for growth *(31,35,38,39)* because the drug would be required to restore the set point ratio for proper cell growth. It would also explain why some paclitaxel-resistant cells display increase sensitivity to depolymerizing agents. If the latter occurred in patients, it may suggest novel therapeutic strategies using a sequence of polymerizing and depolymerizing agents.

It is important to note that a causal link between tubulin mutation and resistance has only been substantiated in a few cases where enforced expression of the mutant tubulin mediates paclitaxel resistance *(32,40)*, production of the putative mutated protein (predicted by cDNA analysis) is documented *(41)*, or the mutant tubulin and/or microtubules that presumably contained the mutant tubulin has altered polymerization properties *(32,34,37)*.

Similar to the way mutations in the epidermal growth factor receptor (EGFR) have been correlated with enhanced sensitivity to an EGFR inhibitor in patients *(42,43)*, one might expect to find mutations in tubulin in resistant patients. One study reported mutations in class I β-tubulin in the serum DNA isolated from 33% of patients with non-small cell lung cancer that were associated with resistance to paclitaxel *(44)*. However, the results have not been confirmed by subsequent studies where DNA or cDNA was obtained from tumor or serum samples *(45–48)*. In addition, no mutations in β-tubulin that encode a different protein structure have been found in 62 human breast cancers *(49)*. The discrepancy between the original report and subsequent studies is likely attributed to the use of nonselective primers used during polymerase chain reaction (PCR) amplification of β-tubulin that would allow hybridization of probes to tubulin pseudogenes present in genomic DNA *(46–48)*. The lack of positive results does not exclude the possibility that clinical resistance to paclitaxel is correlated with mutations in other isomers of α- or β-tubulin.

2.2. Changes in Tubulin Isoform Expression

It is likely that each isomer has different functional properties, and therefore, differential expression could mediate resistance. This is based on numerous experimental findings. *First*, each β-tubulin isotype has a unique pattern of expression in tissue *(50)*. For example, class βII predominates in brain tissue, βIII and IVa are found primarily in neurons, and class I and IVb are constitutively expressed. Based on PCR analysis, 17 human tumor cell lines of diverse origin predominately expressed class βI (range 76.0–99.7%) and class βIII (range: 0.2–11.0 %) *(30)*. In contrast, based on protein analysis using human breast tissue, class βII is the most highly expressed isoform (58% compared with total tubulin derived from classes I, II, and IV), no differences are observed between tumor and breast tissue, and protein expression does not correlate with tubulin mRNA levels using PCR analysis *(51)*. A similar lack of correlation between tubulin isotype protein expression and mRNA levels has been noted in other paclitaxel-resistant cell lines *(41)*. Based on protein expression analysis, human breast, lung, and cervical lung carcinoma cell lines predominately express Kα-1, α6-tubulins (α6-tubulin has a distinct amino acid sequence compared with all the tubulin isoforms mentioned above) *(52,53)*. *Second*, the rate of tubulin polymerization and microtubule dynamics depends on the isotype composition *(54–57)*. In particular, microtubules assembled from purified αβIII isotype (from bovine brain) are more dynamic than microtubules made from αβII or αβIV isotypes *(57)*, and even mixing αβII and αβIII isomers (1:1) behave differently compared with monoisomeric studies. *Third*, changes in isoform expression, particularly in βIII and βIV, are correlated with paclitaxel resistance.

A list of alterations in isoform expression and its association with paclitaxel resistance across approximately 15 paclitaxel-resistant tumor cell lines has been previously summarized *(20)*. In most paclitaxel-selected cell lines, an elevation in the expression of the βIII or βIV isoforms (range: two- to ninefold), which is based on reverse transcription-PCR methodology, is correlated with low-level of paclitaxel resistance (usually under 10-fold) compared with parental cells (*see* Fig. 3C). In addition, the expression level of more than one isoform can be altered. Overexpression of the βIII and βIV isoforms are also found in non-drug-selected, paclitaxel-resistant cell lines. For example, in 17 non-drug-selected cancer cell lines, a significant correlation with paclitaxel resistance is found only with the level of βIII expression ($r^2 = 0.61$, $p < 0.007$) and is not associated with resistance to three depolymerizing agents *(30)*. More importantly, a clinical correlation has been reported by Kavallaris et al., who found a significant increase in classes βI (3.6-fold), III (4.4-fold), and IVa (7.6-fold) isotypes in tumors from paclitaxel resistant patients compared with untreated primary ovarian tumors *(58)*.

One group has reported that changes in α-tubulin may influence paclitaxel resistance because it is overexpressed (along with β-tubulin) in a multidrug resistance protein (MDR)1-expressing H460 lung carcinoma cell line that was 1000-fold resistant to paclitaxel *(59)*. Consistent with this, downregulation of Kα-1 tubulin by antisense methodologies in the drug resistant cell line increases the sensitivity to paclitaxel by 50%, whereas overexpression of Kα-1 in drug parental cells confers approximately a two- to threefold increase in resistance to a few anti microtubule agents including paclitaxel *(59)*.

Does this association with altered β-tubulin isoform expression imply a causal relationship? The evidence is controversial. In favor of this possibility, microtubules composed of βIII or βIV tubulin are less sensitive to the suppressive effects of paclitaxel on microtubule dynamics *(56)*, and bovine brain depleted of βIII tubulin has enhanced sensitivity to paclitaxel *(55)*. In addition, downregulation of βIII tubulin by antisense oligonucleotides in paclitaxel-resistant A549-T24 cells increases the sensitivity to paclitaxel, albeit a modest 1.6-fold *(60)*, whereas moderate overexpression of human βIII tubulin in CHO cells increases resistance to paclitaxel 1.5- to 2-fold *(61)*. Arguing against this relationship are the facts that stable overexpression of class I, II, III (that contained a point mutation), or IVb by transfection methods fails to confer resistance to paclitaxel *(50,62,63)*. The meaning of the negative data remains controversial, because among other problems, tubulin expression is tightly controlled in cells and compensatory changes in response to over- or underexpression of the class II or IV isoforms may confound the analysis *(63)*. Beyond this, many MAPs bind to the variable C-terminal regions of tubulin isoforms, so differential MAP expression may also contribute to resistance. Ultimately, detecting quantitative differences in the expression of tubulin isoforms in patients who may not be responsive to paclitaxel will be a challenge. This is underscored by the work of Dozier et al., who used immunocytochemistry, enzyme-linked immunosorbent assay methodology (to measure protein levels), and PCR methodology (to measure mRNA levels) to assess tubulin isoform expression in normal and tumor breast tissue *(51)*. He found that βIII expression, which is low compared to other isoforms, is predominately isolated to nerve fibers and not tumor cells. In addition, the level of expression of mRNA does not correlate with βIII protein expression.

2.3. Changes in Microtubule-Associated Proteins

MAPs can alter the state of polymerization and therefore, may influence sensitivity to taxanes. Two MAPs, τ and MAP-2, are primarily found in neurons and are not very relevant to the discussion here, although, Veitia et al. report higher τ expression in docetaxel-sensitive tumors (64). MAP-4 is present in all nonneuronal tissue (28). It stabilizes microtubules by increasing the rescue frequency without altering the catastrophe frequency. The protein is localized to mitotic spindle and interphase microtubules. Like other MAPs, phosphorylation of MAP-4 results in loss of binding and stabilization of microtubules and can undergo cell-cycle dependent phosphorylation. Therefore, a decrease in MAP-4 expression or an increase in MAP-4 phosphorylation may shift microtubules to a more destabilized state and therefore, mediate resistance to paclitaxel. Consistent with this hypothesis, an increase in MAP-4 phosphorylation is associated with paclitaxel resistance in paclitaxel-selected ovarian cell lines (65) and an A549 paclitaxel-selected cell line (38). Furthermore, enhanced expression of MAP-4 by transfection methods or as occurring in p53 mutant cells stabilizes microtubules and slightly enhances paclitaxel sensitivity (66). However, contrary to this prediction, overexpression of MAP-4 is found in epothilone-selected leukemic cell lines that are also 15-fold resistant to paclitaxel (36).

In contrast to MAP-4, stathmin destabilizes microtubules. It does so by either sequestering tubulin dimers, which would block the formation of microtubules, or by stimulating microtubule +-end catastrophe (29,67). Stathmin associates longitudinally along the lateral border of tubulin dimers causing a bend in the microtubule that does not allow polymerization (68,69). Consistent with this, stathmin inhibits paclitaxel-induced polymerization of microtubules from purified tubulin (70). The protein is deactivated by phosphorylation mediated by a variety of kinases, including those that participate in G_2/M phase of the cell cycle (29). Therefore, overexpression of stathmin or dephosphorylation of the protein would shift microtubules to a depolymerized state and may mediate resistance to paclitaxel. Experimental data fit this hypothesis. Stathmin levels increase in paclitaxel-selected A549 lung carcinoma cells (by twofold) or in A2780/1A9 ovarian cells (by two- to threefold) that are resistant to paclitaxel or epothilone (38,71). Of course, other changes including mutations in tubulin and changes in MAP-4 levels have been observed in these same cells. Furthermore, downregulation of stathmin by antisense methodologies enhances sensitivity to paclitaxel (72).

Other MAPs may influence paclitaxel sensitivity and are just beginning to be explored. These include the microtubule-based motor proteins, the kinesins and dyneins (73), an apoptotic regulatory protein that binds to microtubules, survivin (see Section 4.) (74), and many recently described microtubule plus-end tracking proteins (75,76).

2.4. Posttranslational Changes

A few associations between changes in posttranslational modifications of tubulin and paclitaxel resistance have been observed. Enhanced acetylation of α-tubulin has been found in a low-level paclitaxel-resistant small cell lung carcinoma cell line (77). Enhanced tyrosinyated α-tubulin coordinated with an increase in total α-tubulin has been observed in an MCF-7/paclitaxel-selected cell line (78). In contrast, tubulin isolated from A549 or HeLa cell lines selected for resistance to paclitaxel and epothilone, respectively, are not extensively posttranslationally modified and even so, little changes in posttranslational modifications of tubulin isoforms exist in resistant cells (41). It remains unclear if posttranslational modifications of tubulin might effect microtubule stability associated with taxane resistance attributable to a direct effect on the microtubule or its interaction with regulatory proteins that might bind in the same region as the posttranslational modification.

3. RESISTANCE TO TAXANES ASSOCIATED WITH TRANSPORTERS

Unlike water-soluble drugs, hydrophobic drugs such as paclitaxel and docetaxel probably diffuse into the cell membrane without the need for any specific carrier protein. However, entry and exit of hydrophobic agents from the cell membrane can be regulated by a variety of ATP-binding cassette (ABC)-transporters. Of the 48 ABC transporters in the human genome, four have been associated with resistance to paclitaxel and docetaxel (79,80). They are P-glycoprotein encoded by MDR1 (according to the ABC classification system, designated ABCB1); sister of P-gylcoprotein (also known as the bile salt export protein, encoded by ABCB11), multidrug resistance protein MRP7 (encoded by ABCC10), and MDR3 (sometimes called MDR2 and encoded by ABCB4). Transfection of cells with ABC11 confers low level of resistance to paclitaxel in one of two reports (81,82). Cells transfected with MDR3, which primarily transports phosphatidylcholine, transports paclitaxel inefficiently and does not display resistance to paclitaxel (83). Recently, Kruh's laboratory reported that transfection of HEK-293 cells with MRP7 mediates approximately 10-fold resistance to docetaxel, threefold resistance to paclitaxel, and vinca alkaloids, but no resistance to doxorubuicin or cisplatin (84). The latter three transporters will not be discussed further.

P-glycoprotein, like many ABC transporters, is composed of two halves, each containing six transmembrane domains and an ATP-binding site, connected by a linker region (Fig. 4). On binding paclitaxel, docetaxel, or a variety of other cancer chemotherapeutic agents, such as vinca alkaloids, anthracyclines, mitoxantrone, and bisantrene to the transmembrane region of P-glycoprotein, ATP hydrolysis is used to expel these agents from cells (79,80). The evidence that P-glycoprotein mediates resistance to paclitaxel and docetaxel in experimental models is strong for the following reasons. First, expression of P-glycoprotein by transfection methods or as it occurs endogenously in tumor cell lines (e.g., certain colon carcinomas) is associated with resistance to paclitaxel or docetaxel. Second, P-glycoprotein expression increases remarkably in numerous tumor cell lines selected for resistance to paclitaxel, docetaxel, or other substrates for P-glycoprotein. The level of P-glycoprotein increases with the amount of resistance to paclitaxel, although there may not be linear relationship. In extreme cases, where resistance to paclitaxel or docetaxel can exceed 1000-fold, P-glycoprotein overexpression is extraordinarily pronounced and is usually mediated by gene amplification. This is aphysiological. However, KB-8-5 HeLa cells (which were selected for resistance to continuous low-level exposure to colchicine) (85), or MES-SA sarcoma cells (which were selected for only 7 d in the presence of 10 nM paclitaxel) (86) have low to moderate P-glycoprotein expression and are 20- to 40-fold resistant to paclitaxel. This is likely to be physiological, because the level of P-glycoprotein expression in KB-8-5 cells is at the upper end of the range found in certain types of tumors (87,88). Remarkably, the growth of tumors derived from KB-8-5 cells in nude mice are completely unresponsive to paclitaxel given at the maximum tolerated dose (and optimal schedule), whereas the growth of tumors derived from KB, parental cells that are treated the same way are completely inhibited by paclitaxel (89). Third, agents that inhibit the function of P-glycoprotein, the so-called reversal agents such as verapamil and cyclosporine A, resensitize P-glycoprotein-expressing cells to paclitaxel, whereas they have little or no effect on cells that do not overexpress P-glycoprotein. Fourth, paclitaxel can be used to enrich for cells that express viral-directed exogenous P-glycoprotein in vivo (90), even many months after insertion of the

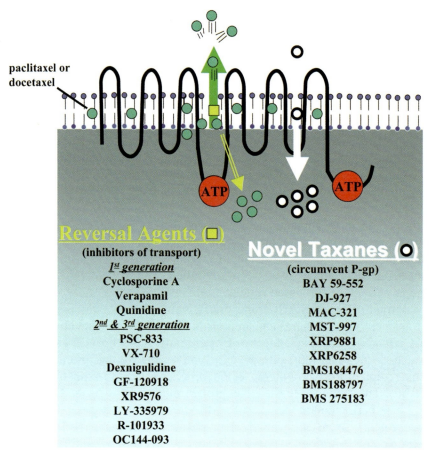

Fig. 4. Resistance to taxanes mediated by P-glycoprotein. P-glycoprotein is an ATP-dependent transporter that is embedded in the plasma membrane. Paclitaxel or docetaxel (both indicated in green), diffuse into the membrane and are actively expelled (green arrow) by P-glycoprotein. Reversal agents (yellow) bind to P-glycoprotein and inhibit the transport of taxanes, thereby increasing the intracellular concentrations of paclitaxel or docetaxel to cytotoxic levels. Certain novel taxanes (white) circumvent P-glycoprotein (P-gp) because they are not effectively expelled by P-glycoprotein.

gene and apparent loss of protein expression *(91)*. Finally, further evidence is obtained in mice where P-glycoprotein has been deleted by genetic methods *(80)*. Normally, P-glycoprotein is expressed at the blood–brain barrier as well as the luminal (apical) surface of cells that line the gastrointestinal tract, the fetal–maternal interface, and hepatobilary interface (in hepatocytes). However, mice that have a deletion of one or more P-glycoprotein isoforms (known as mdr1a and mdr1b) have altered pharmacokinetics of paclitaxel. In particular, the oral bioavailability of paclitaxel increases from 11% in wild-type mice to 35% in the mdr1a knockout mice *(92)*. Furthermore, when paclitaxel is given orally, fecal excretion (the normal route of elimination of paclitaxel) is reduced from 40 (after intravenous administration) and 87% (after oral administration) in wild-type animals compared with <3% observed in knockout animals. Consistent with this, oral absorption of paclitaxel markedly improves if it is coadministered with a P-glycoprotein reversal agent such as cyclosporine A or its derivative, PSZ-833, in mice *(93,94)* and in humans *(95,96)*.

The interaction of P-glycoprotein with docetaxel is not exactly the same as paclitaxel. Similar to paclitaxel, docetaxel can be transported by P-glycoprotein (97,98), cells that overexpress P-glycoprotein can be highly resistant to docetaxel (89,99), and cyclosporine A enhances the bioavailability of docetaxel in patients ninefold (100). However, the bioavailability of docetaxel is increased to 23% in mdr1a/b$^{-/-}$ animals, which is lower compared with paclitaxel (94,101). In addition, total plasma exposure is unchanged for docetaxel, but increases twofold for paclitaxel in the knockout animals compared with wild-type animals. Furthermore, an inhibitor of CYP3A4, ritonavir, which has only minor inhibiting properties of P-glycoprotein, increases the exposure of docetaxel by 50-fold in mice (101). Cyclosporine A also inhibits cytochrome P450 3A4 (102), and therefore, it may inhibit both P-glycoprotein-mediated absorption and one of the two cytochrome P450 enzymes that inactivate paclitaxel or docetaxel (the other enzyme is cytochrome P450 2C8) (103). Therefore, alterations in taxane metabolism may influence drug resistance.

If P-glycoprotein plays an important role in resistance to paclitaxel in patients, then the protein should be overexpressed or have increased functionality in resistant patients. Is this true? In support of this, the highest P-glycoprotein levels are found in many (but not all) colon and renal carcinomas (87,88) that are resistant to paclitaxel or docetaxel. However, expression of P-glycoprotein is much more subtle and variable in breast, lung, and ovarian carcinomas that are 16–55% (104–106), 15–30% (107–110), and 16–47% (111–113) positive for P-expression by immunocytochemical methods, respectively. In a meta-analysis using 31 reports, Trock et al. found that breast cancer patients who are positive for P-glycoprotein expression are three times more likely to fail to respond to chemotherapy (which contained taxanes in some regimens) than patients whose tumors are P-glycoprotein-negative (114). However, the association was not confirmed in a recent study where the expression of P-glycoprotein was compared in greater than 60 breast carcinoma patients before and after chemotherapy (106). Exactly how much P-glycoprotein or what increase in P-glycoprotein functionality is needed to cause patients to failure to respond to paclitaxel is not known. If a small change in expression is relevant, can it be reliably detected with the current histological methods? Despite efforts to standardize the methods (115), they may not be able to discern subtle changes with certainty.

3.1. Reversal of P-Glycoprotein-Mediated Resistance

Assuming P-glycoprotein is relevant in the clinic, then there might be two ways to circumvent such resistance. The first method is to inhibit the expression or function of P-glycoprotein. The second method would be to use chemotherapeutic agents that do not interact with P-glycoprotein. In the first case, numerous P-glycoprotein reversal agents have been coadministered with substrates for P-glycoprotein, including taxanes (see Fig. 4). First-generation reversal agents described in the 1980s, such as verapamil, cyclosporine A, and quinidine, have been followed by second- and third-generation agents that include PSC-833 (valspodar), dexniguldipine, VX-710 (biricodar), GF-120918 (elacridar), XR9576 (tariquidar), LY-335979 (zosuquidar), R-101933 (laniquidar), and OC144-093 (ONT-093) (79,116,117). The latter agents are devoid of unwanted side effects (i.e., calcium channel blocking or immunosuppressive activity) and are more potent than original reversal agents. The agents work by binding to P-glycoprotein and blocking its ability to transport substrates. Trials with reversal agents in patients with acute myelogenous leukemia have been logical starting point, because an inverse relationship has been estab-

lished between P-glycoprotein expression and function with response to chemotherapy *(118–120)*. Whereas addition of cyclosporine A to daunorubicin and cytarabine therapy for acute myelogenous leukemia reduces resistance, improves duration of remission, and enhances overall survival *(121)*, studies with the a nonimmunosuppressive analog of cyclosporine, PSC-833, in combination with the same agents, daunorubicin and etoposide, or mitoxantrone, etoposide, and cytarabine do not produce marked benefit *(122–124)*. In addition, reversal agents combined with cytotoxic agents do not add significant benefit for the treatment of drug-resistant solid tumors *(125)*, including a regimen that used paclitaxel monotherapy combined with PSC-833 in patients with refractory ovarian carcinoma *(126)*. The interpretation of these clinical studies is obscured because in many cases a dose reduction of paclitaxel (as well as other chemotherapeutic agents) is required to achieve acceptable toxicity *(116,127,128)*. This is because of an alteration in the clearance of such agents mediated by P-glycoprotein, other transporters, or metabolizing enzymes as described above *(127–130)*. Beyond this, many of the clinical trials have not determined P-glycoprotein expression levels, nor correlated P-glycoprotein expression levels with response to reversal agent therapy. In theory, P-glycoprotein positive patients would be the only ones to benefit from such therapy. It may be possible to identify these patients and the activity of reversal agents in the tumor using imaging methods *(79)*.

Some of the newer P-glycoprotein reversal agents, such as XR-9576 *(131)*, LY-335979 *(132,133)*, R101933 *(134)*, and OC144-093 *(135)*, which do not influence the plasma pharmocokinetics of clinically used taxanes and/or have reduced interaction with metabolic enzymes involved in taxane metabolism, may prove to be more promising agents. Clinical evaluation of some of these agents is in progress. However, based on the experiments using knockout animals, all reversal agents would be expected to enhance the toxicity of paclitaxel or docetaxel in any cell or compartment expressing P-glycoprotein. It is also important to note that GF120918 also inhibits the ABCG2 transporter *(136)*; this transporter is not involved with taxane transport but its use may confound certain combination studies. Other strategies designed to inhibit P-glycoprotein expression at the mRNA or DNA levels are summarized elsewhere *(117)*.

3.2. Circumventing P-Glycoprotein-Mediated Resistance

An alternative approach to overcome P-glycoprotein-mediated resistance to taxanes is to identify taxanes or taxane-like molecules that do not interact with P-glycoprotein (*see* Fig. 4). Several such taxane analogs exist including SBT-1213, BAY 59-8862 (IDN5109, SB-T-101131, ortataxel) *(137,138)*, DJ-927 *(139)*, MAC-321 (TL-139) *(89)*, MST-997 (TL-909) *(140)*, XRP9881 (RPR 109881A) *(141)*, XRP6258 (RPR 116258A) *(142)*, BMS-184476 and BMS-188797 *(143)*, and BMS-275183 *(144,145)*. Because the structures of these compounds are highly related to paclitaxel or docetaxel (*see* Fig. 1), subtle changes in the structure of taxanes markedly influences their interaction with P-glycoprotein. For example, resistance to MAC-321 *(89)* and MST-997 *(140,146)* is 1- and 40-fold in cells that express low and high-levels of P-glycoprotein (compared with parental cells), whereas resistance to paclitaxel is 20- and 1000-fold in the same cells, respectively. All of these novel taxanes when given intravenously retain antitumor activity in animal models using tumors that overexpress P-glycoprotein and are insensitive to paclitaxel *(89,138–140,146,147)*. Oral activity with BMS-275813, XRP6258, BAY 59-8862, MAC-321, MST-997, and DJ-927 (but not paclitaxel or docetaxel) has been demonstrated in experimental tumor models. This is presumably because of their weak

interaction with P-glycoprotein in the gastrointestinal tract or hepatocytes located at the biliary interface. One of the most advanced agents, XRP9881 *(148)*, demonstrates a 29% partial response rate in metastatic breast cancer patients who have failed previous taxane therapy. A phase III trial in metastatic breast cancer with XRP9881 is underway. BMS-275183*(145)*, BMS-184476*(149,150)*, BMS-188797*(151)*, MAC-321 *(152,153)*, MST-997, BAY 59-8862 *(154–156)*, and DJ927 *(157)* are in phase I or II clinical trials. A variation of this approach is to use novel microtubule polymerizing agents besides taxane analogs that do not interact with P-glycoprotein. Three types of such agents, epothilones *(158)*, discodermolide *(159)*, and laulimalide *(160)*, induce microtubule polymerization, are poor substrates for P-glycoprotein, and retain some activity in paclitaxel-selected cells that have mutations in tubulin *(37,161)*. Epothilone and discodermolide bind to a similar, but distinct, site compared with paclitaxel *(24,35,37)*, whereas laulimalide probably does not because it cannot inhibit the binding of paclitaxel to tubulin *(161)*. Several epothilone analogs are in clinical trials *(159)*.

4. CONTROL OF APOPTOSIS

Because cell division is a highly regulated event, resistance to taxanes could also be mediated by changes in the regulation of cell division beyond microtubules. When the mitotic apparatus is impaired cells can arrest at prometaphase or pass through mitosis without cell division and become aneuploid *(162)*. This signals a cascade of phosphorylation- and caspase-dependent events leading to apoptosis or programmed cell death *(74,163)*. Apoptosis, in turn, is also a highly ordered event orchestrated by multiple pathways that utilize positive and negative regulatory proteins. Therefore, it is conceivable that changes in the activity or expression of proteins that control cell cycle progression and apoptosis can influence sensitivity to taxanes, as well as a variety of other chemotherapeutic drugs.

Mammalian cells use two main pathways to undergo apoptosis: the extrinsic and intrinsic pathways (Fig. 5) *(74)*. The extrinsic signaling pathway is mediated by death receptors (DR) such as subsets of the prototypical tumor necrosis factor (TNF) receptor, which binds TNF-related apoptosis-inducing ligand (TRAIL), also known as TRAIL/ Apo-2L, and Fas/CD95, which binds Fas ligand (FasL) or agonistic anti-Fas antibodies *(164,165)*. Ligand-induced oligomerization of DRs mediates the recruitment and assembly of the adaptor protein, Fas-associated protein with death domain, and cysteine aspartyl-specific proteases (caspase) 8 into a death-inducing signaling complex. Assembly of the death-inducing signaling complex juxtaposes multiple procaspase 8 zymogens, resulting in autocatalytic cleavage and activation of caspase 8, leading to further downstream cleavage of the effector procaspases 3, 6, and 7. Interestingly, there is tantalizing evidence that suggests paclitaxel resistance is associated with TNF-α or TRAIL expression. First, relatively high concentrations of paclitaxel induces TNF-α expression in murine macrophages *(166,167)* associated with apoptosis that is blocked by antibodies against TNF-α *(168)*. Second, nanomolar concentrations of paclitaxel promotes TRAIL-induced apoptosis through Akt inactivation in a renal carcinoma cell line, but not a normal renal epithelial cell line *(169)*. Similarly, TRAIL is ineffective as a single agent but enhances sensitivity to paclitaxel in two ovarian carcinoma cell lines *(170)*. Finally, paclitaxel as well as a variety of chemotherapeutic agents induce DR family members and sensitivity to TRAIL-induced apoptosis in breast cancer cell line grown in vitro or in vivo *(171)*. However, the utility of TRAIL in the clinic (and its association with paclitaxel resistance in patients) needs further exploration.

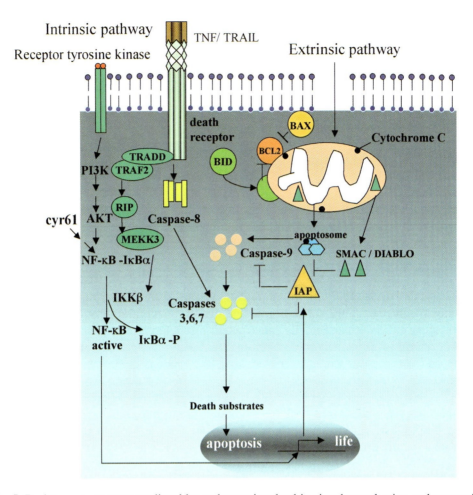

Fig. 5. Resistance to taxanes mediated by pathways involved in signal transduction and apoptosis. Pathways that mediate death and life regulate apoptosis. In the intrinsic pathway, tumore necrosis factor (TNF) or TNF-related apoptosis-inducing ligand (TRAIL) bind to the death receptor. A ligand-bound death receptor activates caspase 8, which in turn activates effector caspases 3, 6, and 7. The same receptor also activates inhibitory (I)κBα kinase (IKK)β, which allows nuclear factor of κB (NF-κB) to move to the nucleus and activate transcription of antiapoptotic genes such as inhibitors of apoptosis proteins (*IAP*) (shown) or Bcl-2 (not shown). NF-κB can also be activated by growth factor receptors (via AKT) or extracellular matrix protein cysteine-rich 61 (Cyr61). In the extrinsic pathway, cell death is regulated when the mitochondrial permeability is inhibited by Bcl-2 or promoted by BAX, thereby controlling the release of cytochrome *c*. Cytoplasmic cytochrome *c* mediates activation of the apoptosome, caspase 9, and ultimately, caspases 3, 6, and 7. Activation of caspases can be in inhibited by IAPs. The mitochondria also can release second mitochondria-derived activator of caspases (SMAC/ DIABLO). SMAC/DIABLO promotes apoptosis by inhibiting IAP. Overexpression or hyperactivation of the NF-κB pathway, IAP, or Bcl-2 can mediate resistance to taxanes. (Adapted with permission from refs. *231* and *232*, respectively. *See* also www.nature.com/reviews).

The mitochondrial or intrinsic pathway is primarily initiated by release of cytochrome *c* and protein factors from the mitochondrial inner membrane space (*see* Fig. 4) *(172)*. These factors include second mitochondria-derived activator of caspases and Omi/HtrA2 (a serine protease) and mediate caspase disinhibtion *(163)*. Accumulation of cytochrome *c* in the cytoplasm results in binding to the scaffolding protein, apoptotic protease activa-

tion factor-1 (Apaf-1), causing a dATP/ATP conformational change that allows binding and autocatalytic cleavage of procaspase 9 *(173)*. The formation of this macromolecular complex, termed the apoptosome, leads to effector procaspases 3, 6, and 7 cleavage and downstream activation of sentinel cell death events.

Within the cytosol, both the extrinsic and intrinsic pathways are regulated by the *Bcl-2* super family of genes, which are defined by the conserved bcl homology domains. Based on their ability to either induce or inhibit the apoptosis cascade, the Bcl-2 proteins can be subdivided into three subfamily members *(174)*. The first subset inhibits apoptosis and includes Bcl-2, Bcl-x_L, and Mcl-1. The second family members, Bax and Bak, translocate into the outer mitochondrial membrane space and oligomerize into voltage-gated pore complexes resulting in the release of cytochrome *c* and other polypeptides (as described above) in the intrinsic pathway. Lastly, Bid, Bim, and Bad are proapoptotic proteins that function primarily as transdominant inhibitors that bind and neutralize Bcl-2 cell survival activity. In addition, activated caspase 8 can cleave Bid at the C terminus (tBid) and facilitate oligomerization of Bax and Bak at the mitochondrial membrane thereby linking the extrinsic and intrinsic death pathways *(174)*. Conversely, antiapoptotic Bcl-2 and Bcl-x_L, can bind and antagonize proapoptotic Bax and Bak, thus preventing dimerization and subsequent pore formation; a salient feature in tumor cell survival. Bcl-2 members are typically regulated posttranslationally by a number of different growth factor and cytokine signaling pathways *(174)*.

Changes in the levels or posttranslational modifications of Bcl-2 family members have been associated with taxane resistance. For example, the primary mechanism of paclitaxel- and docetaxel-induced cell death is hyperphosphorylation of Bcl-2 and Bcl-x_L as well as Bax upregulation *(175–177)*. Moreover, biotinylated paclitaxel can bind and sequester Bcl-2, and therefore suggests that taxane-induced cell death may be mediated by microtubule-independent mechanisms *(178)*. The net effect of hyperphosphorylation of, or direct binding to, these proteins result in the inability of Bcl-2 or Bcl-x_L to antagonize Bak or Bax, thereby leading to apoptosis. Alternatively, upregulation of Bcl-2 or Bcl-x_L by ectopic expression or continuous exposure to paclitaxel can lead to resistance *(179,180)*. The primary mechanism of resistance involves the inhibition of the mitochondrial pathway as increased levels of Bcl-2 sequestered Bax and Bak and prevented cytochrome *c* release *(181)*. Growth factors or hormone driven induction of Bcl-2 can also lead to paclitaxel resistance. For example, exposure to estrogen in estrogen receptor-positive MCF-7 breast carcinoma cell lines leads to an increase in Bcl-2 levels and resistance to paclitaxel-induced apoptosis, whereas cotreatments with antiestrogens restored sensitivity *(182)*. However, whereas the overall levels of Bcl-2 increased, Bax and Bak remained unchanged. At the level of the apoptosome, loss of Apaf-1 expression in Apaf-1$^{-/-}$ cells has also been shown to confer resistance to apoptosis mediated by paclitaxel, whereas ectopic overexpression of Apaf-1 sensitized leukemia cells to paclitaxel-induced apoptosis *(183,184)*. Thus altering the relative ratio of Bcl-2 family members either by overexpression, growth factor induction, or inhibition by paclitaxel itself can lead to a loss of drug sensitivity.

Given that the rate-limiting step in apoptosis is caspase activation, a class of proteins termed inhibitors of apoptosis proteins (IAPs) that directly bind and inhibit caspases, provide another level of regulation *(185)*. This class includes XIAP, cIAP-1, cIAP-2, and survivin, which are linked by conserved baculoviral inhibitor repeats domains that are responsible for caspase inhibition. Survivin is particularly relevant to taxane resistance, because it is localized to the mitotic apparatus and plays a dual role monitoring spindle integrity and regulating cell death *(74)*. More specifically, survivin is upregulated during the G_2/M phase of the cell cycle and is subsequently localized to the centrosome, polymerized microtubules of the metaphase and anaphase spindle, and midbodies *(74)*. Inhibition of phosphorylation of Thr-34 within survivin by purvanalol A (an inhibitor of cyclin dependent kinase 1) or overexpression of dominant negative survivin enhances paclitaxel-induced cell death in vitro and in vivo in MCF7 breast tumor lines *(186,187)*. In addition, ectopic expression of survivin is able to counteract apoptosis induced by paclitaxel in NIH3T3 fibroblasts *(188)*. Moreover, high levels of survivin are associated with advanced ovarian carcinomas that are resistant to paclitaxel/platinum therapy but not nonpaclitaxel-based regimens *(189)*. In the same study, when ovarian carcinoma cells are selected for paclitaxel resistance by continuous exposure, the levels of phosphorylated survivin are elevated implying increased activation *(190)*. Clinically, survivin expression is of prognostic importance, given that it is upregulated in a wide variety of solid and liquid tumor types, it is associated with more-aggressive disease, and in colorectal cancer, decreased 5-yr survival rates are observed in tumors that have elevated levels of survivin *(74)*. Another interesting mediator of taxane resistance is XIAP, which is overexpressed in a variety of tumors including those derived from lung, breast, and colon *(191)*. Moreover, small molecule inhibitors of XIAP that potentiate the toxicity of paclitaxel and other chemotherapeutic agents have been identified *(192)*. Thus, modulating the rate-limiting enzymatic activity of caspases by altering the levels and activity of inhibitors, such as the IAPs, can lead to paclitaxel resistance.

5. ACTIVATION OF TRANSCRIPTION FACTORS

Drug resistance is typically associated with alterations in gene expression by activation or inhibition of transcription factors. For example, pathways that regulate the transcription factor, nuclear factor of κB (NF-κB), plays an important role in governing multiple apoptotic and survival mechanisms *(193)*. NF-κB is often constitutively activated in many types of tumor types. Currently, there are five known members of the NF-κB family members which are distinguished by their reticuloendotheliosis homology domain, the portion of the protein that controls DNA binding and dimerization *(194)*. The most common form observed in many human tumor cells is the p50/p65 heterodimer *(194)*. In its inactive form, NF-κB is sequestered and bound to inhibitor (I)κBα, an endogenous repressor, that is phosphorylated by the IκBα kinase (IKK) complex on stimulation with TNF-α or interleukin (IL)-1β *(195,196)*. Phosphorylation of IκBα leads to degradation by the 26S proteosome complex, thereby liberating NF-κB for nuclear translocation and transcriptional activation of pro- and antiapoptotic genes. The antiapoptotic proteins induced include XIAP, cIAP1 and 2, Bcl-x_L and caspase 8/Fas-associated death domain-like IL-1B-converting enzyme inhibitory protein *(197)*. Thus, aberrant regulation of the NF-κB system would be expected to mediate resistance to a variety of agents that induce apoptosis.

Modulation of NF-κB alters the sensitivity of the cell to paclitaxel. For example, constitutive activation of NF-κB in MDA-MB-231 breast tumor cells renders them resistant to paclitaxel as result of induction of antiapoptotic genes such as *c-IAP2*, manganese superoxide dismutase, TNF receptor-associated factor, and defender against cell death-1 *(198)*. Conversely, downregulation of NF-κB activity either by antisense or ectopic overexpression of an IκBα super repressor or nondegradable mutant protein sensitizes breast cancer cells to paclitaxel *(198–200)*. Furthermore, paclitaxel resistance in human pancreatic tumor cell lines AsPC-1, Capan-1, and Panc-1 is because of paclitaxel-induced upregulation of IKK, downstream activation NF-κB, and subsequent upregulation of Bcl-x$_L$ *(201)*. In addition, ectopic expression of mitogen-activated protein kinase kinase kinase 3, which is upstream of IKK, mediates more than a 25-fold increase in resistance to paclitaxel (albeit from 1 to 25 μ*M*, an aphysiological concentration), as well as other chemotherapeutic agents *(202)*. It is interesting to note that mitogen-activated protein kinase kinase kinase 3 is overexpressed in 39% of breast tumor biopsies compared with matched tissue controls *(202)*. However, it remains to be determined whether its overexpression in tumors in humans has any effect on taxane responsiveness in the clinic.

Recently, a novel non-cytokine-dependent NF-κB pathway was reported in MCF-7 cells that overexpress cysteine-rich extracellular matrix protein (Cyr)61. Cyr61 primarily transmits signals via integrin receptors such as $\alpha_v\beta_1$, $\alpha_{II}\beta_3$, and $\alpha_v\beta_5$ *(203,204)*. These cells are resistant to physiological concentrations of paclitaxel (10–100 n*M*) as a result of NF-κB activation by integrin-dependent PI3/Akt signaling and subsequent induction of XIAP. The later discovery is intriguing given that this is the first example of an extracellular matrix/integrin signaling pathway driving NF-κB-mediated paclitaxel resistance. Moreover, elevated Cyr61 protein and mRNA levels have been detected in breast carcinomas *(205,206)* and positively correlated with more advanced features of breast cancer *(206)*. However, correlations between Cyr61 expression and taxane resistance in patients have not been reported. Collectively, these data suggest that inhibition of the NFκB signaling pathway may selectively enhance the efficacy of paclitaxel in tumor cells.

Other transcription factors such as interferon regulatory factor (IRF)9 can also lead to paclitaxel resistance. For example, Luker and colleagues demonstrated that after single-step selection of MCF-7 breast adenocarcinoma cells in 72-n*M* paclitaxel, transcriptional activation of IRF9 and other interferon-responsive genes occurs, is independent of interferon treatment, and enforced expression of IRF9 mediates 13-fold resistance to paclitaxel *(207)*. Interestingly, approximately 50% of donor-matched breast and uterine tumors overexpress IRF9. However, tumors were not subclassified into paclitaxel-sensitive or -resistant, so it is unclear whether overexpression is associated with resistance. Moreover, the subset of IRF9 target genes that may lead to resistance in vitro remains to be determined. A novel class of nuclear receptors termed xenobiotic receptors represents another family of transcription factors that may be involved in paclitaxel resistance *(208)*. Paclitaxel (but not docetaxel) can bind to xenobiotic receptors, which results in ligand-dependent nuclear translocation and induction of P-glycoprotein and the detoxifying enzyme family of cytochrome p450 *(208)*. This model suggests that resistance to paclitaxel is mediated by a novel feedback mechanism in which drug export or increased taxane metabolism may lead to decreased sensitivity. Thus, it is clear that in various tumor models that alterations in transcription of genes involved in the control apoptosis, cell-cycle, drug efflux pumps, and detoxifying enzyme can lead to taxane resistance.

6. ROLE OF CYTOKINES AND CHEMOKINES IN PACLITAXEL DRUG RESISTANCE

The cytokine IL-6 and chemokine IL-8 are classically recognized as immune regulators during inflammatory responses. However, they may also play a potential role in tumorigeneis, angiogenesis, and resistance *(209,210)*. Indeed, treatment with paclitaxel is associated with an increase in expression of IL-6, IL-8, and the chemokine monocyte

chemoattractant protein 1 in patients with ovarian cancer *(211)*. Moreover, in two independent studies, increases in IL-6, IL-8, and monocyte chemoattractant protein 1 levels
are detected in a 600-gene cDNA array in SKOV-3 ovarian carcinoma cells that acquire
paclitaxel resistance as a result of continuous exposure and selection *(212,213)*. In addition, transfection of IL-6 cDNAs into paclitaxel-sensitive U2-OS human osteosarcoma
cell lines mediates fivefold resistance to paclitaxel *(214)*. The lack of MDR-1, MRP-1,
and lung resistance-related protein overexpression and activity in these IL-6-transfected
lines suggest that the multidrug-resistance phenotype is not a result of increased drug
efflux *(214)*. A possible consequence of increase in IL-6 expression may be a direct
consequence of activation of signal transducer and activator of transcription 3, the effector transcription factor in IL-6 signaling and an important mediator in tumor cell survival
in a number of tumor cell lines *(215)*. Despite the observation that paclitaxel induces IL-
8 in ovarian carcinoma cell lines and elevated serum IL-8 levels in ovarian cancer patients
correlates with more aggressive disease *(211,216)*, there is no evidence to date that IL-
8 contributes directly to paclitaxel resistance.

7. ROLE OF KINASES IN DRUG RESISTANCE

It is well established that networks of constitutively activated kinases governs growth
factor independence in tumor cell proliferation. Therefore, one mechanism in which
tumor cells can become drug resistant is through positive selection for kinases that, as a
result of gain of function mutations or amplification, can subvert the apoptotic response.
For example, increased levels of mitotic kinases that play a role in monitoring spindle
checkpoints can confer drug resistance. One such example is the serine/threonine kinase,
Aurora A or breast-tumor-amplified kinase, which is localized to chromosome 20q13, a
region commonly amplified in human breast and colon tumors and correlates with poor
prognosis *(217,218)*. In addition, Aurora A is overexpressed in ovarian, prostate, neuroblastoma, and cervical cancer lines *(217)*. The primary functions of Aurora A are
centromsome separation, bipolar spindle formation, and chromosomal kinetochore attachment to the mitotic spindle *(219)*. Accordingly, overexpression of Aurora A leads to
centrosome amplification, chromosomal instability, and transformation in epithelial tumor
lines *(220)*. Moreover, it has been demonstrated recently that enforced overexpresssion
of Aurora A in a human epithelial tumor cell line confers resistance to paclitaxel-induced
apoptosis *(221)*. Inhibition of the expression of two other proteins, budding uninhibited
benzimidazole receptor (a kinase) and mitotic arrest deficient 2, which regulate the
spindle assembly checkpoint, have also been associated with paclitaxel resistance *(222)*.

Given that ligand-independent activation of growth factor receptor tyrosine kinases
are critical for oncogenic transformation and tumor cell proliferation, it is conceivable
that gene amplification or overexpression or receptor tyrosine kinases may also generate
drug resistance. The erb/EGFR family members, HER-2/*neu*, and EGFRvIII (an EGFR
variant with a truncated extracellular domain), are amplified and overexpressed in a
primary breast and ovarian carcinomas *(223,224)*, tumors in which taxane treatment is
frequently used. Ectopic expression of EGFRvIII or HER-2/*neu* in NIH3T3 murine
fibroblasts induce transformation and resistance to paclitaxel-mediated cytotoxicty *(225)*.
The mechanism of resistance is not fully understood, although both EGFRvIII- and HER-
2-expressing cells do not overexpress P-glycoprotein, and in one case, have increases in
type IVa β-tubulin isoforms *(225,226)*. Moreover, exogenous expression of HER-2/*neu*
in MDA-MB-435 human breast cancer cells is associated with resistance to paclitaxel-

induced apoptosis *(226)* and inhibition of the cell cycle-regulatory protein p34^{Cdc2}, which controls entry into mitosis and subsequent apoptosis *(227)*. Consistent with this, inhibition of erbB-2 by Herceptin® reverses both p34^{cdc2}-mediated inhibition and paclitaxel resistance *(227)*. It will be interesting to determine whether a causal link exists between EGFR overexpression and paclitaxel resistance by ascertaining the effects of the emerging class of EGFR inhibitors *(228)*, such as gefitinib (Iressa®), in breast, lung, and ovarian cancers patients that have failed previous taxane therapy.

Decreased paclitaxel sensitivity can also be because of increased signal transduction through a number of different cascades as opposed to direct amplification of kinases. For example, numerous extracellular and intracellular oncogenic signals intersect with the phosphatidylinositol 3-kinase (PI3K)/Akt pathway, which is often constitutively activated as a result of decreased expression of the endogenous Akt inhibitor, phosphatase and tensin homolog on chromosome ten, a tumor suppressor gene *(229)*. Indeed, an increase in resistance to paclitaxel in MDA-MB-231 and MDA-MB-435 human breast tumor lines is because of extracellular matrix ligand-dependent activation of β_1 integrin signaling via the PI3K/Akt pathway *(230)*. In addition, the activation status of Akt may be critical for taxane sensitivity because paclitaxel-mediated cytotoxicty is reversed on treatment with the PI3K inhibitor, LY294002, and that HER-2/*neu* and EGFR signal cascades can trigger Akt-mediated control of NF-κB.

8. CLINICAL CORRELATIONS WITH IN VITRO MECHANISMS

One of the greatest challenges facing both researchers and clinician alike is the ability to predict drug resistance in a given population of patients. Which of the mechanisms mentioned above account for resistance in patients, and can the results of this analysis be used to tailor future therapies? Two basic problems limit the answer to these questions. First, methods need to be developed to measure accurately the expression or functionality of individual mechanisms that contribute to resistance. Second, given the cellular heterogeneity in human tumors, it is highly likely that more than one mechanism may contribute to resistance, possibly within the same tumor. Beyond this, it must be recognized that paclitaxel resistance found in patients may not replicate the mechanisms defined, for the most part, by in vitro studies described here. Additional contributing factors that make the analysis complex include (1) greater genetic heterogeneity in tumors compared with cell lines; (2) local environmental factors such as hypoxia, interstitial hypertension, drug delivery; and (3) bioavailability of taxanes related to metabolism, compartmentalization, and formulation. In fact, it was recently reported that a reformulated version of Taxol in a non-cremophor-based vehicle was effective in paclitaxel-resistant patients *(233)*. As with much of the successful oncological therapies to date, empirical investigation in patients with selective agents that inhibit certain transporters, tubulin isoforms, apoptotic regulators, or signal transduction when used alone or in combination with standard taxane therapies will be necessary to bridge the gap between possible mechanisms of taxane resistance in the laboratory and prolonged survival in patients.

ACKNOWLEDGMENTS

A review of this breadth necessarily prohibits a comprehensive review of the field. We apologize to those authors whose contributions were not cited. We thank Dr. Christoph Dehnhardt for translation of the article by Lucas and Dr. Malathi Hari for her critical review. We also thank Drs. Arie Zask and Ayral-Kaloustain for their help summarizing the chemical structures of taxanes.

REFERENCES

1. Lucas H. Ueber ein in den blattern von *Taxus baccata* L. enthaltenes alkaloid (das Taxin) (in German). Arch Pharm 1856; 85:145–149.
2. Hoernel A. The Bower manuscript. In: Dept. of Government Printing. Calcutta, India, 1912.
3. Hartwell J. Plants used against cancer: a survey. Lawrence, MA: Quarterman, 1982.
4. Wani MC, Taylor HL, Wall ME, et al. Plant antitumor agents. VI. The isolation and structure of taxol, a novel antileukemic and antitumor agent from Taxus brevifolia. J Am Chem Soc 1971; 93:2325–2327.
5. Schiff PB, Fant J, Horwitz SB. Promotion of microtubule assembly in vitro by taxol. Nature 1979; 277:665–667.
6. Rowinsky EK, Tolcher AW. Antimicrotubule agents. In: Devita VT Jr, Hellman S, Rosenberg SA, eds. Cancer principles and practice, 6th edition. Philadelphia: Lippincott Williams and Wilkins, 2001:431–452.
7. Rose WC. Taxol: a review of its preclinical in vivo antitumor activity. Anticancer Drugs 1992; 3:311–321.
8. Einzig AI. Review of phase II trials of Taxol (paclitaxel) in patients with advanced ovarian cancer. Ann Oncol 1994; 5:S29–S32.
9. Legha SS, Ring S, Papadopoulos N, et al. A phase II trial of taxol in metastatic melanoma. Cancer 1990; 65:2478–2481.
10. Einzig AI, Gorowski E, Sasloff J, et al. Phase II trial of taxol in patients with metastatic renal cell carcinoma. Cancer Invest 1991; 9:133–136.
11. Oncology/Immunology BMS. Taxol (paclitaxel). In: Physicians' Desk Reference. Montvale: Medical Economics, 2002:1129–1138.
12. Gueritte-Voegelein F, Guenard D, Lavelle F, et al. Relationships between the structure of taxol analogues and their antimitotic activity. J Med Chem 1991; 34:992–998.
13. Bissery MC, Nohynek G, Sanderink GJ, et al. Docetaxel (Taxotere): a review of preclinical and clinical experience. Part I: Preclinical experience. Anticancer Drugs 1995; 6:339–368.
14. Kingston DG. The chemistry of taxol. Pharmacol Ther 1991; 52:1–34.
15. Jordan MA. Mechanism of action of antitumor drugs that interact with microtubules and tubulin. Curr Med Chem Anti-Canc Agents 2002; 2:1–17.
16. Desai A, Mitchison TJ. Microtubule polymerization dynamics. Annu Rev Cell Dev Biol 1997; 13:83–117.
17. Schiff PB, Horwitz SB. Taxol stabilizes microtubules in mouse fibroblast cells. Proc Natl Acad Sci U S A 1980; 77:1561–1565.
18. Nogales E. Structural insight into microtubule function. Annu Rev Biophys Biomol Struct 2001; 30:397–420.
19. Parness J, Horwitz SB. Taxol binds to polymerized tubulin in vitro. J Cell Biol 1981; 91:479–487.
20. Orr GA, Verdier-Pinard P, McDaid H, et al. Mechanisms of taxol resistance related to microtubules. Oncogene 2003; 22:7280–7295.
21. Lowe J, Li H, Downing KH, et al. Refined structure of $\alpha\beta$-tubulin at 3.5 Å resolution. J Mol Biol 2001; 313:1045–1057.
22. Li Y, Poliks B, Cegelski L, et al. Conformation of microtubule-bound paclitaxel determined by fluorescence spectroscopy and REDOR NMR. Biochemistry 2000; 39:281–291.
23. Snyder JP, Nettles JH, Cornett B, et al. The binding conformation of Taxol in β-tubulin: a model based on electron crystallographic density. Proc Natl Acad Sci U S A 2001; 98:5312–536.
24. Nettles JH, Li H, Cornett B, et al. The binding mode of epothilone A on α,β-tubulin by electron crystallography. Science 2004; 305:866–869.
25. Sullivan KF, Cleveland DW. Identification of conserved isotype-defining variable region sequences for four vertebrate β tubulin polypeptide classes. Proc Natl Acad Sci U S A 1986; 83:4327–4331.
26. Stanchi F, Corso V, Scannapieco P, et al. TUBA8: A new tissue-specific isoform of alpha-tubulin that is highly conserved in human and mouse. Biochem Biophys Res Commun 2000; 270:1111–1118.
27. Sullivan KF. Structure and utilization of tubulin isotypes. Annu Rev Cell Biol 1988; 4:687–716.
28. Andersen SS. Spindle assembly and the art of regulating microtubule dynamics by MAPs and Stathmin/Op18. Trends Cell Biol 2000; 10:261–267.
29. Cassimeris L. The oncoprotein 18/stathmin family of microtubule destabilizers. Curr Opin Cell Biol 2002; 14:18–24.

30. Nicoletti MI, Valoti G, Giannakakou P, et al. Expression of β-tubulin isotypes in human ovarian carcinoma xenografts and in a sub-panel of human cancer cell lines from the NCI-Anticancer Drug Screen: correlation with sensitivity to microtubule active agents. Clin Cancer Res 2001; 7:2912–2922.

31. Loganzo F, Annable T, Xingzhi T, et al. Cells made resistant to paclitaxel in the presence of an MDR1-reversal agent express a b-tubulin mutation (Asp26Glu), are less resistant to the novel taxane MAC-321, and are collaterally sensitive to tubulin depolymerizing agents. Proc Am Assoc Cancer Res 2003; 44, 2nd ed:1152.

32. Wang Y, Veeraraghavan S, Cabral F. Intra-allelic suppression of a mutation that stabilizes microtubules and confers resistance to colcemid. Biochemistry 2004; 43:8965–8973.

33. Goncalves A, Braguer D, Kamath K, et al. Resistance to Taxol in lung cancer cells associated with increased microtubule dynamics. Proc Natl Acad Sci U S A 2001; 98:11,737–11,742.

34. Giannakakou P, Sackett DL, Kang YK, et al. Paclitaxel-resistant human ovarian cancer cells have mutant β-tubulins that exhibit impaired paclitaxel-driven polymerization. J Biol Chem 1997; 272:17,118–17,125.

35. He L, Yang C-PH, Horwitz SB. Mutations in β-tubulin map to domains involved in regulation of microtubule stability in epothilone-resistant cell lines. Mol Cancer Ther 2001; 1:3–10.

36. Verrills NM, Flemming CL, Liu M, et al. Microtubule alterations and mutations induced by desoxyepothilone B: implications for drug-target interactions. Chem Biol 2003; 10:597–607.

37. Giannakakou P, Gussio R, Nogales E, et al. A common pharmacophore for epothilone and taxanes: molecular basis for drug resistance conferred by tubulin mutations in human cancer cells. Proc Natl Acad Sci U S A 2000; 97:2904–2909.

38. Martello LA, Verdier-Pinard P, Shen HJ, et al. Elevated levels of microtubule destabilizing factors in a Taxol-resistant/dependent A549 cell line with an alpha-tubulin mutation. Cancer Res 2003; 63:1207–1213.

39. Minotti AM, Barlow SB, Cabral F. Resistance to antimitotic drugs in Chinese hamster ovary cells correlates with changes in the level of polymerized tubulin. J Biol Chem 1991; 266:3987–3994.

40. Gonzalez-Garay ML, Chang L, Blade K, et al. A β-tubulin leucine cluster involved in microtubule assembly and paclitaxel resistance. J Biol Chem 1999; 274:23,875–23,882.

41. Verdier-Pinard P, Wang F, Martello L, et al. Analysis of tubulin isotypes and mutations from taxol-resistant cells by combined isoelectrofocusing and mass spectrometry. Biochemistry 2003; 42:5349–5357.

42. Lynch TJ, Bell DW, Sordella R, et al. Activating mutations in the epidermal growth factor receptor underlying responsiveness of non-small-cell lung cancer to gefitinib. N Engl J Med 2004; 350:2129–2139.

43. Paez JG, Janne PA, Lee JC, et al. EGFR mutations in lung cancer: correlation with clinical response to gefitinib therapy. Science 2004; 304:1497–1500.

44. Monzo M, Rosell R, Sanchez JJ, et al. Paclitaxel resistance in non-small-cell lung cancer associated with β-tubulin gene mutations. J Clin Oncol 1999; 17:1786–1793.

45. Kohonen-Corish MR, Qin H, Daniel JJ, et al. Lack of β-tubulin gene mutations in early stage lung cancer. Int J Cancer 2002; 101:398–399.

46. Sale S, Sung R, Shen P, et al. Conservation of the class I β-tubulin gene in human populations and lack of mutations in lung cancers and paclitaxel-resistant ovarian cancers. Mol Cancer Ther 2002; 1:215–225.

47. Kelley MJ, Li S, Harpole DH. Genetic analysis of the β-tubulin gene, TUBB, in non-small-cell lung cancer. J Natl Cancer Inst 2001; 93:1886–1888.

48. Tsurutani J, Komiya T, Uejima H, et al. Mutational analysis of the β-tubulin gene in lung cancer. Lung Cancer 2002; 35:11–16.

49. Hasegawa S, Miyoshi Y, Egawa C, et al. Mutational analysis of the class I β-tubulin gene in human breast cancer. Int J Cancer 2002; 101:46–51.

50. Burkhart CA, Kavallaris M, Horwitz SB. The role of β-tubulin isotypes in resistance to antimitotic drugs. Biochim Biophys Acta 2001; 1471:1–9.

51. Dozier JH, Hiser L, Davis JA, et al. Beta class II tubulin predominates in normal and tumor breast tissues. Breast Cancer Res 2003; 5:R157–R169.

52. Rao S, Aberg F, Nieves E, et al. Identification by mass spectrometry of a new α-tubulin isotype expressed in human breast and lung carcinoma cell lines. Biochemistry 2001; 40:2096–2103.

53. Verdier-Pinard P, Wang F, Burd B, et al. Direct analysis of tubulin expression in cancer cell lines by electrospray ionization mass spectrometry. Biochemistry 2003; 42:12,019–12,027.

54. Lu Q, Luduena RF. In vitro analysis of microtubule assembly of isotypically pure tubulin dimers. Intrinsic differences in the assembly properties of α β II, α β III, and α β IV tubulin dimers in the absence of microtubule-associated proteins. J Biol Chem 1994; 269:2041–2047.

55. Lu Q, Luduena RF. Removal of β III isotype enhances taxol induced microtubule assembly. Cell Struct Funct 1993; 18:173–182.
56. Derry WB, Wilson L, Khan IA, et al. Taxol differentially modulates the dynamics of microtubules assembled from unfractionated and purified β-tubulin isotypes. Biochemistry 1997; 36:3554–3562.
57. Panda D, Miller HP, Banerjee A, et al. Microtubule dynamics in vitro are regulated by the tubulin isotype composition. Proc Natl Acad Sci U S A 1994; 91:11,358–11,362.
58. Kavallaris M, Kuo DY, Burkhart CA, et al. Taxol-resistant epithelial ovarian tumors are associated with altered expression of specific β-tubulin isotypes. J Clin Invest 1997; 100:1282–1293.
59. Kyu-Ho Han E, Gehrke L, Tahir SK, et al. Modulation of drug resistance by α-tubulin in paclitaxel-resistant human lung cancer cell lines. Eur J Cancer 2000; 36:1565–1571.
60. Kavallaris M, Burkhart CA, Horwitz SB. Antisense oligonucleotides to class III β-tubulin sensitize drug-resistant cells to Taxol. Br J Cancer 1999; 80:1020–1025.
61. Hari M, Yang H, Zeng C, et al. Expression of class III β-tubulin reduces microtubule assembly and confers resistance to paclitaxel. Cell Motil Cytoskeleton 2003; 56:45–56.
62. Blade K, Menick DR, Cabral F. Overexpression of class I, II or IVb β-tubulin isotypes in CHO cells is insufficient to confer resistance to paclitaxel. J Cell Sci 1999; 112(Pt 13):2213–2221.
63. Ranganathan S, McCauley RA, Dexter DW, et al. Modulation of endogenous β-tubulin isotype expression as a result of human beta(III)cDNA transfection into prostate carcinoma cells. Br J Cancer 2001; 85:735–740.
64. Veitia R, Bissery MC, Martinez C, et al. Tau expression in model adenocarcinomas correlates with docetaxel sensitivity in tumour-bearing mice. Br J Cancer 1998; 78:871–877.
65. Poruchynsky MS, Giannakakou P, Ward Y, et al. Accompanying protein alterations in malignant cells with a microtubule-polymerizing drug-resistance phenotype and a primary resistance mechanism. Biochem Pharmacol 2001; 62:1469–1480.
66. Zhang CC, Yang JM, White E, et al. The role of MAP4 expression in the sensitivity to paclitaxel and resistance to vinca alkaloids in p53 mutant cells. Oncogene 1998; 16:1617–1624.
67. Belmont LD, Mitchison TJ. Identification of a protein that interacts with tubulin dimers and increases the catastrophe rate of microtubules. Cell 1996; 84:623–631.
68. Ravelli RB, Gigant B, Curmi PA, et al. Insight into tubulin regulation from a complex with colchicine and a stathmin-like domain. Nature 2004; 428:198–202.
69. Gigant B, Curmi PA, Martin-Barbey C, et al. The 4 Å X-ray structure of a tubulin:stathmin-like domain complex. Cell 2000; 102:809–816.
70. Larsson N, Segerman B, Gradin HM, et al. Mutations of oncoprotein 18/stathmin identify tubulin-directed regulatory activities distinct from tubulin association. Mol Cell Biol 1999; 19:2242–2250.
71. Balachandran R, Welsh MJ, Day BW. Altered levels and regulation of stathmin in paclitaxel-resistant ovarian cancer cells. Oncogene 2003; 22:8924–8930.
72. Iancu C, Mistry SJ, Arkin S, et al. Taxol and anti-stathmin therapy: a synergistic combination that targets the mitotic spindle. Cancer Res 2000; 60:3537–3541.
73. Sharp DJ, Rogers GC, Scholey JM. Microtubule motors in mitosis. Nature 2000; 407:41–47.
74. Altieri DC. Survivin, versatile modulation of cell division and apoptosis in cancer. Oncogene 2003; 22:8581–8589.
75. Carvalho P, Tirnauer JS, Pellman D. Surfing on microtubule ends. Trends Cell Biol 2003; 13:229–237.
76. Howard J, Hyman AA. Dynamics and mechanics of the microtubule plus end. Nature 2003; 422:753–758.
77. Ohta S, Nishio K, Kubota N, et al. Characterization of a taxol-resistant human small-cell lung cancer cell line. Jpn J Cancer Res 1994; 85:290–297.
78. Banerjee A. Increased levels of tyrosinated α-, β(III)-, and β(IV)-tubulin isotypes in paclitaxel-resistant MCF-7 breast cancer cells. Biochem Biophys Res Commun 2002; 293:598–601.
79. Gottesman MM, Fojo T, Bates SE. Multidrug resistance in cancer: role of ATP-dependent transporters. Nat Rev Cancer 2002; 2:48–58.
80. Borst P, Elferink RO. Mammalian ABC transporters in health and disease. Annu Rev Biochem 2002; 71:537–592.
81. Childs S, Yeh RL, Hui D, et al. Taxol resistance mediated by transfection of the liver-specific sister gene of P-glycoprotein. Cancer Res 1998; 58:4160–4167.
82. Lecureur V, Sun D, Hargrove P, et al. Cloning and expression of murine sister of P-glycoprotein reveals a more discriminating transporter than MDR1/P-glycoprotein. Mol Pharmacol 2000; 57:24–35.
83. Smith AJ, van Helvoort A, van Meer G, et al. MDR3 P-glycoprotein, a phosphatidylcholine translocase, transports several cytotoxic drugs and directly interacts with drugs as judged by interference with nucleotide trapping. J Biol Chem 2000; 275:23,530–23,539.

84. Hopper-Borge E, Chen ZS, Shchaveleva I, et al. Analysis of the drug resistance profile of multidrug resistance protein 7 (ABCC10): resistance to docetaxel. Cancer Res 2004; 64:4927–4930.

85. Shen DW, Cardarelli C, Hwang J, et al. Multiple drug-resistant human KB carcinoma cells independently selected for high-level resistance to colchicine, adriamycin, or vinblastine show changes in expression of specific proteins. J Biol Chem 1986; 261:7762–7770.

86. Dumontet C, Duran GE, Steger KA, et al. Resistance mechanisms in human sarcoma mutants derived by single-step exposure to paclitaxel (Taxol). Cancer Res 1996; 56:1091–1097.

87. Goldstein LJ. MDR1 gene expression in solid tumours. Eur J Cancer 1996; 32A:1039–1050.

88. Goldstein LJ, Galski H, Fojo A, et al. Expression of a multidrug resistance gene in human cancers. J Natl Cancer Inst 1989; 81:116–124.

89. Sampath D, Discafani CM, Loganzo F, et al. MAC-321, A novel taxane with greater efficacy than paclitaxel and docetaxel in vitro and in vivo. Mol Cancer Thera 2003; 2:873–994.

90. Sorrentino BP, Brandt SJ, Bodine D, et al. Selection of drug-resistant bone marrow cells in vivo after retroviral transfer of human MDR1. Science 1992; 257:99–103.

91. Licht T, Haskins M, Henthorn P, et al. Drug selection with paclitaxel restores expression of linked IL-2 receptor γ-chain and multidrug resistance (MDR1) transgenes in canine bone marrow. Proc Natl Acad Sci U S A 2002; 99:3123–3128.

92. Sparreboom A, van Asperen J, Mayer U, et al. Limited oral bioavailability and active epithelial excretion of paclitaxel (Taxol) caused by P-glycoprotein in the intestine. Proc Natl Acad Sci U S A 1997; 94:2031–2035.

93. van Asperen J, van Tellingen O, Sparreboom A, et al. Enhanced oral bioavailability of paclitaxel in mice treated with the P-glycoprotein blocker SDZ PSC 833. Br J Cancer 1997; 76:1181–1183.

94. van Asperen J, van Tellingen O, van der Valk MA, et al. Enhanced oral absorption and decreased elimination of paclitaxel in mice cotreated with cyclosporin A. Clin Cancer Res 1998; 4:2293–2297.

95. Britten CD, Baker SD, Denis LJ, et al. Oral paclitaxel and concurrent cyclosporin A: targeting clinically relevant systemic exposure to paclitaxel. Clin Cancer Res 2000; 6:3459–3468.

96. Meerum Terwogt JM, Malingre MM, Beijnen JH, et al. Coadministration of oral cyclosporin A enables oral therapy with paclitaxel. Clin Cancer Res 1999; 5:3379–3384.

97. Wils P, Phung-Ba V, Warnery A, et al. Polarized transport of docetaxel and vinblastine mediated by P-glycoprotein in human intestinal epithelial cell monolayers. Biochem Pharmacol 1994; 48:1528–1530.

98. Shirakawa K, Takara K, Tanigawara Y, et al. Interaction of docetaxel ("Taxotere") with human P-glycoprotein. Jpn J Cancer Res 1999; 90:1380–1386.

99. Loganzo F, Discafani CM, Annable T, et al. HTI-286, a synthetic analogue of the tripeptide hemiasterlin, is a potent antimicrotubule agent that circumvents P-glycoprotein-mediated resistance in vitro and in vivo. Cancer Res 2003; 63:1838–1845.

100. Malingre MM, Richel DJ, Beijnen JH, et al. Coadministration of cyclosporine strongly enhances the oral bioavailability of docetaxel. J Clin Oncol 2001; 19:1160–1166.

101. Bardelmeijer HA, Ouwehand M, Buckle T, et al. Low systemic exposure of oral docetaxel in mice resulting from extensive first-pass metabolism is boosted by ritonavir. Cancer Res 2002; 62:6158–6164.

102. Wacher VJ, Silverman JA, Zhang Y, et al. Role of P-glycoprotein and cytochrome P450 3A in limiting oral absorption of peptides and peptidomimetics. J Pharm Sci 1998; 87:1322–1330.

103. Sparreboom A, van Tellingen O, Nooijen WJ, et al. Preclinical pharmacokinetics of paclitaxel and docetaxel. Anticancer Drugs 1998; 9:1–17.

104. Schneider J, Bak M, Efferth T, et al. P-glycoprotein expression in treated and untreated human breast cancer. Br J Cancer 1989; 60:815–818.

105. Charpin C, Vielh P, Duffaud F, et al. Quantitative immunocytochemical assays of P-glycoprotein in breast carcinomas: correlation to messenger RNA expression and to immunohistochemical prognostic indicators. J Natl Cancer Inst 1994; 86:1539–1545.

106. Rudas M, Filipits M, Taucher S, et al. Expression of MRP1, LRP and Pgp in breast carcinoma patients treated with preoperative chemotherapy. Breast Cancer Res Treat 2003; 81:149–157.

107. Scagliotti GV, Michelotto F, Kalikatzaros G, et al. Detection of multidrug resistance associated P-170 glycoprotein in previously untreated non small cell lung cancer. Anticancer Res 1991; 11:2207–2210.

108. Kreisholt J, Sorensen M, Jensen PB, et al. Immunohistochemical detection of DNA topoisomerase IIalpha, P-glycoprotein and multidrug resistance protein (MRP) in small-cell and non-small-cell lung cancer. Br J Cancer 1998; 77:1469–1473.

109. Chiou JF, Liang JA, Hsu WH, et al. Comparing the relationship of Taxol-based chemotherapy response with P-glycoprotein and lung resistance-related protein expression in non-small cell lung cancer. Lung 2003; 181:267–273.

110. Yeh JJ, Hsu WH, Wang JJ, et al. Predicting chemotherapy response to paclitaxel-based therapy in advanced non-small-cell lung cancer with P-glycoprotein expression. Respiration 2003; 70:32–35.

111. Izquierdo MA, van der Zee AG, Vermorken JB, et al. Drug resistance-associated marker LRP for prediction of response to chemotherapy and prognoses in advanced ovarian carcinoma. J Natl Cancer Inst 1995; 87:1230–1237.

112. Schneider J, Jimenez E, Marenbach K, et al. Co-expression of the MDR1 gene and HSP27 in human ovarian cancer. Anticancer Res 1998; 18:2967–2971.

113. Baekelandt MM, Holm R, Nesland JM, et al. P-glycoprotein expression is a marker for chemotherapy resistance and prognosis in advanced ovarian cancer. Anticancer Res 2000; 20:1061–1067.

114. Trock BJ, Leonessa F, Clarke R. Multidrug resistance in breast cancer: a meta-analysis of MDR1/ gp170 expression and its possible functional significance. J Natl Cancer Inst 1997; 89:917–931.

115. Beck WT, Grogan TM, Willman CL, et al. Methods to detect P-glycoprotein-associated multidrug resistance in patients' tumors: consensus recommendations. Cancer Res 1996; 56:3010–3020.

116. Bates S. Solving the problem of multidrug resistance: ABC transporters in clinical oncology. In: Holland, BI, Cole SPC, Kuchler K, Higgins, CF, eds. ABC proteins: from bacteria to man. London: Academic, 2003:359–3291.

117. Lee CH. Reversing agents for ATP-binding cassette (ABC) transporters: application in modulating multidrug resistance (MDR). Curr Med Chem Anti-Canc Agents 2004; 4:43–52.

118. Campos L, Guyotat D, Archimbaud E, et al. Clinical significance of multidrug resistance P-glycoprotein expression on acute nonlymphoblastic leukemia cells at diagnosis. Blood 1992; 79:473–476.

119. Leith CP, Kopecky KJ, Godwin J, et al. Acute myeloid leukemia in the elderly: assessment of multidrug resistance (MDR1) and cytogenetics distinguishes biologic subgroups with remarkably distinct responses to standard chemotherapy. A Southwest Oncology Group study. Blood 1997; 89:3323–3329.

120. Leith CP, Kopecky KJ, Chen IM, et al. Frequency and clinical significance of the expression of the multidrug resistance proteins MDR1/P-glycoprotein, MRP1, and LRP in acute myeloid leukemia: a Southwest Oncology Group Study. Blood 1999; 94:1086–1099.

121. List AF, Kopecky KJ, Willman CL, et al. Benefit of cyclosporine modulation of drug resistance in patients with poor-risk acute myeloid leukemia: a Southwest Oncology Group study. Blood 2001; 98:3212–3220.

122. Baer MR, George SL, Dodge RK, et al. Phase 3 study of the multidrug resistance modulator PSC-833 in previously untreated patients 60 years of age and older with acute myeloid leukemia: Cancer and Leukemia Group B Study 9720. Blood 2002; 100:1224–1232.

123. Gruber A, Bjorkholm M, Brinch L, et al. A phase I/II study of the MDR modulator Valspodar (PSC 833) combined with daunorubicin and cytarabine in patients with relapsed and primary refractory acute myeloid leukemia. Leuk Res 2003; 27:323–328.

124. Greenberg PL, Lee SJ, Advani R, et al. Mitoxantrone, etoposide, and cytarabine with or without valspodar in patients with relapsed or refractory acute myeloid leukemia and high-risk myelodysplastic syndrome: a phase III trial (E2995). J Clin Oncol 2004; 22:1078–1086.

125. Garraway LA, Chabner B. MDR1 inhibition: less resistance or less relevance? Eur J Cancer 2002; 38:2337–2340.

126. Fracasso PM, Brady MF, Moore DH, et al. Phase II study of paclitaxel and valspodar (PSC 833) in refractory ovarian carcinoma: a gynecologic oncology group study. J Clin Oncol 2001; 19:2975–2982.

127. Patnaik A, Warner E, Michael M, et al. Phase I dose-finding and pharmacokinetic study of paclitaxel and carboplatin with oral valspodar in patients with advanced solid tumors. J Clin Oncol 2000; 18:3677–3689.

128. Fracasso PM, Westervelt P, Fears CL, et al. Phase I study of paclitaxel in combination with a multidrug resistance modulator, PSC 833 (Valspodar), in refractory malignancies. J Clin Oncol 2000; 18:1124–1134.

129. Advani R, Fisher GA, Lum BL, et al. A phase I trial of doxorubicin, paclitaxel, and valspodar (PSC 833), a modulator of multidrug resistance. Clin Cancer Res 2001; 7:1221–1229.

130. Chico I, Kang MH, Bergan R, et al. Phase I study of infusional paclitaxel in combination with the P-glycoprotein antagonist PSC 833. J Clin Oncol 2001; 19:832–842.

131. Mistry P, Stewart AJ, Dangerfield W, et al. In vitro and in vivo reversal of P-glycoprotein-mediated multidrug resistance by a novel potent modulator, XR9576. Cancer Res 2001; 61:749–758.

132. Starling JJ, Shepard RL, Cao J, et al. Pharmacological characterization of LY335979: a potent cyclopropyldibenzosuberane modulator of P-glycoprotein. Adv Enzyme Regul 1997; 37:335–347.

133. Dantzig AH, Law KL, Cao J, et al. Reversal of multidrug resistance by the P-glycoprotein modulator, LY335979, from the bench to the clinic. Curr Med Chem 2001; 8:39–50.

134. van Zuylen L, Sparreboom A, van der Gaast A, et al. The orally administered P-glycoprotein inhibitor R101933 does not alter the plasma pharmacokinetics of docetaxel. Clin Cancer Res 2000; 6:1365–1371.

135. Newman MJ, Rodarte JC, Benbatoul KD, et al. Discovery and characterization of OC144-093, a novel inhibitor of P-glycoprotein-mediated multidrug resistance. Cancer Res 2000; 60:2964–2972.

136. Allen JD, Brinkhuis RF, Wijnholds J, et al. The mouse Bcrp1/Mxr/Abcp gene: amplification and overexpression in cell lines selected for resistance to topotecan, mitoxantrone, or doxorubicin. Cancer Res 1999; 59:4237–4241.

137. Ojima I, Slater JC, Michaud E, et al. Syntheses and structure-activity relationships of the second-generation antitumor taxoids: exceptional activity against drug-resistant cancer cells. J Med Chem 1996; 39:3889–3896.

138. Polizzi D, Pratesi G, Tortoreto M, et al. A novel taxane with improved tolerability and therapeutic activity in a panel of human tumor xenografts. Cancer Res 1999; 59:1036–1040.

139. Shionoya M, Jimbo T, Kitagawa M, et al. DJ-927, a novel oral taxane, overcomes P-glycoprotein-mediated multidrug resistance in vitro and in vivo. Cancer Sci 2003; 94:459–466.

140. Longley RE, Fasciani G, Sander L, et al. In vitro mechanism of action studies with the taxane analog, TL-909 (MST-997). Proc Am Assoc Cancer Res 2004; 45:LB-90.

141. Kurata T, Shimada Y, Tamura T, et al. Phase I and pharmacokinetic study of a new taxoid, RPR 109881A, given as a 1-hour intravenous infusion in patients with advanced solid tumors. J Clin Oncol 2000; 18:3164–3171.

142. Cisternino S, Bourasset F, Archimbaud Y, et al. Nonlinear accumulation in the brain of the new taxoid TXD258 following saturation of P-glycoprotein at the blood-brain barrier in mice and rats. Br J Pharmacol 2003; 138:1367–1375.

143. Rose WC, Fairchild C, Lee FY. Preclinical antitumor activity of two novel taxanes. Cancer Chemother Pharmacol 2001; 47:97–105.

144. Rose WC, Long BH, Fairchild CR, et al. Preclinical pharmacology of BMS-275183, an orally active taxane. Clin Cancer Res 2001; 7:2016–2021.

145. Broker LE, De Vos FY, Gall H, et al. A phase I trial of the novel oral taxane BMS-275183 in patients with advanced solid tumors. ASCO meeting abstract. 2004; abstract no. 2029.

146. Sampath D, Discafani D, Beyer C, et al. MST-997: A novel taxane with superior efficacy that overcomes paclitaxel and docetaxel resistance in vitro and in vivo. EORTC/NCI/AACR meeting, 2004; abstract no. 524.

147. Nicoletti MI, Colombo T, Rossi C, et al. IDN5109, a taxane with oral bioavailability and potent antitumor activity. Cancer Res 2000; 60:842–846.

148. Dieras VC, Limantani SA, Lortholary A, et al. A multicentre, non randomized phase II study with RPR 109881A in metastatic breast cancer (MBC) patients (pts). ASCO meeting. 2004; abstract no. 565.

149. Sessa C, Perotti A, Salvatorelli E, et al. Phase IB and pharmacological study of the novel taxane BMS-184476 in combination with doxorubicin. Eur J Cancer 2004; 40:563–570.

150. Hidalgo M, Aylesworth C, Hammond LA, et al. Phase I and pharmacokinetic study of BMS-184476, a taxane with greater potency and solubility than paclitaxel. J Clin Oncol 2001; 19:2493–2503.

151. Advani R, Fisher GA, Lum BL, et al. Phase I and pharmacokinetic study of BMS-188797, a new taxane analog, administered on a weekly schedule in patients with advanced malignancies. Clin Cancer Res 2003; 9:5187–5194.

152. Brahmer JR, Shapiro M, Carducci K, et al. Phase I trial of a potent novel taxane, TL00139 (MAC-321), in patients with advanced malignant solid tumors. ASCO meeting. 2004: abstract no. 527.

153. Zhu AX, Bukowski R, Lockhart AC, et al. Phase 1 trial of oral MAC-321 in subjects with advanced malignant solid tumors. ASCO meeting. 2004; abstract no. 2040.

154. Cobb PW, Joly F, Venner P, et al. An uncontrolled phase II multi-center trial evaluating anti-tumor efficacy and safety of BAY 59-8862 in patients with advanced renal cell cancer. ASCO meeting. 2004; abstract no. 1640.

155. Amadori D, Santoro A, Hoffken K, et al. A phase II trial of a novel taxane BAY 59-8862 in patients with advanced taxane-resistant breast cancer. ASCO meeting. 2004; abstract no. 176.

156. Gurtler JS, Von Pawel J, Spiridonidis CH, et al. An uncontrolled phase II study evaluating anti-tumor efficacy and safety of ortataxel (BAY 59-8862) in patients with taxane-resistant non-small cell lung cancer. ASCO meeting. 2004; abstract no. 7136.

157. Syed SK, Beeram M, Takimoto CH, et al. Phase I and pharmacokinetics (PK) of DJ-927, an oral taxane, in patients (Pts) with advanced cancers. ASCO meeting. 2004; abstract no. 2028.

158. Altmann KH. Epothilone B and its analogs—a new family of anticancer agents. Mini Rev Med Chem 2003; 3:149–158.
159. Mani S, Macapinlac M Jr, Goel S, et al. The clinical development of new mitotic inhibitors that stabilize the microtubule. Anticancer Drugs 2004; 15:553–558.
160. Mooberry SL, Tien G, Hernandez AH, et al. Laulimalide and isolaulimalide, new paclitaxel-like microtubule-stabilizing agents. Cancer Res 1999; 59:653–660.
161. Pryor DE, O'Brate A, Bilcer G, et al. The microtubule stabilizing agent laulimalide does not bind in the taxoid site, kills cells resistant to paclitaxel and epothilones, and may not require its epoxide moiety for activity. Biochemistry 2002; 41:9109–9115.
162. Woods CM, Zhu J, McQueney PA, et al. Taxol-induced mitotic block triggers rapid onset of a p53-independent apoptotic pathway. Mol Med 1995; 1:506–526.
163. van Loo G, Saelens X, van Gurp M, et al. The role of mitochondrial factors in apoptosis: a Russian roulette with more than one bullet. Cell Death Differ 2002; 9:1031–1042.
164. Schulze-Osthoff K, Ferrari D, Los M, et al. Apoptosis signaling by death receptors. Eur J Biochem 1998; 254:439–459.
165. Ashkenazi A, Dixit VM. Apoptosis control by death and decoy receptors. Curr Opin Cell Biol 1999; 11:255–260.
166. Manthey CL, Brandes ME, Perera PY, et al. Taxol increases steady-state levels of lipopolysaccharide-inducible genes and protein-tyrosine phosphorylation in murine macrophages. J Immunol 1992; 149:2459–2465.
167. Bogdan C, Ding A. Taxol, a microtubule-stabilizing antineoplastic agent, induces expression of tumor necrosis factor alpha and interleukin-1 in macrophages. J Leukoc Biol 1992; 52:119–121.
168. Lanni JS, Lowe SW, Licitra EJ, et al. p53-independent apoptosis induced by paclitaxel through an indirect mechanism. Proc Natl Acad Sci U S A 1997; 94:9679–9683.
169. Asakuma J, Sumitomo M, Asano T, et al. Selective Akt inactivation and tumor necrosis actor-related apoptosis-inducing ligand sensitization of renal cancer cells by low concentrations of paclitaxel. Cancer Res 2003; 63:1365–1370.
170. Vignati S, Codegoni A, Polato F, et al. Trail activity in human ovarian cancer cells: potentiation of the action of cytotoxic drugs. Eur J Cancer 2002; 38:177–183.
171. Singh TR, Shankar S, Chen X, et al. Synergistic interactions of chemotherapeutic drugs and tumor necrosis factor-related apoptosis-inducing ligand/Apo-2 ligand on apoptosis and on regression of breast carcinoma in vivo. Cancer Res 2003; 63:5390–5400.
172. Jiang X, Wang X. Cytochrome c-mediated apoptosis. Annu Rev Biochem 2004; 73:87–106.
173. Budihardjo I, Oliver H, Lutter M, et al. Biochemical pathways of caspase activation during apoptosis. Annu Rev Cell Dev Biol 1999; 15:269–290.
174. Korsmeyer SJ. BCL-2 gene family and the regulation of programmed cell death. Cancer Res 1999; 59:1693s–1700s.
175. Srivastava RK, Srivastava AR, Korsmeyer SJ, et al. Involvement of microtubules in the regulation of Bcl2 phosphorylation and apoptosis through cyclic AMP-dependent protein kinase. Mol Cell Biol 1998; 18:3509–3517.
176. Haldar S, Basu A, Croce CM. Bcl2 is the guardian of microtubule integrity. Cancer Res 1997; 57:229–233.
177. Fan W. Possible mechanisms of paclitaxel-induced apoptosis. Biochem Pharmacol 1999; 57:1215–1221.
178. Rodi DJ, Janes RW, Sanganee HJ, et al. Screening of a library of phage-displayed peptides identifies human bcl-2 as a taxol-binding protein. J Mol Biol 1999; 285:197–203.
179. Ibrado AM, Liu L, Bhalla K. Bcl-xL overexpression inhibits progression of molecular events leading to paclitaxel-induced apoptosis of human acute myeloid leukemia HL-60 cells. Cancer Res 1997; 57:1109–1115.
180. Huang Y, Ibrado AM, Reed JC, et al. Co-expression of several molecular mechanisms of multidrug resistance and their significance for paclitaxel cytotoxicity in human AML HL-60 cells. Leukemia 1997; 11:253–257.
181. Ibrado AM, Kim CN, Bhalla K. Temporal relationship of CDK1 activation and mitotic arrest to cytosolic accumulation of cytochrome C and caspase-3 activity during Taxol-induced apoptosis of human AML HL-60 cells. Leukemia 1998; 12:1930–1936.
182. Huang Y, Ray S, Reed JC, et al. Estrogen increases intracellular p26Bcl-2 to p21Bax ratios and inhibits taxol-induced apoptosis of human breast cancer MCF-7 cells. Breast Cancer Res Treat 1997; 42:73–81.
183. Perkins C, Kim CN, Fang G, et al. Overexpression of Apaf-1 promotes apoptosis of untreated and paclitaxel- or etoposide-treated HL-60 cells. Cancer Res 1998; 58:4561–4566.

184. Perkins CL, Fang G, Kim CN, et al. The role of Apaf-1, caspase-9, and bid proteins in etoposide- or paclitaxel-induced mitochondrial events during apoptosis. Cancer Res 2000; 60:1645–16453.
185. Deveraux QL, Reed JC. IAP family proteins—suppressors of apoptosis. Genes Dev 1999; 13:239–252.
186. O'Connor DS, Wall NR, Porter AC, et al. A p34(cdc2) survival checkpoint in cancer. Cancer Cell 2002; 2:43–54.
187. Wall NR, O'Connor DS, Plescia J, et al. Suppression of survivin phosphorylation on Thr34 by flavopiridol enhances tumor cell apoptosis. Cancer Res 2003; 63:230–235.
188. Li F, Ambrosini G, Chu EY, et al. Control of apoptosis and mitotic spindle checkpoint by survivin. Nature 1998; 396:580–584.
189. Zaffaroni N, Daidone MG. Survivin expression and resistance to anticancer treatments: perspectives for new therapeutic interventions. Drug Resist Updat 2002; 5:65–72.
190. Zaffaroni N, Pennati M, Colella G, et al. Expression of the anti-apoptotic gene survivin correlates with taxol resistance in human ovarian cancer. Cell Mol Life Sci 2002; 59:1406–1412.
191. Tamm I, Kornblau SM, Segall H, et al. Expression and prognostic significance of IAP-family genes in human cancers and myeloid leukemias. Clin Cancer Res 2000; 6:1796–1803.
192. Schimmer AD, Welsh K, Pinilla C, et al. Small-molecule antagonists of apoptosis suppressor XIAP exhibit broad antitumor activity. Cancer Cell 2004; 5:25–35.
193. Richmond A. NF-κ B, chemokine gene transcription and tumour growth. Nat Rev Immunol 2002; 2:664–674.
194. Ghosh S, May MJ, Kopp EB. NF-κ B and Rel proteins: evolutionarily conserved mediators of immune responses. Annu Rev Immunol 1998; 16:225–260.
195. Karin M, Yamamoto Y, Wang QM. The IKK NF-κ B system: a treasure trove for drug development. Nat Rev Drug Discov 2004; 3:17–26.
196. Karin M, Cao Y, Greten FR, et al. NF-κB in cancer: from innocent bystander to major culprit. Nat Rev Cancer 2002; 2:301–310.
197. Arlt A, Schafer H. NFκB-dependent chemoresistance in solid tumors. Int J Clin Pharmacol Ther 2002; 40:336–347.
198. Patel NM, Nozaki S, Shortle NH, et al. Paclitaxel sensitivity of breast cancer cells with constitutively active NF-κB is enhanced by IκBα super-repressor and parthenolide. Oncogene 2000; 19:4159–4169.
199. Huang Y, Fan W. IκB kinase activation is involved in regulation of paclitaxel-induced apoptosis in human tumor cell lines. Mol Pharmacol 2002; 61:105–13.
200. Huang Y, Johnson KR, Norris JS, et al. Nuclear factor-κB/IκB signaling pathway may contribute to the mediation of paclitaxel-induced apoptosis in solid tumor cells. Cancer Res 2000; 60:4426–4432.
201. Dong QG, Sclabas GM, Fujioka S, et al. The function of multiple IκB : NF-κB complexes in the resistance of cancer cells to Taxol-induced apoptosis. Oncogene 2002; 21:6510–6519.
202. Samanta AK, Huang HJ, Bast RC Jr, et al. Overexpression of MEKK3 confers resistance to apoptosis through activation of NFκB. J Biol Chem 2004; 279:7576–7583.
203. Lau LF, Lam SC. The CCN family of angiogenic regulators: the integrin connection. Exp Cell Res 1999; 248:44–57.
204. Lin MT, Chang CC, Chen ST, et al. Cyr61 expression confers resistance to apoptosis in breast cancer MCF-7 cells by a mechanism of NF-κB-dependent XIAP up-regulation. J Biol Chem 2004; 279:24,015–24,023.
205. Sampath D, Winneker RC, Zhang Z. Cyr61, a member of the CCN family, is required for MCF-7 cell proliferation: regulation by 17β-estradiol and overexpression in human breast cancer. Endocrinology 2001; 142:2540–2548.
206. Xie D, Nakachi K, Wang H, et al. Elevated levels of connective tissue growth factor, WISP-1, and CYR61 in primary breast cancers associated with more advanced features. Cancer Res 2001; 61:8917–8923.
207. Luker KE, Pica CM, Schreiber RD, et al. Overexpression of IRF9 confers resistance to antimicrotubule agents in breast cancer cells. Cancer Res 2001; 61:6540–6547.
208. Synold TW, Dussault I, Forman BM. The orphan nuclear receptor SXR coordinately regulates drug metabolism and efflux. Nat Med 2001; 7:584–590.
209. Jee SH, Shen SC, Chiu HC, et al. Overexpression of interleukin-6 in human basal cell carcinoma cell lines increases anti-apoptotic activity and tumorigenic potency. Oncogene 2001; 20:198–208.
210. Li A, Dubey S, Varney ML, et al. IL-8 directly enhanced endothelial cell survival, proliferation, and matrix metalloproteinases production and regulated angiogenesis. J Immunol 2003; 170:3369–3376.

211. Penson RT, Kronish K, Duan Z, et al. Cytokines IL-1β, IL-2, IL-6, IL-8, MCP-1, GM-CSF and TNFα in patients with epithelial ovarian cancer and their relationship to treatment with paclitaxel. Int J Gynecol Cancer 2000; 10:33–41.
212. Duan Z, Feller AJ, Penson RT, et al. Discovery of differentially expressed genes associated with paclitaxel resistance using cDNA array technology: analysis of interleukin (IL) 6, IL-8, and monocyte chemotactic protein 1 in the paclitaxel-resistant phenotype. Clin Cancer Res 1999; 5:3445–3453.
213. Lamendola DE, Duan Z, Yusuf RZ, et al. Molecular description of evolving paclitaxel resistance in the SKOV-3 human ovarian carcinoma cell line. Cancer Res 2003; 63:2200–2205.
214. Duan Z, Lamendola DE, Penson RT, et al. Overexpression of IL-6 but not IL-8 increases paclitaxel resistance of u-2os human osteosarcoma cells. Cytokine 2002; 17:234–242.
215. Bowman T, Garcia R, Turkson J, et al. STATs in oncogenesis. Oncogene 2000; 19:2474–2788.
216. Lee LF, Schuerer-Maly CC, Lofquist AK, et al. Taxol-dependent transcriptional activation of IL-8 expression in a subset of human ovarian cancer. Cancer Res 1996; 56:1303–1308.
217. Zhou H, Kuang J, Zhong L, et al. Tumour amplified kinase STK15/BTAK induces centrosome amplification, aneuploidy and transformation. Nat Genet 1998; 20:189–193.
218. Sen S, Zhou H, White RA. A putative serine/threonine kinase encoding gene BTAK on chromosome 20q13 is amplified and overexpressed in human breast cancer cell lines. Oncogene 1997; 14:2195–2200.
219. Nigg EA. Mitotic kinases as regulators of cell division and its checkpoints. Nat Rev Mol Cell Biol 2001; 2:21–32.
220. Giet R, Prigent C. Aurora/Ipl1p-related kinases, a new oncogenic family of mitotic serine-threonine kinases. J Cell Sci 1999; 112(Pt 21):3591–3601.
221. Anand S, Penrhyn-Lowe S, Venkitaraman AR. AURORA-A amplification overrides the mitotic spindle assembly checkpoint, inducing resistance to Taxol. Cancer Cell 2003; 3:51–62.
222. Sudo T, Nitta M, Saya H, et al. Dependence of paclitaxel sensitivity on a functional spindle assembly checkpoint. Cancer Res 2004; 64:2502–2508.
223. Slamon DJ, Clark GM, Wong SG, Levin WJ, Ulrich A, McGuire WL. Human breast cancer: correlation of relapse and survival with amplification of the HER2/*neu* oncogene. Science 1987; 235:177–182.
224. Moscatello DK, Montgomery RB, Sundareshan P, et al. Transformational and altered signal transduction by a naturally occurring mutant EGF receptor. Oncogene 1996; 13:85–96.
225. Montgomery RB, Guzsman J, O'Rourke DM, et al. Expression of oncogenic epidermal growth factor receptor family kinases induces paclitaxel resistance and alters β-tubulin isotype expression. J Biol Chem 2000; 275:17,358–17,363.
226. Yu D, Liu B, Tan M, et al. Overexpression of c-erbB-2/neu in breast cancer cells confers increased resistance to Taxol via mdr-1-independent mechanisms. Oncogene 1996; 13:1359–1365.
227. Lee S, Yang W, Lan KH, et al. Enhanced sensitization to taxol-induced apoptosis by herceptin pretreatment in ErbB2-overexpressing breast cancer cells. Cancer Res 2002; 62:5703–5710.
228. Arteaga CL. ErbB-targeted therapeutic approaches in human cancer. Exp Cell Res 2003; 284:122–130.
229. Sulis ML, Parsons R. PTEN: from pathology to biology. Trends Cell Biol 2003; 13:478–483.
230. Aoudjit F, Vuori K. Integrin signaling inhibits paclitaxel-induced apoptosis in breast cancer cells. Oncogene 2001; 20:4995–5004.
231. Li Q, Verma IM. NF-κB regulation in the immune system. Nat Rev Immunol 2002; 2:725–734.
232. Altieri DC. Validating survivin as a cancer therapeutic target. Nat Rev Cancer 2003; 3:46–54.
233. Nyman DW, Campbell KJ, Hersh E, et al. Phase I and pharmacokinetics trial of ABI-007, a novel nanoparticle formulation of paclitaxel in patiens with advanced nonhematologic malignancies. J Clin Oncol 2005; 23:7785–7793.

19

CpG Island Methylation and Drug Resistance

Jens M. Teodoridis, PhD and Robert Brown, PhD

CONTENTS

INTRODUCTION
CpG ISLAND METHYLATION AND EPIGENETIC SILENCING
ANALYSIS OF DNA METHYLATION
ABERRANT CpG ISLAND DNA METHYLATION AND DRUG RESISTANCE
INHIBITORS OF DNA METHYLATION
CONCLUSIONS
REFERENCES

SUMMARY

Covalent epigenetic modifications such as DNA hypermethylation and histone posttranslational modifications are associated with transcriptional inactivation of many genes and are important during tumor development and progression. Genes involved in key DNA damage response pathways, such as cell cycle control, apoptosis signaling, and DNA repair, can frequently become methylated and epigenetically silenced in tumors. This may lead to differences in intrinsic sensitivity of tumors to chemotherapy, depending on the specific function of the gene inactivated. Furthermore, chemotherapy itself can exert a selective pressure on epigenetically silenced drug sensitivity genes present in subpopulations of cells, leading to acquired chemoresistance. Since the DNA sequences of epigenetically inactivated genes are not mutated but rather subject to reversible modifications via DNA methyltransferases (DNMTs) or histone modification, it is possible to reverse silencing using small molecule inhibitors. Such compounds show antitumor activity and can increase the sensitivity of drug-resistant preclinical tumor models. Clinical trials of epigenetic therapies are now underway. Epigenetic profiling, using DNA methylation and histone analysis, will provide guidance on optimization of these therapies with conventional chemotherapy and will help identify patient populations who may particularly benefit from such approaches.

Key Words: Methylation; epigenetics; DNMT; histones; CpG islands.

1. INTRODUCTION

DNA methylation, the addition of a methyl group to the carbon 5 position of cytosine residues, is the only common covalent modification of human DNA and occurs almost exclusively at cytosines that are followed immediately by a guanine (so-called CpG dinucleotides). In the bulk of the genome, CpG dinucleotides are relatively rare and are

From: *Cancer Drug Discovery and Development: Cancer Drug Resistance*
Edited by: B. Teicher © Humana Press Inc., Totowa, NJ

nearly always methylated. By contrast, small stretches of DNA, known as CpG islands, are rich in CpG nucleotides and in normal cells, are nearly always methylation-free. These CpG islands are frequently associated with the promoter regions of human genes, and methylation within the islands has been shown to be associated with posttranslational modification of histones, chromatin condensation, and transcriptional inactivation of the associated gene. Aberrant methylation of CpG islands and transcriptional silencing is frequently observed in tumors compared to normal tissue. Moreover, methylation does not occur randomly, as certain CpG islands are consistently methylated in several tumor types, whereas other CpG islands are predominantly methylated in specific tumor types. This is consistent with a model in which methylation of CpG islands at particular genes gives the cancer cell a growth or survival advantage, and so, patterns of methylation emerge depending on the selective pressure for gene silencing in the tumor type examined.

Genes involved in key DNA damage response pathways, such as cell cycle control, apoptosis signaling, and DNA repair, can frequently become epigenetically silenced and methylated in tumors. This may lead to differences in intrinsic sensitivity of tumors to chemotherapy, depending on the specific function of the gene inactivated. Furthermore, it is proposed that chemotherapy itself can exert a selective pressure on epigenetically silenced drug sensitivity genes present in subpopulations of cells, leading to acquired chemoresistance. Because the DNA sequence of epigenetically inactivated genes are not mutated, but rather subject to reversible modifications that can be targeted by therapies that inhibit DNA methyltransferases (DNMTs) or histone modification, it is possible to reverse epigenetic silencing using small molecules. Such inhibitors show antitumor activity and can increase the sensitivity of drug-resistant preclinical tumor models. Clinical trials of epigenetic therapies are now underway, and epigenetic profiling using DNA methylation and histone analysis will provide guidance on optimization of the use of these therapies with conventional chemotherapy, as well as helping to identify patient populations who may particularly benefit from such approaches.

2. CpG ISLAND METHYLATION AND EPIGENETIC SILENCING

Epigenetic change can be defined as a stable change in gene expression inherited through subsequent cell divisions that is not because of a change in DNA sequence. The only known epigenetic modification of DNA itself is the transfer of a methyl group to the carbon 5 position of cytosines, usuall in the context of CpG dinucleotides. This reaction is catalyzed by members of the family of DNMTs: DNMT1, DNMT3a, and DNMT3b (1,2). Two major changes in DNA methylation commonly occur in cancer compared to normal tissue. First, cancer cells show genome-wide hypomethylation, which has been associated with chromosomal instabilities (3,4), as well as activation of normally silenced repetitive DNA elements (5). Secondly, de novo methylation of CpG islands, often associated with the promoters of genes, can occur throughout tumor development. It is estimated that in tumors there are on average 600 CpG islands aberrantly methylated compared to normal tissue, although this can vary widely between tumor types and within particular histological subtypes (6). Moreover, methylation does not occur randomly, as there are CpG islands that are methylated in multiple tumor types, whereas other CpG islands are methylated in certain tumor types (6,7). This is consistent with a model in which methylation of CpG islands at particular genes would give the cancer cell a growth or survival advantage, and so patterns of methylation emerge depending on the selective pressure for gene silencing in the tumor type examined.

During carcinogenesis, most cancers need to develop certain hallmarks such as evasion of apoptosis, insensitivity to antigrowth signals, limitless replicative potential, self-sufficiency in growth signals, sustained angiogenesis, and tissue invasion *(8)*. Many genes that are known to be methylated in cancers can affect these hallmarks of cancer (Table 1), and selection for loss of expression of these genes during tumor development can act as a driving force behind the epigenetic inactivation of specific genes. In addition to methylation and silencing of specific genes involved in tumorigenesis, it has been suggested that tumors may acquire a methylator phenotype *(9)*. Thus, some genes may become methylated by chance and be subsequently coselected during tumor development despite having no immediate effect on tumor phenotype. However, such changes may influence subsequent behavior of the tumor by affecting biological properties, such as propensity to undergo invasion and metastasis, or acquisition of drug resistance.

3. ANALYSIS OF DNA METHYLATION

Originally, the methylation state of individual genes was determined by comparing restriction digests of DNA using methylation sensitive or insensitive isoschizomeres, e.g., HpaII and MspI, and subsequent Southern blotting. Size differences of detected bands indicated methylation at the recognition sites of the restriction enzymes. (For a detailed overview of this and other methods, *see* ref. *10*). This approach has been largely replaced by methods based on bisulfite modification of DNA for which reaction parameters have been described in detail *(11,12)*. Bisulfite treatment of DNA converts unmethylated cytosines into uracils but does not affect methylated cytosines, thereby converting differences in methylation into differences in sequence. One method of analyzing such changes in sequence is methylation-specific polymerase chain reaction ([PCR] MSP) *(13)*. MSP is performed using primers specific for either unmethylated or methylated sequences, thereby allowing the detection of the respective methylation state. (A list of cancer-relevant genes and the primers used is given in Table 1.) Among the advantages of MSP are the simple experimental procedure, the easy signal detection because of its gain-of-signal character, and its high sensitivity, allowing the detection of as little as 0.1% methylation in a DNA sample *(13)*. On the other hand, combined bisulfite restriction analysis (COBRA) uses primers that amplify the template following bisulfite modification, irrespective of its methylation state *(14)*. The PCR product should therefore be heterogeneous and reflect the various methylation states represented in the template. Discrimination of methylation states is achieved by restriction digest using a restriction site whose presence depends on the methylation state of the DNA. COBRA allows the quantification of the methylation, but its disadvantage is that the methylation of one CpG site is not necessarily representative for the methylation state of other CpG sites within the analyzed sequence, and that not all CpG sites can be analyzed with this technique. The highest resolution of the methylation status of a DNA region is achieved by bisulfite sequencing *(15)*. Following bisulfite modification, the DNA is amplified irrespective of its methylation state as in COBRA, but subsequently, methylation at all CpG sites is determined by cloning and sequencing of the PCR product. This method allows determination of methylation at single-nucleotide resolution but is relatively labor-intensive and time-consuming.

Analysis of DNA methylation is also possible on the genome-wide level. Restriction landmark genomic scanning is performed by digesting genomic DNA with the methyla-

Table 1

Primers Used in Studies of Methylation States of Genes

Function	Protein affected	Primers (5'→3')	Method[a]	Reference
Regulation of apoptosis	APAF-1	TTTCGGGTAAAAGGGATAGAATTAGA TATAACGCCCTTCCCCGACGACG	MSP	(35)
	BNIP3	TAGGATTCGTTTCGCGTACG ACCGCGTCGCCCATTAACCGCG	MSP	(65)
	CASP8	TAGGGGATTCGGACATTGCGA CGTATATCTACATTCGAAACGA	MSP	(66)
	DAPK	GGATAGTCGGATCGAGTTAACGTC CCCTCCCAACAGCGCA	MSP	(67)
	DcR1	TTACGCGTACGAATTTAGTTAAC ATCAACGACCGACCGAAACG	MSP	(68)
	DcR2	GGGATAAAGCGTTTCGATC CGACAACAAAACCGCG	MSP	(68)
	DLC-1	CCCAACGAAAAAACCCGACTAACG TTTAAAGATCGAAACGAGGGGAGCG	MSP	(69)
	Fas	AGAAAGGGTAGGGAGGTCG ATCACTCTTACGCGAAATC	MSP	(70)
	p14ARF	GTGTTAAAGGGCGGCGTAGC AAAACCCTCACTCGCGACGA	MSP	(71)
	p53	TTATAGTTTTGGTTTGTAGAAT TAACTCAAAAAAACTCATCAA *TTTTTATTTTTAAAATGTTAGTA* *ATCAAATTCAATCAAAAACTTA*	NaBis[b]	(72)
	p73	GGACGTAGCGAAATCGGGGTTC ACCCCGAACATGCGACGTCCG	MSP	(73)
	SHP1	GAACGTTATTATAGTATAGCGTTC TCACGCATACGAACCCAAACG	MSP	(74)
	TMS1	TTGTAGCGGGGTGAGCGGC AACGTCCATAAACAACAACGCG	MSP	(75)

	Sequence	Method	Ref.
TRAIL-R1	GAGCGTAGCGAGTGGGATAGAG CCGAACCCGAACACTAAATCCG	MSP	(70)
Insensitivity to anti-growth Signals			
WIF-1	GGGCGTTTATTGGGCGTAT AAACCAACAATCAACGAAC	MSP	(76)
XAF1	GTTTAGGTTGGAGTGTAGTGG CATATTCTACTCTCTACAAAC	NaBis	(77)
CRBP1	TTGGGAATTTAGTTGTTCGTCGTTTC AAACAACGACTACCGATACTACGCG	MSP	(78)
CyclinD2	TACGTGTTAGGGTCGATCG CGAAATATCTAACGCTAAACG	MSP	(79)
LOT1	GGGGTAGTCGTGTTTATAGTTTAGTA CGAACACCCAAACACCTACCCTA *ATAGTTTAGTAGCGCGGGGT* *CCTACCCTACGAAACGACGA*	NaBis[b]	(80)
p15INK4[b]	GCGTTCGTATTTTGCGGTT CGTACAATAACCGAACGACCGA	MSP	(13)
p16INK4[a]	TTATTAGAGGGTGGGGCGGATCGC GACCCCGAACCGCGACCGTAA	MSP	(13)
p57KIP2	TTTCGTTTGTAGATAAAGGA CTAACTATCCGATAATAAACTCTTCTA *GGGGGTGGGGAGTGTTGT* *ATATTTTCAATTTCAACAACACCA*	NaBis[b]	(81)
Pax5α	GGGTTTGTATATGGAGATGTTATAGG CAACATCACAAAATATCCCCAAACAC *ATAAAGTTTGGGGCGGCGC* *GCGCCCCAACGCGCCG*	MSP[c]	(82)
Pax5β	AGTTTGTGGGTTGTTTAGTTAATGG CAAAAAATCCCAACCACCAAAACC *GAGTTGAGTTTCGGGCGGC* *GCCGCCGCCGCCGTCG*	MSP[c]	(82)
PTEN	TTCGTTCGTCGTCGTCGTATTT GCCGCTTAACTCTAAACCGCAACCG	MSP	(83)
RARβ2	TGTCGAGAACGGCGAGCGATTC CGACCAATCCAACCGAAACGA	MSP	(78)

(continued)

363

Table 1 (Continued)
Primers Used in Studies of Methylation States of Genes

Function	Protein affected	Primers (5'→3')	Method[a]	Reference
	RASSF1A	CGAGAGCGCGTTTAGTTTCGTT CGATTAAACCCGTACTTCGCTAA	MSP	(84)
	14-3-3σ	TGGTAGTTTTTATGAAAGGCGTC CCTCTAACCGCCCACCACG	MSP	(85)
Limitless replicative potential	CDX1	TTGTTTTTTATTTTAAGTTGGTTATTG AAAAATAAACTAACCAAAACCTAAAAA *TTATTTTTTTTAGGTTTTGGTTAGTT* *CCACCCAAACCTTTATAACTC*	NaBis[d]	(52)
	hTR	GACGTAAAGTTTTTTCGGACG ACCCGATACGCTACCGAACG	MSP	(86)
	pRb	GGGAGTTTCGCGGACGTGAC ACGTCGAAACACGCCCG	MSP	(87)
	SOCS-1	TTCGCGTGTATTTTTAGGTCGGTC CGACACAACTCCTACAAGGACCG	MSP	(88)
	SOCS-3	TATATATTCGCGAGCGCGGTTT CGCTGCGCCCAGATGTT	MSP	(89)
Angiogenesis	THBS1	GGAGAGAGGAGTTTAGATTGGTT AATAAAAATTACTCCTAAAAAAC	COBRA	(90)
	THBS2	TGTATATTTTGATTTGGGA TTACCAACATTTATCTCAAAC *GGGTGATGTTTGAGGTGTGGGAG* *CAAATCCCCTTAATACACACTT*	COBRA[b]	(91)
	VHL	TGGAGGATTTTTTTGCGTACGC GAACCGAACGCCGCGAA	MSP	(13)
Intercellular adhesion and tissue invasion	ADAM23	TTTGTTTTGGATAAATTAAGGTTA CTACAAAAATCAAAACTAAATCTC *GTATGTAAATATAAAGGATTGTAG* *ATAAAATATATCCTCCTAAATAT*	NaBis[b]	(49)
	E-Cadherin	TTAGGTTAGAGGGTTATCGCGT TAACTAAAAATTCACCTACCGAC	MSP	(13)

364

H-Cadherin	TCGCGGGGTTCGTTTTCGC GACGTTTCATTCATTACACGCG	MSP	(53)
Cav-1	GGTATTTTTGTAGGCGCGTC CTAACAACAAAAAACGAAAAACG	MSP	(92)
CLCA2	GGGATTTATTATGTTTTTATTTTTAGAT ATCTACCCACTATAATACCCCTAC	NaBis	(93)
CLDN-7	GACGTTAGGTTATTTTCGGTC AAACGGCGTTTCTAAACGCCG	MSP	(94)
LAMA3	TATAGGAATTATAGAGCGGTGC CCTAAAACGTCCGCTAACTACG	MSP	(95)
LAMB3	ATCGATTAATTTATTTGTTTAGTTTC GAATCTCAAAAATCTAACAACCG	MSP	(95)
LAMC2	AGGTGTGCGTTTTTTCGTTGC TACAAAAATCGCTACCCGACG	MSP	(95)
Maspin	AAAAGAATGGAGATTAGAGTATTTTTTGTG CCTAAAATCACAATTATCCTAAAAAATA	NaBis	(50)
OPCML	GCGCGGTGCGGGTTTATTTTC TCCCGATACCGCCTCGAAACGAACG	MSP	(51)
SLIT2	GGGAGGTGGGATTGTTTAGATATTT CAAAAACTCCTTAAACAACTTTAAAATCCTAAAA	NaBis	(96)
TIMP3	CGTTTCGTTATTTTTTGTTTTCGGTTTC MSP CCGAAAACCCCGCCTCG		(97)
DNA repair BRCA1	GAGTTTCGAGAGACGTTTGG AATCTCAACGAACTCACGCC	MSP	(86)
FancF	TTTTTTGCGTTTGTTGGAGAATCGGGTTTTC ATACACCGCAAACCGCCGACGAACAAAAACG	MSP	(26)
MGMT	TTTCGACGTTCGTAGGTTTTCGC GCACTCTTCCGAAAACGAAACG	MSP	(67)
MLH1	ACGTAGACGTTTTATTAGGGTCGC CCTCATCGTAACTACCCGCG	MSP	(98)
MSH2	TCGTGGTCGGACGTCGTTC CAACGTCTCCTTCGACTACACCG	MSP	(98)

(continued)

Table 1 (*Continued*)
Primers Used in Studies of Methylation States of Genes

Function	Protein affected	Primers (5'→3')	Method[a]	Reference
Drug metabolism, detoxification	CytP4501A1	GTTAGTTGGGGTTAGGTTGAG CATAACCTAACTACCTACCTCC	NaBis	(99)
	GSTp1	TTCGGGGTGTAGCGCTCGTC GCCCCAATACTAAATCACGACG	MSP	(100)
	MDR	CTCTCTAAACCCGCGAACGAT TTGGGGTTTGGTAGCGC	MSP	(101)
	RFC	CCGAATCGCAAATACCGATAAAAAACG GGTTTTGTAAATTTCGGTTCGC	MSP	(101)

[a]MSP, methylation specific polymerase chain reaction (PCR); NaBis, bisulfite sequencing; COBRA, combined restriction analysis.
[b]Two rounds of PCR, first round of amplification with upper primer pair, second round with lower primer pair (italics).
[c]Nested amplification, first round with methylation unspecific primers, second round with methylation specific primers (italics).
[d]Bisulfite sequencing was performed on two overlapping PCR products.

366

tion-sensitive restriction enzyme *Not*I, end-labeling of the resulting DNA fragments, and subsequent digest with two different restriction enzymes and two-dimensional gel electrophoresis *(6)*. Comparison of signal intensities between tumor and normal DNA after autoradiography allows estimation of the number of aberrantly methylated CpG islands in tumor samples, and individual aberrantly methylated CpG islands can be identified by sequencing. Differential methylation hybridization is an alternative means of examining genome-wide methylation patterns that uses restriction digest of genomic DNA and ligation to linkers *(16)*, followed by digestion with a methylation-sensitive restriction enzyme such as *Bst*UI, PCR amplification, and hybridization to arrayed CpG-rich DNA sequences (representing putative CpG islands). Comparison to hybridization signals obtained from undigested linker-ligated DNA allows the identification of aberrantly methylated CpG islands.

4. ABERRANT CpG ISLAND DNA METHYLATION AND DRUG RESISTANCE

4.1. DNA Methylation and Intrinsic Drug Resistance

Variations in patterns of CpG island methylation can occur within the same tumor types. For example, late-stage ovarian cancers can be clustered using unsupervised hierarchical clustering into two groups based on differences in CpG island methylation *(17)*. Increased methylation of a subset of CpG islands in these tumors significantly correlated with worse clinical outcome, as defined by the time of clinical disease recurrence after chemotherapy *(17)*. These types of studies raise the possibility of using methylation profiling to identify which patients may benefit more from existing treatments, or identifying patient populations likely to be suitable for clinical trials of novel agents that target epigenetic mechanisms. Although identification of methylation of CpG islands as prognostic markers at clinical presentation of a patient's tumor has potential for molecular classification of tumor pathology, this does not demonstrate an involvement of DNA methylation in drug resistance. However, a number of recent studies suggest a direct role for epigenetic inactivation of genes, especially those with a role in cellular drug response, in determining tumor chemosensitivity.

The DNA repair enzyme O^6-methylguanine-DNA methyltransferase (MGMT) removes mutagenic alkyl groups from the O^6 position of guanine, which could otherwise lead to G to A transitions after DNA replication *(18)*. The level of MGMT expression is proportional to the resistance of cells to cyclophosphamide in xenografts *(19)*, and glioma cells with reduced MGMT expression are more sensitive to alkylating agents *(20,21)*. Epigenetic inactivation of the *mgmt* gene is frequently observed in colorectal cancer and gliomas *(22)*. Methylation of a CpG island in the *mgmt* promoter is an independent predictor of longer survival for glioblastoma patients treated with a methylating agent (temozolomide), in addition to radiation, in a prospective study *(23)*. Hypermethylation of the *mgmt* promoter also correlated with increased survival of patients with diffuse large B-cell lymphoma after chemotherapy that included cyclophosphamide *(24)*.

Fanconi anemia, complementation group F (FANCF) is crucial for the activation of a DNA repair complex containing BRCA1 and BRCA2. Inactivation of this pathway results in a decreased ability to repair DNA damage and an increased susceptibility to develop cancer *(25)*. In ovarian cancer cell lines, methylation of the *fancf* gene was observed in cells with a defective BRCA2 pathway and increased sensitivity to cisplatin. Treatment with 2'-deoxy-5-azacytidine led to demethylation of the *fancf* gene and reduced sensitivity towards cisplatin in these cell line models *(26)*. Methylation of the *fancf* gene has also been observed in ovarian cancer *(26)*, acute myeloid leukemia *(27)*, and lung and head and neck cancers *(28)*, although the relevance for clinical outcome, following chemotherapy, of methylation of *fancf* is still to be established. A two-step model for the role of the *fancf* gene in tumorigenesis and acquired chemoresistance has been proposed *(26)*. According to this model, epigenetic inactivation of *fancf* is an early event in tumor progression, but subsequent chemotherapy selects for cells in which the *fancf* methylation was reversed and which therefore display higher resistance to platinum-based chemotherapy.

In contrast to the above, where methylation of DNA repair genes during tumor development is proposed to lead to drug sensitivity, methylation of proapoptotic genes could lead to drug resistance. Many proapoptotic genes can become aberrantly methylated in tumors during tumor development (*see* Table 1). For instance, methylation of the DNA mismatch repair gene human mutL homologue 1 (*hMLH1*) and transcriptional silencing occurs in cisplatin-resistant ovarian cell line models. MLH1 has been shown to be necessary for engagement of a variety of downstream cellular responses to alkylating agent and cisplatin-induced DNA damage *(29,30)*. It has been argued that because mismatch repair (MMR) proteins can recognize and bind to certain types of damage in DNA, that this is necessary for MMR-dependent engagement of DNA damage responses such as activation of p53, p73, and other downstream apoptosis-signaling pathways *(30–32)*. Hence, loss of MLH1 expression may lead to reduced engagement of apoptosis either because of reduced cycles of futile repair *(33)* or reduced stalling (or increased bypass) of lesions in DNA during DNA replication *(34)*.

Apoptotic protease activating factor 1 (*apaf1*) represents another gene whose methylation may lead to increased resistance to chemotherapy *(35,36)*. Methylation of *apaf1* in melanoma cells can be reversed be DNMT inhibitors, leading to increased *apaf1* transcription and increased doxorubicin-induced apoptosis *(36)*. Apaf-1 is an adapter molecule that binds to and promotes procaspase 9 activation in the presence of cytochrome *c*. The release of mature caspase 9 activates a caspase cascade required for apoptosis *(37,38)*. Thus, *apaf1* is only one of a network of apoptotic and antiapoptotic genes whose expression can influence sensitivity to chemotherapy *(39)*. Methylation of other members of this network and caspase cascade have the potential to influence apoptosis and hence, chemosensitivity. For instance, caspase 8 is frequently methylated in tumors and again demethylating agents can induce gene reexpression, increased apoptosis, and chemosensitization *(40)*.

It can be seen from the above discussion that there is growing evidence for a potential role of CpG island methylation of genes with a known direct role in drug responses in predicting clinical outcome following chemotherapy. However, there is a need for large, appropriately powered prospective studies to fully validate these initial hypotheses, generating studies and demonstrating the potential to use methylation patterns of known or unknown genes to identify which patients may benefit from particular chemotherapeutic regimes or are appropriate for novel agents that target aberrant methylation. Given the potential of opposing effects depending on which genes are methylated, e.g., methylation of DNA repair genes such as *mgmt* and *fancf* conferring sensitivity, whereas methylation of proapoptotic genes such as *hMLH1* and *apaf1* would confer resistance, it will be important to examine whether particular methylation events are dominant in conferring resistance and whether these markers are independent from each other in clinical studies.

4.2. CpG Island Methylation and Acquired Drug Resistance

Most clinical studies of drug resistance have focused on tumor characteristics at presentation, rather than at relapse. Whereas studies of tumors prechemotherapy are important for identifying prognostic markers and possible mechanisms of intrinsic resistance, they will provide limited information on mechanisms of acquired resistance. Thus, tumors at presentation will be heterogeneous, consisting of chemosensitive and resistant subpopulations, making it difficult to identify the subpopulations that lead to treatment failure of an initially responsive tumor. If the hypothesis is correct that chemotherapy positively selects for resistant subpopulations, analysis of tumors at relapse may allow these subpopulations of cells to become more apparent, and will allow mechanisms of acquired, rather than intrinsic, drug resistance to be identified and analyzed for associations with patient survival.

Matched cell line models of acquired resistance have shown that common patterns of CpG island methylation can be identified as being selected for by chemotherapy in vitro *(41)*. Acquired methylation of specific candidate CpG islands, such as at the *hMLH1* gene, also can be selected for in vitro *(42)*. However, so far the potential role for acquired methylation of CpG islands in matched tumors before and after chemotherapy from the same patient has not been examined. This is partly because of the difficulties in obtaining tumor samples routinely from patients postchemotherapy or at relapse. In order to overcome this practical difficulty, there has been increasing interest in the use of markers in plasma for the prognostication and monitoring of cancer *(43)*. DNA can be detected in plasma from cancer patients with the same characteristic changes, including CpG island methylation, found in the corresponding tumor *(44)*. DNA methylation is particularly suited for such analysis of plasma DNA, because sensitive methylation-specific PCR-based assays require only small amounts of DNA, and methylation of genes frequently aberrantly methylated in tumors is rarely observed in normal tissue, including peripheral blood mononuclear cell DNA that may be present with tumor DNA in plasma *(45)*. Nevertheless, such analysis will have limited sensitivity, as not all patients may have detectable tumor DNA in plasma. Recently, we have examined plasma DNA of patients with epithelial ovarian cancer enrolled in the SCOTROC1 phase III clinical trial for methylation of the *hMLH1* CpG island before carboplatin/taxoid chemotherapy and at relapse *(46)*. Methylation of *hMLH1* is increased at relapse, with 25% (34/138) of relapse samples having *hMLH1* methylation that is not detected in matched prechemotherapy plasma samples. Furthermore, *hMLH1* methylation is significantly associated with increased microsatellite instability in plasma DNA at relapse, providing an independent measure of function of the MMR pathway. Acquisition of *hMLH1* methylation in plasma DNA at relapse predicts poor overall survival of patients, independent from time to progression and age (HR1.99, 95% CI 1.20–3.30, $p = 0.007$). These data support the clinical relevance of acquired *hMLH1* methylation, and concomitant loss of DNA mismatch repair, following chemotherapy of ovarian cancer patients.

5. INHIBITORS OF DNA METHYLATION

Several small molecule inhibitors of DNA methylation that are derivatives of 2′-deoxycytidine are known *(47)*, e.g., 5-aza-2′-deoxycytidine (decitabine), 5-azacytidine arabinosyl-5-azacytosine, and diyhdro-5-azacytidine. Demethylating agents have been proposed to have antitumor properties, because they can activate the expression of epigenetically silenced genes including tumor suppressor genes *(48–53)*. However, in addition, these demethylating agents can restore sensitivity to a range of chemotherapeutic agents including cisplatin, epirubicin, and temozolomide *(42,54)*. These nucleoside DNMT inhibitors are phosphorylated to their nucleotide analogs before being incorporated into DNA. Once incorporated into DNA, they complex with, and inactivate, all three forms of DNA methyltransferases. Nucleoside DNMT inhibitors have been reported to have antitumor activity, especially against hematologic malignancies *(55)*. Like many other novel therapeutics currently being developed against specific targets, demethylating agents are hoped to function in a specific manner, and thus have less side effects than the nonspecific conventional chemotherapy, by reversing repression of tumor suppressor and cell cycle genes aberrantly methylated in tumor cells, leading to inhibition of tumor growth *(56)*. An important consequence of this is that, unlike conventional cytotoxic agents, it may be best to use such drugs at concentrations lower than the maximum tolerated dose. For example, there is an optimal concentration at which analogs of 5-azacytosine induce cellular differentiation; higher concentrations produce less differentiation and more cytotoxicity *(57)*. Thus, in the case of decitabine, although its use at high doses may induce direct toxicity effects because of its incorporation into DNA, prolonged low-dose schedules *(58)* or low doses in combinations with other drugs *(54)* may be more biologically effective in inhibiting DNMT activity with less toxicity.

The combination of decitabine and cisplatin showed a synergistic cytotoxic interaction in many human tumor cell lines. Although a possible underlying mechanism originally suggested is the increased binding of cisplatin to decitabine-substituted DNA that is independent of DNA hypomethylation *(59)*, more-recent studies have focused on the effects of decitabine in reactivating drug sensitivity genes *(54)*. Decitabine was used in vivo to sensitize MMR-deficient, drug-resistant ovarian (A2780/cp70) and colon (SW48) tumor xenografts that are MLH1-negative because of gene promoter hypermethylation. Treatment of tumor-bearing mice with the demethylating agent decitabine at a nontoxic dose induces MLH1 expression, and reexpression of MLH1 was associated with a decrease in *hMLH1* gene promoter methylation. Decitabine treatment alone had no effect on the growth rate of the tumors. However, decitabine treatment sensitized the xenografts to cisplatin, carboplatin, temozolomide, and epirubicin, although this was schedule dependent with decitabine having to be given at least 6 d before the cytotoxic. Decitabine treatment did not sensitize xenografts of HCT116, which lacks MMR because of *hMLH1* mutation, or A2780/cp70 that reexpressed MLH1 because of chromosome transfer.

The human multidrug resistance gene 1 *(MDR1)* encodes P-glycoprotein, a transmembrane protein that acts as a drug efflux pump, reducing intracellular levels of certain anticancer drugs and thus reducing their effectiveness. Increased transcription of the *MDR1* gene in chronic lymphocytic leukemia and bladder cancer following chemotherapy has been shown to be associated with decreased methylation. This would argue that treatment of sensitive tumors with a demethylating agent could lead to resistance to chemotherapy by increased expression of *MDR1*. Indeed, increased resistance of tumor cells after treatment with azacytidine analogs to drugs that are substrates of P-glycoprotein has been observed *(60)*. However, increased sensitization and no effect has also been reported to be induced by DNMT inhibitors for MDR-drugs in different tumor models *(54,61,62)*. This again emphasizes the possibility that these agents will have different effects depending on the pattern of genes methylated in a given tumor and argues that patient stratification depending on their methylation status may be necessary in clinical trials of demethylating agents.

6. CONCLUSIONS

There is accumulating evidence that aberrant CpG island methylation is a clinically relevant driving force behind gene-silencing events that have potential to alter intrinsic and acquired resistance to anticancer drugs. Epigenetic inactivation of genes occurs at a much higher rate than gene mutation *(63)*. Multiple genes, and hence, multiple resistance mechanisms, have the potential to become simultaneously inactivated as tumors acquire methylation of multiple CpG islands. CpG methylation either of specific genes or global patterns has the potential to be used as predictive or prognostic markers *(64)*, but further clinical studies are necessary to substantiate their significance. Methods for the analysis of the methylation states of specific CpG islands and global methylation states exist and have potential to define further patient populations, and in the next 5 yr, DNA methylation patterns will probably become increasingly important in the management of cancer patients. DNA methylation is being examined as a means of early diagnosis of cancer and, the detection of methylation in DNA isolated from body fluids of cancer patients could provide a noninvasive means of diagnosis *(46)*.

Small molecules that allow reversal of aberrant epigenetic modifications are now entering clinical trials. Nucleoside DNMT inhibitors, such as decitabine, have been reported to have antitumor activity, especially against hematologic malignancies. Such demethylating agents have been proposed to reactivate tumor suppressor genes aberrantly methylated in tumor cells, leading to inhibition of tumor growth because of induction of apoptosis or differentiation. An important consequence of this is that, unlike conventional cytotoxic agents, it may be best to use such drugs at concentrations lower than the maximum tolerated dose and in a manner dependent on their demethylating activity. Furthermore, synergistic activity with other types of investigational epigenetic therapies and existing chemotherapies opens the possibility of rational combinations and scheduling of these agents based on their biological activity. Perhaps the combination of epigenetic drugs with existing therapies holds the greatest promise in their clinical use, particularly if prospective studies continue to support CpG island methylation as a clinically relevant mechanism of resistance to chemotherapy. Epigenetic silencing does recur over time in cells where reexpression has been induced by treatment with DNMT inhibitors. Therefore, there is only a specific window of time within which tumor cells will die because of epigenetic reversal of silencing of tumor suppressor genes and subsequent apoptosis or differentiation. However, this window of demethylation can be used for appropriate scheduling of a cytotoxic or other treatment. The ideal scenario will be to have robust means of identifying CpG island methylation and to provide a personalized treatment for that patient based on the methylation profile.

REFERENCES

1. Liu K, Wang YF, Cantemir C, Muller MT. Endogenous assays of DNA methyltransferases: evidence for differential activities of DNMT1, DNMT2, and DNMT3 in mammalian cells in vivo. Mol Cell Biol 2003; 23:2709–2719.
2. Bird AP, Wolffe AP. Methylation-induced repression—belts, braces, and chromatin. Cell 1999; 99(5):451–454.
3. Eden A, Gaudet F, Waghmare A, Jaenisch R. Chromosomal instability and tumors promoted by DNA hypomethylation. Science 2003; 300:455.
4. Gaudet F, Hodgson JG, Eden A, et al. Induction of tumors in mice by genomic hypomethylation. Science 2003; 300:489–492.
5. Walsh CP, Chaillet JR, Bestor TH. Transcription of IAP endogenous retroviruses is constrained by cytosine methylation. Nat Genet 1998; 20:116–117.

6. Costello JF, Fruhwald MC, Smiraglia DJ, et al. Aberrant CpG-island methylation has non-random and tumor-type-specific patterns. Nat Genet 2000; 24:132–138.

7. Esteller M, Herman JG. Cancer as an epigenetic disease: DNA methylation and chromatin alterations in human tumours. J Pathol 2002; 196:1–7.

8. Hanahan D, Weinberg RA. The hallmarks of cancer. Cell 2000; 100:57–70.

9. Toyota M, Ahuja N, Ohe-Toyota M, Herman JG, Baylin SB, Issa JP. CpG island methylator phenotype in colorectal cancer. Proc Natl Acad Sci U S A 1999; 96:8681–8686.

10. Dahl C, Guldberg P. DNA methylation analysis techniques. Biogerontology 2003; 4:233–450.

11. Warnecke PM, Stirzaker C, Song J, Grunau C, Melki JR, Clark SJ. Identification and resolution of artifacts in bisulfite sequencing. Methods 2002; 27:101–107.

12. Grunau C, Clark SJ, Rosenthal A. Bisulfite genomic sequencing: systematic investigation of critical experimental parameters. Nucleic Acids Res 2001; 29:E65–E65.

13. Herman JG, Graff JR, Myohanen S, Nelkin BD, Baylin SB. Methylation-specific PCR: a novel PCR assay for methylation status of CpG islands. Proc Natl Acad Sci U S A 1996; 93:9821–9826.

14. Xiong Z, Laird PW. COBRA: a sensitive and quantitative DNA methylation assay. Nucleic Acids Res 1997; 25:2532–2534.

15. Frommer M, McDonald LE, Millar DS, et al. A genomic sequencing protocol that yields a positive display of 5-methylcytosine residues in individual DNA strands. Proc Natl Acad Sci U S A 1992; 89:1827–1831.

16. Huang TH, Perry MR, Laux DE. Methylation profiling of CpG islands in human breast cancer cells. Hum Mol Genet 1999; 8:459–470.

17. Wei SH, Chen CM, Strathdee G, et al. Methylation microarray analysis of late-stage ovarian carcinomas distinguishes progression-free survival in patients and identifies candidate epigenetic markers. Clin Cancer Res 2002; 8:2246–2252.

18. Gerson SL. MGMT: its role in cancer aetiology and cancer therapeutics. Nat Rev Cancer 2004; 4:296–307.

19. Mattern J, Eichhorn U, Kaina B, Volm M. O^6-methylguanine-DNA methyltransferase activity and sensitivity to cyclophosphamide and cisplatin in human lung tumor xenografts. Int J Cancer 1998; 77:919–922.

20. Silber JR, Bobola MS, Ghatan S, Blank A, Kolstoe DD, Berger MS. O^6-methylguanine-DNA methyltransferase activity in adult gliomas: relation to patient and tumor characteristics. Cancer Res 1998; 58:1068–1073.

21. Silber JR, Blank A, Bobola MS, Ghatan S, Kolstoe DD, Berger MS. O^6-methylguanine-DNA methyltransferase-deficient phenotype in human gliomas: frequency and time to tumor progression after alkylating agent-based chemotherapy. Clin Cancer Res 1999; 5:807–814.

22. Esteller M, Hamilton SR, Burger PC, Baylin SB, Herman JG. Inactivation of the DNA repair gene O^6-methylguanine-DNA methyltransferase by promoter hypermethylation is a common event in primary human neoplasia. Cancer Res 1999; 59:793–797.

23. Hegi ME, Diserens AC, Godard S, et al. Clinical trial substantiates the predictive value of O^6-methylguanine-DNA methyltransferase promoter methylation in glioblastoma patients treated with temozolomide. Clin Cancer Res 2004; 10:1871–1874.

24. Esteller M, Gaidano G, Goodman SN, et al. Hypermethylation of the DNA repair gene O-methylguanine DNA methyltransferase and survival of patients with diffuse large B-cell lymphoma. J Natl Cancer Inst 2002; 94:26–32.

25. Olopade OI, Wei M. FANCF methylation contributes to chemoselectivity in ovarian cancer. Cancer Cell 2003; 3:417–420.

26. Taniguchi T, Tischkowitz M, Ameziane N, et al. Disruption of the Fanconi anemia-BRCA pathway in cisplatin-sensitive ovarian tumors. Nat Med 2003; 9:568–574.

27. Tischkowitz M, Ameziane N, Waisfisz Q, et al. Bi-allelic silencing of the Fanconi anaemia gene FANCF in acute myeloid leukaemia. Br J Haematol 2003; 123:469–471.

28. Marsit CJ, Liu M, Nelson HH, Posner M, Suzuki M, Kelsey KT. Inactivation of the Fanconi anemia/BRCA pathway in lung and oral cancers: implications for treatment and survival. Oncogene 2004; 23:1000–1004.

29. Papouli E, Cejka P, Jiricny J. Dependence of the cytotoxicity of DNA-damaging agents on the mismatch repair status of human cells. Cancer Res 2004; 64:3391–3394.

30. Stojic L, Mojas N, Cejka P, et al. Mismatch repair-dependent G2 checkpoint induced by low doses of SN1 type methylating agents requires the ATR kinase. Genes Dev 2004; 18:1331–1344.

31. Shimodaira H, Yoshioka-Yamashita A, Kolodner RD, Wang JY. Interaction of mismatch repair protein PMS2 and the p53-related transcription factor p73 in apoptosis response to cisplatin. Proc Natl Acad Sci U S A 2003; 100:2420–2425.

32. Duckett DR, Bronstein SM, Taya Y, Modrich P. hMutSα and MutLα dependent phosphorylation of p53 in response to DNA methylator damage. Proc Natl Acad Sci U S A 1999; 96:12,384–12,388.

33. Karran P, Hampson R. Genomic instability and tolerance to alkylating agents. Cancer Surveys 1996; 28:69–85.

34. Moreland NJ, Illand M, Kim YT, Paul J, Brown R. Modulation of drug resistance mediated by loss of mismatch repair by the DNA polymerase inhibitor aphidicolin. Cancer Res 1999; 59:2102–2106.

35. Fu WN, Bertoni F, Kelsey SM, et al. Role of DNA methylation in the suppression of Apaf-1 protein in human leukaemia. Oncogene 2003; 22:451–455.

36. Soengas MS, Capodieci P, Polsky D, et al. Inactivation of the apoptosis effector Apaf-1 in malignant melanoma. Nature 2001; 409:207–211.

37. Slee EA, Adrain C, Martin SJ. Serial killers: ordering caspase activation events in apoptosis. Cell Death Differ 1999; 6:1067–1074.

38. Saleh A, Srinivasula SM, Acharya S, Fishel R, Alnemri ES. Cytochrome c and dATP-mediated oligomerization of Apaf-1 is a prerequisite for procaspase-9 activation. J Biol Chem 1999; 274:17,941–17,945.

39. Pommier Y, Sordet O, Antony S, Hayward RL, Kohn KW. Apoptosis defects and chemotherapy resistance: molecular interaction maps and networks. Oncogene 2004; 23:2934–2949.

40. Fulda S, Kufer MU, Meyer E, van Valen F, Dockhorn-Dworniczak B, Debatin KM. Sensitization for death receptor- or drug-induced apoptosis by re-expression of caspase-8 through demethylation or gene transfer. Oncogene 2001; 20:5865–5877.

41. Wei SH, Brown R, Huang TH. Aberrant DNA methylation in ovarian cancer: is there an epigenetic predisposition to drug response? Ann N Y Acad Sci 2003; 983:243–250.

42. Strathdee G, MacKean M, Illand M, Brown R. A role for methylation of the *hMLH1* promoter in loss of hMLH1 expression and drug resistance in ovarian cancer. Oncogene 1999; 18:2335–2341.

43. Johnson PJ, Lo YMD. Plasma nucleic acids in the diagnosis and management of malignant disease. Clinical Chemistry 2002; 48:1186–1193.

44. Esteller M, Sanchez-Cespedes M, Rosell R, Sidransky D, Baylin SB, Herman JG. Detection of aberrant promoter hypermethylation of tumour suppressor genes in serum DNA from non-small cell lung cancer patients. Cancer Res 1999; 59:67–70.

45. Toyota M, Kopecky KJ, Toyota MO, Jair KW, Willman CL, Issa JP. Methylation profiling in acute myeloid leukemia. Blood 2001; 97:2823–2829.

46. Gifford G, Paul J, Vasey PA, Kaye SB, Brown R. The acquisition of hMLH1 methylation in plasma DNA after chemotherapy predicts poor survival for ovarian cancer patients. Clin Cancer Res 2004; 10:4420–4426.

47. Goffin J, Eisenhauer E. DNA methyltransferase inhibitors-state of the art. Ann Oncol 2002; 13:1699–1716.

48. Arnold CN, Goel A, Boland CR. Role of hMLH1 promoter hypermethylation in drug resistance to 5-fluorouracil in colorectal cancer cell lines. Int J Cancer 2003; 106:66–73.

49. Costa FF, Verbisck NV, Salim AC, et al. Epigenetic silencing of the adhesion molecule ADAM23 is highly frequent in breast tumors. Oncogene 2004; 23:1481–1488.

50. Domann FE, Rice JC, Hendrix MJ, Futscher BW. Epigenetic silencing of maspin gene expression in human breast cancers. Int J Cancer 2000; 85:805–810.

51. Sellar GC, Watt KP, Rabiasz GJ, et al. OPCML at 11q25 is epigenetically inactivated and has tumor-suppressor function in epithelial ovarian cancer. Nat Genet 2003; 34:337–343.

52. Suh ER, Ha CS, Rankin EB, Toyota M, Traber PG. DNA methylation down-regulates CDX1 gene expression in colorectal cancer cell lines. J Biol Chem 2002; 277:35,795–35,800.

53. Toyooka KO, Toyooka S, Virmani AK, et al. Loss of expression and aberrant methylation of the CDH13 (H-cadherin) gene in breast and lung carcinomas. Cancer Res 2001; 61:4556–4560.

54. Plumb JA, Strathdee G, Sludden J, Kaye SB, Brown R. Reversal of drug resistance in human tumor xenografts by 2'-deoxy-5-azacytidine-induced demethylation of the hMLH1 gene promoter. Cancer Res 2000; 60:6039–6044.

55. Lyons J, Bayar E, Fine G, et al. Decitabine: development of a DNA methyltransferase inhibitor for hematological malignancies. Curr Opin Investig Drugs 2003; 4:1442–1450.

56. Issa JP. Decitabine. Curr Opin Oncol 2003; 15:446–451.

57. Taylor SM, Jones PA. Multiple new phenotypes induced in 10T2 and 3T3 cells treated with 5-azacytidine. Cell 1979; 17:771–779.

58. Issa JP, Garcia-Manero G, Giles FJ, et al. Phase 1 study of low-dose prolonged exposure schedules of the hypomethylating agent 5-aza-2'-deoxycytidine (decitabine) in hematopoietic malignancies. Blood 2004; 103:1635–1640.

59. Ellerhorst JA, Frost P, Abbruzzese JL, Newman RA, Chernajovsky Y. 2'-deoxy-5-azacytidine increases binding of cisplatin to DNA by a mechanism independant of DNA hypomethylation. British Journal of Cancer 1993; 67:209–215.

60. Kantharidis P, El-Osta A, deSilva M, et al. Altered methylation of the human MDR1 promoter is associated with acquired multidrug resistance. Clin Cancer Res 1997; 3:2025–2032.

61. Efferth T, Futscher BW, Osieka R. 5-Azacytidine modulates the response of sensitive and multidrug-resistant K562 leukemic cells to cytostatic drugs. Blood Cells Mol Dis 2001; 27:637–648.

62. Ando T, Nishimura M, Oka Y. Decitabine (5-aza-2'-deoxycytidine) decreased DNA methylation and expression of MDR-1 gene in K562/ADM cells. Leukemia 2000; 14:1915–1920.

63. Bhattacharyya NP, Skandalis A, Ganesh A, Groden J, Meuth M. Mutator phenotypes in human colorectal carcinoma cell lines. Proc Natl Acad Sci U S A 1994; 91:6319–6323.

64. Brown R, Strathdee G. Epigenomics and epigenetic therapy of cancer. Trends Mol Med 2002; 8(Suppl):S43–S48.

65. Okami J, Simeone DM, Logsdon CD. Silencing of the hypoxia-inducible cell death protein BNIP3 in pancreatic cancer. Cancer Res 2004; 64:5338–5346.

66. Teitz T, Wei T, Valentine MB, et al. Caspase 8 is deleted or silenced preferentially in childhood neuroblastomas with amplification of MYCN. Nat Med 2000; 6:529–535.

67. Balana C, Ramirez JL, Taron M, et al. O^6-methyl-guanine-DNA methyltransferase methylation in serum and tumor DNA predicts response to 1,3-*bis*(2-chloroethyl)-1-nitrosourea but not to temozolamide plus cisplatin in glioblastoma multiforme. Clin Cancer Res 2003; 9:1461–1468.

68. van Noesel MM, van Bezouw S, Salomons GS, et al. Tumor-specific down-regulation of the tumor necrosis factor-related apoptosis-inducing ligand decoy receptors DcR1 and DcR2 is associated with dense promoter hypermethylation. Cancer Res 2002; 62:2157–2161.

69. Kim TY, Jong HS, Song SH, et al. Transcriptional silencing of the DLC-1 tumor suppressor gene by epigenetic mechanism in gastric cancer cells. Oncogene 2003; 22:3943–3951.

70. Hopkins-Donaldson S, Ziegler A, Kurtz S, et al. Silencing of death receptor and caspase-8 expression in small cell lung carcinoma cell lines and tumors by DNA methylation. Cell Death Differ 2003; 10:356–364.

71. Esteller M, Tortola S, Toyota M, et al. Hypermethylation-associated inactivation of p14(ARF) is independent of p16(INK4a) methylation and p53 mutational status. Cancer Res 2000; 60:129–133.

72. Kang JH, Kim SJ, Noh DY, et al. Methylation in the p53 promoter is a supplementary route to breast carcinogenesis: correlation between CpG methylation in the p53 promoter and the mutation of the p53 gene in the progression from ductal carcinoma in situ to invasive ductal carcinoma. Lab Invest 2001; 81:573–579.

73. Corn PG, Kuerbitz SJ, van Noesel MM, et al. Transcriptional silencing of the p73 gene in acute lymphoblastic leukemia and Burkitt's lymphoma is associated with 5' CpG island methylation. Cancer Res 1999; 59:3352–3356.

74. Oka T, Ouchida M, Koyama M, et al. Gene silencing of the tyrosine phosphatase SHP1 gene by aberrant methylation in leukemias/lymphomas. Cancer Res 2002; 62:6390–6394.

75. Stimson KM, Vertino PM. Methylation-mediated silencing of TMS1/ASC is accompanied by histone hypoacetylation and CpG island-localized changes in chromatin architecture. J Biol Chem 2002; 277:4951–4958.

76. Mazieres J, He B, You L, et al. Wnt inhibitory factor-1 is silenced by promoter hypermethylation in human lung cancer. Cancer Res 2004; 64:4717–4720.

77. Byun DS, Cho K, Ryu BK, et al. Hypermethylation of XIAP-associated factor 1, a putative tumor suppressor gene from the 17p13.2 locus, in human gastric adenocarcinomas. Cancer Res 2003; 63:7068–7075.

78. Esteller M, Guo M, Moreno V, et al. Hypermethylation-associated Inactivation of the cellular retinol-binding-protein 1 gene in human cancer. Cancer Res 2002; 62:5902–5905.

79. Evron E, Umbricht CB, Korz D, et al. Loss of cyclin D2 expression in the majority of breast cancers is associated with promoter hypermethylation. Cancer Res 2001; 61:2782–2787.

80. Abdollahi A, Pisarcik D, Roberts D, Weinstein J, Cairns P, Hamilton TC. LOT1 (PLAGL1/ZAC1), the candidate tumor suppressor gene at chromosome 6q24-25, is epigenetically regulated in cancer. J Biol Chem 2003; 278:6041–6049.

81. Li Y, Nagai H, Ohno T, et al. Aberrant DNA methylation of p57(KIP2) gene in the promoter region in lymphoid malignancies of B-cell phenotype. Blood 2002; 100:2572–2577.

82. Palmisano WA, Crume KP, Grimes MJ, et al. Aberrant promoter methylation of the transcription factor genes PAX5 alpha and beta in human cancers. Cancer Res 2003; 63:4620–4625.

83. Salvesen HB, MacDonald N, Ryan A, et al. PTEN methylation is associated with advanced stage and microsatellite instability in endometrial carcinoma. Int J Cancer 2001; 91:22–26.

84. Honorio S, Agathanggelou A, Wernert N, Rothe M, Maher ER, Latif F. Frequent epigenetic inactivation of the RASSF1A tumour suppressor gene in testicular tumours and distinct methylation profiles of seminoma and nonseminoma testicular germ cell tumours. Oncogene 2003; 22:461–466.

85. Umbricht CB, Evron E, Gabrielson E, Ferguson A, Marks J, Sukumar S. Hypermethylation of 14-3-3 sigma (stratifin) is an early event in breast cancer. Oncogene 2001; 20:3348–3353.

86. Strathdee G, Appleton K, Illand M, et al. Primary ovarian carcinomas display multiple methylator phenotypes involving known tumor suppressor genes. Am J Pathol 2001; 158:1121–1127.

87. Simpson DJ, Hibberts NA, McNicol AM, Clayton RN, Farrell WE. Loss of pRb expression in pituitary adenomas is associated with methylation of the RB1 CpG island. Cancer Res 2000; 60:1211–1216.

88. Yoshikawa H, Matsubara K, Qian GS, et al. SOCS-1, a negative regulator of the JAK/STAT pathway, is silenced by methylation in human hepatocellular carcinoma and shows growth-suppression activity. Nat Genet 2001; 28:29–35.

89. He B, You L, Uematsu K, et al. SOCS-3 is frequently silenced by hypermethylation and suppresses cell growth in human lung cancer. Proc Natl Acad Sci U S A 2003; 100:14,133–14,138.

90. Li Q, Ahuja N, Burger PC, Issa JP. Methylation and silencing of the thrombospondin-1 promoter in human cancer. Oncogene 1999; 18:3284–3289.

91. Whitcomb BP, Mutch DG, Herzog TJ, Rader JS, Gibb RK, Goodfellow PJ. Frequent HOXA11 and THBS2 promoter methylation, and a methylator phenotype in endometrial adenocarcinoma. Clin Cancer Res 2003; 9:2277–2287.

92. Chan TF, Su TH, Yeh KT, et al. Mutational, epigenetic and expressional analyses of caveolin-1 gene in cervical cancers. Int J Oncol 2003; 23:599–604.

93. Li X, Cowell JK, Sossey-Alaoui K. CLCA2 tumour suppressor gene in 1p31 is epigenetically regulated in breast cancer. Oncogene 2004; 23:1474–1480.

94. Kominsky SL, Argani P, Korz D, et al. Loss of the tight junction protein claudin-7 correlates with histological grade in both ductal carcinoma in situ and invasive ductal carcinoma of the breast. Oncogene 2003; 22:2021–2033.

95. Sathyanarayana UG, Toyooka S, Padar A, et al. Epigenetic inactivation of laminin-5-encoding genes in lung cancers. Clin Cancer Res 2003; 9:2665–2672.

96. Dallol A, Krex D, Hesson L, Eng C, Maher ER, Latif F. Frequent epigenetic inactivation of the *SLIT2* gene in gliomas. Oncogene 2003; 22:4611–4616.

97. Bachman KE, Herman JG, Corn PG, et al. Methylation-associated silencing of the tissue inhibitor of metalloproteinase-3 gene suggest a suppressor role in kidney, brain, and other human cancers. Cancer Res 1999; 59:798–802.

98. Herman JG, Umar A, Polyak K, et al. Incidence and functional consequences of hMLH1 promoter hypermethylation in colorectal carcinoma. Proc Natl Acad Sci U S A 1998; 95:6870–6875.

99. Anttila S, Hakkola J, Tuominen P, et al. Methylation of cytochrome P4501A1 promoter in the lung is associated with tobacco smoking. Cancer Res 2003; 63:8623–8628.

100. Lee TL, Leung WK, Chan MW, et al. Detection of gene promoter hypermethylation in the tumor and serum of patients with gastric carcinoma. Clin Cancer Res 2002; 8:1761–1766.

101. Worm J, Kirkin AF, Dzhandzhugazyan KN, Guldberg P. Methylation-dependent silencing of the reduced folate carrier gene in inherently methotrexate-resistant human breast cancer cells. J Biol Chem 2001; 276:39,990–40,000.

20 De Novo and Acquired Resistance to Antitumor Alkylating Agents

Lori A. Hazlehurst, PhD
and William S. Dalton, MD, PhD

Contents

INTRODUCTION
MECHANISMS ASSOCIATED WITH ACQUIRED RESISTANCE
TO ALKYLATING AGENTS
RESISTANCE TO ALKYLATING AGENTS ASSOCIATED WITH DE NOVO
DRUG RESISTANCE
CONCLUSION
REFERENCES

SUMMARY

Delineating mechanisms that mediate *de novo* and acquired resistance to alkylating agents could potentially lead to novel targets for improving the efficacy of this important class of anticancer drugs. *De novo* resistance is likely to contribute to minimal residual disease and the subsequent emergence of a more permanent form of drug resistance referred to as acquired drug resistance. The tumor microenvironment represents a rich source of both soluble factors and components of extracellular matrixes, both of which can favor cell survival following drug exposure. Experimental evidence suggests signals that originate from the tumor microenvironment are likely to contribute to *de novo* resistance and thereby facilitate the emergence of acquired resistance. DNA repair pathways, cell cycle checkpoints, drug metabolism, transporters, and alterations in the apoptotic machinery represent potential mechanisms of resistance to alkylating agents. The role of these pathways in conferring acquired and *de novo* resistance will be discussed in detail this chapter.

Key Words: Antitumor alkylating agents; *de novo* resistance; acquired resistance; glutathione; glutathione *S*-transferase, Fanconi anemia/BRCA1 pathway.

1. INTRODUCTION

The acquisition of drug resistance continues to limit the clinical success of alkylating agents and other chemotherapeutic drugs *(1)*. Often, acquired drug resistance is manifested by multifactorial resistant mechanisms, and therefore is therapeutically difficult to reverse *(2,3)*. Because of the complexity of acquired drug resistance, others and we have started to explore mechanisms contributing to *de novo* resistance. By definition, *de*

From: *Cancer Drug Discovery and Development: Cancer Drug Resistance*
Edited by: B. Teicher © Humana Press Inc., Totowa, NJ

novo resistance is present before drug exposure and selection for drug resistance. Mechanisms associated with *de novo* drug resistance may contribute to the failure to eliminate minimal residual disease and facilitate the emergence of acquired drug resistance. We propose that targeting *de novo* resistance could enhance the efficacy of currently used drugs and reduce the probability of the emergence of acquired clinical drug resistance. Obviously, enhancing initial drug efficacy will reduce tumor burden and potentially prevent minimal residual disease from progressing to drug resistant disease. Specifically, we have shown that cell adhesion of hematopoietic tumor cell lines, as well as primary patient specimens, via β1 integrins causes resistance to wide variety of cytotoxics including alkylating agents *(3–7,8)*. We have referred to the phenomenon as cell adhesion-mediated drug resistance or CAM-DR. This chapter discusses several pathways, including CAM-DR, that may contribute to clinical *de novo* resistance.

In contrast to *de novo* resistance, acquired drug resistance occurs following drug selection. Acquired drug resistance has been modeled in tissue culture by chronic exposure to a cytotoxic agent, until a stable drug resistance phenotype is selected *(9,10)*. Several resistance models to alkylating agents have been developed, and mechanisms associated with these models are discussed in this chapter. These models have been crucial for identifying resistance pathways as well as understanding of the mechanisms of action of alkylating agents. However, it has become apparent that consideration of the tumor microenvironment will be instrumental to understand fully mechanisms of drug resistance. Experimental evidence supporting the concept that the tumor microenvironment could influence drug response, and emergence of drug resistance was first demonstrated by Teicher et al. *(11)*. They showed that treatment of mice bearing EMT-6 tumors with crosslinking agents for 6 mo and the subsequent emergence of drug resistance resulted in a phenotype that was only operative in vivo. These studies emphasized the need to consider the tumor microenvironment as a factor for determining drug response, and contributing to minimal residual disease and the emergence of acquired drug resistance.

2. MECHANISMS ASSOCIATED WITH ACQUIRED RESISTANCE TO ALKYLATING AGENTS

Alkylating agents are considered the first class of chemotherapeutic drugs developed to treat cancer, and were derived from sulfur mustard gas, a compound initially developed for warfare use *(12)*. The lead alkylating compounds derived from sulfur mustards were the nitrogen mustards. Alkylating agents are strong electrophiles and covalently bind nucleophilic targets such as phosphate, amino, sulfhydryl, hydroxyl, carboxyl, and imidazole groups. Thus, DNA, RNA, and proteins all represent potential targets for alkylation. However, the majority of evidence indicates that the primary target is DNA and specifically, the formation of DNA interstrand crosslinks (ICLs) *(13)*. Following the formation of ICLs, the activation of DNA repair pathways and cell cycle checkpoints are critical components in determining cellular fate (Fig. 1). In addition, downstream mediators of the apoptotic pathway can also increase the threshold of ICLs needed to activate cell death. Using cell line models to study acquired drug resistance, several mechanisms have been discovered. These mechanisms include reducing the amount of active drug reaching the nucleus (transport and metabolism), enhanced DNA repair pathways, antiapoptotic machinery, and altered cell cycle checkpoints that could all influence drug response associated with alkylating agents. The following subheading will summarize resistance mechanisms associated with acquired resistance to alkylating agents.

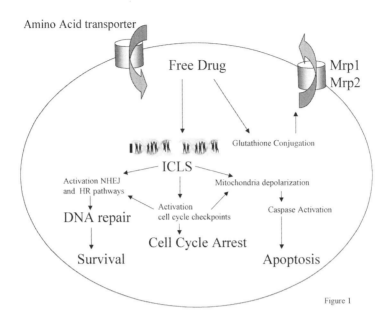

Amino Acid transporter

Free Drug

Mrp1
Mrp2

Glutathione Conjugation

ICLS

Activation NHEJ
and HR pathways

Mitochondria depolarization

DNA repair

Activation
cell cycle checkpoints

Caspase Activation

Survival

Cell Cycle Arrest

Apoptosis

Figure 1

Fig. 1. Multiple mechanisms can confer resistance to alkylating agents. These mechanisms include (a) altered transport, (b) glutathione conjugation, (c) DNA repair, (d) cell cycle checkpoints, and (e) either increased levels of antiapoptotic BCL-2 family members or decreased levels of proapoptotic BCL-2 family members.

2.1. DNA Repair Associated With Acquired Resistance

Recent clinical evidence has shown that repair of ICLs is an important determinant of acquired clinical resistance to alkylating agents. For example, Spanswick et al. showed that myeloma cells derived from relapsed patients repaired 40 to 80% of ICLs by 40 h following ex vivo exposure to melphalan. In contrast, myeloma cells derived from patients who had never been treated with melphalan showed no repair of melphalan induced crosslinks *(14)*. Similarly, Torres-Garcia et al. reported in chronic lymphocytic leukemia (CLL) that previously untreated CLL specimens demonstrated minimal repair of melphalan-induced ICLs. In contrast, lymphocytes derived from resistant CLL patients showed complete repair of melphalan induced ICLs within 24 h *(15)*. Together, these data indicate the importance of repair of interstrand crosslinks in mediating acquired clinical drug resistance, suggesting that further studies are warranted to identify targets associated with repair of ICLs.

As shown in Fig. 2, several DNA repair pathways can contribute to the repair of ICLs induced by alkylating agents. These pathways include nonhomologous end-joining (NHEJ) and homologous recombination. Recent experimental evidence suggests that homologous recombination and specifically, the Fanconi anemia pathway, may be a critical determinant associated with resistance to alkylating agents *(3,16,17)*. Hematopoietic cells derived from Fanconi anemia (FA) patients are characteristically exquisitely hypersensitive to crosslinking agents such as melphalan and mitomycin C *(18)*. In addition, FA cells in culture demonstrate an increased rate of spontaneous chromosomal breakage, and patients are predisposed to cancer including an especially high incidence of acute myelogenous leukemia, squamous cell carcinoma of the head and neck, esophageal, and gynecologic cancers *(19)*. Together, the clinical data suggest that the FA

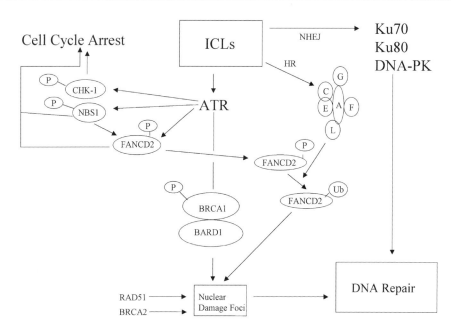

Fig 2. Following the formation of ICLs induced by alkylating agents, cell cycle checkpoints and DNA repair pathways are activated. Coordinated activation of both cell cycle checkpoints and DNA repair pathways allows for time to repair damaged DNA. Both homologous recombination (HR) and nonhomologous end-joining (NHEJ) DNA repair pathways can be activated following the induction of ICLs, and both pathways play a role in determining sensitivity to alkylating agents.

pathway is integral for maintaining genomic integrity. To date, eight members have been cloned and identified as critical components of the FA pathway. Six of the eight FA proteins form a nuclear multiprotein complex consisting of Fanconi anemia (FANC)A, FANCC, FANCG, FANCE, FANCF, and FANCL. The seventh member, FANCD1, was identified as breast cancer (BRCA)2 *(20)*, and the eighth member, FANCD2, becomes activated by monoubiquination at lysine-561 following DNA damage *(21)*. The nuclear multiprotein complex is required for the monoubiquination of FANCD2, and recently, Garcia-Higuera et al. provided several lines of evidence linking the FA and BRCA pathway *(21)*. For example, exposure to DNA damaging agents is known to increase the levels of mono-ubiquinated FANCD2, and furthermore, the mono-ubiquinated form FANCD2 is localized within DNA damage foci containing BRCA1, BRCA2, and Rad51. Moreover, BRCA1 was shown to coimmunoprecipitate with FANCD2. Finally, BRAC1[-/-] cells show reduced formation of foci containing FANCD2, suggesting that BRCA1 stabilized this complex, providing further evidence that BRCA1 and FANCD2 directly interact with each other *(21)*.

Our laboratory showed recently that, using gene expression profiling, selection of 8226 human myleoma cells with melphalan resulted in increased expression levels of FANCF, Rad51c, and decreased levels of BRCA1-associated protein *(3)*. BRCA1-associated protein would effectively sequester BRCA1 in the cytoplasm *(22)* and thus limit the amount of BRCA1 available to form drug-induced DNA damage repair foci. Thus, we identified several changes in gene expression, which would directly affect the FA/BRCA pathway in an acquired melphalan resistant cell line. We recently validated the overexpression of these proteins, and we are currently using small interfering (si)RNA strategies to determine the functional role of each of these changes in mediating resistance to melphalan. Recently, Taniguchi et al. proposed a model for ovarian cancer, where the initial progression of the disease correlates with silencing of FANCF associated with methylation of the promoter followed by demethlyation and increased expression and resistance to *cis*-platinum *(23)*. Together, these data suggest that the FA pathway may be a determinant of both tumor progression and resistance to chemotherapy. This paradigm may apply to other diseases such as myeloma and chronic lymphocytic leukemia, diseases that initially respond well to alkylating agents but invariably develop resistance to further drug treatment. More studies are warranted to determine the pathways that regulate the expression and silencing of FANCF as potentially increased expression of FANCF could contribute to both *de novo* and acquired resistance to alkylating agents.

NHEJ is predominately mediated by DNA-dependent protein kinase (DNA-PK), and evidence suggests that this pathway is critical for the repair of DNA double-strand breaks initiated by ionizing radiation. DNA-PK is a serine/threonine kinase belonging to the phosphoinositide 3 kinase family. The Ku autoantigen, consisting of a Ku80/Ku86 dimer, is required for the recruitment of DNA-PK to a DNA double-strand break (reviewed in ref. *24*). Mutations in DNA-PK result in hypersensitivity to both γ-radiation and crosslinking agent-mediated cell death *(25)*. In addition, Ku80 knockouts show increased sensitivity to alkylating agents *(26)*. Clinical relevance of the DNA-PK pathway was demonstrated by Muller et al., when they showed that resistance of CLL to chlorambucil (CLB) correlated with increased binding of Ku subunits to DNA and increased DNA-PK activity *(27)*. In summary, experimental evidence indicates that both NHEJ and homologous recombination can contribute to resistance associated with alkylating agents, supporting the underlying functional complexity of acquired drug resistance.

2.2. Alterations in Cell Cycle Checkpoints Associated With Acquired Resistance

It has become apparent that cell cycle checkpoints and DNA repair are integrally linked biochemical processes. Following DNA damage and cell cycle arrest, it is currently unclear what combinations of signals lead to repair and survival vs the induction of apoptosis and cell death. However, one of the first biological steps is recognition of the aberrant DNA lesion. To date, the DNA damage sensors appear to be the phosphoinositide 3 kinase family members DNA-PK, ataxia telangiectasia mutated (ATM) kinase, and ATM- and Rad3-related (ATR) kinase. These are serine/threonine kinases that are known to phosphorylate cell cycle checkpoints including CHK1, CHK2, and p53 *(24,28,29)*. Although these family members have similar consensus sequence for phosphorylation, they are not functionally redundant. For example, dominant-negative studies demonstrate that ATR, but not ATM, is critical for DNA damage caused by bulky lesions such as *cis*-platinum and methyl methanesulfonate *(30,31)*. In contrast, knocking out ATM does not sensitize cells to these agents. In addition, recent evidence has linked the DNA damage sensor ATR pathway to the Fanconia anemia pathway. Andreassen et al. showed that silencing of ATR resulted in the attenuation of mitomycin C-induced mono-ubiquination of FANCD2 *(32)*. Moreover, Pichierri and Rosselli showed that ATR directly phosphorylates FANCD2 *(33)*. These investigators also showed that, using siRNA, knocking out ATR resulted in an abrogation of crosslink-induced inhibition of DNA synthesis. In contrast, siRNA directed at CHK1 only partially reversed inhibition of DNA synthesis. In summary, their data showed in addition to CHK1, an ATR-dependent Nijmegen breakage syndrome 1/FA pathway was required to get complete inhibition of DNA synthesis following treatment with crosslinking agents. In contrast to what

Andressen observed, these investigators did not show that ATR-dependent phosphory-lation was required for efficient mono-ubquination of FANCD2, suggesting that at least in some cells, an alternative ATR-independent pathway regulates the formation of crosslink induced formation of FANCD2 foci.

It is also apparent that delaying cell cycle progression in at the G_1/S boundary follow-ing DNA damage can favor cell survival. Evidence supporting this concept includes studies looking at drug sensitivity in cells deficient in cell cycle checkpoints. For example, Fan et al. showed that cells lacking the CDK2 inhibitor p21 demonstrated increased sensitivity to nitrogen mustards (34). Conversely, ectopic overexpression of either the cyclin-dependent kinase (CDK) inhibitor p27[kip1] or p21 is associated with resistance to DNA damaging agents (35,36). It is well known that acquired drug resistant cell lines typically demonstrate reduced growth rates. Our laboratory recently identified several changes in gene expression in the acquired melphalan resistant cell line that would be indicative of longer transit time at G_1. These changes included increased expression of p27[kip1] and p57[kip2] and decreased expression of cyclin D1 and CDC25A (3). The CDK inhibitors p27[kip1] and p57[kip2] are well-described inhibitors of CDK2, and CDK2 activity is required for exit through the G_1/S interphase (37,38). In addition, CDC25A is a phos-phatase that is required for the activation of CDK2 and progression through the G_1/S boundary. Moreover, Mailand et al. showed that overexpression of CDC25A resulted in enhanced DNA damage and decreased survival (39). Together, these data indicate that inhibitors of CDK2 may contribute to acquired drug resistance. However, further studies are warranted to determine the downstream resistance mechanisms associated with alter-ations in G_1/S checkpoints.

2.3. Alterations in Apoptotic Machinery Associated With Acquired Resistance

It is clear that DNA damaging drugs elicit an apoptotic response. However, it is currently unclear what culminations of signals following DNA damage are required to elicit the apoptotic response. Despite this uncertainty, experimental evidence does show that DNA damage causes depolarization of the mitochondria membrane potential and the subsequent activation of effector caspases. Thus, both pro- and antiapoptotic Bcl-2 fam-ily members are critical for defining the threshold of ICLs required to depolarize the mitochondria membrane potential and the subsequent activation of effector caspases (40,41). Bcl-2 family members can be broken down into those proteins that inhibit the depolarization of the mitochondria membrane potential (antiapoptotic) vs proteins that promote the depolarization of the mitochondria membrane potential (proapoptotic). The proapoptotic Bcl-2 family members can be further subdivided into BH3-only domain and multidomain proteins. The multidomain members are comprised of Bax, Bak, Bok, and Bcl-x_S, whereas Bad, Bik, Bid, Hrk, Blk, Bim, Bmf, Noxa, Puma, and Bcl-g constitute the BH3 only group (42,43). Double-knockout studies of Bak- and Bax-depleted cells show resistance to a wide variety of cytotoxic insults. In addition, overexpression of BH3 only members does not result in apoptosis in Bax[-/-], Bak[-/-] cells (44). Together, these results suggest that BH3-only members mechanistically work by either activating Bax or Bak, or by binding and interfering with antiapoptotic family members and displacing Bax/Bak Bcl-2 heterodimers.

Despite the experimental evidence showing that either ectopic expression of antiapoptotic or reduction in proapoptotic molecules is sufficient to cause drug resis-tance, it is currently unclear if alterations in the apoptotic machinery play an important role in acquired drug resistance. For example, our laboratory showed that, using gene expression profiling, the melphalan-acquired drug-resistant cell line showed changes in the apoptotic machinery that was predictive for both cell survival and cell death *(3)*. These apparent functionally opposing changes in gene expression of apoptotic mediators made it impossible to predict what net effect these changes would have on cell survival. This is similar to what Reinhold et al. showed with acquired resistance associated with topotecan selection *(45)*. These investigators proposed a two-step model in which some proapoptotic genes may emerge that have dual roles with respect to cell cycle progression, and thus allow for growth in the presence of drug exposure. Further studies are warranted to validate this two-step model associated with acquired drug resistance, and whether the molecular changes favoring growth at the expense of apoptosis observed in several acquired drug resistant cell lines can be exploited in a therapeutic setting.

2.4. Alterations in Glutathione Metabolism Associated With Acquired Resistance

Alkylating agents are electrophiles, and thus, glutathione conjugation represents a plausible mechanism for detoxification of this class of drugs. Indeed, several investigators have shown that acquired drug-resistant cell lines contain elevated levels of glutathione *(46–50)*. In addition depletion of glutathione levels with L-buthionine-[*S,R*]-sulfoximine is reported to increase the sensitivity of cells to melphalan in several cell line models *(46,51,52)*. We showed recently that, using gene expression profiling, the catalytic subunit of glutamylcysteine synthase is increased in acquired melphalan resistance *(3)*. The gene expression profiling correlated with our earlier finding showing that the acquired myeloma drug resistant cell line demonstrated increased glutathione levels, suggesting that this pathway maybe important for acquired drug resistance *(46)*. Moreover, increased expression of glutamylcysteine synthase is consistent with our previous report showing that L-buthionine-[*S,R*]-sulfoximine partially reversed the resistance to melphalan in the acquired drug resistant cell line. In addition to *de novo* synthesis of enzymes, the conjugation reaction represents another mechanism for detoxification of alkylating agents. For example, Horton et al. showed that the ovarian carcinoma cell line A2780 selected for chlorambucil resistance demonstrated increased expression of glutathione *S*-transferase (GST)-μ, which correlated with a sixfold increase an efficiency of CBL conjugation *(53)*. However, mixed results have been obtained with studies in which either glutamylcysteine synthase or GSTs have been ectopically expressed in cell lines with respect to conferring resistance to alkylating agents *(54,55)*. Thus, overall, the role of glutathione in mediating clinical drug resistance remains controversial, and further studies are needed to define further the role of glutathione conjugation in mediating resistance to alkylating agents. In addition to glutathione detoxification, metallothionein 2 is reported to form covalent bonds with melphalan, and overexpression is reported to confer drug resistance and this pathway represents another potential detoxification mechanism contributing to drug resistance *(56–58)*.

2.5. Acquired Resistance and Drug Transport

Overexpression of drug efflux pumps is a common mechanism associated with acquired multidrug resistance. However, alkylating agents do not show crossresistance in cell lines that overexpress MDR1 or BCRP and appear to be poor substrates for drug transporters *(2,10)*. Recently, multidrug resistance protein (MRP) has shown to be an efficient pump for glutathione-conjugated compounds. Both glutathione-conjugated CLB and melphalan have been shown to be substrates for MRP1 *(59)*. Moreover, there is some evidence that glutathione conjugated CLB is a good substrate for either MRP1 or MRP2 *(60,61)*. Smitherman et al. showed that overexpression of GST A1-1 in cells that overexpress MRP2 increased the resistance associated with CLB treatment *(61)*. Both Melphalan and CLB share structural similarities; however, surprisingly the synergy was only noted with CLB.

Reduced drug uptake is another potential mechanism of drug resistance. Some alkylating agents like melphalan contain a phenylalanine group and are reported to use the L-type amino acid transporter for cellular uptake *(62)*. Indeed, we reported that the 8226-acquired drug resistant myeloma cell line showed a modest reduction in the L-type amino acid transporter *(3)*. However, this modest reduction was not enough to detect differences between drug sensitive and resistant cell lines in the concentration of intracellular melphalan. In summary, acquired resistance to alkylating agents can be mediated by multiple genotypic changes making the reversal of acquired resistance a clinically difficult challenge.

3. RESISTANCE TO ALKYLATING AGENTS ASSOCIATED WITH *DE NOVO* DRUG RESISTANCE

In contrast to acquired drug resistance, *de novo* resistance is not associated with drug selection. The tumor microenvironment is composed of both soluble factors and extracellular matrixes, which can potentially provide survival signals allowing for tumor progression. In fact, the tumor microenvironment represents the first selection pressure to which tumor cells are exposed, and thus, interaction with the tumor microenvironment creates an advantage for tumor cells to survive initial drug exposure. We showed recently that cellular adhesion of hematopoietic tumor cells via $\beta 1$ integrins is sufficient to cause resistance to a multiple drugs, including alkylating agents. We referred to this phenomenon as CAM-DR. Moreover, we validated the CAM-DR phenotype in primary patient specimens were we showed that adhesion of myeloma patient specimens to fibronectin (FN) was sufficient to confer resistance to melphalan *(3)*. However, the tumor microenvironment is also composed of cyctokines and growth factors, and indeed, we have shown via Transwell experiments that soluble factors produced by myeloma cell interactions with stroma cells is sufficient to cause resistance to alkylating agents *(63)*. In summary, both soluble and matrixes that are localized in the tumor microenvironment are factors when defining determinants of *de novo* drug resistance.

3.1. Alterations in Cell Cycle Checkpoints Associated With De Novo Resistance

Changes in cell cycle checkpoints may represent one pathway especially sensitive to regulation by the tumor microenvironment. For example, St. Croix et al. showed that resistance associated with tumor spheroid growth caused increased $p27^{kip1}$ levels and cell cycle arrest. Using antisense to $p27^{kip1}$, they were able to reverse resistance associated with 4-hydroperoxycyclophosphamide *(64)*. In addition, our laboratory has shown that adhesion 8226 myeloma cells to FN resulted in a G_1/S arrest and increased $p27^{kip1}$ levels. Moreover, knocking down $p27^{kip1}$ levels with antisense reversed the drug-resistant phenotype *(5)*. Finally, transforming growth factor (TGF)-β has been shown to cause resistance to alkylating agents in vivo. In this study, Teicher et al. showed that treatment of animals with TGF-β-neutralizing antibodies increased the sensitivity of cyclophosphamid (CTX) in EMT6/Parental and EMT6/CTX-resistant tumor-bearing mice *(65)*. The role of TGF-β in mediating resistance to crosslinking agents was further strengthened by showing that EMT-6 cells ectopically expressing TGF-β were resistant to CTX in an in vivo model *(66)*. Although the downstream target has not been identified, TGF-β in some cell lines is known to cause cell cycle arrest and increased levels of p27^{kip1} *(67)*, and this may contribute to the observed TGF-β-mediated resistance to alkylating agents. In summary, the tumor microenvironment consists of many signals including cytokines, growth factors, and adhesion molecules that can affect cell cycle and drug sensitivity, and these pathways may represent critical targets in mediating *de novo* resistance.

3.2. Alterations in Apoptotic Machinery Associated With De Novo Resistance

We showed recently that the cell adhesion conferred resistance to melphalan-induced depolarization of mitochondria membrane potential, despite similar numbers of melphalan induced interstrand crosslinks *(3)*. Our results suggested that cell adhesion to FN increases the tolerance for melphalan-induced ICLs. The mitochondrial membrane potential is largely regulated by Bcl-2 family members, and we asked whether changes in either the levels of pro- or anti-Bcl-2 family members contributed to the resistance phenotype. Microarray analysis revealed a modest 1.4-fold reduction in the proapoptotic BH3-only Bcl-2 family member Bim. We confirmed this finding at the protein level showing that adhesion of 8226 cells to FN resulted in a pronounced reduction in Bim protein levels *(3)*. We hypothesize that the reduction in Bim levels is contributing to melphalan resistance, and we are currently validating this target with respects to conferring resistance to alkylating agents.

Ectopic overexpresion of antiapoptotic Bcl-2 family members such as Bcl-2 and Bcl-x$_L$ confers resistance to DNA damaging agents *(68–70)*. Thus, activation of intracellular pathways such as signal transducer and activator of transcription 3, which induce Bcl-x$_L$ expression, could contribute to *de novo* drug resistance *(71)*. Activation of signal transducer and activator of transcription 3 can be activated by cytokines, and this represents one potential cytokine-mediated pathway that may contribute to drug resistance. In summary, although the role of Bcl-2 family members is not clearly delineated in acquired resistance, change in expression of these molecules induced by signals originating from the tumor microenvironment may be a critical determinant of *de novo* resistance.

3.3. Cholesterol Metabolism and Drug Resistance

We reported recently that, using gene expression profiling to compare *de novo* and acquired resistance to melphalan, one common convergence was change in expression of genes that regulated cholesterol synthesis *(3)*. Comparing isogenic myeloma cell lines with *de novo* and acquired melphalan resistance, we noted increases in several metabolic enzymes that would positively regulate cholesterol synthesis, including increased expression of 3-hydroxy-3-methylgluatryl coenzyme A reductase (HMG-CoA). HMG-CoA is the rate-liming step in cholesterol synthesis. Evidence supporting the importance of cholesterol in mediating cell death induced by alkylating agents includes a report from Soma et al., where these investigators showed that treatment of primary human glioma cells treated with simvastatin an inhibitor of HMG-CoA and *N,N'-bis*-(2-choroethyl)-*N*-nitosourea demonstrated synergy with respects to cell death *(72)*. We propose that changes in cholesterol metabolism may play an important role in mediating *de novo* resistance, and that this cholesterol functional genomic fingerprint is maintained in acquired drug resistance. More studies are warranted to determine the clinical significance of cholesterol in mediating *de novo* and acquired resistance to alkylating agents.

4. CONCLUSION

In summary, acquired resistance to alkylating agents results in a complex drug resistant phenotype and genotype. For example, our laboratory observed multiple changes in gene expression that could alter DNA repair, cell cycle, glutathione metabolism, and drug transport. Indeed, it would be difficult to reverse pharmacologically all of these mechanisms simultaneously. We are currently using siRNA technology to prioritize these identified targets with respect to potency of reversing the drug resistance phenotype. However, we propose that targeting mechanisms that contribute to *de novo* resistance and minimal residual disease may be more fruitful. Specifically, evidence suggests that components of the tumor microenvironment may be sufficient to protect subpopulations of cells from drug treatment. It is our hypothesis that this transient protection afforded by the microenvironment increases the probability that an acquired stable drug resistant phenotype will emerge. Thus, identification of signaling pathways that regulate expression or function of Bcl-2 family members, cell cycle checkpoints, and DNA repair complexes may represent important targets for inhibiting *de novo* drug resistance.

REFERENCES

1. Dalton WS, Salmon SE. Drug resistance in myeloma: mechanisms and approaches to circumvention. Hematol Oncol Clin North Am 1992; 6:383–393.
2. Hazlehurst LA, Foley NE, Gleason-Guzman MC, et al. Multiple mechanisms confer drug-resistance to mitoxantrone in the human 8226 myeloma cll line. Cancer Res 1999; 59:1021–1028.
3. Hazlehurst LA, Enkemann S, Beam CAR, et al. Genotypic and phenotypic comparisons of *de novo* and acquired melphalan resistance in an isogenic multiple myeloma cell line model. Cancer Res 2003; 56:660–670.
4. Damiano JS, Cress AE, Hazlehurst LA, Shtil AA, Dalton WS. Cell adhesion mediated drug resistance (CAM-DR): Role of integrins and resistance to apoptosis in human myeloma cell lines. Blood 1999; 93:1658–1667.
5. Hazlehurst LA, Damiano JS, Buyuksalm I, Pledger WJ, Dalton WS. Adhesion to fibronectin regulates p27^{kip1} levels and contributes to cell adhesion mediated drug resistance (CAM-DR). Oncogene 2000; 38:4319–4327.
6. Hazlehurst LA, Dalton WS. Mechanisms associated with cell adhesion mediated drug resistance (CAM-DR) in hematopoietic malignancies. Cancer Metastasis Rev 2001; 20:43–50.
7. Hazlehurst LA, Valkov N, Wisner L, et al. Reduction in drug-induced DNA double strand-breaks associated with β1 integrin-mediated adhesion correlates with drug resistance in U937 cells. Blood 2001; 98:1897–1903.
8. Damiano JS, Hazlehurst LA, Dalton WS. Cell adhesion mediated resistance (CAM-DR) protects the K562 chronic myelogenous leukemia cell line from apoptosis induced by BCR/ABL inhibition cyctoxic drugs and γ radiation. Leukemia 2001; 15:1232–1239.
9. Taylor CW, Dalton WS, Parrish PR, et al. Different mechanisms of decreased drug accumulation in doxorubicin and mitoxantrone resistant variants of the MCF7 human breast cancer cell line. Br J Cancer 1991; 63:923–929.
10. Dalton WS, Durie BG, Alberts DS, Gerlach JH, Cress AE. Characterization of a new drug-resistant human myeloma cell line that expresses P-glycoprotein. Cancer Res 1986; 46:5125–5130.
11. Teicher BA, Herman TS, Holden SA, et al. Tumor resistance to alkylating agents conferred by mechanisms operative only in vivo. Science 1990; 247:1457–1460.
12. Gilman A. The initial clinical trial of nitrogen mustard. Am J Surg 1963; 105:574–578.
13. Zwelling LA, Michaels S, Schwartz H, Dobson PP, Kohn KW. DNA cross-linking as an indicator of sensitivity and resistance of mouse L1210 leukemia to *cis*-diamminedichloroplatinum^{II} and L-phenylalanine mustard. Cancer Res 1981; 41:640–649.
14. Spanswick VJ, Craddock C, Sekhar M, et al. Repair of DNA interstrand crosslinks as a mechanism of clinical resistance to melphalan in multiple myeloma. Blood 2002; 100:224–229.

15. Torres-Garcia SJ, Cousineau L, Caplan S, Panasci L. Correlation of resistance to nitrogen mustards in chronic lymphocytic leukemia with enhanced removal of melphalan-induced DNA cross-links. Biochem Pharmacol 1989; 38:3122–3123.

16. D'Andrea AD. The Fanconi Anemia/BRCA signaling pathway: disruption in cisplatin-sensitive ovarian cancers. Cell Cycle 2003; 2:290–292.

17. Olopade OI, Wei M. FANCF methylation contributes to chemoselectivity in ovarian cancer. Cancer Cell 2003; 3:417–420.

18. Ishida R, Buchwald M. Susceptibility of Fanconi's anemia lymphoblasts to DNA-cross-linking and alkylating agents. Cancer Res 1982; 42:4000–4006.

19. D'Andrea AD, Grompe M. Molecular biology of Fanconi anemia: implications for diagnosis and therapy. Blood 1997; 90:1725–1736.

20. Howlett NG, Taniguchi T, Olson S, et al. Biallelic inactivation of BRCA2 in Fanconi anemia. Science 2002; 297:606–609.

21. Garcia-Higuera I, Taniguchi T, Ganesan S, et al. Interaction of the Fanconi anemia proteins and BRCA1 in a common pathway. Mol Cell 2001; 7:249–262.

22. Li S, Ku CY, Farmer AA, Cong YS, Chen CF, Lee WH. Identification of a novel cytoplasmic protein that specifically binds to nuclear localization signal motifs. J Biol Chem 1998; 273:6183–6189.

23. Taniguchi T, Tischkowitz M, Ameziane N, et al. Disruption of the Fanconi anemia-BRCA pathway in cisplatin-sensitive ovarian tumors. Nat Med 2003; 9:568–574.

24. Durocher D, Jackson SP. DNA-PK, ATM and ATR as sensors of DNA damage: variations on a theme? Curr Opin Cell Biol 2001; 13:225–231.

25. Tanaka T, Yamagami T, Oka Y, Nomura T, Sugiyama H. The *scid* mutation in mice causes defects in the repair system for both double-strand DNA breaks and DNA cross-links. Mutat Res 1993; 288:277–280.

26. Muller C, Calsou P, Salles B. The activity of the DNA-dependent protein kinase (DNA-PK) complex is determinant in the cellular response to nitrogen mustards. Biochimie 2000; 82:25–28.

27. Muller C, Christodoulopoulos G, Salles B, Panasci L. DNA-Dependent protein kinase activity correlates with clinical and in vitro sensitivity of chronic lymphocytic leukemia lymphocytes to nitrogen mustards. Blood 1998; 92:2213–2219.

28. Zhao H, Piwnica-Worms H. ATR-mediated checkpoint pathways regulate phosphorylation and activation of human Chk1. Mol Cell Biol 2001; 21:4129–4139.

29. Guo Z, Kumagai A, Wang SX, Dunphy WG. Requirement for Atr in phosphorylation of Chk1 and cell cycle regulation in response to DNA replication blocks and UV-damaged DNA in Xenopus egg extracts. Genes Dev 2000; 14:2745–2756.

30. Cliby WA, Roberts CJ, Cimprich KA, et al. Overexpression of a kinase-inactive ATR protein causes sensitivity to DNA-damaging agents and defects in cell cycle checkpoints. EMBO J 1998; 17:159–169.

31. Wright JA, Keegan KS, Herendeen DR, et al. Protein kinase mutants of human ATR increase sensitivity to UV and ionizing radiation and abrogate cell cycle checkpoint control. Proc Natl Acad Sci U S A 1998; 95:7445–7450.

32. Andreassen PR, D'Andrea AD, Taniguchi T. ATR couples FANCD2 monoubiquitination to the DNA-damage response. Genes Dev 2004; 18:1958–1963.

33. Pichierri P, Rosselli F. The DNA crosslink-induced S-phase checkpoint depends on ATR-CHK1 and ATR-NBS1-FANCD2 pathways. EMBO J 2004; 23:1178–1187.

34. Fan S, Chang JK, Smith ML, Duba D, Fornace AJ Jr, O'Connor PM. Cells lacking *CIP1/WAF1* genes exhibit preferential sensitivity to cisplatin and nitrogen mustard. Oncogene 1997; 14:2127–2136.

35. Eymin B., Haugg M, Droin N, Sordet O, Dimanche-Boitrel MT, Solary E. p27^{Kip1} induces drug resistance by preventing apoptosis upstream of cytochrome c release and procaspase-3 activation in leukemic cells. Oncogene 1999; 18:1411–1418.

36. Ruan S, Okcu FM, Ren JP, et al. Overexpressed WAF1/CIP1 renders glioblastoma cells resistant to chemotherapy agents 1,3-*bis*-(2-chloroethyl)-1-nitrosurea and cisplatin. Cancer Res 1998; 58:1538–1543.

37. Girard FU, Strausfeild A, Fernedez A, Lamb NJ. Cyclin A is required for the onset of DNA replication in mammalian fibroblasts. Cell 1991; 67:1169–1179.

38. Ohtsubo M, Theodoras AM, Schumacher J, Roberts JM, Pagano M. Human cyclin E, a nuclear protein required for the G$_1$ to S phase transition. Mol Cell Biol 1995; 15:2612–2624.

39. Mailand N, Falck J, Lukas C, et al. Rapid destruction of human Cdc25A in response to DNA damage. Science 2000; 288:1425–1429.

40. Pommier Y, Sordet O, Antony S, Hayward RL, Kohn KW. Apoptosis defects and chemotherapy resistance: molecular interaction maps and networks. Oncogene 2004; 23:2934–2949.

41. Green DR, Kroemer G. The pathophysiology of mitochondrial cell death. Science 2004; 305:626–629.
42. Puthalakath H, Strasser A. Keeping killers on a tight leash: transcriptional and post-translational control of the pro-apoptotic activity of BH3-only proteins. Cell Death Differ 2002; 9:505–512.
43. Harada H, Grant S. Apoptosis regulators. Rev Clin Exp Hematol 2003; 7:117–138.
44. Zong WX, Lindsten T, Ross AJ, MacGregor GR, Thompson CB. BH3-only proteins that bind pro-survival Bcl-2 family members fail to induce apoptosis in the absence of Bax and Bak. Genes Dev 2001; 15:1481–1486.
45. Reinhold WC, Kouros-Mehr H, Kohn KW, et al. Apoptotic susceptibility of cancer cells selected for camptothecin resistance: gene expression profiling, functional analysis, and molecular interaction mapping. Cancer Res 2003; 63:1000–1011.
46. Bellamy WT, Dalton WS, Gleason MC, Grogan TM, Trent JM. Development and characterization of a melphalan-resistant human multiple myeloma cell line. Cancer Res 1991; 51:995–1002.
47. Ahmad S, Okine L, Le B, Najarian P, Vistica DT. Elevation of glutathione in phenylalanine mustard-resistant murine L1210 leukemia cells. J Biol Chem 1987; 262:15,048–15,053.
48. Alaoui-Jamali MA, Panasci L, Centurioni GM, Schecter R, Lehnert S, Batist G. Nitrogen mustard-DNA interaction in melphalan-resistant mammary carcinoma cells with elevated intracellular glutathione and glutathione-S-transferase activity. Cancer Chemother Pharmacol 1992; 30:341–347.
49. Colvin OM, Friedman HS, Gamcsik MP, Fenselau C, Hilton J. Role of glutathione in cellular resistance to alkylating agents. Adv Enzyme Regul 1993; 33:19–26.
50. Ozols RF, O'Dwyer PJ, Hamilton TC, Young RC. The role of glutathione in drug resistance. Cancer Treat Rev 1990; 17(Suppl A):A45–A50.
51. Suzukake K, Petro BJ, Vistica DT. Reduction in glutathione content of L-PAM resistant L1210 cells confers drug sensitivity. Biochem Pharmacol 1982; 31:121–124.
52. Somfai-Relle S, Suzukake K, Vistica BP, Vistica DT. Reduction in cellular glutathione by buthionine sulfoximine and sensitization of murine tumor cells resistant to L-phenylalanine mustard. Biochem Pharmacol 1984; 33:485–490.
53. Horton JK, Roy G, Piper JT, et al. Characterization of a chlorambucil-resistant human ovarian carcinoma cell line overexpressing glutathione S-transferase mu. Biochem Pharmacol 1999; 58:693–702.
54. Tipnis SR, Blake DG, Shepherd AG, McLellan LI. Overexpression of the regulatory subunit of γ-glutamylcysteine synthetase in HeLa cells increases γ-glutamylcysteine synthetase activity and confers drug resistance. Biochem J 1999; 337(Pt 3):559–566.
55. Nakagawa K, Saijo N, Tsuchida S, et al. Glutathione-S-transferase pi as a determinant of drug resistance in transfectant cell lines. J Biol Chem 1990; 265:4296–4301.
56. Kondo Y, Woo ES, Michalska AE, Choo KH, Lazo JS. Metallothionein null cells have increased sensitivity to anticancer drugs. Cancer Res 1995; 55:2021–2023.
57. Kelley SL, Basu A, Teicher BA, Hacker MP, Hamer DH, Lazo JS. Overexpression of metallothionein confers resistance to anticancer drugs. Science 1988; 241:1813–1815.
58. Yu X, Wu Z, Fenselau C. Covalent sequestration of melphalan by metallothionein and selective alkylation of cysteines. Biochemistry 1995; 34:3377–3385.
59. Barnouin K, Leier I, Jedlitschky G, et al. Multidrug resistance protein-mediated transport of chlorambucil and melphalan conjugated to glutathione. Br J Cancer 1998; 77:201–209.
60. Paumi CM, Ledford BG, Smitherman PK, Townsend AJ, Morrow CS. Role of multidrug resistance protein 1 (MRP1) and glutathione S-transferase A1-1 in alkylating agent resistance. Kinetics of glutathione conjugate formation and efflux govern differential cellular sensitivity to chlorambucil versus melphalan toxicity. J Biol Chem 2001; 276:7952–7956.
61. Smitherman PK, Townsend AJ, Kute TE, Morrow CS. Role of multidrug resistance protein 2 (MRP2, ABCC2) in alkylating agent detoxification: MRP2 potentiates glutathione S-transferase A1-1-mediated resistance to chlorambucil cytotoxicity. J Pharmacol Exp Ther 2004; 308:260–267.
62. Yanagida O, Kanai Y, Chairoungdua A, et al. Human L-type amino acid transporter 1 (LAT1): characterization of function and expression in tumor cell lines. Biochim Biophys Acta 2001; 1514:291–302.
63. Nefedova Y, Landowski TH, Dalton WS. Bone marrow stromal-derived soluble factors and direct cell contact contribute to de novo drug resistance of myeloma cells by distinct mechanisms. Leukemia 2003; 17:1175–1182.
64. St. Croix B, Florenes VA, Rak JW, et al. Impact of the cyclin-dependent kinase inhibitor p27[Kip1] on resistance of tumor cells to anticancer agents. Nat Med 1996; 2:1204–1210.
65. Teicher BA, Holden SA, Ara G, Chen G. Transforming growth factor-β in in vivo resistance. Cancer Chemother Pharmacol 1996; 37:601–609.

66. Teicher BA, Ikebe M, Ara G, Keyes SR, Herbst RS. Transforming growth factor-β 1 overexpression produces drug resistance in vivo:revresal by decorin. In Vivo 1997; 11:463–472.
67. Polyak K, Kato JY, Solomon MJ, et al. p27Kip1, a cyclin-CDK inhibitor, links transforming growth factor-beta and contact inhibition to cell cycle arrest. Genes Devel 1994; 8:9–22.
68. Zhang Y, Lei XY. Effect of bcl-2 antisense oligodeoxynucleotides on drug sensitivity of leukemic cells. Hematol J 2003; 4:187–197.
69. Miyashita T, Reed JC. bcl-2 gene transfer increases relative resistance of S49.1 and WEHI7.2 lymphoid cells to cell death and DNA fragmentation induced by glucocorticoids and multiple chemotherapeutic drugs. Cancer Res 1992; 52:5407–5411.
70. Minn AJ, Rudin CM, Boise LH, Thompson CB. Expression of bcl-x$_L$ can confer a multidrug resistance phenotype. Blood 1995; 86:1903–1910.
71. Catlett-Falcone R, Landowski TH, Oshiro MM, et al. Constitutive activation of Stat3 signaling confers resistance to apoptosis in human U266 myeloma cells. Immunity 1999; 10:105–115.
72. Soma MR, Baetta R, De Renzis MR, et al. In vivo enhanced antitumor activity of carmustine [*N,N′-bis*-(2-chloroethyl)-*N*-nitrosourea] by simvastatin. Cancer Res 1995; 55:597–602.

21 Resistance to Antiangiogenic Agents

George W. Sledge, Jr., MD,
Kathy D. Miller, MD, *Bryan Schneider,* MD,
and Christopher J. Sweeney, MBBS

CONTENTS

SUMMARY

Because normal endothelial cells are genetically stable, antiangiogenic therapy was initially theorized to be "a treatment resistant to resistance." However, resistance to antiangiogenic therapy is a very real problem. Mechanisms of resistance to the antiangiogenic effects of cytotoxic agents likely also apply to novel antiangiogenic agents. The use of antiangiogenic agents as adjuvant therapy has potential barriers. The toxicity of chronic antiangiogenic therapy remains largely unexplored, as is the toxicity of combinations of chemotherapy with antiangiogenic therapy. Population-specific feasibility studies can identify toxicities that might not be acceptable in an otherwise healthy patient population.

Key Words: Antiangiogenesis; vascular endothelial growth factor; vascular endothelial growth factor receptor; hypoxia; tyrosine kinase inhibitors.

1. INTRODUCTION

Angiogenesis, the process of new blood vessel formation, plays a central role in both local tumor growth and distant metastasis *(1)*. Because normal endothelial cells are genetically stable, antiangiogenic therapy was initially theorized to be "a treatment resistant to resistance" *(2)*. Initial xenograft studies supported these predictions—widespread activity, limited toxicity, no resistance *(3)*. For a time, it was argued that disease control, if not outright cure, was close at hand. Widespread press coverage followed, with commensurate Wall Street stock valuations of companies without commercial products.

From: *Cancer Drug Discovery and Development: Cancer Drug Resistance*
Edited by: B. Teicher © Humana Press Inc., Totowa, NJ

Regrettably, the idea that antiangiogenic therapy was "resistant to resistance" proved to be what Thomas Huxley famously described as "a beautiful theory killed by nasty, brutish facts." Clinical trials with numerous antiangiogenic agents reproducibly demonstrated their failure to eradicate human cancers. Resistance to antiangiogenic therapy is a very real problem. Why is this the case? This chapter reviews potential mechanisms of acquired and *de novo* resistance to antiangiogenic therapy, then suggest strategies to combat such resistance.

2. RESISTANCE TO ANTIANGIOGENIC THERAPY

Substantial preclinical in vitro and in vivo data, as well as emerging clinical data, suggests distinct antiangiogenic activity for several existing, commonly used cytotoxic agents *(4)*. However, these agents fail to cure most malignancies. Mechanisms of resistance to the antiangiogenic effects of cytotoxic agents likely also apply to novel antiangiogenic agents. Theoretical and (often) substantiated mechanisms of acquired and *de novo* resistance to antiangiogenic therapies are described here.

2.1. Endothelial Cell Heterogeneity

An initial assumption underlying antiangiogenic therapy was that endothelial cells, incapable of mutating to a resistant phenotype, should be reproducibly sensitive to antiangiogenic agents. Furthermore, all endothelial cells were presumed similar, if not identical; therefore, antiangiogenic agents were predicted to be equally effective, regardless of the tumor type or anatomic location.

Were these assumptions correct? For if endothelial cells are heterogenous, then the potential for selective sensitivity exists. And selective sensitivity is little more than a synonym for drug resistance. What is the evidence suggesting the existence of endothelial cell heterogeneity?

Normal embryonic development requires endothelial heterogeneity. Developing endothelium is dynamic and capable of differential gene expression based on the physiologic requirements and microenvironment of the associated tissue. For example, endothelia in the brain and testes express high levels of the multidrug resistance protein, thereby limiting exposure to potentially harmful xenobiotics *(5–7)*. The evolutionary advantage of such organ-specific endothelial gene expression is clear. In contrast, the mechanisms that underlie the exquisite time and spatial control of differential endothelial gene expression during development have not been fully elucidated.

Persistent differences in endothelial function become apparent when comparing the results of in vitro studies using different sources of "normal" endothelial cells. Vascular cell adhesion factor 1 expression is induced on human umbilical vein endothelial cells (HUVECs) by both tumor necrosis factor-α and interleukin 1α, whereas only tumor necrosis factor-α induced vascular cell adhesion factor 1 expression on human dermal microvascular endothelial cells *(8)*. The differential response was explained by distinct expression patterns of the CXC chemokine and interleukin 8 receptors.

St. Croix and colleagues compared the gene expression patterns of vascular endothelial cells derived from normal and malignant colorectal tissues. Of 170 transcripts analyzed, almost half (79) were differentially expressed in tumor-associated endothelial cells (TECs) compared to normal endothelium. Similar, but not identical, expression patterns were found in TECs from metastatic lesions and primary tumor sites *(9)*. The human herpesvirus 8, thought to be the etiologic agent for Kaposi's sarcoma, multicentric

Castleman's disease, and AIDS-associated primary effusion lymphoma, alters gene expression in human dermal microvascular endothelial cells *(10)*. Schlaifer et al. found expression of the energy-dependent efflux pump, P-glycoprotein (P-gp) in TECs but not in human umbilical vein endothelial cells *(11,12)*. Vincristine with the P-gp antagonist verapamil, but not vincristine alone, inhibits angiogenesis induced by mouse sarcoma 180 cells suggesting P-gp expression in TECs has functional significance *(13)*.

In addition, some proangiogenic factors display tissue specificity (in essence, intrapatient spatial heterogeneity). A vascular endothelial growth factor (VEGF) isoform, endocrine gland-derived VEGF, induces proliferation, migration and fenestration in capillary endothelial cells derived from endocrine glands (ovary, testis, adrenal, and placenta) but has little effect on other endothelial cell types *(14)*.

As the data above suggest, endothelial cell heterogeneity is a reality. This reality is derived both from evolutionary advantage (the selective, organ- and tissue-specific activation of genes accompanying normal development) and from tumor-induced microenvironmental plasticity. The genetic stability of endothelial cells is both true and irrelevant in this wider context.

2.2. Intrapatient Heterogeneity

Heterogeneity in endothelial cell gene expression is not the only determinant of antiangiogenic resistance in which hosts may differ. Germline DNA may encode an innately more resistant angiogenesis pathway in certain individuals. Rohan and colleagues found up to a 10-fold difference in the response to growth factor-stimulated angiogenesis in the corneal micropocket assay among 12 inbred mouse strains. Even more importantly, differential sensitivity to angiogenesis inhibitors was seen between mouse strains, with one demonstrating complete resistance to both TNP-470 and thalidomide *(15)*. Similarly, Pandey and colleagues found inherited differences in angiogenic versus angiostatic activity in estrogen-induced rat pituitary tumors *(16)*.

Variations in sensitivity because of inherited polymorphisms in genes encoding pro- and antiangiogenic factors represent one potential source of resistance. Polymorphisms, inherited variations in DNA sequence that are present in more than 1% of a population, are distinct from sporadic mutations acquired by tumors. The vast majority of polymorphisms are single-nucleotide polymorphisms (SNPs), but sequence insertions and deletions have been reported *(17)*. Recently it has become apparent that polymorphisms in the host (germline DNA) play an important role in human cancer in both the development of cancer, permissibility of early metastasis and variability in response to therapy *(17,18)*. Polymorphisms may affect drug metabolism or transport, the efficiency of DNA repair, sensitivity to hypoxia, and neovascularization.

Genetic polymorphisms in genes important in the angiogenesis pathway (e.g., hypoxia-inducible factor 1α [*HIF-1α*], *VEGF*, and endothelial nitric oxide synthase [*eNOS*], among others) have been associated with increased or decreased rates of a variety of malignancies and variable clinical outcomes (discussed in detail in Subheading 2.3.). Angiogensis associated with malignancy overlaps extensively with angiogenesis in cardiovascular disease. Many of the polymorphisms in the same genes are also associated with a variety of vascular-related phenomenon, such as acute myocardial infarction and hypertension *(19–23)*. What makes the variability of this process unique is that this actually represents a host-associated variability as opposed to a resistance mechanism derived from mutations occurring in cancer cells. Furthermore, this host-related variability may not only serve as a prognostic factor (e.g., predisposition to disease or predictor of bad outcome after disease acquisition) but may also serve as a therapeutic predictive factor (e.g., predictor of response or resistance to therapy). Polymorphisms in the *eNOS* gene, for example, have been associated with a variable responsiveness to antihypertensive therapy *(24,25)*. If DNA polymorphisms alter response to one class of vascular-targeting agents (antihypertensives), it is reasonable to suspect that they might alter response to another class (antiangiogenics).

The role of DNA polymorphisms in angiogenesis has only recently been recognized and investigated, predominantly in the field of cardiovascular rather than cancer medicine. A sampling of available clinical data follows.

2.3. Vascular Endothelial Growth Factor

At least six polymorphisms have been described in the *VEGF* gene, with a reported frequency of the rare allele ranging from 12 to 48% *(26)*. Specific polymorphisms have been found to correlate with a variety of nonmalignant pathological conditions including acute renal allograft rejection, smoking-related chronic obstructive pulmonary disease, diabetic retinopathy, and sarcoidosis as well as malignancy *(27–30)*. The risk of prostate cancer is partially determined by which *VEGF* polymorphism a patient inherits. Specifically, patients with the $C^{460}T$ variant allele have a higher risk of prostate cancer *(31)*, whereas patients with the $G^{-1154}A$ variant in the promoter region enjoy a reduced risk *(32)*. The same $G^{-1154}A$ polymorphism was associated with thinner tumors in patients with malignant melanoma *(33)*, supporting the hypothesis that this allele is protective. The $C^{936}T$ *VEGF* allele was more common among controls (29.4%) than among breast cancer patients (17.6%), implying a protective effect for this allele as well *(34)*. These polymorphisms correlate with differential protein expression and therefore likely have functional consequence. Peripheral blood mononuclear VEGF protein production correlates with polymorphism at position $+405^{35}$; the common $C^{936}T$ variant correlates with plasma VEGF level *(34,36)*.

2.3.1. ENDOTHELIAL NITRIC OXIDE SYNTHASE

eNOS is important in regulation of vascular homeostasis in both malignant and cardiac vascular pathobiology *(37–41)*. At least three clinically important polymorphisms have been identified in the *eNOS* gene *(42)*, including a SNP in the promoter region ($T^{786}C$), a SNP in exon 7 ($Glu^{298}Asp$), and a variable number of tandem repeats in intron 4 *(42)*. The prevalence of the variant alleles ranges from 4 to 42%, with marked interethnic variability *(43)*. The $T^{786}C$ SNP correlates with a decreased likelihood of lymphovascular invasion in women with early stage breast cancer; further follow-up confirmed the expected likelihood of metastasis *(44)*. Polymorphisms in intron 4 correlate with an increased risk of lung *(45)* and prostate cancer *(46)*, and with a higher stage of ovarian cancer *(47)*. The $Glu^{298}Asp$ SNP has been associated with a higher likelihood of bone metastases in prostate cancer *(48)*. An in vitro study demonstrated *eNOS* gene expression, protein concentrations, and enzyme activity were genotype dependent *(49)*. Genetic polymorphisms in the *eNOS* gene have also been correlated with plasma nitric oxide levels *(50)*.

2.3.2. HYPOXIA-INDUCIBLE FACTOR 1α

Genetic polymorphisms in HIF-1α, , ranging in frequency from 8 to 11%, also appear to play a role in tumorigenesis. Both the $P^{582}S$ and $A^{588}T$ variants have significantly higher transcription activity than the wild type under normoxic and hypoxic conditions. Furthermore, tumors from patients with head and neck cancer with heterozygous alleles (P[582]S or A[588]T) had significantly increased microvascular density compared with tumor homozygous for the wild-type alleles. In addition, all patients with T1 tumors were wild-type, whereas 14 of 47 patients with tumors of T2 were heterozygous for one of the variant alleles *(51)*.

2.3.3. THROMBOSPONDIN

Several thrombospondin polymorphisms have been identified and are clearly important determinants of cardiovascular disease. The T→G substitution in the 3′ untranslated region of thrombospondin 1 is associated with a reduced risk of coronary artery disease *(52,53)*. Conversely, thrombospondin 1 (N[700]S) *(54)* and thrombospondin 4 (A[387]P) polymorphisms *(52,55,56)* have been correlated with an increased risk of coronary artery disease.

2.3.4. ENDOSTATIN

At least two polymorphisms in the endostatin gene that appear to be clinically important in malignancy have been identified. Heterozygosity of the D[104]N SNP (resulting in decreased endostatin function) correlated with a 2.5-fold increased chance of developing prostate cancer compared to wild-type homozygous subjects *(57)*. Similarly, the G→A substitution in exon 42 confers an increased risk of prostate cancer and increased invasiveness in breast cancer *(58)*. Conversely, Zorick et al. *(59)* have recently demonstrated that Down's syndrome patients have increased and high serum endostatin levels because of having an extra copy of collagen XVIII on chromosome 21, and have suggested that the extreme rarity of solid tumor malignancies in such patients may be related to this change.

Collectively, these data suggest that considerable angiogenic heterogeneity is "hardwired" into individual patients, and that polymorphic genes may play an important functional role in angiogenesis, cardiovascular disease, and cancer. Though not yet examined, it is reasonable to expect that these functionally important polymorphisms may also alter treatment responses to antiangiogenic therapies. Therapeutic response to an antiangiogenic agent might well depend on the specific balance of positive and negative regulators of angiogenesis. An excess of host proangiogenic factors, or a relative deficiency in host-generated negative regulators, might well affect the delicate balance and hence the clinical outcome.

2.4. Tumor Cell Heterogeneity

Tumor cell heterogeneity, whether in expression of angiogenic factors or sensitivity to hypoxia, also results in resistance to antiangiogenic therapy *(60)*. Invasive cancers commonly express multiple angiogenic factors, and from a clinical standpoint, this heterogeneity occurs at an early point in time: Relf et al. identified at least six different proangiogenic factors in each of 64 primary breast tumors studied *(61)*. Genetic instability may result in modulation of both the amount and type of proangiogenic factors expressed in a tumor *(62)*.

Given such redundancy, inhibition of a single factor may fail to produce a sustained clinical effect. Indeed, production of a proangiogenic factor does not guarantee the same response to antiangiogenic therapy. Though Wilms' tumor and neuroblastoma both predominantly produce VEGF, preclinical studies suggest that Wilms' tumor is growthinhibited, whereas neuroblastoma is resistant to a VEGF-directed monoclonal antibody *(63)*. The mechanism underlying this resistance has not yet been elucidated.

Tumor heterogeneity may imply more than just heterogeneity of proangiogenic factors. Kerbel et al. have shown that disruption of p53 in tumor cells reduces sensitivity to antiangiogenic metronomic therapy (64). Chronic hypoxia selects p53 mutant tumor cells resistant to hypoxia-induced apoptosis. Indeed, in most long-term xenograft studies of antiangiogenic therapy, tumors eventually progressed (though more slowly than controls) despite continued treatment (65–67). Heterogeneity of p53 is, of course, common in many types of human cancer.

Hypoxia is a key signal for the induction of angiogenesis, often via HIF-1 and HIF-2 (68–70). HIF-1$\alpha^{-/-}$ tumors have decreased hypoxia-induced VEGF expression and are less vascular but (perhaps paradoxically) have accelerated growth in vivo compared to HIF-1$\alpha^{+/+}$ tumors because of decreased hypoxia-induced apoptosis (71). Yu and colleagues isolated tumor cells based on their relative proximity to perfused vessels and compared HIF-1α expression and in vivo growth characteristics (72). In heterogeneous tumors, HIF-1$\alpha^{+/+}$ cells were located in the perivascular areas and were much more highly dependent on proximity to blood vessels for their growth and survival in vivo than the HIF-1$\alpha^{-/-}$ cells (73).

Erythropoietin production is tightly modulated by hypoxia and HIF-1α. Though the principal function of erythropoietin is to stimulate the maturation of erythroid precursors, erythropoietin modulates a host of cellular signal transduction pathways in endothelia and pluripotent stem cells. Erythropoietin stimulates endothelial cell proliferation and migration as well as erythropoiesis and vascular resistance. Erythropoietin inhibits apoptosis through two distinct mechanisms that involve maintenance of genomic DNA integrity and preservation of cellular membrane asymmetry (74).

A VEGF/VEGFR-2 autocrine loop supports the growth and migration of leukemic cells (75). In response to leukemia-derived proangiogenic and proinflammatory cytokines, endothelial cells release increasing amounts of another VEGF family member, VEGF-C. In turn, interaction of VEGF-C with its receptor VEGFR-3 (FLT-4) promotes leukemia survival and proliferation. VEGF-C protected leukemic cells from the apoptotic effects of three chemotherapeutic agents (76,77). VEGF tyrosine kinase receptors have been found on some solid tumor cells as well, suggesting that such autocrine/paracrine loops may have widespread importance (S. Rafii, unpublished data).

2.5. Impact of the Tumor Microenvironment

The belief that antiangiogenic agents might prove "resistant to resistance" was based in large part on the idea that tumor endothelial cells, given their low potential for mutation, would be unable to generate a resistance phenotype. This recognition of the endothelia's genetic stability was both true and irrelevant: in the tumor microenvironment, epigenetic alterations brought on by the complex interactions of cancer cell, endothelial cells, and other stromal cells are sufficient to alter endothelial cell sensitivity to antiangiogenic attack.

To study angiogenesis and tumor growth at a secondary site, Gohongi and colleagues implanted a gel impregnated with basic fibroblast growth factor (bFGF) or Mz-ChA-2 tumor in the cranial windows of mice without tumors, mice with subcutaneous tumors, or mice with orthotopic cholangiocarcinomas. The concentration of TGF-β1) in the plasma of mice with orthotopic cholangiocarcinoma was 300% higher than that in the plasma of mice without tumors or with subcutaneous tumors. Similarly, angiogenesis in the cranial window was substantially inhibited in mice with orthotopic tumors but only minimally affected by subcutaneous tumors *(78)*. In a xenograft pancreatic cancer model, orthotopic pancreatic tumors grew faster, expressed VEGF, and maintained vascular density and hyperpermeability compared to subcutaneous tumors. As in other models, orthotopic, but not subcutaneous, tumors metastasized similar to advanced human pancreatic cancer *(79)*.

The tumor microenvironment protects the endothelial compartment. Medium conditioned by colon cancer cells increases extracellular signal regulated kinase-1/2 phosphorylation and decreases apoptosis of HUVECs compared to medium conditioned by nonmalignant cells *(80)*. The resistant phenotype can be reproduced in vitro by the addition of VEGF and/or bFGF to HUVEC culture systems. HUVEC antiapoptotic pathways stimulated by VEGF and/or bFGF include (but are by no means limited to) p44 mitogen-activated protein kinase, c-Jun-NH$_2$-kinase, phosphoinositide 3-OH kinase, Bcl-2, inhibitors of apoptosis, and survivin *(81–85)*. Pericytes invest mature vasculature and provide critical survival signals to vascular endothelial cells. Differences in pericyte coverage among tumor types have obvious implications for vessel maturation, survival and sensitivity to antiangiogenic therapies *(86)*.

As many pro- and antiangiogenic factors are contained in or released from the extracellular matrix, differential sensitivity based on site of disease may be anticipated. For example, treatment with the matrix metalloproteinase inhibitor batimastat had different effects on tumor progression and growth, depending on the site of tumor implantation *(87)*. Predicting the effect of an individual intervention in such a complicated and interrelated system as the tumor microenvironment is fraught with hazards. The potential for unintended consequences must be kept in mind. For instance, the proteolytic action of the MMPs releases angiostatin from the extracellular matrix thus MMP inhibition may actually increase angiogenesis by decreasing angiostatin release *(88)*.

The tumor microenvironment also affects drug delivery. Pluen and colleagues studied the diffusion of macromolecules and liposomes in tumors growing in cranial windows and dorsal chambers (DCs). For the same tumor types, diffusion of large molecules was significantly faster in cranial windows than in DC tumors. The slower diffusion in DC tumors was associated with a higher density of host stromal cells that synthesize and organize collagen type I *(89)*. These preclinical findings may seem far removed from the clinical setting at first glance. However mixed responses (i.e., regressions in lung metastases but growth in liver metastases within the same patient) have been observed in early phase clinical trials of antiangiogenics *(90–94)*. Though the mechanisms underlying these mixed responses have not been explored in the clinic, their frequency argues for the critical role of the tumor microenvironment.

2.6. Compensatory Responses to Treatment

As chemotherapy induces tumor cell kill, the production of proangiogenic peptides decreases, leading to regression of the tumor-associated vasculature with increasing tumor hypoxia, stimulating an increase in VEGF production *(95,96)*. The increased VEGF production in areas of tumor hypoxia may stimulate brisk angiogenesis, essentially rescuing areas of tumor that are sublethally injured. In an in vivo model with rat 13762 mammary carcinomas, treatment with cyclophosphamide resulted in tumor hypoxia with increased VEGF production and increased tumor CD31 staining detectable within 24 h *(97)*. It seems reasonable to expect VEGF production to increase in response to treatment with the "pure" antiangiogenics as well. Indeed, VEGF levels increased after therapy with doxorubicin and a VEGF receptor tyrosine kinase inhibitor *(98)*.

Such compensatory responses may well reflect an underlying biologic reality. Hypoxia has been faced over and over again throughout evolutionary history, and relative hypoxia is common in many organs. It is especially common, however, in growing tumors. Hypoxia may be chronic because of consumption/diffusion limitations or periodic resulting from transient reductions in tumor blood flow (so-called cyclic hypoxia) *(99)*. In contrast to normal vasculature, tumor microvessels frequently lack complete endothelial linings and basement membranes with arteriovenous shunts and blind ends being common *(100)*. As such, blood flow through tumors tends to be sluggish *(191)*; cyclic hypoxia is quite common (occurring in as many as half of tumor vessels), suggesting that the cancer cell's natural environment is one of recurring hypoxic insults. Tumor cells by definition must evolve mechanisms to resist such cyclic hypoxia merely to survive. Indeed some cancer cells may remain viable for prolonged periods of hypoxia *(102–104)*. It is reasonable to expect that these compensatory responses can and will be invoked by human cancers undergoing antiangiogenic attack.

2.7. Angiogenesis-Independent Tumor Growth

Classic angiogenesis was, until recently, thought to be an absolute requirement for tumor growth. It is now evident that this is not the case. Vessel cooption, growth by intussusception, vascular mimicry, and vasculogenesis may decrease a tumors dependence on classical angiogenesis.

2.7.1. VESSEL COOPTION

Holash and colleagues were the first to document that some tumors initially grow by coopting existing host vessels. Such coopted vasculature did not immediately undergo angiogenesis but instead regressed, leading to a secondarily avascular tumor and massive tumor cell loss. Ultimately, the remaining tumor was rescued by robust angiogenesis at the tumor margin *(195)*. Kunkel and colleagues studied systemic treatment with DC101, a monoclonal antibody against vascular endothelial growth factor receptor (VEGFR-2) in an orthotopic intracerebral glioma model. Tumor volumes and microvessel density in animals treated with DC101 were reduced compared with immunoglobulin G and phosphate-buffered saline controls. Though systemic inhibition of VEGFR-2 blocked angiogenesis and inhibited glioblastoma growth, there was increased cooption of preexisting cerebral vessels with a distinct growth pattern in the residual tumors. In mice treated with DC101, there was a significant increase in small satellite tumors clustered around, but distinct from, the primary tumor. The satellites contained central vessel cores—coopted vessels. Tumor cells often migrated long distances along the coopted host vasculature to reach the surface and spread over the meninges *(106)*.

How applicable is the phenomenon of vessel cooption to human cancer? Passalidou and colleagues described a group of non-small cell lung carcinomas without morphological evidence of neoangiogenesis; neoplastic cells filled the alveoli with the only vessels belonging to the trapped alveolar septa. The vascular phenotype of all the vessels in the nonangiogenic tumors was the same as that of alveolar vessels in normal lung: LH39-positive and $\alpha V\beta 3$-variable or -negative. This pattern was distinct from the vessels in angiogenic tumors *(197)*. More recently, Stessels et al. compared breast and colorectal cancers metastatic to the liver. Whereas the majority (though by no means all) of colorectal cancers followed a classic pattern of metastasis with angiogenesis, breast cancer metastases were virtually all characterized by what the authors called a "replacement growth pattern" of liver involvement, where cancers cells in essence replaced hepatocytes without disrupting the surrounding stroma *(108)*.

Intussusceptive microvascular growth refers to vascular network formation by insertion of interstitial tissue columns, called tissue pillars or posts, into the vascular lumen and subsequent growth of these columns, resulting in partitioning of the vessel lumen. Patan and colleagues used intravital microscopy to observe the growth of the human colon adenocarcinoma (LS174T) in vivo *(109)*. Both intussusception and endothelial sprouting occurred at the tumor periphery. In the central regions, intussusception led to network remodeling and occlusion of vascular segments, interfering with vessel patency and causing heterogeneous perfusion and hypoxia, thus perpetuating angiogenesis *(119)*. Interestingly, in mammary tumors of *neu*T transgenic mice, both sprouting and intussusceptive angiogenesis were observed simultaneously in the same nodules *(111)*.

Vascular mimicry refers to the unique ability of some aggressive tumor cells to form tubular structures and patterned networks in three-dimensional culture, "mimicking" embryonic vasculogenic networks *(112)*. Several adhesion factors were exclusively expressed by highly aggressive (vasculogenic) melanoma cells; downregulation of VE-cadherin expression or restoration of EphA2 ligand binding in the aggressive melanoma cells abrogated their ability to form vasculogenic networks *(113)*. Multiple vascular cell-associated markers were identified by RNase protection assay in invasive ovarian cancer cells that lined the vascular structure. Tumor cells lined 7 to 10% of channels containing red blood cells in patient tumor sections from advanced high-grade ovarian cancers. By comparison, all vascular areas in benign tumors and low-stage cancers were endothelial-lined *(114,115)*.

Postnatal vasculogenesis refers to incorporation of bone marrow derived endothelial progenitor cells (EPCs) into growing adult vasculature. Using transgenic mice constitutively expressing β-galactosidase under the transcriptional regulation of an endothelial cell-specific promoter (Flk-1/LZ or Tie- 2/LZ), Asahara and others have identified EPCs in the neovasculature of developing tumors *(116–118)*. The role of EPCs was further documented by Lyden and colleagues using the angiogenic defective, tumor-resistant immunodeficient (Id) mutant mice. Transplantation of wild-type Barrett metaplasia or VEGF-mobilized stem cells restored tumor angiogenesis and growth; donor-derived EPCs were detected throughout the neovessels of tumors and Matrigel-plugs in an Id1$^{+/-}$ Id3$^{-/-}$ host. Incorporated EPCs were associated with VEGF receptor 1-positive myeloid cells. Targeting either VEGFR1 or VEGFR2 alone partially blocked the growth of tumors in this model; inhibition of both VEGFR1 and VEGFR2 was necessary to completely ablate tumor growth *(119)*. Recent data suggest that inflammatory breast cancer, a rare but highly aggressive form of the disease, relies almost entirely on vasculogenesis as opposed to angiogenesis, apparently because of the inability of the cancer cells to bind endothelial cells *(120)*.

The relative frequency and importance of alternate means of vascular supply in human tumors is unknown. To what extent do these alternative means of establishing circulation affect response to antiangiogenic therapy? For if "classic" angiogenesis is not the predominant mechanism by which a tumor gets its blood supply, can antiangiogenic therapy be expected to succeed? This question needs answering in the clinic, but preclinical models have begun to explore the relative resistance of alternative blood supplies to antiangiogenic agents. Van der Schaft et al. have demonstrated that cancers characterized by "vasculogenic mimicry" are resistant to the antiangiogenic agent endostatin *(121)*. In contrast, bone marrow-derived endothelial cells remain sensitive to VEGF-targeting therapy *(119)*.

2.8. Pharmacokinetic Resistance

Preclinical studies of novel agents often fail to anticipate the dynamic nature of interactions between drug, host, and tumor. It is a peculiar failing of modern science that the study of simple—indeed, simplistic—model systems at the molecular or cellular level is considered more "scientific" than the study of complex, whole systems. And yet, the failure of many antiangiogenic agents clearly occurs at exactly the higher-order levels of complexity seen in whole systems. These failures represent what might be termed "pharmacokinetic resistance": the inability to deliver the right dose of a biologically active agent to the right cells for the right amount of time.

Maximal antiangiogenic therapy typically requires prolonged exposure to low drug concentrations, exactly counter to the maximum tolerated doses administered when optimal tumor cell kill is the goal *(122)*. Three recent reports confirm the importance of dose and schedule. In all three the combination of low-, frequent-dose chemotherapy plus an agent that specifically targets the endothelial cell compartment (so-called metronomic therapy) controlled tumor growth much more effectively than the cytotoxic agent alone *(65,123,124)*.

Dose and schedule may be critical for antiangiogenic efficacy. Constant exposure to low noncytostatic doses of interferon was more effective in downregulating bFGF expression in the laryngeal cancer cell line HlaC79 than high doses *(125)*. Ten thousand units of interferon-α administered daily was more efficacious in inhibiting the growth of bladder cancer in a mouse orthotopic model than the 70,000 U given in two or three divided doses over 1 wk or as one injection per week *(126)*. Daily subcutaneous administration of 5000 or 10,000 U/d produced maximal reduction in tumor vessel density, bFGF, and MMP-9 expression (at both the mRNA and protein levels) and serum levels of bFGF.

What might explain the paradoxical observation that lower-dose interferon is more effective in inhibiting angiogenesis? Interferons bind to receptors on the cytoplasmic membrane and activate the Janus kinase (JAK) family of protein tyrosine kinases. The JAK pathway then activates signal transducer and activator of transcription, which in turn activates multiple genes that control the immune system, growth, and hematopoiesis. A family of proteins termed cytokine-inducible SH2 proteins negatively regulates cytokine signals. Interferon-γ induces the activation of one of the cytokine-inducible SH2 protein family, suppressors of cytokine signaling-1 (SOCS-1). Low, constant doses of interferon may activate the JAK-signal transducer and activator of transcription pathway and downregulate bFGF and MMP-9 without activating the SOCS-1 inhibitor. In contrast, higher doses also activate SOCS-1, shifting the balance to an angiogenic or neutral phenotype *(127)*.

The natural inhibitors of angiogenesis angiostatin and endostatin are cleared rapidly from the circulation when administered as an intravenous bolus *(128,129)*. It is likely that the overall balance of pro- and antiangiogenic factors remains tilted toward angiogenesis for substantial periods with such bolus administration. As expected, the most profound effects in preclinical models maintained constant exposure with continuous infusions *(130–132)*.

3. THWARTING RESISTANCE TO ANTIANGIOGENIC THERAPY

The initial clinical experience with novel antiangiogenic agents confirms the reality of resistance. Whereas some trials have demonstrated modest clinical efficacy *(133–136)*, leading to the approval by the Food and Drug Administration of the VEGF-targeting antibody bevacizumab, results have not lived up to initial expectations. Understanding the potential mechanisms of antiangiogenic resistance suggests several possible means to ameliorate or bypass such resistance.

3.1. Use Standard Therapies With Antiangiogenic Intent

Chemotherapeutic agents were developed based on the concept of maximum tolerated dose, and with the assumption that the cancer cells are the sole—or at least primary—target. Numerous chemotherapeutic agents have antiangiogenic activity at dose levels far lower than those required to kill cancer cells *(4)*. Chronic low-dose chemotherapy (so-called metronomic therapy) may be potently antiangiogenic, though this effect seems most pronounced when the chemotherapeutic agent is combined with a specific endothelial agent *(65,137)*.

3.2. Combine Antiangiogenic Agents With Standard Chemotherapy Regimens

Extensive preclinical data support this combined approach, with multiple antiangiogenic and chemotherapeutic agents having additive or synergistic combinatorial activity *(65,137–140)*. The mechanistic rationale for many of these combinations is poorly understood and not intuitive, as both radiotherapy and chemotherapy depend on an effective blood supply for therapeutic efficacy. A potential explanation may lie in the inherent inefficiency of the tumor vasculature. Antiangiogenic therapy "normalizes" flow initially resulting in improved tissue oxygenation and decreased interstitial pressure, increasing delivery of cytotoxic agents *(101)*.

Potential interactions between VEGF and chemotherapeutic agents have been extensively examined. VEGF is antiapoptotic for endothelial cells via several pathways, including induction of the antiapoptotic proteins Bcl-2 and A1, activation of the phosphoinositide 3 kinase/Akt signaling pathway, stimulation of nitric oxide and PGI_2, and increased focal adhesion kinase tyrosine phosphorylation *(141)*. This survival function may play a role in the protection of tumor endothelial cells against the antiangiogenic effects of commonly used chemotherapeutic agents. For instance, Sweeney and colleagues demonstrated that VEGF protects endothelial cells against docetaxel, an effect reversed by an anti-VEGF monoclonal antibody *(140)*.

The antiapoptotic effects of VEGF may not be limited to endothelial cells. Neuropilin 1, a receptor important in neuronal guidance, is a newly identified coreceptor for VEGF *(142)* and is highly expressed by some tumor cells *(143–145)*. And, as previously described, there is a growing list of human tumors known to contain VEGF receptors. In these tumors, VEGF may act as an antiapoptotic factor, potentially protecting tumor cells against chemotherapeutic agents. It is reasonable to expect that the combination of a chemotherapeutic agent with an agent targeting VEGF will increase therapeutic activity against both the cancer cell and the endothelial cell.

At present, there are little clinical data supporting such effects. Wedam et al. recently demonstrated that the VEGF-targeting agent bevacizumab down-regulates KDR (VEGF R-2) in cancer cells in patients receiving bevacizumab for the treatment of inflammatory breast cancer *(146)*. This represents the first clinical evidence of a direct effect of an antiangiogenic agent on a cancer (as opposed to an endothelial) cell.

3.3. Combine Multiple Antiangiogenic Agents

As tumor progression is associated with expression of increasing numbers of proangiogenic factors, the use of multiple antiangiogenic agents to simultaneously attack this multiply redundant process may thwart resistance to individual agents. This approach is, of course, not unique to antiangiogenic therapy, having previously been used to limit resistance to cytotoxic, antimicrobial, and antiviral therapies. The combination of antiangiogenic agents has been tested in preclinical models with success, e.g., interferon and TNP-1470 *(147)* and angiostatin with endostatin *(148)*.

3.4. Combine Antiangiogenic Agents With Other Biologically Targeted Agents

The epidermal growth factor receptor (EGFR) and HER-2 both regulate VEGF in human tumors; their blockade reduces VEGF production and angiogenesis *(149–155)*. Given the plethora of indirect influences on angiogenesis, might we be able to utilize the combination of biologic agents as a means of inhibiting angiogenesis? Might we be able to combine antiangiogenic agents with antigrowth factor receptor agents as a means of overcoming resistance? This strategy was effective in preclinical tumor models *(156)*, and is currently under clinical investigation with combinations of antiangiogenic agents and trastuzumab in patients with HER-2-positive breast cancer.

Conversely, antiangiogenic agents might offer a means of overcoming resistance to growth factor-targeting agents. Recent data from Viloria-Petit et al. suggest that increased production of VEGF represents one mechanism by which tumor cells escape anti-EGFR monoclonal antibody therapy *(157)*. The combination of a VEGF-targeting agent with an anti-EGFR agent might thereby limit resistance to growth factor receptor therapy.

3.5. Use Antiangiogenic Therapy as Adjuvant Therapy

It is a rare treatment that is more effective for large tumors than for small. Tumor progression results in resistance to all anticancer therapies. One means of thwarting the development of drug resistance associated is to treat cancers when they are small. The adjuvant setting (or similar minimal residual disease setting) is the logical place to accomplish this goal.

The use of antiangiogenics as adjuvant therapy has its own potential barriers. Physicians, companies, and regulatory agencies are loath to use agents in the adjuvant setting until there is evidence of activity in advanced disease. The toxicity of chronic antiangiogenic therapy remains largely unexplored, as is the toxicity of combinations of chemotherapy with antiangiogenic therapy. Though intuitively, the impact of angiogenesis inhibition is expected to be greatest in patients with micrometastatic disease, proof of this concept will require commitment of substantial human and financial resources to randomized adjuvant trials.

Recent studies illustrate the importance of population-specific feasibility trials, especially for agents administered chronically *(159,159)*. Experience gained in patients with advanced disease is meaningful, but even large trials of patients with metastatic disease provide long-term safety data in only a limited number of patients. Population-specific feasibility studies can identify toxicities that might not be acceptable in an otherwise healthy patient population, thereby limiting exposure and avoiding premature closure of a large adjuvant trial *(160)*. A population-specific feasibility trial examining bevacizumab in the setting of adjuvant chemotherapy for early stage breast has recently (2004) been approved in concept by the National Cancer Institute for an Eastern Cooperative Oncology Group trial.

3.6. Use Antiangiogenic Therapy as Targeted Therapy

Antiangiogenic therapy has been applied as a general therapy given on a population basis, rather than as a targeted therapy given to patients with a specific molecular phenotype. It is reasonable to ask whether we can call failure to respond to a therapy "resistance" if the target at which the therapy is aimed is not present in the tumor. If a patient's tumor does not express VEGF and therefore fails to respond to an antiVEGF therapy, is the tumor resistant, or is the therapy merely misguided? As insensitivity because of lack of therapeutic target results in resistance at the *patient* level, proper targeting is a means of overcoming such resistance. Ideal targets are biologically relevant, reproducibly measurable, and definably correlated with clinical benefit. Examples of molecular targets fulfilling such criteria are limited and include estrogen receptor or HER-2 for breast cancer, c-Kit for gastrointestinal stromal tumors, or bcr-abl for chronic myelogenous leukemia.

At present, we are unable to point to any truly targeted antiangiogenic therapy. It is reasonable, if not critical, to perform tissue collection for testing as part of the development of antiangiogenic agents. Though we lack validated assays for most of the antiangiogenic therapeutic targets, the availability of tissues for testing will speed development and validation of appropriate assays.

4. CONCLUSION

Early enthusiasm for antiangiogenic therapy has given way to clinical reality: resistance continues to be a problem in the antiangiogenic era. Acknowledging this fact does not imply pessimism as to the ultimate role of antiangiogenic therapy. Rather, it is to be reminded that the way forward lies in advancing our knowledge of fundamental cancer biology. The "final laboratory" of the clinic is the most challenging place to perform good science. It is also, by its nature, the most rewarding.

ACKNOWLEDGMENTS

Supported in part by grants from the Breast Cancer Research Foundation (G.W.S., K.D.M.), a Faculty Development Award from the Pharmaceutical and Research Manufacturers of America Foundation (C.J.S.), and the Walther Medical Foundation (GWS).

REFERENCES

1. Folkman J. What is the evidence that tumors are angiogenesis dependent? J Natl Cancer Inst 1990; 82:4–6.
2. Kerbel RS. A cancer therapy resistant to resistance [news; comment] [see comments]. Nature 1997; 390:335–336.
3. Boehm T, Folkman J, Browder T, et al. Antiangiogenic therapy of experimental cancer does not induce acquired drug resistance [see comments]. Nature 1997; 390:404–407.
4. Miller K, Sweeney C, Sledge G. Redefining the target: chemotherapeutics as antiangiogenics. J Clin Oncol 2001; 19:1195–1206.
5. Barrand MA, Robertson KJ, von Weikersthal SF. Comparisons of P-glycoprotein expression in isolated rat brain microvessels and in primary cultures of endothelial cells derived from microvasculature of rat brain, epididymal fat pad and from aorta. FEBS Lett 1995; 374:179–183.
6. Regina A, Koman A, Piciotti M, et al. Mrp1 multidrug resistance-associated protein and P-glycoprotein expression in rat brain microvessel endothelial cells. J Neurochem 1998; 71:705–715.
7. Wijnholds J, Scheffer GL, van der Valk M, et al. Multidrug resistance protein 1 protects the oropharyngeal mucosal layer and the testicular tubules against drug-induced damage. J Exp Med 1998; 188:797–808.
8. Gille J, Swerlick RA, Lawley TJ, et al. Differential regulation of vascular cell adhesion molecule-1 gene transcription by tumor necrosis factor α and interleukin-1 α in dermal microvascular endothelial cells. Blood 1996; 87:211–217.
9. St. Croix B, Rago C, Velculescu V, et al. Genes expressed in human tumor endothelium. Science 2000; 289:1197–1202.

10. Poole LJ, Yu Y, Kim PS, et al. Altered patterns of cellular gene expression in dermal microvascular endothelial cells infected with Kaposi's sarcoma-associated herpesvirus. J Virol 2002; 76:3395–3420.

11. Schlaifer D, Laurent G, Chittal S, et al. Immunohistochemical detection of multidrug resistance associated P- glycoprotein in tumour and stromal cells of human cancers [published erratum appears in Br J Cancer 1991 Jan;63(1):164-5]. Br J Cancer 1990; 62:177–182.

12. Toth K, Vaughan MM, Peress NS, et al. MDR1 P-glycoprotein is expressed by endothelial cells of newly formed capillaries in human gliomas but is not expressed in the neovasculature of other primary tumors. Am J Pathol 1996; 149:853–858.

13. Iwahana M, Utoguchi N, Mayumi T, et al. Drug resistance and P-glycoprotein expression in endothelial cells of newly formed capillaries induced by tumors. Anticancer Res 1998; 18:2977–2980.

14. LeCouter J, Kowalski J, Foster J, et al. Identification of an angiogenic mitogen selective for endocrine gland endothelium. Nature 2001; 412:877–884.

15. Rohan RM, Fernandez A, Udagawa T, et al. Genetic heterogeneity of angiogenesis in mice. FASEB J 2000; 14:871–876.

16. Pandey J, Cracchiolo D, Hansen FM, et al. Strain differences and inheritance of angiogenic versus angiostatic activity in oestrogen-induced rat pituitary tumours. Angiogenesis 2002; 5:53–66.

17. Lenz H. The use and development of germline polymorphisms in clinical oncology. J Clin Oncol 2004; 22:2519–2521.

18. Evans W, McLeod H. Pharmacogenomics—drug disposition, drug targets, and side effects. N Engl J Med 2003; 348:538–549.

19. Gorchakova O, Koch W, von Beckerath N, et al. Association of a genetic variant of endothelial nitric oxide synthase with the 1 year clinical outcome after coronary stent placement. Eur Heart J 2003; 24:820–827.

20. Tan J, Zhu Z, Zhu S, et al. Study on the relationship between nitric oxide synthase gene G894T polymorphism and hypertension related risk factors in patients with essential hypertension in Chongqing city. Chung-Hua Liu Hsing Ping Hsueh Tsa Chih Chinese Journal of Epidemiology 2004; 25:158–161.

21. Casas J, Bautista L, Humphries S, et al. Endothelial nitric oxide synthase genotype and ischemic heart disease: meta-analysis of 26 studies involving 23028 subjects. Circulation 2004; 109:1359–1365.

22. Fatini C, Sofi F, Sticchi E, et al. Influence of endothelial nitric oxide synthase gene polymorphisms (G894T, 4a4b, T-786C) and hyperhomocysteinemia on the predisposition to acute coronary syndromes. Am Heart J 2004; 147:516–521.

23. Sharan K, Surrey S, Ballas S, et al. Sandler E. Keller M. Association of T-786C eNOS gene polymorphism with increased susceptibility to acute chest syndrome in females with sickle cell disease. Br J Haematol 2004; 124:240–243.

24. Turner S, Chapman A, Schwartz G, et al. Effects of endothelial nitric oxide synthase, α-adducin, and other candidate gene polymorphisms on blood pressure response to hydrochlorothiazide. Am J Hypertension 2003; 16:843–849.

25. Jachymova M, Horky K, Bultas J, et al. Jachymova M. Horky K. Bultas J. Kozich V. Jindra A. Peleska J. Martasek P. Association of the Glu298Asp polymorphism in the endothelial nitric oxide synthase gene with essential hypertension resistant to conventional therapy. Biochem Biophysi Res Commun 2001; 284:426–430.

26. Brogan I, Khan N, Isaac K, et al. Novel polymorphisms in the promoter and 5' UTR regions of the human vascular endothelial growth factor gene. Hum Immunol 1999; 60:1245–1249.

27. Shahbazi M, Fryer A, Pravica V, et al. Vascular endothelial growth factor gene polymorphisms are associated with acute renal allograft rejection. J Am Soc Nephrol 2002; 13:260–264.

28. Sakao S, Tatsumi K, Hashimoto T, et al. Vascular endothelial growth factor and the risk of smoking-related COPD. Chest 2003; 124:323–327.

29. Awata T, Inoue K, Kurihara S, et al. A common polymorphism in the 5'-untranslated region of the VEGF gene is associated with diabetic retinopathy in type 2 diabetes. Diabetes 2002; 51:1635–1639.

30. Morohashi K, Takada T, Omori K, et al: Vascular endothelial growth factor gene polymorphisms in Japanese patients with sarcoidosis. Chest 2003; 123:1520–1526.

31. Lin C, Wu H, Tsai F, et al. Vascular endothelial growth factor gene-460 C/T polymorphism is a biomarker for prostate cancer. Urology 2003; 62:374–377.

32. McCarron S, Edwards S, Evans P, et al: Influence of cytokine gene polymorphisms on the development of prostate cancer. Cancer Res 2002; 62:3369–3372.

33. Howell W, Bateman A, Turner S, et al. Influence of vascular endothelial growth factor single nucleotide polymorphisms on tumour development in cutaneous malignant melanoma. Genes Immun 2002; 3:229–232.

34. Krippl P, Langsenlehner U, Renner W, et al. A common 936 C/T gene polymorphism of vascular endothelial growth factor is associated with decreased breast cancer risk. Int J Cancer 2003; 106:468–471.
35. Watson C, Webb N, Bottomley M, et al. Identification of polymorphisms within the vascular endothelial growth factor (VEGF) gene: correlation with variation in VEGF protein production. Cytokine 2000; 12:1232–1235.
36. Renner W, Kotschan S, Hoffmann C, et al. A common 936 C/T mutation in the gene for vascular endothelial growth factor is associated with vascular endothelial growth factor plasma levels. J Vasc Res 2000; 37:443–448.
37. Cooke J, Dzau V. Nitric oxide synthase: role in the genesis of vascular disease. Annu Rev Med 1997; 48:489–509.
38. Yoshimura M, Yasue H, Nakayama M, et al. Genetic risk factors for coronary artery spasm: significance of endothelial nitric oxide synthase gene T-786→C and missense Glu298Asp variants. J Invest Med 2000; 48:367–374.
39. Cai H, Wilcken D, Wang X. The Glu-298→Asp (894G→T) mutation at exon 7 of the endothelial nitric oxide synthase gene and coronary artery disease. J Mol Med 1999; 77:511–514.
40. Nakayama M, Yasue H, Yoshimura M, et al: Nakayama M, Yasue H, Yoshimura M, et al. The 5′-flanking region of the endothelial nitric oxide synthase gene is associated with coronary spasm. Circulation 1999; 99:2864–2870,
41. Nakayama M, Yasue H, Yoshimura M, et al. T(-786)→C mutation in the 5′-flanking region of the endothelial nitric oxide synthase gene is associated with myocardial infarction, especially without coronary organic stenosis. Am J Cardiol 2000; 86:628–634.
42. Nadaud S, Bonnardeaux A, Lathrop M, et al. Gene structure, polymorphism and mapping of the human endothelial nitric oxide synthase gene. Biochem Biophys Res Commun 1994; 198:1027–1033.
43. Tanus-Santos J, Desai M, Flockhart D. Effects of ethnicity on the distribution of clinically relevant endothelial nitric oxide variants. Pharmacogenetics 2001; 11:719–725.
44. Ghilardi G, Biondi M, Cecchini F, et al. Vascular invasion in human breast cancer is correlated to T→786C polymorphism of NOS3 gene. Nitric Oxide 2003; 9:118–122.
45. Cheon K, Choi K, Lee H, et al. Gene polymorphisms of endothelial nitric oxide synthase and angiotensin-converting enzyme in patients with lung cancer. Lung 2000; 178:351–360.
46. Medeiros R, Morais A, Vasconcelos A, et al. Endothelial nitric oxide synthase gene polymorphisms and genetic susceptibility to prostate cancer. Eur J Cancer Prev 2002; 11:343–350.
47. Hefler L, Ludwig E, Lampe D, et al. Polymorphisms of the endothelial nitric oxide synthase gene in ovarian cancer. Gynecol Oncol 2002; 86:134–137.
48. Medeiros R, Morais A, Vasconcelos A, et al. Outcome in prostate cancer: association with endothelial nitric oxide synthase Glu-Asp298 polymorphism at exon 7. Clin Cancer Res 2002; 8:3433–3437.
49. Yagihashi N, Kasajima H, Sugai S, et al. Increased in situ expression of nitric oxide synthase in human colorectal cancer. Virchows Arch 2000; 436:109–114.
50. Wang X, Mahaney M, Sim A, et al. Genetic contribution of the endothelial constitutive nitric oxide synthase gene to plasma nitric oxide levels. Arterioscler Thromb Vasc Biol 1997; 17:3147–3153.
51. Tanimoto K, Yoshiga K, Eguchi H, et al. Hypoxia-inducible factor-1α polymorphisms associated with enhanced transactivation capacity, implying clinical significance. Carcinogenesis 2003; 24:1779–1783.
52. Topol E, McCarthy J, Gabriel S, et al. Single nucleotide polymorphisms in multiple novel thrombospondin genes may be associated with familial premature myocardial infarction. Circulation 2001; 104:2641–2644.
53. Boekholdt S, Trip M, Peters R, et al. Thrombospondin-2 polymorphism is associated with a reduced risk of premature myocardial infarction. Arterioscler Thromb Vasc Biol 2002; 22:24–27.
54. Topol EJ, McCarthy J, Gabriel S, et al. Single nucleotide polymorphisms in multiple novel thrombospondin genes may be associated with familial premature myocardial infarction. Circulation 2001; 104:2641–2644.
55. Wessel J, Topol E, Ji M, et al. Replication of the association between the thrombospondin-4 A387P polymorphism and myocardial infarction. Am Heart J 2004; 147:905–909.
56. McCarthy J, Parker A, Salem R, et al. Large scale association analysis for identification of genes underlying premature coronary heart disease: cumulative perspective from analysis of 111 candidate genes. J Med Genet 2004; 41:334–341.
57. Iughetti P, Suzuki O, Godoi P, et al. A polymorphism in endostatin, an angiogenesis inhibitor, predisposes for the development of prostatic adenocarcinoma. Cancer Res 2001; 61:7375–7378.
58. Balasubramanian S, Brown N, Reed M. Role of genetic polymorphisms in tumour angiogenesis. Br J Cancer 2002; 87:1057–1065.

59. Zorick T, Mustacchi Z, Bando S, et al. High serum endostatin levels in Down's syndrome: implications for improved treatment and prevention of solid tumors. Eur J Hum Genet 2001; 9:811–814.

60. Yu JL, Coomber BL, Kerbel RS. A paradigm for therapy-induced microenvironmental changes in solid tumors leading to drug resistance. Differentiation 2002; 70:599–609.

61. Relf M, LeJeune S, Scott PA, et al. Expression of the angiogenic factors vascular endothelial cell growth factor, acidic and basic fibroblast growth factor, tumor growth factor β-1, platelet-derived endothelial cell growth factor, placenta growth factor, and pleiotrophin in human primary breast cancer and its relation to angiogenesis. Cancer Res 1997; 57:963–969.

62. Cahill DP, Kinzler KW, Vogelstein B, et al. Genetic instability and darwinian selection in tumours. Trends Cell Biol 1999; 9:M57–M60.

63. Kim E, Moore J, Huang J, et al. All angiogenesis is not the same: Distinct patterns of response to antiangiogenic therapy in experimental neuroblastoma and Wilms tumor. J Pediatr Surg 2001; 36:287–290. =art&artType=abs&id=ajpsu0360287&target=.

64. Kerbel R. 2001;

65. Klement G, Baruchel S, Rak J, et al. Continuous low-dose therapy with vinblastine and VEGF receptor-2 antibody induces sustained tumor regression without overt toxicity. J Clin Invest 2000; 105:R15–R24.

66. Witte L, Hicklin DJ, Zhu Z, et al. Monoclonal antibodies targeting the VEGF receptor-2 (Flk1/KDR) as an anti-angiogenic therapeutic strategy. Cancer Metastasis Rev 1998; 17:155–161.

67. Filleur S, Volpert OV, Degeorges A, et al. In vivo mechanisms by which tumors producing thrombospondin 1 bypass its inhibitory effects. Genes Dev 2001; 15:1373–1382.

68. Wang GL, Jiang BH, Rue EA, et al. Hypoxia-inducible factor 1 is a basic-helix-loop-helix-PAS heterodimer regulated by cellular O2 tension. Proc Natl Acad Sci U S A 1995; 92:5510–5514.

69. Salceda S, Caro J. Hypoxia-inducible factor 1α (HIF-1α) protein is rapidly degraded by the ubiquitin-proteasome system under normoxic conditions. Its stabilization by hypoxia depends on redox-induced changes. J Biol Chem 1997; 272:22,642–22,647.

70. Jewell UR, Kvietikova I, Scheid A, et al. Induction of HIF-1α in response to hypoxia is instantaneous. Faseb J 2001; 15:1312–1314.

71. Carmeliet P, Dor Y, Herbert JM, et al. Role of HIF-1α in hypoxia-mediated apoptosis, cell proliferation and tumour angiogenesis. Nature 1998; 394:485–490.

72. Yu JL, Rak JW, Carmeliet P, et al. Heterogeneous vascular dependence of tumor cell populations. Am J Pathol 2001; 158:1325–1334.

73. Brown EB, Campbell RB, Tsuzuki Y, et al. In vivo measurement of gene expression, angiogenesis and physiological function in tumors using multiphoton laser scanning microscopy. Nat Med 2001; 7:864–868.

74. Chong ZZ, Kang JQ, Maiese K: Angiogenesis and plasticity: role of erythropoietin in vascular systems. J Hematother Stem Cell Res 2002; 11:863–871.

75. Dias S, Hattori K, Zhu Z, et al. Autocrine stimulation of VEGFR-2 activates human leukemic cell growth and migration. J Clin Invest 2000; 106:511–521.

76. Dias S, Choy M, Alitalo K, et al. Vascular endothelial growth factor (VEGF)-C signaling through FLT-4 (VEGFR-3) mediates leukemic cell proliferation, survival, and resistance to chemotherapy. Blood 2002; 99:2179–2184.

77. Zhu Z, Hattori K, Zhang H, et al. Inhibition of human leukemia in an animal model with human antibodies directed against vascular endothelial growth factor receptor 2. Correlation between antibody affinity and biological activity. Leukemia 2003; 17:604–611.

78. Gohongi T, Fukumura D, Boucher Y, et al. Tumor-host interactions in the gallbladder suppress distal angiogenesis and tumor growth: involvement of transforming growth factor β1. Nat Med 1999; 5:1203–1208.

79. Tsuzuki Y, Carreira CM, Bockhorn M, et al. Pancreas microenvironment promotes vegf expression and tumor growth: novel window models for pancreatic tumor angiogenesis and microcirculation. Lab Invest 2001; 81:1439–1451.

80. Liu W, Davis DW, Ramirez K, et al. Endothelial cell apoptosis is inhibited by a soluble factor secreted by human colon cancer cells. Int J Cancer 2001; 92:26–30.

81. Gupta K, Kshirsagar S, Li W, et al. VEGF prevents apoptosis of human microvascular endothelial cells via opposing effects on MAPK/ERK and SAPK/JNK signaling. Exp Cell Res 1999; 247:495–504.

82. Tran J, Rak J, Sheehan C, et al. Marked induction of the IAP family antiapoptotic proteins survivin and XIAP by VEGF in vascular endothelial cells [In Process Citation]. Biochem Biophys Res Commun 1999; 264:781–788.

83. Tran J, Master Z, Yu JL, et al. A role for survivin in chemoresistance of endothelial cells mediated by VEGF. Proc Natl Acad Sci U S A 2002; 99:4349–4354.

84. Karsan A, Yee E, Poirier GG, et al. Fibroblast growth factor-2 inhibits endothelial cell apoptosis by Bcl-2-dependent and independent mechanisms. Am J Pathol 1997; 151:1775–1784.

85. Gerber HP, Dixit V, Ferrara N. Vascular endothelial growth factor induces expression of the antiapoptotic proteins Bcl-2 and A1 in vascular endothelial cells. J Biol Chem 1998; 273:13,313–13,316.

86. Eberhard A, Kahlert S, Goede V, et al. Heterogeneity of angiogenesis and blood vessel maturation in human tumors: implications for antiangiogenic tumor therapies [published erratum appears in Cancer Res 2000 Jul 1;60(13):3668]. Cancer Res 2000; 60:1388–1393.

87. Low JA, Johnson MD, Bone EA, et al. The matrix metalloproteinase inhibitor batimastat (BB-94) retards human breast cancer solid tumor growth but not ascites formation in nude mice. Clin Cancer Res 1996; 2:1207–1214.

88. Pozzi A, Moberg PE, Miles LA, et al. Elevated matrix metalloprotease and angiostatin levels in integrin α 1 knockout mice cause reduced tumor vascularization. Proc Natl Acad Sci U S A 2000; 97:2202–2207.

89. Pluen A, Boucher Y, Ramanujan S, et al. Role of tumor-host interactions in interstitial diffusion of macromolecules: cranial vs. subcutaneous tumors. Proc Natl Acad Sci U S A 2001; 98:4628–4633.

90. Eder J, Clark J, Supko J, et al. A phase I pharmacokinetic and pharmacodynamic trial of recombinant endostatin. Proc Am Soc Clin Oncol 2001; 20:70a.

91. Herbst R, Tran H, Mullani N, et al. Phase I clinical trial of recombinant human endostatin in patients with solid tumors: pharmcokinetic, safety and efficacy analysis ysing surrogate endpoints of tissue and radiologic response. Proc Am Sco Clin Oncol 2001; 20:3a.

92. Thomas J, Schiller J, Lee F, et al. A phase I pharmacokinetic and pharmacodynamic study of recombinant human endostatin. Proc Am Soc Clin Oncol 2001; 20:70a.

93. Miller K, Haney L, Pribluda V, et al. A phase I safety, pharmacokinetic and pharmacodynamic study of 2-methoxyestradiol in patients with refractory metastatic breast cancer. Proc Am Soc Clin Oncol 2001; 20:43a.

94. Sledge G, Miller K, Novotny W, et al. A phase II trial of single-agent rhuMAb VEGF (recombinant humanized monoclonal antibody to vascular endothelial cell growth factor) in patients with relapsed metastatic breast cancer. Proc Am Soc Clin Oncol 2000; 19:3a.

95. Ghiso N, Rohan RM, Amano S, et al. Suppression of hypoxia-associated vascular endothelial growth factor gene expression by nitric oxide via cGMP. Invest Ophthalmol Vis Sci 1999; 40:1033–1039.

96. Liu W, Ahmad SA, Reinmuth N, et al. Endothelial cell survival and apoptosis in the tumor vasculature. Apoptosis 2000; 5:323–328.

97. Kakeji Y, Maehara Y, Ikebe M, et al. Dynamics of tumor oxygenation, CD31 staining and transforming growth factor-β levels after treatment with radiation or cyclophosphamide in the rat 13762 mammary carcinoma. Int J Radiat Oncol Biol Phys 1997; 37:1115–1123.

98. Overmoyer B, Robertson K, Persons M, et al. A phase I pharmacokinetic and pharmacodynamic study of SU5416 and Adriamycin in inflammatory breast cancer. Breast Cancer Res Treat 2001; 69:284.

99. Durand RE, LePard NE. Contribution of transient blood flow to tumour hypoxia in mice. Acta Oncol 1995; 34:317–323.

100. Brown JM, Giaccia AJ. The unique physiology of solid tumors: opportunities (and problems) for cancer therapy. Cancer Res 1998; 58:1408–1416.

101. Jain RK. Normalizing tumor vasculature with anti-angiogenic therapy: a new paradigm for combination therapy. Nat Med 2001; 7:987–989.

102. Durand RE, Raleigh JA. Identification of nonproliferating but viable hypoxic tumor cells in vivo. Cancer Res 1998; 58:3547–3550.

103. Durand RE, Sham E. The lifetime of hypoxic human tumor cells. Int J Radiat Oncol Biol Phys 1998; 42:711–715.

104. Wouters BG, Koritzinsky M, Chiu RK, et al. Modulation of cell death in the tumor microenvironment. Semin Radiat Oncol 2003; 13:31–41.

105. Holash J, Maisonpierre PC, Compton D, et al. Vessel cooption, regression, and growth in tumors mediated by angiopoietins and VEGF. Science 1999; 284:1994–1998.

106. Kunkel P, Ulbricht U, Bohlen P, et al. Inhibition of glioma angiogenesis and growth in vivo by systemic treatment with a monoclonal antibody against vascular endothelial growth factor receptor-2. Cancer Res 2001; 61:6624–6628.

107. Passalidou E, Trivella M, Singh N, et al. Vascular phenotype in angiogenic and non-angiogenic lung non-small cell carcinomas. Br J Cancer 2002; 86:244–249.

108. Stessels F, Van den Eynden G, Van den Auwera I, et al. Breast adenocarcinoma liver metastases, in contrast to colorectal cancer liver metastases, display a non-angiogenic growth pattern that preserves the stroma and lacks hypoxia. Br J Cancer 2004; 90:1429–1436.

109. Patan S, Munn LL, Jain RK. Intussusceptive microvascular growth in a human colon adenocarcinoma xenograft: a novel mechanism of tumor angiogenesis. Microvasc Res 1996; 51:260–272.

110. Patan S, Tanda S, Roberge S, et al. Vascular morphogenesis and remodeling in a human tumor xenograft: blood vessel formation and growth after ovariectomy and tumor implantation. Circ Res 2001; 89:732–739.

111. Djonov V, Andres AC, Ziemiecki A. Vascular remodelling during the normal and malignant life cycle of the mammary gland. Microsc Res Tech 2001; 52:182–189.

112. Folberg R, Hendrix MJ, Maniotis AJ. Vasculogenic mimicry and tumor angiogenesis. Am J Pathol 2000; 156:361–381.

113. Hendrix MJ, Seftor EA, Meltzer PS, et al. Expression and functional significance of VE-cadherin in aggressive human melanoma cells: Role in vasculogenic mimicry. Proc Natl Acad Sci U S A 2001; 98:8018–8023.

114. Sood AK, Seftor EA, Fletcher MS, et al. Molecular determinants of ovarian cancer plasticity. Am J Pathol 2001; 158:1279–1288.

115. Hendrix MJ, Seftor EA, Kirschmann DA, et al. Molecular biology of breast cancer metastasis. Molecular expression of vascular markers by aggressive breast cancer cells. Breast Cancer Res 2000; 2:417–422.

116. Asahara T, Masuda H, Takahashi T, et al. Bone marrow origin of endothelial progenitor cells responsible for postnatal vasculogenesis in physiological and pathological neovascularization. Circ Res 1999; 85:221–228.

117. Hattori K, Dias S, Heissig B, et al. Vascular endothelial growth factor and angiopoietin-1 stimulate postnatal hematopoiesis by recruitment of vasculogenic and hematopoietic stem cells. J Exp Med 2001; 193:1005–1014.

118. Bolontrade MF, Zhou RR, Kleinerman ES. Vasculogenesis Plays a Role in the Growth of Ewing's Sarcoma in Vivo. Clin Cancer Res 2002; 8:3622–3627.

119. Lyden D, Hattori K, Dias S, et al. Impaired recruitment of bone-marrow-derived endothelial and hematopoietic precursor cells blocks tumor angiogenesis and growth. Nat Med 2001; 7:1194–1201.

120. Alpaugh M, Barsky S. The molecular basis of inflammatory breast cancer. Breast Cancer Res Treat 2001; 69:312.

121. van der Schraft D, et al. The differential effects of angiogenesis inhibitors on vascular network formation by endothelial cells versus aggressive melanoma tumor cells. Proc Am Assoc Cancer Res 2003; 2003:696A.

122. Slaton JW, Perrotte P, Inoue K, et al. Interferon-α-mediated down-regulation of angiogenesis-related genes and therapy of bladder cancer are dependent on optimization of biological dose and schedule. Clin Cancer Res 1999; 5:2726–2734.

123. Browder T, Butterfield CE, Kraling BM, et al. Antiangiogenic scheduling of chemotherapy improves efficacy against experimental drug-resistant cancer [In Process Citation]. Cancer Res 2000; 60:1878–1886.

124. Wild R, Ghosh K, Dings R, et al. Carboplatin differentially induces the VEGF stress response in endothelial cells: potentiation of anti-tumor effects by combination treatment with antibody to VEGF. Proc Am Assoc Canc Res 2000; 41:307.

125. Riedel F, Gotte K, Bergler W, et al. Expression of basic fibroblast growth factor protein and its down-regulation by interferons in head and neck cancer. Head Neck 2000; 22:183–189.

126. Folkman J, Ingber D. Inhibition of angiogenesis. Semin Cancer Biol 1992; 3:89–96.

127. Yasukawa H, Sasaki A, Yoshimura A. Negative regulation of cytokine signaling pathways. Annu Rev Immunol 2000; 18:143–164.

128. Fogler W, Song M, Supko J, et al. Recombinant human endostatin demonstrates consistent and predictable pharmacokinetics following intravenous bolus administration to cancer patients. Proc Am Soc Clin Oncol 2001; 20:69a.

129. DeMoraes E, Fogler W, Grant D, et al. Recombinant human angiostatin: a phase I clinical trial assessing safety, pharmacokinetics and pharmacodynamics. Proc Am Soc Clin Oncol 2001; 20:3a.

130. O'Reilly MS, Holmgren L, Shing Y, et al. Angiostatin: a novel angiogenesis inhibitor that mediates the suppression of metastases by a Lewis lung carcinoma [see comments]. Cell 1994; 79:315–328.

131. O'Reilly MS, Holmgren L, Chen C, et al. Angiostatin induces and sustains dormancy of human primary tumors in mice. Nat Med 1996; 2:689–692.

132. O'Reilly MS, Boehm T, Shing Y, et al. Endostatin: an endogenous inhibitor of angiogenesis and tumor growth. Cell 1997; 88:277–285.

133. Hurwitz H, Fehrenbacher L, Cartwright T, et al. Bevacizumab (a monoclonal antibody to vascular endothelial growth factor) prolongs survival in first-line colorectal cancer (CRC): Results of a phase III trial of bevacizumab in combination with bolus IFL (irinotecan, 5-fluorouracil, leucovorin) as first-line therapy in subjects with metastatic CRC. Proc Am Soc Clin Oncol 2003; 22:abstract 3646.

134. DeVore R, Fehrenbacher L, Herbst R, et al. A randomized phase II trial comparing rhuMAb VEGF (recombinant humanized monoclonal antibody to vascular endothelial growth factor) plus carboplatin/paclitaxel (CP) to CP alone in patients with stage IIIB/IV NSCLC. Proc Am Soc Clin Oncol 2000; 19:485a.

135. Bergsland E, Hurwitz H, Fehrenbacher L, et al. A randomized phase II trial comparing rhuMAb VEGF (recombinant humanized monoclonal antibody to vascular endothelial growth factor) plus 5-fluorouracil/leulovorin (FU/LV) to FU/LV alone in patients with metastatic colorectal cancer. Proc Am Soc Clin Oncol 2000; 19:242a.

136. Barlogie B, Tricot G, Anaissie E. Thalidomide in the management of multiple myeloma. Semin Oncol 2001; 28:577–582.

137. Browder T, Butterfield CE, Kraling BM, et al. Antiangiogenic scheduling of chemotherapy improves efficacy against experimental drug-resistant cancer. Cancer Res 2000; 60:1878–1886.

138. Teicher B, Sotomayor E, Huang Z. Antiangiogenic agents potentiate cytotoxic cancer therapies against primary and metastatic disease. Cancer Res 1992; 52:6702–6704.

139. Teicher BA, Holden SA, Jui-Tsai C, et al. Minocycline as a modulaor of chemoherapy and hyperthermia in vitro and in vivo. Cancer Lett 1994; 82:17–25.

140. Sweeney CJ, Miller KD, Sissons SE, et al. The Antiangiogenic Property of Docetaxel Is Synergistic with a Recombinant Humanized Monoclonal Antibody against Vascular Endothelial Growth Factor or 2-Methoxyestradiol but Antagonized by Endothelial Growth Factors. Cancer Res 2001; 61:3369–3372.

141. Zachary I, Gliki G. Signaling transduction mechanisms mediating biological actions of the vascular endothelial growth factor family. Cardiovasc Res 2001; 49:568–581.

142. Gluzman-Poltorak Z, Cohen T, Herzog Y, et al. Neuropilin-2 is a receptor for the vascular endothelial growth factor (VEGF) forms VEGF-145 and VEGF-165 [corrected]. J Biol Chem 2000; 275:18,040–18,045.

143. Bachelder RE, Crago A, Chung J, et al. Vascular endothelial growth factor is an autocrine survival factor for neuropilin-expressing breast carcinoma cells. Cancer Res 2001; 61:5736–5740.

144. Bagnard D, Vaillant C, Khuth ST, et al. Semaphorin 3A-vascular endothelial growth factor-165 balance mediates migration and apoptosis of neural progenitor cells by the recruitment of shared receptor. J Neurosci 2001; 21:3332–3341.

145. Miao HQ, Lee P, Lin H, et al. Neuropilin-1 expression by tumor cells promotes tumor angiogenesis and progression. Faseb J 2000; 14:2532–2539.

146. Wedam S, Low J, Yang X, et al. A pilot study to evaluate response and angiogenesis after treatment with bevacizumab in patients with inflammatory breast cancer. J Clin Oncol, 2004 ASCO Annual Meetin Proceedings 2004; 22:578.

147. Brem H, Gresser I, Grosfeld J, et al. The combination of antiangiogenic agents to inhibit primary tumor growth and metastasis. J Pediatr Surg 1993; 28:1253–1257.

148. Scappaticci FA, Smith R, Pathak A, et al. Combination angiostatin and endostatin gene transfer induces synergistic antiangiogenic activity in vitro and antitumor efficacy in leukemia and solid tumors in mice. Mol Ther 2001; 3:186–196.

149. Rak J, Yu JL, Klement G, et al. Oncogenes and angiogenesis: signaling three-dimensional tumor growth. J Investig Dermatol Symp Proc 2000; 5:24–33.

150. Petit AM, Rak J, Hung MC, et al. Neutralizing antibodies against epidermal growth factor and ErbB-2/neu receptor tyrosine kinases down-regulate vascular endothelial growth factor production by tumor cells in vitro and in vivo: angiogenic implications for signal transduction therapy of solid tumors. Am J Pathol 1997; 151:1523–1530.

151. Koukourakis MI, Giatromanolaki A, O'Byrne KJ, et al. bcl-2 and c-erbB-2 proteins are involved in the regulation of VEGF and of thymidine phosphorylase angiogenic activity in non-small-cell lung cancer. Clin Exp Metastasis 1999; 17:545–554.

152. Yen L, You X, Al Moustafa A, et al. Heregulin selectively upregulates vascular endothelial growth factor secretion in cancer cells and stimulates angiogenesis. Oncogene 2000; 19:3460–3469.

153. Maity A, Pore N, Lee J, et al. Epidermal growth factor receptor transcriptionally up-regulates vascular endothelial growth factor expression in human glioblastoma cells via a pathway involving phosphatidylinositol 3′-kinase and distinct from that induced by hypoxia. Cancer Res 2000; 60:5879–5886.

154. Clarke K, Smith K, Gullick WJ, et al. Mutant epidermal growth factor receptor enhances induction of vascular endothelial growth factor by hypoxia and insulin-like growth factor-1 via a PI3 kinase dependent pathway. Br J Cancer 2001; 84:1322–1329.

155. Bruns CJ, Solorzano CC, Harbison MT, et al. Blockade of the epidermal growth factor receptor signaling by a novel tyrosine kinase inhibitor leads to apoptosis of endothelial cells and therapy of human pancreatic carcinoma. Cancer Res 2000; 60:2926–2935.

156. Ciardiello F, Caputo R, Bianco R, et al. Inhibition of growth factor production and angiogenesis in human cancer cells by ZD1839 (Iressa), a selective epidermal growth factor receptor tyrosine kinase inhibitor. Clin Cancer Res 2001; 7:1459–1465.

157. Viloria-Petit A, Crombet T, Jothy S, et al. Acquired resistance to the antitumor effect of epidermal growth factor receptor-blocking antibodies in vivo: a role for altered tumor angiogenesis. Cancer Res 2001; 61:5090–5101.

158. Miller KD, Gradishar W, Schuchter L, et al. A randomized phase II pilot trial of adjuvant marimastat in patients with early-stage breast cancer. Ann Oncol 2002; 13:1220–1224.

159. Miller KD, Saphner TJ, Waterhouse DM, et al. A randomized phase II pilot trial of BMS-275291 in patients with early stage breast cancer. Proc Am Assoc Cancer Res 2003; abstract 6353.

160. Bryant J, Smith R, Margolese R, et al. Increased gallbladder adverse events associated with octreotide pa LAR in patients with breast cancer. Proc Am Soc Clin Oncol 2001; 20:abstract 197.

IV The Role of Hormones, Growth Factors, and Oncogenes

22 Resistance to Antiestrogens

Clodia Osipo, PhD and Ruth M. O'Regan, MD

SUMMARY

Discovery of the estrogen receptors (ERs) has been critical for the development of endocrine therapy in breast cancer. Expression of ER-α, the predominant isoform, in breast tumors of both pre- and postmenopausal women is a highly predictive marker for response to antiestrogen treatment. Tamoxifen, an antiestrogen, that competitively blocks the actions of 17β-estradiol (E_2), binds and activates ER-α in breast tumors and is used for treating all stages of breast cancer. Although tamoxifen is effective in reducing recurrence from ER-positive early stage breast cancer, approximately 50% of patients do not benefit from its use, because their breast cancers have intrinsic or *de novo* tamoxifen-resistance. Additionally, most patients that do initially benefit from tamoxifen, will develop acquired resistance to the drug during the treatment regimen. Despite increasing use of the aromatase inhibitors as breast cancer therapies, tamoxifen remains the hormonal therapy of choice in premenopausal women, and is the only hormonal therapy approved for breast cancer prevention. Therefore, a current goal in breast cancer research is to elucidate the mechanisms of both intrinsic and acquired resistance to tamoxifen and other antiestrogens in order to develop new therapeutic strategies to prevent and/or treat resistant breast cancer.

Key Words: Antiestrogen; resistance, tamoxifen; breast cancer; estrogen receptor; aromatase inhibitors; growth factors.

1. INTRODUCTION TO ANTIESTROGENS

In 1962, Jensen and colleagues discovered estrogen receptor (ER)-α. Jensen demonstrated that 17β-estradiol (E_2), the circulating female hormone that promoted breast cancer growth, binds to diverse tissue sites around a woman's body, but is retained in

From: *Cancer Drug Discovery and Development: Cancer Drug Resistance*
Edited by: B. Teicher © Humana Press Inc., Totowa, NJ

estrogen-target tissues, for example, the uterus and vagina. The identification of the ER-α as the target of E_2 action in the breast, and the discovery that antiestrogens blocked the binding of E_2 to the ER-α, provided a therapeutic target and an approach for the treatment of breast cancer. Nonsteroidal antiestrogens were initially developed as contraceptives in the 1960s. Walpole and colleagues synthesized tamoxifen (termed ICI 46, 474), a potent antiestrogen with antifertility properties in rats. However, in humans, tamoxifen induced ovulation in subfertile women, and consequently, its development as a contraceptive was discontinued. Fortunately, Walpole also patented the application of tamoxifen as a drug treatment for hormone-dependent cancers.

Although many antiestrogens were discovered and tested during the 1960s and 1970s, only tamoxifen was considered safe enough for extensive clinical evaluation (2). Clinical trials were started to evaluate tamoxifen compared to the standard endocrine treatment at the time, diethylstilbestrol (DES), for the treatment of advanced breast cancer in postmenopausal women. Tamoxifen was as effective as DES for the treatment of advanced breast cancer, but with fewer side effects. This advantage in side effect profile of tamoxifen compared to DES was crucial for its subsequent development as a treatment for all stages of breast cancer.

Further clinical trials demonstrated that tamoxifen was truly a targeted therapy; it was highly effective in patients with tumors expressing hormone receptors, but ineffective when neither ER nor progesterone receptor (PR) were expressed (4). Following its approval as a treatment for advanced breast cancer, tamoxifen was evaluated as an adjuvant therapy in early stage breast cancer, and was demonstrated to reduce recurrence rates by 50% (5). Five years of adjuvant tamoxifen treatment was found to be more effective than less than 5 yr in improving time to tumor recurrence and overall survival (5). In contrast to the beneficial effects of tamoxifen as a treatment for breast cancer, both laboratory and clinical results demonstrated that tamoxifen acted as an estrogen agonist on the uterus, and increased the risk of endometrial cancer by 0.1% (5–7). These results strongly suggested that tamoxifen was not a pure antiestrogen, but had selective functions depending on the target tissue. Tamoxifen was demonstrated to reduce the incidence of contralateral breast cancer, in patients with ER-positive breast tumors (5). Based on this observation, and its acceptable side effect profile (5), tamoxifen was evaluated as a breast cancer preventive in high-risk women (8), and was approved for this indication in 1998.

2. MECHANISMS OF ACTION

2.1. Selective ER Modulators

The concept of selective estrogen receptor modulators (SERMs) was first recognized in the 1980s from research that investigated the pharmacological properties of tamoxifen at distinct tissue locations around a woman's body (Fig. 1A). For example, tamoxifen has estrogen-like properties on bone in ovariectomized rats (10), is both a partial estrogen and an antiestrogen on the uterus (7), and an antiestrogen/antitumor agent in the rat mammary gland (11). In athymic mice bitransplanted with human breast cancers and endometrial cancers, tamoxifen inhibits growth of the breast cancers, while simultaneously stimulating growth of the endometrial cancers (7). This concept of the selective actions by nonsteroidal antiestrogens first recognized in the laboratory was then applied to clinical drug development (12). Tamoxifen maintains bone density and lowers circulating cholesterol levels in postmenopausal women (13). More importantly, tamoxifen lowers the

SERM
(Tamoxifen)

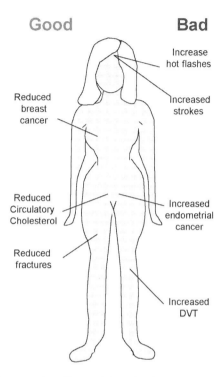

Fig. 1. Differential agonist/antagonist effects of the selective estrogen receptor modulator (SERM) tamoxifen on different tissues around a woman's body.

recurrence of ER-positive breast cancer and decreases the incidence of contralateral breast by 50%, whereas it causes a modest increase in the risk of endometrial cancer by 0.1% in postmenopausal women *(5,8)*. The beneficial effects of tamoxifen around a woman's body were used to justify the evaluation of tamoxifen as an adjuvant treatment for ductal carcinoma *in situ (14)*, and as a preventive in high-risk pre- and postmenopausal women *(8)*.

To date, there is no definitive explanation as to why tamoxifen has differential agonist and antagonist effects at different target tissues. As this chapter outlines, possible explanations include differential expression of ER subtypes, and/or coregulatory proteins, in different target tissues.

2.1.1. ACTIVATION OF ER

An understanding of the selective nature of antiestrogens in patients first requires an understanding of the function of ER at the molecular level. Human ER is a member of the nuclear receptor family of ligand-inducible transcription factors *(15)*. The classical model of ER activation involves the binding of the ligand E_2 to the ligand-binding domain (LBD) of the nuclear ER in target tissues that induces a conformational change in the three-dimensional structure of the complex. The E_2–ER complex dimerizes and subse-

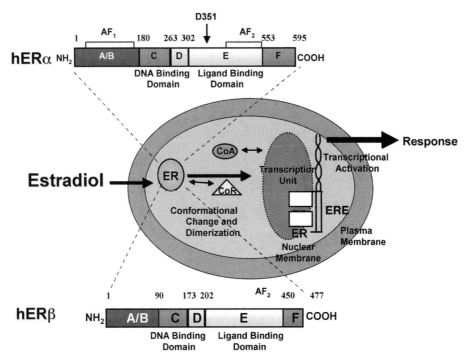

Fig. 2. Comparison of structures of estrogen receptor (ER)-α and ER-β. Depending on the expression of coregulators of the ER, gene transcription is activated or inhibited.

quently binds to DNA sequences referred to as estrogen response elements (EREs) *(16)*. These EREs are *cis*-acting enhancer elements located within regulatory regions of target genes. The DNA-bound ER interacts with the preinitiation transcriptional machinery either directly or indirectly via coregulatory proteins (Fig. 2).

In contrast, the nonclassical or tethered pathway for activation of the ER involves the indirect interaction of the nuclear E_2–ER complex with transcription factors including Jun/Fos (activating protein [AP]-1) or specificity protein (Sp)1 and subsequent activation of AP-1 or Sp1-driven genes, respectively *(17)*. Thus, the ER can regulate the transcription of a wide variety of genes by both classical and nonclassical pathways. It is also now apparent that ER-α can exist both in the nucleus and in the cytoplasm, and can have differential effects on gene transcription, for example at AP-1 sites, depending on its cellular location *(18)*.

2.1.2. ER-α AND ER-β

The identification of different ER isoforms is a recognized method in pharmacology for developing tissue-selective drugs. The discovery of two genetically distinct ERs, ER-α and ER-β *(19–21)*, provides a possible explanation for the tissue selective nature of antiestrogens. The two receptors have some degree of homology in that both receptors have a LBD and DNA-binding domain *(see* Fig. 2) *(22)*. However, there are notable differences in the two activating functions (AFs). First, ER-β does not have an AF1 region but retains an AF2 region. These differences in the AF regions alter the activity of the antiestrogen–ER complex, resulting in increased or decreased estrogenic activity. For example, tamoxifen is more antiestrogenic when it is complexed with ER-β *(23,24)*.

However, to date, little is known about the role of ER-β in antiestrogen action. What is known from mRNA expression profiles is that ER-β is expressed in a wide variety of tissues, including the breast and uterus (20,21,25). However, the existence of significant levels of ER-β protein in all mRNA-expressing tissues has been more difficult to interpret and requires further investigation. Studies in vitro indicate that both ER-α and ER-β activate transcription in response to E_2 at estrogen-response elements (ERE)-containing promoters, with ER-α being a more efficient transcriptional activator than ER-β. However, when both receptors are expressed in cells, a splice variant of ER-β decreases the activity of ER-α and decreases the overall sensitivity of agonists (26). The mechanism is not known, and little in vivo data exist showing competition between the two receptors for the same DNA-sequence and/or heterodimerization of ER-β with ER-α. In cells where tamoxifen activates ER-α-mediated, ERE-driven transcriptional activity, coexpression of ER-β completely suppresses this activity (27). Thus, expression levels of ER-β might regulate the magnitude of the tamoxifen–ER-α complex on ERE-driven genes, but only if the ratio of receptors was appropriate. In AP-1-containing elements/ ER-α systems, where ER-α binds indirectly to AP-1 promoters by interaction with AP-1, estrogens activate transcription and antiestrogens display a range of activities from partial to full agonists (23). In contrast, estrogens antagonize and all antiestrogens-tested activate transcription in cells expressing AP-1–ER-β systems (23). However, demonstration of the physiological significance of the AP-1–ER interaction in vivo has yet to be shown. Studies in vitro have demonstrated that tamoxifen appears to inhibit E_2-activated transcription by both ER-α and ER-β (23). However, in some cell and promoter contexts, the tamoxifen–ER-α complex manifests partial agonist activity. Therefore, it remains to be explained how the same ER-α–ligand complex can be recognized differently in different cells.

There is accumulating evidence to suggest that both ERs exist, not only in the nucleus, but in the cytoplasm, under specific conditions, and that their functions in response to estrogen may differ depending on their location (Fig. 3) (18,28,29). Nongenomic actions of ER-α have been demonstrated to activate mitogen-activated protein kinase (MAPK), in response to estrogen, resulting in cell proliferation (18). Additionally, binding of estrogen to cytoplasmic ER-α has been demonstrated to activate AP-1 sites, whereas AP-1 activation is inhibited by binding of estrogen to nuclear ER-α (18). It is possible that location of ER-α in the cell may contribute to differential effects of tamoxifen on different target tissues.

2.1.3. COREGULATORS OF ER

Another explanation for the selective activities of antiestrogens in different cell types is the expression pattern of coregulatory proteins (30). ERs directly or indirectly activate or repress target genes by binding to hormone response elements in promoter or enhancer regions (see Fig. 2). Modulation of transcription by ERs requires the recruitment of coregulators. Coregulators are transcription modifiers that can either activate or repress the activity of the ER complex (see Fig. 3). A basic mechanism for the switching of target genes from off to on requires a ligand-dependent exchange of corepressors for coactivators. The family of steroid receptor coactivators ([SRC]-1, -2, and -3) compliment the activity of the ER (31–37). Ligand-dependent recruitment of coactivators is dependent on the AF-2 region within the C terminus of the LBD of both ER-α and ER-β. The precise region of the coactivators that interacts with the AF-2 region of the ER is an LXXLL domain, where "L" represents a leucine, and "X" represents any amino acid

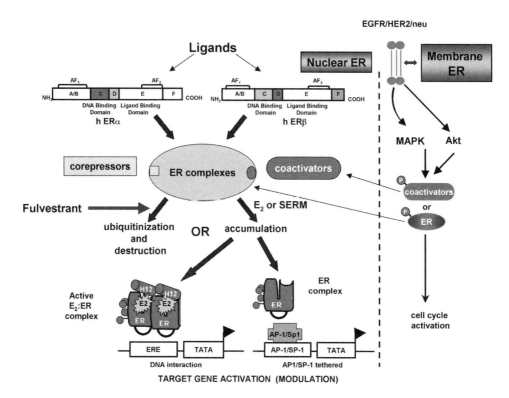

Fig. 3. Comparison of nuclear and nongenomic estrogen receptor (ER) pathways. Activation of nuclear ER pathways can result in classical or nonclassical gene transcription. Activation on nongenomic ER results in activation of mitogen-activated protein kinase (MAPK) or phosphatidylinositol 3 kinase pathways.

(38). The ER–coactivator complex functions to stabilize the preinitiation transcriptional machinery and promotes chromatin remodeling by recruiting histone acetyltransferases at the promoter region of the target gene *(39).* Thereafter, transcription of the target gene is either activated or repressed, depending on the promoter and cellular context. More than 30 additional putative coactivators have been identified to date *(40).* Thus, expression levels of coactivators might explain the selective actions of antiestrogens in different cells. The estrogen-like activity of the tamoxifen–ER complex has been shown to be because of higher levels of SRC-1 in endometrial cancer cells vs MCF-7 breast cancer cells, where the tamoxifen–ER complex is mostly antiestrogenic *(41).*

ER-α and ER-β also play critical roles by repressing gene transcription. They function as ligand-independent repressors on some target genes or ligand-dependent repressors on others *(42).* Corepressors are coregulators that repress the activity of both ER-α and ER-β. The known corepressors are N-CoR, SMRT, and REA *(42–48).* These coregulators contain multi-independent repressor domains that interact with histone deacetylases to mediate deacetylation of histones and promote condensation of chromatin repressing transcription of the target gene. The ER–corepressor complex prevents the interaction of the ligandless ER to the transcriptional machinery resulting in transcriptional repression *(see* Fig. 3). Transcriptional repression of target genes by antiestrogen–ER complexes might depend on the structure of the selective antiestrogen, the three-dimensional structure of the antiestrogen–ER complex, and the availability of corepressors vs coactivators.

In summary, the mechanism resulting in differential effects of SERMs on different target tissues is not definitely known. Differential expression of coregulators in different target tissues probably plays a role in this process.

3. RESISTANCE TO ANTIESTROGENS

3.1. Overview

Tamoxifen is widely used for all stages of breast cancer. Approximately 50% of patients with hormone receptor-positive breast cancer respond to tamoxifen treatment (49). Unfortunately, the other 50% of patients do not respond, and many who initially respond will eventually experience disease relapse. Therefore, a major problem with the use of tamoxifen therapy is that many breast tumors will either be resistant (intrinsic or *de novo*) before endocrine treatment or become resistant (acquired) during therapy. Considerable research has examined possible mechanisms responsible for the tamoxifen-resistant phenotype. Examples of this research include loss of the *ER-α* gene and/or protein in tumors during short-term and long-term treatment, identification of mutations within the *ER-α* gene, changes in the pharmacologic response of resistant breast cancer cells to tamoxifen, activation of ER-α-mediated gene transcription in the absence of ligand, modifications in gene transcription by changes in interactions between ER-α and coregulators, and the development of enhanced surface-to-intracellular signaling crosstalk between growth factor receptors and ER-α. Current evidence suggests that tamoxifen resistance (both intrinsic and acquired) is likely multifactorial.

3.1.1. HORMONE RECEPTOR-NEGATIVE BREAST CANCER AND RESISTANCE

Breast cancers initially lacking expression of ER and/or PR have intrinsic resistance to endocrine therapy. In addition, loss of ER-α expression on recurrence of breast cancer during tamoxifen therapy has been reported in 25% of tumors (50–52). However, most of acquired resistance occurring during tamoxifen treatment is not because of changes in ER-α expression, and most tamoxifen-resistant breast tumors retain ER-α, and, therefore, may respond to secondary endocrine treatments. In summary, absence of ER-α does predict for *de novo* tamoxifen resistance, but does not appear to be a major mechanism for acquired resistance.

3.1.2. ER-α AND ER-β MUTATIONS

Several mutant forms of both ER-α and ER-β have been identified and previously reviewed (53–55). However, the functional significance of these mutants as a mechanism of antiestrogen resistance is yet to be elucidated. Most of the data demonstrate existence of splice variants for ER-α and ER-β mRNA, without evidence of translation into functional proteins. In most cases, breast tumors express both mutant and wild-type ER, with the wild-type being the predominant species. A single point mutation in the LBD of ER-α has been reported (D351Y) that converts tamoxifen and raloxifene from antiestrogen to estrogens in in vivo and in vitro models of antiestrogen-stimulated MCF-7 tumor cells (56,57). However, the D351Y ER-α mutant has yet to be detected in either *de novo* or acquired resistant breast tumors from patients. In addition, mutations in the F-region of the ER have been shown to affect the activities of both E_2 and 4-hydroxytamoxifen (4OHT), the active metabolite of tamoxifen (58). In summary, the clinical relevance of ER mutants is unclear to date as a mechanism of resistance to antiestrogens. However, an understanding of ER mutations in response to antiestrogens may lead to the development of better antiestrogens or other drugs for breast cancer treatment.

3.1.3. Role of Nongenomic ER

There is increasing evidence to support the existence of ERs outside the nucleus. Nongenomic actions of estradiol have only been recognized recently (*see* Fig. 3), and encompass activation of MAPK, Ras, Raf-1, phosphokinase C and phosphokinase A *(59,60)*. Santen et al. *(28)* have suggested that estradiol binds to an ER near or in the cell membrane, initiating binding of Shc, and resultant association with Grb-2 and Sos. Ultimately, this series of events results in activation of Ras and MAPK, resulting in cell proliferation *(28)*. Therefore, it seems possible that two estradiol-regulated pathways exist, a genomic pathway where binding to nuclear ER results in gene transcription, and a nongenomic pathway, that results in cell proliferation through MAPK. Santen et al. have also demonstrated that estrogen deprivation of breast cancer cells in vitro results in hypersensitivity to estradiol *(61)*. Treatment of these estrogen-deprived cells with estradiol resulted in an increase in MAPK phosphorylation in minutes because of activation of nongenomic ER *(28)*. Hypersensitivity to estradiol may occur in tamoxifen-exposed breast cancers, and may explain the activity of aromatase inhibitors, which reduce circulating estrogen levels in postmenopausal women, in tamoxifen-refractory breast tumors. Therefore, increasing evidence suggests that activation of nongenomic ER pathways, perhaps associated with an increase in growth factor expression, may play a role in tamoxifen-resistance.

3.1.4. Role of PR

PR has been demonstrated to play an important role in determining sensitivity of breast cancer cells to tamoxifen. Horwitz demonstrated that patients with metastatic breast cancers expressing both ER and PR were more likely to respond to tamoxifen, than breast tumors expressing only ER *(4)*. Additionally, they showed that patients with metastatic breast tumors that were ER-negative, but PR-positive, were more likely to respond to tamoxifen compared to patients with ER-positive, PR-negative tumors *(4)*. There are less data available regarding the predictive value of PR to tamoxifen in the adjuvant setting. The Oxford Overview analysis *(5)* does not correlate patient outcome specifically with PR-status, because many of the trials do not report PR-status at all, or report it independent of ER-status. However, over the past 12 mo, there has been renewed interest in PR as a predictor for outcome from tamoxifen.

The Arimidex®, Tamoxifen, Alone or in Combination trial randomized 9000 postmenopausal patients with early-stage breast cancer to the aromatase inhibitor, anastrozole, alone, tamoxifen alone, or to a combination of the two drugs, each given for 5 yr. Overall, at a follow-up of 4 yr, patients treated with anastrozole were significantly less likely to have a disease recurrence compared to patients treated with tamoxifen *(62)*. A retrospective analysis *(63)* of this trial evaluated the role of PR in predicting outcome from the individual therapies, in a large subset of patients enrolled in the trial. This analysis revealed no statistically significant difference in disease-free survival between anastrozole and tamoxifen, in patients with ER-positive, PR-positive breast cancers *(63)*. In contrast, patients with ER-positive, PR-negative tumors treated with anastrozole had a highly statistically significantly improved disease-free survival, with a relative improvement of 50%, compared to patients with the same tumor phenotype treated with tamoxifen *(63)*. In the small amount of patients with ER-negative, PR-positive breast cancers, there was no significant difference in outcome between treatment groups *(63)*. Therefore, it appears the absence of PR is associated with a decrease in sensitivity to tamoxifen, and/or an increase in sensitivity to aromatase inhibitors.

PR exists in two isoforms, PRA and PRB, resulting from posttranslationally modifications. Commercially available PR antibodies, used in immunohistochemistry, detect either isoform, but are unable to differentiate between them. Using Western blot analysis, however, the two distinct isoforms can be detected based on size. Fuqua et al. recently correlated expression of PRA and PRB with 5-yr disease-free survival in patients with early-stage breast cancer treated with tamoxifen *(64)*. They demonstrated that the majority of breast cancers express both isoforms in varying ratios *(64)*. Tumors with higher expression of PRB, compared to PRA, were associated with a significantly improved 5-yr disease-free survival compared to tumors with higher expression of PRA, to PRB *(64)*.

To date, it remains unclear as to why the absence of PR, or higher expression of PRA to PRB, results in likely *de novo* resistance to tamoxifen. It is possible that the absence of PR allows a nongenomic ER pathway to be more dominant, which may in turn result in increased activation of the MAPK, and/or Akt pathways, leading to increased cell proliferation, and/or inhibition of apoptosis. These hypotheses are being actively researched, and may lead to new therapeutic possibilities in patients with tumors expressing ER, but lacking PR.

3.1.5. ROLE OF COREGULATORS IN RESISTANCE

The recruitment of coactivators or corepressors (coregulators) to the ER determines the switch between ER activation and repression (*see* Fig. 3). In addition, the coordinated action of ligand, ER, and coregulators determines that genes are transcribed or repressed depending on the cellular context, and thus, which cells will or will not proliferate. Available data suggest that intricate modulation of the ER-to-coregulator ratio in breast cancer cells could determine whether a breast cancer cell is sensitive or resistant to antiestrogens. For example, the coactivator SRC-1 activates ER in a ligand-independent manner while increasing 4OHT's agonist activity *(65)*. On the other hand, the corepressor SMRT blocks the agonist activity of 4OHT-induced by SRC-1 *(65)*. The other member of the p160 coactivator family is amplified in breast cancer (AIB1, SRC-3, RAC3). AIB1 mRNA was found to be amplified in 60% of breast cancers, and its protein product was found to be overexpressed in about 10% of tumors. Recently, an association was discovered between high AIB1 and HER-2/*neu*, a member of the epidermal growth factor receptor (EGFR) family of receptor tyrosine kinases, and tamoxifen-resistant breast cancers *(66)*. The potential mechanism for this resistance requires activation of the MAPK signaling cascade by HER-2/*neu*, which in turn potentially phosphorylates and activates AIB1 (*see* Fig. 3). Activated AIB1 in turn can convert 4OHT from an antiestrogen to an estrogen with regard to ER-α activity. In contrast, low levels of N-CoR mRNA, a corepressor, have been associated with tamoxifen resistance *(67)*. In summary, the specific expression of coregulators in breast cancer cells could well determine, at least in part, whether a patient is likely to benefit from tamoxifen, or other antiestrogens. Based on available data, it would seem reasonable to consider measuring levels of coregulators, particularly AIB1, in breast tumors, before initiating tamoxifen therapy. Additionally, the identification of abnormally expressed coregulators will probably assist in the design of future therapies that improve the efficacy of endocrine treatment without the development of resistance.

3.1.6. EGFR AND HER-2/*NEU* AND ANTIESTROGEN RESISTANCE

Several laboratory and clinical studies suggest that overexpression and/or aberrant activity of the HER-2/*neu* (ErbB2) signaling pathway is associated with antiestrogen resistance in breast cancer *(68–70)*. The HER-2/*neu* receptor is a member of the EGFR family of receptor tyrosine kinases, which include HER-3 (ErbB3) and HER-4 (ErbB4) *(71–74)*. Ligand (i.e., EGF, transforming growth factor-α, heregulin, or HB-EGF) binding to EGFR, HER-3, or HER-4 results in homodimerization of individual receptors or heterodimerization with the preferred partner, HER-2/*neu*. On dimerization, the tyrosine kinase domains-located within the COOH-terminal regions of receptors are activated by an autophosphorylation cascade on specific tyrosine residues. The phosphotyrosine residues recruit SH_2 domain-containing intracellular adaptor molecules, including Shc, Grb-2, and the p85 subunit of phosphatidylinositol 3 kinase (PI3-K), that in turn activate downstream effectors such as MAPK and Akt that promote cellular proliferation, survival, transformation, and inhibit apoptosis. HER-2/*neu* has been suggested to be a proto-oncogene, which when overexpressed, transforms normal mammary epithelial cells. HER-2/*neu* is overexpressed and/or amplified in 25–30% of breast tumors and is associated with a more aggressive phenotype and poor prognosis *(75)*. HER-2/*neu* was first noted to be associated with tamoxifen resistance, when transfection of HER-2/*neu* into MCF7 cells rendered the cells resistant to the inhibitory effects of tamoxifen *(76)*. Subsequently, retrospective analyses of trials in which patients with metastatic breast cancer yielded conflicting results on whether HER-2/*neu* predicted for a worse outcome with tamoxifen *(69)*. In the neoadjuvant setting, clinical response rates to tamoxifen have been noted to be lower in patients with HER-2/*neu*-overexpressing breast cancers *(70,77)*. Based on these data, one possible mechanism for *de novo* resistance to tamoxifen is overexpression of HER-2/*neu* in ER-α-positive breast cancers. However, as outlined here, a recent study suggests that overexpression of HER-2/*neu* alone is not sufficient to produce the tamoxifen resistant phenotype. This retrospective study of patients treated with adjuvant tamoxifen demonstrated that high levels of HER-2/*neu* alone was associated with a similar 5-yr disease-free survival compared to patients with breast cancers with low levels of HER-2/*neu* expression *(66)*. However, patients with tumors expressing high levels of HER-2/*neu* along with high levels of the coactivator AIB1, had a significantly shorter disease-free survival *(66)*.

Expression of HER-2/*neu* also appears to play a role in acquired resistance to tamoxifen. Several groups have demonstrated an increase in expression of HER-2/*neu* in SERM-resistant tumors compared to wild-type tumors *(78,79)*. We have observed an increase in both HER-2/*neu* and EGFR in tamoxifen and raloxifene-resistant breast cancers compared to tamoxifen-sensitive breast cancers *(79)*. Iressa® (ZD1839, gefitinib), an EGFR-specific tyrosine kinase inhibitor has been shown to inhibit growth of breast cancer cell lines in vitro that are resistant to tamoxifen *(80)*. Osborne et al. have noted an increase in EGFR in tamoxifen-resistant tumors in vivo, and have demonstrated that gefitinib, a tyrosine kinase inhibitor that targets EGFR, can inhibit the growth of these tamoxifen-resistant breast cancers, and can delay the onset of tamoxifen resistance *(81)*. This finding is being evaluated in clinical trials. Therefore, it appears that increased expression of EGFR and HER-2/*neu* may play a role in acquired SERM resistance.

Based on these findings, clinical trials are being developed using agents in combination that target the ER and the EGFR pathways. Strategies used to target EGFR and HER-2/*neu* include the use of humanized monoclonal antibodies to the receptors *(82)*, tyrosine kinase inhibitors that block reduction of ATP to ADP + P_i, and receptor antisense molecules *(83)*. Trastuzumab (Herceptin®) is a humanized monoclonal antibody directed against the ectodomain of the HER-2/*neu* receptor. It has been shown to restore breast cancer cell sensitivity to tamoxifen in HER-2/*neu*-overexpressing cells *(76)*. One small clinical trial *(84)* evaluated the use of trastuzumab with the aromatase inhibitor, letrozole, in patients with tamoxifen-refractory, HER-2/*neu*-positive metastatic breast cancer. Response rates were not notably different from historical trials utilizing the agents separately *(84)*. EGFR and/or HER-2/*neu* inhibitors may prove to be beneficial in preventing and/or treating tamoxifen-resistant breast cancer.

3.1.7. Role of MAPK

MAPK is a serine/threonine kinase that is activated by phosphorylation cascades originating from GTP-bound Ras, a downstream effector of EGFR and HER-2/*neu* (*see* Fig. 3). MAPK has been shown to be hyperactivated in MCF-7 breast cancer cells overexpressing either EGFR or HER-2/*neu (76,85,86)*. This increased activity of MAPK promotes an enhanced association of ER-α with coactivators and decreased interaction with corepressors, thereby enhancing hormone-dependent gene transcription and possibly leading to tamoxifen resistant breast cancer (*see* Fig. 3). The role of the MAPK signaling pathway in tamoxifen resistance has been demonstrated primarily in vitro using specific inhibitors, such as U0126 (MAPK kinase, MAPK kinase/extracellular signal-related kinase 1/2 inhibitor), AG1478 (EGFR and HER-2/*neu* inhibitors) and PD98059 (MAPK, extracellular signal-related kinase 1/2 inhibitor) *(76,85,86)* . The exact mechanism by which hyperactivated MAPK converts the antiestrogenic activity of the tamoxifen–ER-α complex to more estrogenic in resistant breast cancer cells is yet unclear. However, it has been demonstrated that activation of the Ras/MAPK pathway by EGFR/ HER-2/*neu* receptor activation could phosphorylate Ser-118 in the AF-1 domain of ER-α, thus promoting ligand-independent transcription of the ER-α and possibly loss of tamoxifen-induced inhibition of ER-α-mediated gene transcription *(25,87)*. Conversely, there is increasing evidence to suggest that nongenomic ER plays a role in MAPK phosphorylation. There is evidence in vitro that estrogen can bind to nongenomic ER, and result in MAPK phosphorylation *(28)*. Based on these preclinical data, several clinical trials are underway to determine whether treating patients with EGFR inhibitors (for example, gefitinib) and/or MAPK-specific inhibitors (for example, U0126) can effectively treat and/or prevent antiestrogen resistance in breast tumors.

3.1.8. Role of PI3-K/AKT Signaling

PI3-K is a heterodimer complex consisting of a regulatory subunit, p85, and a catalytic subunit, p110. The regulatory subunit p85 is phosphorylated by either receptor tyrosine kinases such as EGFR/HER-2/*neu* or intracellular adapter kinases such as Shc or Src, and thereafter interacts and activates the catalytic subunit p110 *(88)*. Activated PI3-K subsequently activates downstream effector kinases such as Akt (phosphokinase B), a serine/ threonine kinase (*see* Fig. 3). Akt has been shown to activate, either directly or indirectly, proteins responsible for survival and inhibition of apoptosis in cancer cells. Several reports indicate that the PI3-K/Akt pathway interacts with the ER-α pathway resulting in bidirectional crosstalk. It has been shown that PI3-K/Akt can mediate E_2-induced transcription of cyclin D1 and entry of MCF-7 breast cancer cells into S phase (*see* Fig. 3) *(89)*. In addition, the PI3-K/Akt pathway can induce ER-α phosphorylation on Ser-167 to promote ER-α-mediated transcription, thereby, protecting cells against tamoxifen-induced apoptosis *(90)*. Accumulating data suggest that ER-α-positive breast tumors with alterations of PI3-K and Akt signaling, whether dependent or independent of EGFR/ HER-2/*neu*, might be insensitive to antiestrogens and thus lead to resistance. Future studies are needed to confirm whether blocking PI3-K and/or Akt signaling in ER-α-positive breast cancer will be beneficial in subverting resistance to antiestrogens.

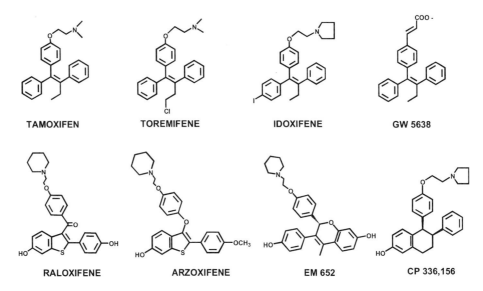

Fig. 4. Structures of available selective estrogen receptor modulators.

4. NEW ANTIESTROGENS

New drug discovery for SERMs is currently driven by the known side effects of tamoxifen, which include the increase in the incidence of endometrial cancer, and the development of resistance. Additionally, recent reports of the lack of efficacy of hormone-replacement therapy on coronary heart disease, and its association with increased breast cancer risk, have led to a search for "the ideal SERM" *(91)*. Several approaches are being pursued including altering the antiestrogenic side chain or improving the pharmacokinetics of existing SERMs. Several novel antiestrogenic compounds have been developed as treatments for ER-α-positive breast cancer, without the agonist effects associated with tamoxifen. These new compounds have the potential to be at least as effective as tamoxifen, possibly without the development of acquired resistance during therapy, and may offer a reduction in incidence of endometrial cancer. These newer agents can be broadly divided into two groups, newer SERMs, which include tamoxifen-like, triphenylethylene, agents such as toremifene (Farneston®), idoxifene, and GW 5638 (Fig. 4A), and the fixed-ring compounds (benzothiophenes) such as raloxifene (Evista®), arzoxifene, EM 652, and CP 336,156 (Fig. 4B); and selective estrogen receptor downregulators (SERDs) such as ICI 182,780 (fulvestrant, Faslodex®) (Fig. 5), SR 16234, and ZK 191703. Both of these classes of newer agents act directly on nuclear ER. The new SERMs, like tamoxifen, bind to ER-α, but result in incomplete receptor dimerization. SERDs also bind to the ER-α, destabilize the protein structure, and induce ubiquitin-mediated degradation of the protein, resulting in marked down-regulation of the receptor *(92,93)*. In phase II trials that enrolled patients with tamoxifen-resistant metastatic breast cancer, the new SERMs all showed low response rates (0–15%), suggesting crossresistance to tamoxifen *(94)*. Additionally, phase III trials that randomized over 1500 patients with metastatic breast cancer to either toremifene and idoxifene first line, or to tamoxifen, no significant difference in outcome was observed in patients treated with the new SERMs compared to tamoxifen *(96)*. Based on these results, toremifene is approved in the United States as an alternative treatment to tamoxifen in patients with hormone-

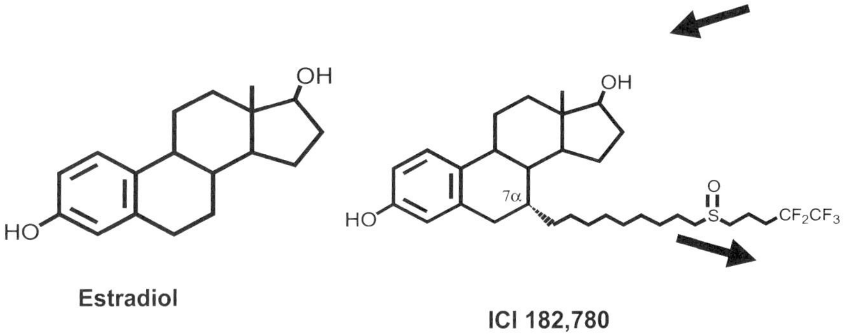

Fig. 5. Structure of fulvestrant (ICI 182,780) compared to estradiol.

responsive metastatic breast cancer. Few clinical trials have evaluating the effectiveness of the fixed-ring compounds in patients with breast cancer. Buzdar et al *(97)* demonstrated minimal activity of raloxifene in patients with tamoxifen-resistant metastatic breast cancer, and its development as a breast cancer therapy was subsequently abandoned. Raloxifene, based on its estrogenic effects on bone mineral density, is approved for the prevention and treatment of osteoporosis in postmenopausal women in the United States *(97)*. Currently, raloxifene is being compared to tamoxifen as a breast cancer preventive in the Study of Tamoxifen and Raloxifene trial *(98)*. Raloxifene, based on preclinical studies *(99)*, has been demonstrated to be less estrogenic than tamoxifen on the uterus, and it is hoped that there will be no increase in uterine cancer in patients taking the drug for osteoporosis or prevention. We have demonstrated that raloxifene stimulates the growth of tamoxifen-resistant breast and uterine cancers in vivo *(100)*, and therefore, it is not recommended that raloxifene be used after adjuvant tamoxifen.

Fulvestrant and other SERDs have been shown to have high affinity for the ER compared to tamoxifen, with none of the agonist activities. Unlike the currently available hormonal agents, fulvestrant has poor oral bioavailability and must be given by intramuscular injection. In clinical trials, fulvestrant showed promise for the treatment of advanced tamoxifen-refractory breast cancer *(101)*. However, in a phase III clinical trial where patients were randomized to fulvestrant or tamoxifen as first-line therapy of advanced breast cancer, fulvestrant did not demonstrate superiority to tamoxifen in terms of disease progression *(102)*. When only patients with hormone receptor-positive breast cancer were evaluated, progression-free survival was identical in patients randomized to tamoxifen or to fulvestrant *(102)* Currently, fulvestrant is approved for the treatment of antiestrogen-resistant advanced breast cancer in the United States. However, it is not clear as yet where it fits in the sequencing of hormonal therapies for metastatic breast cancer. Additionally, it is not clear that its current dosing frequency of 250 mg monthly is the most effective. Trials are ongoing to address these issues. Finally, oral SERDs are currently in preclinical development.

5. AROMATASE INHIBITORS

An alternate strategy for treating hormone-responsive breast cancer is to inhibit binding of E_2 to ER by inhibiting the production of E_2 by blocking the cytochrome p450 aromatase enzyme, the rate-limiting enzyme that converts androgens (i.e., testosterone and androstenedione) to estrogens (i.e., E_2 and estrone) in the adrenal gland, adipose

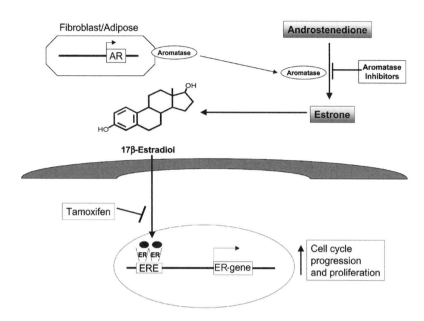

Fig. 6. Comparison of mechanisms of action and sites of activity of aromatase inhibitors to those of tamoxifen.

tissue, and other tissues in postmenopausal women, as well as in the stroma surrounding, breast tumors (Fig. 6). The main drugs of this type are aromatase inhibitors that include type I (steroidal) (Fig. 7A) or type II (nonsteroidal) (Fig. 7B). The steroidal inhibitors are competitive-substrate mimics of androstenedione. These include formestane and exemestane, which are irreversible inhibitors that bind with high affinity to the binding site of aromatase and become converted to a covalently bound intermediate. Nonsteroidal inhibitors include the first-generation aromatase inhibitor aminoglutethimide and the third-generation compounds anastrozole and letrozole. The nonsteroidal aromatase inhibitors act by binding reversibly to the enzyme and competitively inhibiting binding of the substrate, androstenedione. The benefits of using aromatase inhibitors over tamoxifen are believed to be the complete deprivation of E_2 and perhaps better efficacy for ER-α-positive breast cancer *(103)*. Recent clinical data have demonstrated that anastrozole *(104)*, letrozole *(105)*, and exemestane *(106)* are more effective than tamoxifen as first-line treatments for metastatic breast cancer. Based on these clinical results *(104,105)* currently both anastrozole and letrozole are approved as first-line treatment for post-menopausal ER-α-positive advanced breast cancer.

These encouraging results from the metastatic disease setting led to a number of trial examining aromatase inhibitors as adjuvant therapies for early stage breast cancer. These adjuvant trials have two different designs, head-to-head comparisons of the aromatase inhibitors and tamoxifen; aromatase inhibitors after some duration of tamoxifen. The first head-to-head trial to report efficacy data to date is the Arimidex, Tamoxifen, Alone or in Combination trial. This trial randomized over 9000 postmenopausal patients with early stage breast cancer to anastrozole, tamoxifen, or the combination for 5 yr. As outlined in Subheading 3.1.4., after 4 yr of follow-up *(62)*, the absolute difference in recurrence rate in favor of patients treated with anastrozole, compared to tamoxifen, is 2.7% in patients with known hormone receptor-positive tumors. Although anastrozole was approved as

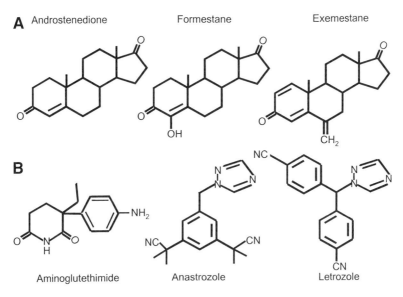

Fig. 7. Structures of steroidal and nonsteroidal aromatase inhibitors.

an adjuvant therapy for hormone receptor-positive breast cancer in postmenopausal patients, no survival data are available as yet from this trial. Data from several other head-to-head trials are awaited.

Continuing tamoxifen for more than 5 yr has not been demonstrated to improve outcome in patients with node-negative early-stage breast cancer *(107)*. The MA-17 trial evaluated the use of letrozole after 5 yr of tamoxifen. At a follow-up of 30 mo, patients treated with letrozole had a significantly improved disease-free survival compared to patients treated with placebo *(108)*. Additionally, patients treated with letrozole had a significantly improved survival compared to those treated with placebo *(108)*. Letrozole was recently approved for extended adjuvant therapy after 5 yr of tamoxifen. The Intergroup Exemestane trial evaluated the use of exemestane after 2 to 3 yr of adjuvant tamoxifen. Disease-free survival was significantly better in patients who switched to exemestane after 2 to 3 yr of tamoxifen, compared to patients who remained on tamoxifen for the remainder of the 5 yr *(109)*. The results of several other trials, evaluating the optimal way of sequencing aromatase inhibitors after tamoxifen, are awaited.

Preliminary data from these trials suggest that aromatase inhibitors may be as effective as tamoxifen for treating all stages of breast cancer. Additionally, the adjuvant trials have demonstrated that the aromatase inhibitors are superior to tamoxifen in reducing the incidence of contralateral breast cancers *(62,109,110)*, and are, therefore, being examined as breast cancer preventives. To date, the safety profile of these agents seems at least as good as tamoxifen. Decreases in bone mineral density, with resulting increases in fractures have been demonstrated *(62)*, secondary to the lack of estrogenic effects of the aromatase inhibitors on bones. Additionally, long-term safety with these agents is unknown.

5.1. Mechanisms of Resistance to Aromatase Inhibitors

As outlined, patients who experience disease relapse after tamoxifen can benefit from aromatase inhibitors *(111,112)*. First-line trials comparing the aromatase inhibitors to tamoxifen in patients with advanced breast cancer have demonstrated that the aromatase inhibitors are more effective to tamoxifen, suggesting that estrogen deprivation may be more effective than tamoxifen in delaying resistance. However, patients with advanced breast cancer treated with aromatase inhibitors will eventually experience disease relapse, indicating the development of resistance. To date, it is unclear whether similar mechanisms identified for tamoxifen resistance are also involved in resistance to aromatase inhibitors. Patients treated with aromatase inhibitors clearly benefit from second-line endocrine therapy, suggesting that ER-α continues to be expressed and functional. Although the exact mechanisms contributing to aromatase inhibitor resistance have yet to be elucidated fully, in vitro studies have identified mutations within the aromatase gene that confer resistance (113). However, these mutations have not yet been identified in human breast carcinomas (114). Other studies have demonstrated that estrogen deprivation supersensitizes breast cancer cells to low levels of estrogen, thus creating a hypersensitive environment to overcome estrogen deprivation resulting in resistance (115–118). In addition, results suggest that there is increased crosstalk between growth factor receptor signaling pathways and ER-α. ER-α has been shown to become activated and supersensitized by several different intracellular kinases, including MAPKs, insulin-like growth factors, and the PI3-K/Akt pathway (90,119–121). Therefore, the data suggest that the ER-α continues to be an integral part of the breast cancer cell-signaling pathway, even after resistance to aromatase inhibitors has developed.

6. FUTURE RESEARCH AND THERAPEUTICS

It is clear that the central regulator of growth for ER-α-positive breast tumors is ER-α. ER signaling does not appear to be independent of other cellular signaling pathways. Research studies have demonstrated that there is bidirectional crosstalk between EGFR/HER-2/neu, MAPK, PI3-K/Akt, and ER-α that ultimately affects the cellular response of a cell to estrogens and mitogens. ER-α integrates numerous signals from hormones, growth factors, and intracellular kinases along with the array of coregulators to modulate cellular physiology and tumor pathology. The first generation antiestrogen/SERM, tamoxifen, has been effective at increasing overall survival of patients with ER-α-positive breast cancer. However, the eventual development of resistance to tamoxifen is common because of the multiple signaling networks affecting the function of the ER-α. As a result of this limitation, intense research over the last 25 yr has revealed the need for alternate treatment strategies to tamoxifen such as newer and better SERMs with less agonist activity in the uterus while being full antagonists in the breast.

In addition to SERMs, other therapeutic approaches have emerged, such as the use of aromatase inhibitors to prevent the synthesis of E_2, and thus, deprive breast cancer cells and other cells of E_2. Estrogen deprivation, however, may result in resistance, bone loss, and possibly decreases in cognitive brain function. The long-term effects of estrogen deprivation have not been realized, but with longer follow-up in the adjuvant aromatase inhibitor clinical trials, the consequences of using aromatase inhibitors will hopefully be clearer.

Therapeutic opportunities also exist from research studies investigating the role of growth factor receptors, EGFR and HER-2/neu, and their intracellular signaling communicators, MAPK and PI3-K/Akt, in the development of tamoxifen resistance. Trastuzumab, the HER-2/neu-specific antibody, has been shown to be highly effective at treating breast tumors-overexpressing HER-2/neu. Moreover, research data indicate a role for HER-2/neu in antiestrogen resistance demonstrating a rationale for using trastuzumab to treat or prevent antiestrogen-resistant breast cancer. Gefitinib and other receptor tyrosine kinase inhibitors may also prove to be beneficial in preventing resistance when given in combination with tamoxifen or other SERMs or SERDs, such as fulvestrant.

In addition to EGFR and HER-2/*neu* as important modulators of tamoxifen action, dissecting the specific interrelationship between ER-α and its coregulators may open the door for novel therapeutics. An understanding of how ER-α-mediated gene transcription is dysregulated in breast cancer and how this changes in resistance during endocrine therapy will hopefully lead to improved strategies for the use of current and future antiestrogen therapies.

REFERENCES

1. Jensen EV J, HI. Basic Guides to the mechanism of estrogen action. Recent Prog Horm Res 1962; 18:387–414.
2. Jordan VC, Dowse LJ. Tamoxifen as an anti-tumour agent: effect on oestrogen binding. J Endocrinol 1976; 68:297–303.
3. Cole MP, Jones CT, Todd ID. A new anti-oestrogenic agent in late breast cancer. An early clinical appraisal of ICI46474. Br J Cancer 1971; 25:270–275.
4. Horwitz KB MW, Pearson OH, et al. Predicting response to endocrine therapy in human breast cancer. Science 1975; 189:726–727.
5. Early Breast Cancer Trialists' Collaborative Group. Tamoxifen for early breast cancer: an overview of the randomised trials [*see* comment]. Lancet 1998; 351:1451–1467.
6. Fisher B, Costantino JP, Redmond CK, Fisher ER, Wickerham DL, Cronin WM. Endometrial cancer in tamoxifen-treated breast cancer patients: findings from the National Surgical Adjuvant Breast and Bowel Project (NSABP) B-14. J Natl Cancer Inst 1994; 86:527–537.
7. Gottardis MM, Robinson SP, Satyaswaroop PG, Jordan VC. Contrasting actions of tamoxifen on endometrial and breast tumor growth in the athymic mouse. Cancer Res 1988; 48:812–815.
8. Fisher B, Costantino JP, Wickerham DL, et al. Tamoxifen for prevention of breast cancer: report of the National Surgical Adjuvant Breast and Bowel Project P-1 Study. J Natl Cancer Inst 1998; 90:1371–1388.
9. Fisher B, Costantino JP, Wickerham DL, et al. Tamoxifen for prevention of breast cancer: report of the National Surgical Adjuvant Breast and Bowel Project P-1 Study [*see* comment]. J Natl Cancer Inst 1998; 90:1371–1388.
10. Jordan VC, Phelps E, Lindgren JU. Effects of anti-estrogens on bone in castrated and intact female rats. Breast Cancer Res Treat 1987; 10:31–35.
11. Jordan VC, Lababidi MK, Langan-Fahey S. Suppression of mouse mammary tumorigenesis by long-term tamoxifen therapy. J Natl Cancer Inst 1991; 83:492–496.
12. Jordan VC. Selective estrogen receptor modulation: a personal perspective. Cancer Res 2001; 61:5683–5687.
13. Love RR, Wiebe DA, Feyzi JM, Newcomb PA, Chappell RJ. Effects of tamoxifen on cardiovascular risk factors in postmenopausal women after 5 years of treatment. J Natl Cancer Inst 1994; 86:1534–1539.
14. Fisher B, Dignam J, Wolmark N, et al. Tamoxifen in treatment of intraductal breast cancer: National Surgical Adjuvant Breast and Bowel Project B-24 randomised controlled trial [*see* comment]. Lancet 1999; 353:1993–2000.
15. Mangelsdorf DJ, Thummel C, Beato M, et al. The nuclear receptor superfamily: the second decade. Cell 1995; 83:835–839.
16. Klinge CM. Estrogen receptor interaction with estrogen response elements. Nucleic Acids Res 2001; 29:2905–2919.
17. Kushner PJ, Agard DA, Greene GL, et al. Estrogen receptor pathways to AP-1. J Steroid Biochem Mol Biol 2000; 74:311–317.
18. Bjornstrom L, Sjoberg M. Estrogen receptor-dependent activation of AP-1 via non-genomic signalling. Nucl Recept 2004; 2:3.
19. Green S, Walter P, Greene G, et al. Cloning of the human oestrogen receptor cDNA. J Steroid Biochem 1986; 24:77–83.
20. Kuiper GG, Enmark E, Pelto-Huikko M, Nilsson S, Gustafsson JA. Cloning of a novel receptor expressed in rat prostate and ovary. Proc Natl Acad Sci U S A 1996; 93:5925–5930.
21. Mosselman S, Polman J, Dijkema R. ER beta: identification and characterization of a novel human estrogen receptor. FEBS Lett 1996; 392:49–53.

22. Kumar V, Green S, Stack G, Berry M, Jin JR, Chambon P. Functional domains of the human estrogen receptor. Cell 1987; 51:941–951.

23. Paech K, Webb P, Kuiper GG, et al. Differential ligand activation of estrogen receptors ERα and ERβ at AP1 sites. Science 1997; 277:1508–1510.

24. Tonetti DA, Rubenstein R, DeLeon M, et al. Stable transfection of an estrogen receptor β cDNA isoform into MDA-MB-231 breast cancer cells. J Steroid Biochem Mol Biol 2003; 87:47–55.

25. Kato S, Endoh H, Masuhiro Y, et al. Activation of the estrogen receptor through phosphorylation by mitogen-activated protein kinase. Science 1995; 270:1491–1494.

26. Palmieri C, Cheng GJ, Saji S, et al. Estrogen receptor β in breast cancer. Endocr Relat Cancer 2002; 9:1–13.

27. Omoto Y, Eguchi H, Yamamoto-Yamaguchi Y, Hayashi S. Estrogen receptor (ER) β1 and ERβcx/β2 inhibit ERα function differently in breast cancer cell line MCF7. Oncogene 2003; 22:5011–5020.

28. Santen RJ, Song RX, Zhang Z, et al. Adaptive hypersensitivity to estrogen: mechanism for superiority of aromatase inhibitors over selective estrogen receptor modulators for breast cancer treatment and prevention. Endocr Relat Cancer 2003; 10:111–130.

29. Kumar R, Wang RA, Mazumdar A, et al. A naturally occurring MTA1 variant sequesters oestrogen receptor-α in the cytoplasm. Nature 2002; 418:654–657.

30. Hall JM, Couse JF, Korach KS. The multifaceted mechanisms of estradiol and estrogen receptor signaling. J Biol Chem 2001; 276:36,869–36,872.

31. Anzick SL, Kononen J, Walker RL, et al. AIB1, a steroid receptor coactivator amplified in breast and ovarian cancer. Science 1997; 277:965–968.

32. Chen H, Lin RJ, Schiltz RL, et al. Nuclear receptor coactivator ACTR is a novel histone acetyltransferase and forms a multimeric activation complex with P/CAF and CBP/p300. Cell 1997; 90:569–5680.

33. Li H, Gomes PJ, Chen JD. RAC3, a steroid/nuclear receptor-associated coactivator that is related to SRC-1 and TIF2. Proc Natl Acad Sci U S A 1997; 94:8479–8484.

34. Suen CS, Berrodin TJ, Mastroeni R, Cheskis BJ, Lyttle CR, Frail DE. A transcriptional coactivator, steroid receptor coactivator-3, selectively augments steroid receptor transcriptional activity. J Biol Chem 1998; 273:27,645–27,653.

35. Onate SA, Tsai SY, Tsai MJ, O'Malley BW. Sequence and characterization of a coactivator for the steroid hormone receptor superfamily. Science 1995; 270:1354–1357.

36. Hong H, Kohli K, Garabedian MJ, Stallcup MR. GRIP1, a transcriptional coactivator for the AF-2 transactivation domain of steroid, thyroid, retinoid, and vitamin D receptors. Mol Cell Biol 1997; 17:2735–2744.

37. Voegel JJ, Heine MJ, Zechel C, Chambon P, Gronemeyer H. TIF2, a 160 kDa transcriptional mediator for the ligand-dependent activation function AF-2 of nuclear receptors. EMBO J 1996; 15:3667–3675.

38. Heery DM, Kalkhoven E, Hoare S, Parker MG. A signature motif in transcriptional co-activators mediates binding to nuclear receptors. Nature 1997; 387:733–736.

39. DiRenzo J, Shang Y, Phelan M, et al. BRG-1 is recruited to estrogen-responsive promoters and cooperates with factors involved in histone acetylation. Mol Cell Biol 2000; 20:7541–7549.

40. Rosenfeld MG, Glass CK. Coregulator codes of transcriptional regulation by nuclear receptors. J Biol Chem 2001; 276:36,865–36,868.

41. Shang Y, Brown M. Molecular determinants for the tissue specificity of SERMs. Science 2002; 295:2465–2468.

42. Huang HJ, Norris JD, McDonnell DP. Identification of a negative regulatory surface within estrogen receptor α provides evidence in support of a role for corepressors in regulating cellular responses to agonists and antagonists. Mol Endocrinol 2002; 16:1778–1792.

43. Shang Y, Hu X, DiRenzo J, Lazar MA, Brown M. Cofactor dynamics and sufficiency in estrogen receptor-regulated transcription. Cell 2000; 103:843–852.

44. Webb P, Nguyen P, Kushner PJ. Differential SERM effects on corepressor binding dictate ERα activity in vivo. J Biol Chem 2003; 278:6912–6920.

45. Wei LN, Hu X, Chandra D, Seto E, Farooqui M. Receptor-interacting protein 140 directly recruits histone deacetylases for gene silencing. J Biol Chem 2000; 275:40,782–40,787.

46. Oesterreich S, Zhang Q, Hopp T, et al. Tamoxifen-bound estrogen receptor (ER) strongly interacts with the nuclear matrix protein HET/SAF-B, a novel inhibitor of ER-mediated transactivation. Mol Endocrinol 2000; 14:369–381.

47. Johansson L, Thomsen JS, Damdimopoulos AE, Spyrou G, Gustafsson JA, Treuter E. The orphan nuclear receptor SHP inhibits agonist-dependent transcriptional activity of estrogen receptors ERα and ERβ. J Biol Chem 1999; 274:345–353.

48. Montano MM, Ekena K, Delage-Mourroux R, Chang W, Martini P, Katzenellenbogen BS. An estrogen receptor-selective coregulator that potentiates the effectiveness of antiestrogens and represses the activity of estrogens. Proc Natl Acad Sci U S A 1999; 96:6947–6952.
49. Fisher B, Redmond C, Brown A, et al. Adjuvant chemotherapy with and without tamoxifen in the treatment of primary breast cancer: 5-year results from the National Surgical Adjuvant Breast and Bowel Project Trial. J Clin Oncol 1986; 4:459–471.
50. Kuukasjarvi T, Kononen J, Helin H, Holli K, Isola J. Loss of estrogen receptor in recurrent breast cancer is associated with poor response to endocrine therapy. J Clin Oncol 1996; 14:2584–2589.
51. Bachleitner-Hofmann T, Pichler-Gebhard B, et al. Pattern of hormone receptor status of secondary contralateral breast cancers in patients receiving adjuvant tamoxifen. Clin Cancer Res 2002; 8:3427–3432.
52. Johnston SR, Saccani-Jotti G, Smith IE, et al. Changes in estrogen receptor, progesterone receptor, and pS2 expression in tamoxifen-resistant human breast cancer. Cancer Res 1995; 55:3331–3338.
53. Hopp TA, Fuqua SA. Estrogen receptor variants. J Mammary Gland Biol Neoplasia 1998; 3:73–83.
54. Murphy LC, Dotzlaw H, Leygue E, Coutts A, Watson P. The pathophysiological role of estrogen receptor variants in human breast cancer. J Steroid Biochem Mol Biol 1998; 65:175–180.
55. Fuqua SA. The role of estrogen receptors in breast cancer metastasis. J Mammary Gland Biol Neoplasia 2001; 6:407–417.
56. Jiang SY, Langan-Fahey SM, Stella AL, McCague R, Jordan VC. Point mutation of estrogen receptor (ER) in the ligand-binding domain changes the pharmacology of antiestrogens in ER-negative breast cancer cells stably expressing complementary DNAs for ER. Mol Endocrinol 1992; 6:2167–2174.
57. Liu H, Park WC, Bentrem DJ, et al. Structure-function relationships of the raloxifene-estrogen receptor-α complex for regulating transforming growth factor-α expression in breast cancer cells. J Biol Chem 2002; 277:9189–9198.
58. Schwartz JA, Zhong L, Deighton-Collins S, Zhao C, Skafar DF. Mutations targeted to a predicted helix in the extreme carboxyl-terminal region of the human estrogen receptor-α alter its response to estradiol and 4-hydroxytamoxifen. J Biol Chem 2002; 277:13,202–13,209.
59. Kelly MJ, Lagrange AH, Wagner EJ, Ronnekleiv OK. Rapid effects of estrogen to modulate G protein-coupled receptors via activation of protein kinase A and protein kinase C pathways. Steroids 1999; 64:64–75.
60. Migliaccio A, Di Domenico M, Castoria G, et al. Tyrosine kinase/p21ras/MAP-kinase pathway activation by estradiol-receptor complex in MCF-7 cells. EMBO J 1996; 15:1292–1300.
61. Song RX, Mor G, Naftolin F, et al. Effect of long-term estrogen deprivation on apoptotic responses of breast cancer cells to 17β-estradiol. J Natl Cancer Inst 2001; 93:1714–1723.
62. Baum M, Buzdar A, Cuzick J, et al. Anastrozole alone or in combination with tamoxifen versus tamoxifen alone for adjuvant treatment of postmenopausal women with early-stage breast cancer: results of the ATAC (Arimidex, Tamoxifen Alone or in Combination) trial efficacy and safety update analyses. Cancer 2003; 98:1802–1810.
63. Dowsett M, Group obotAT. Analysis of time to recurrence in the ATAC (arimidex, tamoxifen, alone or in combination) trial according to estrogen and progesterone receptor status. Breast Cancer Res Treat 2003; 82(Suppl 1):S7.
64. Hopp TA, Weiss HL, Hilsenbeck SG, et al. Breast cancer patients with progesterone receptor PR-A-rich tumors have poorer disease-free survival rates. Clin Cancer Res 2004; 10:2751–2760.
65. Smith CL, Nawaz Z, O'Malley BW. Coactivator and corepressor regulation of the agonist/antagonist activity of the mixed antiestrogen, 4-hydroxytamoxifen. Mol Endocrinol 1997; 11:657–666.
66. Osborne CK, Bardou V, Hopp TA, et al. Role of the estrogen receptor coactivator AIB1 (SRC-3) and HER-2/neu in tamoxifen resistance in breast cancer. J Natl Cancer Inst 2003; 95:353–361.
67. Girault I, Tozlu S, Lidereau R, Bieche I. Expression analysis of DNA methyltransferases 1, 3A, and 3B in sporadic breast carcinomas. Clin Cancer Res 2003; 9:4415–4422.
68. Kurokawa H, Arteaga CL. ErbB (HER) receptors can abrogate antiestrogen action in human breast cancer by multiple signaling mechanisms. Clin Cancer Res 2003; 9(Pt 2):511S–515S.
69. De Laurentis M, Bianco AR, De Placido S. A meta-analysis of the interaction between HER2 expression and response to endocrine treatment in advanced breast cancer. Biol Ther Breast Cancer 2000; 2:11–14.
70. Ellis MJ, Coop A, Singh B, et al. Letrozole is more effective neoadjuvant endocrine therapy than tamoxifen for ErbB-1- and/or ErbB-2-positive, estrogen receptor-positive primary breast cancer: evidence from a phase III randomized trial [see comment]. J Clin Oncol 2001; 19:3808–3816.
71. Yarden Y, Sliwkowski MX. Untangling the ErbB signalling network. Nat Rev Mol Cell Biol 2001; 2:127–137.

72. Yarden Y. The EGFR family and its ligands in human cancer. signalling mechanisms and therapeutic opportunities. Eur J Cancer 2001; 37(Suppl 4):S3–S8.
73. Yarden Y. Biology of HER2 and its importance in breast cancer. Oncology 2001; 61(Suppl 2):S1–S13.
74. Rubin I, Yarden Y. The basic biology of HER2. Ann Oncol 2001; 12(Suppl 1):S3–S8.
75. Spigel DR, Burstein HJ. HER2 overexpressing metastatic breast cancer. Curr Treat Options Oncol 2002; 3:163–174.
76. Benz CC, Scott GK, Sarup JC, et al. Estrogen-dependent, tamoxifen-resistant tumorigenic growth of MCF-7 cells transfected with HER2/neu. Breast Cancer Res Treat 1993; 24:85–95.
77. Smith I, Dowsett M, Trialists ObotI. Comparison of anastrozole versus tamoxifen alone and in combination as neoadjuvant treatment of estrogen receptor-positive (ER+) operable breast cancer in postmenopausal women: the IMPACT trial. Breast Cancer Res Treat 2003; 82(Suppl 1):S6.
78. Shou J, Massarweh S, Osborne CK, et al. Mechanisms of tamoxifen resistance: increased estrogen receptor-HER2/neu cross-talk in ER/HER2-positive breast cancer. J Natl Cancer Inst 2004; 96:926–935.
79. Osipo C, Liu H, Gajdos C, Jordan VC. HER2/neu and EGFR mRNA expression in tamoxifen resistant breast cancer. Proc Am Assoc Cancer Res 2002; 43.
80. Morris C. The role of EGFR-directed therapy in the treatment of breast cancer. Breast Cancer Res Treat 2002; 75(Suppl 1):S51–S55; discussion S57–S59.
81. Shao W, Brown M. Advances in estrogen receptor biology: prospects for improvements in targeted breast cancer therapy. Breast Cancer Res 2004; 6:39–52.
82. Slamon DJ, Leyland-Jones B, Shak S, et al. Use of chemotherapy plus a monoclonal antibody against HER2 for metastatic breast cancer that overexpresses HER2. N Engl J Med 2001; 344:783–792.
83. Nahta R, Hortobagyi GN, Esteva FJ. Growth factor receptors in breast cancer: potential for therapeutic intervention. Oncologist 2003; 8:5–17.
84. Wong ZW, Isaacs C, Harris L, Ellis M. A phase II trial of letrozole and trastuzumab for ER and/or PR and HER positive metastatic breast cancer. Breast Cancer Res Treat 2003; 82(Suppl 1):S106.
85. Kurokawa H, Lenferink AE, Simpson JF, et al. Inhibition of HER2/neu (erbB-2) and mitogen-activated protein kinases enhances tamoxifen action against HER2-overexpressing, tamoxifen-resistant breast cancer cells. Cancer Res 2000; 60:5887–5894.
86. Oh AS, Lorant LA, Holloway JN, Miller DL, Kern FG, El-Ashry D. Hyperactivation of MAPK induces loss of ERα expression in breast cancer cells. Mol Endocrinol 2001; 15:1344–1359.
87. Bunone G, Briand PA, Miksicek RJ, Picard D. Activation of the unliganded estrogen receptor by EGF involves the MAP kinase pathway and direct phosphorylation. EMBO J 1996; 15:2174–2183.
88. Fry MJ. Phosphoinositide 3-kinase signalling in breast cancer: how big a role might it play? Breast Cancer Res 2001; 3:304–312.
89. Castoria G, Migliaccio A, Bilancio A, et al. PI3-kinase in concert with Src promotes the S-phase entry of oestradiol-stimulated MCF-7 cells. EMBO J 2001; 20:6050–6059.
90. Campbell RA, Bhat-Nakshatri P, Patel NM, Constantinidou D, Ali S, Nakshatri H. Phosphatidylinositol 3-kinase/AKT-mediated activation of estrogen receptor α: a new model for anti-estrogen resistance. J Biol Chem 2001; 276:9817–9824.
91. Rossouw JE, Anderson GL, Prentice RL, et al. Risks and benefits of estrogen plus progestin in healthy postmenopausal women: principal results From the Women's Health Initiative randomized controlled trial. JAMA 2002; 288:321–333.
92. Dauvois S, White R, Parker MG. The antiestrogen ICI 182780 disrupts estrogen receptor nucleocytoplasmic shuttling. J Cell Sci 1993; 106(Pt 4):1377–1388.
93. Dauvois S, Danielian PS, White R, Parker MG. Antiestrogen ICI 164,384 reduces cellular estrogen receptor content by increasing its turnover. Proc Natl Acad Sci U S A 1992; 89:4037–4041.
94. Pukkala E, Kyyronen P, Sankila R, Holli K. Tamoxifen and toremifene treatment of breast cancer and risk of subsequent endometrial cancer: a population-based case-control study. Int J Cancer 2002; 100:337–341.
95. Holli K. Tamoxifen versus toremifene in the adjuvant treatment of breast cancer. Eur J Cancer 2002; 38(Suppl 6):S37–S38.
96. Howell SJ, Johnston SR, Howell A. The use of selective estrogen receptor modulators and selective estrogen receptor down-regulators in breast cancer. Best Pract Res Clin Endocrinol Metab 2004; 18:47–66.
97. Buzdar AU, Marcus C, Holmes F, Hug V, Hortobagyi G. Phase II evaluation of Ly156758 in metastatic breast cancer. Oncology 1988; 45:344–345.
98. Kelminski A. The Study of Tamoxifen and Raloxifene (STAR trial) for the prevention of breast cancer. Hawaii Med J 2002; 61:209–210.

99. Black LJ, Sato M, Rowley ER, et al. Raloxifene (LY139481 HCI) prevents bone loss and reduces serum cholesterol without causing uterine hypertrophy in ovariectomized rats. J Clin Invest 1994; 93:63–69.

100. O'Regan RM, Gajdos C, Dardes RC, et al. Effects of raloxifene after tamoxifen on breast and endometrial tumor growth in athymic mice [*see* comment]. J Natl Cancer Inst 2002; 94:274–283.

101. Osborne CK, Wakeling A, Nicholson RI. Fulvestrant: an oestrogen receptor antagonist with a novel mechanism of action. Br J Cancer 2004; 90(Suppl 1):S2–S6.

102. Howell A, Robertson JF, Abram P, et al. Comparison of fulvestrant versus tamoxifen for the treatment of advanced breast cancer in postmenopausal women previously untreated with endocrine therapy: a multinational, double-blind, randomized trial. J Clin Oncol 2004; 22:1605–1613.

103. Johnston SR, Dowsett M. Aromatase inhibitors for breast cancer: lessons from the laboratory. Nat Rev Cancer 2003; 3:821–831.

104. Bonneterre J, Buzdar A, Nabholtz JM, et al. Anastrozole is superior to tamoxifen as first-line therapy in hormone receptor positive advanced breast carcinoma. Cancer 2001; 92:2247–2258.

105. Mouridsen H, Gershanovich M, Sun Y, et al. Superior efficacy of letrozole versus tamoxifen as first-line therapy for postmenopausal women with advanced breast cancer: results of a phase III study of the International Letrozole Breast Cancer Group. J Clin Oncol 2001; 19:2596–2606.

106. Paridaens R, Dirix L, Lohrisch C, et al. Mature results of a randomized phase II multicenter study of exemestane versus tamoxifen as first-line hormone therapy for postmenopausal women with metastatic breast cancer. Ann Oncol 2003; 14:1391–1398.

107. Fisher B, Dignam J, Bryant J, Wolmark N. Five versus more than five years of tamoxifen for lymph node-negative breast cancer: updated findings from the National Surgical Adjuvant Breast and Bowel Project B-14 randomized trial [*see* comment]. J Natl Cancer Inst 2001; 93:684–690.

108. Goss PE. Final results of MA-17 trial. Special Presentation ASCO 2004.

109. Coombes RC, Hall E, Gibson LJ, et al. A randomized trial of exemestane after two to three years of tamoxifen therapy in postmenopausal women with primary breast cancer. N Engl J Med 2004; 350:1081–1092.

110. Goss PE, Ingle JN, Martino S, et al. A randomized trial of letrozole in postmenopausal women after five years of tamoxifen therapy for early-stage breast cancer [*see* comment]. N Engl J Med 2003; 349:1793–1802.

111. Buzdar A, Jonat W, Howell A, et al. Anastrozole, a potent and selective aromatase inhibitor, versus megestrol acetate in postmenopausal women with advanced breast cancer: results of overview analysis of two phase III trials. Arimidex Study Group. J Clin Oncol 1996; 14:2000–2011.

112. Dombernowsky P, Smith I, Falkson G, et al. Letrozole, a new oral aromatase inhibitor for advanced breast cancer: double-blind randomized trial showing a dose effect and improved efficacy and tolerability compared with megestrol acetate. J Clin Oncol 1998; 16:453–461.

113. Kao YC, Cam LL, Laughton CA, Zhou D, Chen S. Binding characteristics of seven inhibitors of human aromatase: a site-directed mutagenesis study. Cancer Res 1996; 56:3451–3460.

114. Sourdaine P, Parker MG, Telford J, Miller WR. Analysis of the aromatase cytochrome P450 gene in human breast cancers. J Mol Endocrinol 1994; 13:331–337.

115. Masamura S, Santner SJ, Heitjan DF, Santen RJ. Estrogen deprivation causes estradiol hypersensitivity in human breast cancer cells. J Clin Endocrinol Metab 1995; 80:2918–2925.

116. Santen R, Jeng MH, Wang JP, et al. Adaptive hypersensitivity to estradiol: potential mechanism for secondary hormonal responses in breast cancer patients. J Steroid Biochem Mol Biol 2001; 79:115–125.

117. Chan CM, Martin LA, Johnston SR, Ali S, Dowsett M. Molecular changes associated with the acquisition of oestrogen hypersensitivity in MCF-7 breast cancer cells on long-term oestrogen deprivation. J Steroid Biochem Mol Biol 2002; 81:333–341.

118. Martin LA, Farmer I, Johnston SR, Ali S, Marshall C, Dowsett M. Enhanced estrogen receptor (ER) α, ERBB2, and MAPK signal transduction pathways operate during the adaptation of MCF-7 cells to long term estrogen deprivation. sJ Biol Chem 2003; 278:30,458–30,468.

119. Jeng MH, Yue W, Eischeid A, Wang JP, Santen RJ. Role of MAP kinase in the enhanced cell proliferation of long-term estrogen deprived human breast cancer cells. Breast Cancer Res Treat 2000; 62:167–175.

120. Shim WS, Conaway M, Masamura S, et al. Estradiol hypersensitivity and mitogen-activated protein kinase expression in long-term estrogen deprived human breast cancer cells in vivo. Endocrinology 2000; 141:396–405.

121. Stephen RL, Shaw LE, Larsen C, Corcoran D, Darbre PD. Insulin-like growth factor receptor levels are regulated by cell density and by long term estrogen deprivation in MCF7 human breast cancer cells. J Biol Chem 2001; 276:40,080–40,086.

23 Mechanisms of Glucocorticoid Actions and Resistance in Multiple Myeloma

Varsha Gandhi, PhD and Beatriz Sanchez-Vega, PhD

CONTENTS

SUMMARY

Glucocorticoids are lipophilic compounds derived from cholesterol and are used in the treatment of some hematological malignancies such as multiple myeloma. Alternative splicing gives rise to numerous glucocorticoid receptor isoforms. The molecular basis of glucocorticoid resistance is poorly understood. Resistance can involve alterations in the glucocorticoid receptors or receptor-associated proteins, such as chaperones, that affect cellular response. Alternatively, glucocorticiods may be effluxed from cells, or there may be enhanced expression of proteins involved in cell survival, defective apoptosis machinery, or altered expression of adhesion molecules that can result in drug resistance.

Key Words: Glucocorticoids; resistance; receptor protein; apoptosis; myeloma; isoforms; posttranslation modification.

1. INTRODUCTION: GLUCOCORTICOIDS

Glucocorticoids (GCs) are lipophilic compounds derived from cholesterol that have a wide range of biological activities. In addition to their physiological roles, GCs are

From: *Cancer Drug Discovery and Development: Cancer Drug Resistance*
Edited by: B. Teicher © Humana Press Inc., Totowa, NJ

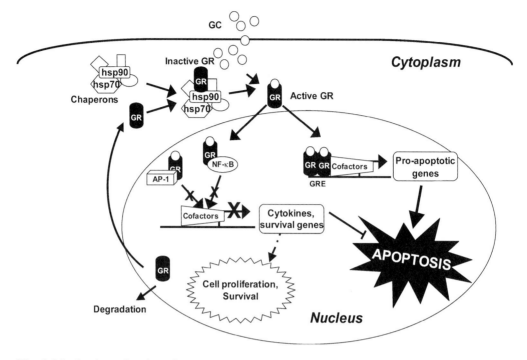

Fig. 1. Mechanism of action of glucocorticoids. The glucocorticoids (GCs) enter into the cell by passive diffusion through the cytoplasmic membrane and bind to the glucocorticoid receptor (GR) that is located in the cytoplasm associated with heat shock proteins. Upon ligand binding, the heat shock protein/GR complex dissociates, and the receptor is phosphorylated and translocated into the nucleus, where it exerts its action by interacting with other transcription factors, cofactors, and DNA. Finally, after dissociating from DNA, GR is exported into the cytoplasm, becoming again fully competent for ligand binding and signal transduction.

among the most widely prescribed class of drugs in the world for inflammation, arthritis, and cancer *(1)*. GCs induce apoptosis and play an important role in the treatment of a number of hematological malignances such as multiple myeloma (MM) *(2)*. MM is a relatively rare clonal B-cell malignancy characterized by the accumulation of terminally differentiated, antibody-producing plasma cells in the bone marrow (BM) *(3)*. Although GCs are highly effective in MM treatment, some patients do not respond, and those that do respond eventually develop resistance to this therapy *(4,5)*.

2. GR MECHANISMS OF ACTION

Most of the glucocorticoid hormone effects are mediated by the glucocorticoid receptor (GR). GR is a member of the nuclear hormone receptor super family of ligand-activated transcription factors, participates in numerous signaling pathways leading to altered gene expression in target cells and tissues, is ubiquitously expressed, and is essential for life *(6)*. In the absence of GC hormones, GR is retained in the cytoplasm in association with chaperone and heat shock proteins *(7–9)*. This association keeps the receptor in a conformation that can bind steroid but is transcriptionally inactive *(10)*.

The most accepted mechanism for GCs entry to a cell is through passive diffusion, facilitated by their relative small size and lipophilic nature *(11)*, although some transporter proteins of the MDR family are recognized to transport GC *(12)*. After diffusion through the cell membrane, the steroid molecules bind to GR. Upon ligand binding, the heat shock protein/GR complex dissociates, and the receptor is phosphorylated and translocated into the nucleus where it exerts its action by interacting with other transcription factors, cofactors, and DNA (Fig. 1).

The interaction of GR with other transcription factors results in a mutual inhibition of their activities. Most of the actual evidences indicate that two transcription factors appear to be the most likely targets of GC-induced repression, nuclear factor (NF-κB, p50/p65) (13–17) and activating protein (AP-1) (18–20).

In addition to a direct interaction with other regulatory proteins, GR is able to induce or repress the expression of specific target genes by binding to GC response elements (GREs) located in the promoter regions of GC-responsive genes (1). A consensus GRE consists of a palindromic 15-mer: 5'-GGTACAnnnTGTTCT-3'(21), although it is now becoming clear that a variety of combinations of half-sites and related sequences are often present in promoter sites. GR can repress gene transcription by binding to DNA sequences called negative GREs in the promoters of specific genes (22), or to DNA elements that consist of a nonoverlapping GRE and a binding site for a different transcription factor (composite GREs) (23).

Finally, after dissociating from DNA, GR is exported into the cytoplasm, becoming again fully competent for ligand binding and signal transduction (24). The mechanism by which GR is exported to the cytoplasm is not completely known. However, the calcium-calreticulin-mediated, a nuclear export signal-independent nuclear export system, was reported to be involved in the nuclear export and cytoplasmic retention of GR (25,26). In addition, removal of the ligand-binding domain (LBD) from GR resulted in constitutive localization in the nucleus (27). Also, endogenous 14-3-3σ helps localize ligand-free GR-α in the cytoplasm and contributes to nuclear export of GR-α after withdrawal of ligand (28). Regulation of nuclear translocation has previously been implicated in the regulation of transcription factor activity (29).

GR also takes part in a crosstalk with other signal transduction pathways (30). Although it is clear that steroid receptors exert their primary influence by altering gene transcription, receptor effects on RNA stability and protein turnover have also been observed (31,32).

3. THE GR GENE

There is only one known GR gene, but several GR isoforms arose as a result of alternative splicing events (33). The human GR gene is located on chromosome 5q31 (34) and consists of nine exons. In addition, the GR gene contains at least three promoters whose utilization gives rise to at least five separate transcripts containing different untranslated first exons (Fig. 2) (35). Initial studies of the human GR gene characterized a promoter region located 3 kb upstream from exon 2 that is associated with an untranslated exon (exon 1C) (36,37), and demonstrated several binding sites for the ubiquitous transcription factors specificity protein (SP-1) and activating protein (AP-2) (35,38), AP-1 (39), and the transcription factor Ying Yang 1 (YY-1) (40). Promoter C lacks both TATA and CCAAT boxes and contains a CpG island characteristic of housekeeping genes. Furthermore, this promoter also contains a GR enhancing factor-binding element sequence (41). There is also a tumor necrosis factor (TNF)-responsive NF-κB DNA-binding site in this promoter (42).

The second promoter discovered on the GR gene is the promoter B that resides over 1000 nucleotides upstream of the exon 1C start site and is preceding the exon 1B. Like promoter C, promoter B lacks consensus TATA or CAAT boxes, but contains regions

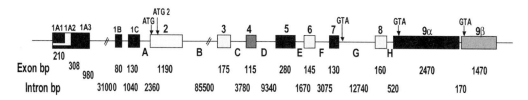

Fig. 2. Glucocorticoid receptor gene structure. The glucocorticoid gene comprises fourteen different exons: five alternative exons 1 (1A1, 1A2, 1A3, 1B, and 1C) that correspond to different 5′ untranslated regions, seven coding exons (exons 2–8), and two alternative exons 9 that codify for the C-terminal part of the protein and also contain the 3′ untranslated region. The numbers denote the size in base pairs of each exon and intron.

that are GC rich, and binding sites for YY-1 *(40)* and SP-1 *(43)*. The GR promoter B can drive transcription in the absence of promoter C *(40)*.

Finally, the promoter A is located approximately 31 kb upstream of the coding sequence, and contains a TATA box-like sequence, a sequence resembling a CAAT box, and a NF-κB-binding site. There is an intraexonic site in exon 1A that is an apparent half-GRE that can bind the GR-β isoform. In addition, promoter A contains a putative interferon regulatory factor-binding element and a sequence resembling a GRE *(35)*. The exon 1A region utilizes three separate splice donor sites generating three alternative exons A (1A1, 1A2, and 1A3).

The five alternative exons 1 (1A1, 1A2, 1A3, 1B, and 1C) and the first part of exon 2 contain the 5′ untranslated region (UTR), exons 2-9α or 2-9β the coding sequences, and the final part of the two alternative exons 9 the 3′UTR *(44)* (Fig. 2). None of the alternative exons 1 is predicted to alter the amino acid sequence because there is an in-frame stop codon preceding the translation initiation site in exon 2 that is common to all mRNA variants. It has been suggested that promoter usage may regulate the differential GR expression in response to GCs *(45)*, the expression of specific membrane or intracellular receptor isoforms *(46)*, or even direct GR mRNA translation *(47)*.

Thus, GR expression, although considered ubiquitous, is regulated by a variety of transcription factors binding to their response elements within the promoter. This regulation clearly provides the potential to translate into both cell type- and tissue-specific expression of this gene *(40)*. Transcriptional regulation from the three known GR promoter regions is complex and influenced by developmental and hormonal factors *(35,48)*.

4. GR ISOFORMS

Alternative splicing gives rise to numerous GR isoforms. These isoforms are named GR-α, GR-β, GR-P, GR-γ, GR-A, and GR-B (Fig. 3).

4.1. Glucocorticoid Receptor-α

The effects of GC are mediated through the GR-α isoform, which resides in the cytoplasm in absence of hormone and is composed of a single polypeptide chain of 777 amino acids *(34)*. GR-α is translated from two transcripts of 7 and 5.5 kb generated from alternative polyadenylation sites in the 3′UTR of exon 9α. Reductions in the number of GR-α molecules per cell have been shown to reduce glucocorticoid sensitivity *(49–53)*.

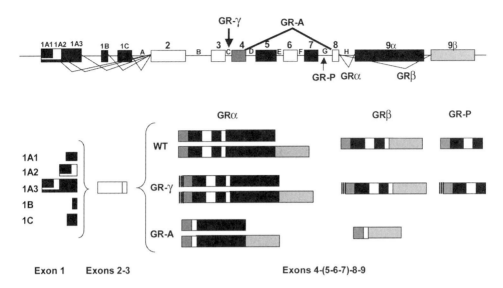

Fig. 3. Structure and transcriptional isoforms of the human glucocorticoid (GR) gene. (**A**) Schematic representation of the different exons composing the human GR gene. 1A1, 1A2, 1A3, 1B, and 1C represent the different alternative untranslated first exons. (**B**) Different isoforms generated by alternative splicing of the human GR gene. Each isoform can be expressed from one of the five alternative untranslated first exons. Exons 2–4 are common to all isoforms. When the exon 9α is present on the transcript, independently of the presence or absence of exon 9β, the GR-α isoform is generated. GR-β is produced when exon 9β is joined to exon 8. When the splicing event that joins exon 7 with exon 8 fails, another GR isoform is produced, the GR-P isoform, that ends at intron G. GR-α, GR-β, and GR-P represent the three major 3′ ends of the GR. Another GR isoform, GR-γ, is created when in the splicing junction between exons 3 and 4, three additional bases are kept; its 3′ end can be exons 9α, 9β, or intron G. The elimination of exons 5, 6, and 7 by alternative splicing give rise to the GR-A isoform, and its C-terminal region can be coded by exons 9α or 9β.

4.2. Glucocorticoid Receptor-β

GR-β is translated from a transcript of 4.3 kb generated by alternative splicing of exon 9. GR-β is a single polypeptide chain of 90 kDa composed of 742 amino acids. Although identical through amino acid 727, the 15 C-terminal amino acids in GR-β are unique, and replace the C-terminal 50 amino acids in GR-α. GR-β fails to bind hormone or activate gene transcription, has an increased half-life compared to GR-α *(42,54)*, and is located in the nucleus in the absence of ligand *(55)*. GR-β is capable of binding to heat shock protein (hsp90), although with less stability as compared with GR-α *(56)*. In addition, it binds a GRE with greater capacity than GR-α in the absence of GC and this binding is not affected by GC *(56)*. The observation of highly variable cell and tissue expression profiles suggests an important role for GR-β in human GC physiology.

4.3. Glucocorticoid Receptor-P

Another isoform, GR-P, first described in tumor cells from a GC-resistant myeloma patient *(57,58)*, is 676 amino acids and is encoded by exons 2–7 and part of intron 7 (intron G) as a unique C-terminal tail. This truncated isoform lacks a large part of the LBD, including the domains for silencing of the receptor in the absence of hormone and the transactivation domain, τ2. The GR-P isoform seems to be present in several hematological tumor cells as well as in normal lymphocytes.

4.4. Glucocorticoid Receptor-γ

GR-γ is the result of the retention of three base pairs between exon 3 and 4 because of the use of an alternative splice donor site. Consequently, an mRNA coding for an additional amino acid (arginine) located at amino acid 452 of the DNA-binding domain is produced. GR-γ is a ligand-dependent transcription factor with reduced transactivating activity (59). GR-γ seems rather ubiquitously expressed, although its function is presently unknown.

4.5. Glucocorticoid Receptor-A

Moalli et al. described the GR-A isoform, which presents an internal deletion in the first portion of the LBD including a region important in the phenomenon of hormone down-regulation, nuclear localization, and transactivation of target genes (57). In GR-A mRNA, exons 5, 6, and 7 are precisely excised because of an alternate splicing event. The mRNA and protein encoded by this mutant are 555 base pairs and 185 amino acids, respectively, smaller than the wild type.

4.6. Glucocorticoid Receptor-B

In addition to the transcriptional isoforms described above, various isoforms are also produced by alternative translation initiation (60). The major protein product, termed GR-A, has an apparent molecular mass of 94 kDa, and represents translation from the first initiator AUG codon. However, this start codon lies within a weak Kozak translation initiation consensus sequence, which appears to result in leaky ribosomal scanning (61) and translation initiation from a downstream AUG codon. The next downstream start codon (Met-27) results in the production of a 91-kDa protein, termed GR-B. The shorter GR-B species is nearly twice as efficient in GRE-mediated transactivation as the longer GR-A isoform, but has a similar efficacy in repression of NF-κB transactivation.

Interestingly, although GR is primarily expressed as a nuclear receptor, a cell membrane-associated receptor has been described recently (62). However, little is known about its function or its mechanism of action.

5. THE GR PROTEIN

The structural organization of GR is well known (63,64). GR contains three functional domains: the N-terminal part or modulating domain, also known as the immunogenic domain that is involved in modulation of gene transcription (65); the DNA-binding domain (DBD), consisting of two zinc fingers followed by an amphipathic α-helix (66) and is involved in DNA binding, homo- and heterodimerization (67) and gene transcription enhancement (68); and the LBD at the carboxyl terminus that controls the activity of the receptor as a whole through its interaction with heat shock proteins (69) and chaperones (inactive receptor) or with GCs and coactivators (active receptor) (Fig. 4). In addition to ligand binding, the LBD contains a receptor dimerization function (70,71), as well as domains for silencing of the receptor in the absence of the hormone (72,73). This suggests that the actual function of the LBD is inactivating the receptor, which can be disinhibited by ligand binding.

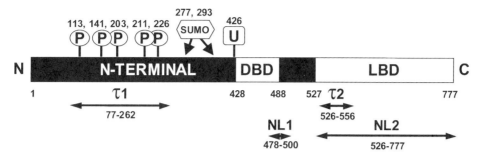

Fig. 4. Glucocorticoid receptor protein structure. The glucocorticoid receptor contains three functional domains: the N-terminal part or modulating domain, involved in modulation of gene transcription; the DNA-binding domain (DBD) that is involved in DNA binding, dimerization and gene transcription enhancement; and the ligand-binding domain (LBD) that interact with glucocorticoids, heat shock proteins, and coactivators. NL1 and NL2, nuclear localization signals; τ1 and τ2, transactivation domains; P, phosphorylation sites; SUMO, sumoylation sites; U, ubiquitination site. The numbers represent the amino acid positions where the domains are located.

Two domains in GR have been found to be involved in nuclear localization (NL). The first, NL1, is located in the C-terminal part of the DBD and extends into the hinge between DBD and LBD (amino acids 478–500) *(74)*. The function of NL1 is inhibited by the LBD, and ligand binding can abolish this inhibition *(75)*. Two regions (amino acids 600–626 and 696–777) appear to be involved in the LBD-dependent inhibition. The first region shows little inhibitory effect on NL1 function, but the presence of the second region fully inhibits nuclear localization of the unliganded GR *(76)*. The second nuclear localization signal, NL2, is located in the LBD *(77)*, but its exact localization is unknown. NL1 catalyzes rapid transport of GR through the nuclear pore, employing the importing-mediated pathway, whereas NL2 contributes to a slower traffic via as yet unknown hormone-dependent mechanisms *(78)*.

Two domains in GR have been found to be crucial for optimal transactivation of target genes *(79)*. The first, τ1, is located in the N terminus of the receptor, between amino acids 77 and 262. Its function is hormone independent, in contrast to the transactivation properties of τ2, which is located in the LBD, between amino acids 526 and 556. Hormone binding is required for the activity of τ2 *(80)*.

6. POSTTRANSLATION MODIFICATIONS OF GR PROTEIN

Different posttranslational modifications such as phosphorylation, acetylation, ubiquitination, and sumoylation are important in GR function and GC-induced receptor down-regulation and hence resistance to GCs.

6.1. Phosphorylation

GR is phosphorylated in the absence of hormone and become hyperphosphorylated after hormone-induced activation *(81–83)*. There are five putative phosphorylation sites in the human GR; these are all serines located in one of the transactivation regions in the N-terminal part of the receptor (at positions 113, 141, 203, 211, and 226). Mutation of all these sites in the human GR does not affect the transactivation properties of the receptor *(84)*. There also appears to be a strong cell-cycle dependency of GR phosphorylation *(85)*, as well as a potential role of phosphorylation in nuclear-cytoplasmic transport *(86)*.

Basal phosphorylation is almost three times higher in G_2/M than in S phase of the cell cycle. GC treatment fails to hyperphosphorylate GR in the G_2/M phase, but doubles the phosphorylated status in S phase. As well, protein kinase A is able to interact with GR and enhance its transactivation activity *(87)*. GR phosphorylation has been implicated with mechanism of GC resistance *(85,88,89)*.

6.2. Ubiquitination

The ubiquitin pathway implies the covalent binding of ubiquitin molecules, a polypeptide of 76 amino acids, to certain lysine residues in target genes. Polyubiquitination of a protein acts as a signal for protein recognition and degradation by the proteasome. GR is a substrate for the ubiquitin–proteasome degradative pathway, playing a role in GR downregulation induced by hormone, and Lys-426 of GR is implicated in this mechanism *(90)*. Interestingly, the τ1 domain present in the N terminus of GR was described as an acidic region *(84)*, and such domains specifically signal ubiquitin-mediated proteolysis of activated transcription factors *(91)*. Thus, it is possible that GR is targeted for degradation once transcriptionally activated, which provides an efficient way to limit in time and intensity the glucocorticoid action.

6.3. Sumoylation

Another related posttranslational modification of GR is sumoylation, or the covalent addition of small ubiquitin-related modifier 1 (SUMO1) peptide *(92)*. Sumoylation does not signal proteolysis, but appears to play multiple roles in subcellular protein translocation, nuclear body formation, protein stabilization, and modulation of the transcriptional activity of several transcription factors *(93,94)*. GR can be sumoylated on Lys-277 and -293. As a result, both GR protein degradation and GR transcriptional activation are enhanced *(92,95)*.

Thus, the complexity of GC biology lies more in the variety of receptors themselves rather than in the ligands to which they bind. Assuming that there are four or perhaps more GR isoforms in a cell, combined with up to eight phosphorylation sites, at least one ubiquilation site, and perhaps several sumoylation sites, the capacity to generate dozens of unique GRs in a single cell presents an enormous potential for signaling diversity.

7. GR DOWN/UPREGULATION BY HORMONES

The level of expression of GR is an important determinant of the type and magnitude of the cellular response to the hormone *(96)*. Consequentially, processes that regulate the expression of the human GR gene are important and must be tightly regulated. It is known that GR must be present at sufficient levels in the cell to modulate the transcription of target genes *(96,97)*, and that different thresholds of effective GR levels may exist for GC-suppressed genes *(98)*.

In most cells tested to date, GR is downregulated in response to hormone treatment, and the cells remain viable *(48,99,100)*. This reduction in cellular receptor levels leads to insensitivity to subsequent hormone administrations. In sharp contrast, in immature thymocytes, and T-lymphoblasts, GR mRNA, and protein are upregulated by hormone treatment, which is followed by apoptosis *(101–103)*.

The mechanism of downregulation is poorly understood. However, it has been shown that downregulation takes place at both mRNA and protein levels, and that multiple mechanisms play a role *(82,99,104–107)*. At the level of RNA, both transcriptional repression *(99)* and mRNA destabilization *(108,109)* seems to contribute to homologous downregulation and sequences in the LBD (amino acids 550–697) of GR appear to be essential for the initiation of this response. However, GC-mediated downregulation of receptor mRNA does not require ongoing mRNA or protein synthesis, suggesting that a GC-inducible protein is not involved in receptor autoregulation *(104,110)*. In addition, two sequences have been found in the human GR promoter (between –2838 and –1476) that are homologous to the negative GREs found in the promoter of the pro-opiomelanocortin gene that are required for hormone-dependent repression of the transcription of this gene *(111)*. However, whether this region is involved in GR downregulation is not known. Another mechanism that may be implicated in GR downregulation by GCs could be the use of different promoters. In this sense, exon 1A containing transcripts are more regulated by GCs than exon 1B- and exon 1C-containing transcripts *(35,112)*.

Hormone treatment has also been shown to decrease the stability of the GR protein *(105,106)*, and the proteasome complex seems to be involved in this downregulation *(90)*.

8. APOPTOSIS

The distinguishing characteristic of GC-induced apoptosis is the initiation at the transcriptional level and the involvement of the proteasome *(113–118)* and calcium *(119,120)*. The process of GC-induced apoptosis can be arbitrarily subdivided into three stages: an initiation stage that involves GR activation and GR-mediated gene regulation; a decision stage that involves the counterbalancing influence of prosurvival and proapoptotic factors; and the execution stage, which involves caspase and endonuclease activation *(2,121)*.

8.1. Initiation Stage

The initiation stage is the sequence of events leading up to and including direct regulation of gene transcription by GR. Both positive and negative effects on transcription have been demonstrated in response to steroid treatment *(122)*. Once in the nucleus, transcription is activated *(123)* or repressed *(22,124,125)* through a complicated mechanism that is not fully understood. The transcriptional activity of GR depends on coactivators that facilitate recruitment of the basal transcription machinery or remodel chromatin *(71,126–128)*. GR interacts with many coactivators and corepressors, and almost all of these coactivators interact with the τ2 transactivation domain when the hormone is present. The most known GR cofactors are AP-1 *(19,20)* and NF-κB *(16,17,129)*. Other known cofactors that interact with GR are the transcription factor IID complex *(130)*, signal transduction and transcription activators STAT5 *(131)*, STAT3 *(131,132)*, and the coactivators with histone acetyl transferase activity, cAMP response element-binding protein (CREB)/p300 *(133,134)*, and steroid receptor coactivator 1 *(135)*. Other proteins that can associate with GR-α and act as coactivators are proteins from the vitamin D3 receptor-interacting protein complex of proteins *(136)*, and brahma-related gene 1, the function of which is to remove histone H1 from the chromatin, allowing general transcription factors such as NF-1 and TATA box-binding protein to access their binding sites *(127)*.

The target genes whose activation or repression initiates the apoptosis process remain uncertain, but there is a theory proposing that apoptosis is initiated via positive regulation of genes that induce cell death or/and negative modulation of cytokines or so-called survival genes. However, although as yet no GR-inducible proapoptotic genes have been identified, many proteins are modulated by GC at the transcriptional and posttranscriptional level when cells undergo GC-induced apoptosis. Thereby, it has been demonstrated that GCs trigger early transient induction of genes involved in cell defense and repair, followed by induction of genes known to mediate apoptosis *(137)*.

8.2. Decision Stage

Crosstalk between other signaling pathways and the GR signaling pathway modulates GC-induced apoptosis and is as a major determinant of the decision to live or die when a cell is exposed to GC. There are two ways by which signaling crosstalk might regulate apoptosis; one is that the activation of prosurvival signaling pathways may repress GC-induced apoptosis *(138–141)*. Alternatively, GCs may repress prosurvival signaling pathways *(142–147)*. In each case, GC-induced lymphocytolysis requires ongoing protein synthesis *(15,148,149)*. The GR pathway can interact with the Raf/Ras/mitogen-activated protein kinase (MAPK) *(145,150)*, the cAMP/protein kinase A *(87)*, MAPK and phosphatidylinositol 3-kinase *(140,142,151)*, and the c-jun N-terminal kinase (JNK) *(141,152)* pathways.

GC-induced apoptosis is regulated both positively and negatively by members of the Bcl-2 protein family *(153)*. Bcl-2 over expression inhibits events associated with GC-induced apoptosis, including caspase activation and mitochondrial dysfunction *(154,155)*. There is some evidence that suggests that Bcl-2 might work upstream of caspase activation to inhibit commitment to cell death and not at the level of caspase inhibition *(156)*. Furthermore, Bcl-2 may also function by regulating proteasome-mediated degradation of prosurvival transcription factors *(14,114)*.

Proapoptotic members of the Bcl-2 family, such as Bim, Bak, Bax, or Bad, may trigger the caspase cascade or regulate degradation of cell cycle factors and transcription factors by the proteasome *(121,157,159)*.

8.3. Execution Stage

Most of the morphological changes of apoptosis are caused by caspases, a family of cysteine proteases that cleave substrates at aspartate residues *(160)*. The data available today suggest that there may be more than one pathway to GC-induced apoptosis *(45,161)*. The prevailing pathway to GC-induced apoptosis appears to be caspase 9-dependent and caspase 3-independent. This pathway involves activation of caspase 9 (the initiator caspase), followed by the sequential activation of caspases 1 and 6 (the effector caspases) *(162)*. An alternative pathway that is caspase 9 independent and caspase 3 dependent may also exist, but is less well-defined *(121)*. In addition, the fact that caspase inhibitors only delay GC-mediated cell death and do not affect long-term survival suggests that caspases are neither the sole nor the direct targets of GC action *(45)*.

The role of mitochondria in GC-induced apoptosis is uncertain, but it seems that mitochondrial dysfunction does not appear to be a central step in the initiation of the cell death pathway in GC-induced apoptosis. Although GC treatment induces loss of mitochondrial membrane potential *(163)*, it appears to occur downstream of caspase activation and may be induced by caspase activity *(164)*. In GC-treated MM cells, second mitochondrial-derived activator of caspases (SMAC) is released into the cytosol, where it activates caspase 9 without the simultaneous release of cytochrome *c* and oligomerization of apoptotic protease activating factor 1 (APAF-1) *(165,166)*.

9. RESISTANCE

The molecular basis of GC resistance is still poorly understood. The mechanism of GC resistance may affect all aspects of GC action, thus involving defects at the GC, GR, and

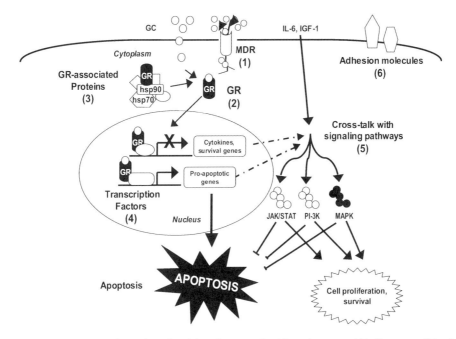

Fig. 5. Potential mechanisms involved in glucocorticoid resistance. (1) One possible factor involved in the modulation of glucocorticoid (GC) response is the export of GC out of the cell by the overexpression of multidrug resistance (MDR) proteins. (2) In the absence of glucocorticoid hormones, the glucocorticoid receptor (GR) is retained in the cytoplasm in association with chaperone proteins that keeps the receptor in a conformation that can bind steroid but is transcriptionally inactive. Other mechanism of GC resistance could be the altered expression of the GR chaperon proteins. (3) A lower number of GR-α receptors per cell are associated with a decrease in GC sensitivity. In addition, mutations in the GR gene, albeit rare, have been detected in several GC resistance malignances. The expression of some of the GR isoforms could have a role in the development of GC resistance. (4) Molecular mechanisms such us enhanced expression of activating protein 1 and nuclear factor-κB, the main targets of GR action, may be involved in GC resistance, inducing gene expression of survival genes and cytokines. (5) The crosstalk between other signaling pathways and the GR signaling pathway modulates GC-induced apoptosis. Thus, in order to induce an apoptotic signal, the GCs should repress prosurvival signaling pathways. The signaling pathways triggered by interleukin (IL-6) are the most important, because this cytokine activates several survival pathways in multiple myeloma (MM) cells that are able to block GC-induced apoptosis. (6) Adhesion of MM cells to bone marrow stromal cells induces the secretion of IL-6 and other growth factors from the stromal cells, these growth factors mediate MM growth, survival, and drug resistance. The upregulation of cell-adhesion molecules has been related to resistance of MM cells to the treatment with several drugs.

GR-associated proteins level, or may interfere with individual GC responses such as induction of apoptosis, cell cycle arrest, and so on. In the latter case, the defect could be localized at the level of transcription factors, GR-target genes, or imbalance with other signaling pathways (Fig. 5).

9.1. MDR Proteins

The first requirement of GC action is the entry of GCs into the cell and the maintenance of drug levels inside the cell the time needed for the drug to induce apoptosis. Because the most accepted mechanism by which GCs enter the cell is through passive diffusion facilitated by their relative small size and lipophilic nature *(11)*, one possible factor involved in the modulation of GC response is the export of GC out of the cell. It has been shown that multidrug-resistant protein 1 (MDR1), a member of the ATP-binding cassette (ABC) family of transporters, is capable of transporting some GCs. Dexamethasone (DEX), prednisolone, cortisol, and triancinolone can be transported by an Abcb1b/Abcb1a transporter (MDR1 and MDR3, respectively) *(12)*. Moreover, studies using human myeloma cell lines have shown that the overexpression of MDR1 is responsible for conferring drug resistance to natural products and GCs *(167,168)*. Thus, the expression of these MDR proteins could be one mechanism by which GC resistance occurs.

9.2. Binding of GC to GR

After diffusion through the cell membrane, the steroid molecules bind to GR. Thus, the second requirement for GC action is the presence of GR, at enough levels and in an adequate conformation to bind GCs.

9.2.1. CHAPERONE PROTEINS

In the absence of glucocorticoid hormones, GR is retained in the cytoplasm in association with chaperone proteins *(7–9)*. This association keeps the receptor in a conformation that can bind steroid but is transcriptionally inactive *(10)*. Multiple molecular chaperones interact with steroid receptors to promote functional maturation and stability of receptor complexes. These chaperones include hsp90 and hsp70 as essential and abundant components, and Hop, hsp40, and p23 as nonessential cochaperones that are present in much lower abundance in cells. In addition, the immunophilin cochaperones, cyclophilin 40, FK506-binding protein 51 kDa and -52 kDa, and the serine/threonine protein phosphatase PP5 have been implicated as modulators of steroid receptor function through their association with hsp90, the molecular chaperone with a key role in steroid hormone signaling *(169–172)*. One mechanism of GC resistance could be the altered expression of GR chaperon proteins *(173,174)*. Observations of glucocorticoid resistance in New World primates, attributed to FK506-binding protein 51 kDa overexpression and incorporation into glucocorticoid receptor complexes, have provided the first evidence that these chaperones can control hormone-binding affinity *(175)*.

9.2.2. GLUCOCORTICOID RECEPTOR

Prior studies demonstrated that the lack of responsiveness to DEX in MM cells was coupled with significantly low levels of GR-α *(137,176)*. In addition, mutations in the GR gene, albeit rare, have been detected in several GC resistance malignances *(177)*.

9.2.2.1. GR Gene Mutations

Numerous mutations in the GR gene have been described including mutations that render receptors unable to bind hormone *(5,178-180)*, with altered affinity *(181,182)*, and deficient in nuclear transfer *(4,5)*. Most of these mutations are clustered in the LBD and DBD. (A review of the GR gene mutations *[177]* or http://nrr.georgetown.edu/GRR/mutation/mutation.html provides additional information.) However, somatic GR mutations responsible for the acquisition of GC resistance in malignant human cells have only been demonstrated in cultured cells *(178,179,183–186)*. Furthermore, the analysis of leukemia cell samples obtained from GC-resistant patients with chronic lymphocyte leukemia has not revealed any GR point mutations *(187)*. Thus, whether GR mutations are the major GC resistance mechanism in vivo is still unresolved.

9.2.2.2. Decreased GR Expression

A large number of studies about the relationship between GR expression and the clinical response to GC therapy found that a lower number of GR-α receptors per cell was associated with a decrease in GC sensitivity *(49–53)*, but this was not always confirmed *(188)*. Thus, basal expression levels of GR may be only part of the history, and clinical resistance to GCs may probably be because of more subtle changes in receptor properties or to defects further downstream in the apoptotic pathway. Kofler proposed the hypothesis that autoinduction of GR is a prerequisite for GC-induced apoptosis *(45)*. Early studies have shown a correlation between GC-sensitivity and GR autoinduction in myeloma *(189)* and lymphoblastic leukemia *(101,190)*.

9.2.2.3. GR Isoforms

As outlined before, various GR isoforms resulting from alternative splicing, polyadenylation, or translational initiation have been described. The splice variant GR-β has been proposed to have a dominant-negative effect on the actions of GR-α that could be attributable to the formation of heterodimers GR-α/GR-β *(56)*, to sequestration of an essential factor needed by GR-α for transcriptional activity *(191,192)*, or to a competition with GR-α for GRE sites *(193)*. However, the last mechanism seems unlikely, because androgen receptor- and progesterone receptor-induced transactivation on GRE-driven promoters is not inhibited by GR-β *(56)*. Recently, it has been demonstrated that the 15 amino acids encoded by exon 9β not only prevents ligand binding, but are also essential for the inhibitory effect of GR-β on GR-α *(192)*. Most clinical evidence that GR-β is capable of decreasing GC sensitivity of target cells has been obtained in respiratory medicine *(194)*, ulcerative colitis *(195)*, and rheumatoid arthritis patients *(196)*. However, there is still much controversy concerning the functional significance of GR-β, especially with respect to its putative inhibiting activities on GR-α *(197)*. On the other hand, it was suggested that the relative levels of the two isoforms may play a role in the occurrence of resistance in tumor cells during the treatment of hematological malignances with GC *(198,199)*. However, the low levels of GR-β compared to GR-α suggest at least in physiological conditions, that GR-β is not expressed at levels sufficient to inhibit GR-α function.

As with the GR-β isoform, there is controversy about the role of GR-P in GC sensitivity, with reports suggesting that it might contribute to the resistant phenotype *(58)*, and others providing evidence that GR-P can increase the activity of GR-α in some cells *(200)*. Another isoform, GR-A, was detected in a GC-resistant cell line but not in its sensitive counterpart *(57)*. However, whether expression of the different GR variants affects sensitivity to GC-induced apoptosis in lymphoid malignances is unknown.

9.3. Transcription Factors

The mechanism by which GCs induce apoptosis is an extremely complex signaling pathway, and it is unlikely that one single mechanism accounts for the immunosuppressive, anti-inflammatory, and cytotoxic effects mediated by the GCs. The initiation stage on the GC-induced apoptosis is the sequence of events leading up to and including direct regulation of gene transcription by the GR.

As mentioned before, two transcription factors appear to be the most likely targets of GC-induced repression, NF-κB, and AP-1. It has been shown that NF-κB plays a critical role in DNA synthesis and protection against DEX-induced apoptosis in MM cells *(201)*. Thus, molecular mechanisms such us enhanced AP-1 and NF-κB expression may be involved in GC resistance inducing gene expression of survival genes and cytokines.

Alternatively, the inhibitory effects of GC on NF-κB activity can be counterbalanced by the cytokines IL-2 and IL-4, which are reported to rescue lymphocytes from GC-induced apoptosis by inhibiting inhibitory-κB (IκB) induction by DEX *(15,149)*. In addition, interferon (IFN-α) and IL-6 can inhibit DEX-induced apoptosis in MM cells, inhibition that is concurrent with the induction of AP-1 binding activity *(202)*.

9.4. Crosstalk With Other Signaling Pathways

The crosstalk between other signaling pathways and the GR signaling pathway modulates GC-induced apoptosis. Thus, in order to induce an apoptotic signal, the GCs should repress prosurvival signaling pathways. The interference with the signaling pathways triggered by IL-6 is the most important, because this cytokine activates several survival pathways in MM cells that are able to block GC-induced apoptosis *(139)*. DEX has also been reported to regulate negatively IL-6 gene expression *(203)*.

IL-6 can activate Janus kinase/STAT *(131,204,205)*, phosphoinositol 3 kinase *(142,151,176,206)*, and MAPK *(143)* survival pathways, protecting MM cells from DEX-induced apoptosis. Several studies have shown that GR activity can be inhibited by the activation of the MAPK pathway members JNK *(88,141,152)* and p38 *(89,207)*. In addition, DEX-induced apoptosis is mediated by activation of related adhesion focal tyrosine kinase (RAFTK) *(144)*. RAFKT is a member of the focal adhesion kinase subfamily that interacts with, and regulates, several signaling proteins, including p38 MAPK *(208)*, and JNK and Src kinases *(209)*. IL-6 induces activation of Src homology 2-containing phosphotyrosine phosphatase, a tyrosine phosphatase which dephosphorylates RAFTK, thereby blocking DEX-induced apoptosis and promoting MM cell survival *(176)*.

IL-6 is also able to activate STAT3, which in turn induces the expression of antiapoptotic members of the Bcl-2 family *(205)*. Similarly, activation of STAT6 with subsequent inhibition of GR has been shown to be responsible for GC resistance after IL-4 exposure *(210)*. In addition, increased expression of STAT5 may also be implicated in GC resistance because STAT5 binds to the GC/GR complex, sequestering the latter and preventing its action *(131)*. STAT5 is a member of the family of transcription factors that are activated by receptors of the cytokines *(204)*.

Other growth factors in MM cells are insulin-like growth factor (IGF-1) and IFN-α. IGF-1 also activates phosphoinositol 3 kinase and MAPK pathways *(211)*, and is able to block DEX-induced apoptosis *(212)*. Similarly, IFN-α inhibits GC-mediated apoptosis and promotes the survival, but not the proliferation, of myeloma cells *(138)*. In addition, the proinflammatory cytokines tumor necrosis factor-α and IL-1 can regulate human glucocorticoid receptor gene expression and seem to interfere with GC-induced apoptosis by changing the GR-α/GR-β ratio *(42)*.

Together, IL-6 and IGF-1 represent a significant obstacle for the treatment of MM, because they are able to activate signaling pathways that blocks GC-induced apoptosis. Thus, treatments that combine GC with agents that inhibit survival pathways may improve the GC-sensitivity and the development of resistance.

On the other hand, GC-induced apoptosis is regulated both positively and negatively by members of the Bcl-2 protein family *(153)*. The expression of antiapoptotic Bcl-2 family members has been associated with resistance to anticancer drugs. Moreover, overexpression of Bcl-2 is associated with DEX resistance in MM cells *(213)*. In a MM cell line, Bcl-2 antisense oligonucleotides alone had no effect on cell survival, but induced apoptosis synergistically with DEX *(214)*. Furthermore, inhibition of the antiapoptotic member of the Bcl-2 family, MCL-1, also sensitizes MM cells to DEX-induced apoptosis *(214)*.

In addition, the data available today suggest that there may be more than one pathway to GC-induced apoptosis at the level of the final executor molecules of apoptosis. These executor molecules are caspase 8 and 9 that lead to caspase 3 activation and the morphological changes of apoptosis. An upregulation of the protein hsp27, a protein able to inhibit the release of SMAC of caspases from the mitochondria, is associated with GC resistance *(215)*.

9.5. Adhesion

The microenvironment has been shown to influence tumor cell phenotype with respect to growth, metastasis, and response to chemotherapy. There is a multidrug-resistant phenotype that is associated with cell-cell adhesion or adhesion to extracellular matrices *(216,217)*. The molecular mechanism associated with the cell adhesion-mediated drug resistance phenotype includes alteration in intracellular distribution of the drug target *(218)*, increased $p27^{KIP1}$ levels *(219)*, increased expression of antiapoptotic molecules *(220)*, and activation of NF-κB (RelB/p50) *(221)*. Cell adhesion-mediated drug resistance is particularly relevant in hematological malignancies such as multiple myeloma, where myeloma cells localize in the bone marrow and interact with stroma and stromal cells, initiating the production of proteins that stimulate or support tumor survival. The upregulation of cell-adhesion molecules like integrin β1, very late-activating antigen 4 (VLA-4), very late-activating antigen 5 (VLA-5), syndecan-1, and integrin β2 have been related with resistance of MM cells to the treatment with several drugs *(222,223)*. In addition, MM cells adhered to fibronectin are less susceptible to the effects of doxorubicin and melphalan compared with the same cells growth in suspension *(216)*.

Adhesion of MM cells to bone marrow stromal cells induces the secretion of IL-6 and other growth factors from the stromal cells; these growth factors mediate MM growth, survival, and drug resistance *(206)*.

In addition, a proliferation-inducing ligand (APRIL) was involved in the survival of MM primary cells cultured with their bone-marrow environment, and protected them from DEX-induced apoptosis *(224)*.

Although GCs are highly effective in MM treatment, some patients do not respond, and those that do respond eventually develop resistance to this therapy. The molecular basis of GC resistance is still poorly understood, and it may affect all aspects of GC action or may interfere with individual GC responses. In the former case, the export of GC out of the cell, an altered expression of the GR or the chaperones that stabilize it, an unbalance in the expression of the different GR isoforms, or an unfunctional GR may be involved. In the latter case, an enhanced expression of proteins involved in cell survival, a defective apoptotic machinery or an altered expression of adhesion molecules could be responsible for drug resistance. Mechanistic-based combinations with GCs may serve as avenues to combat GC resistance. Similarly, novel agents that initiate cytotoxicity through GC-independent pathways provide alternative strategies to treat GC resistance in MM.

ACKNOWLEDGMENTS

This work was supported in part by grants CA57629 and CA85915 from the National Cancer Institute, Department of Health and Human Services.

REFERENCES

1. Newton R. Molecular mechanisms of glucocorticoid action: what is important? Thorax 2000; 55:603–613.
2. Greenstein S, Ghias K, Krett NL, Rosen ST. Mechanisms of glucocorticoid-mediated apoptosis in hematological malignancies. Clin Cancer Res 2002; 8:1681–1694.
3. Anderson KC, Shaughnessy JD Jr, Barlogie B, Harousseau JL, Roodman GD. Multiple myeloma. Hematology (Am Soc Hematol Educ Program) 2002; 1:214–240.
4. Hillmann AG, Ramdas J, Multanen K, Norman MR, Harmon JM. Glucocorticoid receptor gene mutations in leukemic cells acquired in vitro and in vivo. Cancer Res 2000; 60:2056–2062.
5. Moalli PA, Rosen ST. Glucocorticoid receptors and resistance to glucocorticoids in hematologic malignancies. Leuk Lymphoma 1994; 15:363–374.
6. Cole TJ, Blendy JA, Monaghan AP, et al. Targeted disruption of the glucocorticoid receptor gene blocks adrenergic chromaffin cell development and severely retards lung maturation. Genes Dev 1995; 9:1608–1621.
7. Miyata Y, Yahara I. Cytoplasmic 8 S glucocorticoid receptor binds to actin filaments through the 90-kDa heat shock protein moiety. J Biol Chem 1991; 266:8779–8783.
8. Prima V, Depoix C, Masselot B, Formstecher P, Lefebvre P. Alteration of the glucocorticoid receptor subcellular localization by non steroidal compounds. J Steroid Biochem Mol Biol 2000; 72:1–12.
9. Freeman BC, Yamamoto KR. Continuous recycling: a mechanism for modulatory signal transduction. Trends Biochem Sci 2001; 26:285–290.
10. Cadepond F, Schweizer-Groyer G, Segard-Maurel I, et al. Heat shock protein 90 as a critical factor in maintaining glucocorticosteroid receptor in a nonfunctional state. J Biol Chem 1991; 266:5834–5841.
11. Furu K, Kilvik K, Gautvik KM, Haug E. The mechanism of [3H]dexamethasone uptake into prolactin producing rat pituitary cells (GH3 cells) in culture. J Steroid Biochem 1987; 28:587–591.
12. Webster JI, Carlstedt-Duke J. Involvement of multidrug resistance proteins (MDR) in the modulation of glucocorticoid response. J Steroid Biochem Mol Biol 2002; 82:277–288.
13. De Bosscher K, Vanden Berghe W, Vermeulen L, Plaisance S, Boone E, Haegeman G. Glucocorticoids repress NF-κB-driven genes by disturbing the interaction of p65 with the basal transcription machinery, irrespective of coactivator levels in the cell. Proc Natl Acad Sci U S A 2000; 97:3919–3924.
14. Feinman R, Koury J, Thames M, Barlogie B, Epstein J, Siegel DS. Role of NF-κB in the rescue of multiple myeloma cells from glucocorticoid-induced apoptosis by bcl-2. Blood 1999; 93:3044–3052.
15. Xie H, Seward RJ, Huber BT. Cytokine rescue from glucocorticoid induced apoptosis in T cells is mediated through inhibition of IκBα. Mol Immunol 1997; 34:987–994.
16. McKay LI, Cidlowski JA. Cross-talk between nuclear factor-κ B and the steroid hormone receptors: mechanisms of mutual antagonism. Mol Endocrinol 1998; 12:45–56.
17. Nissen RM, Yamamoto KR. The glucocorticoid receptor inhibits NFκB by interfering with serine-2 phosphorylation of the RNA polymerase II carboxy-terminal domain. Genes Dev 2000; 14:2314–2329.
18. Jehn BM, Osborne BA. Gene regulation associated with apoptosis. Crit Rev Eukaryot Gene Expr 1997; 7:179–193.
19. Jonat C, Rahmsdorf HJ, Park KK, et al. Antitumor promotion and antiinflammation: down-modulation of AP-1 (Fos/Jun) activity by glucocorticoid hormone. Cell 1990; 62:1189–1204.
20. Yang-Yen HF, Chambard JC, Sun YL, et al. Transcriptional interference between c-Jun and the glucocorticoid receptor: mutual inhibition of DNA binding due to direct protein-protein interaction. Cell 1990; 62:1205–1215.
21. Beato M, Chalepakis G, Schauer M, Slater EP. DNA regulatory elements for steroid hormones. J Steroid Biochem 1989; 32:737–747.
22. Cairns C, Cairns W, Okret S. Inhibition of gene expression by steroid hormone receptors via a negative glucocorticoid response element: evidence for the involvement of DNA-binding and agonistic effects of the antiglucocorticoid/antiprogestin RU486. DNA Cell Biol 1993; 12:695–702.
23. Pearce D, Yamamoto KR. Mineralocorticoid and glucocorticoid receptor activities distinguished by nonreceptor factors at a composite response element. Science 1993; 259:1161–1165.
24. Hache RJ, Tse R, Reich T, Savory JG, Lefebvre YA. Nucleocytoplasmic trafficking of steroid-free glucocorticoid receptor. J Biol Chem 1999; 274:1432–1439.
25. Holaska JM, Black BE, Love DC, Hanover JA, Leszyk J, Paschal BM. Calreticulin is a receptor for nuclear export. J Cell Biol 2001; 152:127–140.
26. Holaska JM, Black BE, Rastinejad F, Paschal BM. Ca^{2+}-dependent nuclear export mediated by calreticulin. Mol Cell Biol 2002; 22:6286–6297.

27. Kino T, Stauber RH, Resau JH, Pavlakis GN, Chrousos GP. Pathologic human GR mutant has a transdominant negative effect on the wild-type GR by inhibiting its translocation into the nucleus: importance of the ligand-binding domain for intracellular GR trafficking. J Clin Endocrinol Metab 2001; 86:5600–5608.

28. Kino T, Souvatzoglou E, De Martino MU, Tsopanomihalu M, Wan Y, Chrousos GP. Protein 14-3-3sigma interacts with and favors cytoplasmic subcellular localization of the glucocorticoid receptor, acting as a negative regulator of the glucocorticoid signaling pathway. J Biol Chem 2003; 278:25,651–25,656.

29. Carmo-Fonseca M. The contribution of nuclear compartmentalization to gene regulation. Cell 2002; 108:513–5121.

30. Horwitz KB, Jackson TA, Bain DL, Richer JK, Takimoto GS, Tung L. Nuclear receptor coactivators and corepressors. Mol Endocrinol 1996; 10:1167–1177.

31. Petersen DD, Koch SR, Granner DK. 3' noncoding region of phosphoenolpyruvate carboxykinase mRNA contains a glucocorticoid-responsive mRNA-stabilizing element. Proc Natl Acad Sci U S A 1989; 86:7800–7804.

32. Seene T, Alev K. Effect of glucocorticoids on the turnover rate of actin and myosin heavy and light chains on different types of skeletal muscle fibres. J Steroid Biochem 1985; 22:767–771.

33. Yudt MR, Cidlowski JA. The glucocorticoid receptor: coding a diversity of proteins and responses through a single gene. Mol Endocrinol 2002; 16:1719–1726.

34. Hollenberg SM, Weinberger C, Ong ES, et al. Primary structure and expression of a functional human glucocorticoid receptor cDNA. Nature 1985; 318:635–641.

35. Breslin MB, Geng CD, Vedeckis WV. Multiple promoters exist in the human GR gene, one of which is activated by glucocorticoids. Mol Endocrinol 2001; 15:1381–1395.

36. Zong J, Ashraf J, Thompson EB. The promoter and first, untranslated exon of the human glucocorticoid receptor gene are GC rich but lack consensus glucocorticoid receptor element sites. Mol Cell Biol 1990; 10:5580–5585.

37. Govindan MV, Pothier F, Leclerc S, Palaniswami R, Xie B. Human glucocorticoid receptor gene promotor-homologous down regulation. J Steroid Biochem Mol Biol 1991; 40:317–323.

38. Nobukuni Y, Smith CL, Hager GL, Detera-Wadleigh SD. Characterization of the human glucocorticoid receptor promoter. Biochemistry 1995; 34:8207–8214.

39. Wei P, Vedeckis WV. Regulation of the glucocorticoid receptor gene by the AP-1 transcription factor. Endocrine 1997; 7:303–310.

40. Breslin MB, Vedeckis WV. The human glucocorticoid receptor promoter upstream sequences contain binding sites for the ubiquitous transcription factor, Yin Yang 1. J Steroid Biochem Mol Biol 1998; 67:369–381.

41. Warrior N, Page N, Govindan MV. Expression of human glucocorticoid receptor gene and interaction of nuclear proteins with the transcriptional control element. J Biol Chem 1996; 271:18,662–18,671.

42. Webster JC, Oakley RH, Jewell CM, Cidlowski JA. Proinflammatory cytokines regulate human glucocorticoid receptor gene expression and lead to the accumulation of the dominant negative β isoform: a mechanism for the generation of glucocorticoid resistance. Proc Natl Acad Sci U S A 2001; 98:6865–6870.

43. Nunez BS, Vedeckis WV. Characterization of promoter 1B in the human glucocorticoid receptor gene. Mol Cell Endocrinol 2002; 189:191–199.

44. Encio IJ, Detera-Wadleigh SD. The genomic structure of the human glucocorticoid receptor. J Biol Chem 1991; 266:7182–7188.

45. Kofler R. The molecular basis of glucocorticoid-induced apoptosis of lymphoblastic leukemia cells. Histochem Cell Biol 2000; 114:1–7.

46. Chen F, Watson CS, Gametchu B. Association of the glucocorticoid receptor alternatively-spliced transcript 1A with the presence of the high molecular weight membrane glucocorticoid receptor in mouse lymphoma cells. J Cell Biochem 1999; 74:430–446.

47. Diba F, Watson CS, Gametchu B. 5'UTR sequences of the glucocorticoid receptor 1A transcript encode a peptide associated with translational regulation of the glucocorticoid receptor. J Cell Biochem 2001; 81:149–161.

48. Kalinyak JE, Dorin RI, Hoffman AR, Perlman AJ. Tissue-specific regulation of glucocorticoid receptor mRNA by dexamethasone. J Biol Chem 1987; 262:10,441–10,444.

49. Mastrangelo R, Malandrino R, Riccardi R, Longo P, Ranelletti FO, Iacobelli S. Clinical implications of glucocorticoid receptor studies in childhood acute lymphoblastic leukemia. Blood 1980; 56:1036–1040.

50. Costlow ME, Pui CH, Dahl GV. Glucocorticoid receptors in childhood acute lymphocytic leukemia. Cancer Res 1982; 42:4801–4806.

51. Iacobelli S, Marchetti P, De Rossi G, Mandelli F, Gentiloni N. Glucocorticoid receptors predict response to combination chemotherapy in patients with acute lymphoblastic leukemia. Oncology 1987; 44:13–16.
52. Pui CH, Dahl GV, Rivera G, Murphy SB, Costlow ME. The relationship of blast cell glucocorticoid receptor levels to response to single-agent steroid trial and remission response in children with acute lymphoblastic leukemia. Leuk Res 1984; 8:579–585.
53. Quddus FF, Leventhal BG, Boyett JM, Pullen DJ, Crist WM, Borowitz MJ. Glucocorticoid receptors in immunological subtypes of childhood acute lymphocytic leukemia cells: a Pediatric Oncology Group Study. Cancer Res 1985; 45(Pt 1):6482–6486.
54. Oakley RH, Sar M, Cidlowski JA. The human glucocorticoid receptor β isoform. Expression, biochemical properties, and putative function. J Biol Chem 1996; 271:9550–9559.
55. Oakley RH, Webster JC, Sar M, Parker CR Jr, Cidlowski JA. Expression and subcellular distribution of the β-isoform of the human glucocorticoid receptor. Endocrinology 1997; 138:5028–5038.
56. Oakley RH, Jewell CM, Yudt MR, Bofetiado DM, Cidlowski JA. The dominant negative activity of the human glucocorticoid receptor β isoform. Specificity and mechanisms of action. J Biol Chem 1999; 274:27,857–27,866.
57. Moalli PA, Pillay S, Krett NL, Rosen ST. Alternatively spliced glucocorticoid receptor messenger RNAs in glucocorticoid-resistant human multiple myeloma cells. Cancer Res 1993; 53:3877–3879.
58. Krett NL, Pillay S, Moalli PA, Greipp PR, Rosen ST. A variant glucocorticoid receptor messenger RNA is expressed in multiple myeloma patients. Cancer Res 1995; 55:2727–2729.
59. Rivers C, Levy A, Hancock J, Lightman S, Norman M. Insertion of an amino acid in the DNA-binding domain of the glucocorticoid receptor as a result of alternative splicing. J Clin Endocrinol Metab 1999; 84:4283–4286.
60. Yudt MR, Cidlowski JA. Molecular identification and characterization of a and b forms of the glucocorticoid receptor. Mol Endocrinol 2001; 15:1093–1103.
61. Kozak M. Adherence to the first-AUG rule when a second AUG codon follows closely upon the first. Proc Natl Acad Sci U S A 1995; 92:2662–2666.
62. Gametchu B, Chen F, Sackey F, Powell C, Watson CS. Plasma membrane-resident glucocorticoid receptors in rodent lymphoma and human leukemia models. Steroids 1999; 64:107–119.
63. Giguere V, Hollenberg SM, Rosenfeld MG, Evans RM. Functional domains of the human glucocorticoid receptor. Cell 1986; 46:645–652.
64. Weinberger C, Hollenberg SM, Rosenfeld MG, Evans RM. Domain structure of human glucocorticoid receptor and its relationship to the v-erb-A oncogene product. Nature 1985; 318:670–672.
65. Wright AP, Zilliacus J, McEwan IJ, et al. Structure and function of the glucocorticoid receptor. J Steroid Biochem Mol Biol 1993; 47:11–19.
66. Luisi BF, Xu WX, Otwinowski Z, Freedman LP, Yamamoto KR, Sigler PB. Crystallographic analysis of the interaction of the glucocorticoid receptor with DNA. Nature 1991; 352:497–505.
67. Tao Y, Williams-Skipp C, Scheinman RI. Mapping of glucocorticoid receptor DNA binding domain surfaces contributing to transrepression of NF-κ B and induction of apoptosis. J Biol Chem 2001; 276:2329–2332.
68. Miesfeld R, Godowski PJ, Maler BA, Yamamoto KR. Glucocorticoid receptor mutants that define a small region sufficient for enhancer activation. Science 1987; 236:423–427.
69. Dalman FC, Scherrer LC, Taylor LP, Akil H, Pratt WB. Localization of the 90-kDa heat shock protein-binding site within the hormone-binding domain of the glucocorticoid receptor by peptide competition. J Biol Chem 1991; 266:3482–3490.
70. Dahlman-Wright K, Wright AP, Gustafsson JA. Determinants of high-affinity DNA binding by the glucocorticoid receptor: evaluation of receptor domains outside the DNA-binding domain. Biochemistry 1992; 31:9040–9044.
71. Bledsoe RK, Montana VG, Stanley TB, et al. Crystal structure of the glucocorticoid receptor ligand binding domain reveals a novel mode of receptor dimerization and coactivator recognition. Cell 2002; 110:93–105.
72. Hollenberg SM, Giguere V, Segui P, Evans RM. Colocalization of DNA-binding and transcriptional activation functions in the human glucocorticoid receptor. Cell 1987; 49:39–46.
73. Godowski PJ, Rusconi S, Miesfeld R, Yamamoto KR. Glucocorticoid receptor mutants that are constitutive activators of transcriptional enhancement. Nature 1987; 325:365–368.
74. Brink M, Humbel BM, De Kloet ER, Van Driel R. The unliganded glucocorticoid receptor is localized in the nucleus, not in the cytoplasm. Endocrinology 1992; 130:3575–3581.
75. Baumann H, Paulsen K, Kovacs H, et al. Refined solution structure of the glucocorticoid receptor DNA-binding domain. Biochemistry 1993; 32:13,463–13,4671.

76. Cadepond F, Gasc JM, Delahaye F, et al. Hormonal regulation of the nuclear localization signals of the human glucocorticosteroid receptor. Exp Cell Res 1992; 201:99–108.
77. Picard D, Yamamoto KR. Two signals mediate hormone-dependent nuclear localization of the glucocorticoid receptor. EMBO J 1987; 6:3333–3340.
78. Savory JG, Hsu B, Laquian IR, et al. Discrimination between NL1- and NL2-mediated nuclear localization of the glucocorticoid receptor. Mol Cell Biol 1999; 19:1025–1037.
79. Hollenberg SM, Evans RM. Multiple and cooperative trans-activation domains of the human glucocorticoid receptor. Cell 1988; 55:899–906.
80. Danielian PS, White R, Lees JA, Parker MG. Identification of a conserved region required for hormone dependent transcriptional activation by steroid hormone receptors. EMBO J 1992; 11:1025–1033.
81. Hu JM, Bodwell JE, Munck A. Cell cycle-dependent glucocorticoid receptor phosphorylation and activity. Mol Endocrinol 1994; 8:1709–1713.
82. Hoeck W, Rusconi S, Groner B. Down-regulation and phosphorylation of glucocorticoid receptors in cultured cells. Investigations with a monospecific antiserum against a bacterially expressed receptor fragment. J Biol Chem 1989; 264:14,396–14,402.
83. Orti E, Mendel DB, Smith LI, Munck A. Agonist-dependent phosphorylation and nuclear dephosphorylation of glucocorticoid receptors in intact cells. J Biol Chem 1989; 264:9728–9731.
84. Almlof T, Wright AP, Gustafsson JA. Role of acidic and phosphorylated residues in gene activation by the glucocorticoid receptor. J Biol Chem 1995; 270:17,535–17,540.
85. Bodwell JE, Webster JC, Jewell CM, Cidlowski JA, Hu JM, Munck A. Glucocorticoid receptor phosphorylation: overview, function and cell cycle-dependence. J Steroid Biochem Mol Biol 1998; 65:91–99.
86. DeFranco DB, Qi M, Borror KC, Garabedian MJ, Brautigan DL. Protein phosphatase types 1 and/or 2A regulate nucleocytoplasmic shuttling of glucocorticoid receptors. Mol Endocrinol 1991; 5:1215–1228.
87. Doucas V, Shi Y, Miyamoto S, West A, Verma I, Evans RM. Cytoplasmic catalytic subunit of protein kinase A mediates cross-repression by NF-κ B and the glucocorticoid receptor. Proc Natl Acad Sci U S A 2000; 97:11,893–11,898.
88. Rogatsky I, Logan SK, Garabedian MJ. Antagonism of glucocorticoid receptor transcriptional activation by the c-Jun N-terminal kinase. Proc Natl Acad Sci U S A 1998; 95:2050–2055.
89. Irusen E, Matthews JG, Takahashi A, Barnes PJ, Chung KF, Adcock IM. p38 mitogen-activated protein kinase-induced glucocorticoid receptor phosphorylation reduces its activity: role in steroid-insensitive asthma. J Allergy Clin Immunol 2002; 109:649–657.
90. Wallace AD, Cidlowski JA. Proteasome-mediated glucocorticoid receptor degradation restricts transcriptional signaling by glucocorticoids. J Biol Chem 2001; 276:42,714–42,721.
91. Salghetti SE, Muratani M, Wijnen H, Futcher B, Tansey WP. Functional overlap of sequences that activate transcription and signal ubiquitin-mediated proteolysis. Proc Natl Acad Sci U S A 2000; 97:3118–3123.
92. Tian S, Poukka H, Palvimo JJ, Janne OA. Small ubiquitin-related modifier-1 (SUMO-1) modification of the glucocorticoid receptor. Biochem J 2002; 367(Pt 3):907–911.
93. Melchior F. SUMO—nonclassical ubiquitin. Annu Rev Cell Dev Biol 2000; 16:591–626.
94. Muller S, Hoege C, Pyrowolakis G, Jentsch S. SUMO, ubiquitin's mysterious cousin. Nat Rev Mol Cell Biol 2001; 2:202–210.
95. Le Drean Y, Mincheneau N, Le Goff P, Michel D. Potentiation of glucocorticoid receptor transcriptional activity by sumoylation. Endocrinology 2002; 143:3482–3489.
96. Vanderbilt JN, Miesfeld R, Maler BA, Yamamoto KR. Intracellular receptor concentration limits glucocorticoid-dependent enhancer activity. Mol Endocrinol 1987; 1:68–74.
97. Okret S, Dong Y, Bronnegard M, Gustafsson JA. Regulation of glucocorticoid receptor expression. Biochimie 1991; 73:51–59.
98. Vig E, Barrett TJ, Vedeckis WV. Coordinate regulation of glucocorticoid receptor and c-jun mRNA levels: evidence for cross-talk between two signaling pathways' at the transcriptional level. Mol Endocrinol 1994; 8:1336–1346.
99. Burnstein KL, Bellingham DL, Jewell CM, Powell-Oliver FE, Cidlowski JA. Autoregulation of glucocorticoid receptor gene expression. Steroids 1991; 56:52–58.
100. Rosewicz S, McDonald AR, Maddux BA, Goldfine ID, Miesfeld RL, Logsdon CD. Mechanism of glucocorticoid receptor down-regulation by glucocorticoids. J Biol Chem 1988; 263:2581–2584.
101. Denton RR, Eisen LP, Elsasser MS, Harmon JM. Differential autoregulation of glucocorticoid receptor expression in human T- and B-cell lines. Endocrinology 1993; 133:248–256.
102. Eisen LP, Elsasser MS, Harmon JM. Positive regulation of the glucocorticoid receptor in human T-cells sensitive to the cytolytic effects of glucocorticoids. J Biol Chem 1988; 263:12,044–12,048.

103. Ramdas J, Liu W, Harmon JM. Glucocorticoid-induced cell death requires autoinduction of glucocorticoid receptor expression in human leukemic T cells. Cancer Res 1999; 59:1378–1385.

104. Burnstein KL, Jewell CM, Sar M, Cidlowski JA. Intragenic sequences of the human glucocorticoid receptor complementary DNA mediate hormone-inducible receptor messenger RNA down-regulation through multiple mechanisms. Mol Endocrinol 1994; 8:1764–1773.

105. Dong Y, Poellinger L, Gustafsson JA, Okret S. Regulation of glucocorticoid receptor expression: evidence for transcriptional and posttranslational mechanisms. Mol Endocrinol 1988; 2:1256–1264.

106. McIntyre WR, Samuels HH. Triamcinolone acetonide regulates glucocorticoid-receptor levels by decreasing the half-life of the activated nuclear-receptor form. J Biol Chem 1985; 260:418–427.

107. Vedeckis WV, Ali M, Allen HR. Regulation of glucocorticoid receptor protein and mRNA levels. Cancer Res 1989; 49(Suppl):2295s–2302s.

108. Alksnis M, Barkhem T, Stromstedt PE, et al. High level expression of functional full length and truncated glucocorticoid receptor in Chinese hamster ovary cells. Demonstration of ligand-induced down-regulation of expressed receptor mRNA and protein. J Biol Chem 1991; 266:10,078–10,085.

109. Meyer AS, Schmidt TJ. Potential mechanisms underlying autoregulation of glucocorticoid receptor mRNA levels in the DHD/K12/PROb rat colonic adenocarcinoma cell line. J Steroid Biochem Mol Biol 1995; 55:219–228.

110. Okret S, Poellinger L, Dong Y, Gustafsson JA. Down-regulation of glucocorticoid receptor mRNA by glucocorticoid hormones and recognition by the receptor of a specific binding sequence within a receptor cDNA clone. Proc Natl Acad Sci U S A 1986; 83:5899–5903.

111. Drouin J, Trifiro MA, Plante RK, Nemer M, Eriksson P, Wrange O. Glucocorticoid receptor binding to a specific DNA sequence is required for hormone-dependent repression of pro-opiomelanocortin gene transcription. Mol Cell Biol 1989; 9:5305–5314.

112. Pedersen KB, Vedeckis WV. Quantification and glucocorticoid regulation of glucocorticoid receptor transcripts in two human leukemic cell lines. Biochemistry 2003; 42:10,978–10,990.

113. Grimm LM, Goldberg AL, Poirier GG, Schwartz LM, Osborne BA. Proteasomes play an essential role in thymocyte apoptosis. EMBO J 1996; 15:3835–3844.

114. He H, Qi XM, Grossmann J, Distelhorst CW. c-Fos degradation by the proteasome. An early, Bcl-2-regulated step in apoptosis. J Biol Chem 1998; 273:25,015–25,019.

115. Grassilli E, Benatti F, Dansi P, et al. Inhibition of proteasome function prevents thymocyte apoptosis: involvement of ornithine decarboxylase. Biochem Biophys Res Commun 1998; 250:293–297.

116. Gil-Gomez G, Berns A, Brady HJ. A link between cell cycle and cell death: Bax and Bcl-2 modulate Cdk2 activation during thymocyte apoptosis. EMBO J 1998; 17:7209–7218.

117. Yang Y, Fang S, Jensen JP, Weissman AM, Ashwell JD. Ubiquitin protein ligase activity of IAPs and their degradation in proteasomes in response to apoptotic stimuli. Science 2000; 288:874–877.

118. Dallaporta B, Pablo M, Maisse C, et al. Proteasome activation as a critical event of thymocyte apoptosis. Cell Death Differ 2000; 7:368–373.

119. Distelhorst CW, Dubyak G. Role of calcium in glucocorticosteroid-induced apoptosis of thymocytes and lymphoma cells: resurrection of old theories by new findings. Blood 1998; 91:731–734.

120. Jayaraman T, Marks AR. T cells deficient in inositol 1,4,5-trisphosphate receptor are resistant to apoptosis. Mol Cell Biol 1997; 17:3005–3012.

121. Distelhorst CW. Recent insights into the mechanism of glucocorticosteroid-induced apoptosis. Cell Death Differ 2002; 9:6–19.

122. Almawi WY, Abou Jaoude MM, Li XC. Transcriptional and post-transcriptional mechanisms of glucocorticoid antiproliferative effects. Hematol Oncol 2002; 20:17–32.

123. Yamamoto KR, Alberts BM. Steroid receptors: elements for modulation of eukaryotic transcription. Annu Rev Biochem 1976; 45:721–746.

124. Drouin J, Charron J, Gagner JP, et al. Pro-opiomelanocortin gene: a model for negative regulation of transcription by glucocorticoids. J Cell Biochem 1987; 35:293–304.

125. Adcock IM, Nasuhara Y, Stevens DA, Barnes PJ. Ligand-induced differentiation of glucocorticoid receptor (GR) trans-repression and transactivation: preferential targetting of NF-κB and lack of I-κB involvement. Br J Pharmacol 1999; 127:1003–1011.

126. Jenkins BD, Pullen CB, Darimont BD. Novel glucocorticoid receptor coactivator effector mechanisms. Trends Endocrinol Metab 2001; 12:122–126.

127. Fryer CJ, Archer TK. Chromatin remodelling by the glucocorticoid receptor requires the BRG1 complex. Nature 1998; 393:88–91.

128. McKenna NJ, O'Malley BW. Nuclear receptors, coregulators, ligands, and selective receptor modulators: making sense of the patchwork quilt. Ann N Y Acad Sci 2001; 949:3–5.

129. Scheinman RI, Gualberto A, Jewell CM, Cidlowski JA, Baldwin AS Jr. Characterization of mechanisms involved in transrepression of NF-κB by activated glucocorticoid receptors. Mol Cell Biol 1995; 15:943–953.

130. Ford J, McEwan IJ, Wright AP, Gustafsson JA. Involvement of the transcription factor IID protein complex in gene activation by the N-terminal transactivation domain of the glucocorticoid receptor in vitro. Mol Endocrinol 1997; 11:1467–1475.

131. Stocklin E, Wissler M, Gouilleux F, Groner B. Functional interactions between Stat5 and the glucocorticoid receptor. Nature 1996; 383:726–728.

132. De Miguel F, Lee SO, Onate SA, Gao AC. Stat3 enhances transactivation of steroid hormone receptors. Nucl Recept 2003; 1:3.

133. Chakravarti D, LaMorte VJ, Nelson MC, et al. Role of CBP/P300 in nuclear receptor signalling. Nature 1996; 383:99–103.

134. Kamei Y, Xu L, Heinzel T, et al. A CBP integrator complex mediates transcriptional activation and AP-1 inhibition by nuclear receptors. Cell 1996; 85:403–414.

135. Yao TP, Ku G, Zhou N, Scully R, Livingston DM. The nuclear hormone receptor coactivator SRC-1 is a specific target of p300. Proc Natl Acad Sci U S A 1996; 93:10,626–10,631.

136. Rachez C, Lemon BD, Suldan Z, et al. Ligand-dependent transcription activation by nuclear receptors requires the DRIP complex. Nature 1999; 398:824–828.

137. Chauhan D, Auclair D, Robinson EK, et al. Identification of genes regulated by dexamethasone in multiple myeloma cells using oligonucleotide arrays. Oncogene 2002; 21:1346–1358.

138. Ferlin-Bezombes M, Jourdan M, Liautard J, Brochier J, Rossi JF, Klein B. IFN-α is a survival factor for human myeloma cells and reduces dexamethasone-induced apoptosis. J Immunol 1998; 161:2692–2699.

139. Hardin J, MacLeod S, Grigorieva I, et al. Interleukin-6 prevents dexamethasone-induced myeloma cell death. Blood 1994; 84:3063–3070.

140. Ogawa M, Nishiura T, Oritani K, et al. Cytokines prevent dexamethasone-induced apoptosis via the activation of mitogen-activated protein kinase and phosphatidylinositol 3-kinase pathways in a new multiple myeloma cell line. Cancer Res 2000; 60:4262–4269.

141. Xu FH, Sharma S, Gardner A, et al. Interleukin-6-induced inhibition of multiple myeloma cell apoptosis: support for the hypothesis that protection is mediated via inhibition of the JNK/SAPK pathway. Blood 1998; 92:241–251.

142. Hideshima T, Nakamura N, Chauhan D, Anderson KC. Biologic sequelae of interleukin-6 induced PI3-K/Akt signaling in multiple myeloma. Oncogene 2001; 20:5991–6000.

143. Chauhan D, Kharbanda S, Ogata A, et al. Interleukin-6 inhibits Fas-induced apoptosis and stress-activated protein kinase activation in multiple myeloma cells. Blood 1997; 89:227–234.

144. Chauhan D, Hideshima T, Pandey P, et al. RAFTK/PYK2-dependent and -independent apoptosis in multiple myeloma cells. Oncogene 1999; 18:6733–6740.

145. Widen C, Zilliacus J, Gustafsson JA, Wikstrom AC. Glucocorticoid receptor interaction with 14-3-3 and Raf-1, a proposed mechanism for cross-talk of two signal transduction pathways. J Biol Chem 2000; 275:39,296–39,2301.

146. Jamieson CA, Yamamoto KR. Crosstalk pathway for inhibition of glucocorticoid-induced apoptosis by T cell receptor signaling. Proc Natl Acad Sci U S A 2000; 97:7319–7324.

147. Asada A, Zhao Y, Kondo S, Iwata M. Induction of thymocyte apoptosis by Ca²⁺-independent protein kinase C (nPKC) activation and its regulation by calcineurin activation. J Biol Chem 1998; 273:28,392–28,398.

148. Bansal N, Houle A, Melnykovych G. Apoptosis: mode of cell death induced in T cell leukemia lines by dexamethasone and other agents. FASEB J 1991; 5:211–216.

149. Ramdas J, Harmon JM. Glucocorticoid-induced apoptosis and regulation of NF-κB activity in human leukemic T cells. Endocrinology 1998; 139:3813–3821.

150. Rowley M, Van Ness B. Activation of N-ras and K-ras induced by interleukin-6 in a myeloma cell line: implications for disease progression and therapeutic response. Oncogene 2002; 21:8769–8775.

151. Tai YT, Podar K, Mitsiades N, et al. CD40 induces human multiple myeloma cell migration via phosphatidylinositol 3-kinase/AKT/NF-κB signaling. Blood 2003; 101:2762–2769.

152. Hideshima T, Hayashi T, Chauhan D, Akiyama M, Richardson P, Anderson K. Biologic sequelae of c-Jun NH-terminal kinase (JNK) activation in multiple myeloma cell lines. Oncogene 2003; 22:8797–8801.
153. Adams JM, Cory S. The Bcl-2 protein family: arbiters of cell survival. Science 1998; 281:1322–1326.
154. McColl KS, He H, Zhong H, Whitacre CM, Berger NA, Distelhorst CW. Apoptosis induction by the glucocorticoid hormone dexamethasone and the calcium-ATPase inhibitor thapsigargin involves Bcl-2 regulated caspase activation. Mol Cell Endocrinol 1998; 139:229–238.
155. Camilleri-Broet S, Vanderwerff H, Caldwell E, Hockenbery D. Distinct alterations in mitochondrial mass and function characterize different models of apoptosis. Exp Cell Res 1998; 239:277–292.
156. Brunet CL, Gunby RH, Benson RS, Hickman JA, Watson AJ, Brady G. Commitment to cell death measured by loss of clonogenicity is separable from the appearance of apoptotic markers. Cell Death Differ 1998; 5:107–115.
157. Hsu YT, Wolter KG, Youle RJ. Cytosol-to-membrane redistribution of Bax and Bcl-X_L during apoptosis. Proc Natl Acad Sci U S A 1997; 94:3668–3672.
158. Mok CL, Gil-Gomez G, Williams O, et al. Bad can act as a key regulator of T cell apoptosis and T cell development. J Exp Med 1999; 189:575–586.
159. Bouillet P, Metcalf D, Huang DC, et al. Proapoptotic Bcl-2 relative Bim required for certain apoptotic responses, leukocyte homeostasis, and to preclude autoimmunity. Science 1999; 286:1735–1738.
160. Cohen GM. Caspases: the executioners of apoptosis. Biochem J 1997; 326(Pt 1):1–16.
161. Miyashita T, Nagao K, Krajewski S, et al. Investigation of glucocorticoid-induced apoptotic pathway: processing of caspase-6 but not caspase-3. Cell Death Differ 1998; 5:1034–1041.
162. Komoriya A, Packard BZ, Brown MJ, Wu ML, Henkart PA. Assessment of caspase activities in intact apoptotic thymocytes using cell-permeable fluorogenic caspase substrates. J Exp Med 2000; 191:1819–1828.
163. Zamzami N, Marchetti P, Castedo M, et al. Sequential reduction of mitochondrial transmembrane potential and generation of reactive oxygen species in early programmed cell death. J Exp Med 1995; 182:367–377.
164. Hakem R, Hakem A, Duncan GS, et al. Differential requirement for caspase 9 in apoptotic pathways in vivo. Cell 1998; 94:339–352.
165. Chauhan D, Pandey P, Ogata A, et al. Cytochrome c-dependent and -independent induction of apoptosis in multiple myeloma cells. J Biol Chem 1997; 272:29,995–29,997.
166. Chauhan D, Hideshima T, Rosen S, Reed JC, Kharbanda S, Anderson KC. Apaf-1/cytochrome c-independent and Smac-dependent induction of apoptosis in multiple myeloma (MM) cells. J Biol Chem 2001; 276:24,453–24,456.
167. Dalton WS. Detection of multidrug resistance gene expression in multiple myeloma. Leukemia 1997; 11:1166–1169.
168. Bourgeois S, Gruol DJ, Newby RF, Rajah FM. Expression of an mdr gene is associated with a new form of resistance to dexamethasone-induced apoptosis. Mol Endocrinol 1993; 7:840–851.
169. Nelson GM, Prapapanich V, Carrigan PE, Roberts PJ, Riggs DL, Smith DF. The hsp70 cochaperone hip enhances functional maturation of glucocorticoid receptor. Mol Endocrinol 2004; 18:1620–1630.
170. Morishima Y, Kanelakis KC, Murphy PJ, et al. The hsp90 cochaperone p23 is the limiting component of the multiprotein hsp90/hsp70-based chaperone system in vivo where it acts to stabilize the client protein: hsp90 complex. J Biol Chem 2003; 278:48,754–48,763.
171. Ratajczak T, Ward BK, Minchin RF. Immunophilin chaperones in steroid receptor signalling. Curr Top Med Chem 2003; 3:1348–1357.
172. Wikstrom AC, Widen C, Erlandsson A, Hedman E, Zilliacus J. Cytosolic glucocorticoid receptor-interacting proteins. Ernst Schering Res Found Workshop 2002; 177–196.
173. Kojika S, Sugita K, Inukai T, et al. Mechanisms of glucocorticoid resistance in human leukemic cells: implication of abnormal 90 and 70 kDa heat shock proteins. Leukemia 1996; 10:994–999.
174. Kanelakis KC, Morishima Y, Dittmar KD, et al. Differential effects of the hsp70-binding protein BAG-1 on glucocorticoid receptor folding by the hsp90-based chaperone machinery. J Biol Chem 1999; 274:34,134–34,140.
175. Scammell JG, Denny WB, Valentine DL, Smith DF. Overexpression of the FK506-binding immunophilin FKBP51 is the common cause of glucocorticoid resistance in three New World primates. Gen Comp Endocrinol 2001; 124:152–165.
176. Chauhan D, Pandey P, Hideshima T, et al. SHP2 mediates the protective effect of interleukin-6 against dexamethasone-induced apoptosis in multiple myeloma cells. J Biol Chem 2000; 275:27,845–27,850.
177. Bray PJ, Cotton RG. Variations of the human glucocorticoid receptor gene (NR3C1): pathological and in vitro mutations and polymorphisms. Hum Mutat 2003; 21:557–568.

178. Powers JH, Hillmann AG, Tang DC, Harmon JM. Cloning and expression of mutant glucocorticoid receptors from glucocorticoid-sensitive and -resistant human leukemic cells. Cancer Res 1993; 53:4059–4065.
179. Strasser-Wozak EM, Hattmannstorfer R, Hala M, et al. Splice site mutation in the glucocorticoid receptor gene causes resistance to glucocorticoid-induced apoptosis in a human acute leukemic cell line. Cancer Res 1995; 55:348–353.
180. Thompson EB, Harmon JM. Glucocorticoid receptors and glucocorticoid resistance in human leukemia in vivo and in vitro. Adv Exp Med Biol 1986; 196:111–127.
181. Smets L, Metwally EA, Knol E, Martens M. Potentiation of glucocorticoid-induced lysis in refractory and resistant leukemia cells by inhibitors of ADP-ribosylation. Leuk Res 1988; 12:737–743.
182. Nagano M, Nakamura T, Niimi S, et al. Substitution of arginine for cysteine 643 of the glucocorticoid receptor reduces its steroid-binding affinity and transcriptional activity. Cancer Lett 2002; 181:109–114.
183. Ashraf J, Thompson EB. Identification of the activation-labile gene: a single point mutation in the human glucocorticoid receptor presents as two distinct receptor phenotypes. Mol Endocrinol 1993; 7:631–642.
184. Geley S, Hartmann BL, Hala M, Strasser-Wozak EM, Kapelari K, Kofler R. Resistance to glucocorticoid-induced apoptosis in human T-cell acute lymphoblastic leukemia CEM-C1 cells is due to insufficient glucocorticoid receptor expression. Cancer Res 1996; 56:5033–5038.
185. Hala M, Hartmann BL, Bock G, Geley S, Kofler R. Glucocorticoid-receptor-gene defects and resistance to glucocorticoid-induced apoptosis in human leukemic cell lines. Int J Cancer 1996; 68:663–668.
186. Karkera JD, Taymans SE, Turner G, Yoshikawa T, Detera-Wadleigh SD, Wadleigh RG. Deletion of a consensus oestrogen response element half-site in the glucocorticoid receptor of human multiple myeloma. Br J Haematol 1997; 99:372–374.
187. Soufi M, Kaiser U, Schneider A, Beato M, Westphal HM. The DNA and steroid binding domains of the glucocorticoid receptor are not altered in mononuclear cells of treated CLL patients. Exp Clin Endocrinol Diabetes 1995; 103:175–183.
188. Csoka M, Bocsi J, Falus A, et al. Glucocorticoid-induced apoptosis and treatment sensitivity in acute lymphoblastic leukemia of children. Pediatr Hematol Oncol 1997; 14:433–442.
189. Gomi M, Moriwaki K, Katagiri S, Kurata Y, Thompson EB. Glucocorticoid effects on myeloma cells in culture: correlation of growth inhibition with induction of glucocorticoid receptor messenger RNA. Cancer Res 1990; 50:1873–1878.
190. Barrett TJ, Vig E, Vedeckis WV. Coordinate regulation of glucocorticoid receptor and c-jun gene expression is cell type-specific and exhibits differential hormonal sensitivity for down- and up-regulation. Biochemistry 1996; 35:9746–9753.
191. Bamberger CM, Bamberger AM, de Castro M, Chrousos GP. Glucocorticoid receptor β, a potential endogenous inhibitor of glucocorticoid action in humans. J Clin Invest 1995; 95:2435–2441.
192. Yudt MR, Jewell CM, Bienstock RJ, Cidlowski JA. Molecular origins for the dominant negative function of human glucocorticoid receptor β. Mol Cell Biol 2003; 23:4319–4330.
193. Leung DY, Hamid Q, Vottero A, et al. Association of glucocorticoid insensitivity with increased expression of glucocorticoid receptor β. J Exp Med 1997; 186:1567–1574.
194. Hamid QA, Wenzel SE, Hauk PJ, et al. Increased glucocorticoid receptor β in airway cells of glucocorticoid-insensitive asthma. Am J Respir Crit Care Med 1999; 159(Pt 1):1600–1604.
195. Honda M, Orii F, Ayabe T, et al. Expression of glucocorticoid receptor β in lymphocytes of patients with glucocorticoid-resistant ulcerative colitis. Gastroenterology 2000; 118:859–866.
196. Derijk RH, Schaaf MJ, Turner G, et al. A human glucocorticoid receptor gene variant that increases the stability of the glucocorticoid receptor β-isoform mRNA is associated with rheumatoid arthritis. J Rheumatol 2001; 28:2383–2388.
197. Gagliardo R, Vignola AM, Mathieu M. Is there a role for glucocorticoid receptor β in asthma? Respir Res 2001; 2:1–4.
198. de Castro M, Elliot S, Kino T, et al. The non-ligand binding β-isoform of the human glucocorticoid receptor (hGR β): tissue levels, mechanism of action, and potential physiologic role. Mol Med 1996; 2:597–607.
199. Shahidi H, Vottero A, Stratakis CA, et al. Imbalanced expression of the glucocorticoid receptor isoforms in cultured lymphocytes from a patient with systemic glucocorticoid resistance and chronic lymphocytic leukemia. Biochem Biophys Res Commun 1999; 254:559–565.
200. de Lange P, Segeren CM, Koper JW, et al. Expression in hematological malignancies of a glucocorticoid receptor splice variant that augments glucocorticoid receptor-mediated effects in transfected cells. Cancer Res 2001; 61:3937–3941.

201. Hideshima T, Chauhan D, Richardson P, et al. NF-κ B as a therapeutic target in multiple myeloma. J Biol Chem 2002; 277:16,639–16,647.
202. Liu P, Oken M, Van Ness B. Interferon-α protects myeloma cell lines from dexamethasone-induced apoptosis. Leukemia 1999; 13:473–480.
203. Shiao RT, McLeskey SB, Khera SY, Wolfson A, Freter CE. Mechanisms of inhibition of IL-6-mediated immunoglobulin secretion by dexamethasone and suramin in human lymphoid and myeloma cell lines. Leuk Lymphoma 1996; 21:293–303.
204. Biola A, Lefebvre P, Perrin-Wolff M, Sturm M, Bertoglio J, Pallardy M. Interleukin-2 inhibits glucocorticoid receptor transcriptional activity through a mechanism involving STAT5 (signal transducer and activator of transcription 5) but not AP-1. Mol Endocrinol 2001; 15:1062–1076.
205. Catlett-Falcone R, Landowski TH, Oshiro MM, et al. Constitutive activation of Stat3 signaling confers resistance to apoptosis in human U266 myeloma cells. Immunity 1999; 10:105–115.
206. Chauhan D, Anderson KC. Mechanisms of cell death and survival in multiple myeloma (MM): Therapeutic implications. Apoptosis 2003; 8:337–343.
207. Hideshima T, Akiyama M, Hayashi T, et al. Targeting p38 MAPK inhibits multiple myeloma cell growth in the bone marrow milieu. Blood 2003; 101:703–705.
208. Pandey P, Avraham S, Kumar S, et al. Activation of p38 mitogen-activated protein kinase by PYK2/related adhesion focal tyrosine kinase-dependent mechanism. J Biol Chem 1999; 274:10,140–10,144.
209. Tokiwa G, Dikic I, Lev S, Schlessinger J. Activation of Pyk2 by stress signals and coupling with JNK signaling pathway. Science 1996; 273:792–794.
210. Biola A, Andreau K, David M, et al. The glucocorticoid receptor and STAT6 physically and functionally interact in T-lymphocytes. FEBS Lett 2000; 487:229–233.
211. Ge NL, Rudikoff S. Insulin-like growth factor I is a dual effector of multiple myeloma cell growth. Blood 2000; 96:2856–2861.
212. Xu F, Gardner A, Tu Y, Michl P, Prager D, Lichtenstein A. Multiple myeloma cells are protected against dexamethasone-induced apoptosis by insulin-like growth factors. Br J Haematol 1997; 97:429–440.
213. Gazitt Y, Fey V, Thomas C, Alvarez R. Bcl-2 overexpression is associated with resistance to dexamethasone, but not melphalan, in multiple myeloma cells. Int J Oncol 1998; 13:397–405.
214. Derenne S, Monia B, Dean NM, et al. Antisense strategy shows that Mcl-1 rather than Bcl-2 or Bcl-x(L) is an essential survival protein of human myeloma cells. Blood 2002; 100:194–199.
215. Chauhan D, Li G, Hideshima T, et al. Hsp27 inhibits release of mitochondrial protein Smac in multiple myeloma cells and confers dexamethasone resistance. Blood 2003; 102:3379–3386.
216. Damiano JS, Cress AE, Hazlehurst LA, Shtil AA, Dalton WS. Cell adhesion mediated drug resistance (CAM-DR): role of integrins and resistance to apoptosis in human myeloma cell lines. Blood 1999; 93:1658–1667.
217. Green SK, Frankel A, Kerbel RS. Adhesion-dependent multicellular drug resistance. Anticancer Drug Des 1999; 14:153–168.
218. Hazlehurst LA, Dalton WS. Mechanisms associated with cell adhesion mediated drug resistance (CAM-DR) in hematopoietic malignancies. Cancer Metastasis Rev 2001; 20:43–50.
219. Hazlehurst LA, Damiano JS, Buyuksal I, Pledger WJ, Dalton WS. Adhesion to fibronectin via β1 integrins regulates p27kip1 levels and contributes to cell adhesion mediated drug resistance (CAM-DR). Oncogene 2000; 19:4319–4327.
220. Shain KH, Landowski TH, Dalton WS. Adhesion-mediated intracellular redistribution of c-Fas-associated death domain-like IL-1-converting enzyme-like inhibitory protein-long confers resistance to CD95-induced apoptosis in hematopoietic cancer cell lines. J Immunol 2002; 168:2544–2553.
221. Landowski TH, Olashaw NE, Agrawal D, Dalton WS. Cell adhesion-mediated drug resistance (CAM-DR) is associated with activation of NF-κ B (RelB/p50) in myeloma cells. Oncogene 2003; 22:2417–2421.
222. Dalton WS. The tumor microenvironment: focus on myeloma. Cancer Treat Rev 2003; 29(Suppl 1):11–19.
223. Damiano JS, Dalton WS. Integrin-mediated drug resistance in multiple myeloma. Leuk Lymphoma 2000; 38:71–81.
224. Moreaux J, Legouffe E, Jourdan E, et al. BAFF and APRIL protect myeloma cells from apoptosis induced by interleukin 6 deprivation and dexamethasone. Blood 2004; 103:3148–3157.

24 Herceptin Resistance

Ingrid A. Mayer, MD and Carlos L. Arteaga, MD

CONTENTS

INTRODUCTION
INSULIN GROWTH FACTOR I RECEPTOR SIGNALING
THE PI3K/AKT PATHWAY
CELL CYCLE AND P27
OTHER POTENTIAL MECHANISMS
CONCLUSIONS
ACKNOWLEDGMENTS
REFERENCES

SUMMARY

Finding the appropriate patients and ensuring that molecular therapeutics are delivered to the tumor in biologically relevant doses are the backbone of targeted therapies. This chapter reviews mechanisms of resistance to trastuzumab (Herceptin®), an important targeted therapy in breast cancer management. Monoclonal antibodies that target the HER-2/*neu* ectodomain sensitize HER-2/*neu* activation and HER-2/*neu*-dependent gene expression, resulting in cell cycle progression and cellular differentiation. Trastuzumab activation of Akt is downregulated even in trastuzumab-resistant clones of breast cancer cells. The main mechanisms of resistance to trasuzumab known to date seem to evolve around complex interactions involving mainly the insulin growth factor receptor, phosphatidylinositol 3 kinase/Akt, and cell cycle regulatory pathways.

Key Words: Herceptin; estrogen receptor; epithelial growth factor receptor; HER-2; ErbB2.

1. INTRODUCTION

Finding the appropriate patients and ensuring that molecular therapeutics are delivered to the tumor in biologically relevant doses are the backbone of targeted therapies. Lately, the development of new strategies for the treatment of breast cancer has not only focused on target identification, but also on understanding the expression, regulation, and function of critical signaling pathways involved in breast cancer initiation and progression. It is well established now that therapy for breast cancer should be guided by biologic features of the tumor, such as hormone-receptor positivity or HER-2/*neu* overexpression. The purpose of this chapter is to review mechanisms of resistance of trastuzumab (Herceptin®), an important targeted therapy in breast cancer management.

From: *Cancer Drug Discovery and Development: Cancer Drug Resistance*
Edited by: B. Teicher © Humana Press Inc., Totowa, NJ

HER-2/*neu* is a 185-kDa oncoprotein (p185), which is overexpressed in about 30% of invasive breast cancers *(1,2)*. HER-2/*neu* overexpression is not only associated with resistance to cytotoxic and endocrine therapy, but also with an aggressive biological behavior that translates into shorter disease-free interval and overall survival in patients with early and advanced breast cancer *(3)*. The HER-2/*neu* molecule is composed of an extracellular ligand-binding domain, an amphipathic transmembrane region, and an intracellular tyrosine kinase domain, which contains a carboxy tail with five major autophosphorylation sites *(4)*. To date, no direct ligand has been identified for HER-2/*neu*. Abundant experimental evidence indicates that the HER-2/*neu* transmembrane protein acts as a coreceptor that leads to formation of homo- and heterodimeric receptor complexes with other members of the HER (ErbB) family, into which HER-2/*neu* is recruited as a preferential dimerization partner *(5)*. This process is followed by intrinsic tyrosine kinase-mediated autophosphorylation and mutual phosphorylation/activation of the respective dimerization partners *(6,7)*. In vitro studies have identified distinct receptor heterodimers that are associated with the malignant phenotype of several human breast cancer cell lines, and that might also play a significant role in malignant transformation in vivo. Combinations that have most often been associated with malignant behavior include EGFR-HER-2/*neu*, EGFR-HER-3, and HER-2/*neu*-HER-3. Alternatively, in vitro HER-2/*neu* activation has also been demonstrated to occur as a result of spontaneous cleavage of its extracellular domain (ECD), thereby resulting in the production of a truncated membrane-bound fragment (p95) with tyrosine kinase activity. Because the p95 fragment has also been detected in breast cancer specimens, it has been suggested that shedding of the ECD may represent an alternative activation mechanism of HER-2/*neu* in vivo *(8,9)*.

Monoclonal antibodies that target the HER-2/*neu* ectodomain sensitize HER-2/*neu* overexpressing cells to apoptotic stimuli by interfering with HER-2/*neu* activation and HER-2/*neu*-dependent gene expression, resulting in cell cycle progression and cellular differentiation. Trastuzumab is a humanized antibody against HER-2/*neu* (murine monocolonal antibody 4D5 combined with a human immunoglobulin-G) that is now a fundamental part of the therapy for patients with metastatic HER-2/*neu*-overexpressing breast cancers. Some of trastuzumab's mechanisms of action identified to date include:

1. G_1 arrest via upregulation of the cyclin-dependent kinase (CDK) inhibitor p27 *(10–14)*.
2. Induction of antibody-dependent cellular cytotoxicity through interaction with CD16-positive immune effector cells *(10–12)*.
3. Receptor downregulation from the tumor cell surface *(11,12)*.
4. Stimulation of HER-2 homodimerization and hence prevention of heterodimer formation *(11)*.
5. Inhibition of postreceptor downstream signal transduction *(10,12,15)*.
6. Inhibition of the production of angiogenic factors such as vascular endothelial growth factor *(11,15)*.
7. Inhibition of constitutive HER-2 cleavage/shedding mediated by metalloproteases, which results in the release of soluble ECD and constitutive activation of the remaining membrane-associated HER-2 domain (the truncated receptor known as p95) *(8,9,11,12,16)*.

A landmark randomized phase III trial comparing first-line standard chemotherapy (adriamycin-cyclophosphamide or paclitaxel) with or without trastuzumab in 469 women with HER-2/*neu*-overexpressing metastatic breast cancer showed that the trastuzumab-based combination therapy not only reduced the relative risk of death by 20% at a median follow-up of 30 mo, but also significant increased the time to disease progression, rates of response, duration of responses and time to treatment failure. Nevertheless, the concurrent use of trastuzumab with the anthracycline regimen significantly increased the risk of cardiac dysfunction to unacceptable levels. The increase in overall survival seen with trastuzumab and first-line chemotherapy for women with HER-2/*neu*-overexpressing metastatic breast cancer has made its use standard of care in this setting *(17)*. For women who cannot or are not willing to receive cytotoxic chemotherapy for metastatic breast cancer, the use of trastuzumab as single-agent in first-line treatment is a valid option. In women with HER-2/*neu*-overexpressing 3+ tumors verified by immunohistochemistry or those with *HER-2/neu* gene amplification as detected by fluorescent *in situ* hybridization, the response rate is about 35%. About 50% of responders are free of progression after 1 yr. The median survival in patients with HER-2-overxpressing tumors is about 24 mo, suggesting that patients do not incur a major survival disadvantage if they receive trastuzumab alone as first-line therapy for metastatic disease *(18)*.

Despite these encouraging results, the response rate to trastuzumab is ≤40% as single agent in first-line treatment of metastatic breast cancer, and the median duration of response is between 9 and 12 mo *(18–20)*. This suggests that both *de novo* and acquired resistance to trastuzumab occur, although very little is known on possible mechanisms of resistance to trastuzumab. No mechanism of resistance has yet been proven in the clinical setting, and most of the hypotheses discussed in this chapter derive from preclinical data.

2. INSULIN GROWTH FACTOR I RECEPTOR SIGNALING

Higher levels of circulating insulin growth factor (IGF)-I are associated with increased risk of several cancers including breast cancer. In addition, preclinical data supports evidence that the IGF signaling pathway is aberrantly activated breast cancer cells *(21–24)*. IGF-I signaling is known to activate several pathways involved in mitogenesis and cell survival *(25,26)*.

Lu et al. *(27)* demonstrated that an increased level of IGF-I receptor (IGF-IR) signaling interferes with trastuzumab's action on cell growth. These investigators used two human breast cancer cell lines complementary in terms of IGF-IR expression: MCF-7/HER-2-18 cells, which overexpress HER-2 by transfection and activated endogenous IGF-IRs, and SKBR3 cells, which exhibit *HER-2* gene amplification and low levels of IGF-IRs. In MCF-7/HER-2-18 cells, trastuzumab inhibited growth only when IGF-IR signaling was blocked by cotreatment with the anti-IGF-IR antibody α-IR3 or IGF-binding protein 3. Unlike the MCF-7/HER-2-18 cells, which were resistant to trastuzumab, the SKBR3 cells, which have a low level of IGF-IR expression, were sensitive to trastuzumab. Furthermore, the SKBR3 cells became resistant to trastuzumab when cells were genetically altered to overexpress IGF-IRs (SKBR3/IGF-IR). The addition of IGF-binding protein 3, which decreased IGF-IR signaling, restored the ability of trastuzumab to suppress growth. Thus, in breast cancer cells that overexpress HER-2, the increased levels of IGF-IR signaling interferes with the antitumor action of trastuzumab.

The same group (Lu et al. *[28]*) then proceeded to elucidate the underlying mechanism of trastuzumab resistance associated with IGF signaling. They reasoned that the interaction between IGF-IR signaling and trastuzumab occurred at the level of cell-cycle regulators, based on the fact that both IGF-I signaling (that causes upregulation of cyclins, cyclin-associated Cdk activity and downregulation of p27 *[29,30]*) and trastuzumab involve the Cdk inhibitor p27 *(11,13)*. SKBR3/neo cells (expressing few IGF-I receptors) and SKBR3/IGF-IR cells (overexpressing transfected IGF-I receptors) were used. In cells overexpressing IGF-IR, the increase in p27 induced by trastuzumab was attenuated by IGF-I. This was accompanied by an increase in Skp2 expression and an increase in the association of p27 with Skp2. Skp2 is an ubiquitin ligase for p27 and is required for its ubiquitination and subsequent degradation in the proteasome (31–33). LLnL, a highly specific proteasome inhibitor, completely blocked the ability of IGF-I to reduce p27 protein levels in trastuzumab-treated cells. Treatment with IGF-I decreased the association of p27 with Cdk2, markedly increased Cdk2 activity, and released cells from G_1 arrest, which had been suppressed by trastuzumab in the IGF-IR-overexpressing breast cancer cell line. Therefore, Lu et al. (28) concluded that the IGF-I-induced antagonism of trastuzumab-induced G_1 arrest involves targeting of p27 to the ubiquitin/proteasome degradation machinery.

To investigate the role of the Ras/Raf/mitogen-activated protein kinase (MAPK)/ MAPK extracellular signal-related kinase pathway and the phosphatidylinositol 3 kinase (PI3K) pathway in linking IGF-IR signaling to antagonism of trastuzumab action, Lu et al. (28) used PD98059 and LY294002, specific inhibitors of MAPK extracellular signal-related kinase pathway and PI3K, respectively. PD98059 reduced IGF-I-induced phosphorylation of MAPK, whereas LY294002 reduced IGF-I-induced phosphorylation of AKT in IGF-IR-overexpressing cells. MAPK inhibition did not influence the basal level of p27 or the trastuzumab-induced increase in p27 levels. IGF-I treatment still diminished the trastuzumab-induced increase in p27 in IGF-IR-overexpressing cells. However, blockade of the PI3K pathway increased the basal level of p27, whereas treatment with IGF-I did not attenuate the trastuzumab-induced increase in the p27. This provides evidence for an important role of the PI3K pathway in the action of IGF-I as an attenuator of trastuzumab-induced accumulation of p27. They also examined the roles of MAPK and PI3K on the effects of IGF-I-mediated Skp2 modulation. Trastuzumab reduced Skp2 levels. Consistent with the above-mentioned results, MAPK inhibition failed to influence the IGF-I-induced increase in Skp2, whereas PI3K inhibition eliminated this increase. This result suggests that the IGF-I-induced decrease in p27 is associated with a PI3K pathway-dependent increase in IGF-I-induced Skp2.

In summary, these findings suggest that trastuzumab leads to growth inhibition in cells where HER-2/neu is overexpressed. This inhibition can be compensated for by increased IGF-IR signaling, resulting in resistance to trastuzumab. IGF-IR-mediated resistance to trastuzumab treatment appears to involve the PI3K pathway, leading to enhanced degradation of p27. Future clinical studies combining trastuzumab with IGF signaling inhibitors will address the contribution of the latter pathway to trastuzumab resistance.

3. THE PI3K/AKT PATHWAY

Both genetic and biochemical data suggest that activation of the PI3K/Akt survival pathway contributes to breast cancer development and tumorigenesis:

1. Breast cancer predisposition is found in patients with familial syndromes characterized by germ-line phosphatase and tensin homologue deleted in chromosome ten ([PTEN]a 3-phosphoinositide-specific phosphatase) mutations (Cowden's, Bannayan-Zonana) (34,35). In spontaneous breast cancers, PTEN mutations are found in approx 5% of samples, and loss of heterozygosity of the PTEN locus is present in 40% (36–38).

2. In vitro transfection of wild-type PTEN into PTEN-negative breast cancer cells has been shown to decrease Akt activity and cause cell cycle arrest, apoptosis, or anoikis *(39,40)*.

3. Overexpression of constitutively active Akt in transgenic mice under the control of the mammary-specific Moloney murine tumor virus promoter results in mammary hyperplasia and/or is required for breast cancer formation in transgenic mice expressing Polyomavirus middle T antigen or IGF-II in the mammary gland *(41,42)*.

Akt is a downstream target of many receptor-stimulated pathways involved in breast cancer, including estrogen receptor (ER)-α, IGF-IR, epidermal growth factor receptor, and ErbB2 *(41,42)*. Amplification of the *Akt2* gene is found in 3% of spontaneous breast cancers *(43)*, and an inverse relationship between ER status and Akt3 activity has been described in both breast cancer cell lines and tumor specimens *(44)*.

Using a small molecule inhibitor of the PI3K/Akt pathway (LY294002) and transfection of Akt mutants, Clark et al. *(45)* demonstrated that Akt promotes breast cancer cell survival and resistance to trastuzumab. Using phosphospecific antibodies and in vitro kinase assays, they showed that Akt is constitutively active in four of six breast cancer cell lines that varied in ErbB2 and ER status, and that Akt activity was associated with mutant PTEN status or ErbB2 overexpression. Inhibition of the PI3K/Akt pathway with LY294002 or dominant-negative mutant Akt increased apoptosis, suggesting that HER-2-overexpressing breast cancer cells' survival is dependent on the PI3K/Akt pathway. LY294002 also potentiated apoptosis caused by trastuzumab, which suggests that the PI3K/Akt pathway plays a major role in regulating response to this therapeutic agent in HER-2-overexpressing breast cancer cells.

Yakes et al. *(46)* examined the role of PI3K/Akt on the antitumor effect of trastuzumab. They demonstrated that inhibition of PI3K and Akt is required for the antitumor action of trastuzumab against HER-2-overexpressing breast cancer cells. Several experiments corroborated this hypothesis:

1. In HER-2-overexpressing trastuzumab-sensitive cell lines, treatment with the antibody was associated with inhibition of active MAPK and active Akt.

2. Treatment of HER-2-overexpressing/trastuzumab-sensitive cells with trastuzumab also eliminated PI3K activity, as measured by the formation of PIP_3 in vitro.

3. The PI3K/Akt inhibitor LY294002 caused cell growth inhibition in a similar fashion as trastuzumab, suggesting a link between the inhibition of PI3K-Akt and the antiproliferative effect of trastuzumab.

4. Transduction of HER-2-overexpressing/trastuzumab-sensitive cells with an adenovirus-encoding active (myristoylated) Akt, but not with a β-galactosidase control adenovirus, prevented trastuzumab-induced inhibition of the cell proliferation and apoptosis of HER-2-overexpressing cells.

Taken altogether, these data imply that the disabling of the PI3K/Akt pathway is a key component for the antitumor effects of trastuzumab, and that constitutively activated/forced expression of Akt could be associated with resistance to trastuzumab in HER-2-overexpressing breast cancer cells.

4. CELL CYCLE AND P27

The Cdk inhibitor p27 is involved in regulating cell proliferation. p27 is a distal downstream effector of multiple converging growth factor receptor pathways including EGFR, HER-2, and IGF-IR. Trastuzumab increases the half-life of p27 by decreasing cyclin E/cdk2-mediated phosphorylation of p27 and blocking subsequent p27 ubiquitin-dependent degradation *(47)*. Trastuzumab also increases association between p27 and cdk2 complexes resulting in G_1 arrest *(13)*.

Nahta et al. *(48)* demonstrated that HER-2-overexpressing trastuzumab-resistant cells have low p27 levels, low p27/Cdk2 complexes and, thus, increased Cdk2 activity and proliferation rate. By flow cytometry, trastuzumab-resistant cells were found to have an increased S-phase fraction and reduced doubling time. When p27 levels and cdk2 kinase activity were examined in trastuzumab-resistant cells, they found that p27 was reduced irrespective of the increase in S phase, and cdk2 kinase activity was increased. Upon forcing p27 expression in trastuzumab-resistant cells via transfection or pharmacological induction with a proteasome inhibitor, they demonstrated that trastuzumab sensitivity was restored. These data suggest that a threshold level of Cdk2-associated p27 is important for the antitumor effect of trastuzumab.

Further evidence supports Akt-mediated regulation of p27:

1. Akt inhibits p27 protein levels *(49)* and AFX-mediated transcription of p27 *(50)* by phosphorylating fork head transcription factors and thus, excluding them from the nucleus.
2. Ectopic expression of PTEN *(51)* results in inhibition of PI3K and Akt, increase in p27 levels, and growth arrest *(52,53)*. Conversely, loss of PTEN function leads to derepression of Akt activity, down-regulation of p27, and cellular transformation *(54)*.
3. Akt can phosphorylate p27 directly in Thr-157; this modification results in cytoplasmic retention of p27 where it does not associate with Cdk2 *(55)*.

Consistent with the above data that implicates Akt in p27 regulation, Yakes et al. *(46)* demonstrated that treatment with either trastuzumab or LY294002 increased the levels of p27 in the nucleus>cytosol, thus increasing the ratio of p27:cdk2 in the nucleus and inhibiting cdk2 activity and cell proliferation. Transduction with an adenovirus encoding active prevented trastuzumab- or LY294002-induced downregulation of cyclin D1 and phosphorylation of GSK-3β and prevented the accumulation of p27 in the nucleus and cytosol. These data further corroborate that Akt inhibition is at least partially responsible for the changes in cell cycle- and apoptosis-regulatory molecules after HER-2 blockade with trastuzumab. Interestingly, Kute et al. *(56)* demonstrated that trastuzumab activation of Akt is downregulated even in trastuzumab-resistant clones of breast cancer cells. They found that there is a lower basal association of p27 with cdk2 in trastuzumab-resistant cells compared to trastuzumab-sensitive cells, and the addition of trastuzumab did not affect the p27/cdk2 association in resistant cells. Hence, resistance to trastuzumab appears to correlate with either low levels and/or cytosolic localization of p27.

5. OTHER POTENTIAL MECHANISMS

It is conceivable that other mechanisms of resistance to trastuzumab may have an important role, possibly in conjunction with better-defined pathway interactions. One could speculate that alterations in the HER-2 receptor or in downstream signaling pathways that mediate some of the trastuzumab's known mechanisms of action or are linked in a way to the HER-family pathway, may be responsible for resistance to trastuzumab *(57)*. To name a few, the presence of truncated HER-2 receptors that cannot bind antibodies, mutation of important downstream molecules associated with cell proliferation or apoptosis (e.g., members of the PI3k and MAPK pathways), a decrease in patient's immune effector function, overexpression of COX-2, heterodimerization with other members of the HER family, could all contribute at different levels for primary or acquired resistance to trastuzumab *(58)*.

6. CONCLUSIONS

The main mechanisms of resistance to trastuzumab known to date seem to evolve around complex interactions involving mainly the IGF-IR, PI3K/Akt and cell cycle regulatory (namely p27) pathways. Trastuzumab is known to downregulate Akt activity, increasing both phosphorylation and nuclear translocation of p27. This last step results in inhibition of cdk2 activity and the cells then remain in the G_1 phase of the cell cycle. Because the disabling of the PI3K/Akt pathway is a key component for the antitumor effects of trastuzumab, constitutively activated/forced expression of Akt could be associated with resistance to trastuzumab in HER-2-overexpressing breast cancer cells. Low levels and/or cytosolic localization of p27 could also account for trastuzumab resistance with or without associated downregulation of Akt activity. Trastuzumab associated inhibition in cells where HER-2 is overexpressed can be compensated for by increased IGF-IR signaling. This process predominantly involves the PI3K pathway, leading to enhanced degradation of p27, which ultimately could result in resistance to trastuzumab.

Despite many unanswered questions regarding mechanisms of resistance to trastuzumab, some progress has been made in developing and understanding HER-2-targeted therapies. In looking for ways to counteract trastuzumab resistance, it is conceivable that associations of trastuzumab with PI3K/Akt pathway inhibitors (e.g., mammalian target of rapamycin inhibitors), or cell cycle regulators (e.g., proteasome inhibitors) or IGF-I inhibitors (e.g., tyrosine kinase inhibitors) should be explored in a clinical setting. Another approach likely to be informative is rebiopsing HER-2-overexpressing accessible tumor tissues that escape therapy with trastuzumab after an initial response. In the meantime, preclinical studies will continue to be paramount in helping the design of successful clinical studies.

ACKNOWLEDGMENTS

Supported in part by R01 CA80195 (CLA), Breast Cancer Specialized Program of Research Excellence (SPORE) Grant P50 CA98131, and Vanderbilt-Ingram Cancer Center Support Grant P30 CA68485.

REFERENCES

1. Schechter AL, et al. The neu oncogene: an erb-B-related gene encoding a 185,000-Mr tumour antigen. Nature 1984; 312(5994):513–516.
2. Olayioye MA, et al. The ErbB signaling network: receptor heterodimerization in development and cancer. EMBO J 2000; 19(13):3159–3167.
3. Slamon DJ, et al. Human breast cancer: correlation of relapse and survival with amplification of the HER-2/neu oncogene. Science 1987; 235(4785):177–182.
4. Ullrich A, Schlessinger J. Signal transduction by receptors with tyrosine kinase activity. Cell 1990; 61(2):203–212.
5. Graus-Porta D, et al. ErbB-2, the preferred heterodimerization partner of all ErbB receptors, is a mediator of lateral signaling. EMBO J 1997; 16(7):1647–1655.
6. Segatto O, et al. The role of autophosphorylation in modulation of erbB-2 transforming function. New Biol 1990; 2(2):187–195.

7. Tzahar E, et al. A hierarchical network of interreceptor interactions determines signal transduction by Neu differentiation factor/neuregulin and epidermal growth factor. Mol Cell Biol 1996; 16(10):5276–5287.

8. Christianson TA, et al. NH2-terminally truncated HER-2/neu protein: relationship with shedding of the extracellular domain and with prognostic factors in breast cancer. Cancer Res 1998; 58(22):5123–5129.

9. Molina MA, et al. Trastuzumab (herceptin), a humanized anti-Her2 receptor monoclonal antibody, inhibits basal and activated Her2 ectodomain cleavage in breast cancer cells. Cancer Res 2001; 61(12):4744–4749.

10. Arteaga CL, Chinratanalab W, Carter MB. Inhibitors of HER2/neu (erbB-2) signal transduction. Semin Oncol 2001; 28(6 Suppl 18):30–35.

11. Baselga J, Albanell J. Mechanism of action of anti-HER2 monoclonal antibodies. Ann Oncol 2001; 12 Suppl 1:S35–S41.

12. Baselga J, et al. Mechanism of action of trastuzumab and scientific update. Semin Oncol 2001; 28(5 Suppl 16):4–11.

13. Lane HA, et al. Modulation of p27/Cdk2 complex formation through 4D5-mediated inhibition of HER2 receptor signaling. Ann Oncol 2001; 12 Suppl 1:S21–S22.

14. Sliwkowski MX, et al. Nonclinical studies addressing the mechanism of action of trastuzumab (Herceptin). Semin Oncol 1999; 26(4 Suppl 12):60–70.

15. Petit AM, et al. Neutralizing antibodies against epidermal growth factor and ErbB-2/neu receptor tyrosine kinases down-regulate vascular endothelial growth factor production by tumor cells in vitro and in vivo: angiogenic implications for signal transduction therapy of solid tumors. Am J Pathol 1997; 151(6):1523–1530.

16. Codony-Servat J, et al. Cleavage of the HER2 ectodomain is a pervanadate-activable process that is inhibited by the tissue inhibitor of metalloproteases-1 in breast cancer cells. Cancer Res 1999; 59(6):1196–1201.

17. Slamon DJ, et al. Use of chemotherapy plus a monoclonal antibody against HER2 for metastatic breast cancer that overexpresses HER2. N Engl J Med 2001; 344(11):783–792.

18. Vogel CL, et al. Efficacy and safety of trastuzumab as a single agent in first-line treatment of HER2-overexpressing metastatic breast cancer. J Clin Oncol 2002; 20(3):719–726.

19. Baselga J. Clinical trials of Herceptin(R) (trastuzumab). Eur J Cancer 2001; 37 Suppl 1:18–24.

20. Burstein HJ, et al. Clinical activity of trastuzumab and vinorelbine in women with HER2-overexpressing metastatic breast cancer. J Clin Oncol 2001; 19(10):2722–2730.

21. Hankinson SE, et al. Circulating concentrations of insulin-like growth factor-I and risk of breast cancer. Lancet 1998; 351(9113):1393–1396.

22. Holly J. Insulin-like growth factor-1 and risk of breast cancer. Lancet 1998; 352(9137):1388.

23. Nickerson T, Huynh H, Pollak M. Insulin-like growth factor binding protein-3 induces apoptosis in MCF7 breast cancer cells. Biochem Biophys Res Commun 1997; 237(3):690–693.

24. Yu H, et al. Insulin-like growth factor-binding protein-3 and breast cancer survival. Int J Cancer 1998; 79(6):624–628.

25. LeRoith D, et al. Molecular and cellular aspects of the insulin-like growth factor I receptor. Endocr Rev 1995; 16(2):143–63.

26. O'Connor R, Fennelly C, Krause D. Regulation of survival signals from the insulin-like growth factor-I receptor. Biochem Soc Trans 2000; 28(2):47–51.

27. Lu Y, et al. Insulin-like growth factor-I receptor signaling and resistance to trastuzumab (Herceptin). J Natl Cancer Inst 2001; 93(24):1852–1857.

28. Lu Y, Zi X, Pollak M. Molecular mechanisms underlying IGF-I-induced attenuation of the growth-inhibitory activity of trastuzumab (Herceptin) on SKBR3 breast cancer cells. Int J Cancer 2004; 108(3):334–341.

29. Dupont J, Karas M, LeRoith D. The potentiation of estrogen on insulin-like growth factor I action in MCF-7 human breast cancer cells includes cell cycle components. J Biol Chem 2000; 275(46):35,893–35,901.

30. Reiss K, et al. Insulin-like growth factor-1 receptor and its ligand regulate the reentry of adult ventricular myocytes into the cell cycle. Exp Cell Res 1997; 235(1):198–209.

31. Carrano AC, et al. SKP2 is required for ubiquitin-mediated degradation of the CDK inhibitor p27. Nat Cell Biol 1999; 1:193–199.

32. Nakayama K, et al. Targeted disruption of Skp2 results in accumulation of cyclin E and p27Kip1, polyploidy and centrosome overduplication. EMBO J 2000; 19:2069–2081.

33. Tsvetkov LM, et al. p27Kip1 ubiquitination and degradation is regulated by the SCF(Skp2) complex through phosphorylated Thr187 in p27. Curr Biol 1999; 9:661–664.

34. Lali FV, et al. The pyridinyl imidazole inhibitor SB203580 blocks phosphoinositide-dependent protein kinase activity, protein kinase B phosphorylation, and retinoblastoma hyperphosphorylation in interleukin-2-stimulated t cells independently of p38 mitogen-activated protein kinase. J Biol Chem 2000; 275:7395–7402.

35. Marsh DJ, et al. Germline mutations in PTEN are present in Bannayan-Zonana syndrome. 1997; 16:333–334.

36. Feilotter HE, et al. Analysis of the 10q23 chromosomal region and the PTEN gene in human sporadic breast carcinoma. Br J Cancer 1999; 79:718–723.

37. Rhei E, et al. Mutation analysis of the putative tumor suppressor gene PTEN/MMAC1 in primary breast carcinomas. Cancer Res 1997; 57:3657–3659.

38. Singh B, Ittmann MM, Krolewski JJ. Sporadic breast cancers exhibit loss of heterozygosity on chromosome segment 10q23 close to the Cowden disease locus. Genes Chromosomes Cancer 1998; 21:166–171.

39. Li J, et al. The PTEN/MMAC1 tumor suppressor induces cell death that is rescued by the AKT/protein kinase B oncogene. Cancer Res 1998; 58:5667–5672.

40. Lu Y, et al. The PTEN/MMAC1/TEP tumor suppressor gene decreases cell growth and induces apoptosis and anoikis in breast cancer cells. Oncogene 1999; 18:7034–7045.

41. Hutchinson J, et al. Activation of Akt (Protein Kinase B) in Mammary Epithelium Provides a Critical Cell Survival Signal Required for Tumor Progression. Mol Cell Biol 2001; 21:2203–2212.

42. Moorehead RA, et al. Inhibition of mammary epithelial apoptosis and sustained phosphorylation of Akt/PKB in MMTV-IGF-II transgenic mice. Cell Death Differ 2001; 8:16–29.

43. Bellacosa A, et al. Molecular alterations of the AKT2 oncogene in ovarian and breast carcinomas. Int J Cancer 1995; 64:280–285.

44. Nakatani K, et al. Up-regulation of Akt3 in Estrogen Receptor-deficient Breast Cancers and Androgen-independent Prostate Cancer Lines. J Biol Chem 1995; 274:21,528–21,532.

45. Clark AS, et al. Constitutive and inducible Akt activity promotes resistance to chemotherapy, trastuzumab, or tamoxifen in breast cancer cells. Mol Cancer Ther 2002; 1(9):707–717.

46. Yakes FM, et al. Herceptin-induced inhibition of phosphatidylinositol-3 kinase and Akt Is required for antibody-mediated effects on p27, cyclin D1, and antitumor action. Cancer Res 2002; 62(14):4132–4141.

47. Le XF, et al. The role of cyclin-dependent kinase inhibitor p27Kip1 in anti-HER2 antibody-induced G1 cell cycle arrest and tumor growth inhibition. J Biol Chem 2003; 278(26):23,441–23,450.

48. Nahta R, et al. P27(kip1) down-regulation is associated with trastuzumab resistance in breast cancer cells. Cancer Res 2004; 64(11):3981–3986.

49. Collado M, et al. inhibition of the phosphoinositide 3-kinase pathway induces a senescence-like arrest mediated by p27Kip1. J Biol Chem 2000; 275:21,960–21,968.

50. Medema RH, et al. AFX-like Forkhead transcription factors mediate cell-cycle regulation by Ras and PKB through p27kip1. Nature (Lond) 2000; 404:782–787.

51. Cantley LC, Neel BG. New insights into tumor suppression: PTEN suppresses tumor formation by restraining the phosphoinositide 3-kinase/AKT pathway. PNAS 1999; 96:4240–4245.

52. Li DM, Sun H. PTEN/MMAC1/TEP1 suppresses the tumorigenicity and induces G1 cell cycle arrest in human glioblastoma cells. Proc Natl Acad Sci U S A 1998; 95(26):15,406–15,411.

53. Sun H, et al. PTEN modulates cell cycle progression and cell survival by regulating phosphatidylinositol 3,4,5,-trisphosphate and Akt/protein kinase B signaling pathway. Proc Natl Acad Sci U S A 1999; 96(11):6199–6204.

54. Di Cristofano A, et al. Pten and p27KIP1 cooperate in prostate cancer tumor suppression in the mouse. Nat Genet 2001; 27(2):222–624.

55. Yakes FM, et al. Oncogene-activated Akt directly phosphorylates the cyclin-dependent kinase (Cdk) inhibitor p27kip1 and mediates cell cycle progression. Proc Am Assoc Cancer Res 2001; 238.

56. Kute T, et al. Development of Herceptin resistance in breast cancer cells. Cytometry 2004; 57A(2):86–93.

57. Albanell J, Baselga J. Unraveling resistance to trastuzumab (Herceptin): insulin-like growth factor-I receptor, a new suspect. J Natl Cancer Inst 2001; 93(24):1830–1832.

58. Cardoso F, et al. Resistance to trastuzumab: a necessary evil or a temporary challenge? Clin Breast Cancer 2002; 3(4):247–257; discussion 258–259.

25 Role of TGF-β in Tumor Progression and Metastasis

Jan Pinkas, *PhD* and Beverly A. Teicher, *PhD*

SUMMARY

The development of cancer has been shown to occur through a process of malignant transformation that involves a series of genetic changes that provide a selective advantage over normal cells, and research over the past few decades has identified numerous genes and pathways involved in all stages of tumor progression. These genetic changes invariably disrupt fundamental cellular processes controlling proliferation, apoptosis, differentiation, and genome stability, and it is the combinatorial effect of these genetic changes that result in malignant transformation. Proliferating hematopoietic and epithelial cell populations are particularly susceptible to accumulation of a series of genetic changes required for full-blown malignancy, and nearly 90% of all human solid tumors arise from epithelial cells. The majority of patients who succumb to cancer die as a result of metastatic disease progression rather than from the primary tumor. The process of metastasis is extremely complex, and involves many steps including dissemination of tumor cells from the primary tumor through the vascular and lymphatic system coupled with the ability to colonize selectively distant tissues and organs. The pleiotropic cytokine transforming growth factor-β and its signaling effectors have been shown to be involved at numerous steps in the development of cancer. The role of transforming growth factor-β signaling in cancer is complex, with biphasic functions as a tumor suppressor in normal tissue and early-stage lesions and as a prometastatic agent in late-stage disease.

Key Words: Transforming growth factor-β; transforming growth factor-β receptor; Smad; osteoclasts; fibrosis.

From: *Cancer Drug Discovery and Development: Cancer Drug Resistance*
Edited by: B. Teicher © Humana Press Inc., Totowa, NJ

1. INTRODUCTION

The development of cancer has been shown to occur through a process of malignant transformation that involves a series of genetic changes that provide a selective advantage over normal cells, and research over the past few decades has identified numerous genes and pathways involved in all stages of tumor progression *(1)*. These genetic changes invariably disrupt fundamental cellular processes controlling proliferation, apoptosis, differentiation, and genome stability, and it is the combinatorial effect of these genetic changes that result in malignant transformation *(1)*. Proliferating hematopoietic and epithelial cell populations are particularly susceptible to accumulation of a series of genetic changes required for full-blown malignancy, and nearly 90% of all human solid tumors arise from epithelial cells *(2)*. The majority of patients who succumb to cancer die as a result of metastatic disease progression rather than from the primary tumor *(3)*. The process of metastasis is extremely complex, and involves many steps including dissemination of tumor cells from the primary tumor through the vascular and lymphatic system coupled with the ability to colonize selectively distant tissues and organs *(4)*. The pleiotropic cytokine transforming growth factor-β (TGF-β) and its signaling effectors have been shown to be involved at numerous steps in the development of cancer, and the complex role of TGF-β in transformation and metastasis represent the focus of this chapter.

2. SIGNAL TRANSDUCTION BY TGF-β

2.1. TGF-β *Ligands and Receptors*

The TGF-β signal transduction pathway controls numerous cellular, developmental and homeostatic processes including proliferation, differentiation, apoptosis, cell fate specification, and extracellular matrix (ECM) production in species ranging from flies to mammals *(5)*. TGF-β was initially identified in culture supernatants from Moloney sarcoma virus-transformed mouse fibroblasts *(6)*, and was subsequently characterized as a 24-kDa homodimeric signaling molecule *(7–9)*. It became readily apparent that TGF-β ligands belonged to a superfamily of structurally related proteins including the activins and the bone morphogenetic proteins, and greater then 40 members of the TGF-β superfamily have been identified to date *(5)*.

Three mammalian TGF-β isoforms (TGF-β1, 2, and 3) have been identified that exhibit similar activities in in vitro cell-based assays, but gene deletion experiments clearly demonstrate distinct phenotypes for animals lacking any of the TGF-β ligands in vivo *(10)*. The TGF-β ligands are synthesized as homodimeric pro-proteins that are cleaved by furin-type proteases in the trans Golgi generating the mature TGF-β 24-kDa dimer noncovalently associated with the latency associated protein (LAP), and latent TGF-β-binding protein is frequently linked to LAP through disulfide bonds before the entire latent complex is secreted *(11)*. The latent TGF-β-binding protein is a member of the fibrillin family of structural proteins *(12)* that target and sequester latent TGF-β in the ECM. The latent TGF-β complex may represent an important safety measure against unintentional activation, and could provide a pool of TGF-β that could be rapidly activated without the need for protein synthesis.

A number of different mechanisms including protease activation, conformational changes, and reactive oxygen species have been described to activate latent TGF-β *(11)*. Tumor and endothelial cell lines frequently express elevated levels of components of the urokinase-type plasminogen activator system that can produce the protease plasmin *(13)*, and cell-based studies demonstrated that plasmin can directly activate latent TGF-β in vitro *(14)*. In addition, members of the metalloprotease family, matrix metalloproteinases 2 and 9, implicated in mediating the invasiveness of malignant cells *(15)* can also activate latent TGF-β *(16)*. This suggests that active TGF-β is released at sites of cell invasion and migration during angiogenesis and tumor development.

The activation of latent TGF-β can also be accomplished through nonproteolytic mechanisms. The extracellular matrix glycoprotein thrombospondin 1, which responds to alterations in matrix homeostasis, can activate latent TGF-β in addition to modulating cell adhesion, stimulating angiogenesis and reconstruction of the matrix during wound repair *(17)*. The $\alpha_v\beta_6$ integrin heterodimer that is expressed on the surface of epithelial cells in response to wounding or inflammation has been identified as an activator of latent TGF-β through a mechanism involving a conformational change in the TGF-β/LAP complex *(18)*. Reactive oxygen species produced in the mammary gland in vivo after irradiation are potent activators of latent TGF-β1 *(19)*. The bone matrix is rich in latent TGF-β *(20)*, and the acidic environment generated by osteoclasts during bone resorption can denature LAP and release active TGF-β *(21)*. Many of these mechanisms of latent TGF-β activation have been co-opted by tumors and their associated stroma, and should be available to induce signaling in the tumor cells.

Active TGF-β ligand stimulates signaling by binding to a heteromeric complex of single-pass transmembrane proteins, known as the type I and type II receptors. Additional levels of complexity are possible because vertebrates have seven type I and five type II receptors that are expressed in a developmentally regulated and tissue-specific manner that mediates signaling by the superfamily of TGF-β ligands *(5)*. In addition, there is a transmembrane proteoglycan with no intrinsic signaling capacity known as the type III receptor that binds with high affinity to all three TGF-β isoforms. It is thought that binding of TGF-β to the type III receptor increases the local concentration of ligand and enhances presentation of ligand to the type II receptor that has a lower intrinsic binding affinity for TGF-β *(22)*. Active ligand initially binds either to the type III receptor that presents TGF-β to the type II receptor or binds directly to the type II receptor. Binding of ligand then induces association with the type I receptor and allows the constitutively active type II receptor to transphosphorylate the type I receptor that activates its kinase domain *(5)*. The importance of the TGF-β signal transduction pathway is made clear by the numerous mechanisms that exist to control extracellular signaling by regulating the availability and activation of ligand, the interaction of active ligand with numerous heteromeric receptor complexes expressed in developmentally regulated and tissue-specific fashion, and the internalization and vesicular trafficking of activated receptors.

2.2. Mothers Against Decapentaplegic Homolog-Dependent Signal Transduction

There are eight vertebrate mothers against decapentaplegic homolog (Smad) proteins in three distinct classes that mediate signaling downstream of TGF-β, activin, and bone morphogenetic protein receptors *(23)*. The activated TGF-β type I receptor initiates intracellular signaling by carboxy-terminal phosphorylation of receptor-activated Smads (R-Smads), Smad2 and Smad3. Enhanced membrane targeting of R-Smads by the by the Smad anchor for receptor activation (SARA) auxiliary protein has been shown to facilitate recognition by the activated receptor complex. Receptor-mediated activation of Smad2/3 occurs at the plasma membrane, but the process is more efficient in early endosomes enriched in SARA *(24)*. The pathways regulating internalization of TGF-β receptors remain unclear, but the receptors have been shown to be internalized in a clathrin-dependent mechanism *(25)* and in cholesterol-rich lipid rafts containing caveolin 1

(26). Recently, an elegant study demonstrated that receptor activation can be regulated at the level of receptor internalization via vesicle trafficking *(27)*. Internalization of TGF-β receptors into early endosome antigen 1-positive endosomes enriched in SARA promoted signaling, and in contrast, receptor turnover was enhanced after internalization through the caveolin 1-rich lipid raft pathway *(27)*.

Phosphorylated R-Smads are then released from the active type I receptor and form heteromeric complexes with a common Smad4. The stoichiometry of the oligomeric Smad complex has been the subject of intense debate, and studies have demonstrated that both heterotrimers and heterodimers can be formed *(28)*. Phosphorylated R-Smads then translocate to the nucleus, where they can regulate gene transcription. Continuous receptor activation is required to maintain active Smads in the nucleus, because dephosphorylated Smads are rapidly exported to the cytoplasm *(28)*, but the nuclear phosphatase responsible for Smad dephosphorylation has not yet been identified. In the nucleus, heteromeric Smad complexes can mediate transcriptional activation or repression of target genes containing a minimal Smad-binding element in a cell-type-specific fashion through interactions with other DNA-binding factors, corepressors, and coactivators *(23)*. In addition, Smads have also been shown to be substrates for phosphorylation by components of the mitogen-activated protein kinase (MAPK) *(29)*, c-Jun N-terminal kinase *(30)*, and protein kinase C *(31)* pathways, and the functional consequences of these modifications are still being elucidated. It is evident that Smad-mediated regulation of gene transcription in response to TGF-β is highly cell-type specific and context dependent.

2.3. Smad-Independent Signal Transduction

More recently, TGF-β has been shown to activate other Smad-independent signal transduction cascades, including the ERK, c-Jun N-terminal kinase, and p38 MAPK pathways. Studies utilizing mutated type I receptors that are defective in Smad phosphorylation demonstrated that p38 MAPK is still activated in response to TGF-β *(32)*. In addition, TGF-β-induced activation of MAPK pathways can also enhance transcriptional activity through phosphorylation of either Smad *(30)* or of interacting activating transcription factor 2 and c-Jun transcription factor complexes *(33,34)*. TGF-β-induced activation of the Ras/MAPK pathway can also stimulate TGF-β1 expression resulting in amplification of responses *(35)*. The ability of TGF-β to coordinately activate Smads and MAPK signaling has been shown to mediate epithelial to mesenchymal transformation (EMT) *(36,37)*, and cellular responses to TGF-β depend on the balance between direct activation of Smads and MAPK pathways.

Several Rho-like GTPases have also been shown to be activated by TGF-β through Smad-independent mechanisms. TGF-β enhanced the expression of RhoB by increasing protein stability through inhibition of its proteosomal degradation *(38)*, and TGF-β-mediated induction of the NET1 guanine nucleotide exchange factor stimulated the activation of RhoA *(39,40)*. These Rho-like GTPases have been shown to mediate TGF-β-induced changes in cytoskeletal organization that are associated with stress fiber formation *(37)* and EMT *(39,41)*. Recently, a novel Smad independent and Rho-like GTPase dependent pathway has been identified in fibroblast cells that regulate morphologic transformation. p21-activated kinase 2 was shown to be activated in a panel of fibroblast cell lines but not in epithelial cells in response to TGF-β signaling, and the activation of p21-activated kinase 2 was regulated by the Rac1 and Cdc42 GTPases *(42)*. These results demonstrate that TGF-β signaling can activate cell-type-specific Rho GTPases to mediate morphologic transformation of epithelial and fibroblast cells through Smad-independent mechanisms.

TGF-β-induced activation of the type I receptor can also stimulate signaling through protein phosphatase 2A (PP2A) and the phosphatidylinositol 3 kinase (PI3K) pathways. The inhibitory Bα regulatory subunit of PP2A can associate with the activated type I receptor, and this interaction results in the release of the active catalytic domain of PP2A *(43)*. Active PP2A can dephosphorylate and inactivate p70[S6K], leading to growth arrest through a Smad-independent mechanism *(44)*. The PI3K effector protein kinase B (PKB) has also been shown to be phosphorylated and activated in response to TGF-β resulting in enhanced cell survival. The activation of PKB in response to TGF-β can be either direct *(45)* or indirect through increased TGF-α expression and consequent EGF receptor stimulation *(46)*. In addition, it was recently reported that in response to insulin signaling PKB can interact with unphosphorylated Smad3 and sequester it outside the nucleus *(47,48)*. This interaction resulted in the inhibition of Smad3-mediated transcription and attenuation of TGF-β-induced apoptosis, and the ratio of Smad3 to PKB correlated with the sensitivity of cells to TGF-β-induced apoptosis *(47,48)*. These results clearly demonstrate that numerous mechanisms exist to integrate signals from growth factor and TGF-β-mediated pathways in a highly cell-type-specific fashion.

3. TGF-β IN CANCER

3.1. Multifunctional Role of TGF-β in Cancer

The role of TGF-β signaling in cancer is complex, with biphasic functions as a tumor suppressor in normal tissue and early-stage lesions and as a prometastatic agent in late-stage disease. During normal development and tissue homeostasis, TGF-β signaling functions to restrain proliferation through induction of cytostatic and apoptotic gene expression programs *(49)*. The tumor-suppressive ability of TGF-β has been clearly demonstrated both in experimental model systems as well as in studies of human malignancies. The TGF-β-induced cytostatic gene expression program has primarily been elucidated in studies with epithelial and lymphoid cells and minimally includes activation of cyclin-dependent kinase inhibitors p15[INK4B] and p21[WAF1] and repression/growth-enhancing transcription factors c-Myc and ID1-3 *(50)*. The growth suppressive effects of TGF-β have also been clearly demonstrated in animal models. Transgenic expression of TGF-β1 in mammary gland *(51,52)*, skin *(53)*, pancreas *(54)*, and liver *(55,56)* promoted growth arrest and in some settings enhanced apoptosis. Furthermore, coexpression of TGF-β1 markedly suppressed mammary tumor development induced by transgenic expression of TGF-α or carcinogen treatment *(57)*. These in vitro and in vivo studies provided evidence that TGF-β can function as a tumor suppressor through induction of antiproliferative and apoptotic gene expression programs.

Conversely, attenuation of TGF-β signaling has been correlated with tumor progression and enhanced metastatic potential in both animal models and human patient samples. Transgenic expression of dominant-negative TGF-βII receptor enhanced carcinogen-induced lung *(58)* and mammary tumorigenesis *(59)*. Mice with ablation of the *Tgf-β1* or the *Smad3* genes develop adenomas in the colon that progress to frank carcinomas *(60,61)*. In addition, mice heterozygous for the *Tgf-β1* gene that only express ~10–25% of normal protein levels demonstrate enhanced carcinogen-induced tumor development *(62)*. Germline or sporadic mutation of components of the TGF-β signal transduction pathway has also been shown to occur in human cancers. Inactivating mutations in the TGF-βII receptor have been identified in a subset of sporadic and hereditary colon cancers characterized by microsatellite instability (MSI), and reconstitution of TGF-βII receptor expression in colorectal carcinoma cell lines with MSI reversed transformation *(63)*. Inactivating mutations in the *Smad2* and *Smad4* genes have also been identified in colorectal and pancreatic carcinomas *(64,65)*. Sporadic mutations in the TGF-βI receptor have been identified at low frequency in breast *(66)*, ovarian *(67)*, and pancreatic *(68)* carcinomas. The incidence of germline or sporadic mutations in components of the TGF-β signal transduction pathway in solid malignancies appears to occur at low frequency, with the exception of pancreatic carcinoma and MSI colorectal carcinoma. Recently, polymorphisms in the *TGF-β1* gene have been associated with decreased 5-yr survival in a study of breast cancer patients *(69)*, and multiple polymorphisms in the *TGFBRI* gene have correlated with an increased risk of breast and ovarian cancer as well as hematologic malignancies *(70,71)*, but not with disease progression in prostate cancer *(72)*. The functional consequences of these polymorphisms on TGF-β signaling remain unclear and await further study.

The majority of cancers retain TGF-βI/II receptors but have attenuated growth-inhibitory responses to TGF-β through subversion of the normal cytostatic gene expression program and activation of the PI3K and Ras signal transduction pathways. With the loss of antimitogenic effects of TGF-β, tumor cells demonstrate increased motility and elevated matrix protease activity *(37,73)*, and many tumors and their associated stromal cells increase their production of TGF-β *(74)*, which is a potent regulator of fibroblast-mediated ECM expression *(75)*. Elevated TGF-β levels have been shown to induce an EMT of normal and transformed epithelial cells, which can result in enhanced migratory ability *(76)*. The increased migratory capacity of epithelial cells that have undergone EMT is mediated by repression of the cell–cell adhesion protein, E-cadherin, and induction of fibroblast-specific markers *(77)*. Multiple signal transduction pathways have been implicated in TGF-β-induced EMT, and the process requires both Smad-dependent and -independent signals *(78)*. A potent synergy has been demonstrated between the TGF-β and Ras/MAPK pathways in promoting EMT and enhancing the invasive and metastatic properties of malignant cells *(77,79)*.

Strong evidence exists from animal models that residual TGF-β signaling can promote late-stage tumor progression and enhance metastasis. Studies with mice heterozygous for the *Tgf-β1* gene demonstrated enhanced carcinogen-induced tumorigenesis, and tumors that developed retained the remaining wild-type *Tgf-β1* allele indicating that there was no selective pressure to abrogate completely TGF-β signaling *(62)*. In addition, transgenic mice expressing TGF-β1 in keratinocytes developed fewer carcinogen-induced benign papillomas in the skin, but the rate of conversion of benign lesions into invasive spindle cell carcinomas was dramatically increased in the TGF-β1 transgenic mice *(80)*. These results demonstrate the multifunctional activity of TGF-β as both a tumor suppressor and as a prometastatic agent.

TGF-β has also been shown to act as a potent suppressive cytokine with effects on normal hematopoietic homeostasis as well as attenuating host antitumor immune responses *(74,81–83)*. Studies with genetically engineered mice identified a critical role for TGF-β1 in homeostasis of T-lymphocytes. Genetic deletion of the *Tgf-β1* gene *(84–87)*, abrogation of signaling through transgenic expression of dominant-negative TGF-βII receptor in T-cells *(88)*, or reconstitution of lethally irradiated mice with dominant-negative TGF-βII receptor-transduced bone marrow *(89)* resulted in the development of a lethal, multifocal inflammatory disease. These studies highlight the important role that

TGF-β1 plays in limiting T-cell proliferation during normal tissue homeostasis. It has been hypothesized that expression of TGF-β1 by malignant epithelial cells or associated stromal cells in the tumor microenvironment mediate tumor progression through suppressive effects on a number immune effector cell populations.

The ability of the host immune system to induce tumor-specific T-cells in patients with advanced cancer has been well documented *(90–92)*, but the eradication of established tumors by endogenous immune responses is rare. It is clear that tumors can tolerize host immune responses raised against the malignant lesion *(93)*, and recent evidence has implicated regulatory T-cells (Treg cells) as key players in tumor-mediated immunosuppression *(94)*. Elevated levels of Treg cells have been identified in the blood and tumor tissue of cancer patients *(95–98)*. A recent study revealed a strong predictive correlation between increasing intratumoral Treg cell numbers and reduced survival in patients with ovarian carcinoma *(99)*, and numerous studies have demonstrated that Treg cells can potently suppress the activation of CD4+ and CD8+ T-cells *(95,100–103)* and natural killer (NK) cells *(95)*. Furthermore, TGF-β1 has been shown to regulate directly the development of Treg cells in vitro and in vivo *(104–106)*, and this may represent a major mechanism by which TGF-β1 promotes tumor progression. Several experiments with mouse lymphoma, melanoma, and prostate carcinoma tumor models have validated the hypothesis that inhibition of TGF-β1-mediated immunosuppression can have strong therapeutic potential in the treatment of cancer. Transgenic mice expressing dominant-negative TGF-β type II receptor in T-cells mounted potent antitumor immune responses after inoculation of EL-4 lymphoma or B16-F10 melanoma cells in contrast to control mice that were unable to activate CD4+ and CD8+ T-cell antitumor immune responses and rapidly succumbed to tumor growth *(107)*. Mice reconstituted with dominant-negative TGF-β type II receptor-transduced bone marrow that were insensitive to TGF-β-mediated suppression of T-cell responses survived challenge with B16-F10 melanoma or TRAMP-C2 metastatic prostate carcinoma cells as compared to control mice *(108)*. In addition, studies with a mouse fibrosarcoma tumor model have identified a novel mechanism that can suppress CD8+ T-cell antitumor immune responses independent of Treg cell function. A nonlymphoid splenic cell of the myeloid lineage has been described that can be induced to secrete TGF-β1 and directly suppress antitumor activity of cytolytic T-cells *(109,110)*. These studies suggest that elevated TGF-β levels in tumor-bearing animals can suppress host T-cell responses raised against the malignant lesion through a number of different mechanisms.

In addition to its well-described role in suppression of cytolytic T-cell responses, TGF-β has also been shown to inhibit the activation of NK cells in cancer patients. Plasma TGF-β1 levels were significantly elevated in human lung and colorectal carcinoma patients as compared to normal volunteers, and cell surface expression of the NK cell activation marker NKG2D was inversely correlated with plasma TGF-β1 levels *(111)*. Incubation of NK cells with plasma isolated from cancer patients or exogenous TGF-β1 specifically reduced cell surface levels of NKG2D, without modulating expression of other NK cell receptors *(111)*. TGF-β1 has also been shown to downregulate the expression of NKp30, which represents the major receptor involved in NK-mediated cell killing of immature dendritic cells (DCs), and it has been hypothesized that this could inhibit the selection of DCs undergoing maturation *(112)*. These results indicate that TGF-β1 impairs multiple NK cell functions through downregulation of specific cell surface receptors. Immunosuppression in cancer patients can also be mediated through direct effects on DCs *(113)*, which are specialized antigen-presenting cells that initiate primary immune responses, and manipulating DC function is an area of intense investigation for the active immunotherapy of cancer *(114)*. TGF-β1 can interfere with DC function through down-regulation of cell surface class I and class II major histocompatibility complex antigens, costimulatory molecules, and chemokine receptors in vitro *(115–117)*, and tumor-derived TGF-β1 has been shown to reduce the efficacy of DC vaccines in mouse tumor models *(118,119)*. These studies demonstrate clearly that TGF-β can act as a potent immunosuppressive cytokine on cells from multiple lineages to attenuate antitumor immune responses.

3.2. Breast Cancer

The role of TGF-β signaling in the development and progression of breast cancer has been studied extensively, and as in other systems, TGF-β has been shown to play a dual role as a potent growth inhibitor in early-stage disease and as a pro-oncogenic factor in late-stage disease *(120)*. The majority of breast cancers express elevated levels of TGF-β1 ligand in the tumor microenvironment associated with either malignant epithelial cells *(121,122)*, stromal cells *(123)* or both. A recent study of a large panel of breast cancers (456 cases) demonstrated that more then 90% of the tumors expressed phosphorylated Smad2, indicating that TGF-β signaling was intact *(124)*, but it is possible that other signal transduction pathways can modulate the phosphorylation status of Smad2 in these tumors. In addition, numerous studies have identified a strong correlation between elevated plasma TGF-β1 levels and disease progression in breast cancer *(123,125,126)*. Pre- and postoperative plasma TGF-β1 levels associated tightly with clinical outcome in a small study of newly diagnosed breast cancer patients *(123)*. Patients whose plasma TGF-β1 levels normalized after resection of the tumor had a favorable prognosis, and patients with persistently elevated levels of TGF-β1 in the plasma had an increased risk of lymph node metastases and disease progression *(123)*. These studies suggest that plasma TGF-β1 levels might be a useful prognostic factor for advanced disease.

Furthermore, increased immunoreactivity for TGF-β protein has been correlated with an adverse prognosis *(121,127,128)* and increased lymph node involvement *(122)*. Elevated expression of TGF-β was associated with resistance to therapy with the antiestrogen tamoxifen *(129)*. Studies with human MCF-7 breast carcinoma cells demonstrated significant induction in expression of components of the TGF-β signal transduction pathway after culture in the absence of estrogen *(130–132)*. Clonal MCF-7 cell lines expressing elevated levels of TGF-β1 promoted tumor development in the absence of estrogens *(133)*, and tumor development was attenuated after combination therapy with tamoxifen and an antibody that neutralizes all three active TGF-β isoforms, but not after treatment with either agent alone *(133,134)*. Recently, a highly significant association was identified between TGF-β type II receptor expression and reduced disease-free survival in estrogen receptor-negative breast cancer patients *(135)*, suggesting that tumor promoting functions of TGF-β are involved in disease progression.

Several recent studies elegantly elucidated the dual tumor suppressive and prometastatic functions of TGF-β signaling using bitransgenic mouse models of breast cancer. Transgenic expression of the *neu* oncogene driven by the mouse mammary tumor virus long-terminal repeat produces multifocal mammary adenocarcinomas that are metastatic to lung *(136,137)*, and this is a highly relevant model, because amplification of the *Her-2/neu* epidermal growth factor tyrosine kinase gene is a frequent event in human breast cancer *(138–140)*. Transgenic mice expressing constitutively activated and dominant-negative TGF-β receptors were developed to determine the role of TGF-β signaling in modulating Neu-induced mammary tumorigenesis and metastasis *(141)*. Coexpression of constitutively activated TGF-β type I receptor significantly increased the latency of Neu-induced primary mammary tumors, and conversely, transgenic expression of dominant-negative TGF-β type II receptor decreased the latency of tumor development *(141)*. These studies clearly demonstrated the tumor-suppressive functions of TGFβ in Neu-induced mammary tumorigenesis. In contrast, the prometastatic abilities of TGF-β signaling were also revealed in these bitransgenic models of breast cancer. Mice coexpressing activated TGF-β type I receptor *(141)* or activated TGF-β1 *(142)* and Neu had an increased incidence of extravascular metastatic foci in the lung. These studies demonstrated that abrogation of TGF-β signaling could inhibit late-stage tumor development and metastasis.

Furthermore, studies utilizing a doxycycline (DOX)-inducible transgenic promoter provided additional evidence supporting a role for TGF-β1 as a prometastatic factor in a mouse model of breast cancer *(143)*. Previous studies demonstrated that transgenic expression of polyoma virus middle T oncogene (PyMT) driven by mouse mammary tumor virus long-terminal repeat potently induced multifocal mammary tumors that were metastatic to lung *(144)*. The role of TGF-β1 in tumor progression and metastasis was determined by generating triple transgenic mice where DOX-inducible active TGF-β1 could be expressed in PyMT-transformed mammary epithelial cells in a temporal and spatial fashion *(143)*. Mice with palpable mammary tumors were treated with DOX to induce expression of active TGF-β1 resulting in no effect on the growth kinetics of the primary mammary tumors, but induction for as little as 2 wk resulted in a more then 10-fold increase in metastatic lesions in the lung *(143)*. Several lines of evidence suggested that active TGF-β1 mediated these prometastatic effects through a direct effect on the mammary tumor cells rather than by paracrine effects on associated tumor stromal, endothelial, and immune cells. Elevated levels of active TGF-β1 and phosphorylated Smad2 were primarily found in PyMT-expressing mammary epithelium, but a threefold elevation in serum TGF-β1 levels were seen in animals after induction with DOX, suggesting that paracrine or systemic effects could contribute to the increased lung metastasis *(143)*. It will be technically challenging to design studies to determine the exact contribution of TGF-β1-mediated autocrine versus paracrine/systemic effects that contribute to increased metastasis.

Numerous studies have provided evidence that attenuation of TGF-β signaling can modulate tumor progression and metastasis in a cell autonomous fashion. Expression of dominant-negative TGF-β type II receptor in a series of genetically related cell lines derived from nontransformed MCF-10A human mammary epithelial cells could cooperate with Ras to enhance tumorigenesis of a premalignant cell line *(145)*. Conversely, dominant-negative TGF-β type II receptor expression in a high-grade metastatic cell line had no effect on primary tumor development, but markedly inhibited metastatic capability *(145)*. The TGF-β pathway has also been shown to play a critical role in tissue-specific metastasis of breast cancer cells to bone. Human breast cancers frequently metastasize to bone, resulting in significant clinical symptoms such as pathologic fractures and pain because of osteolytic bone destruction *(146–148)*. Studies with human breast carcinoma cell lines in a mouse bone tumor model have identified a molecular basis for this tissue tropism. Inoculation of MDA-MB-23-231 human breast carcinoma cells into the left ventricle of nude mice seeds cells into the arterial circulation and consistently produces osteolytic bone lesions and visceral metastases with short latency *(149)*. Tumor cells growing in the bone microenvironment have been shown to express elevated levels of parathyroid hormone-related peptide (PTHrP) *(150)*, which can potently stimulate activation of osteoclasts and bone resorption *(151,152)*. Constitutively activated TGF-β type I receptor enhanced the expression of PTHrP in MDA-MB-23-231 cells in vitro and promoted increased osteolytic bone destruction in vivo *(152)*, and expression of dominant-negative TGF-β type II receptor inhibited PTHrP expression and osteolytic bone tumor development *(153)*. Recently, an elegant study elucidated a multigenic expression program activated by TGF-β that regulates bone- *(154)* and adrenal gland-specific *(155)* metastasis of MDA-MB-23-231 human breast carcinoma cells. These studies clearly link dysregulated TGF-β signaling with the growth of osteolytic breast cancer metastases, and suggest that this may represent an important point for therapeutic intervention in advanced breast cancer.

3.3. Prostate Cancer

Elevated levels of TGF-β1 are consistently found in prostate cancer as compared to normal prostate tissue from human patients *(156–160)*. Furthermore, expression of TGF-β1 appeared to be an early event in prostate cancer *(161)*, with expression increasing during tumor progression and metastasis *(157,159,160,162)*. Patients with hormone refractory and recurrent prostate cancer frequently present with osteoblastic bone lesions that are thought to be stimulated by TGF-β released from tumor microenvironment or the bone matrix *(147,148)*. No consistent role for TGF-β2 or -3 in prostate cancer has yet been clearly identified *(158,163)*, but a recent study demonstrated that prostate-specific antigen could specifically activate latent TGF-β2, suggesting that alternate mechanisms exist for autocrine regulation of TGF-β activation in prostate cancer *(164)*. In addition, several studies have identified a strong correlation between elevated preoperative plasma TGF-β1 levels and prostate cancer progression and metastasis in patients undergoing radical prostatectomy for locally advanced disease *(165–167)*. Elevated postoperative plasma TGF-β1 levels were predictive for disease recurrence and metastasis *(167)*, indicating that micrometastatic lesions were already established at the time of surgical resection of the primary tumor. Recently, a microarray analyses of a panel of prostate carcinomas identified a gene expression signature that correlated with tumor stage as measured by Gleason score *(168,169)*. The expression of TGF-β type II receptor was consistently downregulated during disease progression in several independent panels of prostate carcinomas *(168,169)* in agreement with previous reports in the literature *(157,170–172)*, but the expression of several TGF-β-induced genes involved in ECM deposition (collagen 1A) and bone-specific metastasis (osteopontin) were significantly elevated and correlated with increasing Gleason grade *(168)*. These results suggest that tumor cells loose growth inhibitory responses to TGF-β1 while maintaining prometastatic activities during disease progression in prostate cancer.

Studies with prostate epithelial cell lines demonstrated that loss of growth inhibitory responses to TGF-β mediated by reduced expression of the type I and II receptors correlated with malignant transformation *(173,174)*, and malignant cells frequently increased expression of TGF-β1 *(173)*. This reduction in sensitivity to TGF-β1-mediated growth inhibition was also seen in prostate carcinoma cell lines growing in vitro as compared to nontumorigenic prostate epithelial cells *(63,175,176)*. Androgen-independent prostate carcinoma cells, DU145, PC-3, and LNCaP, which are resistant to chemotherapy, secreted elevated levels of TGF-β1 into the culture medium when grown in vitro, and animals bearing tumor xenografts of these cell lines had increased plasma levels of TGF-β1 *(177)*. In addition, treatment of animals bearing prostate carcinoma xenografts with cytotoxic chemotherapy led to a time dependent induction of plasma TGF-β1 that correlated with the degree of drug resistance of the tumor cell lines *(177)*. This study provides data supporting the hypothesis that TGF-β1 expression can contribute to drug resistance of prostate carcinoma.

A strong mechanistic connection between TGF-β1 expression and metastatic ability has been demonstrated utilizing a rat prostate carcinoma cell line. Overexpression of TGF-β1 in the Dunning R3327 MATLyLu rat prostate carcinoma cell line resulted in enhanced primary tumor growth rate and metastasis to the lung and lymph node after subcutaneous implantation *(161,178)*, and conversely, reduction of TGF-β1 levels by stably expressing an antisense oligonucleotide in the MATLyLu prostate carcinoma cell line inhibited primary tumor growth and metastasis *(179)*. These studies clearly demonstrate that TGF-β1 expression can enhance the metastatic capacity of rat prostate carcinoma cell lines, but it is unclear whether this prometastatic activity is mediated through autocrine effects on the prostate carcinoma cells or through paracrine effects on associated stromal, endothelial, and immune cells.

Numerous studies have demonstrated that the stroma plays a significant role in tumorigenesis in the prostate *(180, 183)*, but the role of TGF-β in this process has not been clearly defined. Carcinoma-associated fibroblasts (CAF) derived from prostate carcinomas can stimulate tumor progression of nontransformed prostate epithelial cells in an in vivo tissue recombination system *(184)*. In addition, TGF-β1 expression was significantly higher in CAF than in fibroblasts derived from normal human prostate, and increasing levels of TGF-β1 expression correlated with the capacity of CAF to promote malignant transformation of normal prostate epithelial cells *(185)*. Furthermore, normal human prostate fibroblasts could be converted to CAF in vitro by exposure to TGF-β1 in the culture medium, suggesting that prostate carcinoma cell-derived TGF-β1 could support the development of reactive stroma *(181)*. However, it is unclear whether CAF influence tumor development by secretion of factors that promote a reactive ECM and enhance angiogenesis or that directly stimulate proliferation of tumor cells. The role of stromal cells in prostate tumorigenesis was addressed using a coculture xenograft model. LNCaP prostate carcinoma cells formed tumors very inefficiently when implanted as xenografts into immune compromised mice, and mixing tumor cells with tumor-derived ECM components (Matrigel) promoted tumor incidence *(186)* in agreement with previous studies in the literature *(187,188)*. Tumor incidence could be dramatically increased by cotransplanting LNCaP carcinoma cells with CAF and Matrigel, and the xenograft tumors constructed this way had significantly enhanced angiogenesis as measured by a more then 10-fold increase in microvessel density *(186)*. Inclusion of LAP to neutralize TGF-β during the generation of the LNCaP differential reactive stroma tumor xenografts reduced microvessel density 3.5-fold and tumor weight by nearly 50% *(189)*, but it is unclear whether the TGF-β1 is being secreted from the prostate carcinoma cells, the CAF or both. These studies clearly demonstrate that TGF-β produced in the tumor microenvironment can have direct effects on prostate epithelial cells as well as paracrine effects on tumor associated stromal and endothelial cells.

4. THERAPEUTIC INTERVENTION

Several approaches are being pursued to develop TGF-β antagonists primarily for the treatment of fibrotic disorders and cancer *(190,191)*. The most advanced of these approaches focuses on the development of large molecule inhibitors, which include monoclonal antibodies, soluble receptors, and antisense oligonucleotides. Multiple human and mouse monoclonal and rabbit polyclonal antibodies that neutralize active TGF-β isoforms by blocking ligand access to the receptors have been described. Phage display technology was utilized to develop recombinant human antibodies that selectively neutralize specific TGF-β isoforms, and these antibodies are currently being evaluated in a number of clinical trials for the treatment of fibrotic disorders. A human monoclonal antibody, CAT-152, which neutralizes TGF-β2, is currently in phase III trials for prevention of scarring induced by glaucoma surgery *(192)*, and a second recombinant human monoclonal antibody, CAT-192, which selectively targets TGF-β1 *(193)*, was examined in a phase I/II trial for the treatment of scleroderma. Two pan-neutralizing mouse monoclonal antibodies, 1D11 *(194)* and 2G7 *(195)*, have been utilized extensively to demonstrate the therapeutic potential of TGF-β antagonism in mouse tumor models. Mouse and human tumor cell lines frequently secrete elevated levels of TGF-β isoforms in vitro and in vivo *(74,196)* and have been useful models to examine the therapeutic potential of TGF-β antagonists. The growth of MDA-MB-23-231 human breast carcinoma cells implanted intra-abdominally was significantly reduced after treatment with 2G7, and antitumor activity correlated with enhanced cell killing mediated by splenic NK cells *(133)*.

Several reports have demonstrated that tumor resistance to chemotherapy in vitro and in vivo can be reversed with TGF-β antagonist treatment. Tamoxifen-resistant LCC2 breast carcinoma cells express elevated levels of TGF-β2 as compared to the tamoxifen-sensitive cell line LCC1, and combination treatment with tamoxifen and the pan-neutralizing TGF-β antibody 2G7 inhibited the growth of LCC2 human breast carcinoma xenografts as compared to treatment with either agent alone *(134)*. In addition, a critical role for NK cells in mediating antitumor activity was identified supporting a role for tumor-derived TGF-β in suppressing host immune surveillance *(134)*. Studies with MDA-MB-23-231 cells grown three-dimensionally as spheroids in vitro demonstrated that treatment with 2G7 enhanced cell killing by the alkylating agent cisplatin (CDDP), suggesting that tumor-derived TGF-β may contribute to drug resistance of malignant cells *(197)*. Drug-resistant sublines of the EMT6 mouse mammary carcinoma cell line were generated in vivo by treatment of tumor-bearing animals with alkylating agents cyclophosphamide (CTX) and CDDP over a 6-mo period *(198)*. Treatment of animals bearing drug-resistant tumors with TGF-β neutralizing antibodies *(199)* or the leucine-rich proteoglycan decorin *(200)* increased the sensitivity of the EMT6-CTX tumors to CTX and the EMT6-CDDP tumors to CDDP. These studies reveal a role for TGF-β in contributing to drug resistance in vitro and in vivo, and suggest that TGF-β antagonists may be effective in the treatment of drug resistant tumors.

Several large molecule protein therapeutics have been developed to neutralize active TGF-β isoforms *(190,191)*. The extracellular ligand-binding domain of the TGF-β type II receptor has been fused to the Fc domain of human IgG$_1$ (abbreviated Fc: TβRII or SR2F) to produce a high-affinity and stable antagonist capable of neutralizing TGF-β1 and -β3 isoforms *(201,202)*. Transgenic expression of high levels of systemic SR2F did not result in significant pathology as was seen in the TGF-β1$^{-/-}$ gene deletion mice, but it did suppress spontaneous metastasis from primary mammary tumors *(203)*. In addition, studies utilizing purified Fc: TβRII protein demonstrated an inhibition of spontaneous lung metastasis from orthotopically implanted 4T1 and EMT6 mammary carcinomas *(204)*. A recent study identified CD8$^+$ T cells as key mediators of Fc: TβRII mediated antitumor activity in a syngeneic model of malignant mesothelioma *(205)*. Antibodies designed to neutralize active TGF-β isoforms have potent antitumor activities in rodent models of melanoma *(206)*, multiple myeloma *(207)*, and prostate carcinoma *(189)*.

Small-molecule inhibitors have also been developed that target the serine/threonine kinase activity of the TGF-β type I receptor and inhibit the phosphorylation of Smad-2/3 *(208–210)*. These compounds have proven to be effective against TGF-β-induced EMT of normal mammary epithelial cells *(208)* and migration and invasion phenotype of pancreatic carcinoma cells *(211)*. Recently, the SD-208 inhibitor was shown to inhibit the growth of intracranial gliomas in a syngeneic mouse model, and antitumor efficacy correlated strongly with increased infiltration of NK cells, CD8[+] T cells, and macrophages into the tumor *(212)*. However, many of the small molecules have also been shown to inhibit other TGF-β type I receptors such as ALK4, resulting in the modulation of activin-dependent Smad activation *(209)*. The significance of this activity against other TGF-β type I receptors in addition to ALK5 is unclear.

5. SUMMARY AND CONCLUSIONS

The TGF-β signal transduction pathway has been shown to play a critical role in normal development and tissue homeostasis by inhibiting aberrant cellular proliferation through induction of cytostatic and apoptotic gene expression programs. TGF-β signaling exerts a biphasic role in cancer, with dual functions as a tumor suppressor in normal tissue and early stage lesions and as a prometastatic agent in late-stage disease. The molecular mechanisms that control the conversion of TGF-β from a tumor suppressor to a tumor promoter are poorly understood, and additional studies utilizing preclinical tumor models will be required to elucidate the complex role of TGF-β in tumor–host interactions. Numerous studies have clearly demonstrated the ability of TGF-β to enhance the migratory and invasive capacity of tumor cells, to generate a reactive stromal compartment, to promote angiogenesis and to suppress antitumor immune responses. This multifactorial activity of TGF-β in cancer makes it an extremely attractive target for therapeutic intervention, and the next several years will produce exciting data on the initial clinical application of neutralizing antibody and small molecule therapeutics in oncology and fibrotic disorders.

REFERENCES

1. Vogelstein B, Kinzler KW. Cancer genes and the pathways they control. Nature Medicine 2004; 10:789–799.
2. Birchmeier C, Birchmeier W, Brand-Saberi B. Epithelial-mesenchymal transitions in cancer progression. Acta Anat 1996; 156:217–226.
3. Ahmad A, Hart IR. Mechanisms of metastasis. Crit Rev Oncol Hematol 1997; 26:163–173.
4. Chambers AF, Groom AC, MacDonald IC. Dissemination and growth of cancer cells in metastatic sites. Nat Rev Cancer 2002; 2:563–572.
5. Shi Y, Massague J. Mechanisms of TGF-β signaling from cell membrane to the nucleus. Cell 2003; 113:685–700.
6. de Larco JE, Todaro GJ. Growth factors from murine sarcoma virus-transformed cells. Proc Natl Acad Sci U S A 1978; 75:4001–4005.
7. Assoian RK, Komoriya A, Meyers CA, et al. Transforming growth factor-β in human platelets. Identification of a major storage site, purification, and characterization. J Biol Chem 1983; 258:7155–7160.
8. Frolik CA, Dart LL, Meyers CA, et al. Purification and initial characterization of a type β transforming growth factor from human placenta. Proc Natl Acad Sci U S A 1983; 80:3676–3680.
9. Roberts AB, Frolik CA, Anzano MA, et al. Transforming growth factors from neoplastic and nonneoplastic tissues. Fed Proc 1983; 42:2621–2626.

10. Doetschman T. Interpretation of phenotype in genetically engineered mice. Lab Anim Sci 1999; 49:137–143.

11. Annes JP, Munger JS, Rifkin DB. Making sense of latent TGFβ activation. J Cell Sci 2003; 116:217–224.

12. Ramirez F, Pereira L. The fibrillins. Int J Biochem Cell Biol 1999; 31:255–259.

13. Andreasen PA, Kjoller L, Christensen L, et al. The urokinase-type plasminogen activator system in cancer metastasis: a review. Int J Cancer 1997; 72:1–22.

14. Sato Y, Rifkin DB. Inhibition of endothelial cell movement by pericytes and smooth muscle cells: activation of a latent transforming growth factor-β 1-like molecule by plasmin during co-culture. J Cell Biol 1989; 109:309–315.

15. Stamenkovic I. Matrix metalloproteinases in tumor invasion and metastasis. Semin Cancer Biol 2000; 10:415–433.

16. Yu Q, Stamenkovic I. Cell surface-localized matrix metalloproteinase-9 proteolytically activates TGF-β and promotes tumor invasion and angiogenesis. Genes Dev 2000; 14:163–176.

17. Crawford SE, Stellmach V, Murphy-Ullrich JE, et al. Thrombospondin-1 is a major activator of TGF-β1 in vivo. Cell 1998; 93:1159–1170.

18. Munger JS, Huang X, Kawakatsu H, et al. The integrin α v β 6 binds and activates latent TGF β 1: a mechanism for regulating pulmonary inflammation and fibrosis. Cell 1999; 96:319–328.

19. Ewan KB, Shyamala G, Ravani SA, et al. Latent transforming growth factor-β activation in mammary gland: regulation by ovarian hormones affects ductal and alveolar proliferation. Am J Pathol 2002; 160:2081–2093.

20. Oursler MJ. Osteoclast synthesis and secretion and activation of latent transforming growth factor β. J Bone Miner Res 1994; 9:443–452.

21. Teitelbaum SL. Bone resorption by osteoclasts. Science 2000; 289:1504–1508.

22. Lopez-Casillas F, Wrana JL, Massague J. Bglycan presents ligand to the TGF β signaling receptor. Cell 1993; 73:1435–1444.

23. Derynck R, Zhang YE. Smad-dependent and Smad-independent pathways in TGF-β family signalling. Nature 2003; 425:577–584.

24. Hayes S, Chawla A, Corvera S. TGF β receptor internalization into EEA1-enriched early endosomes: role in signaling to Smad2. J Cell Biol 2002; 158:1239–1249.

25. Ehrlich M, Shmuely A, Henis YI. A single internalization signal from the di-leucine family is critical for constitutive endocytosis of the type II TGF-β receptor. J Cell Sci 2001; 114:1777–1786.

26. Razani B, Zhang XL, Bitzer M, et al. Caveolin-1 regulates transforming growth factor (TGF)-β/SMAD signaling through an interaction with the TGF-β type I receptor. J Biol Chem 2001; 276:6727–6738.

27. Di Guglielmo GM, Le Roy C, Goodfellow AF, et al. Distinct endocytic pathways regulate TGF-β receptor signalling and turnover. Nat Cell Biol 2003; 5:410–421.

28. Inman GJ, Hill CS. Stoichiometry of active smad-transcription factor complexes on DNA. J Biol Chem 2002; 277:51,008–51,016.

29. Kretzschmar M, Doody J, Timokhina I, et al. A mechanism of repression of TGFβ/ Smad signaling by oncogenic Ras. Genes Dev 1999; 13:804–816.

30. Engel ME, McDonnell MA, Law BK, et al. Interdependent SMAD and JNK signaling in transforming growth factor-β-mediated transcription. J Biol Chem 1999; 274:37,413–37,420.

31. Yakymovych I, Ten Dijke P, Heldin CH, et al. Regulation of Smad signaling by protein kinase C. FASEB J 2001; 15:553–555.

32. Yu L, Hebert MC, Zhang YE. TGF-β receptor-activated p38 MAP kinase mediates Smad-independent TGF-β responses. EMBO J 2002; 21:3749–3759.

33. Hanafusa H, Ninomiya-Tsuji J, Masuyama N, et al. Involvement of the p38 mitogen-activated protein kinase pathway in transforming growth factor-β-induced gene expression. J Biol Chem 1999; 274:27,161–27,167.

34. Hocevar BA, Brown TL, Howe PH. TGF-β induces fibronectin synthesis through a c-Jun N-terminal kinase-dependent, Smad4-independent pathway. EMBO J 1999; 18:1345–1356.

35. Yue J, Mulder KM. Activation of the mitogen-activated protein kinase pathway by transforming growth factor-β. Methods Mol Biol 2000; 142:125–131.

36. Zavadil J, Bitzer M, Liang D, et al. Genetic programs of epithelial cell plasticity directed by transforming growth factor-β. Proc Natl Acad Sci U S A 2001; 98:6686–6691.

37. Bakin AV, Rinehart C, Tomlinson AK, et al. p38 mitogen-activated protein kinase is required for TGFβ-mediated fibroblastic transdifferentiation and cell migration. J Cell Sci 2002; 115:3193–3206.

38. Engel ME, Datta PK, Moses HL. RhoB is stabilized by transforming growth factor β and antagonizes transcriptional activation. J Biol Chem 1998; 273:9921–9926.
39. Bhowmick NA, Ghiassi M, Bakin A, et al. Transforming growth factor-β1 mediates epithelial to mesenchymal transdifferentiation through a RhoA-dependent mechanism. Mol Biol Cell 2001; 12:27–36.
40. Shen X, Li J, Hu PP, et al. The activity of guanine exchange factor NET1 is essential for transforming growth factor-β-mediated stress fiber formation. J Biol Chem 2001; 276:15,362–15,368.
41. Edlund S, Landstrom M, Heldin CH, et al. Transforming growth factor-β-induced mobilization of actin cytoskeleton requires signaling by small GTPases Cdc42 and RhoA. Mol Biol Cell 2002; 13:902–914.
42. Wilkes MC, Murphy SJ, Garamszegi N, et al. Cell-type-specific activation of PAK2 by transforming growth factor β independent of Smad2 and Smad3. Mol Cell Biol 2003; 23:8878–8889.
43. Griswold-Prenner I, Kamibayashi C, Maruoka EM, et al. Physical and functional interactions between type I transforming growth factor β receptors and Bα, a WD–40 repeat subunit of phosphatase 2A. Mol Cell Biol 1998; 18:6595–6604.
44. Petritsch C, Beug H, Balmain A, et al. TGF-β inhibits p70 S6 kinase via protein phosphatase 2A to induce G(1) arrest. Genes Dev 2000; 14:3093–3101.
45. Bakin AV, Tomlinson AK, Bhowmick NA, et al. Phosphatidylinositol 3-kinase function is required for transforming growth factor β-mediated epithelial to mesenchymal transition and cell migration. J Biol Chem 2000; 275:36,803–36,810.
46. Vinals F, Pouyssegur J. Transforming growth factor β1 (TGF-β1) promotes endothelial cell survival during in vitro angiogenesis via an autocrine mechanism implicating TGF-α signaling. Mol Cell Biol 2001; 21:7218–7230.
47. Remy I, Montmarquette A, Michnick SW. PKB/Akt modulates TGF-β signalling through a direct interaction with Smad3. Nat Cell Biol 2004; 6:358–365.
48. Conery AR, Cao Y, Thompson EA, et al. Akt interacts directly with Smad3 to regulate the sensitivity to TGF-β induced apoptosis. Nat Cell Biol 2004; 6:366–372.
49. Siegel PM, Massague J. Cytostatic and apoptotic actions of TGF-β in homeostasis and cancer. Nat Rev Cancer 2003; 3:807–821.
50. Kang Y, Chen CR, Massague J. A self-enabling TGFβ response coupled to stress signaling: Smad engages stress response factor ATF3 for Id1 repression in epithelial cells. Mol Cell 2003; 11:915–926.
51. Pierce DF Jr, Johnson MD, Matsui Y, et al. Inhibition of mammary duct development but not alveolar outgrowth during pregnancy in transgenic mice expressing active TGF-β 1. Genes Dev 1993; 7:2308–2317.
52. Jhappan C, Geiser AG, Kordon EC, et al. Targeting expression of a transforming growth factor β 1 transgene to the pregnant mammary gland inhibits alveolar development and lactation. EMBO J 1993; 12:1835–1845.
53. Cui W, Fowlis DJ, Cousins FM, et al. Concerted action of TGF-β 1 and its type II receptor in control of epidermal homeostasis in transgenic mice. Genes Dev 1995; 9:945–955.
54. Lee MS, Gu D, Feng L, et al. Accumulation of extracellular matrix and developmental dysregulation in the pancreas by transgenic production of transforming growth factor-β 1. Am J Pathol 1995; 147:42–52.
55. Sanderson N, Factor V, Nagy P, et al. Hepatic expression of mature transforming growth factor β 1 in transgenic mice results in multiple tissue lesions. Proc Natl Acad Sci U S A 1995; 92:2572–2576.
56. Bottinger EP, Factor VM, Tsang ML, et al. The recombinant proregion of transforming growth factor β1 (latency-associated peptide) inhibits active transforming growth factor β1 in transgenic mice. Proc Natl Acad Sci U S A 1996; 93:5877–5882.
57. Pierce DF, Jr., Gorska AE, Chytil A, et al. Mammary tumor suppression by transforming growth factor β 1 transgene expression. Proc Natl Acad Sci U S A 1995; 92:4254–4258.
58. Bottinger EP, Jakubczak JL, Haines DC, et al. Transgenic mice overexpressing a dominant-negative mutant type II transforming growth factor β receptor show enhanced tumorigenesis in the mammary gland and lung in response to the carcinogen 7,12-dimethylbenz-[a]-anthracene. Cancer Res 1997; 57:5564–5570.
59. Gorska AE, Jensen RA, Shyr Y, et al. Transgenic mice expressing a dominant-negative mutant type II transforming growth factor-β receptor exhibit impaired mammary development and enhanced mammary tumor formation. Am J Pathol 2003; 163:1539–1549.
60. Engle SJ, Hoying JB, Boivin GP, et al. Transforming growth factor β1 suppresses nonmetastatic colon cancer at an early stage of tumorigenesis. Cancer Res 1999; 59:3379–3386.
61. Zhu Y, Richardson JA, Parada LF, et al. Smad3 mutant mice develop metastatic colorectal cancer. Cell 1998; 94:703–714.

62. Tang B, Bottinger EP, Jakowlew SB, et al. Transforming growth factor-β1 is a new form of tumor suppressor with true haploid insufficiency. Nat Med 1998; 4:802–807.

63. Markowitz S, Wang J, Myeroff L, et al. Inactivation of the type II TGF-β receptor in colon cancer cells with microsatellite instability. Science 1995; 268:1336–1338.

64. Eppert K, Scherer SW, Ozcelik H, et al. MADR2 maps to 18q21 and encodes a TGFβ-regulated MAD-related protein that is functionally mutated in colorectal carcinoma. Cell 1996; 86:543–552.

65. Hahn SA, Schutte M, Hoque AT, et al. DPC4, a candidate tumor suppressor gene at human chromosome 18q21.1. Science 1996; 271:350–353.

66. Chen T, Carter D, Garrigue-Antar L, et al. Transforming growth factor β type I receptor kinase mutant associated with metastatic breast cancer. Cancer Res 1998; 58:4805–4810.

67. Wang D, Kanuma T, Mizunuma H, et al. Analysis of specific gene mutations in the transforming growth factor-β signal transduction pathway in human ovarian cancer. Cancer Res 2000; 60:4507–4512.

68. Goggins M, Shekher M, Turnacioglu K, et al. Genetic alterations of the transforming growth factor β receptor genes in pancreatic and biliary adenocarcinomas. Cancer Res 1998; 58:5329–5332.

69. Shu XO, Gao YT, Cai Q, et al. Genetic polymorphisms in the TGF-β 1 gene and breast cancer survival: a report from the Shanghai Breast Cancer Study. Cancer Res 2004; 64:836–839.

70. Kaklamani VG, Hou N, Bian Y, et al. TGFBR1*6A and cancer risk: a meta-analysis of seven case-control studies. J Clin Oncol 2003; 21:3236–3243.

71. Pasche B, Kaklamani V, Hou N, et al. TGFBR1*6A and cancer: a meta-analysis of 12 case-control studies. J Clin Oncol 2004; 22:756–758.

72. Kaklamani V, Baddi L, Rosman D, et al. No major association between TGFBR1*6A and prostate cancer. BMC Genet 2004; 5:28.

73. Hojo M, Morimoto T, Maluccio M, et al. Cyclosporine induces cancer progression by a cell-autonomous mechanism. Nature 1999; 397:530–534.

74. Wojtowicz-Praga S. Reversal of tumor-induced immunosuppression by TGF-β inhibitors. Invest New Drugs 2003; 21:21–32.

75. Blobe GC, Schiemann WP, Lodish HF. Role of transforming growth factor β in human disease. N Engl J Med 2000; 342:1350–1358.

76. Miettinen PJ, Ebner R, Lopez AR, et al. TGF-β induced transdifferentiation of mammary epithelial cells to mesenchymal cells: involvement of type I receptors. J Cell Biol 1994; 127:2021–2036.

77. Oft M, Peli J, Rudaz C, et al. TGF-β1 and Ha-Ras collaborate in modulating the phenotypic plasticity and invasiveness of epithelial tumor cells. Genes Dev 1996; 10:2462–2477.

78. Itoh S, Thorikay M, Kowanetz M, et al. Elucidation of Smad requirement in transforming growth factor-β type I receptor-induced responses. J Biol Chem 2003; 278:3751–3761.

79. Janda E, Lehmann K, Killisch I, et al. Ras and TGF[β] cooperatively regulate epithelial cell plasticity and metastasis: dissection of Ras signaling pathways. J Cell Biol 2002; 156:299–313.

80. Cui W, Fowlis DJ, Bryson S, et al. TGFβ1 inhibits the formation of benign skin tumors, but enhances progression to invasive spindle carcinomas in transgenic mice. Cell 1996; 86:531–542.

81. Letterio JJ, Roberts AB. Regulation of immune responses by TGF-β. Annu Rev Immunol 1998; 16:137–161.

82. Letterio JJ, Roberts AB. TGF-β: a critical modulator of immune cell function. Clin Immunol Immunopathol 1997; 84:244–250.

83. Gorelik L, Flavell RA. Transforming growth factor-β in T-cell biology. Nat Rev Immunol 2002; 2:46–53.

84. Letterio JJ, Geiser AG, Kulkarni AB, et al. Autoimmunity associated with TGF-β1-deficiency in mice is dependent on MHC class II antigen expression. J Clin Invest 1996; 98:2109–2119.

85. Kulkarni AB, Ward JM, Yaswen L, et al. Transforming growth factor-β 1 null mice. An animal model for inflammatory disorders. Am J Pathol 1995; 146:264–275.

86. Yaswen L, Kulkarni AB, Fredrickson T, et al. Autoimmune manifestations in the transforming growth factor-β 1 knockout mouse. Blood 1996; 87:1439–1445.

87. Shull MM, Ormsby I, Kier AB, et al. Targeted disruption of the mouse transforming growth factor-β1 gene results in multifocal inflammatory disease. Nature 1992; 359:693–699.

88. Gorelik L, Flavell RA. Abrogation of TGFβ signaling in T cells leads to spontaneous T cell differentiation and autoimmune disease. Immunity 2000; 12:171–181.

89. Shah AH, Tabayoyong WB, Kimm SY, et al. Reconstitution of lethally irradiated adult mice with dominant negative TGF-β type II receptor-transduced bone marrow leads to myeloid expansion and inflammatory disease. J Immunol 2002; 169:3485–3491.

90. Meidenbauer N, Zippelius A, Pittet MJ, et al. High frequency of functionally active Melan-a-specific T cells in a patient with progressive immunoproteasome-deficient melanoma. Cancer Res 2004; 64:6319–6326.

91. Zippelius A, Batard P, Rubio-Godoy V, et al. Effector function of human tumor-specific CD8 T cells in melanoma lesions: a state of local functional tolerance. Cancer Res 2004; 64:2865–2873.

92. Housseau F, Langer DA, Oberholtzer SD, et al. Tumor-specific CD8+ T lymphocytes derived from the peripheral blood of prostate cancer patients by in vitro stimulation with autologous tumor cell lines. Int J Cancer 2002; 98:57–62.

93. Pardoll D. Does the immune system see tumors as foreign or self? Annu Rev Immunol 2003; 21:807–839.

94. Terabe M, Berzofsky JA. Immunoregulatory T cells in tumor immunity. Curr Opin Immunol 2004; 16:157–162.

95. Wolf AM, Wolf D, Steurer M, et al. Increase of regulatory T cells in the peripheral blood of cancer patients. Clin Cancer Res 2003; 9:606–612.

96. Woo EY, Yeh H, Chu CS, et al. Cutting edge: Regulatory T cells from lung cancer patients directly inhibit autologous T cell proliferation. J Immunol 2002; 168:4272–4276.

97. Woo EY, Chu CS, Goletz TJ, et al. Regulatory CD4(+)CD25(+) T cells in tumors from patients with early-stage non-small cell lung cancer and late-stage ovarian cancer. Cancer Res 2001; 61:4766–4772.

98. Liyanage UK, Moore TT, Joo HG, et al. Prevalence of regulatory T cells is increased in peripheral blood and tumor microenvironment of patients with pancreas or breast adenocarcinoma. J Immunol 2002; 169:2756–2761.

99. Curiel TJ, Coukos G, Zou L, et al. Specific recruitment of regulatory T cells in ovarian carcinoma fosters immune privilege and predicts reduced survival. Nat Med 2004; 10:942–949.

100. Read S, Powrie F. CD4(+) regulatory T cells. Curr Opin Immunol 2001; 13:644–649.

101. Shevach EM, Piccirillo CA, Thornton AM, et al. Control of T cell activation by CD4+CD25+ suppressor T cells. Novartis Found Symp 2003; 252:24–36; discussion 36–44, 106–114.

102. Piccirillo CA, Shevach EM. Cutting edge: control of CD8+ T cell activation by CD4+CD25+ immunoregulatory cells. J Immunol 2001; 167:1137–1140.

103. Somasundaram R, Jacob L, Swoboda R, et al. Inhibition of cytolytic T lymphocyte proliferation by autologous CD4+/CD25+ regulatory T cells in a colorectal carcinoma patient is mediated by transforming growth factor-β. Cancer Res 2002; 62:5267–5272.

104. Huber S, Schramm C, Lehr HA, et al. Cutting edge: TGF-β signaling is required for the in vivo expansion and immunosuppressive capacity of regulatory CD4+CD25+ T cells. J Immunol 2004; 173:6526–6531.

105. Schramm C, Huber S, Protschka M, et al. TGFβ regulates the CD4+CD25+ T-cell pool and the expression of Foxp3 in vivo. Int Immunol 2004; 16:1241–1249.

106. Fantini MC, Becker C, Monteleone G, et al. Cutting edge: TGF-β induces a regulatory phenotype in CD4+CD25- T cells through Foxp3 induction and down-regulation of Smad7. J Immunol 2004; 172:5149–5153.

107. Gorelik L, Flavell RA. Immune-mediated eradication of tumors through the blockade of transforming growth factor-β signaling in T cells. Nat Med 2001; 7:1118–1122.

108. Shah AH, Tabayoyong WB, Kundu SD, et al. Suppression of tumor metastasis by blockade of transforming growth factor β signaling in bone marrow cells through a retroviral-mediated gene therapy in mice. Cancer Res 2002; 62:7135–7138.

109. Terabe M, Matsui S, Noben-Trauth N, et al. NKT cell-mediated repression of tumor immunosurveillance by IL–13 and the IL-4R-STAT6 pathway. Nat Immunol 2000; 1:515–520.

110. Terabe M, Matsui S, Park JM, et al. Transforming growth factor-β production and myeloid cells are an effector mechanism through which CD1d-restricted T cells block cytotoxic T lymphocyte-mediated tumor immunosurveillance: abrogation prevents tumor recurrence. J Exp Med 2003; 198:1741–1752.

111. Lee JC, Lee KM, Kim DW, et al. Elevated TGF-β1 secretion and down-modulation of NKG2D underlies impaired NK cytotoxicity in cancer patients. J Immunol 2004; 172:7335–7340.

112. Castriconi R, Cantoni C, Della Chiesa M, et al. Transforming growth factor β 1 inhibits expression of NKp30 and NKG2D receptors: consequences for the NK-mediated killing of dendritic cells. Proc Natl Acad Sci U S A 2003; 100:4120–4125.

113. Gabrilovich D. Mechanisms and functional significance of tumour-induced dendritic-cell defects. Nat Rev Immunol 2004; 4:941–952.

114. O'Neill DW, Adams S, Bhardwaj N. Manipulating dendritic cell biology for the active immunotherapy of cancer. Blood 2004; 104:2235–2246.

115. Takayama T, Morelli AE, Onai N, et al. Mammalian and viral IL–10 enhance C-C chemokine receptor 5 but down-regulate C-C chemokine receptor 7 expression by myeloid dendritic cells: impact on chemotactic responses and in vivo homing ability. J Immunol 2001; 166:7136–7143.

116. Sato K, Kawasaki H, Nagayama H, et al. TGF-β 1 reciprocally controls chemotaxis of human peripheral blood monocyte-derived dendritic cells via chemokine receptors. J Immunol 2000; 164:2285–2295.

117. Wu RS, Kobie JJ, Besselsen DG, et al. Comparative analysis of IFN-γ B7.1 and antisense TGF-β gene transfer on the tumorigenicity of a poorly immunogenic metastatic mammary carcinoma. Cancer Immunol Immunother 2001; 50:229–240.

118. Kao JY, Gong Y, Chen CM, et al. Tumor-derived TGF-β reduces the efficacy of dendritic cell/tumor fusion vaccine. J Immunol 2003; 170:3806–3811.

119. Kobie JJ, Wu RS, Kurt RA, et al. Transforming growth factor β inhibits the antigen-presenting functions and antitumor activity of dendritic cell vaccines. Cancer Res 2003; 63:1860–1864.

120. Roberts AB, Wakefield LM. The two faces of transforming growth factor β in carcinogenesis. Proc Natl Acad Sci U S A 2003; 100:8621–8623.

121. Gorsch SM, Memoli VA, Stukel TA, et al. Immunohistochemical staining for transforming growth factor β 1 associates with disease progression in human breast cancer. Cancer Res 1992; 52:6949–6952.

122. MacCallum J, Bartlett JM, Thompson AM, et al. Expression of transforming growth factor β mRNA isoforms in human breast cancer. Br J Cancer 1994; 69:1006–1009.

123. Kong FM, Anscher MS, Murase T, et al. Elevated plasma transforming growth factor-β 1 levels in breast cancer patients decrease after surgical removal of the tumor. Ann Surg 1995; 222:155–162.

124. Xie W, Mertens JC, Reiss DJ, et al. Alterations of Smad signaling in human breast carcinoma are associated with poor outcome: a tissue microarray study. Cancer Res 2002; 62:497–505.

125. Li C, Wilson PB, Levine E, et al. TGF-β1 levels in pre-treatment plasma identify breast cancer patients at risk of developing post-radiotherapy fibrosis. Int J Cancer 1999; 84:155–159.

126. Ivanovic V, Todorovic-Rakovic N, Demajo M, et al. Elevated plasma levels of transforming growth factor-β 1 (TGF-β 1) in patients with advanced breast cancer: association with disease progression. Eur J Cancer 2003; 39:454–461.

127. Travers MT, Barrett-Lee PJ, Berger U, et al. Growth factor expression in normal, benign, and malignant breast tissue. Br Med J (Clin Res Ed) 1988; 296:1621–1624.

128. MacCallum J, Keen JC, Bartlett JM, et al. Changes in expression of transforming growth factor β mRNA isoforms in patients undergoing tamoxifen therapy. Br J Cancer 1996; 74:474–478.

129. Thompson AM, Kerr DJ, Steel CM. Transforming growth factor β 1 is implicated in the failure of tamoxifen therapy in human breast cancer. Br J Cancer 1991; 63:609–614.

130. Lafon C, Mazars P, Guerrin M, et al. Early gene responses associated with transforming growth factor-β 1 growth inhibition and autoinduction in MCF-7 breast adenocarcinoma cells. Biochim Biophys Acta 1995; 1266:288–295.

131. Herman ME, Katzenellenbogen BS. Alterations in transforming growth factor-α and -β production and cell responsiveness during the progression of MCF-7 human breast cancer cells to estrogen-autonomous growth. Cancer Res 1994; 54:5867–5874.

132. Sun L, Wu G, Willson JK, et al. Expression of transforming growth factor β type II receptor leads to reduced malignancy in human breast cancer MCF-7 cells. J Biol Chem 1994; 269:26,449–26,455.

133. Arteaga CL, Hurd SD, Winnier AR, et al. Anti-transforming growth factor (TGF)-β antibodies inhibit breast cancer cell tumorigenicity and increase mouse spleen natural killer cell activity. Implications for a possible role of tumor cell/host TGF-β interactions in human breast cancer progression. J Clin Invest 1993; 92:2569–2576.

134. Arteaga CL, Koli KM, Dugger TC, et al. Reversal of tamoxifen resistance of human breast carcinomas in vivo by neutralizing antibodies to transforming growth factor-β. J Natl Cancer Inst 1999; 91:46–53.

135. Buck MB, Fritz P, Dippon J, et al. Prognostic significance of transforming growth factor β receptor II in estrogen receptor-negative breast cancer patients. Clin Cancer Res 2004; 10:491–498.

136. Muller WJ, Sinn E, Pattengale PK, et al. Single-step induction of mammary adenocarcinoma in transgenic mice bearing the activated c-neu oncogene. Cell 1988; 54:105–115.

137. Guy CT, Webster MA, Schaller M, et al. Expression of the neu protooncogene in the mammary epithelium of transgenic mice induces metastatic disease. Proc Natl Acad Sci U S A 1992; 89:10,578–10,582.

138. Slamon DJ, Clark GM, Wong SG, et al. Human breast cancer: correlation of relapse and survival with amplification of the HER-2/neu oncogene. Science 1987; 235:177–182.

139. Slamon DJ, Godolphin W, Jones LA, et al. Studies of the HER-2/neu proto-oncogene in human breast and ovarian cancer. Science 1989; 244:707–712.

140. Slamon DJ. Studies of the HER-2/neu proto-oncogene in human breast cancer. Cancer Invest 1990; 8:253.
141. Siegel PM, Shu W, Cardiff RD, et al. Transforming growth factor β signaling impairs Neu-induced mammary tumorigenesis while promoting pulmonary metastasis. Proc Natl Acad Sci U S A 2003; 100:8430–8435.
142. Muraoka RS, Koh Y, Roebuck LR, et al. Increased malignancy of Neu-induced mammary tumors overexpressing active transforming growth factor β1. Mol Cell Biol 2003; 23:8691–8703.
143. Muraoka-Cook RS, Kurokawa H, Koh Y, et al. Conditional overexpression of active transforming growth factor β1 in vivo accelerates metastases of transgenic mammary tumors. Cancer Res 2004; 64:9002–9011.
144. Guy CT, Cardiff RD, Muller WJ. Induction of mammary tumors by expression of polyoma virus middle T oncogene: a transgenic mouse model for metastatic disease. Mol Cell Biol 1992; 12:954–961.
145. Tang B, Vu M, Booker T, et al. TGF-β switches from tumor suppressor to prometastatic factor in a model of breast cancer progression. J Clin Invest 2003; 112:1116–1124.
146. Guise TA, Chirgwin JM. Transforming growth factor-β in osteolytic breast cancer bone metastases. Clin Orthop 2003; 4/5 Suppl.:S32–S38.
147. Boyce BF, Yoneda T, Guise TA. Factors regulating the growth of metastatic cancer in bone. Endocr Relat Cancer 1999; 6:333–347.
148. Roodman GD. Mechanisms of bone metastasis. N Engl J Med 2004; 350: 1655–1664.
149. Arguello F, Baggs RB, Frantz CN. A murine model of experimental metastasis to bone and bone marrow. Cancer Res 1988; 48:6876–6881.
150. Guise TA. Parathyroid hormone-related protein and bone metastases. Cancer 1997; 80:1572–1580.
151. Guise TA, Yin JJ, Taylor SD, et al. Evidence for a causal role of parathyroid hormone-related protein in the pathogenesis of human breast cancer-mediated osteolysis. J Clin Invest 1996; 98:1544–1549.
152. Kakonen SM, Selander KS, Chirgwin JM, et al. Transforming growth factor-β stimulates parathyroid hormone-related protein and osteolytic metastases via Smad and mitogen-activated protein kinase signaling pathways. J Biol Chem 2002; 277:24,571–24,578.
153. Yin JJ, Selander K, Chirgwin JM, et al. TGF-β signaling blockade inhibits PTHrP secretion by breast cancer cells and bone metastases development. J Clin Invest 1999; 103:197–206.
154. Kang Y, Siegel PM, Shu W, et al. A multigenic program mediating breast cancer metastasis to bone. Cancer Cell 2003; 3:537–549.
155. Minn AJ, Kang Y, Serganova I, et al. Distinct organ-specific metastatic potential of individual breast cancer cells and primary tumors. J Clin Invest 2005; 115:44–55.
156. Bello-DeOcampo D, Tindall DJ. TGF-β1/Smad signaling in prostate cancer. Curr Drug Targets 2003; 4:197–207.
157. Gerdes MJ, Larsen M, McBride L, et al. Localization of transforming growth factor-β1 and type II receptor in developing normal human prostate and carcinoma tissues. J Histochem Cytochem 1998; 46:379–388.
158. Perry KT, Anthony CT, Steiner MS. Immunohistochemical localization of TGF β 1, TGF β 2, and TGF β 3 in normal and malignant human prostate. Prostate 1997; 33:133–140.
159. Eastham JA, Truong LD, Rogers E, et al. Transforming growth factor-β 1: comparative immunohistochemical localization in human primary and metastatic prostate cancer. Lab Invest 1995; 73:628–635.
160. Shariat SF, Menesses-Diaz A, Kim IY, et al. Tissue expression of transforming growth factor-β1 and its receptors: correlation with pathologic features and biochemical progression in patients undergoing radical prostatectomy. Urology 2004; 63:1191–1197.
161. Steiner MS, Zhou ZZ, Tonb DC, et al. Expression of transforming growth factor-β 1 in prostate cancer. Endocrinology 1994; 135:2240–2247.
162. Wikstrom P, Stattin P, Franck-Lissbrant I, et al. Transforming growth factor β1 is associated with angiogenesis, metastasis, and poor clinical outcome in prostate cancer. Prostate 1998; 37:19–29.
163. Djonov V, Ball RK, Graf S, et al. Transforming growth factor-β 3 is expressed in nondividing basal epithelial cells in normal human prostate and benign prostatic hyperplasia, and is no longer detectable in prostate carcinoma. Prostate 1997; 31:103–109.
164. Dallas SL, Zhao S, Cramer SD, et al. Preferential production of latent transforming growth factor β-2 by primary prostatic epithelial cells and its activation by prostate-specific antigen. J Cell Physiol 2005; 202:361–370.
165. Adler HL, McCurdy MA, Kattan MW, et al. Elevated levels of circulating interleukin-6 and transforming growth factor-β1 in patients with metastatic prostatic carcinoma. J Urol 1999; 161:182–187.

166. Kattan MW, Shariat SF, Andrews B, et al. The addition of interleukin-6 soluble receptor and transforming growth factor β1 improves a preoperative nomogram for predicting biochemical progression in patients with clinically localized prostate cancer. J Clin Oncol 2003; 21:3573–3579.

167. Shariat SF, Kattan MW, Traxel E, et al. Association of pre- and postoperative plasma levels of transforming growth factor β(1) and interleukin 6 and its soluble receptor with prostate cancer progression. Clin Cancer Res 2004; 10:1992–1999.

168. Singh D, Febbo PG, Ross K, et al. Gene expression correlates of clinical prostate cancer behavior. Cancer Cell 2002; 1:203–209.

169. Holzbeierlein J, Lal P, LaTulippe E, et al. Gene expression analysis of human prostate carcinoma during hormonal therapy identifies androgen-responsive genes and mechanisms of therapy resistance. Am J Pathol 2004; 164:217–227.

170. Guo Y, Jacobs SC, Kyprianou N. Down-regulation of protein and mRNA expression for transforming growth factor-β (TGF-β1) type I and type II receptors in human prostate cancer. Int J Cancer 1997; 71:573–579.

171. Williams RH, Stapleton AM, Yang G, et al. Reduced levels of transforming growth factor β receptor type II in human prostate cancer: an immunohistochemical study. Clin Cancer Res 1996; 2:635–640.

172. Kim IY, Ahn HJ, Zelner DJ, et al. Loss of expression of transforming growth factor β type I and type II receptors correlates with tumor grade in human prostate cancer tissues. Clin Cancer Res 1996; 2:1255–1261.

173. Lee C, Sintich SM, Mathews EP, et al. Transforming growth factor-β in benign and malignant prostate. Prostate 1999; 39:285–290.

174. Tang B, de Castro K, Barnes HE, et al. Loss of responsiveness to transforming growth factor β induces malignant transformation of nontumorigenic rat prostate epithelial cells. Cancer Res 1999; 59:4834–4842.

175. Jakowlew SB, Moody TW, Mariano JM. Transforming growth factor-β receptors in human cancer cell lines: analysis of transcript, protein and proliferation. Anticancer Res 1997; 17:1849–1860.

176. Webber MM, Quader ST, Kleinman HK, et al. Human cell lines as an in vitro/in vivo model for prostate carcinogenesis and progression. Prostate 2001; 47:1–13.

177. Teicher BA, Kakeji Y, Ara G, et al. Prostate carcinoma response to cytotoxic therapy: in vivo resistance. In Vivo 1997; 11:453–461.

178. Steiner MS, Barrack ER. Transforming growth factor-β 1 overproduction in prostate cancer: effects on growth in vivo and in vitro. Mol Endocrinol 1992; 6:15–25.

179. Matthews E, Yang T, Janulis L, et al. Down-regulation of TGF-β1 production restores immunogenicity in prostate cancer cells. Br J Cancer 2000; 83:519–525.

180. Cunha GR, Hayward SW, Wang YZ. Role of stroma in carcinogenesis of the prostate. Differentiation 2002; 70:473–485.

181. Tuxhorn JA, Ayala GE, Smith MJ, et al. Reactive stroma in human prostate cancer: induction of myofibroblast phenotype and extracellular matrix remodeling. Clin Cancer Res 2002; 8:2912–2923.

182. Ayala G, Tuxhorn JA, Wheeler TM, et al. Reactive stroma as a predictor of biochemical-free recurrence in prostate cancer. Clin Cancer Res 2003; 9:4792–4801.

183. Bhowmick NA, Neilson EG, Moses HL. Stromal fibroblasts in cancer initiation and progression. Nature 2004; 432:332–337.

184. Olumi AF, Grossfeld GD, Hayward SW, et al. Carcinoma-associated fibroblasts direct tumor progression of initiated human prostatic epithelium. Cancer Res 1999; 59:5002–5011.

185. San Francisco IF, DeWolf WC, Peehl DM, et al. Expression of transforming growth factor-β 1 and growth in soft agar differentiate prostate carcinoma-associated fibroblasts from normal prostate fibroblasts. Int J Cancer 2004; 112:213–218.

186. Tuxhorn JA, McAlhany SJ, Dang TD, et al. Stromal cells promote angiogenesis and growth of human prostate tumors in a differential reactive stroma (DRS) xenograft model. Cancer Res 2002; 62:3298–3307.

187. Kleinman HK, McGarvey ML, Hassell JR, et al. Basement membrane complexes with biological activity. Biochemistry 1986; 25:312–318.

188. Swarm RL. Transplantation of a chondrosarcoma in mice of different inbred strains. J Natl Cancer Inst 1963; 31:953–975.

189. Tuxhorn JA, McAlhany SJ, Yang F, et al. Inhibition of transforming growth factor-β activity decreases angiogenesis in a human prostate cancer-reactive stroma xenograft model. Cancer Res 2002; 62:6021–6025.

190. Dumont N, Arteaga CL. Targeting the TGF β signaling network in human neoplasia. Cancer Cell 2003; 3:531–536.

191. Yingling JM, Blanchard KL, Sawyer JS. Development of TGF-β signalling inhibitors for cancer therapy. Nat Rev Drug Discov 2004; 3:1011–1022.

192. Mead AL, Wong TT, Cordeiro MF, et al. Evaluation of anti-TGF-β2 antibody as a new postoperative anti-scarring agent in glaucoma surgery. Invest Ophthalmol Vis Sci 2003; 44:3394–3401.

193. Benigni A, Zoja C, Corna D, et al. Add-on anti-TGF-β antibody to ACE inhibitor arrests progressive diabetic nephropathy in the rat. J Am Soc Nephrol 2003; 14:1816–1824.

194. Dasch JR, Pace DR, Waegell W, et al. Monoclonal antibodies recognizing transforming growth factor-β. Bioactivity neutralization and transforming growth factor β 2 affinity purification. J Immunol. 1989; 142:1536–1541.

195. Lucas C, Bald LN, Fendly BM, et al. The autocrine production of transforming growth factor-β 1 during lymphocyte activation. A study with a monoclonal antibody-based ELISA. J Immunol 1990; 145:1415–1422.

196. Teicher BA. Malignant cells, directors of the malignant process: role of transforming growth factor-β. Cancer Metastasis Rev 2001; 20:133–143.

197. Ohmori T, Yang JL, Price JO, et al. Blockade of tumor cell transforming growth factor-βs enhances cell cycle progression and sensitizes human breast carcinoma cells to cytotoxic chemotherapy. Exp Cell Res 1998; 245:350–359.

198. Teicher BA, Herman TS, Holden SA, et al. Tumor resistance to alkylating agents conferred by mechanisms operative only in vivo. Science 1990; 247:1457–1461.

199. Teicher BA, Holden SA, Ara G, et al. Transforming growth factor-β in in vivo resistance. Cancer Chemother Pharmacol 1996; 37:601–609.

200. Teicher BA, Ikebe M, Ara G, et al. Transforming growth factor-β 1 overexpression produces drug resistance in vivo: reversal by decorin. In Vivo 1997; 11:463–472.

201. Komesli S, Vivien D, Dutartre P. Chimeric extracellular domain type II transforming growth factor (TGF)-β receptor fused to the Fc region of human immunoglobulin as a TGF-β antagonist. Eur J Biochem 1998; 254:505–513.

202. George J, Roulot D, Koteliansky VE, et al. In vivo inhibition of rat stellate cell activation by soluble transforming growth factor β type II receptor: a potential new therapy for hepatic fibrosis. Proc Natl Acad Sci U S A 1999; 96:12,719–12,724.

203. Yang YA, Dukhanina O, Tang B, et al. Lifetime exposure to a soluble TGF-β antagonist protects mice against metastasis without adverse side effects. J Clin Invest 2002; 109:1607–1615.

204. Muraoka RS, Dumont N, Ritter CA, et al. Blockade of TGF-β inhibits mammary tumor cell viability, migration, and metastases. J Clin Invest 2002; 109:1551–1559.

205. Suzuki E, Kapoor V, Cheung HK, et al. Soluble type II transforming growth factor-β receptor inhibits established murine malignant mesothelioma tumor growth by augmenting host antitumor immunity. Clin Cancer Res 2004; 10:5907–5918.

206. Wojtowicz-Praga S, Verma UN, Wakefield L, et al. Modulation of B16 melanoma growth and metastasis by anti-transforming growth factor β antibody and interleukin-2. J Immunother Emphasis Tumor Immunol 1996; 19:169–175.

207. Urashima M, Ogata A, Chauhan D, et al. Transforming growth factor-β1: differential effects on multiple myeloma versus normal B cells. Blood 1996; 87:1928–1938.

208. Ge R, Rajeev V, Subramanian G, et al. Selective inhibitors of type I receptor kinase block cellular transforming growth factor-β signaling. Biochem Pharmacol 2004; 68:41–50.

209. Inman GJ, Nicolas FJ, Callahan JF, et al. SB-431542 is a potent and specific inhibitor of transforming growth factor-β superfamily type I activin receptor-like kinase (ALK) receptors ALK4, ALK5, and ALK7. Mol Pharmacol 2002; 62:65–74.

210. Sawyer JS, Anderson BD, Beight DW, et al. Synthesis and activity of new aryl- and heteroaryl-substituted pyrazole inhibitors of the transforming growth factor-β type I receptor kinase domain. J Med Chem 2003; 46:3953–3956.

211. Subramanian G, Schwarz RE, Higgins L, et al. Targeting endogenous transforming growth factor β receptor signaling in SMAD4-deficient human pancreatic carcinoma cells inhibits their invasive phenotype1. Cancer Res 2004; 64:5200–5211.

212. Uhl M, Aulwurm S, Wischhusen J, et al. SD-208, a novel transforming growth factor β receptor I kinase inhibitor, inhibits growth and invasiveness and enhances immunogenicity of murine and human glioma cells in vitro and in vivo. Cancer Res 2004; 64:7954–7961.

26

p53-Based Immunotherapy of Cancer

Albert B. DeLeo, PhD

SUMMARY

In recent years, there has been an increasing awareness that the immune system, in particular the T-cell component, plays a significant role in tumor eradication. Advances in molecular immunology and identification of T-cell-defined human tumor antigens have accelerated the development of vaccines to promote T-cell-mediated antitumor immune responses. In general, many shared human tumor antigens are derived from proteins overexpressed or derepressed in tumors relative to normal cells. Alteration in the tumor suppressor gene product, p53, is one of the most common events in human cancers, but mutant p53-based immunotherapy would require "custom-made" vaccines for use in relatively few patients. Because most mutations in *p53* are associated with accumulation or "overexpression" of mutant p53 in the cytosol, the protein is more readily available for antigenic processing and presentation than are the low levels of p53 molecules expressed in normal cells. A vaccine targeting wild-type sequence (wt) or nonmutant sequence peptides derived from altered p53 molecules, therefore, is a more attractive approach for developing broadly applicable cancer vaccines.

Extensive preclinical murine tumor model studies using peptide-based and DNA vaccines have demonstrated that wt p53-based vaccines can induce tumor eradication in the absence of deleterious antitumor autoimmune side effects. Like any T-cell-based immunotherapy, effective p53-based immunotherapy will be dependent on patients' responsiveness to wt p53 peptides and the ability of their tumors to present these peptides for T-cell recognition. These and other issues and concerns related to p53-based

From: *Cancer Drug Discovery and Development: Cancer Drug Resistance*
Edited by: B. Teicher © Humana Press Inc., Totowa, NJ

vaccines are discussed together with a brief summary of the initial clinical trials of p53-based immunotherapy.

Key Words: p53; immunotherapy; vaccines; dendritic cells; CTL; Th; peptides; immunoselection; immunotherapy.

1. INTRODUCTION

The *p53* tumor suppressor gene product was identified 25 yr ago as a transformation-related antigen, using antibodies present in the sera of mice immunized against chemically induced sarcomas *(1)*. It was characterized as being expressed at elevated levels in murine tumors induced with irradiation, RNA and DNA viruses, and chemical carcinogens. Of the nontransformed cells/tissues tested for expression, only thymocytes and mitogen-activated lymphocytes showed low but detected levels of the antigen *(2)*. Since then, genetic events leading to loss of function of p53 have been identified as the most frequently occurring event associated with oncogenesis *(3–5)*. Whereas genetic alterations of the *p53* gene, namely missense mutations, are considered the primary cause leading to loss of its function, alterations in gene products of several pathways that are critical for regulation of p53 can also result in loss of its function. Several approaches for restoring the normal p53 function of regulating the cell cycle and reversing the transformation phenotype of cancer cells are being actively pursued. They involve focusing on *p53* gene replacement, identifying pharmacological agents capable of restoring mutated p53 to its normal conformation and functional activities, and viruses that are lytic to cells harboring mutant p53 *(6–8)*. Another approach can be traced to the origins of the identification of p53, namely that as a tumor antigen, p53 could be targeted with cancer vaccines.

2. CANCER VACCINES

Preclinical murine and clinical evidence indicates that the immune system plays a major role in host defense against progressive tumor growth and drives the concept of developing immunotherapy to augment the antitumor immune responsiveness of patients with cancer in order to eradicate their tumors *(9)*. Although all elements of the immune system are involved in tumor eradication, it has been shown to be primarily dependent on T-cell-mediated antitumor responses. Whereas CD8+ cytotoxic T-lymphocytes (CTLs) are considered the critical effectors for tumor eradication, CD4+ T-lymphocytes or T-helper (Th) cells have been shown to be required for expansion and maintenance of these effectors *(10–13)*. Both T-cell subsets recognize short peptides or "epitopes" derived from proteins that are presented on the cell surface in association with class I or II human leukocyte antigen (HLA) molecules *(14,15)*. A major focus of cancer immunotherapy, therefore, has been to develop vaccines that would induce and/or expand CTL-mediated antitumor immune responses.

2.1. T-Cell-Defined Tumor-Associated Antigens

Nearly all the human tumor antigens being used in developing cancer vaccines are "shared" tumor-associated determinants. They represent nonmutated peptides derived from three distinct groups of proteins *(16)*. One group is derived from proteins that are expressed in the testes, but not normal cells. Epigenetic and/or genetic events result in activation of genes encoding these "cancer–testes" or "cancer germline" proteins. Their lack of expression on normal cells and inappropriate expression in wide range of tumors makes them immunologically "nonself" in nature and enhances their potential for use in cancer vaccines. The other two groups of tumor-associated antigen (TAAs) are "self-antigens," and can be distinguished by their patterns of expression in tumors and normal adult cells. One group consists of tissue-specific or differentiation antigens that are overexpressed in tumors relative to normal cells, whereas the other represents antigens derived from a variety of gene products involved in cell cycle regulation. Loss of their functional activities is a critical event in transformation. Many of these proteins are products of oncogenes or tumor suppressor genes; p53 is a prime example of the latter group of gene products. The identification of melanoma-associated antigens and the development and clinical introduction of melanoma vaccines has accelerated the effort to develop vaccines for more widely occurring types of cancer, namely carcinomas of the breast, colon, and lung. An obvious candidate for such vaccines is p53.

2.2. p53: A TAA

Following the serological identification of p53 as a transformation-related murine tumor antigen (1), a subsequent study by Crawford and colleagues identified anti-p53 immunoglobulin (Ig)G antibodies in the sera of some patients with cancer (17). Because an IgG response against a protein like p53 requires the participation of CD4+ Th cells as well as B-cells, that study and subsequent others have established the immunogenicity of p53 in humans and the presence, in some patients, of T-cell-mediated anti-p53 responses (18–21).

A key function of p53 is to prevent DNA replication following DNA damage because of a genotoxic event, such as irradiation (3). It does so by blocking replication until DNA repair has occurred. In normal cells, therefore, wild-type (wt) p53 molecules are sequestered in the nucleus and have a relatively short half-life. Genetic alterations in p53, which result in loss of p53 function, have been shown to be the most frequently occurring genetic event associated with human cancer (5). At least 50% of all human tumors analyzed contain genetic alterations in p53. Most are missense mutations, in exons 5–8, which encode the DNA binding region of the molecule. In studies in which all the p53 exons (exons 2–11) as well as intron/exon junctions have been analyzed, as was recently done for a group of squamous cell carcinoma of the head and neck (SCCHN) tumors (22,23), the incidence of genetic defects can approach 80%. Missense mutation of p53, however, is frequently associated with stabilization (increased half-life) of mutated p53 molecules, resulting in accumulation or "overexpression" in the cytosol of tumors (24). As the accumulation of mutated p53 in tumors resembles the overexpression or derepression phenotype associated with many shared tumor-associated tissue/differentiation melanoma antigens targeted with vaccines (10,17), it was hypothesized that the accumulation of mutant p53 molecules in the tumor cytosol would enhance processing and presentation of p53-derived peptides for CTL recognition and eradication (24).

2.3. Two Classes of T-Cell-Defined p53 Peptides

In contrast to most other tumor associated antigens (TAAs), however, two classes of epitopes can de derived from a mutant p53 molecule can be presented, an epitope containing the missense mutation, which would be nonself and a unique tumor-specific antigen and an array of epitopes composed of nonmutated, wt peptide sequences derived from the rest of the mutant molecule (Fig. 1). The latter would be "self-TAAs." Although mutant peptides should be highly immunogenic and induce robust antitumor responses, the constraints of antigen processing and presentation limit their presentation to tumors

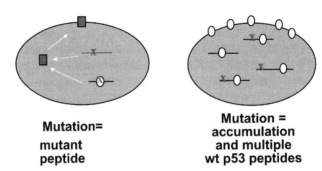

■ **mutant sequence peptide / unique**

○ **wild-type (wt) sequence peptide / shared TAA**

Fig. 1. Two classes of cytotoxic T-lymphocyte (CTL)/defined p53 tumor peptides.

of only a few individuals that express the appropriate class I HLA molecules capable of presenting the mutation. Consequently, vaccines targeting a mutant peptide would essentially need to be "custom-made" for an individual patient and of limited applicability. In contrast, due the polymorphisms of HLA molecules, there is a much greater probability that one or more wt p53 peptides can be presented for T-cell recognition by tumors expressing any given class I HLA allele. These wt p53 peptides represent shared TAAs, and vaccines targeting them would be broadly applicable *(24,25)*. Although they would be targeting self-epitopes and presumably would induce less robust antitumor responses than the mutant p53 epitopes, wt p53-based vaccines represent a practical approach to developing a broadly applicable cancer vaccine.

3. PRECLINICAL MURINE STUDIES OF P53-BASED IMMUNOTHERAPY

The demonstration that a wt p53 peptide-based dendritic cell vaccine induced rejection of a transplanted chemically induced tumor established the potential efficacy of p53-based vaccines as broadly applicable for use in immunotherapy of cancer. Since then, studies utilizing mice and murine tumor models have been continually used to evaluate the efficacies of various types of p53-based vaccines, including DNA vaccines, as well as the roles that tolerance to "self-p53" peptides and the potential of inducing autoimmune might have in vaccine-induced, anti-p53 immune responses.

3.1. p53-Based Immunotherapy of Mice Bearing Transplanted Tumors

The study by Majordomo et al. *(25)*, which used the same tumor model systems that were used to serologically identify p53, was the first to demonstrate the ability of a wt p53 peptide to induce tumor rejection of a chemically induced tumor in mice. The study was also one of the first studies that established dendritic cells, considered the professional antigen-presenting cell, as the vehicle of choice for tumor peptide based vaccines. Furthermore, no "antiself" autoimmune side effects were detected in wt p53-immunized mice. As in any vaccine development program, optimization of the immunogen and vaccine vehicle are critical. A wide range of p53-based vaccines and immunization protocols has been evaluated in the past decade. Murine studies have shown that effective anti-wt p53 T-cell-mediated antitumor responses could be induced by: (1) wt p53 peptides or recombinant p53 protein admixed with chemical adjuvants or pulsed onto bone marrow-derived dendritic cells (DCs) *(25,26)*, as well as (2) DCs transfected with nonviral plasmids or viruses encoding intact p53 or fragments *(27,28)*. In addition, p53 nonviral plasmids DNA vaccines biolistically (gene gun) delivered as well as recombinant viral vectors expressing p53 have shown to be effective in inducing antitumor immunity *(29,30)*.

Comparisons of the anti-wt p53 CTL responses of wt mice and p53 null mice to mouse and human p53 have been critical in demonstrating the extent of tolerance that exists to self-wt p53 peptides, and reducing fears that anti-wt p53 antitumor immune responses might be associated with deleterious autoimmune responses as well *(31,32)*. The finding that anti-wt p53 CTL responses in p53$^{+/+}$ mice display a low-to-intermediate affinity, whereas those generated in p53 null mice are of high affinity was a clear indication of the extent to which tolerance to self-p53 epitopes exists in mice. The fact that antihuman p53 CTLs generated in normal and HLA-A2-transgenic mice display higher affinities for their ligands than do antimouse p53 CTLs induced in the same mice further demonstrated the level of tolerance to wt p53 epitopes in mice. Subsequently, adoptive transfer of high-affinity anti-wt p53 CTLs derived from p53 null mice to tumor-bearing p53$^{+/+}$ mice showed that these effectors were very effective in inducing tumor eradication *(33–35)*. Although the high-affinity anti-p53 CTLs were capable of recognizing mitogen-activated T-cells, there was no evidence of autoimmunity in the treated mice. More recently, several reports employing administration of anti-CD40 antibody and/or cytosine-phosphate-guanine oligonucleotides in combination with wt p53-based vaccines have demonstrated that these agents can enhance the induction/expansion of anti-wt p53 CTLs, but not their avidity *(36–38)*.

3.2. p53-Based Immunotherapy of Mice Bearing Primary Chemically Induced Tumors

As insightful as the murine tumor model studies using transplantable tumor were, they did not mimic the relatively long-term tumor-immune system interactions that occur in hosts bearing primary tumors. Methylcholanthrene (MCA) is one of several polycyclic hydrocarbons that have been used routinely to induce tumors in experimental laboratory animals, especially inbred strains of mice and rats. It is also a major environmental pollutant and has been implicated as a causative agent in human cancers. MCA induces murine tumors within 6 mo of exposure. These tumors have a high incidence of genetic alterations in p53, and many are sensitive to wt p53-specific CTLs *(25)*. In addition to being a carcinogen, MCA is also as an immunosuppressive effect on the mice, which is prominent within weeks of its administration and persists for approx 3 mo *(39–41)*.

We recently reported the results of p53-based immunization of MCA-treated mice employing peptide-pulsed DC and DNA vaccines administered in protection, therapy, and combination protection/therapy protocols *(42)*. The results indicate that the efficacy of p53-based immunization relative to reducing tumor incidence was severely compromised by vaccine-induced "tumor escape." As compared to tumors induced in nonimmunized mice, a higher incidence of "epitope-loss" tumors was detected in tumors from the immunized mice. The increase in tumor escape arose as a consequence of either increased frequencies of mutations within/flanking p53 epitope-coding regions and/or downregulation of expression of H2 molecules, the class I major histocompatibility complex molecules that present these epitopes for CTL recognition. One must note that the conditions of immunizing and inducing anti-p53 immune response in the presence of a potent carcinogen are ideal for promoting immunoselection of epitope-loss tumors. These findings are consistent with current views of immunoselection occurring in patients receiving tumor peptide-based immunotherapy and warrant further evaluation of p53-based immunization in the MCA and other primary murine tumor model systems.

4. PRECLINICAL DEVELOPMENT OF p53-BASED IMMUNOTHERAPY

Development of p53-based immunotherapy has greatly benefited from the knowledge and insights gained from many of the preclinical studies in murine tumor model systems. In the course of a decade, it has progressed from identification of the first CTL-defined wt p53 peptide to clinical introduction of several types of wt p53-based vaccines. The use of high-affinity anti-wt p53 T-cells derived from p53 null mice and HLA-A2.1-transgenic p53 null mice has been shown to be very effective in inducing tumor eradication. Although of high-affinity, these cells do not react with normal cells and did not induce any detectable evidence of autoimmunity. Consequently, the concept of genetically engineering high-affinity anti-p53 human T-cell effectors by transfecting peripheral blood mononuclear cells (PBMCs), with cDNA encoding the T-cell receptor (TCR) derived from antihuman p53 murine CTLs is being actively pursued *(43)*.

4.1. CTL-Defined Human wt p53 Peptides

Unlike many of the presently identified CTL-defined human tumor peptides, nearly all of the wt p53 peptides have been identified by "reverse immunology," namely using algorithm-predictions of putative class I HLA-binding peptides *(44)* and immunizing HLA transgenic mice and/or in vitro stimulation (IVS) of PBMCs obtained from normal donors *(45–53)*. The majority of those identify are HLA-A*0201 (HLA-A2)-restricted epitopes, although an HLA-A24-restricted wt p53 has also been identified. In this manner, wt $p53_{65–73}$, wt $p53_{149–157}$, wt $p53_{189–196}$, wt $p53_{217–225}$, and wt $p53_{264–173}$ epitopes were identified. Several of these peptides are being use in p53-based vaccine trials for cancer patients expressing the *HLA-A2.1* allele.

4.2. Th Cell-Defined wt p53 Peptides

The identification of anti-p53 IgG antibodies in the sera of some patients with cancer is indicative of anti-p53 CD4+ Th cell responses having been induced in these individuals. Unfortunately, it is also associated with a poor prognosis, which might be attributable to a predominating Th2 antitumor immune response in these patients rather than the Th1-biased response that is generally associated with tumor eradication. Preclinical studies have demonstrated that vaccines employing Th- as well as CTL-defined epitopes derived from the same tumor antigen show enhanced efficacy because of the established role of the antigen-specific CD4+ T-cells in the induction and maintenance of effective antitumor immunity *(54,55)*. Consequently, the identification of Th cell-defined p53 peptides would be useful not only for enhancing the efficacy of p53-based immunization, but also to possibly "reverse" the Th2-biased responses of p53 sero-positive patients. Several in vitro-based studies have focused on proliferative T-cell-mediated responses to intact p53 protein or p53 peptides relative to anti-p53 antibody production in patients with cancer *(19–22,56)*, but none identified the T-cell-defined epitopes. The study of Fujita et al. *(57)* identified several immunogenic HLA class II-restricted wt p53 peptides. The abilities of these peptides to be naturally presented, however, were not established in their study. In our recent study, which utilized recombinant wt p53 protein-pulsed DCs as the antigen presenting cell and algorithm-predicted HLA-DRB1*0401-binding 15-mer peptides *(58)*, we identified wt p53$_{110-124}$ peptide as a naturally presented HLA-DRB1*0401-restricted epitope *(59)*. In in vitro-based experiments using the autologous PCI-13 SCCHN system available in our laboratory, the addition of anti-wt p53$_{110-124}$ CD4$^+$ T-cells to PBMCs was shown to increase the total number CD8+ T-cells in the IVS cultures and, more relevantly, enhance the induction of anti-PCI 13 effectors. This effect was dependent on the ratio PBMC/CD4 cells in the cultures. These results are consistent with the concept of developing a multiepitope p53 vaccine that would employ Th-defined as well as CTL-defined p53 peptides to maximize its efficacy.

5. CRITICAL ISSUES AND CONCERNS THAT CONFRONT THE CLINICAL INTRODUCTION OF p53-BASED CANCER VACCINES

Successful development of p53-based immunotherapy needs not only to overcome the general issues and concerns that conform any immunization targeting a self-TAA, but also several which are unique because of the complexity of this molecule and its role as a tumor suppressor. The two critical concerns of any tumor antigen-specific immunization are (1) the responsiveness of the patient to the immunization and (2) the ability of the patient's tumor to present the targeted antigen *(10)*. In addition to a general impairment of immunocompetency, which characterizes many patients with cancer, the issue of tolerance/anergy to wt p53 epitopes needs to be taken into account. Second, there is concern of knowing whether (a) tumor(s) being targeted with a p53-based vaccine can present the targeted wt p53 epitopes. In addition to direct mutation/deletion in p53 exons, which can influence processing and presentation of p53-derived epitopes *(60)*, defects in any of the pathways involved in posttranslational modification and degradation of p53 promote "loss of p53 function" as well as processing and presentation of p53 epitopes *(6,7)*. Finally, loss of function of p53 is considered an early event in an oncogenic process that can occur over decades. The induction of an anti-p53 antitumor immune response, during the early stages of oncogenesis even if it is not robust, could readily promote over a long period of time the immunoselection of p53 epitope-loss tumors *(61–63)*. This would mimic the outgrowth of epitope loss: tumors that were enhanced in p53-immunized mice bearing primary chemically induced tumors *(43)*, and might be particularly relevant to the concept of p53-based immunization of "high risk" individuals to prevent cancer.

5.1. Immunological Tolerance and Autoimmunity

Effective immunity against self-tumor antigens, such as wt p53 peptides, must breach the fine line that separates an antitumor immune response from a potentially deleterious autoimmune response. This subtle distinction is particularly important in the case of wt p53 epitopes. Most self-TAAs, such as those derived from tissue-specific or differentiation antigens, have limited tissue distribution, and immune responses to them are governed by peripheral tolerance. In contrast, p53 is expressed by all nucleated cells and readily available in the thymus for induction of tolerance to wt p53 epitopes *(2)*. Based on in vitro-based immunological studies involving PBMCs, it is apparent that only a subset of normal donors and patients with cancer are responsive IVS with autologous DCs pulsed with wt p53 peptides or transfected with adeno/wt p53 construct *(48,64)*. The DCs were chosen for this assay as they are considered the only antigen-presenting cell capable of inducing antigen-specific responses from naive T-cells. The induced/expanded anti-wt p53 CTLs display a low-to-intermediate affinity for their ligands and a limited repertoire of TCR usage *(48,65,66)*. The latter is quite evident following an analysis of TCRVβ usage of anti-wt p53$_{264-272}$ CTLs. Despite the vast TCR repertoires theoretically available for any immunogen, a TCRVβ immunoscope analysis of anti-wt p53$_{264-272}$ CTLs generated from PBMCs from HLA-A2$^+$ individuals showed restrictions in TCRVβ family usage *(66)*. Whether the weak immunogenicity of wt p53 peptides reflects deletion or anergy of anti-wt p53 T-cells is an open question, but preclinical murine studies have clearly demonstrated that the anti-wt p53 CTLs induced in p53 null mice are high affinity relative to those induced in normal p53$^{+/+}$ mice *(32,33)*. Despite their increased affinity, their adoptive transfer into normal mice did not result in deleterious autoimmune side effects, indicating that even the biochemical detectable levels of p53 expressed in some normal cells in the mice *(2)* are not sufficient to sensitize them to anti-p53 CTLs *(25,67)*.

5.2. "Optimized" p53 Peptides

In many instances, the immunogenicity of a weakly immunogenic peptide can be enhanced by an amino acid exchange in the peptide sequence, which both increases its binding to HLA molecules and/or interaction with the TCR and results in an increased stabilization of the HLA/peptide/TCR complex. Ultimately, this results in an increase in the expansion of T-cells capable of recognizing the parental peptide *(68–71)*. This approach was successful in optimizing the immunogenicity of the wt p53$_{264-272}$ and p53$_{149-157}$ peptides. In the case of the wt p53$_{264-272}$ peptide (LLGRNSFEV), which contains a favorable amino acid (leucine) at anchor positions 2 and 9, the exchange of tryptophan for phenylalanine at position 7 of the peptide, F270W, did not increase its binding to HLA-A2.1 molecules, but did increase its immunogenicity. Presumably, this was because of enhanced stability of the HLA/peptide/TCR complex, and was evidenced by an increased affinity for the parental peptide of anti-wt p53$_{264-272}$ CTLs induced using the optimized peptide. The amino acid exchange of a favorable anchor amino acid (leucine) for an unfavorable anchor amino acid (threonine) in position 2 of the wt p53$_{149-157}$ peptide (STPPPGTRV) increased its binding affinity to HLA-A2.1 molecules and its immunogenicity *(72)*.

5.3. Parameters Influencing Tumor Presentation of wt p53 Peptides for T-Cell Recognition

In addition to defects in antigen processing and presentation *(73)*, which confront any T-cell-based immunotherapy, the ability of tumors to present CTL-defined wt p53 peptides appears to be more complicated than of any other shared TAA (Fig. 2). It first arose with the differences in the sensitivities of three SCCHN cell lines to HLA-A2-restricted, anti-wt p53$_{264-272}$ CTLs *(45,46,48)*. The PCI-13 SCCHN cell line, which displays the "classic" phenotype of accumulation of mutant p53 (E286K) associated with presentation of wt p53$_{264-272}$ peptide, was sensitive to anti-wt p53$_{264-272}$ CTLs. In contrast, SCC-9, which expresses a deletion in *p53* and does not accumulate p53, was sensitive to lysis by the CTLs, whereas SCC-4, which displays the classic phenotype of accumulating mutant p53 (P151M), was not. Subsequently, Theobald et al. established that the commonly occurring p53 R273H mutation blocked processing of the wt p53$_{264-272}$ peptide, and that MCF7 cells, which accumulate wt p53, presumably because of defects in pathways regulating p53, did present the peptide *(46,60)*. Further confounding the situation is the demonstration by Vierboom et al. *(67)* that cells expressing the

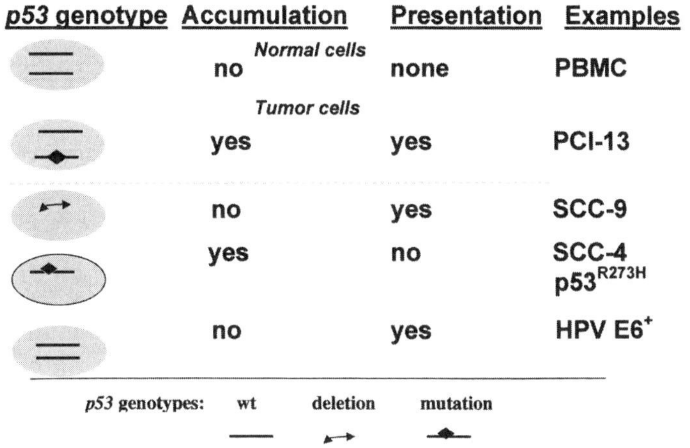

Fig. 2. Presentation of wild-type (wt) p53$_{264-272}$ peptide for cytotoxic T-lymphocyte recognition by tumor cells is associated with several distinct *p53* genotypes and properties.

oncogenic human papillomavirus (HPV) E6 protein, which functions by enhancing the degradation of p53 leading to "loss of function," have a wt p53$^+$/accumulation$^-$ phenotype, yet are sensitive to anti-wt p53 CTLs. The interaction of p53 with heat shock protein, which is apparently dependent on the conformation of the p53 molecules, influences proteasomal degradation of mutant p53 in tumors cells, and represents another set of parameters that can impact on wt p53 CTL-recognition of tumors. Clearly, a major focus of future research is to better assess the ability of tumors to present wt p53 peptides for T-cell recognition.

5.4. Implication of Immunoselection of p53 Epitope-Loss Tumors

Nearly 18,000 human tumors have been analyzed for genetic alterations in *p53*, most of which are missense mutations *(22)*. The class I HLA haplotypes of the patients from which these tumors were obtained from, however, are essentially unknown. One, therefore, is unable to readily assess whether a relationship exists between sites/nature of p53 mutations and the host's class I HLA haplotype. Several years ago, the results of an analysis by Wiedenfeld et al. indicated the possible increase in the incidence of p53 epitope loss in lung tumors of HLA-A2$^+$ individuals *(62)*. An analysis of the sites of p53 missense mutations expressed in 27 SSCHN obtained from HLA-A2$^+$ patients, 8/13 occurred within or immediately flanking one of three known CTL-defined wt p53 epitopes *(74)*. Six of the missense mutations within CTL-defined epitopes, p53$_{149-157}$, p53$_{217-225}$, and p53$_{264-273}$, and one was a mutation at codon 273, which is known to block processing of the p53$_{264-272}$ peptide *(60)*. The eighth missense mutation was in codon 226, the codon immediately flanking the wt p53$_{217-225}$ epitope, which may also function like the R273H mutation in blocking epitope processing. Mutations in the p53$_{217-225}$ epitope at codon 220 were detected in 2/27 tumors. Codons 273 and 220 are considered p53 mutational "hot spots." Mutation at p53 codon 273 is the most frequently detected p53 mutation in human cancers (~12%), whereas mutation at codon 220 ranks sixth, with a frequency of approx 1% *(5)*. These values are independent of tumor type and do not take into account the HLA haplotypes of the tumors. The frequency of mutations at p53 codon 220 in the HLA-A2$^+$ SCCHN we analyzed is well above its frequency in all the human tumors that have been analyzed. Obviously, more-extensive analyses of the HLA/p53 phenotypes of SCCHN and other types of cancers need to be done to determine the true significance of this observation. Three distinct missense mutations in the $p53_{149-157}$ epitope were detected in the study. Two of these were nonconserved amino acid exchanges at the anchor positions of the peptide. Whether these mutations yield T-cell-defined mutant p53 epitopes is under investigation.

Overall, the skewed pattern of p53 missense mutation in the tumors of HLA-A2$^+$ patients with SCCHN (74) is highly suggestive of possible immunoselection that promotes the outgrowth of p53 epitope-loss tumors. It also implies that wt p53 peptides, although "self-antigens," are surprising immunogenic. Given that mutation of p53 is considered an early event in development of SCCHN, the immunological pressure exerted over long periods by anti-wt p53 CTLs combined with the inherent genetic instability and heterogeneity of tumors could readily promote the outgrowth of p53 epitope-loss tumors in some patients.

A further implication that p53-related immunoselection in patients with cancer occurs is the inverse correlation between the frequencies of anti-wt $p53_{264-272}$ tetramer$^+$ CD8$^+$ T-cells present in PBMCs obtained from HLA-A2$^+$ patients with SCCHN and the mutational site/level of p53 expressed in their tumors (74). The results obtained from the 27 patients divide these individuals into two groups, low tetramer$^+$ T-cell frequency/IVS nonresponsive vs high tetramer$^+$ T-cell frequency/IVS responsive. When this distinction was correlated to p53 immunohistochemistry and genotyping, the tumors of nonresponsive patients had a p53 phenotype traditionally consistent with a tumor's ability to present the wt $p53_{264-272}$ peptide (accumulation of mutant p53), whereas the responders had tumors expressing normal levels of wt p53 and, presumably, a low potential to present the epitope (see Fig. 2). Whereas these results are strongly supportive of immunoselection of epitope-loss tumors, they also are consistent with the possibility that the SCCHN tumors expressing wt p53 and associated with high frequencies of anti-wt p53 CTLs might also be HPV$^+$. The expression of HPV E6 enhances the degradation of wt and mutant p53 and presentation of peptides derived from these molecules (67,75). The ability of an HPV$^+$ tumor to present the $p53_{264-272}$ peptide for CTL recognition, therefore, need not require accumulation of p53. Obviously, the role of HPV in presentation of p53-derived epitopes required further investigation.

6. CLINICAL TRIALS OF p53-BASED IMMUNOTHERAPY OF PATIENTS WITH CANCER

In vitro-based studies using PBMCs obtained from normal donors and patients have shown the utility of peptide or protein-pulsed DCs (36,47,60) or DCs transfected with recombinant adenoviral constructs expressing p53 for induction/expansion of anti-wt p53 CTLs and Th cells (68). As a result of these experiments, the concept of genetically engineering high-affinity anti-p53 human T-cell effectors by transfecting PBMCs with cDNA encoding the TCR derived from antihuman p53 murine CTLs is also being actively pursued (70). A number of p53-based vaccine clinical trails have been introduced in Europe and the United States for patients with breast, colon, or ovarian carcinoma. The initial findings of four of these trials have been reported. Vaccines consisting of p53 peptides admixed with chemical adjuvants or DC, recombinant viral vectors expressing wt p53 as well as DCs transfected with adenoviral construct-expressing wt p53 were employed in these trials. The concept of replacing mutant p53 in a patient's tumor with functional wt p53 delivered using a recombinant adenoviral/wt p53 construct preceded its use in p53-based immunotherapy. An unreported aspect of replacement adeno/p53 gene therapy trials is whether "bystander" antitumor immune responses are induced in the patients receiving this gene therapy *(76)*. Induction of bystander anti-p53 immune responses has been shown to occur as a result of other types of cancer therapies not directly targeting p53, which also warrants further study *(77,78)*.

Two HLA-A2-restricted wt p53 peptide-based vaccine trials have been initiated using peptide-pulsed DCs and/or peptides admixed with chemical adjuvants. The NCI p53 vaccine trial is for HLA-A2$^+$ patients with low-burden ovarian cancer *(79)*. In this trial, one group of five patients received multiple monthly immunizations of the peptide pulsed onto autologous DCs and administered intravenously, whereas the second group of six patients received the peptide admixed with ISA-51 and GM-CSF and given subcutaneously. Both groups of patients also received low dose interleukin 2 for 10 d, beginning with cycle 3 of the vaccination protocol. Immunological monitoring, using enzyme-linked immunosorbent and tetramer assays, showed the induction in individuals of both groups of anti-wt p53 CTL responses. This was accompanied by increased progression-free survival times. The other p53 peptide-pulsed DC trial was for HLA-A2$^+$ patients with advanced breast cancer *(80)*. It consisted of a multiple p53 peptide-pulsed DC vaccine, which included three wt p53 epitopes mixed with three modified or "optimized" peptides, in addition to a generic pan-DR-binding protein peptide. The vaccine was administered together with interleukin 2. The immunological monitoring of PBMCs obtained from six patients receiving up to 10 immunizations was reported. The results show sporadic anti-p53 CTL responses and 1/6 patient showed a clinical response.

An advantage of using recombinant protein or viral vectors encoding p53 as immunogen is that it permits multiple CTL and Th epitopes to be presented, and gives the investigator the option of monitoring the trial for identified HLA class I-restricted p53 epitopes or not. The initial results of the immunological monitoring of phase I/II immunization trials of patients using either a recombinant adenovirus or canarypox virus encoding wt p53 have been reported. Theobald et al. chose to focus on the responses of HLA-A2$^+$ patients treated with a recombinant adeno/p53 vaccine to the wt p53$_{264-272}$ peptide *(81)*. Although antiviral responses were detected, no significant CTL-responses to the epitope were detected. In contrast, entry criteria for patients with advanced colon carcinoma recruited for a clinical vaccine trial of canary pox virus encoding wt p53 was independent of their class I HLA haplotype. No deleterious autoimmune side effects were noted for monkeys treated with this p53 viral construct. The regimen was found to induce or augment humoral anti-p53 IgG responses in 3/16 patients and anti-p53 T-cell proliferative responses in 4/16 *(83,84)*. A clear distinction between the two trials is that the anti-p53 T-cell responses in the latter trial were not restricted to a defined wt p53 peptide; instead, they were detected using mixtures of overlapping wt p53 peptides to stimulate the T-cells. The assays were independent of the patients' HLA haplotypes and identity of the p53 epitopes. According to the National Cancer Institute, a third viral-based vaccine trial for patients with lung cancer modeled on murine studies using adenoviral/p53-transfected dendritic cell vaccine *(28)* is in progress.

7. SUMMARY

Advances in molecular immunology combined with improved and more detailed immunological monitoring of patients are enhancing the development of cancer vaccines. Compared to many of the other tumor antigens being targeted, p53 is unique in many respects. It is truly a self-antigen. It is expressed in all nucleated cells. Despite this, no evidence of deleterious autoimmune reactions has been detected in preclinical experimental laboratory animal studies and, more importantly, in patients with cancer participating in early phase p53-based immunotherapy trials. This is because of the high level of tolerance that exists to p53 and the low levels of expression and rapid turnover of p53 in normal cells. Whether an "autoimmune response," such as those that signal the efficacy of some melanoma vaccines, will be eventually evident in patients receiving extensive and prolonged p53-based immunotherapeutic regimens is a critical unknown. Furthermore, p53 seems to have the ability to readily "dodge the immunological bullet." The very nature of the genetic instability that is initiated by loss of function of p53 coupled with the pressure of immunoselection/editing as a result of anti-p53 immune responses represent a combination of influences that promotes tumor escape and is, at the very least, challenging. Whether vaccine-induced immunoselection will occur in patients, as it does in mice bearing primary tumors, needs to be monitored. Nonetheless, p53-based vaccines appear to have a high potential for developing into a broadly applicable immunotherapy for cancer. Whereas nothing is impossible, development of p53-based immunotherapy is certainly more difficult that initially envisioned.

ACKNOWLEDGMENTS

Grant support: NIH Grant PO-1 DE-12321.

REFERENCES

1. DeLeo AB, Jay G, Appella E, Dubois GC, Law LW, Old LJ. Detection of a transformation-related antigen in chemically induced sarcomas and other transformed cells of the mouse. Proc Natl Acad Sci U S A 1979; 76:2420–2424.
2. Jay G, DeLeo, AB, Appella E, DuBois GC, Law LW, Khoury G, Old, LJ. A common transformation-related protein in murine sarcomas and leukemias, Cold Spring Harbor Sym Quant Biol. 1980; 44:659–664.
3. Harris CC. Structure and function of the p53 tumor suppressor gene: clues for rational cancer therapeutic strategies. J Natl Cancer Inst 1996; 88:1442–1455.
4. Hollstein M, Shomer B, Greenblatt M, et al. Somatic point mutations in the p53 gene of human tumors and cell lines: updated compilation. Nucleic Acids Res 1996; 24:141–146.
5. Oliver M, Eeles R, Hollstein, M, Khan MA, Harris CC, Hainaut P. TP53 Database: new online mutation analysis and recommendations to users. Hum Mutat 2002; 19:607–614.
6. Lane D. p53 from pathway to therapy. Carcinogenesis 2004; 25:1077–1081.
7. Li M, Brooks CL, Kon N, Gu W. A dynamic role of HAUSP in the p53-Mdm2 pathway. Mol Cell 2004; 13:879–886.
8. McCormick F. Cancer-specific viruses and the development of ONYX-015. Cancer Biol Ther 2003; 2:S157–S160.
9. Sogn JA. Tumor immunology: the glass is half full. Immunity 1998; 9:757–763.
10. Rosenberg SA. Shedding light on immunotherapy for cancer. N Engl J Med 2004; 350:1461–1463.
11. Toes RE, Ossendorp F, Offringa Melief CJM. CD4 T cells and their role in antitumor immune responses. J Exp Med 1999; 189:753–756.
12. Hung K. Hayashi R, Lafond-Walker A, Lowenstein C, Pardoll D, Levitsky H. The central role of CD4(+) T cells in the antitumor immune response. J Exp Med 1998; 188:2357–2368.
13. Ossendorp F, Mengede E, Camps M, Filius R, Melief CJM. Specific T helper cell requirement for optimal induction of cytotoxic T lymphocytes against major histocompatibility complex class II negative tumors. J Exp Med 1998; 187:693–702.

14. Rotzschke O, Falk K, Deres K, et al. Isolation and analysis of naturally processed viral peptides as recognized by cytotoxic T cells. Nature 1990; 348:252–254.
15. Falk K, Rotzschke O, Stevanovic S, Jung G, Rammensee HG. Allele-specific motifs revealed by sequencing of self-peptides eluted from MHC molecules. Nature 1991; 351:290–296.
16. Renkvist N, Castelli C, Robbins PF, Parmiani G. A listing of human tumor antigens recognized by T cells. Cancer Immunol Immunother 2001; 50:3–15.
17. Crawford LV, Pim DC, Bulbrook RD. Detection of antibodies against the cellular protein p53 in sera from patients with breast cancer. Int J Cancer 1982; 30:403–408.
18. Bourhis J, Lubin R, Roche B, et al. Analysis of p53 serum antibodies in patients with head and neck squamous cell carcinoma. J Natl Cancer Inst 1996; 88:1228–1233.
19. Soussi T. p53 Antibodies in the sera of patients with various types of cancer: a review. Cancer Res 2000; 60:1777–1788.
20. Houbiers JG, van der Burg SH, van de Watering LM, et al. Antibodies against p53 are associated with poor prognosis of colorectal cancer. Br J Cancer 1995; 72:637–641.
21. van der Burg SH, de Cock K, Menon AG, et al. Long lasting p53-specific T cell memory responses in the absence of anti-p53 antibodies in patients with resected primary colorectal cancer. Eur J Immunol 2001; 31:146–155.
22. Hauser U, Balz V, Carey TE, et al. Reliable detection of p53 aberrations in squamous cell carcinomas of the head and neck requires transcript analysis of the entire coding region. Head Neck 2002; 24:868–873.
23. Balz V, Scheckenbach K, Gotte K, Bockmuhl U, Petersen I, Bier H. Is the p53 inactivation frequency in squamous cell carcinomas of the head and neck underestimated? Analysis of p53 exons 2-11 and human papillomavirus 16/18 E6 transcripts in 123 unselected tumor specimens. Cancer Res 2003; 63:1188–1191.
24. Nijman,HW, Van der Burg SH. Vierboom MP, Houbiers JG, Kast WM, Melief CJ. p53, a potential target for tumor-directed T cells. Immunol Lett 1994; 40:171–178.
25. Mayordomo JI, Loftus DJ, Sakamoto H, et al. Therapy of murine tumors with p53 wild-type and mutant sequence peptide-based vaccines. J Exp Med 1996; 183:1357–1365.
26. Hilburger Ryan M, Abrams SI. Characterization of CD8+ cytotoxic T lymphocyte/tumor cell interactions reflecting recognition of an endogenously expressed murine wild-type p53 determinant. Cancer Immunol Immunother 2001; 49:603–612.
27. Tuting T, DeLeo AB, Lotze MT, Storkus WJ. Genetically modified bone marrow-derived dendritic cells expressing tumor-associated viral or "self" antigens induce antitumor immunity in vivo. Eur J Immunol 1997; 27:2702–2707.
28. Nikitina EY, Chada S, Muro-Cacho C, et al. An effective immunization and cancer treatment with activated dendritic cells transduced with full-length wild-type p53. Gene Ther 2002; 9:345–352.
29. Tuting T, Gambotto A, Robbins PD, Storkus WJ, DeLeo AB. Co-delivery of T helper 1-biasing cytokine genes enhances the efficacy of gene gun immunization of mice: studies with the model tumor antigen beta-galactosidase and the BALB/c Meth A p53 tumor-specific antigen. Gene Ther 1999; 6:629–636.
30. Putzer BM, Bramson JL, Addison CL, et al. Combination therapy with interleukin-2 and wild-type p53 expressed by adenoviral vectors potentiates tumor regression in a murine model of breast cancer. Hum Gene Ther 1998; 9:707–718.
31. Theobald M, Biggs J, Hernandez J, Lustgarten J, Labadie C, Sherman LA. Tolerance to p53 by A2.1-restricted cytotoxic T lymphocytes. J Exp Med 1997; 185:833–841.
32. Hernandez J, Lee PP, Davis MM, Sherman LA. The use of HLA A2.1/p53 peptide tetramers to visualize the impact of self tolerance on the TCR repertoire. J Immunol 2000; 164:596–602.
33. Vierboom MP, Nijman HW, Offringa R, et al. Tumor eradication by wild-type p53-specific cytotoxic T lymphocytes. J Exp Med 1997; 186:695–704.
34. Zwaveling S, Vierboom MP, Ferreira Mota SC, et al. Antitumor efficacy of wild-type p53-specific CD4(+) T-helper cells. Cancer Res 2002; 62:6187–6193.
35. McCarty TM, Liu X, Sun JY, Peralta EA, Diamond DJ, Ellenhorn JD. Targeting p53 for adoptive T-cell immunotherapy. Cancer Res 1998; 58:2601–2605.
36. Hernandez J, Ko A, Sherman LA. CTLA-4 blockade enhances the CTL responses to the p53 self-tumor antigen. J Immunol 2001; 166:3908–3914.
37. Espenschied J, Lamont J, Longmate J, et al. CTLA-4 blockade enhances the therapeutic effect of an attenuated poxvirus vaccine targeting p53 in an established murine tumor model. J Immunol 2003; 170:3401–3407.

38. Daftarian P, Song GY, Ali S, et al. Two distinct pathways of immuno-modulation improve potency of p53 immunization in rejecting established tumors. Cancer Res 2004; 64:5407–5414.
39. Wojdani A, Alfred LJ. Alterations in cell-mediated immune functions induced in mouse splenic lymphocytes by polycyclic aromatic hydrocarbons. Cancer Res 1984; 44:942–945.
40. Burchiel SW, Luster MI. Signaling by environmental polycyclic aromatic hydrocarbons in human lymphocytes. Clin Immunol 2001; 98:2–10.
41. Lutz CT, Browne G, Petzold CR. Methylcholanthrene causes increased thymocyte apoptosis. Toxicology 1998; 128:151–167.
42. Cicinnati VR Dworacki G, Albers A, et al. Impact of p53-based immunization on primary chemically induced tumors. Int J Cancer 2004; 113:961–970.
43. Liu, X, Peralta, EA, Ellenhorn JD, Diamond DJ. Targeting of human p53-overexpressing tumor cells by an HLA A*0201-restricted murine T-cell receptor expressed in Jurkat T cells. Cancer Res 2000; 60:693–701.
44. Rammensee H, Bachmann J, Emmerich NP, Bachor OA, Stevanovic S. SYFPEITHI: database for MHC ligands and peptide motifs. Immunogenetics 1991; 50:213–219.
45. Ropke M, Hald J, Guldberg P, et al. Spontaneous human squamous cell carcinomas are killed by a human cytotoxic T lymphocyte clone recognizing a wild-type p53-derived peptide. Proc Natl Acad Sci U S A 1996; 93:14,704–14,707.
46. Theobald M, Biggs J, Dittmer D, Levine AJ, Sherman LA. Targeting p53 as a general tumor antigen. Proc Natl Acad Sci U S A 1995; 92:11,993–11,997.
47. Gnjatic S, Cai Z, Viguier M, Chouaib S, Guillet JG, Choppin J. Accumulation of the p53 protein allows recognition by human CTL of a wild-type p53 epitope presented by breast carcinomas and melanomas. J Immunol 1998; 160:328–333.
48. Chikamatsu K, Nakano K, Storkus WJ, et al. Generation of anti-p53 cytotoxic T lymphocytes from human peripheral blood using autologous dendritic cells. Clin Cancer Res 1999; 5:1281–1288.
49. Eura M, Chikamatsu K, Katsura F, et al. A wild-type sequence p53 peptide presented by HLA-A24 induces cytotoxic T lymphocytes that recognize squamous cell carcinomas of the head and neck. Clin Cancer Res 2000; 6:979–986.
50. McArdle SE, Rees RC, Mulcahy KA, Saba J, McIntyre CA, Murray AK. Induction of human cytotoxic T lymphocytes that preferentially recognise tumour cells bearing a conformational p53 mutant. Cancer Immunol Immunother 2000; 49:417–425.
51. Barfoed AM, Petersen TR, Kirkin AF, Thor Straten P, Claesson MH, Zeuthen J. Cytotoxic T-lymphocyte clones, established by stimulation with the HLA-A2 binding p5365-73 wild type peptide loaded on dendritic cells in vitro, specifically recognize and lyse HLA-A2 tumour cells overexpressing the p53 protein. Scand J Immunol 2000; 51:128–133.
52. Schirle M, Keilholz W, Weber B, et al. Identification of tumor-associated MHC class I ligands by a novel T cell-independent approach. Eur J Immunol 2000; 30:2216–2225.
53. Wurtzen PA, Pedersen LO, Poulsen HS, Claesson MH. Specific killing of P53 mutated tumor cell lines by a cross-reactive human HLA-A2-restricted P53-specific CTL line. Int J Cancer 2001; 93:855–861.
54. Casares N, Lasarte JJ, de Cerio AL, et al. Immunization with a tumor-associated CTL epitope plus a tumor-related or unrelated Th1 helper peptide elicits protective CTL immunity. Eur J Immunol 2001; 31:1780–1789.
55. Wang L, Miyahara Y, Kato T, Aota T, Kuribayashi K, Shiku H. Essential roles of tumor-derived helper T cell epitopes for an effective peptide-based tumor vaccine. Cancer Immun 2003; 3:16.
56. Tilkin AF, Lubin R, Soussi T, et al. Primary proliferative T cell response to wild-type p53 protein in patients with breast cancer. Eur J Immunol 1995; 25:1765–1769.
57. Fujita H, Senju S, Yokomizo H, et al. Evidence that HLA class II-restricted human CD4+ T cells specific to p53 self peptides respond to p53 proteins of both wild and mutant forms. Eur J Immunol 1998; 28:305–316.
58. Brusic V, Rudy G, Honeyman, G, Hammer J, Harrison L. Prediction of MHC class II-binding peptides using an evolutionary algorithm and artificial neural network. Bioinformatics 1998; 14: 121–130.
59. Chikamatsu K, Albers A, Stanson J, et al. P53(110-124)-specific human CD4+ T-helper cells enhance in vitro generation and antitumor function of tumor-reactive CD8+ T cells. Cancer Res 2003; 63:3675–3681.
60. Theobald M, Ruppert T, Kuckelkorn U, et al. The sequence alteration associated with a mutational hotspot in p53 protects cells from lysis by cytotoxic T lymphocytes specific for a flanking peptide epitope. J Exp Med 1998; 188:1017–1028.

61. Wiedenfeld E A, Fernandez-Vina M, Berzofsky JA, Carbone DP. Evidence for selection against human lung cancers bearing p53 missense mutations which occur within the HLA A*0201 peptide consensus motif. Cancer Res 1994; 54:1175–1177.

62. Dunn GP, Bruce AT, Ikeda H, Old LJ, Schreiber RD. Cancer immunoediting: from immunosurveillance to tumor. Nat Immunol 2002; 3:991–998.

63. Khong HT, Restifo NP. Natural selection of tumor variants in the generation of "tumor escape" phenotypes. Nat Immunol 2002; 3:999–1005.

64. Nikitina EY, Clark JI, Van Beynen J, et al. Dendritic cells transduced with full-length wild-type p53 generate antitumor cytotoxic T lymphocytes from peripheral blood of cancer patients. Clin Cancer Res 2001; 7:127–135.

65. Hoffmann TK, Nakano K, Elder EM, et al. Generation of T cells specific for the wild-type sequence p53(264-272) peptide in cancer patients: implications for immunoselection of epitope loss variants. J Immunol 2000; 165:5938–5944.

66. Hoffmann TK, Loftus DJ, Nakano K, et al. The ability of variant peptides to reverse the nonresponsiveness of T lymphocytes to the wild-type sequence p53(264-272) epitope. J Immunol 2002; 168:1338–1347.

67. Vierboom MP, Zwaveling S, Bos GMJ, et al. High steady-state levels of p53 are not a prerequisite for tumor eradication by wild-type p53-specific cytotoxic T lymphocytes. Cancer Res 2000; 60:5508–5513.

68. Boehncke WH, Takeshita T, Pendleton CD, et al. The importance of dominant negative effects of amino acid side chain substitution in peptide-MHC molecule interactions and T cell recognition. J Immunol 1993; 150:331–341.

69. Zaremba S, Barzaga E, Zhu M, Soares N, Tsang KY, Schlom J. Identification of an enhancer agonist cytotoxic T lymphocyte peptide from human carcinoembryonic antigen. Cancer Res 1997; 57:4570–4577.

70. Rivoltini L, Squarcina P, Loftus DJ, et al. A superagonist variant of peptide MART1/Melan A27-35 elicits anti-melanoma CD8+ T cells with enhanced functional characteristics: implication for more effective immunotherapy. Cancer Res 1999; 59:301–306.

71. Slansky JE, Rattis, FM, Boyd LF, et al. Enhanced antigen-specific antitumor immunity with altered peptide ligands that stabilize the MHC-peptide-TCR complex. Immunity 2000; 13:529–538.

72. Petersen TR, Buus S, Brunak S, Nissen MH, Sherman LA, Claesson MH. Identification and design of p53-derived HLA-A2-binding peptides with increased CTL immunogenicity. Scand J Immunol 2001; 53:357–364.

73. Marincola FM, Jaffee EM, Hicklin DJ, Ferrone S. Escape of human solid tumors from T-cell recognition: molecular mechanisms and functional significance. Adv Immunol 2000; 74:181–273.

74. Hoffmann TK, Donnenberg AD, Finkelstein SD, et al. Frequencies of tetramer+ T cells specific for the wild-type sequence p53(264-272) peptide in the circulation of patients with head and neck cancer. Cancer Res 2002; 62:3521–3529.

75. McKaig RG, Baric RS, Olshan AF. Human papillomavirus and head and neck cancer: epidemiology and molecular biology. Head Neck 1998; 20:250–265.

76. Waku T, Fujiwara T, Shao J, et al. Contribution of CD95 ligand-induced neutrophil infiltration to the bystander effect in p53 gene therapy for human cancer. J Immunol 2000; 165:5884–5890.

77. Disis ML, Goodell V, Schiffman K, Knutson KL. Humoral epitope-spreading following immunization with a her-2/neu Peptide based vaccine in cancer patients. J Clin Immunol 2004; 24:571–578.

78. Chakraborty M, Abrams SI, Coleman CN, Camphausen K, Schlom J, Hodge JW. External beam radiation of tumors alters phenotype of tumor cells to render them susceptible to vaccine-mediated T-cell killing. Cancer Res 2004; 64:4328–4337.

79. Herrin V, Behrens RJ, Achtar M, et al. Wild type p53 peptide vaccine can generate a specific immune response in low burden ovarian adenocarcinoma. 2003; ASCO Chicago, IL, U S A Abstract 67846.

80. Svane IM, Pedersen AE, Johnsen HE, et al. Vaccination with p53-peptide-pulsed dendritic cells, of patients with advanced breast cancer: report from a phase I study. Cancer Immunol Immunother 2004; 53:633–641.

81. Kuball J, Schuler M, Antunes Ferreira E, et al. Generating p53-specific cytotoxic T lymphocytes by recombinant adenoviral vector-based vaccination in mice, but not man. Gene Ther 2002; 9:833–843.

82. Rosenwirth B, Kuhn EM, Heeney JL, et al. Safety and immunogenicity of ALVAC wild-type human p53 (vCP207) by the intravenous route in rhesus macaques. Vaccine 2001; 19:1661–1670.

83. van der Burg SH, Menon AG, Redeker A, et al. Induction of p53-specific immune responses in colorectal cancer patients receiving a recombinant ALVAC-p53 candidate vaccine. Clin Cancer Res 2002; 8:1019–1027.

84. Menon AG, Kuppen PJ, van der Burg SH, et al. Safety of intravenous administration of a canarypox virus encoding the human wild-type p53 gene in colorectal cancer patients. Cancer Gene Ther 2003; 10:509–517.

27

Response and Resistance to Ionizing Radiation

Paul Dent, PhD, Adly Yacoub, PhD, Michael P. Hagan, MD, PhD, and Steven Grant, MD

SUMMARY

For many years, the impact of ionizing radiation on cell biology and survival was not fully understood, and thought to be solely dependent on the levels of DNA damage caused following radiation exposure. Similarly, the mechanisms by which growth factors and cytokines modulate cell behavior were largely unknown. In the mid-1980s, with the discovery of the first mitogen-activated protein kinase (MAPK) pathway and with subsequent discoveries of other MAPK family pathways in the early 1990s, our understanding of the hormonal control of cell biology was provided with a greater degree of molecular underpinning. In light of these findings, the ability of ionizing radiation to control the activity of MAPK family (and other) signaling pathways was first investigated in the mid-1990s. It was discovered that ionizing radiation in a cell type-dependent manner simultaneously activates multiple intracellular signal transduction pathways: the activation of some pathways has been reported to be DNA-damage dependent, that of others by generation of lipids such as ceramide, whereas others have been noted to be dependent on mitochondria-derived reactive oxygen/nitrogen species and the activation of growth factor receptor tyrosine kinases. The precise roles of growth factor receptors and signal transduction pathways in cellular responses to radiation exposure are presently under intense investigation.

Key Words: Radiation; signaling; kinase; phosphatase; reactive oxygen/nitrogen species; receptor.

From: *Cancer Drug Discovery and Development: Cancer Drug Resistance*
Edited by: B. Teicher © Humana Press Inc., Totowa, NJ

1. INTRODUCTION

For many years, the impact of ionizing radiation on cell biology and survival was not fully understood, and thought to be solely dependent on the levels of DNA damage caused following radiation exposure. Similarly, the mechanisms by which growth factors and cytokines modulate cell behavior were largely unknown. In the mid-1980s, with the discovery of the first mitogen-activated protein kinase (MAPK) pathway and with subsequent discoveries of other MAPK family pathways in the early 1990s, our understanding of the hormonal control of cell biology was provided with a greater degree of molecular underpinning. In light of these findings, the ability of ionizing radiation to control the activity of MAPK family (and other) signaling pathways was first investigated in the mid-1990s. It was discovered that ionizing radiation in a cell type-dependent manner simultaneously activates multiple intracellular signal transduction pathways: the activation of some pathways has been reported to be DNA-damage dependent, that of others by generation of lipids such as ceramide, whereas others have been noted to be dependent on mitochondria-derived reactive oxygen/nitrogen species and the activation of growth factor receptor tyrosine kinases. The precise roles of growth factor receptors and signal transduction pathways in cellular responses to radiation exposure are presently under intense investigation. Generally, in a cell type and dose-dependent manner; inhibition of the extracellular-regulated kinase (ERK)1/2, and to a greater extent, phosphatidylinositol 3 kinase (PI3K)/Akt, pathways can enhance radiosensitivity. The modulation of radiosensitivity by the ERK1/2 and Akt pathways has been correlated, in part, to the expression of both mutant active Ras isoforms and to growth factor receptors of the ErbB and insulin/insulin-like growth factor (IGF) families. The activation of the c-Jun NH_2-terminal kinase (JNK)1/2, ERK1/2, and PI3K/Akt pathways in tumor cells has also been linked to the expression of paracrine ligands such as transforming growth factor (TGF)-α, ligands that can promote cell growth and survival after irradiation and that are generally only expressed at high levels in transformed cells. This chapter discusses the signal transduction pathways activated by ionizing radiation, the roles each pathway can potentially play in cellular responses after irradiation, and the molecular approaches being taken to radiosensitize tumor cells in vitro and in vivo.

1.1. A Brief Overview of MAPK Signaling Pathways and the Affect of Ionizing Radiation on Pathway Activity

Ionizing radiation has been shown to simultaneously activate multiple signal transduction pathways; the specific cassettes of pathways that are activated is cell type dependent. In the following subheadings, the roles of growth factor receptors, MAPK pathways, PI3 kinase/Akt, and nuclear factor (NF)-κB in cell survival after irradiation are described.

1.1.1. The "Classic" MAPK Pathway, ERK1/2

"MAP-2 kinase" was first reported by the laboratory of Dr. Thomas Sturgill in 1986 (1). This protein kinase was originally described as a 42-kDa insulin-stimulated protein kinase activity whose tyrosine phosphorylation increased after insulin exposure, and which phosphorylated the cytoskeletal protein MAP-2. Contemporaneous studies from the laboratory of Dr. Melanie Cobb identified an additional 44-kDa isoform of this enzyme, termed ERK1 (2). Because many growth factors and mitogens could activate these enzymes, the acronym for this enzyme was subsequently changed to denote *mito-gen-activated protein*, or MAP kinase. Additional studies demonstrated that the p42

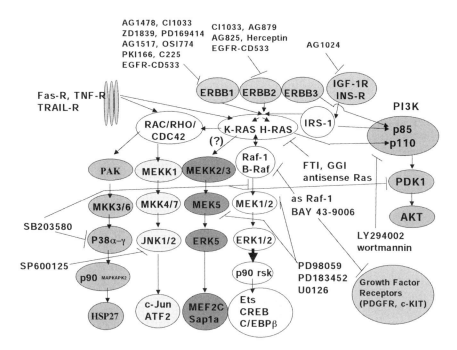

Fig. 1. Some of the characterized signal transduction pathways in mammalian cells. Growth factor receptors, e.g., the ErbB family and insulin receptors, can transmit radiation-induced signals down through GTP-binding proteins into multiple intracellular signal transduction pathways. Predominant among these pathways are the mitogen-activated protein (MAP) kinase superfamily of cascades (extracellular regulated kinase [ERK]1/2, ERK5, JNK, p38) and the phosphatidylinositol 3 kinase (PI3K) pathway. Growth factor receptors, Ras proteins, and downstream pathways are often partially or constitutively activated in tumor cells, and inhibitors have been developed to block the function of these molecules, thereby slowing cell growth and promoting cell death responses. Multiple inhibitors for the ErbB family receptors have been developed. Inhibitors of Ras farnesylation (and geranylgeranylation) are in clinical trials as are inhibitors of the ERK1/2/5 pathway. It should be noted that MAP kinase extracellular-regulated kinase (MEK)1/2 inhibitors also are capable of inhibiting the "Big" MAP kinase pathway via blocking activation of MEK5.

(ERK2) and p44 (ERK1) MAP kinases regulated another protein kinase activity (p90[rsk]) *(3)*, and that they were themselves regulated by protein kinase activities designated MAPK kinase (MKK)1/2 (MAP2K), also termed MAPK extracellular-regulated kinase (MEK)1/2 *(4–7)*. MKK1 and MKK2 were also regulated by reversible phosphorylation *(8)*. The protein kinase responsible for catalyzing MKK1/2 activation was initially described as the proto-oncogene Raf-1 *(9,10)*. This was soon followed by another MEK1/2 activating kinase, termed MEKK1, which was a mammalian homologue with similarity to the yeast *Ste11* and *Byr2* genes *(11)*. However, further studies have shown that the primary function of MEKK1 is to regulate the JNK1/2, rather than the ERK1/2, pathway *(12)* (*see* the JNK1/2 pathway, Subheading 1.1.2.). More-recent studies have suggested that other enzymes at the level of MKK1/2 can also phosphorylate and activate ERK1/2, e.g., RIP2 *(13)*, which plays a role in tumor necrosis factor (TNF)-α-induced, but not EGF-induced, ERK1/2 activation.

Plasma membrane receptors transduce signals through the membrane to its inner leaflet, leading to the recruitment and activation of guanine nucleotide exchange factors, which increases the amount of GTP bound to membrane-associated GTP-binding proteins, in particular Ras family proteins *(14–16)* (Fig. 1). There are four widely recognized isoforms of Ras: Harvey (H), Kirsten (K4A, K4B), and neuroblastoma (N) *(17)*. Receptor-stimulated guanine nucleotide exchange of Ras to the GTP-bound form permits Raf proteins and P110 PI3K to associate with Ras, resulting in kinase translocation to the plasma membrane environment, where activation of these kinases takes place. Ras contains a GTPase activity that converts bound GTP to GDP, resulting in inactivation of the Ras molecule. Mutation of Ras results in a loss of GTPase activity, generating a constitutively active Ras molecule that can lead to elevated activity within downstream signaling pathways.

Raf-1 is a member of a family of serine–threonine protein kinases comprising also B-Raf and A-Raf. All Raf family members can phosphorylate MKK1/2 and activate the ERK1/2 pathway *(18)*. Thus, the Raf kinases act at the level of a MAPK kinase kinase (MAP3K). The NH_2 domain of Raf-1 can reversibly interact with Ras family members in the plasma membrane, and the ability of Raf-1 to associate with Ras is dependent on the Ras molecule being in the GTP-bound state *(19,20)*. Additional protein serine/threonine and tyrosine phosphorylation(s) are also known to play a role increasing Raf-1 activity when in the plasma membrane environment *(21–24)*. Protein kinase C (PKC) isoforms, which can be activated by radiation, have been proposed to be Raf-1-activating kinases *(25–27)*. The initial biochemical analyses of purified Raf-1 demonstrated constitutive Y340-Y341 phosphorylation when the protein was coexpressed with Src. PI3 kinase-dependent phosphorylation of S338 may facilitate Raf-1 tyrosine phosphorylation by Src family members, leading to full activation of Raf-1 *(26,28)*. In this regard, ionizing radiation, compared to epidermal growth factor (EGF), potently enhances tyrosine phosphorylation of Raf-1 *(29)*. Radiation activates Raf-1 but not B-Raf; B-Raf is not tyrosine phosphorylated. Of note, activating B-Raf mutations have been shown to play a role in tumorigenesis in melanoma, thyroid, colorectal and cholangiocarcinoma *(30,31)*.

Phosphorylation of Raf-1 at S259 by either Akt or the cAMP-dependent protein kinase (PKA) can inhibit Raf-1 activity and its activation by upstream stimuli *(32–35)*. Phosphorylation of Raf-1 at S43 by PKA inhibits the interaction of Raf-1 with Ras molecules, thereby blocking Raf-1 translocation to the plasma membrane and its Ras-dependent activation *(36)*. In contrast to Raf-1, the B-Raf isoform does not contain an equivalent to S43, but contains multiple sites of Akt-mediated (and potentially PKA-mediated) phosphorylation in addition to the B-Raf equivalent of S259 *(37)*. B-Raf can be activated by both Ras and by cAMP via the RAP1 GTPase *(38,39)*. Thus, the regulation of the MEK1/2-ERK1/2 pathway is very complex, and in some cell types, may be both inhibited by cAMP/PKA, through Raf-1, as well as being stimulated by cAMP/RAP1, through B-Raf *(40)*.

Gene deletion studies suggest additional complexity that may have significant implications for therapeutic interventions: loss of Raf-1 function was embryonically lethal because of weak placental angiogenesis and hepatoblast apoptosis *(41,42)*. In Raf-1-null hepatocytes, ERK1/2 was activated by B-Raf rather than Raf-1, which suggests (1) fetal hepatocytes may utilize different Raf molecules to activate the ERK1/2 pathway in comparison to adult hepatocytes, and (2) deletion of Raf-1 caused the hepatocytes to survive by recruiting in compensation B-Raf as the MAP3K activator for ERK1/2, which will tend to promote growth arrest over proliferation. With reference to (1), the relative ability of Raf-1 and B-Raf to activate the ERK1/2 pathway in primary hepatocytes and established HepG2 and HuH7 hepatoma cells is also different: in primary hepatocytes and HepG2 cells, ERK1/2 pathway activation by growth factors is dependent on Raf-1 and inhibited by cAMP *(43)*, whereas in HuH7 cells B-Raf, and ERK1/2 activation can be enhanced by cAMP (P. Dent, unpublished data). This implies primary and fetal hepatocytes, and established cell lines can have very different signaling behavioral characteristics. Thus, inhibition of one Raf family member, e.g., by a specific antisense approach, will be unlikely to have a profound prolonged growth inhibitory or radiosensitizing effect on tumor cells because of a compensatory utilization of another Raf family member. In light of this, whereas antisense oligonucleotides to Raf-1 have been shown in vitro and in vivo to enhance the radiosensitivity of tumors cells *(44)*, such studies have been largely abandoned in the clinic because of poor response rates.

In addition to playing a role in the activation of the ERK1/2 pathway, it is important to note that Raf-1 may act on substrates other than MEK1/2, such as the myosin phosphatase-binding protein *(45)*. In this instance, radiation-stimulated Raf-1 was shown to regulate this process. Raf-1 has been proposed to act as an inhibitor of apoptosis signaling kinase 1 (ASK1) by binding to ASK1: the inhibitory actions of Raf-1 were reported to be independent of Raf-1 protein kinase activity *(46)*.

Several groups have shown that the epidermal growth factor receptor ([EGFR], also called ErbB1 and Her-1) is activated in response to irradiation of various carcinoma cell types *(47–50)*. Radiation exposure in the range of 1 to 2 Gy, via activation of ErbB1, can activate the ERK1/2 pathway to a level similar to that observed by physiologic, growth stimulatory, EGF concentrations (~0.1 nM). Recent publications argue that radiation-induced reactive oxygen and nitrogen species (ROS/RNS) appear to play an important role in the activation of ErbB family receptors and the ERK1/2 pathway *(51,52)*. The primary target of ROS/RNS is likely to be protein tyrosine phosphatases, each of which contain an ROS/RNS sensitive cysteine residue within their active sites, and which is a residue that is essential for phosphatase activity *(53)*.

The actions of ErbB receptor autocrine ligands have also been shown to play important roles in the activation of the ERK1/2 pathway after radiation exposure. TGF-α has been shown to mediate secondary activation of ErbB1 and the downstream ERK1/2 and JNK1/2 pathways after irradiation of several carcinoma cell lines *(54,55)*. Radiation caused an ERK1/2-dependent cleavage of pro-TGF-α in the plasma membrane within 2 h that led to its release into the growth media *(56)*. Increasing the radiation dose from 2 up to 10 Gy enhanced both the secondary activation of ErbB1 and the secondary activation of the ERK1/2 and JNK1/2 pathways, suggesting that radiation can promote a dose-dependent increase in the cleavage of pro-TGF-α that reaches a plateau at ~10 Gy *(54,56)*. It should be noted that in contrast to the secondary activation, primary activation of the receptor and signaling pathways appeared to have come to a plateau at 3–5 Gy. In addition, signaling by Ras proteins ERK1/2 and p53, the activities of which can be increased following radiation exposure, has been shown over many hours/days in a variety of cell systems to increase the expression of autocrine factors such as heparin-binding EGF and epiregulin *(57)*. More-recent findings from our group have shown that loss of mutant active K-Ras expression in HCT116 cells not only causes a reduction in epiregulin expression *(57)*, but also causes a compensatory increase in heregulin expression, resulting in a switch from radiation-induced ERK1/2 signaling to radiation-induced PI3K/Akt signaling in this cell type *(58)*. These findings argue that the activation of ErbB family receptors and the ERK1/2 pathway by radiation will be influenced by both the Ras and p53 status (mutant or wild type) of a given tumor cell.

1.1.2. THE c-JUN KINASE AND STRESS-ACTIVATED PATHWAY, JNK1/2/3

JNK1 and JNK2 were initially described biochemically to be stress-induced protein kinase activities that phosphorylated the NH$_2$-terminus of the transcription factor c-Jun; hence, the pathway is often called the stress-activated protein kinase pathway *(59–61)*.

Multiple stresses increase JNK1/2 (and the subsequently discovered JNK3) activity including UV- and γ-irradiation, cytotoxic drugs, bile acids, and ROS (e.g., H_2O_2). Phosphorylation of the NH_2-terminal sites Ser-63 and Ser-73 in c-Jun increases its ability to transactivate activating protein 1 enhancer elements in the promoters of many genes *(62,63)*. It has been suggested that JNK1/2 can phosphorylate the NH_2-terminus of c-Myc, potentially playing a role in both proliferative and apoptotic signaling *(64)*. In a similar manner to the previously described ERK1/2 MAPK pathway, JNK1/2 activities were regulated by dual threonine and tyrosine phosphorylation, which were found to be catalyzed by a protein kinase analogous to MKK1/2, termed stress-activated extracellular-regulated kinase 1, also called MKK4 *(65,66)*. An additional isoform of MKK4, termed MKK7, was subsequently discovered *(65,66)*. As in the case of MKK1 and MKK2, MKK4 and MKK7 were regulated by dual-serine phosphorylation. Recent studies have also indicated that Akt can phosphorylate and inhibit the activity of MKK4, demonstrating crosstalk between the PI3 kinase and JNK pathways *(67)*.

In contrast to the ERK1/2 pathway, however, which appears to primarily utilize the 3 protein kinases of the Raf family to activate MKK1/2, at least 10 protein kinases are known to phosphorylate and activate MKK4/7, including the Ste11/Byr2-homologues MKKK1–4, as well as proteins such as TGF-β-activated protein kinase 1 and tumor progression locus 2 *(11,68,69)*. Cleavage of MEKK1 by caspase molecules into a constitutively active molecule may play an amplifying role in the execution of apoptotic processes *(69,70)*.

Upstream of the MAP3K enzymes is another layer of JNK1/2 pathway protein kinases, e.g., Ste20-homologues and low-molecular-weight GTP-binding proteins of the Rho family, in particular CDC42 and RAC1 (*see* Fig. 1) *(25,71–73)*. It is not clear how growth factor receptors, e.g. ErbB1, activate the Rho family low-molecular-weight GTP-binding proteins; one mechanism may be via the Ras proto-oncogene, whereas others have suggested via PI3K and/or PKC isoforms *(74)*. In addition, others have shown that agonists acting through the TNF-α and fatty acid synthase receptors, via sphingomyelinase enzymes generating the messenger ceramide, can activate the JNK1/2 pathway by mechanisms that may act through Rho family GTPases (*see* e.g., ref. 75).

Thus, there appear to be at least three distinct mechanisms by which ionizing radiation activates the JNK1/2 pathway. Initial reports demonstrated that radiation-induced ceramide generation, and that the clustering of death receptors on the plasma membrane of cells played an important role in JNK1/2 activation *(76–79)*. This was linked to a proapoptotic role for JNK1/2 signaling following irradiation of cells. Other studies have argued that radiation-induced JNK1/2 activation was dependent on the ataxia telagectasia mutated (ATM) and c-Abl proteins *(80–82)*. Studies by our group of laboratories have shown that low dose radiation activates JNK1/2 in two waves in carcinoma cells *(54)*. The first wave of JNK1/2 activation was dependent on activation of the TNF-α receptor, whereas the second wave of JNK1/2 activity was dependent on ErbB1 and autocrine TGF-α. In HCT116 cells, radiation also activates JNK1/2 in two waves; however, in these cells the second wave of activation is most likely dependent on autocrine epiregulin *(58)*. Finally, it is also possible that radiation-induced JNK1/2 activation could be a secondary event to the activation of effector procaspases: cleavage of the upstream activator MEKK1 can lead to constitutive activation of this enzyme and the downstream JNK1/2 pathway, which, in some cell types, plays a key role in full commitment to apoptotic cell death *(83–85)*.

1.1.3. THE STRESS-ACTIVATED PATHWAY P38

The p38 MAPK pathway was originally described as a mammalian homologue to a yeast osmolarity-sensing pathway *(86)*. It was soon discovered that many cellular stresses activated the p38 MAPK pathway, in a manner similar to that described for the JNK pathway *(65)*. Rho family GTPases appear to play an important role as upstream activators of the p38 MAPK pathway, and via several MAP3K enzymes, e.g., the PAK family *(87)*, regulate the MAP2K enzymes MKK3 and MKK6 *(65,88)*. At least four isoforms of p38 MAPK exist, termed p38-α,, -β, -γ, and -δ *(89)*. There are several protein kinases downstream of p38 MAPK enzymes that are activated following phosphorylation by p38 isoforms including p90^{MAPKAPK2} *(90)* and mitogen- and stress-activated protein kinase 1/2 *(91)*. P90^{MAPKAPK2} phosphorylates and activates HSP27, whereas mitogen- and stress-activated protein kinase 1/2 can phosphorylate and activate transcription factors that regulate survival such as cyclic-AMP response element binding protein *(92)*.

The role of p38 MAPK signaling in cellular responses is diverse, depending on the cell type and stimulus. For example, p38 MAPK signaling has been shown to both promote cell death as well as enhance cell growth and survival *(93–95)*. The ability of ionizing radiation to regulate p38 MAPK activity appears to be highly variable, with different groups reporting no activation *(96)*, weak activation *(97)*, or strong activation *(98,99)*. This is in contrast to the ERK1/2 and JNK1/2 pathways where radiation-induced activation has been observed by many groups, in diverse cell types, in response to low and high radiation doses.

In studies where p38 MAPK activation has been observed following exposure to ionizing radiation, the p38-γ isoform has been proposed to play an essential role in causing radiation-induced G$_2$/M arrest *(99)*. In these studies, p38-γ signaling was dependent on expression of a functional ATM protein. In support of this finding, overexpression of constitutively active MKK6 also enhanced cell numbers in G$_2$/M phase. Other groups have argued that p38-α also plays a role in UV radiation-induced G$_2$/M arrest *(100)*. Collectively, these findings suggest that specific inhibitors of p38-γ may have therapeutic benefit.

1.1.4. THE "BIG" MAPK PATHWAY, ERK5

The "big MAP kinase" pathway was first described in 1995 *(101)*. The term "big" derives from the fact that whereas the molecular masses of ERK1/2 and JNK1/2 are 42/44 and 46/54 kDa, respectively, ERK5 has a mass of ~90 kDa. The upstream activators of ERK5, the MEK5 isoforms, have a similar molecular mass to other MAP2K molecules *(102,103)* and display different subcellular locations. The response of the MEK5-ERK5 pathway to growth factors such as EGF is similar to that of the MEK1/2-ERK1/2 pathway, including in many, but not all cell types, a dependency on Ras signaling *(102–106)*. Furthermore, MEK5 is also partially inhibited by the MEK1/2 inhibitors PD98059 and U0126. PD98059 acts as inhibitor of Raf-mediated phosphorylation of MEK1/2/5 molecules, but it is neither a kinase domain inhibitor of Raf proteins nor of activated MEK1: in cells PD98059 is a relatively good inhibitor of MEK1 and MEK5 (IC$_{50}$ ~5 μM) but a much poorer inhibitor of MEK2 (IC$_{50}$ ~40 μM) *(107–110)*. U0126 is reported as a more equipotent inhibitor of MEK1/2/5 that blocks both activating phosphorylations on the MEK1/2/5 proteins as well as their kinase domain activity, with IC$_{50}$s in the ~0.5 μM range *(111,112)*. The clinically used MEK1/2 inhibitor PD184352 (CI1040) acts in a similar manner to U0126, and at concentrations below 10 μM, has shown specificity for

MEK1/2 over MEK5 *(113–115)*; its use may be a useful tool to demarcate between MEK1/2-ERK1/2 and MEK5-ERK5 signaling dependencies.

The MAP3K enzymes recently shown to phosphorylate MEK5, MEKK2, and MEKK3 have been previously linked to signaling through the JNK1/2 pathway *(116)*. ERK5 has been proposed to phosphorylate and activate the transcription factors MEF2C, SAP 1a, and c-Myc *(106,107)*. In a similar manner to the ERK1/2 pathway, the ERK5 cascade has been proposed to play a key role in growth factor-stimulated cell growth and in cell survival processes (*see* Fig. 1). In growth factor-deprived PC12 cells, the ERK1/2 and ERK5 pathways appeared to each contribute ~50% of a PD98059/U0126-inhibitable survival signal *(117)*. The ability of ionizing radiation to activate MEK5-ERK5 is unknown. Based on the fact that ErbB1/Ras signaling can promote MEK5-ERK5 activation, and radiation also activates these molecules, it seems likely this pathway will be stimulated following exposure of cells to ionizing radiation. One report has shown in drug-resistant MCF-7 cells that MEK5 is overexpressed and plays a protective role against chemotherapeutic agents and death receptor activation *(118)*. Thus, it is possible that inhibition of the MEK5-ERK5 signaling module may promote radiation-induced death.

1.2. A Brief Overview of PI3 Kinase/Akt Signaling, the Affect of Radiation on Pathway Activity, and the Interactions of PI3K/Akt Signaling With Raf/ERK1/2 Pathway Signaling

PI3K enzymes consist of two subunits, a catalytic p110 subunit and a regulatory subunit, p85; several different classes of PI3K enzymes exist *(119,120)*. The p85 subunit of PI3K enzymes contains a phosphotyrosine-binding domain *(121)*. The major catalytic function of the phosphatidyl inositol 3 kinase enzymes is in the p110 subunit that acts to phosphorylate inositol phospholipids (phosphatidyl inositol 4,5 bis-phosphate) at the 3 position within the inositol sugar ring. Mitogens such as TGF-α and heregulin stimulate tyrosine phosphorylation of ErbB family receptors, providing acceptor sites for the phosphotyrosine domain of p85 *(122,123)*. Binding of p85 to active ErbB receptors (predominantly ErbB3) results in p110 PI3K activation. Other studies have suggested that mutant oncogenic H-Ras, or serpentine receptors that are stimulated by mitogens in which the p110 subunit of PI3K can directly bind to Ras-GTP, lead to catalytic activation of the kinase *(124–126)* (*see* Fig. 1).

The molecule inositol 3,4,5 trisphosphate is an acceptor site in the plasma membrane for molecules that contain a plecstrin-binding domain, in particular, the protein kinases phosphoinositide-dependent kinase (PDK)1 and Akt (also called protein kinase B) *(127)*. PDK1 is proposed to phosphorylate and activate Akt. Signaling by PDK1 to Akt and by PDK1 and Akt downstream to other protein kinases such as PKC isoforms, GSK3, mTOR, p70^{S6K}, and p90^{rsk}, has been shown to play a key role in mitogenic and metabolic responses of cells as well as protection of cells from noxious stresses *(128–132)*.

The antiapoptotic role of the PI3K/Akt pathway has been well documented by many investigators in response to numerous noxious stimuli, and in some cell types, the antiapoptotic effects of ErbB signaling have been attributed to activation of the PI3K/Akt pathway *(133,134)*. ErbB signaling to PI3K/Akt has been proposed to enhance the expression of the mitochondrial antiapoptosis proteins BCL-X$_L$, MCL-1, and caspase inhibitor proteins such as c-FLIP isoforms *(135–137)*. Enhanced expression of BCL-X$_L$ and MCL-1 will protect cells from apoptosis via the intrinsic/mitochondrial pathway, whereas expression of c-FLIP isoforms will block killing from the extrinsic pathway via death receptors *(138)*. In addition, Akt has been shown to phosphorylate Bcl2-antagonist of cell death and human procaspase 9, thereby rendering these proteins inactive in apoptotic processes *(139,140)*. Inhibitors of ErbB signaling have been shown to decrease the activity of the PI3K/Akt pathway in a variety of cell types and to increase the sensitivity of cells to a wide range of toxic stresses including cytotoxic drugs and radiation *(141)*. Activation of Akt was shown to protect cells from death in the presence of ErbB receptor inhibition *(142)*. These findings strongly argue that PI3K/Akt signaling is a key cytoprotective response in many cell types downstream of ErbB family receptors.

Inhibition of PI3 kinase signaling in cells has been achieved by use of several drugs, notably wortmannin and LY294002. Wortmannin inhibits PI3K isoforms with IC_{50} values in the low-anomolar range and LY294002 with IC_{50} values in the low-micromolar range *(143)*. Concentrations of 10 µ*M* or less of either drug is sufficient to block PI3K signaling *(133–137)*. The therapeutic usefulness of PI3K inhibitors is limited because of systemic toxicities, e.g., wortmannin was noted to cause hemorrhages, and the development of effective PI3K inhibitors without dose-limiting side effects is being undertaken by many pharmaceutical companies.

1.3. Modulation of Receptor Ras and Signaling Pathway Function to Achieve Radiosensitization

1.3.1. INHIBITION OF GROWTH FACTOR RECEPTORS

Signaling by ErbB family of receptors is, in general, believed to be proproliferative and cytoprotective *(144,145)*. In some cell types, however, signaling by ErbB1 is known to promote growth arrest and apoptosis (see, e.g., refs. *146* and *147*). Because both receptor expression as well as autocrine growth factor levels are often increased in carcinoma cells compared to normal tissue, many laboratories have studied signaling by the ErbB family in tumor cell growth and survival control. Thus, it has been discovered that when signaling from ErbB family receptors is blocked, either by use of inhibitory antibodies (e.g., C225, 4D5 Herceptin®, monoclonal antibody 806), small-molecular-weight inhibitors of receptor tyrosine kinases (e.g., PD183805 [also called CI1033], PKI166, AG1478, PD153035, ZD1839, PD169414, OSI774, AG825, AG879), dominant-negative truncated receptors (e.g., dominant-negative EGFR-CD533, dominant-negative ErbB2) or antisense approaches (antisense EGFR), that tumor cell growth can be reduced, and the sensitivity of these cells to being killed by noxious stresses increased *(148–163)* (*see* Fig. 1).

The antibodies C225 and 4D5 Herceptin bind to the extracellular portions of ErbB1 and ErbB2, respectively *(164,165)*. In the instance of ErbB1, C225 appears to bind to the portion of the molecule that associates with growth factor ligands such as EGF and TGF-α *(166)*. Thus the ability of growth factors, in the presence of receptor bound C225, to stimulate ErbB1 receptor function is abolished (*see* Fig. 1). C225 does not block the primary activation of the receptor or ERK1/2 following irradiation, in general agreement with the ligand-independent nature of this process. The antiproliferative and antisurvival mechanisms of action of Herceptin appear to be more complex, in as much as whereas Herceptin binds to ErbB2, this receptor has no known ligand. Instead, it appears that Herceptin acts by causing the internalization and degradation of ErbB2, as well as by blocking ErbB2 heterodimerization with other ErbB family members *(167)*. Both C225 and Herceptin have been shown to individually kill cells, and to interact in a synergistic fashion in combination with standard therapeutic regimens such as ionizing radiation, cisplatin and taxol to reduce tumor cell survival both in vitro and in vivo *(168–171)*. Both C225 and Herceptin are entering the clinic and it is likely, despite setbacks for C225 in Food and Drug Administration approval, that both agents will become standard tools in the treatment of epithelial cell cancers. More-recent studies have used monoclonal antibodies to target truncated forms of ErbB1, e.g., EGFR VIII *(150,172)*. In these studies, a novel monoclonal antibody, 806, was found to potently inhibit truncated forms of ErbB1 and more weakly inhibit full-length receptors *(172)*. The inhibition of receptor function correlated with reduced tumor cell growth in vitro and in vivo. Of note, however, it is presently unclear whether all of the antitumor effects of anti-ErbB receptor antibodies are mediated solely via receptor inhibition or by a combination of receptor inhibition and enhanced immunological reactivity in vivo because of the Fc portion of the antibody.

Small-molecule inhibitors of the tyrosine kinase domains of the ErbB family of receptors have been used with some success in blocking tumor cell growth and survival both in vitro and in vivo. The inhibitors AG1478, ZD1839 (Iressa®), PD153035 (also called AG1517), PKI166, OSI774, CI1033 (PD183805), and PD169414 (an irreversible inhibitor), all bind to the catalytic kinase domain of ErbB1 and inhibit tyrosine kinase activity *(151–159,173–175)*. Some studies have suggested that CI1033 binds to, and inhibits, all ErbB kinase domains. Inhibition of ErbB1 kinase activity not only blocks phosphorylation of ErbB1 itself in response to the growth factors that it binds, but also inhibits the transphosphorylation of other ErbB family members by ErbB1. In addition to inhibiting ErbB1, the tyrphostin AG1478 has been shown to inhibit ErbB4 *(142)*. The tyrphostin inhibitors AG825 and AG879 are ErbB2 inhibitors with apparently weaker kinase specificity than AG1478 for ErbB1/4, and they can inhibit Trk receptors *(158,159)*. Thus, AG825 / AG879, together with AG1478, have the potential to not only impact on EGF/ TGFα signaling through ErbB1, but also neuregulin/heregulin signaling through ErbB4 and ErbB3 *(176)*. Small-molecular-weight ErbB inhibitors are currently in clinical trials, both as stand-alone agents and in combination with ionizing radiation and other standard chemotherapeutic agents (*see*, e.g., refs. *177*, *178*, *179*, and *180*).

In addition to use of antibodies and small-molecular-weight inhibitors, the ErbB family of receptors has been inhibited by the use of dominant-negative and antisense approaches. In particular, expression of truncated forms of ErbB1 (EGFR-CD533), ErbB2 and ErbB3 in a variety of cell types has been shown to reduce proliferation and survival of both normal and tumor cells in vitro and in vivo *(160,181–185)*. The dominant-negative approaches are believed to act by blocking homo- and heterodimerization of ErbB family members, reducing receptor transphosphorylation and thus, downstream signaling by the receptors. Initial studies demonstrated that radiation could activate ErbB1 *(181)* and subsequent investigations using dominant-negative EGFR-CD533 demonstrated that it could block this effect *(182–185)*. Whether such adenoviral approaches, which lack a true "bystander effect" on uninfected tumor cells, can be translated into the clinic, is unknown.

In addition to the ErbB family, other growth factor and cytokine receptors are believed to play an important role in cellular radiation responses, such as IGF1R *(186)*. Prolonged exposure of MCF-7 cells to tamoxifen results in the development of a cell line that expresses high levels of ErbB1 and its ligand TGF-α *(187)*. Exposure of these cells to ZD1839 (Iressa), results in the development of a cell line resistant to the anti-proliferative and cytotoxic effects of tamoxifen and ErbB receptor inhibitors, but that has become sensitive to inhibitors of the IGF1R such as AG1024 *(188)*. Radiation can enhance tyrosine phosphorylation of the IGF1R, and can radiosensitize tumor cells *(186)*.

Cytokines such as TNF-α, interleukin-6, urokinase-type plasminogen activator, and TGF-β have also been proposed to control cell survival responses following irradiation *(189–192)*. Radiation has been shown to cause rapid activation of the TNF-α receptor and in addition, radiation stimulated signaling modules such as the classical MAPK and p38 pathways are known to enhance the synthesis of TNF-α ligand *(193)*. TNF-α signaling following irradiation may lead to the activation of both procaspase enzymes as well as the cytoprotective transcription factor NF-κB *(194)*. Thus, the cellular outcome of radiation-induced TNF-α receptor signaling will be a complex summation of opposing cellular signals.

TGF-β in nontransformed cells can cause growth arrest and differentiation *(195)*. In tumor cells, TGF-β has been shown to cause in a cell-type-dependent manner either cytoprotection or apoptosis *(196)*. In some cells, TGF-β appears to confer a protective effect via ERK1/2 signaling and potentially the expression of molecules such as heparin-binding EGF and BCL-X_L *(197–199)*. In contrast, TGF-β in other cell types appears to protect cells in a Ras- and ERK1/2-independent manner that is dependent on PI3K signaling *(200)*. Thus, multiple cytokines, in addition to those that bind to ErbB family receptor, play a role in the radiation responses of both nontransformed as well as tumor cells.

1.5.2. INHIBITION OF RAS FUNCTION

Mutated active *H-Ras* was one of the first oncogenes discovered, in bladder cancer cells *(201)*, and approximately one third of human cancers have *Ras* mutations, primarily the *K-Ras* isoforms. Early studies examining Ras transformation noted that Ras proteins were prenylated and proteolytically processed, causing their translocation into the plasma membranes of cells *(202)*. Ras proteins that could not be prenylated were not located in membranes and could not cause transformation. Subsequently, pharmaceutical companies developed inhibitors of Ras prenylation (farnesyltransferase and geranylgeranyltransferase inhibitors) that block the prenylation of Ras proteins as well as other small GTP-binding proteins including RAC/Rho/CDC42 *(203)*. Antisense techniques have also been used to manipulate Ras expression *(204)*. Inhibition of small GTP-binding protein prenylation has been shown to both growth arrest and radiosensitize tumor cells in a mutated active Ras-independent fashion, arguing that Ras may not be the primary target of this therapeutic approach *(205)*. In the clinic, as single agents, farnesyltransferase inhibitors have not proven highly successful and the long-term future of such agents remains unclear.

1.5.3. INHIBITION OF RAF/MEK/ERK1/2 AND PI3 KINASE/AKT FUNCTION

Data from several groups supports the argument that a key radioprotective pathway downstream of plasma membrane receptors is the PI3K pathway. Inhibition of p110 PI3K function by use of the inhibitors LY294002 and wortmannin radiosensitzes tumor cells expressing mutant Ras molecules or wild-type Ras molecules that are constitutively active *(206–209)*. It is possible that these inhibitors may exert a portion of their radiosensitizing properties by inhibiting proteins with PI3K-like kinase domains such as ATM, ATM–Rad3-related, and DNA-PK. Expression of a constitutively active p110 PI3K molecule was able to recapitulate partially the expression of mutant H-Ras in protecting cells from radiation toxicity in these studies. In the same studies that PI3K p110 inhibitors were shown to radiosensitize cells, p38 inhibitors, e.g., SB203580, were used at concentrations that also have been shown to blunt PDK1 and Akt activity *(210–212)*, did not radiosensitize cells. Recent data have also suggested that antisense PDK1 oligo-nucleotides do not radiosensitize cells *(213)*. In contrast, dominant-negative Akt radiosensitizes HCT116 cells expressing mutant active H-Ras *(58)*. Thus, LY294002 and wortmannin may sensitize tumor cells to radiation through PI3K-dependent, PDK1-independent pathway(s). Of note, in these cell lines and culture conditions, inhibition of the ERK1/2 pathway did not appear to alter the radiosensitivity of cells.

The cytotoxic effects of drugs, as well as radiation, can be magnified by inhibition of ErbB receptors that is paralleled by a reduced ability of cells to activate the ERK1/2 and PI3K pathways *(214)*. For example, expression of dominant-negative EGFR–CD533 enhanced apoptosis and radiosensitized MDA-MB-231 mammary carcinoma cells that were dependent on, at least in part, inhibition of radiation-induced ERK1/2 signaling: neither basal activity nor activation of PI3K/Akt was blocked under these conditions *(215)*. Expression of this dominant-negative ErbB1 molecule could also radiosensitize glioblastoma cells that correlated with both reduced basal ERK1/2 activity and radiation-induced ERK1/2 activation *(216)*.

In many cell types, ERK1/2 signaling does not appear to play a role in controlling radiosensitivity. In those cells where effects have been observed, the abilities of MEK1/2 inhibitors to enhance cell killing by radiation was originally linked to a derangement of radiation-induced G_2/M growth arrest and enhanced apoptosis *(164,217)*. Although others have not noted this finding, despite observing radiosensitization *(218)*. In general agreement with this notion, other groups have argued that prolonged activation of the ERK1/2 pathway in fibroblasts following irradiation promotes radiosensitivity in some cell types by abrogating the G_2/M checkpoint *(219,220)*. In agreement with this concept, and of particular note, we have recently shown that the G_2/M checkpoint abrogator UCN-01 potently activates the ERK1/2 pathway *(221)*. MEK1/2 inhibitors synergize with UCN-01 to promote cell death, but radiation does not further enhance the apoptotic response of these cells, indicative that MEK1/2 inhibitors require an intact G_2/M checkpoint to enhance radiation-induced apoptosis. The dual positive and negative nature of ERK1/2 signaling in the control of cell survival has also been observed for other DNA damaging agents such as adriamycin and UV radiation *(222–224)*.

An additional example of this dual nature of ERK1/2 signaling is displayed by DU145 human prostate cancer cells. These cells secrete the ErbB1 ligand TGF-α that confers autocrine growth through ERK1/2 signaling. Ionizing radiation markedly increases the release of TGF-α providing a growth stimulus that is at odds with cellular repair mechanisms. If ErbB1-ERK1/2 signaling is *transiently* blocked either by the tyrphostin AG1478 or by a MEK1/2 inhibitor before irradiation, then DU145 cell growth is retarded and radiation-induced cell killing is decreased. Moreover, if ErbB1 is strongly activated by EGF or TGF-α immediately after irradiation, then cell killing is increased, as would be expected, i.e., transient inhibition of radiation-induced ERK1/2 signaling or suprastimulation of ERK1/2 activity at the time of irradiation radiosensitizes tumor cells. Removal of MEK1/2 inhibitor from the growth media 24 and 48 h after irradiation results in a null effect on DU145 cell radiosensitivity. Similar data were also obtained in A431 squamous carcinoma cells *(225)*. On the other hand, we have previously reported that following irradiation, *prolonged* inhibition of ERK1/2 ($\geq$72 h) can significantly increase the apoptotic response of DU145 and A431 cells and reduce clonogenic survival *(226–228)*. Therefore, the interruption of ERK1/2 signaling can either enhance or degrade carcinoma cell survival depending on its timing and duration.

The transcription factor NF-κB has been shown to be downstream of ErbB and TNF-α receptors and was proposed to act in radioprotection *(229)*. However, other studies have argued against NF-κB as a direct radioprotective factor *(230)*. Several manuscripts have suggested that NF-κB signaling is regulated by the PI3K pathway *(231)*, whereas others have suggested ERK1/2 signaling can regulate this transcription factor through autocrine mechanisms, e.g., enhanced TNF-α expression *(232–235)*. Radiation-induced inhibitory κB kinase activation has been argued to be PI3K-independent *(236)*. ERK1/2 signaling has the potential to inhibit expression of the protein PAR4 that is downstream of mutant Ras molecules *(237,238)*. Proteinase-activated receptor (PAR)4 is a protein inhibitor of PKC-ζ and NF-κB function *(239–243)*. More recently, PAR4 has been shown to radiosensitize prostate tumor cells *(242)*. This may be, in part, because of enhanced signaling from death receptors *(243)*. Thus, PAR4 may be a link between ERK1/2 signaling, NF-κB, function, and radiosensitivity. Hence in a cell-type-dependent manner, PI3K, NF-κB, or ERK1/2 signaling, downstream of receptors and Ras molecules, or a combination of these signals, may play a radioprotective role.

2. FUTURE DIRECTIONS: THE RATIONAL COMBINATION OF SIGNALING MODULATORS IN RADIOTHERAPY

Tumor samples isolated from patients by fine-needle aspiration are often subjected to a battery of tests to determine some of the molecular characteristics known to predispose tumor cells to invasion and chemotherapy/radiation resistance, e.g., ErbB2 expression, Ras protein levels, and estrogen/progesterone receptor expression. Based on knowledge gained in the last 10 yr, it should be straightforward to utilize such samples to also determine the expression of other growth factor receptors, e.g., IGF1R; paracrine ligands, e.g., TGF-α; and the activity status of pathways such as ERK1/2 and PI3K/Akt. Armed with such knowledge, it should then be possible to design rationally therapeutic strategies that are tailored to the malignancy in each individual.

REFERENCES

1. Sturgill TW, Ray LB. Muscle proteins related to microtubule associated protein-2 are substrates for an insulin-stimulatable kinase. Biochem Biophys Res Commun 1986; 134:565–571.
2. Boulton TG, Cobb MH. Identification of multiple extracellular signal-regulated kinases (ERKs) with antipeptide antibodies. Cell Regul 1991; 2:357–371.
3. Sturgill TW, Ray LB, Erikson E, Maller JL. Insulin-stimulated MAP-2 kinase phosphorylates and activates ribosomal protein S6 kinase II. Nature 1988; 334:715–718.
4. Haystead CM, Wu J, Gregory P, Sturgill TW, Haystead TA. Functional expression of a MAP kinase kinase in COS cells and recognition by an anti-STE7/byr1 antibody. FEBS Lett 1993; 317:12–16.
5. Robbins DJ, Zhen E, Owaki H, et al. Regulation and properties of extracellular signal-regulated protein kinases 1 and 2 in vitro. J Biol Chem 1993; 268:5097–5106.
6. Wu J, Michel H, Rossomando A, et al. Renaturation and partial peptide sequencing of mitogen-activated protein kinase (MAP kinase) activator from rabbit skeletal muscle. Biochem J 1992; 285:701–705.
7. Wu J, Harrison JK, Dent P, Lynch KR, Weber MJ, Sturgill TW. Identification and characterization of a new mammalian mitogen-activated protein kinase kinase, MKK2. Mol Cell Biol 1993; 13:4539–4548.
8. Rossomando AJ, Dent P, Sturgill TW, Marshak DR. Mitogen-activated protein kinase kinase 1 (MKK1) is negatively regulated by threonine phosphorylation. Mol Cell Biol 1994; 14:1594–1602.
9. Dent P, Haser W, Haystead TA, Vincent LA, Roberts TM, Sturgill TW. Activation of mitogen-activated protein kinase kinase by v-Raf in NIH 3T3 cells and in vitro. Science 1992; 257:1404–1407.
10. Kyriakis JM, App H, Zhang XF, Banerjee P, Brautigan DL, Rapp UR, Avruch J. Raf-1 activates MAP kinase-kinase. Nature 1992; 358:417–421.
11. Lange-Carter CA, Pleiman CM, Gardner AM, Blumer KJ, Johnson GL. A divergence in the MAP kinase regulatory network defined by MEK kinase and Raf. Science 1993; 260:315–319.
12. Yan M, Dai T, Deak JC, et al. Activation of stress-activated protein kinase by MEKK1 phosphorylation of its activator SEK1. Nature 1994; 37:2798–2800.
13. Navas TA, Baldwin DT, Stewart TA. RIP2 is a Raf1-activated mitogen-activated protein kinase kinase. J Biol Chem 1999; 274:33,684–33,690.

14. Li W, Liang X, Kellendonk C, Poli V, Taub R. STAT3 contributes to the mitogenic response of hepatocytes during liver regeneration. J Biol Chem 2002; 277:28,411–28,417.

15. Okumura K, ShiRasawa S, Nishioka M, Sasazuki T. Activated Ki-Ras suppresses 12-O-tetradecanoylphorbol-13-acetate-induced activation of the c-Jun NH2-terminal kinase pathway in human colon cancer cells. Cancer Res 1999; 59:2445–2450.

16. Olivier JP, Raabe T, Henkemeyer M, et al. A Drosophila SH2-SH3 adaptor protein implicated in coupling the sevenless tyrosine kinase to an activator of Ras guanine nucleotide exchange. Sos Cell 1993; 73:179–191.

17. Reuther GW, Der CJ. The Ras branch of small GTPases: Ras family members don't fall far from the tree. Curr Opin Cell Biol 2000; 12:157–165.

18. Tombes RM, Auer KL, Mikkelsen R, et al. The mitogen-activated protein (MAP) kinase cascade can either stimulate or inhibit DNA synthesis in primary cultures of rat hepatocytes depending upon whether its activation is acute/phasic or chronic. Biochem J 1998; 330:1451–1460.

19. Moodie SA, Willumsen BM, Weber MJ, Wolfman A. Complexes of Ras.GTP with Raf-1 and mitogen-activated protein kinase kinase. Science 1993; 260:1658–1661.

20. Van Aelst L, Barr M, Marcus S, Polverino A, Wigler M. Complex formation between Ras and Raf and other protein kinases. Proc Natl Acad Sci U S A 1993; 90:6213–6217.

21. Dent P, Jelinek T, Morrison DK, Weber MJ, Sturgill TW. Reversal of Raf-1 activation by purified and membrane-associated protein phosphatases. Science 1995; 268:1902–1906.

22. Dent P, Reardon DB, Morrison DK, Sturgill TW. Regulation of Raf-1 and Raf-1 mutants by Ras-dependent and Ras-independent mechanisms in vitro. Mol Cell Biol 1995b; 15:4125–4135.

23. Fabian JR, Daar IO, Morrison DK. Critical tyrosine residues regulate the enzymatic and biological activity of Raf-1 kinase. Mol Cell Biol 1993; 13:7170–7179.

24. Marais R, Light Y, Paterson HF, Mason CS, Marshall CJ. Differential regulation of Raf-1, A-Raf, and B-Raf by oncogenic ras and tyrosine kinases. J Biol Chem 1997; 272:4378–4383.

25. Cai H, Smola U, Wixler V, et al. Role of diacylglycerol-regulated protein kinase C isotypes in growth factor activation of the Raf-1 protein kinase. Mol Cell Biol 1997; 17:732–741.

26. Schonwasser DC, Marais RM, Marshall CJ, Parker PJ. Activation of the mitogen-activated protein kinase/extracellular signal-regulated kinase pathway by conventional, novel, and atypical protein kinase C isotypes. Mol Cell Biol 1998; 18:790–798.

27. Stravitz RT, Rao YP, Vlahcevic ZR, Gurley EC, Jarvis WD, Hylemon PB. Hepatocellular protein kinase C activation by bile acids: implications for regulation of cholesterol 7 α-hydroxylase. Am J Physiol 1996; 271:G293–G303.

28. King AJ, Wireman RS, Hamilton M, Marshall MS. Phosphorylation site specificity of the Pak-mediated regulation of Raf-1 and cooperativity with Src. FEBS Lett 2001; 497:6–14.

29. Kavanagh BD, Dent P, Schmidt-Ullrich RK, Chen P, Mikkelsen RB. Calcium-dependent stimulation of mitogen-activated protein kinase activity in A431 cells by low doses of ionizing radiation. Radiation Res 1998; 149:579–587.

30. Kimura ET, Nikiforova MN, Zhu Z, Knauf JA, Nikiforov YE, Fagin JA. High prevalence of BRaf mutations in thyroid cancer: genetic evidence for constitutive activation of the RET/PTC-Ras-BRaf signaling pathway in papillary thyroid carcinoma. Cancer Res 2003; 63:1454–1457.

31. Tannapfel A, Sommerer F, Benicke M, et al. Mutations of the BRaf gene in cholangiocarcinoma but not in hepatocellular carcinoma. Gut 2003; 52:706–712.

32. Dhillon AS, Pollock C, Steen H, Shaw PE, Mischak H, Kolch W. Cyclic AMP-dependent kinase regulates Raf-1 kinase mainly by phosphorylation of serine 259. Mol Cell Biol 2002; 22:3237–3246.

33. Reusch HP, Zimmermann S, Schaefer M, Paul M, Moelling K. Regulation of Raf by Akt controls growth and differentiation in vascular smooth muscle cells. J Biol Chem 2001; 276:33,630–33,637.

34. Yip-Schneider MT, Miao W, Lin A, Barnard DS, Tzivion G, Marshall MS. Regulation of the Raf-1 kinase domain by phosphorylation and 14-3-3 association. Biochem J 2000; 351:151–159.

35. Zimmermann S, Moelling K. Phosphorylation and regulation of Raf by Akt (protein kinase B). Science 1999; 286:1741–1744.

36. Wu J, Dent P, Jelinek T, Wolfman A, Weber MJ, Sturgill TW. Inhibition of the EGF-activated MAP kinase signaling pathway by adenosine 3′,5′-monophosphate. Science 1993b; 262:1065–1069.

37. Guan KL, Figueroa C, Brtva TR, et al. Negative regulation of the serine/threonine kinase B–Raf by Akt. J Biol Chem 2000; 275:27,354–23,759.

38. Klinger M, Kudlacek O, Seidel MG, Freissmuth M, Sexl V. MAP kinase stimulation by cAMP does not require RAP1 but Src family kinases. J Biol Chem 2002; 277:32,490–32,497.

39. York RD, Molliver DC, Grewal SS, Stenberg PE, McCleskey EW, Stork PJ. Role of phosphoinositide 3-kinase and endocytosis in nerve growth factor-induced extracellular signal-regulated kinase activation via Ras and Rap1. Mol Cell Biol 2000; 20:8069–8083.

40. Brummer T, Shaw PE, Reth M, Misawa Y. Inducible gene deletion reveals different roles for B-Raf and Raf-1 in B-cell antigen receptor signalling. EMBO J 2002; 21:5611–5622

41. Huser M, Luckett J, Chiloeches A, et al. MEK kinase activity is not necessary for Raf-1 function. EMBO J 2001; 20:1940–1951.

42. Mikula M, Schreiber M, Husak Z, et al. Embryonic lethality and fetal liver apoptosis in mice lacking the c-raf-1 gene. EMBO J 2001; 20:1952–1962.

43. Auer KL, Spector MS, Tombes RM, et al. Alpha-adrenergic inhibition of proliferation in HepG2 cells stably transfected with the α1B-adrenergic receptor through a p42MAPkinase/p21Cip1/WAF1-dependent pathway. FEBS Lett 1998a; 436:131–138.

44. Gokhale PC, Zhang C, Newsome JT, et al. Pharmacokinetics, toxicity, and efficacy of ends-modified raf antisense oligodeoxyribonucleotide encapsulated in a novel cationic liposome. Clin Cancer Res 2002; 11:3611–21.

45. Broustas CG, Grammatikakis N, Eto M, Dent P, Brautigan DL, Kasid U. Phosphorylation of the myosin-binding subunit of myosin phosphatase by Raf-1 and inhibition of phosphatase activity. J Biol Chem 2002; 277:3053–3059.

46. Chen J, Fujii K, Zhang L, Roberts T, Fu H. Raf-1 promotes cell survival by antagonizing apoptosis signal-regulating kinase 1 through a MEK-ERK independent mechanism. Proc Natl Acad Sci U S A 2001; 98:7783–7788.

47. Schmidt-Ullrich RK, Mikkelsen RB, Dent P, et al. Radiation-induced proliferation of the human A431 squamous carcinoma cells is dependent on EGFR tyrosine phosphorylation. Oncogene 1997; 15:1191–1197.

48. Carter S, Auer KL, Birrer M, et al. "Inhibition of mitogen activated protein kinase cascade potentiates cell killing by low dose ionizing radiation in A431 human squamous carcinoma cells". Oncogene 1998; 16:2787–2796.

49. Kavanagh BD, Dent P, Schmidt-Ullrich RK, Chen P, Mikkelsen RB. Calcium-dependent stimulation of mitogen-activated protein kinase activity in A431 cells by low doses of ionizing radiation". Radiation Res 1998; 149:579–587.

50. Balaban N, Moni J, Shannon M, Dang L, Murphy E, Goldkorn T. "The effect of ionizing radiation on signal transduction: antibodies to EGF receptor sensitize A431 cells to radiation." Biochim Biophys Acta 1996; 1314:147–156.

51. Leach JK, Van Tuyle G, Lin PS, Schmidt-Ullrich R, Mikkelsen RB. Ionizing radiation-induced, mito-chondria-dependent generation of reactive oxygen/nitrogen. Cancer Res 2001; 61:3894–3901.

52. Leach JK, Black SM, Schmidt-Ullrich RK, Mikkelsen RB. Activation of constitutive nitric-oxide synthase activity is an early signaling event induced by ionizing radiation. J Biol Chem 2002; 277:15,400–15,406.

53. Mikkelsen RB, Wardman P. Biological chemistry of reactive oxygen and nitrogen and radiation-induced signal transduction mechanisms. Oncogene 2003; 22:5734–5754.

54. Dent P, Reardon DB, Park JS, et al. Radiation-induced release of transforming growth factor alpha activates the epidermal growth factor receptor and mitogen-activated protein kinase pathway in carcinoma cells, leading to increased proliferation and protection from radiation-induced cell death. Mol Biol Cell 1999; 8:2493–2506.

55. Hagan M, Wang L, Hanley JR, Park JS, Dent P. Ionizing radiation-induced mitogen-activated protein (MAP) kinase activation in DU145 prostate carcinoma cells: MAP kinase inhibition enhances radiation-induced cell killing and G2/M-phase arrest. Radiat Res 2000; 153:371–383.

56. Yacoub, A Dent P, Hagan M. Ionizing radiation causes a dose-dependent release of the growth factor TGF-α in vitro, from irradiated Xenografts, and during the palliative treatment of patients suffering from hormone refractory prostate carcinoma. Clin Cancer Res 2004; 10:5724–5731.

57. Baba I, Shirasawa S, Iwamoto R, et al. Involvement of deregulated epiregulin expression in tumorigenesis in vivo through activated Ki-Ras signaling pathway in human colon cancer cells. Cancer Res 2000; 60:6886–6889.

58. Caron R, Yacoub A, Zhu X, et al. Heregulin/ErbB3 signaling plays an essential role in H-Ras / PI3K-induced radioresistance in colon cancer cells. Mol Cancer Therap 2004; 4:243–255.

59. Derijard B, Hibi M, Wu IH, et al. JNK1: a protein kinase stimulated by UV light and Ha-Ras that binds and phosphorylates the c-Jun activation domain. Cell 1994; 76:1025–1037.

60. Derijard B, Raingeaud J, Barrett T, Wu IH, Han J, Ulevitch RJ, Davis RJ. Independent human MAP-kinase signal transduction pathways defined by MEK and MKK isoforms. Science 1995; 267:682–685.

61. Hibi M, Lin A, Smeal T, Minden A, Karin M. Identification of an oncoprotein- and UV-responsive protein kinase that binds and potentiates the c-Jun activation domain. Genes Dev 1993; 7:2135–2148.

62. Davis RJ. Signal transduction by the c-Jun N-terminal kinase. Biochem Soc Symp 1999; 64:1–12.

63. Eferl R, Sibilia M, Hilberg F, et al. Functions of c-Jun in liver and heart development. J Cell Biol 1999; 145:1049–1061.

64. Noguchi K, Kitanaka C, Yamana H, Kokubu A, Mochizuki T, Kuchino Y. Regulation of c-Myc through phosphorylation at Ser-62 and Ser-71 by c-Jun N-terminal kinase. J Biol Chem 1999; 274:32,580–32,587.

65. Lin A, Minden A, Martinetto H, Claret FX, et al. Identification of a dual specificity kinase that activates the Jun kinases and p38-Mpk2. Science 1995; 268:286–290.

66. Tournier C, Whitmarsh AJ, Cavanagh J, Barrett T, Davis RJ. The MKK7 gene encodes a group of c-Jun NH2-terminal kinase kinases. Mol Cell Biol 1999; 19:1569–1581.

67. Park HS, Kim MS, Huh SH, et al. Akt (protein kinase B) negatively regulates SEK1 by means of protein phosphorylation. J Biol Chem 2002; 277:2573–2578.

68. Schlesinger TK, Bonvin C, Jarpe MB, et al. Apoptosis stimulated by the 91-kDa caspase cleavage MEKK1 fragment requires translocation to soluble cellular compartments. J Biol Chem 2002; 277:10,283–10,291.

69. Yan M, Dai T, Deak JC, et al. Activation of stress-activated protein kinase by MEKK1 phosphorylation of its activator SEK1. Nature 1994; 37:2798–2800.

70. Widmann C, Gerwins P, Johnson NL, Jarpe MB, Johnson GL. MEK kinase 1, a substrate for DEVD-directed caspases, is involved in genotoxin-induced apoptosis. Mol Cell Biol 1998; 18:2416–2429.

71. Frost JA, Xu S, Hutchison MR, Marcus S, Cobb MH. Actions of Rho family small G proteins and p21-activated protein kinases on mitogen-activated protein kinase family members. Mol Cell Biol 1996; 16:3707–3713.

72. Graves JD, Draves KE, Gotoh Y, Krebs EG, Clark EA. Both phosphorylation and caspase-mediated cleavage contribute to regulation of the Ste20-like protein kinase Mst1 during CD95/Fas-induced apoptosis. J Biol Chem 2001; 276:14,909–14,915.

73. Yustein JT, Li D, Robinson D, Kung HJ. KFC, a Ste20-like kinase with mitogenic potential and capability to activate the SAPK/JNK pathway. Oncogene 2000; 19:710–718.

74. Timokhina I, Kissel H, Stella G, Besmer P. Kit signaling through PI 3-kinase and Src kinase pathways: an essential role for Rac1 and JNK activation in mast cell proliferation. EMBO J 1998; 17:6250–6262.

75. Lu Y, Settleman J. The role of rho family GTPases in development: lessons from Drosophila melanogaster. Mol Cell Biol Res Commun 1999; 1:87–94.

76. Rosette C, Karin M. Ultraviolet light and osmotic stress: activation of the JNK cascade through multiple growth factor and cytokine receptors. Science 1996; 274:1194–1197.

77. Cremesti A, Paris F, Grassme H, et al. Ceramide enables fas to cap and kill. J Biol Chem 2001; 276:23,954–23,961.

78. Verheij M, Bose R, Lin XH, et al. Requirement for ceramide-initiated SAPK/JNK signaling in stress-induced apoptosis. Nature 1996; 380:75–79.

79. Herr I, Wilhelm D, Bohler T, Angel P, Debatin KM. Activation of CD95 (APO-1/Fas) signaling by ceramide mediates cancer therapy-induced apoptosis. EMBO J 1997; 16:6200–6208.

80. Kharbanda S, Yuan ZM, Weichselbaum R, Kufe D. Determination of cell fate by c-Abl activation in the response to DNA damage. Oncogene 1998; 17:3309–3318.

81. Bar-Shira A, Rashi-Elkeles S, Zlochover L, et al. ATM-dependent activation of the gene encoding MAP kinase phosphatase 5 by radiomimetic DNA damage. Oncogene 2002; 21:849–855.

83. Zhang Y, Ma WY, Kaji A, Bode AM, Dong Z. Requirement of ATM in UVA-induced signaling and apoptosis. J Biol Chem 2002; 277:3124–3131.

84. Widmann C, Johnson NL, Gardner AM, Smith RJ, Johnson GL. Potentiation of apoptosis by low dose stress stimuli in cells expressing activated MEK kinase 1. Oncogene 1997; 15:2439–2447.

85. Widmann C, Gerwins P, Johnson NL, Jarpe MB, Johnson GL. MEK kinase 1, a substrate for DEVD-directed caspases, is involved in genotoxin-induced apoptosis. Mol Cell Biol 1998; 18:2416–2429.

86. Schlesinger TK, Bonvin C, Jarpe MB, et al. Apoptosis stimulated by the 91-kDa caspase cleavage MEKK1 fragment requires translocation to soluble cellular compartments. J Biol Chem 2002; 277:10,283–10,291.

87. Han J, Lee JD, Bibbs L, Ulevitch RJ. A MAP kinase targeted by endotoxin and hyperosmolarity in mammalian cells. Science 1994; 265:808–811.

88. Holbrook NJ, Liu Y, Fornace AJ. Signaling events controlling the molecular response to genotoxic stress. EXS 1996; 77:273–288.

89. Han J, Lee JD, Jiang Y, Li Z, Feng L, Ulevitch RJ. Characterization of the structure and function of a novel MAP kinase kinase (MKK6). J Biol Chem 1996; 271:2886–2891.

90. Kyriakis JM, Avruch J. Mammalian mitogen-activated protein kinase signal transduction pathways activated by stress and inflammation. Physiol Rev 2001; 81:807–869.

91. Maizels ET, Mukherjee A, Sithanandam G, et al. Developmental regulation of mitogen-activated protein kinase-activated kinases-2 and -3 (MAPKAPK-2/-3) in vivo during corpus luteum formation in the rat. Mol Endocrinol 2001; 15:716–733.

92. Deak MM, Clifton AD, Lucocq LM, Alessi DR. Mitogen- and stress-activated protein kinase-1 (MSK1) is directly activated by MAPK and SAPK2/p38, and may mediate activation of CREB. EMBO J 1998; 17:4426–4441.

93. Wiggin GR, Soloaga A, Foster JM, Murray-Tait V, Cohen P, Arthur JS. MSK1 and MSK2 are required for the mitogen- and stress-induced phosphorylation of CREB and ATF1 in fibroblasts. Mol Cell Biol 2002; 22:2871–2881.

94. Juretic N, Santibanez JF, Hurtado C, Martinez J. ERK 1,2 and p38 pathways are involved in the proliferative stimuli mediated by urokinase in osteoblastic SaOS-2 cell line. J Cell Biochem 2001; 83:92–98.

95. Liu, H, Lo, CR, Czaja, MJ. NF-κB inhibition sensitizes hepatocytes to TNF-induced apoptosis through a sustained activation of JNK and c-Jun Hepatology 2002; 35:772–778.

96. Yosimichi G, Nakanishi T, Nishida T, Hattori T, Takano-Yamamoto T, Takigawa M. CTGF/Hcs24 induces chondrocyte differentiation through a p38 mitogen-activated protein kinase (p38MAPK), and proliferation through a p44/42 MAPK/extracellular-signal regulated kinase (ERK). Eur J Biochem 2001; 268:6058–6065.

97. Kim SJ, Ju JW, Oh CD, et al. ERK-1/2 and p38 kinase oppositely regulate nitric oxide-induced apoptosis of chondrocytes in association with p53, caspase-3, and differentiation status. J Biol Chem 2002; 277:1332–1339.

98. Taher MM, Hershey CM, Oakley JD, Valerie K. Role of the p38 and MEK-1/2/p42/44 MAP kinase pathways in the differential activation of human immunodeficiency virus gene expression by ultraviolet and ionizing radiation. Photochem Photobiol 2000; 71:455–459.

99. Lee YJ, Soh JW, Dean NM, et al. Protein kinase Cδ overexpression enhances radiation sensitivity via extracellular regulated protein kinase 1/2 activation, abolishing the radiation-induced G(2)-M arrest. Cell Growth Differ 2002; 13:237–246.

100. Wang X, McGowan CH, Zhao M, et al. Involvement of the MKK6-p38γ cascade in γ-radiation-induced cell cycle arrest. Mol Cell Biol 2000; 20:4543–4552.

101. Bulavin DV, Amundson SA, Fornace AJ. p38 and Chk1 kinases: different conductors for the G(2)/M checkpoint symphony. Curr Opin Genet Dev 2002; 12:92–97.

102. Zhou G, Bao ZQ, Dixon JE. Components of a new human protein kinase signal transduction pathway. J Biol Chem 1995; 270:12,665–12,669.

103. English JM, Vanderbilt CA, Xu S, Marcus S, Cobb MH. Isolation of MEK5 and differential expression of alternatively spliced forms. J Biol Chem 1995; 270:28,897–28,902.

104. English JM, Pearson G, Hockenberry T, Shivakumar L, White MA, Cobb MH. Contribution of the ERK5/MEK5 pathway to Ras/Raf signaling and growth control. J Biol Chem 1999; 274:31,588–31,592.

105. Kamakura S, Moriguchi T, Nishida E. Activation of the protein kinase ERK5/BMK1 by receptor tyrosine kinases. Identification and characterization of a signaling pathway to the nucleus. J Biol Chem 1999; 274:26,563–26,571.

106. Kato Y, Kravchenko VV, Tapping RI, Han J, Ulevitch RJ, Lee JD. BMK1/ERK5 regulates serum-induced early gene expression through transcription factor MEF2C. EMBO J 1997; 16:7054–7066.

107. Kato Y, Tapping RI, Huang S, Watson MH, Ulevitch RJ, Lee JD. Bmk1/Erk5 is required for cell proliferation induced by epidermal growth factor. Nature 1998; 395:713–716.

108. Zhao W, Goswami PC, Robbins ME. Radiation-induced up-regulation of Mmp2 involves increased mRNA stability, redox modulation, and MAPK activation. Radiat Res 2004; 161:418–429.

109. Wiesenauer CA, Yip-Schneider MT, Wang Y, Schmidt CM. Multiple anticancer effects of blocking MEK-ERK signaling in hepatocellular carcinoma. J Am Coll Surg 2004; 198:410–421.

110. Alessi DR, Cuenda A, Cohen P, Dudley DT, Saltiel AR. PD 098059 is a specific inhibitor of the activation of mitogen-activated protein kinase kinase in vitro and in vivo. J Biol Chem 1995; 270:27,489–27,494.

111. King AJ, Wireman RS, Hamilton M, Marshall MS. Phosphorylation site specificity of the Pak-mediated regulation of Raf-1 and cooperativity with Src. FEBS Lett 2001; 497:6–14.

112. Favata MF, Horiuchi KY, Manos EJ, et al. Identification of a novel inhibitor of mitogen-activated protein kinase kinase. J Biol Chem 1998; 273:18,623–16,632.

113. Wityak J, Hobbs FW, Gardner DS, et al. Beyond U0126. Dianion chemistry leading to the rapid synthesis of a series of potent MEK inhibitors. Bioorg Med Chem Lett 2004; 14:1483–1486.

114. Mody N, Leitch J, Armstrong C, Dixon J, Cohen P. Effects of MAP kinase cascade inhibitors on the MKK5/ERK5 pathway. FEBS Lett 2001; 502:21–24.

115. Osada S, Saji S, Osada K. Critical role of extracellular signal-regulated kinase phosphorylation on menadione (vitamin K3) induced growth inhibition. Cancer 2001; 91:1156–1165.

116. Allen LF, Sebolt-Leopold J, Meyer MB. CI-1040 (PD184352), a targeted signal transduction inhibitor of MEK (MAPKK). Semin Oncol 2003; 30(5 Suppl 16):105–116.

117. Sun W, Kesavan K, Schaefer BC, et al. MEKK2 associates with the adapter protein Lad/RIBP and regulates the MEK5-BMK1/ERK5 pathway J Biol Chem 2001; 276:5093–5100.

118. Suzaki Y, Yoshizumi M, Kagami S, et al. Hydrogen peroxide stimulates c-Src-mediated big mitogen-activated protein kinase 1 (BMK1) and the MEF2C signaling pathway in PC12 cells: potential role in cell survival following oxidative insults. J Biol Chem 2002; 277:9614–9621.

119. Weldon CB, Scandurro AB, Rolfe KW, et al. Identification of mitogen-activated protein kinase kinase as a chemoresistant pathway in MCF-7 cells by using gene expression microarray. Surgery 2002; 132:293–301.

120. Vanhaesebroeck B, Alessi DR. The PI3K-PDK1 connection: more than just a road to PKB. Biochem J 2000; 346:561–576.

121. Wymann MP, Pirola L. Structure and function of phosphoinositide 3-kinases. Biochim Biophys Acta 1998; 1436:127–150.

122. Ching TT, Lin HP, Yang CC, Oliveira M, Lu PJ, Chen CS. Specific binding of the C-terminal Src homology 2 domain of the p85α subunit of phosphoinositide 3-kinase to phosphatidylinositol 3,4,5-trisphosphate. Localization and engineering of the phosphoinositide-binding motif. J Biol Chem 2001; 276:43,932–43,938.

123. Lee H, Akita RW, Sliwkowski MX, Maihle NJ. A naturally occurring secreted human ErbB3 receptor isoform inhibits heregulin-stimulated activation of ErbB2, ErbB3, and ErbB4. Cancer Res 2001; 61:4467–4473.

124. Yu CF, Roshan B, Liu ZX, Cantley LG. ERK regulates the hepatocyte growth factor-mediated interaction of Gab1 and the phosphatidylinositol 3- kinase. J Biol Chem 2001; 276:32,552–32,558.

125. Van-Weering DH, de Rooij J, Marte B, Downward J, Bos JL, Burgering BM. Protein kinase B activation and lamellipodium formation are independent phosphoinositide 3-kinase-mediated events differentially regulated by endogenous Ras. Mol Cell Biol 1998; 18:1802–1811.

126. Gu H, Maeda H, Moon JJ, et al. New role for Shc in activation of the phosphatidylinositol 3-kinase/ Akt pathway. Mol Cell Biol 2000; 20:7109–7120.

127. Rubio I, Rodriguez-Viciana P, Downward J, Wetzker R. Interaction of Ras with phosphoinositide 3-kinase gamma. Biochem J 1997; 326:891–895.

128. Filippa N, Sable CL, Hemmings BA, Van Obberghen E. Effect of phosphoinositide-dependent kinase 1 on protein kinase B translocation and its subsequent activation. Mol Cell Biol 2000; 20:5712–5721.

129. Balendran A, Hare GR, Kieloch A, Williams MR, Alessi DR. Further evidence that 3-phosphoinositide-dependent protein kinase-1 (PDK1) is required for the stability and phosphorylation of protein kinase C (PKC) isoforms. FEBS Lett 2000; 484:217–223.

130. Cross DA, Alessi DR, Cohen P, Andjelkovich M, Hemmings BA. Inhibition of glycogen synthase kinase-3 by insulin mediated by protein kinase B. Nature 1995; 378:785–789.

131. Alessi DR, Caudwell FB, Andjelkovic M, Hemmings BA, Cohen P. Molecular basis for the substrate specificity of protein kinase B; comparison with MAPKAP kinase-1 and p70 S6 kinase. FEBS Lett 1996; 399:333–338.

132. Podsypanina K, Lee RT, Politis C, et al. An inhibitor of mTOR reduces neoplasia and normalizes p70/S6 kinase activity in Pten± mice. Proc Natl Acad Sci U S A 2001; 98:10,320–10,325.

133. Dickson LM, Lingohr MK, McCuaig J, et al. Differential activation of protein kinase B and p70(S6)K by glucose and insulin-like growth factor 1 in pancreatic β-cells (INS-1). J Biol Chem 2001; 276:21,110–21,120.

134. Kainulainen V, Sundvall M, Maatta JA, Santiestevan E, Klagsbrun M, Elenius K. A natural ErbB4 isoform that does not activate phosphoinositide 3-kinase mediates proliferation but not survival or chemotaxis. J Biol Chem 2000; 275:8641–8649.

135. Daly JM, Olayioye MA, Wong AM, et al. NDF/heregulin-induced cell cycle changes and apoptosis in breast tumour cells: role of PI3 kinase and p38 MAP kinase pathways. Oncogene 1999; 18:3440–3451.

136. Leverrier Y, Thomas J, Mathieu AL, Low W, Blanquier B, Marvel J. Role of PI3-kinase in Bcl-X induction and apoptosis inhibition mediated by IL-3 or IGF-1 in Baf-3 cells. Cell Death Differ 1999; 6:290–296.

137. Kuo ML, Chuang SE, Lin MT, Yang SY. The involvement of PI 3-K/Akt-dependent up-regulation of Mcl-1 in the prevention of apoptosis of Hep3B cells by interleukin-6. Oncogene 2001; 20:677–685.

138. Panka DJ, Mano T, Suhara T, Walsh K, Mier JW. Phosphatidylinositol 3-kinase/Akt activity regulates c-FLIP expression in tumor cells. J Biol Chem 2001; 276:6893–6896.

139. Suhara T, Mano T, Oliveira BE, Walsh K. Phosphatidylinositol 3-kinase/Akt signaling controls endothelial cell sensitivity to Fas-mediated apoptosis via regulation of FLICE-inhibitory protein (FLIP). Circ Res 2001; 89:13–19.

140. Li Y, Tennekoon GI, Birnbaum M, Marchionni MA, Rutkowski JL. Neuregulin signaling through a PI3K/Akt/Bad pathway in Schwann cell survival. Mol Cell Neurosci 2001;17:761–767.

141. Fujita E, Jinbo A, Matuzaki H, Konishi H, Kikkawa U, Momoi T. Akt phosphorylation site found in human caspase-9 is absent in mouse caspase-9. Biochem Biophys Res Commun 1999; 264:550–555.

142. Pianetti S, Arsura M, Romieu-Mourez R, Coffey RJ, Sonenshein GE. Her-2/neu overexpression induces NF-κappaB via a PI3-kinase/Akt pathway involving calpain-mediated degradation of IκB-α that can be inhibited by the tumor suppressor PTEN. Oncogene 2001; 20:1287–1299.

143. Cuello M, Ettenberg SA, Clark AS, et al. Down-regulation of the ErbB-2 receptor by trastuzumab (herceptin) enhances tumor necrosis factor-related apoptosis-inducing ligand-mediated apoptosis in breast and ovarian cancer cell lines that overexpress ErbB-2. Cancer Res 2001; 61:4892–4900.

144. Cuenda A, Alessi DR. Use of kinase inhibitors to dissect signaling pathways. Methods Mol Biol 2000; 99:161–175.

145. Grant S, Qiao L, Dent P. Roles of ErbB family receptor tyrosine kinases, and downstream signaling pathways, in the control of cell growth and survival. Front Biosci 2002; 7:d376–d389.

146. Schmidt–Ullrich RK, Dent P, Grant S, Mikkelsen RB, Valerie K. Signal transduction and cellular radiation responses. Radiat Res 2000; 153:245–257.

147. Jakus J, Yeudall WA. Growth inhibitory concentrations of EGF induce p21 (WAF1/Cip1) and alter cell cycle control in squamous carcinoma cells. Oncogene 1996; 12:2369–2376.

148. Fong WF, Leung CH, Lam W, Wong NS, Cheng SH. Epidermal growth factor induces Gadd45 (growth arrest and DNA damage inducible protein) expression in A431 cells. Biochim Biophys Acta 2001; 1517:250–256.

149. Mendelsohn J. The epidermal growth factor receptor as a target for cancer therapy. Endocr Relat Cancer 2001; 8:3–9.

150. Ross JS, Fletcher JA. The HER-2/neu oncogene in breast cancer: prognostic factor, predictive factor, and target for therapy. Stem Cells 1998; 16:413–428.

151. Mishima K, Johns TG, Luwor RB, et al. Growth suppression of intracranial xenografted glioblastomas overexpressing mutant epidermal growth factor receptors by systemic administration of monoclonal antibody (mAb) 806, a novel monoclonal antibody directed to the receptor. Cancer Res 2001; 61:5349–5354.

152. Erlichman C, Boerner SA, Hallgren CG, et al. The HER tyrosine kinase inhibitor CI1033 enhances cytotoxicity of 7-ethyl-10-hydroxycamptothecin and topotecan by inhibiting breast cancer resistance protein-mediated drug efflux. Cancer Res 2001; 61:739–748.

153. Bruns CJ, Solorzano CC,. Harbison MT, et al. Blockade of the epidermal growth factor receptor signaling by a novel tyrosine kinase inhibitor leads to apoptosis of endothelial cells and therapy of human pancreatic carcinoma. Cancer Res 2000; 60:2926–2935.

154. Suzuki K, Kodama S, Watanabe M. K. Extremely low-dose ionizing radiation causes activation of mitogen-activated protein kinase pathway and enhances proliferation of normal human diploid cells. Cancer Res 2001; 61:5396–5401.

155. Wakita H, Takigawa M. Activation of epidermal growth factor receptor promotes late terminal differentiation of cell-matrix interaction-disrupted keratinocytes. J Biol Chem 1999; 274:37,285–37,291.

156. Barker AJ, Gibson KH, Grundy W, et al. Studies leading to the identification of ZD1839 (IRESSA): an orally active, selective epidermal growth factor receptor tyrosine kinase inhibitor targeted to the treatment of cancer. Bioorg Med Chem Lett 2001; 11:1911–1914.

157. Vincent PW, Bridges AJ, Dykes DJ, et al. Anticancer efficacy of the irreversible EGFr tyrosine kinase inhibitor PD0169414 against human tumor xenografts. Cancer Chemother Pharmacol 2000; 45:231–238.

158. Hidalgo M, Siu LL, Nemunaitis J, et al. Phase I and pharmacologic study of OSI-774, an epidermal growth factor receptor tyrosine kinase inhibitor, in patients with advanced solid malignancies. J Clin Oncol 2001; 19:3267–3279.

159. Fernandes A, Hamburger AW, Gerwin BI. ErbB-2 kinase is required for constitutive stat 3 activation in malignant human lung epithelial cells. Int J Cancer 1999; 83:564–570.

160. Yeh S, Lin HK, Kang HY, Thin TH, Lin MF, Chang C. From HER2/Neu signal cascade to androgen receptor and its coactivators: a novel pathway by induction of androgen target genes through MAP kinase in prostate cancer cells. Proc Natl Acad Sci U S A 1999; 96:5458–5463.

161. Reardon DB, Contessa JN, Mikkelsen RB, et al. Dominant negative EGFR-CD533 and inhibition of MAPK modify JNK1 activation and enhance radiation toxicity of human mammary carcinoma cells. Oncogene 1999; 18:4756–4766.

162. Jones FE, Stern DF, Expression of dominant-negative ErbB2 in the mammary gland of transgenic mice reveals a role in lobuloalveolar development and lactation. Oncogene 1999; 18:3481–3490.

163. Ram TG, Schelling ME, Hosick HL. Blocking HER-2/HER-3 function with a dominant negative form of HER-3 in cells stimulated by heregulin and in breast cancer cells with HER-2 gene amplification. Cell Growth Differ 2000; 11:173–183.

164. Mendelsohn J, Baselga J. The EGF receptor family as targets for cancer therapy. Oncogene 2000; 19:6550–6565.

165. Yarden Y, Sliwkowski MX. Untangling the ErbB signalling network. Nat Rev Mol Cell Biol 2001; 2:127–137.

166. Herbst RS, Langer CJ. Epidermal growth factor receptors as a target for cancer treatment: the emerging role of IMC-C225 in the treatment of lung and head and neck cancers. Semin Oncol 2002; 29:27–36.

167. Baselga J, Albanell J. Mechanism of action of anti-HER2 monoclonal antibodies. Ann Oncol 2001; 12:S35–S41.

168. Burstein HJ, Kuter I, Campos SM, et al. Clinical activity of trastuzumab and vinorelbine in women with HER2-overexpressing metastatic breast cancer. J Clin Oncol 2001; 19:2722–2730.

169. Pegram MD, Lopez A, Konecny G, Slamon DJ. Trastuzumab and chemotherapeutics: drug interactions and synergies. Semin Oncol 2000; 27:21–25.

170. Nasu S, Ang KK, Fan Z, Milas L. C225 antiepidermal growth factor receptor antibody enhances tumor radiocurability. Int J Radiat Oncol Biol Phys 2001; 51:474–477.

171. Baselga J, Pfister D, Cooper MR, et al. Phase I studies of anti-epidermal growth factor receptor chimeric antibody C225 alone and in combination with cisplatin. J Clin Oncol 2000; 18:904–914.

172. Luwor RB, Johns TG, Murone C, et al. Monoclonal antibody 806 inhibits the growth of tumor xenografts expressing either the de2-7 or amplified epidermal growth factor receptor (EGFR) but not wild-type EGFR. Cancer Res 2001; 61:5355–5361.

173. Denny WA. The 4-anilinoquinazoline class of inhibitors of the ErbB family of receptor tyrosine kinases. Farmaco 2001; 56:51–56.

174. Bridges AJ. The rationale and strategy used to develop a series of highly potent, irreversible, inhibitors of the epidermal growth factor receptor family of tyrosine kinases. Curr Med Chem 1999; 6:825–843.

175. Bos M, Mendelsohn J, Kim YM, Albanell J, Fry DW, Baselga J. PD153035, a tyrosine kinase inhibitor, prevents epidermal growth factor receptor activation and inhibits growth of cancer cells in a receptor number-dependent manner. Clin Cancer Res 1997; 3:2099–2106.

176. Pinkas-Kramarski R, Lenferink AE, et al. The oncogenic ErbB-2/ErbB-3 heterodimer is a surrogate receptor of the epidermal growth factor and βcellulin. Oncogene 1998; 16:1249–1258.

177. Tsai CM, Chang KT, Chen JY, Chen YM, Chen MH, Perng RP. Enhancement of chemosensitivity by tyrphostin AG825 in high-p185(neu) expressing non-small cell lung cancer cells. Cancer Res 1996; 56:1068–1074.

178. Rao GS, Murray S, Ethier SP. Radiosensitization of human breast cancer cells by a novel ErbB family receptor tyrosine kinase inhibitor. Int J Radiat Oncol Biol Phys 2000; 48:1519–1528.

179. Nelson JM, Fry DW. Akt, MAPK (Erk1/2), and p38 act in concert to promote apoptosis in response to ErbB receptor family inhibition. J Biol Chem 2001; 276:14,842–14,847.

180. Sirotnak FM, Zakowski MF, Miller VA, Scher HI, Kris MG. Efficacy of cytotoxic agents against human tumor xenografts is markedly enhanced by coadministration of ZD1839 (Iressa), an inhibitor of EGFR tyrosine kinase. Clin Cancer Res 2000; 6:4885–4892.

181. Schmidt-Ullrich RK, Valerie K, Fogleman PB, Walters J. Radiation-induced autophosphorylation of epidermal growth factor receptor in human malignant mammary and squamous epithelial cells. Radiat Res 1996; 145:81–85.

182. Contessa JN, Reardon DB, Todd D, et al. The inducible expression of dominant-negative epidermal growth factor receptor-CD533 results in radiosensitization of human mammary carcinoma cells. Clin Cancer Res 1999; 5:405–411.

183. Lammering G, Hewit TH, Hawkins WT, et al. Epidermal growth factor receptor as a genetic therapy target for carcinoma cell radiosensitization. J Natl Cancer Inst 2001; 93:921–929.

184. Lammering G, Valerie K, Lin PS, et al. Radiosensitization of malignant glioma cells through overexpression of dominant-negative epidermal growth factor receptor. Clin Cancer Res 2001; 7:682–690.

185. Ciardiello F, Caputo R, Troiani T, et al. Antisense oligonucleotides targeting the epidermal growth factor receptor inhibit proliferation, induce apoptosis, and cooperate with cytotoxic drugs in human cancer cell lines. Int J Cancer 2001; 93:172–178.

186. Macaulay VM, Salisbury AJ, Bohula EA, Playford MP, Smorodinsky NI, Shiloh Y. Downregulation of the type 1 insulin-like growth factor receptor in mouse melanoma cells is associated with enhanced radiosensitivity and impaired activation of Atm kinase. Oncogene 2001; 20:4029–4040.

187. Hutcheson IR, Knowlden JM, Madden TA, et al. Oestrogen receptor-mediated modulation of the EGFR/MAPK pathway in tamoxifen-resistant MCF-7 cells. Breast Cancer Res Treat 2003; 81:81–93.

188. Wen B, Deutsch E, Marangoni E, et al. Tyrphostin AG 1024 modulates radiosensitivity in human breast cancer cells. Br J Cancer 2001; 85:2017–2021.

189. Eichholtz-Wirth H. Sagan D. Altered signaling of TNFα-TNFR1 and SODD/BAG4 is responsible for radioresistance in human HT-R15 cells. Anticancer Res 2002; 22(1A):235–240.

190. Legue F, Guitton N, Brouazin-Jousseaume V, Colleu-Durel S, Nourgalieva K, Chenal C. IL-6 a key cytokine in in vitro and in vivo response of sertoli cells to external gamma irradiation. Cytokine 2001; 16:232–238.

191. Ma Z, Webb DJ, Jo M, Gonias SL. Endogenously produced urokinase-type plasminogen activator is a major determinant of the basal level of activated ERK/MAP kinase and prevents apoptosis in MDA-MB-231 breast cancer cells. J Cell Sci 2001; 114:3387–3396.

192. Iyer R, Lehnert BE. Factors underlying the cell growth-related bystander responses to alpha particles. Cancer Res 2000; 60:1290–1298.

193. Rutault K, Hazzalin CA, Mahadevan LC. Combinations of ERK and p38 MAPK inhibitors ablate tumor necrosis factor-α (TNF-α) mRNA induction. Evidence for selective destabilization of TNF-α transcripts. J Biol Chem 2001; 276:6666–6674.

194. Basu S, Rosenzweig KR, Youmell M, Price BD. The DNA-dependent protein kinase participates in the activation of NF κ B following DNA damage. Biochem Biophys Res Commun 1998; 247:79–83.

195. Baxter GF, Mocanu MM, Brar BK, Latchman DS, Yellon DM. Cardioprotective effects of transforming growth factor-β1 during early reoxygenation or reperfusion are mediated by p42/p44 MAPK. J Cardiovasc Pharmacol 2001; 38:930–939.

196. Muraoka RS, Dumont N, Ritter CA, et al. Blockade of TGF-β inhibits mammary tumor cell viability, migration, and metastases. J Clin Invest 2002; 109:1551–1559.

197. Bulus N, Barnard JA. Heparin binding epidermal growth factor-like growth factor is a transforming growth factor β-regulated gene in intestinal epithelial cells. Biochem Biophys Res Commun 1999; 264:808–812.

198. Saile B, Matthes N, El Armouche H, Neubauer K, Ramadori G. The bcl, NFκB and p53/p21WAF1 systems are involved in spontaneous apoptosis and in the anti-apoptotic effect of TGF-β or TNF-α on activated hepatic stellate cells. Eur J Cell Biol 2001; 80:554–561.

199. Lehmann K, Janda E, Pierreux CE, et al. Raf induces TGFβ production while blocking its Apoptotic but not invasive responses: a mechanism leading to increased malignancy in epithelial cells. Genes Dev 2000; 14:2610–2622.

200. Chen RH, Su YH, Chuang RL, Chang TY. Suppression of transforming growth factor-β-induced apoptosis through a phosphatidylinositol 3-kinase/Akt-dependent pathway. Oncogene 1998; 17:1959–1968.

201. Feramisco JR, Clark R, Wong G, Arnheim N, Milley R, McCormick F. Transient reversion of ras oncogene-induced cell transformation by antibodies specific for amino acid 12 of ras protein. Nature 1985; 314:639–642.

202. Willumsen BM, Papageorge AG, Hubbert N, Bekesi E, Kung HF, Lowy DR. Transforming p21 ras protein: flexibility in the major variable region linking the catalytic and membrane-anchoring domains. EMBO J 1985; 4:2893–2896.

203. Zhu K, Hamilton AD, Sebti SM. Farnesyltransferase inhibitors as anticancer agents: current status. Curr Opin Investig Drugs 2003; 4:1428–1435.

204. Stahel RA, Zangemeister-Wittke U. Antisense oligonucleotides for cancer therapy-an overview. Lung Cancer 2003; 41:S81–S88.

205. Lebowitz PF, Prendergast GC. Non-Ras targets of farnesyltransferase inhibitors: focus on Rho. Oncogene 1998; 17:1439–1445.

206. Gupta AK, Bakanauskas VJ, Cerniglia GJ, et al. The Ras radiation resistance pathway. Cancer Res 2001; 61:4278–4782.

207. Gupta AK, McKenna WG, Weber CN, et al. Local recurrence in head and neck cancer: relationship to radiation resistance and signal transduction. Clin Cancer Res 2002; 8:885–892.

208. Gupta AK, Bernhard EJ, Bakanauskas VJ, Wu J, Muschel RJ, McKenna WG. Ras-Mediated radiation resistance is not linked to MAP kinase activation in two bladder carcinoma cell lines. Clin Cancer Res 2002; 154:64–72.

209. Grana TM, Rusyn EV, Zhou H, Sartor CI, Cox AD. Ras mediates radioresistance through both phosphatidylinositol 3-kinase-dependent and Raf-dependent but mitogen-activated protein kinase/extracellular signal-regulated kinase kinase-independent signaling pathways. Cancer Res 2002; 62:4142–4150.

210. Lali FV, Hunt AE, Turner SJ, Foxwell BM. The pyridinyl imidazole inhibitor SB203580 blocks phosphoinositide-dependent protein kinase activity, protein kinase B phosphorylation, and retinoblastoma hyperphosphorylation in interleukin-2-stimulated T cells independently of p38 mitogen-activated protein kinase. J Biol Chem 2000; 275:7395–7402.

211. Rane MJ, Coxon PY, Powell DW, et al. p38 Kinase-dependent MAPKAPK-2 activation functions as 3-phosphoinositide-dependent kinase-2 for Akt in human neutrophils. J Biol Chem 2001; 276:3517–3523.

212. Zhang Y, Dong Z, Nomura M, et al. Signal transduction pathways involved in phosphorylation and activation of p70S6K following exposure to UVA irradiation. J Biol Chem 2001; 276:20,913–20,923.

213. Nakamura JL, Arvold ND, Haas-Kogan DA. Abstract 1207 Proceedings of the 44th annual ASTRO meeting 2002; p177.

214. Munster PN, Marchion DC, Basso AD, Rosen N. Degradation of HER2 by Ansamycins Induces Growth Arrest and Apoptosis in Cells with HER2 Overexpression via a HER3, Phosphatidylinositol 3'-Kinase-AKT-dependent Pathway. Cancer Res 2002; 62:3132–3137.

215. Contessa JN, Hampton J, Lammering G, et al. Ionizing radiation activates Erb-B receptor dependent Akt and p70 S6 kinase signaling in carcinoma cells. Oncogene 2002; 21:4032–4041.

216. Lammering G, TH Hewit, WT Hawkins, et al. J Natl Cancer Inst 2001; 93:921–929.

217. Abbott DW, Holt JT. Mitogen-activated protein kinase kinase 2 activation is essential for progression through the G2/M checkpoint arrest in cells exposed to ionizing radiation. J Biol Chem 1999; 274:2732–2742.

218. Kurland JF, Voehringer DW, Meyn RE. The MEK/ERK pathway acts upstream of NF κ B1 (p50) homodimer activity and Bcl-2 expression in a murine B-cell lymphoma cell line. MEK inhibition restores radiation-induced apoptosis. J Biol Chem 2003; 278:32,465–32,470.

219. Lee YJ, Soh JW, Dean NM, et al. Protein kinase Cδ overexpression enhances radiation sensitivity via extracellular regulated protein kinase 1/2 activation, abolishing the radiation-induced G(2)-M arrest. Cell Growth Differ 2002; 13:237–246.

220. Warenius HM, Jones MD, Thompson CC. Exit from G2 phase after 2 Gy gamma irradiation is faster in radiosensitive human cells with high expression of the Raf1 proto-oncogene. Radiat Res 1996; 146:485–493.

221. McKinstry R, Qiao L, Yacoub A, et al. Inhibitors of MEK1/2 interact with UCN-01 to induce apoptosis and reduce colony formation in mammary and prostate carcinoma cells. Cancer Biol Ther 2002; 1:243–253.

222. Pardo OE, Arcaro A, Salerno G, Raguz S, Downward J, Seckl MJ. Fibroblast growth factor-2 induces translational regulation of Bcl-XL and Bcl-2 via a MEK-dependent pathway: correlation with resistance to etoposide-induced apoptosis. J Biol Chem 2002; 277:12,040–12,046.

223. Tang D, Wu D, Hirao A, et al. ERK activation mediates cell cycle arrest and apoptosis after DNA damage independently of p53. J Biol Chem. 2002; 277:12,710–12,717.

224. Kitagawa D, Tanemura S, Ohata S, et al. Activation of extracellular signal-regulated kinase by ultraviolet is mediated through Src-dependent epidermal growth factor receptor phosphorylation. Its implication in an anti-apoptotic function. J Biol Chem 2002; 277:366–371.

225. Qiao L, Yacoub A, McKinstry R, et al. Pharmacologic inhibitors of the mitogen activated protein kinase cascade have the potential to interact with ionizing radiation exposure to induce cell death in carcinoma cells by multiple mechanisms. Cancer Biol Ther 2002; 1:168–176.

226. Hagan M, Wang L, Hanley JR, Park JS, and Dent P. Ionizing radiation-induced mitogen-activated protein (MAP) kinase activation in DU145 prostate carcinoma cells: MAP kinase inhibition enhances radiation-induced cell killing and G2/M-phase arrest. Radiat Res 2000; 153:371–381.

227. Yacoub A, Park JS, Qiao L, Dent P, Hagan MP. MAPK dependence of DNA damage repair: ionizing radiation and the induction of expression of the DNA repair genes XRCC1 and ERCC1 in DU145 human prostate carcinoma cells in a MEK1/2 dependent fashion. Int J Radiat Biol 2001; 77:1067–1078.

228. Yacoub A, McKinstry R, Hinman D, et al. Epidermal growth factor and ionizing radiation up-regulate the DNA repair genes XRCC1 and ERCC1 in DU145 and LNCaP prostate carcinoma through MAPK signaling. Radiat Res 2003; 159:439–452.

229. Jung M, Dritschilo A. NF-κ B signaling pathway as a target for human tumor radiosensitization. Semin Radiat Oncol 2001; 11:346–351.

230. Russell JS, Raju U, Gumin GJ, et al. Inhibition of radiation-induced nuclear factor-κB activation by an anti-Ras single-chain antibody fragment: lack of involvement in radiosensitization. Cancer Res 2002; 62:2318–2326.

231. Sizemore N, Lerner N, Dombrowski N, Sakurai H, Stark GR. Distinct roles of the Iκ B kinase alpha and beta subunits in liberating nuclear factor κ B (NF-κ B) from Iκ B and in phosphorylating the p65 subunit of NF-κ B. J Biol Chem 2002; 277:3863–3869.

232. Chen BC, Lin WW. PKC- and ERK-dependent activation of I κ B kinase by lipopolysaccharide in macrophages: enhancement by P2Y receptor-mediated CaMK activation. Br J Pharmacol 2001; 134:1055–1065.

233. Bhat-Nakshatri P. Sweeney CJ, Nakshatri H. Identification of signal transduction pathways involved in constitutive NF-κB activation in breast cancer cells. Oncogene 2002; 21:2066–2078.

234. Troppmair J, Hartkamp J, Rapp UR. Activation of NF-κ B by oncogenic Raf in HEK 293 cells occurs through autocrine recruitment of the stress kinase cascade. Oncogene 1998; 17:685–690.

235. Tuyt LM, Dokter WH, Birkenkamp K, et al. Extracellular-regulated kinase 1/2, Jun N-terminal kinase, and c-Jun are involved in NF-κ B-dependent IL-6 expression in human monocytes. J Immunol 1999; 162:4893–4902.

236. Shao R, Tsai EM, Wei K, et al. E1A inhibition of radiation-induced NF-κB activity through suppression of IKK activity and IκB degradation, independent of Akt activation. Cancer Res 2001; 61:7413–7416.

237. Barradas M, Monjas A, Diaz-Meco MT, Serrano M, Moscat J. The downregulation of the pro-apoptotic protein Par-4 is critical for Ras-induced survival and tumor progression. EMBO J 1999; 18:6362.

238. Qiu SG, Krishnan S, el-Guendy N, Rangnekar VM. Negative regulation of Par-4 by oncogenic Ras is essential for cellular transformation. Oncogene 1999; 18:7115–7123.

239. Camandola S, Mattson MP. Pro-apoptotic action of PAR-4 involves inhibition of NF-κB activity and suppression of BCL-2 expression. J Neurosci Res 2000; 61:134–139.

240. Diaz-Meco MT, Lallena MJ, Monjas A, Frutos S, Moscat J. Inactivation of the inhibitory κB protein kinase/nuclear factor κB pathway by Par-4 expression potentiates tumor necrosis factor alpha-induced apoptosis. J Biol Chem 1999; 274:19,606–19,612.

241. Wang YM, Seibenhener ML, Vandenplas ML, Wooten MW. Atypical PKC zeta is activated by ceramide, resulting in coactivation of NF-κB/JNK kinase and cell survival. J Neurosci Res 1999; 55:293–302.

242. Chendil D, Das A, Dey S, Mohiuddin M, Ahmed MM. Par-4, a pro-apoptotic gene, inhibits radiation-induced NF κ B activity and Bcl-2 expression leading to induction of radiosensitivity in human prostate cancer cells PC-3. Cancer Biol Ther 2002; 1(2):152–160.

243. Chakraborty SG, Qiu KM, Vasudevan VM. Rangnekar, Par-4 drives trafficking and activation of Fas and Fasl to induce prostate cancer cell apoptosis and tumor regression. Cancer Res 2001; 61:7255–7263.

28

Amplification in DNA Copy Numbers as a Mechanism of Acquired Drug Resistance

M. Jim Yen, Ie-Ming Shih, MD, PhD,
Victor E. Velculescu, MD, PhD,
and Tian-Li Wang, PhD

CONTENTS

SUMMARY

Resistance to chemotherapeutic agents represents a chief cause of mortality in cancer patients with advanced disease. Gene amplification has been shown to be one of the molecular mechanisms for tumors to escape the effect of chemotherapeutic drugs. The amplification and subsequent overexpression of the chemoresistant gene product are likely the results of tumor cell clonal expansion under the selective pressure of chemotherapeutic agents. In the past few decades, researchers have correlated the amplification of several target genes to drug resistance status in in vitro cell culture models. Although it is possible for gene amplification to be a widespread mechanism of chemoresistance in cancer patients, only a few well-studied examples are presently available. Therefore, the future application of new advances in molecular genetic technology holds promise for the discovery of novel amplified chemoresistant genes, which may significantly affect our understanding of how tumors become chemoresistant as well as provide a molecular platform for customized treatment of cancer patients.

Key Words: Amplification; drug resistance; chromosome instability; fluorescence *in situ* hybridization; comparative genomic hybridization; digital karyotyping.

From: *Cancer Drug Discovery and Development: Cancer Drug Resistance*
Edited by: B. Teicher © Humana Press Inc., Totowa, NJ

1. INTRODUCTION

Tumor resistance to chemotherapeutic agents has been a major problem, compromising the efficacy of chemotherapy in the clinical setting, and is a chief cause of mortality in cancer patients with advanced disease. Several possible mechanisms underlying chemoresistance include decreased drug accumulation in cells, increased inactivation of drug, failure to convert the prodrug to an active form, altered amounts or activity of target proteins, enhanced DNA repair, and resistance to apoptosis *(1)*.

Understanding the molecular mechanisms of chemoresistance will help to develop a tailored therapy that will ideally avoid cytotoxic drug administration to which a cancer is already resistant and employ the use of efficacious drugs to which a cancer is sensitive. This can achieve the goal of maximizing chemotherapy efficacy, while minimizing adverse effects. It has been recognized that gene amplification is associated with resistance to a variety of cancer therapies. Gene amplification can be manifested as multiple extra copies of a subchromosomal region of an amplicon, termed extrachromosomal double-minute chromosomes (DMs), or as chromosomally integrated homogenous staining regions (HSRs). Amplification and consequent overexpression of genes involved in drug resistance confer a selective advantage to cancer cells. Mammalian cells cultured under conditions of incrementally increased doses of cytotoxic drug have been observed to acquire gene amplifications *(2)*. This suggests that cancer cells in patients can acquire drug resistance through amplification of genes related to chemoresistance.

This chapter first reviews the mechanisms of gene amplification and then focuses on the correlation between amplification of certain genes and specific chemoresistance in cancer patients. The current effort of characterizing amplified genomic loci associated with cisplatin-resistance is discussed.

2. MECHANISM OF GENE AMPLIFICATION

In humans, gene amplification is a molecular genetic feature that has been mainly associated with cancer cells. In samples of mitotic chromosome spreads, amplifications usually appear as either expanded HSRs or small, extrachromosomal DMs. Chromosome instability is a prerequisite for gene amplification, which can result from loss of cell cycle control because of a defective checkpoint pathway *(3)*. Using amplification of dihydrofolate reductase (DHFR) as a model in Chinese hamster cells, researchers have found that DHFR amplification is first initiated by chromosome breaks distal to the *DHFR* gene, followed by repeated bridge-breakage-fusion cycles that generate large intrachromosomal repeats. This molecular event ultimately results in HSRs *(4)*. DMs can also be generated by an initial HSR, followed by its breakage into exchromosomal repeating units *(5)*. It has been observed that some tumors preferentially maintain amplicons in DMs, whereas others maintain amplicons in HSRs. DMs and HSRs are both initiated by DNA breaks, but the way by which the extra repeat sequences are processed and maintained appears to depend on tumor type.

Because of increased gene dosage, gene amplification usually results in overexpression of the encoded gene products. Gene amplification may reflect an underlying genomic instability and can initially be a random event. The result of genomic instability such as gene amplification permits cells to acquire growth advantages under a selective pressure such as the presence of a chemotherapeutic drug. Increased protein expression (from amplified genes) may equip the cancer cells with new molecular machinery to better survive and progress during chemotherapy. As a result, the clone with amplification of target genes expands and ultimately predominates in the tumor.

2.1. Gene Amplification Models In Vitro

The association between gene amplification and chemoresistance in tumor cell lines has been observed since the late 1970s *(2)*. Gene amplification of the target for methotrexate (MTX), DHFR, is a well-documented example of a mechanism for acquired drug resistance *(6)*. Exposing parental cells to increasing stepwise concentrations of MTX in vitro has resulted in cell variants that are resistant to MTX. Subsequent analysis of cellular DNA content has demonstrated *DHFR* gene amplification in these resistant clone variants. In most cases, amplified *DHFR* sequences were located in unstable, extrachromosomal DMs.

In vitro-derived multidrug-resistant (MDR) cell lines have lead to the identification of P-glycoprotein, a protein product of the multidrug resistance gene *(MDR1) (7)*. MDR1-positive cell lines can be derived in vitro following incubation with increasing doses of antineoplastic drugs. Researchers have identified *MDR1* gene amplification and protein overexpression in many MDR cell lines *(8)*. MDR1 is a transmembrane protein that shares sequence homology with several bacterial proteins involved in active membrane transport. It functions as an energy-dependent efflux pump responsible for the removal of drugs from MDR cells.

2.2. Detection of Amplified Target Genes in Clinical Tumors

Although amplification of drug resistant genes has been well illustrated in vitro, detection of amplified target genes in clinical tumors was rarely reported in the past. Only a few cases of DHFR amplification and almost no cases of MDR1 amplification were observed in tumors surgically removed from cancer patients *(9–12)*. However, recent studies have demonstrated a higher prevalence of *DHFR* gene amplification in tumor samples because of refined techniques and a larger number of samples examined. Amplifications of target genes involved in chemoresistance have also been associated with resistance against three other antineoplastic compounds including 5-fluorouracil (5-FU), antiandrogen agents, and imatinib (Gleevec®). Furthermore, cisplatin resistance was found to be associated with some of the subchromosomal aberrations. In the following subheadings, we describe those examples occurring in relapsed tumors.

2.2.1. Methotrexate

MTX acts by inhibiting DHFR, thus reducing the metabolism of folates and dihydrofolates to tetrahydrofolates. Tetrahydrofolates serve as the carriers for one-carbon groups essential in DNA synthesis, and inhibition of its synthesis by antagonizing DHFR decreases DNA synthesis, resulting in cell growth suppression. MTX has been used in the treatment of a variety of cancers including lymphoma, osteosarcoma, choriocarcinoma, and carcinomas of breast, head and neck, lung, and gastrointestinal tract. In 1995, a research group from Memorial Sloan-Kettering Cancer Center reported on the incidence of DHFR amplification in the clinical setting. Twenty-nine relapsed patients with acute lymphoblastic leukemia were studied, and it was found that 31% ($^9/_{29}$) had low-level *DHFR* gene amplification (two to four gene copies). In addition, the amplification was associated with increased levels of *DHFR* mRNA and enzyme activity, indicating low-copy number amplification may be an important cause of MTX resistance *(6)*. Furthermore, low-copy number *DHFR* amplification was found to be correlated with p53 mutations, strengthening the concept that mutations in the *p53* gene can lead to gene amplification as a result of defective cell cycle control and increased genetic instability. It is interesting to note that nearly all the amplified cases display low-level gain, rather than amplification in the forms of HSRs and DMs commonly observed in *DHFR* amplifications in vitro. This indicates that the mechanism for *DHFR* gene amplification in vivo is unique from those in vitro, owing possibly to selection pressures or cellular microenvironment differences.

2.2.2. 5-Fluorouracil

5-FU is a pyrimidine antimetabolite used in treating carcinomas of the breast, colon, head and neck, pancreas, rectum, and stomach. 5-FU irreversibly inhibits thymidylate synthase (TYMS), an enzyme normally responsible for conversion of deoxyuridine monophosphate to deoxythymidine monophosphate *(13)*. This process generates the sole *de novo* source of thymidylate, which is an essential precursor to DNA synthesis and therefore, inhibition of TYMS leads to DNA damage and blocks DNA replication and repair. In addition to its effects on DNA synthesis, metabolites of 5-FU can be incorporated into RNA, thereby disrupting normal RNA processing and function.

In colorectal cancer, many patients initially respond to 5-FU based therapy, but unfortunately, most develop recurrences and ultimately die of the disease *(14,15)*. Despite numerous studies using both in vitro models and clinical samples, the molecular mechanisms of 5-FU resistance have not yet been completely elucidated. Some researchers have suggested that TYMS protein overexpression correlates with worse clinical outcome; however, these study results have not been reproducible in terms of ability to predict treatment response based on protein expression. One reason for inconsistency among different studies is the difficulty of measuring gene expression accurately. Recently, a genome-wide technology, digital karyotyping, has been applied to reveal whole-genome alterations in colorectal cancers which are resistant to 5-FU *(16)*. In this study, *TYMS* gene amplification was initially identified in two of four 5-FU-resistant tumors. Further investigation using fluorescence *in situ* hybridization (FISH) analyses on an independent and larger set of colorectal carcinoma samples demonstrated *TYMS* gene amplification in approximately 23% of 5-FU-treated cancers. In contrast, no amplification was observed in patients without 5-FU treatment. Interestingly, patients with metastases containing *TYMS* amplification were found to have substantially shorter median survival lengths than those without amplification. These data provide cogent evidence that genetic amplification of *TYMS* is one of the mechanisms of 5-FU resistance in vivo, and have implications for the management of colorectal cancer patients with recurrent disease.

2.2.3. Antiandrogen Hormone Therapy

Prostate cancer is the second most common cause of cancer death in men. Prostate cancer tumor growth is regulated by the binding of androgens to the androgen receptor (AR), which can be inhibited by androgen antagonists. Antiandrogen hormone therapy, which focuses on attenuating the stimulating effects of androgen, has been the mainstay of treatment for advanced prostate cancer disease *(17)*. Although antiandrogen therapy offers a favorable response rate of 70–80%, the majority of patients eventually develop antiandrogen resistance. AR amplification, overexpression, mutations, and activation have been implicated as mechanisms underlying the antiandrogen resistance in prostate cancer *(18)*.

Several clinical studies have detected *AR* gene amplification by FISH analysis in hormone-refractory prostate carcinomas, and this gene amplification has been correlated with overexpression of AR at the protein level *(18–20)*. The frequency of *AR* gene amplification has been reported to be 20–38% in hormone-refractory tumors, compared to 0–2% in hormone-sensitive tumors and benign prostate hyperplastic tissue *(18–24)*.

2.2.4. IMATINIB

Imatinib (Gleevec) is an antineoplastic tyrosine kinase inhibitor used to treat chronic myelogenous leukemia (CML) and gastrointestinal stromal tumors. Imatinib acts by inhibiting Bcr-Abl, the oncogenic tyrosine kinase fusion protein involved in the pathogenesis of CML, and c-KIT, the tyrosine kinase frequently activated in gastrointestinal stromal tumors *(25)*. In CML, the *abl* gene fuses to the *bcr* gene through chromosomal translocation. This rearranged "Philadelphia" chromosome 22 occurs in almost all cases of CML *(26)*. Imatinib offers a specific and target-based therapy capable of inducing remissions in Philadelphia chromosome-positive leukemia *(26)*.

Clinical trials have shown that imatinib is highly effective in treating CML, with 18-mo complete response rates of 95% or greater. The emergence of drug resistance however, has raised concern regarding the ultimate usefulness of imatinib. At the time of relapse, reappearance of active Bcr-Abl protein could be detected in most patients. The possible cellular mechanisms of imatinib resistance include *bcr-abl* gene amplification, mutations in the Bcr-Abl catalytic domains and incomplete Bcr-Abl inhibition. The link between imatinib resistance and *bcr-abl* gene amplification was initially observed in a cell line generated by culturing cells with increasing concentrations of imatinib *(27)*. Subsequently, several studies have detected *bcr-abl* gene amplification by FISH analysis at rates of 6–27% in tumor cells obtained from patients with imatinib-resistant CML *(26,28–29)*. One case report described a patient who died from imatinib-resistant disease and had a 25-fold *bcr-abl* gene amplification with multiple DMs in the leukemia cells *(30)*. Point mutation of *bcr-abl* is a more frequent event than *bcr-abl* amplification and was found to occur in ~44% of relapsed cases. Because clinical relapse of CML has mainly been associated with recurrence of Bcr-Abl activity *(31)*, this finding indicates that resistant CML remains dependent on Bcr-Abl, rather than developing a Bcr-Abl-independent pathway for resistance *(26)*.

2.2.5. CISPLATIN

Cisplatin is a platinum derivative that acts by forming DNA crosslinks, which inhibit DNA synthesis and activate signal transduction leading to apoptosis. It is one of the most potent antitumor agents, and displays cytotoxicity against a wide variety of solid tumors including neuroblastoma, Hodgkin's, and non-Hodgkin's lymphoma as well as head and neck, breast, testicular, ovarian, and lung cancers. Its efficacy however, is mainly limited by tumor chemoresistance. In ovarian cancers for example, the initial response rate to cisplatin is 70%, but the tumors gradually become resistant to the drug as chemotherapy proceeds *(32)*.

Cisplatin resistance has been reported to be a result of apoptotic signal suppression, decreased drug uptake, increased drug inactivation, and increased DNA adduct repair activity. In order to explore cisplatin resistance at the molecular genetic level, researchers have used comparative genomic hybridization (CGH) and array CGH to identify chromosomal alterations associated with cisplatin resistance in tumors. Using these methods, several candidate chromosomal regions have been identified that could be related to cisplatin resistance. These include a study in multiple myeloma using CGH to show the presence of a high-level gain at 1q12-q22 harboring a gene named PDZ domain-containing 1 *(PDZK1)* in cisplatin-resistant cells. Cell lines with *PDZK1* amplification exhibited resistance to cisplatin, melphalan, and vincristine-induced cell death compared to cell lines without amplification. Complementary to these amplification studies, antisense oligonucleotides that downregulate PDZK1 expression have been shown to sensitize cell lines to cisplatin. These results indicate that PDZK1 is likely to be a target of 1q12-q22 amplification and may be associated with resistance to cisplatin, as well as melphalan and vincristine in multiple myeloma *(33)*.

A different research group has also applied CGH to profile the chromosomal changes in cisplatin-resistant and paclitaxel-resistant human ovarian cancer cell lines. Increased copy number at 6q21-25 and decreased copy number at 7q21-36 and 10q12-15 were observed in cisplatin-resistant cell lines *(34)*. In addition, using quantitative microsatellite analysis with 10 markers at seven different chromosomes, Makhija et al. identified a decreased copy number of a region in chromosome 6 that was significantly related to platinum resistance *(35)*.

Overall, a subchromosomal region that is consistently related to cisplatin resistance has not yet been identified. Therefore, future studies should be directed towards validating these candidate genes as well as continuing to search for additional areas, which may be more frequently associated with cisplatin resistance.

2.3. Genome-Wide Analysis to Identify Gene Amplification Associated With Chemoresistance

As mentioned, increased DNA copy number plays an important role in chemoresistance; however, it is not known whether this mechanism is involved in resistance to chemotherapeutic agents in addition to those discussed. Exploration of cancer genomes using advanced technologies including CGH *(36)*, array CGH *(37)*, and more recently, digital karyotyping *(38)* is expected to facilitate the discovery of novel amplified genes that participate in chemoresistance. Conventional CGH is based on competitive hybridization of normal DNA and tumor DNA on a normal human metaphase spread. It has been widely employed to identify chromosomal imbalances in cancer; however, its relatively low mapping resolution (5–20 Mb) has limited its use as a discovery tool for novel gene amplification in drug resistance *(36)*. On the other hand, array-based CGH applies the technique of conventional CGH to arrayed genomic components of cDNA, bacterial artificial chromosomes, and phage artificial chromosomes. Because thousands of genomic targets representing different genomic locations can be analyzed simultaneously, the assay resolution is greatly enhanced in comparison to conventional CGH.

Digital karyotyping is a recently developed method that can also provide high-resolution quantitative analysis of DNA copy number changes in cancer *(38)*. The principle of the technique is based on isolation and counting of short (21 bp) sequence tags derived from tumor genomic DNA. Digital enumeration of these tags and mapping of these tags to the human genome offers a means for systematic detection of DNA copy number changes on a genomic scale. Digital karyotyping provides unbiased gene dosage readout, as it measures the direct tag count in contrast to the analog signal generated by hybridization that is associated with CGH or array CGH. Using digital karyotyping, investigators have demonstrated that whole-chromosome changes, gains, or losses of chromosomal arms, and interstitial amplifications or deletions can be readily detected. As compared to conventional CGH, digital karyotyping has a much higher resolution in detecting amplifications and deletions; an example of this is shown in Fig. 1. This technology was used to reveal *TYMS* gene amplification in 5-FU-resistant tumors as described in the previous subheading.

3. CONCLUSION

Alteration in gene copy number has been recognized as a molecular mechanism of resistance to chemotherapeutic drugs in vitro *and* in vivo. The purpose of identifying

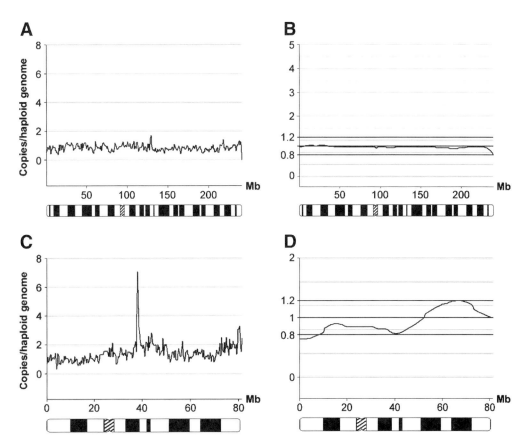

Fig. 1. Detection of chromosomal amplification by digital karyotyping. Digital karyotyping and comparative genomic hybridization (CGH) were performed in an ovarian cancer cell line, SKOV3. Absence of amplification or deletion in chromosome 2 shown by digital karyotyping analysis (**A**) correlates with CGH analysis (**B**). A discrete amplification at chromosome 17q harboring the *HER-2/neu* oncogene was detected by digital karyotyping (**C**); however, conventional CGH performed on the same cell line has missed the distinct amplicon (**D**).

amplified chemoresistant genes is manifold. First, the amplified genes that play a causal role in chemoresistance can provide a valuable indicator for medical oncologists to develop target-based therapies, thereby maximizing therapeutic efficacy, while minimizing adverse effects. Second, inhibition of the function or expression level of the amplified genes may significantly reduce chemoresistance and improve patient survival. Third, detection of amplified genes can predict treatment response and clinical outcome. Finally, characterization of amplified genes will shed light on the molecular mechanisms underlying chemoresistance.

Currently, target gene amplification has been detected in patients treated with chemotherapeutic agents including methotrexate, 5-FU, antiandrogens, and imatinib. These data have provided compelling evidence that DNA copy number alterations play a significant role in acquired drug resistance in cancer patients. The fact that target gene amplification is almost exclusively observed in patients after chemotherapy suggests that the amplification of chemoresistant genes is the result of Darwinian selection (induced by chemotherapeutic agents) of many subclones generated by genomic instability and

Table 1
Examples of Target Gene Amplification in Resistant Clinical Samples

Drug	Effective cancer types	Amplified target gene	Rate of amplification in relapsed cancers	References
Methotrexate	Lymphocytic leukemias, lymphomas, osteosarcoma, choriocarcinoma, trophoblastic neoplasms, and carcinomas of the breast, head and neck, lung, gastrointestinal tract, esophagus, and testes	Dihydrofolate reductase (*DHFR*)	31%	*(6)*
5-Fluorouracil	Carcinomas of the breast, colon, head and neck, pancreas, rectum, and stomach	Thymidylate synthetase (*TYMS*)	23%	*(16)*
Antiandrogen	Prostate cancer	Androgen receptor (*AR*)	20–30%	*(18–24)*
Imatinib	Chronic myelogenous leukemia (CML) and gastrointestinal stromal tumors (GIST)	*bcr-abl*	6–27%	*(26,28–29)*

clonal expansion. Therefore, molecular targeting of the pathways involved in controlling genomic instability or selective killing of cells that carry chromosomal imbalances may have a major impact on the clinical management of cancer.

As summarized in Table 1, the prevalence of chemoresistant gene amplification ranges from 5 to 30% in clinical samples. This is a significant number and warrants the use of such information for the benefit of cancer patients undergoing routine chemotherapy. In particular, because FISH analysis to detect gene amplification is a sensitive and straightforward approach and can be routinely applied to formalin-fixed, paraffin-embedded tissues, it could be readily performed on biopsies of recurrences in patients. If target gene amplification is detected by FISH, we would suggest that those patients should not be treated with the same regimen, because it will likely add toxicity without efficacy. Instead, alternative regimens including many of the newer second-line therapies undergoing clinical trials should be considered. Furthermore, understanding gene amplification as a drug resistance mechanism should stimulate efforts to develop compounds that specifically target cancers with amplified genes *(39)*. The recent advance in new molecular technologies and the success of the Human Genome Project will provide new discovery tools to identify and characterize novel amplified genes involved in chemoresistance. The findings of future studies are expected to offer new targets for disease intervention and improve the clinical management of cancer patients.

ACKNOWLEDGMENTS

We thank Dr. Michael R. Speicher and his research group in providing the CGH figure, and members in our laboratory for critical reading of the manuscript.

REFERENCES

1. Yasui K, Mihara S, Zhao C, et al. Alteration in copy numbers of genes as a mechanism for acquired drug resistance. Cancer Res 2004; 64:1403–1410.
2. Schimke RT. Gene amplification in cultured cells. J Biol Chem 1988; 263:5989–5892.

3. Gollin SM. Chromosomal instability. Curr Opin Oncol 2004; 16:25–31.

4. Ma C, Martin S, Trask B, Hamlin JL. Sister chromatid fusion initiates amplification of the dihydrofolate reductase gene in Chinese hamster cells. Genes Dev 1993; 7:605–620.

5. Singer MJ, Mesner LD, Friedman CL, Trask BJ, Hamlin JL. Amplification of the human dihydrofolate reductase gene via double minutes is initiated by chromosome breaks. Proc Natl Acad Sci U S A 2000; 97:7921–7926.

6. Goker E, Waltham M, Kheradpour A, et al. Amplification of the dihydrofolate reductase gene is a mechanism of acquired resistance to methotrexate in patients with acute lymphoblastic leukemia and is correlated with p53 gene mutations. Blood 1995; 86:677–684.

7. Roninson IB. Molecular mechanism of multidrug resistance in tumor cells. Clin Physiol Biochem 1987; 5:140–51.

8. Reeve JG, Rabbitts PH, Twentyman PR. Amplification and expression of *mdr1* gene in a multidrug resistant variant of small cell lung cancer cell line NCI-H69. Br J Cancer 1989; 60:339–342.

9. Carman MD, Schornagel JH, Rivest RS, et al. Resistance to methotrexate due to gene amplification in a patient with acute leukemia. J Clin Oncol 1984; 2:16–20.

10. Horns RC, Jr., Dower WJ, Schimke RT. Gene amplification in a leukemic patient treated with methotrexate. J Clin Oncol 1984; 2:2–7.

11. Trent JM, Buick RN, Olson S, Horns RC Jr, Schimke RT. Cytologic evidence for gene amplification in methotrexate-resistant cells obtained from a patient with ovarian adenocarcinoma. J Clin Oncol 1984; 2:8–15.

12. Merkel DE, Fuqua SA, McGuire WL. P-glycoprotein in breast cancer. Cancer Treat Res 1989; 48:97–105.

13. Longley DB, Harkin DP, Johnston PG. 5-fluorouracil: mechanisms of action and clinical strategies. Nat Rev Cancer 2003; 3:330–338.

14. Giacchetti S, Perpoint B, Zidani R, et al. Phase III multicenter randomized trial of oxaliplatin added to chronomodulated fluorouracil-leucovorin as first-line treatment of metastatic colorectal cancer. J Clin Oncol 2000; 18:136–147.

15. de Gramont A, Figer A, Seymour M, et al. Leucovorin and fluorouracil with or without oxaliplatin as first-line treatment in advanced colorectal cancer. J Clin Oncol 2000; 18:2938–2947.

16. Wang TL, Diaz LA Jr, Romans K, et al. Digital karyotyping identifies thymidylate synthase amplification as a mechanism of resistance to 5-fluorouracil in metastatic colorectal cancer patients. Proc Natl Acad Sci U S A 2004; 101:3089–3094.

17. Goktas S, Ziada A, Crawford ED. Combined androgen blockade for advanced prostatic carcinoma. Prostate Cancer Prostatic Dis 1999; 2:172–179.

18. Edwards J, Krishna NS, Grigor KM, Bartlett JM. Androgen receptor gene amplification and protein expression in hormone refractory prostate cancer. Br J Cancer 2003; 89:552–556.

19. Linja MJ, Savinainen KJ, Saramaki OR, Tammela TL, Vessella RL, Visakorpi T. Amplification and overexpression of androgen receptor gene in hormone-refractory prostate cancer. Cancer Res 2001; 61:3550–3555.

20. Ford OH III, Gregory CW, Kim D, Smitherman AB, Mohler JL. Androgen receptor gene amplification and protein expression in recurrent prostate cancer. J Urol 2003; 170:1817–1821.

21. Brown RS, Edwards J, Dogan A, et al. Amplification of the androgen receptor gene in bone metastases from hormone-refractory prostate cancer. J Pathol 2002; 198:237–244.

22. Visakorpi T, Hyytinen E, Koivisto P, et al. In vivo amplification of the androgen receptor gene and progression of human prostate cancer. Nat Genet 1995; 9:401–406.

23. Koivisto P, Kononen J, Palmberg C, et al. Androgen receptor gene amplification: a possible molecular mechanism for androgen deprivation therapy failure in prostate cancer. Cancer Res 1997; 57:314–319.

24. Bubendorf L, Kononen J, Koivisto P, et al. Survey of gene amplifications during prostate cancer progression by high-throughout fluorescence in situ hybridization on tissue microarrays. Cancer Res 1999; 59:803–806.

25. Hochhaus A, La Rosee P. Imatinib therapy in chronic myelogenous leukemia: strategies to avoid and overcome resistance. Leukemia 2004; 18:1321–1331.

26. Gambacorti-Passerini CB, Gunby RH, Piazza R, Galietta A, Rostagno R, Scapozza L. Molecular mechanisms of resistance to imatinib in Philadelphia-chromosome-positive leukaemias. Lancet Oncol 2003; 4:75–85.

27. le Coutre P, Tassi E, Varella-Garcia M, et al. Induction of resistance to the Abelson inhibitor STI571 in human leukemic cells through gene amplification. Blood 2000; 95:1758–1766.

28. Gorre ME, Mohammed M, Ellwood K, et al. Clinical resistance to STI-571 cancer therapy caused by BCR-ABL gene mutation or amplification. Science 2001; 293:876–880.

29. Hochhaus A, Kreil S, Corbin AS, et al. Molecular and chromosomal mechanisms of resistance to imatinib (STI571) therapy. Leukemia 2002; 16:2190–2196.

30. Morel F, Bris MJ, Herry A, et al. Double minutes containing amplified *bcr-abl* fusion gene in a case of chronic myeloid leukemia treated by imatinib. Eur J Haematol 2003; 70:235–239.

31. Gambacorti-Passerini CB, Rossi F, Verga M, et al. Differences between in vivo and in vitro sensitivity to imatinib of Bcr/Abl[+] cells obtained from leukemic patients. Blood Cells Mol Dis 2002; 28:361–372.

32. Ozols RF. Current status of chemotherapy for ovarian cancer. Semin Oncol 1995; 22(Suppl 12):S61–S66.

33. Inoue J, Otsuki T, Hirasawa A, et al. Overexpression of PDZK1 within the 1q12-q22 amplicon is likely to be associated with drug-resistance phenotype in multiple myeloma. Am J Pathol 2004; 165:71–81.

34. Takano M, Kudo K, Goto T, Yamamoto K, Kita T, Kikuchi Y. Analyses by comparative genomic hybridization of genes relating with cisplatin-resistance in ovarian cancer. Hum Cell 2001; 14:267–271.

35. Makhija S, Sit A, Edwards R, et al. Identification of genetic alterations related to chemoresistance in epithelial ovarian cancer. Gynecol Oncol 2003; 90:3–9.

36. Kallioniemi A, Kallioniemi OP, Sudar D, et al. Comparative genomic hybridization for molecular cytogenetic analysis of solid tumors. Science 1992; 258:818–821.

37. Pinkel D, Segraves R, Sudar D, et al. High resolution analysis of DNA copy number variation using comparative genomic hybridization to microarrays. Nat Genet 1998; 20:207–211.

38. Wang TL, Maierhofer C, Speicher MR, et al. Digital karyotyping. Proc Natl Acad Sci U S A 2002; 99:16,156–16,161.

39. Neuteboom ST, Karjian PL, Boyer CR, et al. Inhibition of cell growth by NB1011 requires high thymidylate synthase levels and correlates with p53, p21, bax, and GADD45 induction. Mol Cancer Ther 2002; 1:377–384.

V CLINICAL ASPECTS OF RESISTANCE

29 Cancer Chemotherapy

Clinical Evidence for Drug Resistance

Mika A. Sovak, MD, PhD
and David R. Spriggs, MD

SUMMARY

The most informative clinical trials are those in which correlative measurements are being done to determine if the intended target is, in fact, being affected as expected by the treatment being delivered. This chapter focuses on selected mechanisms of acquired drug resistance that have been the targets of novel therapies in the treatment of solid tumors.

Key Words: Clinical drug resistance; biomarkers; response criteria; combination chemotherapy; surrogate markers.

1. INTRODUCTION

Clinical resistance to chemotherapy is the major limiting factor in our efforts to cure cancer. The intricacies of the molecular mechanics underlying drug resistance are detailed in previous chapters. As we progress from the more experimentally controlled environment of the laboratory to the clinical care of patients, the challenge is to identify the significance of each of these defined pathways in a specific disease or patient population. Drug development can take the path of mass screening of compounds and development of those with demonstrable cytotoxic activity, with identification of relevant targets as clinical drug development ongoing, or the synthesis of compounds that specifically target abnormalities in the tumor. In the latter instances, experience is revealing that

From: *Cancer Drug Discovery and Development: Cancer Drug Resistance*
Edited by: B. Teicher © Humana Press Inc., Totowa, NJ

the most informative clinical trials are those in which correlative measurements are being done to determine if the intended target is, in fact, being affected as expected by the treatment being delivered. As drug development continues in the future, we may see a shift towards the use of such correlative assays in the evaluation of all drugs. In this chapter, we focus on selected mechanisms of acquired drug resistance that have been the targets of novel therapies in the treatment of solid tumors; it is not meant to be a comprehensive review. Studies of resistance to cisplatin and methotrexate have provided the foundations of our understanding for certain mechanisms of chemoresistance, and analogs to these two drugs are discussed as illustration. Other pathways of resistance are reviewed briefly to clarify the rational behind their development, and we discuss correlative studies that have increased our understanding of the underlying mechanisms and the overall clinical experience with these agents.

2. CISPLATIN AND METHOTREXATE RESISTANCE AS MODELS

Cisplatin exerts its cytotoxic effects through formation of intrastrand DNA–platinum adducts and is a widely used agent in the treatment of solid tumors. However, the use of cisplatin is restricted by both its toxicity and the emergence of resistance. There is a substantial body of knowledge regarding the mechanisms involved in cisplatin resistance and include reduced intracellular accumulation of available drug (currently attributed to the copper efflux transporter ATP7A [11]), inactivation of drug via interactions with intracellular thiols, alterations in DNA–adduct repair pathways, and changes in downstream signaling pathways (reviewed in ref. 2). Carboplatin was developed for more favorable toxicity profile and similar efficacy in most types of solid tumors, but has a similar resistance profile to cisplatin. Other platinum analogs have been developed for their activity in cisplatin-resistant cells and have entered the arena of clinical development. Satraplatin (JM216/BMS-182751) is an oral, lipophilic platinum analog that had demonstrable preclinical activity in cisplatin-resistant tumor models (3). Studies suggest that satraplatin might overcome platinum resistance mediated by decreased drug accumulation, although this area remains controversial (3,4). Phase I and II trials demonstrated tolerable toxicity but variable efficacy (5–8). ZD0473 (AMD473) is an amino-dichloroplatinum complex with decreased susceptibility to inactivation by intracellular thiol and in vitro activity in cisplatin-resistant cells that has entered early phase clinical trials (9,10). Oxaliplatin (Eloxatin®) has a different activity and toxicity profile from cisplatin and carboplatin, and early data demonstrated activity in cisplatin-resistant scenarios (reviewed in ref. 11). Oxaliplatin is approved for the treatment of colon cancer in combination with 5-fluorouracil (FU)/Leucovorin®, and is used in the treatment of many solid tumors. Structurally, oxaliplatin has a bulky diaminocyclohexane side group. Current theory suggests that oxaliplatin retains activity in cisplatin resistance because of its ability to bypass mismatch repair enzyme monitoring. When cisplatin forms DNA adducts, DNA repair enzymes identify these adducts, and futile attempts to repair the DNA damage results in downstream signaling resulting in apoptosis. Resistance to cisplatin can arise through acquired aberrations in repair enzyme activity, namely either increased repair ability as demonstrated by increased excision repair ability (12) or complete loss of activity and thus increased tolerance of DNA adducts. The mismatch repair (MMR) enzymes are actively involved in the identification of cisplatin–DNA adducts and subsequent stimulation of apoptosis. Preclinical data demonstrate that loss of MMR activity is associated with cisplatin and carboplatin resistance (reviewed in ref. *13*). However in vitro data suggest that oxaliplatin–DNA adducts are not recognized by MMR, and thus, oxaliplatin maintains activity in cisplatin-resistant settings because of a loss of MMR activity *(14,15)*. Clinically colorectal cancers are not susceptible to treatment with cisplatin or carboplatin, but the use of combination therapies with oxaliplatin have become standard of care in advanced disease. The fact that many colorectal cancers have a deficiency in MMR may explain their selective susceptibility to different platinum agents.

Folate metabolism is essential to cellular metabolism and is the target of antimetabolite chemotherapeutics such as methotrexate (MTX) and 5-FU. There are three main enzymes targeted by these drugs: dihydrofolate reductase (DHFR), which is involved in maintenance of reduced intracellular folate pools; thymidylate synthase (TS), which catalyzes the *de novo* synthesis of thymidylate (deoxythymidine monophosphate) from deoxythymidine monophosphate; and glycinamide ribonucleotide transformylase, which uses methylene tetrahydrofolate in the synthesis of *de novo* purine synthesis. MTX inhibits DHFR, whereas its active metabolite, polyglutamated MTX, can target all three enzymes. 5-FU inhibits TS. The clinical usage of these drugs is limited by acquired resistance. In vivo mechanisms of resistance to MTX can be conceived as resistance to membrane transport, decreased polyglutamated MTX, and an increase in the activity of the target enzymes *(16)*, though clear demonstration of these mechanisms in humans is sparse. However, MTX analogs able to withstand presumed pathways of resistance have entered clinical trials. Both folates and antifolates such as MTX are transported across the extracellular membrane by the reduced folate–MTX carrier system (RFC) or to a lesser extent by the membrane-associated folate-binding protein. Defective transport has been seen in numerous preclinical models as a mechanism of MTX resistance (reviewed in ref. *17*). Rationally designed MTX derivatives such as 10-propargyl-10-deazaaminopterins (PDX) are more effectively transported across the RFC and demonstrated significant antitumor preclinical activity. PDX was well tolerated in a phase I study, and demonstrated promising activity in non-small cell lung cancer (NSCLC) in a phase II trial *(18,19)*. Early correlative data demonstrated that patients who had stable disease had higher levels of RFC RNA levels than patients who progressed, although full evaluation was not able to be completed *(18)*. Further trials combining PDX with other chemotherapeutic agents are planned. Edatrexate was developed as a methotrexate analog with a superior therapeutic index attributed to increased polyglutamation within malignant cells compared to MTX. Numerous phase I trials have been conducted in patients with solid tumors demonstrating tolerability of edatrexate *(20,21)*. Phase II trials using combination therapies with edatrexate in mesothelioma and NSCLC have demonstrated minimal activity or significant toxicity *(22,23)*. Pemetrexate (Alimta®) is an antifolate that targets all three enzymes mentioned above, DHFR, TS, and glycinamide ribonucleotide formyltransferase, and takes a more drastic approach to inhibiting folate metabolism. Indeed, pemetrexed plus cisplatin demonstrated significant activity in patients with mesothelioma compared to the platinum alone, and is the only drug approved by the Food and Drug Administration (FDA) for the treatment of mesothelioma *(24)*. A randomized phase III trial of pemetrexed compared to docetaxel demonstrated clinically equal outcomes and less toxicity, leading to approval of pemetrexed for recurrent NSCLC.

3. MULTIDRUG RESISTANCE

Multidrug resistance is characterized by crossresistance to a broad spectrum of chemotherapeutic agents that themselves may have only minimal structural similarities. This phenotype is conferred by membrane transport proteins that belong to the ATP-binding cassette (ABC) transporter family of proteins. P-glycoprotein (P-gp), also known as ABCB1, is encoded by the multidrug resistance gene 1 (*MDR1*) and is perhaps the most extensively studied member of this family. Other members of this family were discovered when it was observed that some cells with this resistance phenotype did not express P-gp *(25–27)*, and include multidrug-resistant-related protein and breast cancer resistance protein. These ABC proteins form ion or transport channels that are ATP-dependent and act as efflux pumps. The teleologic role of these transport channels is to prevent accumulation of toxic substances within the cell. In cancer therapy, these proteins decrease the potential accumulation of chemotherapy within the cell, thus limiting their effectiveness. Overexpression of MDR proteins, often achieved through gene amplification, has been implicated in resistance to anthracyclins, vinca alkaloids, epipodophyllotoxins, and taxanes *(28)*.

There have been numerous attempts at reversing the activity of MDR to overcome drug resistance in the clinical setting. The earliest inhibitors targeting P-gp included cyclosporin A (CsA) and the calcium-channel blocker, verapamil. These drugs were tested in various combinations with chemotherapy in colon and refractory ovarian cancer *(29,30)*. Yahanda et al. *(31)* performed a phase I study evaluating the toxicity of etoposide and CsA given on days 1–3. Pharmacokinetic analysis of etoposide levels were performed and demonstrated that a 50% decrease in the dose of etoposide was required in order to maintain a tolerable regimen *(32)*. No clinical benefit was observed by the addition of CsA. Several studies evaluating the use of verapamil in combination with chemotherapy have been published, some with initial favorable outcomes *(33,34)*. However, the use of CsA and verapamil at serum concentrations able to reverse P-gp activity were limited by the significant increase in toxicity, including cases of complete heart block, prompting the search for less toxic inhibitors.

Second-generation MDR inhibitors have also undergone clinical evaluation. Valspodar (PSC 833) is a derivative of cyclosporin D, and was evaluated in a phase I/II trial in patients with recurrent ovarian cancer who had failed prior platinum and anthracyclin therapy *(35)*. Valspodar was given for 3 d before treatment with cisplatin and doxorubicin in an attempt to reverse acquired drug resistance from prior therapy. In these patients, an overall response rate of 15% was seen with acceptable toxicity. These data prompted a randomized phase III trial of 762 patients with advanced ovarian cancer, comparing standard doses of carboplatin and paclitaxel to the experimental combination of standard dose carboplatin, reduced-dose paclitaxel, and valspodar *(36)*. More hematologic toxicity was observed in the experimental arm without a significant difference in median time to progression (13.2 mo in the experimental arm vs 13.5 mo, $p = 0.6678$) or overall survival ($p = 0.3817$). Because of lack of demonstrable efficacy, further evaluation of valspodar was not pursued. Another MDR inhibitor currently undergoing evaluation is biricodar (VX-710). A phase II study in patients with locally advanced or metastatic breast cancer refractory to paclitaxel was performed. Again, an attempt at reversing acquired drug resistance in this refractory population was done by first delivering a 24-h continuous infusion of biricodar 3 h before giving paclitaxel (80 mg/m^2). An 11% response rate was observed, albeit accompanied by a 40% incidence of grade 4 neutropenia. In a similarly heavily pretreated population of patients with taxol-refractory ovarian cancer, 6% of patients had a partial response, and 30% had stable disease *(37)*. The difference in effectiveness in these early trials between valspodar and biricodar may be because of clinical trial design. As MDR proteins are involved in resistance to taxanes but not platinums, it is possible that valspodar may have demonstrated efficacy had it been tested in combination with a taxane alone.

More-promising data is available for so-called third-generation MDR converters such as GF120918, which inhibits P-gp and breast cancer resistance protein. Early phase I data using GF120918 with intravenous doxorubicin revealed significant increases in the doxorubicin metabolite, doxorubicinol, in patients treated with the combination therapy compared to either drug alone, suggesting that the goal of increasing drug availability through reversal of MDR activity was achieved *(38)*. Significant toxicities included neutropenia and mild cardiac toxicity, likely because of the chemotherapy and its metabolite. Another interesting use of GF120918 is in combination with oral chemotherapeutics, with the aim of increasing their bioavailability. The rationale behind this is that high expression of MDR proteins in the gut lumen prevents absorption of chemotherapy, and reversal of this mechanism has the potential to reduce the often low and variable oral bioavailability of drugs. Kruijtzer et al. have demonstrated increased bioavailability of oral topotecan when given with oral GF120918 as compared to topotecan alone, without any apparent differences in toxicity *(39)*. Other studies combining GF120918 with paclitaxel are ongoing *(40)*. Perhaps MDR inhibitors could best be used in the prevention, rather than the reversal of, chemotherapeutic resistance, a possibility raised by in vitro analysis *(41)*. Further studies will be needed to determine whether these agents can be incorporated into routine clinical care.

4. GLUTATHIONE AND GLUTATHIONE *S*-TRANSFERASE

The glutathione-*S*-transferase (GST) family of enzymes catalyzes the reaction between glutathione (GSH) and electrophilic toxins. This process results in detoxification of not just environmental mutagens, but also chemotherapeutic agents including alkylating agents and platinum compounds. Both GST and GSH are believed to play a significant role in acquired chemotherapy resistance. In vitro data demonstrate increasing levels of GST activity in cells undergoing selection for chemotherapy resistance (reviewed in ref. *42*). Thus, the use of drugs that inhibit GST activity or GSH levels in combination with chemotherapeutic agents is a valid approach to combat chemotherapeutic resistance. Here, we discuss two clinical trials developed along these lines of reasoning, and finally, focus upon a drug that relies upon these acquired mechanism of drug resistance for its own activity.

Buthionine sulfoximine is an irreversible inhibitor of γ-glutamylcysteine synthetase, the limiting enzyme in GSH synthesis. Phase I studies of buthionine sulfoximine in combination with melphalan established that this combination was well tolerated, with correlative studies demonstrating a decrease in GSH activity, as expected, in peripheral mononuclear cells *(43)*. Ethacrynic acid is one known inhibitor of GST activity that has been studied in combination with thiotepa. A phase I study of ethacrynic acid and thiotepa in patients with advanced malignancy was relatively well tolerated, with myelosuppression correlating with thiotepa levels *(44)*. Correlative studies revealed that transient decreases in GST activity in peripheral mononuclear cells was observed after ethacrynic acid treatment, and measurement of area under the ccurve of thiotepa and its main metabolite revealed that ethacrynic acid was effective in decreasing metabolism of thiotepa as hypothesized. However, further clinical development of ethacrynic acid was limited by the expected side effect of diuresis. Perhaps one of the more interesting drugs to take advantage of the imbalance seen in this pathway in cancer cells is TLK286. TLK286 is a glutathione analog, the metabolites of which induce apoptosis, possibly through activation of the mitogen-activated protein kinase pathway. What is most interesting about this drug is that it is cleaved into its active product by GST. Thus, the activity of TLK286 should hypothetically be limited to resistant cancers that have increased the activity of this pathway to overcome chemotherapeutic toxicity. A phase I study of TLK286 in solid tumors demonstrated tolerable toxicities as well as early indication of drug activity (45). Several phase II studies of TLK286 in heavily pretreated patients, some with demonstrable resistance to platinum and taxanes, with ovarian, lung, and breast cancer have demonstrated promising response rates (46–48). In an ongoing phase III trial, patients with platinum-resistant ovarian cancer who have progressed through second line therapy with either topotecan or liposomal doxorubicin are being randomized to either TLK286 or liposomal doxorubicin/topotecan (whichever drug they did not previously received). If the findings of this trial demonstrate an increased benefit for TLK286, approval of this drug could be forthcoming.

5. ABERRANT REGULATION OF APOPTOSIS

Induction of the p53-dependent mitochondrial apoptotic pathway is the final common pathway induced by most chemotherapeutic agents. The regulation of apoptosis by upstream regulatory pathways is extremely complex, and the exact role of each controlling entity controversial. However, there is ample evidence that defects in the apoptotic pathway can result in failure of cells to undergo apoptosis, and this is manifest clinically as multidrug resistance to numerous chemotherapeutics including cisplatin (49). Many therapeutic approaches have focused upon the restoration or activation of alternative pathways to result in apoptosis and overcome resistance. Upstream pathways of interest include those involving the transcription factors nuclear factor (NF)-κB and Bcl-2, the phosphoinositide 3 Kinase (PI3)/Akt pathway, all of which when activated can protect cells from undergoing apoptosis. Here, we focus upon these specific pathways and discuss the rational drug designs targeted at these pathways.

Perhaps the most successful drug to emerge from pharmacological targeting of the apoptotic pathway is the proteasome inhibitor bortezomib (Velcade®/PS341), which was approved for marketing in the United States by the FDA in 2003 for the treatment of multiple myeloma. The ultimate target of bortezomib is NF-κB. NF-κB is a transcription factor whose downstream targets include genes involved in cell proliferation, apoptosis, cell adhesion, and angiogenesis (reviewed in ref. 50). NF-κB is thought to play a central role in oncogenic transformation and in both innate and acquired resistance to chemotherapy. Overexpression of NF-κB results in cell resistance to apoptosis (51–54), and is overexpressed in numerous tumor types including breast (55,56), lung (57), ovarian, and colon cancer (58) (reviewed in ref. 59). The activity of NF-κB is controlled by the inhibitor of κB (IκB), which binds to NF-κB, keeping it in an inactive state in the cytoplasm. Activation of NF-κB requires phosphorylation, ubiquitination, and subsequent degradation of IκB by proteasomes. Bortezomib binds to and inhibits proteasome activity, thus preventing degradation of IκB and hence activation of NF-κB. Therefore, bortezomib could theoretically result in downregulation of NF-κB, with consequent induction of apoptosis. Preclinical data demonstrated significant antitumor activity of bortezomib in a variety of solid tumors *(60)*. Early phase trials were performed in both solid and hematologic toxicities and demonstrated a tolerable toxicity profile *(61,62)*. In addition, Aghajanian et al. measured 20S proteasome activity in peripheral blood samples as a pharmacodynamic measurement of proteasome inhibition by bortezomib. They were able to demonstrate reversible activity of the drug that was predictive of dose escalation. The pivotal trial that lead to FDA approval of bortezomib was a large, multicenter phase II trial in patients with relapsed/refractory multiple myeloma *(63)*. Single-agent bortezomib demonstrated a 35% response rate with a 6% near-complete response and overall survival of 17.8 mo in this heavily pretreated population for whom no proven therapy existed. Additional phase I and II trials are ongoing in ovarian, prostate, colorectal, lung, and gastric carcinoma *(64–68)*. Of significant interest in these studies are the correlative analyses being performed. Aghajanian et al. are measuring NF-κB activity in blood samples of patients with recurrent ovarian cancer who are being treated with carboplatin, with and without bortezomib, to determine the effect of each drug both individually and in combination on NF-κB activity *(68)*. Ocean et al. are analyzing NF-κB levels of expression in peripheral blood lymphocytes pre- and posttreatment to determine if there is any correlation with toxicity *(65)*. Patterns of gene expression pre- and posttreatment in patients with gastric cancer were also analyzed, although results have not yet been published *(64)*. The only other proteasome inhibitor currently undergoing clinical evaluation is PS-519, which was well tolerated in healthy human volunteers *(69)*. Many different agents have been used to block NF-κB activity directly in vitro, but as yet, none has entered clinical trials in solid tumors *(70,71)*. These studies with NF-κB are indicative of the direction in which the field is moving: as more targeted therapies enter development, concomitant correlative studies evaluating response of the intended target may become crucial in further development.

Members of the Bcl-2 family of proteins are one of the downstream targets of NF-κB, and play an integral role in the regulation of the mitochondrial apoptotic pathway. Preclinical data have demonstrated that Bcl-2 overexpression can protect cells from undergoing apoptosis *(72,73)*, and numerous types of solid tumors including colorectal tumors, non-small cell and small cell lung carcinoma, breast, and melanoma have all been demonstrated to overexpress Bcl-2 *(74–78)*. Genasense® (oblimersen sodium/G3139) is an antisense oligonucleotide that binds the first six codons of human *bcl-2* mRNA and results in its degradation. Preclinical studies demonstrated that Genasense was able to induce apoptosis in a variety of cancer models (reviewed in ref. *79*). A randomized phase III clinical trial of Genasense plus dacarbazine vs dacarbazine alone in patients with advanced malignant melanoma was performed and final results presented at American Society of Clinical Oncology 2004 *(80)*. A significant improvement in both response rate and time to progression was observed, although the primary end point of overall survival was not statistically significant. Inability to meet their primary end point led to the rejection of this drug by the FDA. Despite this setback, additional clinical trials are ongoing in lung, breast, and prostate cancer to determine the benefit of this drug in other tumor types *(75,81,82)*.

Akt is a serine/threonine kinase that is activated by the second messenger phosphatidylinositol-3,4,5-triphosphate (PIP$_3$), generated as a result of PI3 kinase (PI3K) activity. Akt is the human homolog of the viral oncogene, v-AKT. Similar to NF-κB, downstream targets of Akt include proteins involved in regulation of apoptosis and cell proliferation, including NF-κB itself. The majority of Akt-regulated pathways are targeted toward cell survival: phosphorylation and suppression of the proapoptotic activity of procaspase 9, Bcl2-antagonist of cell death, and fork head transcription factor, induction of NF-κB activity through phosphorylation and degradation of IκB, and activation of mammalian target of rapamycin (mTOR), a protein kinase involved in control of cell growth and proliferation. It may come as no surprise that the PI3/Akt survival pathway is overactive in many tumor types. PI3K activity is increase in ovarian and cervical carcinoma (83,84), and *akt* gene amplification or RNA expression can be seen in breast, ovarian, and pancreatic tumors (85,86). phosphatase and tensin homolog deleted on chromosome ten, which suppresses PI3 kinase activity and thus, Akt activity, is mutated in a more than 50% of melanomas and prostate cancers, 30–50% of endometrial cancers and glioblastomas, and 10% of breast cancers [S1] (71). Much preclinical evidence exists demonstrating that manipulation of the PI3/Akt pathway can alter sensitivity to chemotherapy (reviewed in refs 71 and 87). There are numerous drugs currently in development that target this pathway. Direct PI3 kinase inhibition by LY294002 or wortmanin has demonstrated increased sensitivity to cisplatin therapy, and these drugs are in preclinical development at this time, although their toxicity may limit their utility (88,89). Another upstream regulator of Akt activity is the heat shock protein (Hsp)90. Hsp90 is a chaperone protein that activates Akt activity. Natural inhibitors of Hsp90 include the ansamycin geldanamycin as well as radicicol derivatives, both of which were too toxic to be considered for clinical development. Several inhibitors of Hsp90 are currently in early stage clinical trials, including the ansamycin 17-allylamino-17-demothoxygeldanamycin. However, this compound was deemed to have significant toxicity and problems with solubility that have limited further clinical development (90,91). Thus, a second-generation, purely synthetic ansamycin, 17-dimethylaminoethylamino-17-demethoxygeldanamycin, has been developed and in early phase clinical trials. Downstream of Akt is mTOR, and inhibitors of this kinase are currently in clinical trials. One such inhibitor, CCI-779, is in phase I and II clinical trials, has tolerable toxicity, and antitumor activity in patients with renal cell carcinoma (92–94). RAD001 (everolimus) is another mTOR inhibitor that is currently undergoing clinical evaluation (95–99).

6. TYROSINE KINASE ACTIVITY

The epidermal growth factor receptor (EGFR) contains an intracellular tyrosine kinase domain that phosphorylates downstream targets involved in cellular growth and proliferation. This pathways are aberrantly activated in many tumor types as a result of receptor overexpression (100), mutated and thus constitutively active receptors (100,101), and crosscommunication with other activating pathways (102) (reviewed in refs. 103 and 104). Extensive preclinical data suggest that activation of this receptor pathway can results in escape from apoptosis (104,105), and thus, targeting this pathway using either monoclonal antibodies (MAbs) against the receptors themselves or tyrosine kinase inhibitors has become an active area of research (105).

The MAbs currently under clinical evaluation include cetuximab (Erbitux®/IMC-C225) (105), ABX-EGF (106,107), and EMD72000 (108). Cetuximab binds to the EGFR, both preventing ligand-induced activation of kinase activity and causing internalization of the receptor[S2] . Cetuximab with irinotecan was demonstrated to have a significant response rate (22%) in irinotecan-refractory colon cancers, and in February 2004 was approved for marketing in the United States for this patient population (109). Ongoing trials continue to evaluate the use of this MAb alone and in combination with standard chemotherapeutics in other cancers. The evaluation of small-molecule tyrosine kinase inhibitors has also led to the drug approval. Early phase trials demonstrated that 250 or 500 mg of gefitinib (Iressa/ZD1839) were both well tolerated, and both doses were further evaluated in randomized phase II trials that demonstrated a significant response rates in patients with advanced NSCLC resistant to cisplatin and taxanes *(110–115)*. No difference was seen between the 250- and 500-mg doses with respect to disease outcome. These trials lead to approval of single-agent gefitinib for patients with platinum and taxane refractory NSCLC in May 2003. Erlotinib (Tarceva®/OSI-779) has demonstrated activity and resulted in an overall survival benefit in patients with NSCLC *(116)*, and is currently under review by the FDA for drug approval in the United States. While undergoing evaluation, it was noted that that patients had either a dramatic response (often, women who had never smoked) to gefitinib or essentially none at all. As 40–80% of NSCLC are known to overexpress EGFR, the known target of gefitinib, this clinical observation was puzzling. Similarly, EGFR is overexpressed in a significant percentage of glioblastoma cells, however these tumors do not exhibit significant responses to Iressa *(117)*. Molecular analyses of the EGFR have provided a key towards understanding these discrepancies. Two recent publications have analyzed the nucleotide sequence analysis of the EGFR in patients who responded to gefitinib compared to nonresponders *(118,119)*. Lynch et al. demonstrated that eight out of nine patients with NSCLC who responded to gefitinib contained a mutation in the ATP-binding tyrosine kinase domain of EGFR, the same area targeted by gefitinib. In vitro functional studies revealed that this mutation resulted in increased and prolonged activation of EGFR activity when ligand was introduced into the system, and that the mutated receptors were more sensitive to prevention of ligand-induced activation by gefitinib than wild-type receptors. [S3] In patients with glioblastoma mutations in the EGFR are also observed; however, these mutations are most commonly seen in the extracellular domain that would not be expected to confer the same susceptibility to Iressa *(120)*. These data once again demonstrate that as targeted drug development continues, we need to be vigilant in characterizing our targets and using correlative markers to monitoring response at the expected site of action.

Gastrointestinal stromal tumors (GISTs) are characterized by cell-surface expression of the transmembrane receptor KIT that is the protein product of the *kit* oncogene. In GIST tumors, a gain-of-function mutation in the *c-kit* DNA between the transmembrane and tyrosine kinase domains results in constitutive activation of receptor kinase activity, with resultant uncontrolled cell proliferation and resistance to apoptosis *(121,122)*. Imatinib (Gleevec®/STI571) is an ATP-competitive inhibitor that blocks the activity of several tyrosine kinases, specifically KIT, the Bcr-Abl fusion protein that displays constitutive activity in chronic myelogenous leukemia (CML), and platelet-derived growth factor receptor. Early data demonstrating imatinib antitumor activity in CML prompted study of this drug in GISTs *(123)*. Even in phase I studies imatinib had significant activity against GISTs, and was well tolerated in this population *(124)*. A randomized phase II study in patients with GIST demonstrating a response rate to imatinib of over 50% led to FDA approval of the drug for this indication *(125)*. However, the emergence of resistance is seen clinically in certain patients who have rapidly progressive disease after a near complete response. In GISTs, this rapid progression can be observed in individual tumor implants that are physically amenable to biopsy. Chen et al. took advantage of this tumor biology and compared the DNA sequence of KIT from tumors before imatinib treatment, in stable/quiescent tumors, and in rapidly progressing tumors *(126)*. They describe an identical novel mutation in the tyrosine kinase domain of KIT that was only seen in rapidly progressing tumors. Moreover, this mutation is found exclusively on the allele carrying the original KIT mutation that is the target of imatinib, suggesting that locoregional genetic instability may be conferred by the original mutation. In CML, clinical resistance to imatinib has also been attributed to a mutation in the Bcr-Abl kinase domain *(127)*. Studies in CML revealed that most mutations in the Bcr-Alb kinase domain seen in resistant disease interfere with the conformation-specific binding of imatinib to the kinase *(128)*. This information has led to the screening of tyrosine kinase inhibitors with less stringent requirements for drug binding. Although not yet in clinical trials, BMS-354825 is one such drug. BMS-354825 is an inhibitor of Src-family kinases that in animal models has activity in imatinib-resistant, Bcr-Abl-driven hematopoietic disease *(129)*. This scenario demonstrates a dynamic model illustrating how the continual interaction between science and clinical observations are necessary to truly understand how best to improve the development of novel drugs for cancer therapy.

REFERENCES

1. Samimi G, Safaei R, Katano K, et al. Increased expression of the copper efflux transporter ATP7A mediates resistance to cisplatin, carboplatin, and oxaliplatin in ovarian cancer cells. Clin Cancer Res 2004; 10:4661–4669.
2. Siddik ZH. Cisplatin: mode of cytotoxic action and molecular basis of resistance. Oncogene 2003; 22:7265–7279.
3. Kelland LR, Abel G, McKeage MJ, et al. Preclinical antitumor evaluation of bis-acetato-ammine-dichloro-cyclohexylamine platinum(IV): an orally active platinum drug. Cancer Res 1993; 53:2581–2586.
4. Fokkema E, Groen HJ, Helder MN, de Vries EG, Meijer C. JM216-, JM118-, and cisplatin-induced cytotoxicity in relation to platinum-DNA adduct formation, glutathione levels and p53 status in human tumour cell lines with different sensitivities to cisplatin. Biochem Pharmacol 2002; 63:1989–1996.
5. Trudeau M, Stuart G, Hirte H, et al. A phase II trial of JM–216 in cervical cancer: an NCIC CTG study. Gynecol Oncol 2002; 84:327–331.
6. Beale P, Raynaud F, Hanwell J, et al. Phase I study of oral JM216 given twice daily. Cancer Chemother Pharmacol 1998; 42:142–148.
7. Fokkema E, Groen HJ, Bauer J, Uges DR, Weil C, Smith IE. Phase II study of oral platinum drug JM216 as first-line treatment in patients with small-cell lung cancer. J Clin Oncol 1999; 17:3822–3827.
8. McKeage MJ, Raynaud F, Ward J, et al. Phase I and pharmacokinetic study of an oral platinum complex given daily for 5 days in patients with cancer. J Clin Oncol 1997; 15:2691–2700.
9. Kelland LR. Preclinical perspectives on platinum resistance. Drugs 2000; 59 Suppl 4:1–8; discussion 37–38.
10. Beale P, Judson I, O'Donnell A, et al. A Phase I clinical and pharmacological study of cis-diamminedichloro(2-methylpyridine) platinum II (AMD473). Br J Cancer 2003; 88:1128–1134.
11. Raymond E, Chaney SG, Taamma A, Cvitkovic E. Oxaliplatin: a review of preclinical and clinical studies. Ann Oncol 1998; 9:1053–1071.
12. Dabholkar M, Vionnet J, Bostick-Bruton F, Yu JJ, Reed E. Messenger RNA levels of XPAC and ERCC1 in ovarian cancer tissue correlate with response to platinum-based chemotherapy. J Clin Invest 1994; 94:703–708.
13. Fink D, Aebi S, Howell SB. The role of DNA mismatch repair in drug resistance. Clin Cancer Res 1998; 4:1–6.
14. Fink D, Nebel S, Aebi S, et al. The role of DNA mismatch repair in platinum drug resistance. Cancer Res 1996; 56:4881–4886.
15. Vaisman A, Varchenko M, Umar A, et al. The role of hMLH1, hMSH3, and hMSH6 defects in cisplatin and oxaliplatin resistance: correlation with replicative bypass of platinum-DNA adducts. Cancer Res 1998; 58:3579–3585.
16. Zhao R, Goldman ID. Resistance to antifolates. Oncogene 2003; 22:7431–7457.
17. Peters GJ, Resistance to Antimetabolites, in Principles of Antineoplastic Drug Development and Pharmacology, Schilsky RL, Milano, GA, Ratain, MJ, Editor. 1996, Marcel Dekker, Inc.: New York, 543–585.
18. Krug LM, Azzoli CG, Kris MG, et al. 10-propargyl-10-deazaaminopterin: an antifolate with activity in patients with previously treated non-small cell lung cancer. Clin Cancer Res 2003; 9:2072–2078.

19. Krug LM, Ng KK, Kris MG, et al. Phase I and pharmacokinetic study of 10-propargyl-10-deazaaminopterin, a new antifolate. Clin Cancer Res 2000; 6:3493–3498.

20. Kuriakose P, Gandara DR, Perez EA. Phase I trial of edatrexate in advanced breast and other cancers. Cancer Invest 2002; 20:473–479.

21. Laurie SA, Pfister DG, Kris MG, et al. Phase I and pharmacological study of two schedules of the antifolate edatrexate in combination with cisplatin. Clin Cancer Res 2001; 7:501–509.

22. Kindler HL, Belani CP, Herndon JE, 2nd, Vogelzang NJ, Suzuki Y, Green MR. Edatrexate (10-ethyl-deaza-aminopterin) (NSC #626715) with or without leucovorin rescue for malignant mesothelioma. Sequential phase II trials by the cancer and leukemia group B. Cancer 1999; 86:1985–1991.

23. Colon-Otero G, Niedringhaus RD, Hillman SH, et al. A phase II trial of edatrexate, vinblastine, adriamycin, cisplastin, and filgrastim (EVAC/G-CSF) in patients with non-small-cell carcinoma of the lungs: a North Central Cancer Treatment Group Trial. Am J Clin Oncol 2001; 24:551–555.

24. Vogelzang NJ, Rusthoven JJ, Symanowski J, et al. Phase III study of pemetrexed in combination with cisplatin versus cisplatin alone in patients with malignant pleural mesothelioma. J Clin Oncol 2003; 21:2636–2644.

25. Barrand MA, Heppell-Parton AC, Wright KA, Rabbitts PH, Twentyman PR. A 190-kilodalton protein overexpressed in non-P-glycoprotein-containing multidrug-resistant cells and its relationship to the MRP gene. J Natl Cancer Inst 1994; 86:110–117.

26. Cole SP, Bhardwaj G, Gerlach JH, et al. Overexpression of a transporter gene in a multidrug-resistant human lung cancer cell line. Science 1992; 258:1650–1654.

27. McGrath T, Latoud C, Arnold ST, Safa AR, Felsted RL, Center MS. Mechanisms of multidrug resistance in HL60 cells. Analysis of resistance associated membrane proteins and levels of mdr gene expression. Biochem Pharmacol 1989; 38:3611–3619.

28. Biedler JL. Genetic aspects of multidrug resistance. Cancer 1992; 70:1799–1809.

29. Ozols RF, Cunnion RE, Klecker RW Jr, et al. Verapamil and adriamycin in the treatment of drug-resistant ovarian cancer patients. J Clin Oncol 1987; 5:641–647.

30. Verweij J, Herweijer H, Oosterom R, et al. A phase II study of epidoxorubicin in colorectal cancer and the use of cyclosporin-A in an attempt to reverse multidrug resistance. Br J Cancer 1991; 64:361–364.

31. Yahanda AM, Alder KM, Fisher GA, et al. Phase I trial of etoposide with cyclosporine as a modulator of multidrug resistance. J Clin Oncol 1992; 10:1624–1634.

32. Lum BL, Kaubisch S, Yahanda AM, et al. Alteration of etoposide pharmacokinetics and pharmaco-dynamics by cyclosporine in a phase I trial to modulate multidrug resistance. J Clin Oncol 1992; 10:1635–1642.

33. Belpomme D, Gauthier S, Pujade-Lauraine E, et al. Verapamil increases the survival of patients with anthracycline-resistant metastatic breast carcinoma. Ann Oncol 2000; 11:1471–1476.

34. Millward MJ, Cantwell BM, Munro NC, Robinson A, Corris PA, Harris AL. Oral verapamil with chemotherapy for advanced non-small cell lung cancer: a randomised study. Br J Cancer 1993; 67:1031–1035.

35. Baekelandt M, Lehne G, Trope CG, et al. Phase I/II trial of the multidrug-resistance modulator valspodar combined with cisplatin and doxorubicin in refractory ovarian cancer. J Clin Oncol 2001; 19:2983–2993.

36. Joly F, Joly C, Mangioni C, et al. A phase 3 study of PSC 833 in combination with paclitaxel and carboplatin (PC-PSC) versus paclitaxel and carboplatin (PC) alone in patients with stage IV or suboptimally debulked stage III epithelial ovarian cancer or primary canre of the peritoneum (Abstract). 2002: 806.

37. Seiden MV, Swenerton KD, Matulonis U, et al. A phase II study of the MDR inhibitor biricodar (INCEL, VX–710) and paclitaxel in women with advanced ovarian cancer refractory to paclitaxel therapy. Gynecol Oncol 2002; 86:302–310.

38. Planting AS, Sonneveld P, Van Der Gaast A, et al. A phase I and pharmacologic study of the MDR converter GF120918 in combination with doxorubicin in patients with advanced solid tumors. Cancer Chemother Pharmacol 2005; 55:91–99.

39. Kruijtzer CM, Beijnen JH, Rosing H, et al. Increased oral bioavailability of topotecan in combination with the breast cancer resistance protein and P-glycoprotein inhibitor GF120918. J Clin Oncol 2002; 20:2943–2950.

40. Malingre MM, Beijnen JH, Rosing H, et al. Co-administration of GF120918 significantly increases the systemic exposure to oral paclitaxel in cancer patients. Br J Cancer 2001; 84:42–47.

41. Cocker HA, Tiffin N, Pritchard-Jones K, Pinkerton CR, Kelland LR. In vitro prevention of the emergence of multidrug resistance in a pediatric rhabdomyosarcoma cell line. Clin Cancer Res 2001; 7:3193–3198.

42. Batist G, Schecter RL, Alaoui-Jamali MA. The Glutathione System and Drug Resistance, in Principles of Antineoplastic Drug Development and Pharmacology, Schilsky RL, Milano, GA, Ratain, MJ, Editor. 1996, Marcel Dekker, Inc.: New York, 503–521.

43. O'Dwyer PJ, Hamilton TC, LaCreta FP, et al. Phase I trial of buthionine sulfoximine in combination with melphalan in patients with cancer. J Clin Oncol 1996; 14:249–256.

44. O'Dwyer PJ, LaCreta F, Nash S, et al. Phase I study of thiotepa in combination with the glutathione transferase inhibitor ethacrynic acid. Cancer Res 1991; 51:6059–6065.

45. Rosen LS, Brown J, Laxa B, et al. Phase I study of TLK286 (glutathione S-transferase P1-1 activated glutathione analogue) in advanced refractory solid malignancies. Clin Cancer Res 2003; 9:1628–1638.

46. Washington D, Miller K, Budd GT. Phase 2 study of TLK286 (GST P1-1 activated glutathione) as ≥ third-line therapy in patients with advanced metastatic breast cancer (MBC). Abstr 61 in Proc Am Soc Clin Oncol 2003. Chicago, IL.

47. Papadimitrakopoulou V, Figlin L, Garland G. Phase 2 study of TLK286 (GST P1-1 activated glutathione analog) administered weekly in patients with non-small cell lung cancer (NSCLC) who failed prior platinum-based regimens. Abstr 2636 in Proc Am Soc Clin Oncol 2003. Chicago, IL.

48. Kavanagh JJ, Gershenson DM, Choi H, et al. Multi-institutional phase 2 study of TLK286 (TELCYTA, a glutathione S-transferase P1-1 activated glutathione analog prodrug) in patients with platinum and paclitaxel refractory or resistant ovarian cancer. Int J Gynecol Cancer 2005; 15:593–600.

49. Johnstone RW, Ruefli AA, Lowe SW. Apoptosis: a link between cancer genetics and chemotherapy. Cell 2002; 108:153–164.

50. Orlowski RZ, Baldwin AS Jr. NF-kappaB as a therapeutic target in cancer. Trends Mol Med 2002; 8:385–389.

51. Chu ZL, McKinsey TA, Liu L, Gentry JJ, Malim MH, Ballard DW. Suppression of tumor necrosis factor-induced cell death by inhibitor of apoptosis c-IAP2 is under NF-kappaB control. Proc Natl Acad Sci U S A 1997; 94:10057–10062.

52. Van Antwerp DJ, Martin SJ, Verma IM, Green DR. Inhibition of TNF-induced apoptosis by NF-κ B. Trends Cell Biol 1998; 8:107–111.

53. Beg AA, Baltimore D. An essential role for NF-kappaB in preventing TNF-α-induced cell death. Science 1996; 274:782–784.

54. Wang CY, Mayo MW, Baldwin AS Jr. TNF- and cancer therapy-induced apoptosis: potentiation by inhibition of NF-kappaB. Science 1996; 274:784–787.

55. Cogswell PC, Guttridge DC, Funkhouser WK, Baldwin AS Jr. Selective activation of NF-kappa B subunits in human breast cancer: potential roles for NF-kappa B2/p52 and for Bcl-3. Oncogene 2000; 19:1123–1131.

56. Sovak MA, Bellas RE, Kim DW, et al. Aberrant nuclear factor-kappaB/Rel expression and the pathogenesis of breast cancer. J Clin Invest 1997; 100:2952–2960.

57. Mukhopadhyay T, Roth JA, Maxwell SA. Altered expression of the p50 subunit of the NF-kappa B transcription factor complex in non-small cell lung carcinoma. Oncogene 1995; 11:999–1003.

58. Bours V, Dejardin E, Goujon-Letawe F, Merville MP, Castronovo V. The NF-kappa B transcription factor and cancer: high expression of NF-kappa B- and I kappa B-related proteins in tumor cell lines. Biochem Pharmacol 1994; 47:145–149.

59. Rayet B, Gelinas C. Aberrant rel/nfkb genes and activity in human cancer. Oncogene 1999; 18:6938–6947.

60. Adams J. The proteasome: a suitable antineoplastic target. Nat Rev Cancer 2004; 4:349–360.

61. Orlowski RZ, Stinchcombe TE, Mitchell BS, et al. Phase I trial of the proteasome inhibitor PS–341 in patients with refractory hematologic malignancies. J Clin Oncol 2002; 20:4420–4427.

62. Aghajanian C, Soignet S, Dizon DS, et al. A phase I trial of the novel proteasome inhibitor PS341 in advanced solid tumor malignancies. Clin Cancer Res 2002; 8:2505–2511.

63. Berenson JR, Jagannath S, Barlogie B, et al. Experience with long-term therapy using the proteasome inhibitor, bortezomib, in advanced multiple myeloma (MM). Abstr 2337 in Proc Am Soc Clin Oncol 2003. Chicago, IL.

64. Ocean AJ, Lane ME, Xiang Z. Genetic analysis of proteasome-related pathways in patients with advanced gastric adenocarcinomas (AGA) treated on a phase II study with PS–341 (bortezomib) with or without irinotecan. Abstr 9717 in Proc Am Soc Clin Oncol 2004. New Orleans, LA.

65. Stevenson JP, Nho CW, Johnson, SW. Effects of bortezomib (PS–341) on NF-κB activation in peripheral blood mononuclear cells (PBMCs) of advanced non-small cell lung cancer (NSCLC) patients: A phase II/pharmacodynamic trial. Abstr 7145 in Proc Am Soc Clin Oncol 2004. New Orleans, LA.

66. Dreicer R, Roth B, Petrylak D. Phase I / II trial of bortezomib plus docetaxel in patients with advanced androgen-independent prostate cancer. Abstr 4654 in Proc Am Soc Clin Oncol 2004. New Orleans, LA.

67. Dragovich T, Lenz HJ, Rocha Lima CMS. Bortezomib ± irinotecan in relapsed / refractory colorectal cancer (CRC): Interim analysis results from phase (ph) 2b study. Abstr 3591 in Proc Am Soc Clin Oncol 2004. New Orleans, LA.

68. Aghajanian C, Dizon DS, Sabbatini P, Raizer JJ, Dupont J, Spriggs DR. Phase I trial of bortezomib and carboplatin in recurrent ovarian or primary peritoneal cancer. J Clin Oncol 2005; 23:5943–5949.

69. Shah IM, Lees KR, Pien CP, Elliott PJ. Early clinical experience with the novel proteasome inhibitor PS-519. Br J Clin Pharmacol 2002; 54:269–276.

70. Karin M, Yamamoto Y, Wang QM. The IKK NF-kappa B system: a treasure trove for drug development. Nat Rev Drug Discov 2004; 3:17–26.

71. Pommier Y, Sordet O, Antony S, Hayward RL, Kohn KW. Apoptosis defects and chemotherapy resistance: molecular interaction maps and networks. Oncogene 2004; 23:2934–2949.

72. Fisher TC, Milner AE, Gregory CD, et al. bcl-2 modulation of apoptosis induced by anticancer drugs: resistance to thymidylate stress is independent of classical resistance pathways. Cancer Res 1993; 53:3321–3326.

73. Miyashita T, Reed JC. Bcl-2 oncoprotein blocks chemotherapy-induced apoptosis in a human leukemia cell line. Blood 1993; 81:151–157.

74. Bhatavdekar JM, Patel DD, Ghosh N, et al. Coexpression of Bcl-2, c-Myc, and p53 oncoproteins as prognostic discriminants in patients with colorectal carcinoma. Dis Colon Rectum 1997; 40:785–790.

75. Herbst RS, Frankel SR. Oblimersen sodium (Genasense bcl-2 antisense oligonucleotide): a rational therapeutic to enhance apoptosis in therapy of lung cancer. Clin Cancer Res 2004; 10:4245s–4248s.

76. Higashiyama M, Doi O, Kodama K, Yokouchi H, Tateishi R. Bcl-2 oncoprotein expression is increased especially in the portion of small cell carcinoma within the combined type of small cell lung cancer. Tumour Biol 1996; 17:341–344.

77. Soengas MS, Lowe SW. Apoptosis and melanoma chemoresistance. Oncogene 2003; 22:3138–3151.

78. Krajewski S, Thor AD, Edgerton SM, Moore DH 2nd, Krajewska M, Reed JC. Analysis of Bax and Bcl-2 expression in p53-immunopositive breast cancers. Clin Cancer Res 1997; 3:199–208.

79. Klasa RJ, Gillum AM, Klem RE, Frankel SR. Oblimersen Bcl-2 antisense: facilitating apoptosis in anticancer treatment. Antisense Nucleic Acid Drug Dev 2002; 12:193–213.

80. Millward MJ, Bedikian AY, Conry RM, et al. Randomized multinational phase 3 trial or dacarbazine (DTIC) with or without Bcl-2 antisense (oblimersen sodium) in patients with advanced malignanat melanoma (MM): Analysis of long-term survival. Abstr 7505 in Proc Am Soc Clin Oncol 2004. New Orleans, LA.

81. Marshall J, Chen H, Yang D, et al. A phase I trial of a Bcl-2 antisense (G3139) and weekly docetaxel in patients with advanced breast cancer and other solid tumors. Ann Oncol 2004; 15:1274–1283.

82. Tolcher AW, Kuhn J, Schwartz G, et al. A phase I pharmacokinetic and biological correlative study of oblimersen sodium (genasense, g3139), an antisense oligonucleotide to the bcl-2 mRNA, and of docetaxel in patients with hormone-refractory prostate cancer. Clin Cancer Res 2004; 10:5048–5057.

83. Shayesteh L, Lu Y, Kuo WL, et al. PIK3CA is implicated as an oncogene in ovarian cancer. Nat Genet 1999; 21:99–102.

84. Ma YY, Wei SJ, Lin YC, et al. PIK3CA as an oncogene in cervical cancer. Oncogene 2000; 19:2739–2744.

85. Ruggeri BA, Huang L, Wood M, Cheng JQ, Testa JR. Amplification and overexpression of the AKT2 oncogene in a subset of human pancreatic ductal adenocarcinomas. Mol Carcinog 1998; 21:81–86.

86. Bellacosa A, de Feo D, Godwin AK, et al. Molecular alterations of the AKT2 oncogene in ovarian and breast carcinomas. Int J Cancer 1995; 64:280–285.

87. Fresno Vara JA, Casado E, de Castro J, Cejas P, Belda-Iniesta C, Gonzalez-Baron M. PI3K/Akt signalling pathway and cancer. Cancer Treat Rev 2004; 30:193–204.

88. Altomare DA, Wang HQ, Skele KL, et al. AKT and mTOR phosphorylation is frequently detected in ovarian cancer and can be targeted to disrupt ovarian tumor cell growth. Oncogene 2004; 23:5853–5857.

89. Akimoto T, Nonaka T, Harashima K, Ishikawa H, Sakurai H, Mitsuhashi N. Selective inhibition of survival signal transduction pathways enhanced radiosensitivity in human esophageal cancer cell lines in vitro. Anticancer Res 2004; 24:811–819.

90. Solit DB, Zheng FF, Drobnjak M, et al. 17-Allylamino-17-demethoxygeldanamycin induces the degradation of androgen receptor and HER-2/neu and inhibits the growth of prostate cancer xenografts. Clin Cancer Res 2002; 8:986–993.

91. Solit DB, Basso AD, Olshen AB, Scher HI, Rosen N. Inhibition of heat shock protein 90 function downregulates Akt kinase and sensitizes tumors to Taxol. Cancer Res 2003; 63:2139–2144.

92. Punt CJ, Boni J, Bruntsch U, Peters M, Thielert C. Phase I and pharmacokinetic study of CCI–779, a novel cytostatic cell-cycle inhibitor, in combination with 5-fluorouracil and leucovorin in patients with advanced solid tumors. Ann Oncol 2003; 14:931–937.

93. Raymond E, Alexandre J, Faivre S, et al. Safety and pharmacokinetics of escalated doses of weekly intravenous infusion of CCI–779, a novel mTOR inhibitor, in patients with cancer. J Clin Oncol 2004; 22:2336–2347.

94. Atkins MB, Hidalgo M, Stadler WM, et al. Randomized phase II study of multiple dose levels of CCI–779, a novel mammalian target of rapamycin kinase inhibitor, in patients with advanced refractory renal cell carcinoma. J Clin Oncol 2004; 22:909–918.

95. Dancey JE. Inhibitors of the mammalian target of rapamycin. Expert Opin Investig Drugs 2005; 14:313–328.

96. O'Donnell A, Faivre S, Judson I. A phase I study of the oral mTOR inhibitor RAD001 as monotherapy to identify the optimal biologically effective dose using toxicity, pharmacokinetic (PK) and pharmacodynamic (PD) endpoints in patients with solid tumours. Abstr 803 in Proc Am Soc Clin Oncol 2003. Chicago, IL.

97. Van Oosterom AT, Dumez H, Desai J. Combination Signal transduction inhibition: A phase I / II trial of the oral mTOR-inhibitor everolimus (E, RAD001) and imatinib mesylate (IM) in patients (pts) with gastrointestinal stromal tumor (GIST) refractory to IM. Abstr 3002 in Proc Am Soc Clin Oncol 2004. New Orleans, LA.

98. DiCosimo S, Matar P, Rojo F. Schedule-dependent effects of the epidermal growth factor receptor (EGFR) tyrosine kinase inhibitor gefitinib in combination with the mammalian target of rapamycin (mTOR) inhibitor everolimus (RAD001). Abstr 3074 in Proc Am Soc Clin Oncol 2004. New Orleans, LA.

99. Pacey S, Rea N, Steven N. Results of phase 1 clinical trial investigating a combination of the oral mTOR-inhibitor Everolimus (E, RAD001) and Gemcitabine (GEM) in patients (pts) with advanced cancers. Abstr 3120 in Proc Am Soc Clin Oncol 2004. New Orleans, LA.

100. Hirsch FR, Varella-Garcia M, Bunn PA Jr, et al. Epidermal growth factor receptor in non-small-cell lung carcinomas: correlation between gene copy number and protein expression and impact on prognosis. J Clin Oncol 2003; 21:3798–3807.

101. Moscatello DK, Holgado-Madruga M, Godwin AK, et al. Frequent expression of a mutant epidermal growth factor receptor in multiple human tumors. Cancer Res 1995; 55:5536–5539.

102. Prenzel N, Zwick E, Daub H, et al. EGF receptor transactivation by G-protein-coupled receptors requires metalloproteinase cleavage of proHB-EGF. Nature 1999; 402:884–888.

103. Salomon DS, Brandt R, Ciardiello F, Normanno N. Epidermal growth factor-related peptides and their receptors in human malignancies. Crit Rev Oncol Hematol 1995; 19:183–232.

104. Mendelsohn J. Targeting the epidermal growth factor receptor for cancer therapy. J Clin Oncol 2002; 20:1S–13S.

105. El-Rayes BF, LoRusso PM. Targeting the epidermal growth factor receptor. Br J Cancer 2004; 91:418–424.

106. Hecht JR, Patnaik A, Malik, I. ABX-EGF monotherapy in patients (pts) with metastatic colorectal cancer (mCRC): An updated analysis. Proc Am Soc Clin Oncol 2004. New Orleans, LA.

107. Rowinsky EK, Schwartz GH, Gollob JA, et al. Safety, pharmacokinetics, and activity of ABX-EGF, a fully human anti-epidermal growth factor receptor monoclonal antibody in patients with metastatic renal cell cancer. J Clin Oncol 2004; 22:3003–3015.

108. Vallbohmer D, Lenz HJ. Epidermal growth factor receptor as a target for chemotherapy. Clin Colorectal Cancer 2005; 5 Suppl 1:S19–S27.

109. Cunningham D, Humblet Y, Siena S, et al. Cetuximab monotherapy and cetuximab plus irinotecan in irinotecan-refractory metastatic colorectal cancer. N Engl J Med 2004; 351:337–345.

110. Baselga J, Pfister D, Cooper MR, et al. Phase I studies of anti-epidermal growth factor receptor chimeric antibody C225 alone and in combination with cisplatin. J Clin Oncol 2000; 18:904–914.

111. Fukuoka M, Yano S, Giaccone G, et al. Multi-institutional randomized phase II trial of gefitinib for previously treated patients with advanced non-small-cell lung cancer. J Clin Oncol 2003; 21:2237–2246.

112. Herbst RS, Maddox AM, Rothenberg ML, et al. Selective oral epidermal growth factor receptor tyrosine kinase inhibitor ZD1839 is generally well-tolerated and has activity in non-small-cell lung cancer and other solid tumors: results of a phase I trial. J Clin Oncol 2002; 20:3815–3825.

113. Kris MG, Natale RB, Herbst RS, et al. Efficacy of gefitinib, an inhibitor of the epidermal growth factor receptor tyrosine kinase, in symptomatic patients with non-small cell lung cancer: a randomized trial. JAMA 2003; 290:2149–2158.

114. Nakagawa K, Tamura T, Negoro S, et al. Phase I pharmacokinetic trial of the selective oral epidermal growth factor receptor tyrosine kinase inhibitor gefitinib ('Iressa', ZD1839) in Japanese patients with solid malignant tumors. Ann Oncol 2003; 14:922–930.

115. Ranson M, Hammond LA, Ferry D, et al. ZD1839, a selective oral epidermal growth factor receptor-tyrosine kinase inhibitor, is well tolerated and active in patients with solid, malignant tumors: results of a phase I trial. J Clin Oncol 2002; 20:2240–2250.

116. Tsao MS, Sakurada A, Cutz JC, et al. Erlotinib in lung cancer—molecular and clinical predictors of outcome. N Engl J Med 2005; 353:133–144.

117. Rich JN, Reardon DA, Peery T, et al. Phase II trial of gefitinib in recurrent glioblastoma. J Clin Oncol 2004; 22:133–142.

118. Paez JG, Janne PA, Lee JC, et al. EGFR mutations in lung cancer: correlation with clinical response to gefitinib therapy. Science 2004; 304:1497–1500.

119. Lynch TJ, Bell DW, Sordella R, et al. Activating mutations in the epidermal growth factor receptor underlying responsiveness of non-small-cell lung cancer to gefitinib. N Engl J Med 2004; 350:2129–2139.

120. Frederick L, Wang XY, Eley G, James CD. Diversity and frequency of epidermal growth factor receptor mutations in human glioblastomas. Cancer Res 2000; 60:1383–1387.

121. Hirota S, Isozaki K, Moriyama Y, et al. Gain-of-function mutations of c-kit in human gastrointestinal stromal tumors. Science 1998; 279:577–580.

122. Lux ML, Rubin BP, Biase TL, et al. KIT extracellular and kinase domain mutations in gastrointestinal stromal tumors. Am J Pathol 2000; 156:791–795.

123. Druker BJ, Talpaz M, Resta DJ, et al. Efficacy and safety of a specific inhibitor of the BCR-ABL tyrosine kinase in chronic myeloid leukemia. N Engl J Med 2001; 344:1031–1037.

124. van Oosterom AT, Judson I, Verweij J, et al. Safety and efficacy of imatinib (STI571) in metastatic gastrointestinal stromal tumours: a phase I study. Lancet 2001; 358:1421–1423.

125. Demetri GD, von Mehren M, Blanke CD, et al. Efficacy and safety of imatinib mesylate in advanced gastrointestinal stromal tumors. N Engl J Med 2002; 347:472–480.

126. Chen LL, Trent JC, Wu EF, et al. A missense mutation in KIT kinase domain 1 correlates with imatinib resistance in gastrointestinal stromal tumors. Cancer Res 2004; 64:5913–5919.

127. Gorre ME, Mohammed M, Ellwood K, et al. Clinical resistance to STI–571 cancer therapy caused by BCR-ABL gene mutation or amplification. Science 2001; 293:876–880.

128. Shah NP, Nicoll JM, Nagar B, et al. Multiple BCR-ABL kinase domain mutations confer polyclonal resistance to the tyrosine kinase inhibitor imatinib (STI571) in chronic phase and blast crisis chronic myeloid leukemia. Cancer Cell 2002; 2:117–125.

129. Shah NP, Tran C, Lee FY, Chen P, Norris D, Sawyers CL. Overriding imatinib resistance with a novel ABL kinase inhibitor. Science 2004; 305:399–401.

30 Molecular Profiling in Breast Cancer

Genomic Approaches Toward Tailored Cancer Therapies

Kristin Kee, PhD and Jeffrey E. Green, MD

CONTENTS

SUMMARY

Since the declaration of the "war on cancer" three decades ago, an improved understanding of molecular mechanisms behind malignant disease has led to the discovery of novel targets for cancer therapy. Despite such great efforts, many compounds that have performed well in the preclinical setting have failed in clinical trials. This may be because of the dynamic nature of cancer, where cells continuously acquire a series of genetic alterations that allow them to escape the constraints of normal cell proliferation and to develop resistance to various drug therapies. Therefore, it is crucial to understand how these genetic changes are involved in the etiology of cancer development and progression, and to identify the molecular mechanisms responsible for resistance to chemotherapeutic drugs. In recent years, the emergence of new genomic technologies has allowed us to address these fundamental issues. Because cellular and molecular heterogeneity of breast tumors involve many genes in pathways that control cell growth, death, and differentiation, the utility of microarray technology for genomic profiling of human breast cancer has provided remarkable insights into the multiple genetic alterations that are involved in the disease that may dictate clinical outcome. Examination of gene expression patterns are being correlated with tumor sensitivities or resistance to particular pharmacological agents. Taken together, microarray technology has led to more definitive classification of breast cancer, identification of signature markers for diagnosis and prognosis, and potential predictive response to clinical treatments that should greatly improve and individualize patient therapies.

Key Words: Breast cancer; gene expression profiling; microarray; oligonucleotide array sequence analysis; genomics; therapeutic targets.

From: *Cancer Drug Discovery and Development: Cancer Drug Resistance*
Edited by: B. Teicher © Humana Press Inc., Totowa, NJ

1. INTRODUCTION: BACKGROUND

Despite increased awareness of breast cancer risk factors and advances in therapy over the past decade, breast cancer remains the most frequently diagnosed cancer in women, and ranks second among cancer mortality in the female population of the United States. It was estimated that 215,990 new cases of invasive breast cancer were identified in 2004 and an estimated 40,100 women died of this disease *(1)*. In addition to invasive breast carcinoma, an estimated 59,390 new cases of *in situ* carcinoma were diagnosed during 2004, of which 85% are ductal carcinoma *in situ* (DCIS) *(1)*. Several risk factors are associated with an increased susceptibility of developing breast cancer: specific genetic alterations, familial history, age, duration of menarche, obesity after menopause, hormonal factors (contraceptives and postmenopausal therapy), preexisting benign lesions, and environmental influences *(1–3)*. Whereas genetic factors account for 35% of breast cancer cases, sporadic breast neoplasias are more prevalent as a result of nongenetic factors and/or environmental insults that contribute to the accumulation of mutations in essential genes *(4,5)*. These mutations initiate cancer development that is thought to progress in a multistage process involving genetic alterations that activate proto-oncogenes and inactivate tumor suppressor genes that normally inhibit tumorigenesis *(6)*.

The relatively few known genetic factors identified in sporadic breast cancer suggest an underlying gap in our knowledge of the etiology and genetics of breast cancer. Pathologic evaluation of tumor specimens has long been the standard of diagnosis and treatment of breast cancer. The recent emergence of gene expression microarray and other genomic technologies provides an opportunity to perform more detailed profiling of the disease in order to more accurately classify, predict outcome, and choose appropriate therapy for improved management (Fig. 1). The focus of this chapter is to highlight recent advances in breast cancer research using microarray technology to (1) establish more precise molecular profiles for tumor classification, (2) correlate expression profiles to clinical outcome, (3) identify critical genes and pathways of oncogenesis in order to identify novel biomarkers and candidate targets for intervention, and (4) predict response of breast tumors to therapies. In addition, approaches to using genomic profiling to examine the pharmacogenomic effects of therapeutic agents on particular tumor types are also considered. The overall goal of these approaches is to gain further insight to breast cancer biology, identify potential new therapeutic targets, and uncover mechanisms of drug action and resistance, so that more selective and less toxic personalized treatments of breast cancer can be identified.

2. STANDARD APPROACHES TO CLINICAL DIAGNOSIS

Pathological and clinical classifications of breast cancer have mainly depended on a combination of morphologic and histologic observations of known prognostic and predictive factors including TNM staging, histologic grade and type, mitotic figure counts, and hormone receptor status *(7)*. The TNM system remains the most important predictor of tumor behavior in breast cancer, in that the stage of the disease is determined from the size of the tumor (T), the involvement of regional lymph nodes (N), and the status of distant metastases (M). Whereas tumor staging indicates breast cancer recurrence and overall survival *(8,9)*, histological grading has better prognostic value because there is an assessment of morphologic and cellular features that include tubule formation, nuclear pleomorphism, cytology, and mitotic count *(7,10)*. Mitotic index, for instance, is a particu-

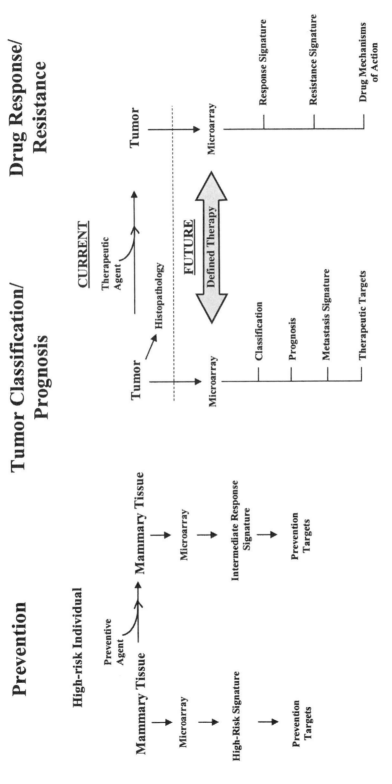

Fig. 1. Utility of microarray technology for chemoprevention studies, tumor classification, prognosis, and drug response and resistance.

larly valuable aspect of the grading classification, because rapidly proliferating cells are readily inhibited by chemotherapeutic agents such as paclitaxel, anthracycline, cyclophosphamide, methotrexate, and fluorouracil. However, because of the morbidity associated with chemotherapy and tumor recurrence following chemotherapy, histological grading alone is an insufficient predictive factor. Clearly, better biological and molecular markers associated with the clinical course of the disease are required to provide a more precise prognosis and predictive response to therapy.

The immunohistological presence or absence of the estrogen receptor (ER)-α, progesterone receptor (PR), and ErbB2 (also known as HER-2/*neu*) proteins has been the foundation of the current molecular classification system of breast cancer *(7)*. ER$^+$ tumors, ErbB2$^+$ tumors, and tumors negative for all the markers have been integrated into the diagnosis and treatment schema and have been used to stratify the risk of recurrence in breast cancer patients. Other biomarkers utilized in breast cancer include the tumor suppressor gene *p53*, cell proliferation markers (*Ki*-67 antigen and proliferating cell nuclear antigen), and angiogenesis factors (vascular endothelial growth factor, CD31, and CD34 antigens, factor VIII-related antigens, and type IV collagen). Whereas these parameters have demonstrated usefulness in diagnosis and perhaps predicting the clinical course of the disease, their utility has been limited in stratifying patients into groups that respond to particular therapeutic regimens.

Unlike standard methodologies in pathology, gene expression profiling collects thousands of data points, and can be used to find clusters of genes whose combined expression behavior corresponds to genotypic and phenotypic differences among large tumor sets *(11)*. Hence, the application of gene expression analysis by microarray to study breast cancer not only will more precisely define tumor classification into improved subcategories, but also has the potential to reveal new prognostic markers, and possibly predict therapeutic outcome.

3. GENE EXPRESSION PROFILING OF BREAST CANCER

It is apparent that molecular alterations in breast cancer are complex and involve interactions between multiple cellular signaling pathways. The completion of the human genome sequence has laid the foundation for the development of genomic technologies to identify tens of thousands of genes in a high-throughput manner. Several platforms for gene expression studies as well as the technical aspects of their approaches have been extensively reviewed in the scientific literature *(12,13)*. On account of the abundance of genes and the intricacies of their interactions, gene expression microarrays have been extensively used to study breast cancer *(14–18)* to delineate the expression patterns of the entire genome and regulatory networks associated with the oncogenic process of multiple clinical samples. There are two frequently used approaches for analyzing gene expression microarray data from tumor samples: *unsupervised analysis* and *supervised analysis*. Typically, *unsupervised analysis* involves clustering of clinical samples that are related statistically and significantly in terms of their gene expression profiles, without knowledge of the biological status of the samples. Analysis of the hierarchal clusters and the distinguishable patterns of gene expression between them can be further used to define their biological differences. Alternatively, *supervised analysis* involves hierarchal clustering of groups of samples with known biological information to guide the clustering algorithm to search for genes that distinguish the groups. The *supervised* analytical method is powerful in that it provides not only lists of relevant genes pertaining

Table 1
Classification of Human Breast Tumor by Gene Expression Signatures

Discriminatory gene signatures (ref.)	*Highlighted features*
Hereditary breast cancer	
176 genes distinguish BRCA1 mutation-positive from BRCA2 mutation-positive tumors *(33)*	Mutations in *BRCA1* or *BRCA2* gene results in gene expression signatures that differ from each other and distinct from sporadic tumors
51 genes distinguish BRCA1 mutation-positive, BRCA2 mutation-positive, and sporadic tumors *(33)*	
60 genes distinguish two classes of non-BRCA1/2 (termed BRCAx) hereditary breast cancer: BRCAx-Group A and BRCAx-Group B *(34)*	BRCA1 mutation leads to gene signature of stress-type state: DNA repair and apoptosis BRCAx-Group A had increased expression of ribosomal genes compared with BRCAx-Group B Observed that Group A had later age of onset and less aggressive tumors
Sporadic breast cancer	
100 genes differentiated ER^+ from ER^- primary tumors *(17)*	Discriminate primary tumors according to ER and LN metastasis status
100 genes predicted ER^+ and ER^- status *(36)*	ER^+ and ER^- tumors display distinct gene expression signatures
476 cDNA intrinsic gene set classified tumors into major groups *(14,15)*: ER^-/basal-like ER^-/ErbB2$^+$ Normal breast-like ER^+/luminal-like: Luminal A Luminal B$^+$C	Identified two novel distinctive types of ER^- tumors: basal-like and ErbB2$^+$ Identified novel subclasses of ER^+/luminal-type tumors: luminal A, luminal B and luminal C TP53 mutations highly expressed in basal-like, ErbB2$^+$ and luminal subtype B$^+$C
606-gene set segregated ER^+ and ER^- breast tumors *(40)*	ER^- cluster had higher percentage of high-grade tumor than ER^+ cluster
137-gene set distinguished high-grade and intermediate-/low-grade breast tumors *(40)*	Further identified subclasses of ER^-
706-gene set classified ER^- subgroups of basal tumors (basal 1 and basal 2) and ErbB2$^+$ overexpression *(40)*	

ER, estrogen receptor; LN, lymph node.

to the group, but also leads to the generation of predictive algorithms by utilizing the expression levels of selected genes to assign new test specimens to the proper group. Both methods are thoroughly reviewed by Quackenbush *(19)* and Simon et al. *(20)*. These methodologies are often implemented to derive specific breast cancer signatures and gene expression patterns (Tables 1 and 2).

3.1. Revised Breast Cancer Classification by Gene Expression Profiling

Genomic classifications based on microarray analyses have been performed on many types of malignancies. Extensive array datasets using breast cancers from different stages and biologic characteristics have been profiled using various microarray platforms (*see* Table 1). Two major types of breast cancer are hereditary and sporadic breast tumors. Familial breast cancers only account for 5–10% of all breast cancers, though it has been

Table 2
Clinical Outcome Gene Expression Signatures for Human Breast Cancer

Discriminatory gene signatures (refs.)	Highlighted features
264-cDNA clone set correlated with survival *(15)*	Luminal A sub-type had a good clinical prognosis whereas, basal-like, ErbB2$^+$, and luminal B$^+$C had a poorer clinical outcome
93-gene set associated with relapse-free survival and predicts clinical outcome *(40)*	Luminal-like subgroup has advantage over basal/ErbB2$^+$ subclasses for overall relapse-free and breast cancer survival
5000 genes that classified tumors into 2 dominant ER$^+$ and ER$^-$ groups *(18)* **231 "classifier" gene set** predict clinical outcome *(18)* **Specific 70 classifier genes** identified as prognostic signature *(16,18)*	Classifier gene sets capable of differentiating between "good" and "poor" prognosis and predict clinical outcome Metastatic capacity may be acquired early during tumorigenesis and intrinsic to the primary tumor
128 genes that distinguished metastatic adenocarcinomas from primary tumors *(45)* **17 unique metastases-associated gene signature** predicted Kaplan-Meier survival analysis *(45)*	Gene expression pattern associated with metastases seem to be present in primary tumors 17-gene signature has predictive ability for metastasis
92-gene set distinguished chemosensitive and chemoresistance patients to neoadjuvant docetaxel treatment *(53)*	Gene signature can predict response to chemotherapeutic treatment

ER, estrogen receptor.

estimated that hereditary factors may play an important role in up to one third of breast cancer cases *(5)*. Thus, a majority of breast cancers are considered sporadic, caused by unknown factors or complex genetic interactions.

3.1.1. HEREDITARY BREAST CANCER GENES 1 AND 2 MUTATION CARRIERS

Common germline mutations of the breast cancer genes 1 and 2 (*BRCA1* and *BRCA2*) are associated with a high penetrance of breast cancer, but they only account for 15–20% of women with a family history of the disease and less than 5% of overall breast cancer cases *(4)*. The lifetime breast cancer risk for females carrying the *BRCA1* and *BRCA2* mutations is estimated to be 60–80% *(21,22)* and 60–85% *(23,24)*, respectively. The *BRCA1* gene, encoding a nuclear protein containing a zinc-finger RING motif at the N-terminal region and an acid-rich C-terminal region, is involved in downstream transcriptional coactivation of p53-responsive genes, such as *p21$^{waf1/cip1}$*, murine double mutant 2, and *bcl-x*. BRCA1 binds to BRCA2, p53, and Rad51 proteins, which are involved in cell cycle regulation and DNA-damage response *(25)*. Although the structural protein motifs and cellular functions of BRCA2 are not fully elucidated *(26)*, BRCA2 has been shown to associate with BRCA1 and Rad51, suggesting its involvement in recombination-mediated repair of double-stranded breaks and the maintenance of chromosome integrity *(27)*. Homozygous BRCA2 knockout mice are small with abnormal tissue differentiation, absence of germ cells, and tendency to develop thymic lymphomas *(28,29)*. Moreover, mouse embryo fibroblasts of BRCA2-null cells display chromosomal segregation abnormalities, suggesting an involvement of BRCA2 in genomic stability *(30,31)*. Tumors with BRCA mutations are generally ER⁻ and PR⁻, have lymphocyte infiltration, and exhibit an aggressive clinical course *(32)*.

Hedenfalk and colleagues *(33)* were the first to report the use of transcriptional profiling to obtain unique molecular signatures of tumors from BRCA1- and BRCA2-mutation-carrying patients. The gene expression profiles were used to determine which genes were differentially expressed by three groups of tumors, with each containing seven specimens: BRCA1-mutation-positive tumors, BRCA2-mutation-positive tumors, and sporadic tumors (BRCA1/2 negative). Using a cDNA microarray containing 5361 genes, the authors identified 176 genes that were differentially expressed in tumors positive for BRCA1 mutations and BRCA2 mutations. Of the genes selected, BRCA1 mutations appear to affect genes in the DNA repair and apoptotic pathways that participate in the activation of cellular response to stress, suggesting that BRCA1 mutations may be involved in cellular pathways distinct from those observed in sporadic tumors. Further analyses (using a modified *F*-test) yielded a subset of 51 genes whose variance among all samples best discriminated between the three types of tumors. Nine genes were differentially expressed between BRCA1-mutation-positive and BRCA1-mutation-negative tumors, whereas 11 genes were differentially expressed between BRCA2-positive and BRCA2-negative tumors. The authors also used a class-prediction method to determine if gene expression profiles can correctly classify BRCA1- and BRCA2-mutation-positive tumors. The test correctly identified all BRCA1-mutation-positive tumors (seven of seven), and 14 of 15 were correctly classified as not having BRCA1 mutations. Only one tumor was misclassified as having a BRCA1 mutation that subsequently was found to have low BRCA1 expression because of hypermethylation of the BRCA1 promoter region, indicative of the posttranscriptional inactivation of BRCA1. In addition, five of eight tumors with BRCA2 mutations and 13 of 14 tumors without BRCA2 mutations were correctly categorized. Even though the accuracy of their classifications was significant, the authors concluded that the analysis of a larger number of samples and larger gene sets would be required to improve the robustness of the class prediction test.

In a subsequent study, Hedenfalk et al. *(34)* identified two novel classes of non-BRCA1/2 breast cancer families (termed BRCAx) that differs from those of breast tumors from the BRCA1 and BRCA2 mutation carriers. Based on cDNA microarray analysis, the authors identified 60 genes that could distinguish two distinct groups subgroups within the 16 tumor specimens from eight BRCAx families, each composed of seven and nine samples, respectively. Interestingly, group A had an increased expression of ribosomal genes compared to group B, possibly indicating their differences in capacity for protein biosynthesis. In a previous study on ovarian cancer, an upregulation of ribosomal genes correlated with the downregulation of a cluster of proliferative genes, which was associated with a less aggressive phenotype *(35)*. Although not statistically significant, the individuals in group A tended to have a later onset of disease with the tumors having a low percentage of cells in S phase, perhaps indicating a less aggressive phenotype. This observation is in agreement with those of Welsh et al. *(35)*. Moreover, groups A and B also showed significant differences in expression of the *CYP1A1* gene, a phase I cytochrome P450 enzyme centrally involved in metabolism of a range of compounds (including steroids), and therefore, suggesting its role in carcinogenesis or in therapeutic response in these tumors. To test further the robustness of their class analysis, they included tumors from known BRCA1 and BRCA2 mutation carriers and found that neither BRCA1 nor BRCA2 tumors clustered with the BRCAx samples using the 60-gene set.

Taken together, the results from these studies demonstrated that gene expression profiles of BRCA1, BRCA2, or BRCAx tumors are generally distinct from each other as well as sporadic tumors, allowing for a better molecular classification of hereditary breast cancer.

3.1.2. Sporadic Breast Cancer

Sporadic breast cancer is dynamic, given that it is thought to arise from an accumulation of multiple genetic mutations or alterations in the expression of important cell regulatory genes, such as *erbB2/her2*, *c-myc*, epidermal growth factor receptor, and *p53*, which affect multiple cellular pathways. Oncogenesis is a process that results not from the dysregulation or mutation of a single gene, but ultimately, from alterations in the regulation of networks of genes. Microarray analysis has become a powerful method to examine the associated expression of thousands of genes, which may lead to more precise tumor classification and predictions of clinical outcome.

3.1.2.1. Estrogen Receptor Classification

Because a major classification of breast cancer is based on ERα status by immunohistochemistry, microarray gene expression profiling has been analyzed to distinguish ER$^+$ from ER$^-$ tumors *(17,18,36)*. Expression data from these studies invariably demonstrated that ER status is associated with distinctive gene expression patterns. West et al. *(17)* used invasive ductal carcinomas with known ER and PR status (13 ER$^+$/lymph node [LN]$^+$, 12 ER$^-$/LN$^+$, 12 ER$^+$/LN$^-$, and 12 ER$^-$/LN$^-$ tumors), and performed a supervised analysis of microarray data to obtain a set of 100 genes that separated ER$^+$ from ER$^-$ tumors. Of the 49 tumors classified by microarray, only five cases had conflicting results based on immunohistochemistry or protein immunoblotting for ERα. The 100-gene set that separated the ER$^+$ and ER$^-$ tumors suggested associations between particular genes and ER status. Importantly, these sets of genes included several that function in the ER pathway, genes that encode proteins that have inverse relationships with ER$^+$ function, such as maspin and glutathione *S*-transferase-π, and genes that are known to function in concert with ER, such as those encoding hepatocyte nuclear factor 3α and androgen receptor. The authors further crossvalidated their prediction model using the 100-gene set with a test set of samples, and found that 34 of 38 unknown samples could be correctly classified regarding their ER statuses. Thus, their study was not only able to identify a set of genes related to ER status, but this set could also be used as a predictor of ER status. In addition, the top 100 genes with the highest correlation to ER status were also used to discriminate LN status according to expression profiles of primary tumors. This classification was closely correlated to ER status, suggesting the use of such a gene-based algorithm might be useful to predict the potential of a primary tumor to metastasize to axillary LNs.

To investigate the gene expression patterns that could stratify tumors into ER$^+$ and ER$^-$ groups, Gruvberger et al. analyzed gene expression profiles of breast cancers from 58 node-negative patients, of which 23 were ER$^+$ and 24 were ER$^-$. Gene expression data from cDNA microarrays containing 6728 genes revealed 3389 genes whose expression was significantly different between the two groups. When these genes were subjected to a training analysis using an artificial neural network algorithm *(37)* and hierarchical clustering techniques, the authors defined a subset of genes whose expression pattern correctly predicted tumor ER status. The *ER* α gene appeared as the top-ranked gene and was closely followed closely by GATA-binding protein 3, a transcription factor often associated with ER$^+$ tumors *(38)*. To test the robustness of the gene signature model for tumor classification, 11 blinded test samples (five ER$^+$ and six ER$^-$) were subjected to the analysis, resulting in the prediction of ER status with 100% accuracy. To examine the relationship between ER function and genes discriminating ER$^+$ and ER$^-$ tumors, the authors compared their results with serial analysis of gene expression data reported for MCF-7 cells treated with estrogen *(39)*. Several genes that belonged to the ER$^+$ set of signature genes in tumors were not directly regulated by estrogen signaling, suggesting that other regulatory pathways may be involved in the expression of those genes *(37)*. Alternatively, estrogen may affect gene expression of stromal cells that could not be demonstrated in an in vitro MCF-7 study *(39)*, or cultured cells may simply respond differently than mammary epithelial cells in vivo.

3.1.2.2. Classification of New Subtypes of Breast Cancer

In addition to classification based on ER hierarchical clustering, a set of approximately 500 genes by Perou et al. *(14)* led to a classification of sporadic breast tumors. This microarray data included 65 surgical specimens taken from 42 individuals with infiltrating ductal carcinomas, lobular tumor, DCIS, fibroadenoma, and normal breast tissues. Twenty of the tumors were matched pairs of breast tumors taken before and after a 16-wk course of doxorubicin chemotherapy, and two tumors were paired with a lymph metastasis from the same patient. The authors consistently found similar gene expression patterns in the two tumor samples from the same individual. They first obtained a data set of 1753 genes (22% of the 8102 genes) with transcripts that varied by at least fourfold in abundance in the sample set. Hierarchical clustering of these genes provided a distinctive molecular profile of each tumor that can be classified into subtypes based solely on differences in expression patterns. Notably, the authors were the first to report two distinctive subtypes of ER$^-$ tumors that are subcategorized into basal-like and ErbB2$^+$, suggesting that these represent two different disease categories. In order to subclassify tumors, another 496 "intrinsic" gene set was selected to show differences between tumors from different patients as opposed to paired tumor samples of pre- and postdoxorubicin therapy from the same patient. The tumors were categorized into four major groups based on their expression pattern of the 496 intrinsic gene set: (1) ER$^-$/basal-like: expressing keratin 5/6 and 17, integrin-β4 and laminin; (2) ER$^-$/ErbB2$^+$ cluster: expressing high levels of ErbB2 and several genes in the ErbB2 amplicon at 17q22.24; (3) normal breast-like: expressing genes characteristic of normal breast tissue such those of adipose tissue and other nonepithelial cell types; and (4) ER$^+$/luminal cell-like: expressing high levels of ER, LIV-1 protein, and various transcription factors, including GATA-binding protein 3, X-box binding protein 1, hepatocyte nuclear factor 3.

In a more extensive study entailing 78 breast tumors, three fibroadenomas, and four normal breast samples, Sorlie et al. *(15)* determined whether a correlation exists between microarray-based tumor classification and clinical outcome. Analysis of the intrinsic subset of 476 genes in these samples revealed a similar pattern of separation of tumors as initially described by Perou et al. *(14)*. However, in the expanded data set that incorporated more tumors, Sorlie et al. reported that the previous ER$^+$/luminal subtype *(14)* was further categorized into two major subgroups with distinctive expression profiles: (1) luminal type A, with high levels of ERα expression along with GATA-binding protein 3, X-box binding protein 1, trefoil factor 3, hepatocyte nuclear factor 3α, and the estrogen-regulated LIV-1; and (2) luminal type B and C, where type B had low to moderate expression of luminal-specific genes included in the ER cluster, and type C had features similar to basal-like and the ErbB2 subtypes but with high expression of a novel set of genes with unknown coordinated function. To test the robustness of classification, the authors incorporated an additional 51 carcinomas from a prospective study on a patient cohort with locally advanced breast cancer who had undergone doxorubicin monotherapy before surgery and received adjuvant tamoxifen based on ER⁺ and/or PR status. The grouping of the five subtypes were robust with >75% accuracy. Because the status of p53 mutation and ErbB2 overexpression in tumors are often associated with poor clinical outcome and poor response to systemic therapy, the authors also evaluated these tumor subtypes for disease-free and overall survival. Using patients from the prospective study, the authors reported that the 71% of basal epithelial-like (five of seven) and 82% ErbB2⁺ subtypes (nine of eleven) that harbored mutations for p53 had shorter survival times and relapse-free survival compared to 13% in the luminal A subtype (four of thirty) with fewer p53 mutations. Interestingly, luminal types B and C had poorer outcome compared to luminal type A, because they have characteristics similar to ER⁻ tumors in the basal-like and ErbB2⁺ subtypes. This suggests that the five expression-based subclasses of breast tumors will have different patient outcomes.

The new classification of basal tumors, i.e., ER⁻ group, by gene expression microarray is an important finding because there are no clinically associated markers to define the group. As indicated, this group of tumors has a poor prognosis like ErbB2⁺ tumors, perhaps because of mutations of p53 *(15)*. However, unlike ErbB2⁺ tumors, basal tumors display a distinct molecular signature of high expression of keratin 5/6, metallothionein 1X, fatty acid binding protein 7, c-Kit, Myc, and secreted frizzled-related protein 1, a modulator of Wnt signaling *(14,15,40)*.

Similar to the findings by Sorlie et al. *(15)*, Sortiriou et al. *(40)* used unsupervised hierarchical clustering analysis to segregate tumors into two main clusters based on basal (ER⁻) and luminal (ER⁺) features. Further subclustering within the basal group established two new classes of basal tumors with distinctive gene signatures—basal 1 subgroup had increased expression of matrix metalloproteinase 7 and cell cycle and growth-related genes, such as topoisomerase IIα, proliferating cell nuclear antigen, BUB1, and CDC2, suggesting a signature for a high rate of proliferation, and the basal 2 subgroup had high expression of transcription factors c-Fos, c-Jun, and Fos B, and overexpression of activating transcription factor 3, transforming growth factor-β receptor II, caveolin 1 and 2, and hepatocyte growth factor. They also defined a new subgroup distinct from the basal-like group in the ER⁻ subset with a high rate of HER-2/*neu* overexpression. The HER-2/*neu* subgroup has a gene profile that includes higher expression of multidrug resistance 1, S100 calcium-binding protein P, fatty acid synthase, and syndecan 1, and lower expression of c-Kit and c-Myc. Taken together, the gene expression signatures obtained from these studies *(14,15,40)* revealed a new classification system for breast tumors that may have important clinical implications.

3.2. Prediction of Outcome by Gene Expression Profiling

One of the greatest challenges in evaluation and clinical management of cancer patients is the ability to predict the clinical behavior of their disease. Because gene expression profiling can survey thousands of genes simultaneously, it will likely be superior to currently used parameters in predicting disease outcome. A pioneering study that made use of gene expression signatures to predict good versus poor prognosis was reported by van't Veer and colleagues *(18)*. The cohort studied were patients under 55 yr of age, without LN involvement, received only radical mastectomy or lumpectomy plus radiation therapy, and had a follow-up of at least 5 yr. Of the 98 primary breast tumors, 34 developed distant metastasis within 5 yr, 44 remained disease-free after a period of at least 5 yr, 18 had BRCA1 germline mutations, and two were BRCA2 carriers. Using oligonucleotide microarrays consisting of 25,000 genes, approximately 5000 genes were regulated in a manner that led to the classification of the tumors into two distinct groups, each containing 62 and 36 tumors, respectively. Most of the tumors in the first group retained ER expression and had a "good" prognosis, with only 34% of the tumors displaying distant metastasis within 5 yr. In contrast, the second group that contained ER-negative tumors had a "poor" prognosis with lymphocytic infiltration. Seventy percent of the patients with sporadic tumors in the second group had progressive disease. Additionally, 16 of the 18 BRCA1 carriers grouped with the sporadic tumor cluster, were ER⁻, and had higher lymphocytic infiltration. The two BRCA2 samples clustered with ER⁺ sporadic tumors and did not display similarities with BRCA1 tumors. Of the 5000 significantly regulated genes, a subset of 231 genes appeared to be associated with disease outcome and was used to further define an optimal "classifier" gene set capable of correctly differentiating between "good" and "poor" prognosis. A poor prognosis signature includes increased expression of genes regulating cell cycle, invasion and metastasis, angiogenesis, and signal transduction. A defined prognostic signature of 70 classifier genes was implemented to predict outcome of 78 sporadic LN-negative patients. Although the 70-gene optimum set managed to predict correctly the actual outcome of disease for 83% of the patients (65 out of 78), it misclassified three tumors with poor prognosis as having good prognosis and 12 tumors from disease-free patients into the poor prognosis group (18). This observation suggests that small primary tumors negative for node metastases can display a poor prognosis signature and may already be programmed for metastasis.

van't Veer and colleagues have demonstrated the predictive power and robustness of a breast cancer prognosis classification using the 70 optimal marker genes. In a follow-up study, van de Vijver et al. further validated the 70-gene set on 295 patients, and found that the patients were stratified into groups where 180 had a poor prognosis signature, and 115 had a good prognosis signature, with an overall 10-yr survival rate of approximately 54 and 95%, respectively (16). In addition, the authors concluded that individuals with a poor-prognostic signature had approximately a 50% chance of remaining disease-free of distant metastasis at 10 yr, whereas those with good prognostic signature had a 85% chance of remaining free of disease (16).

Based on overlapping genes with the van't Veer study (18), Sotiriou and colleagues identified 93 gene elements that were significantly associated with relapse-free survival and demonstrated the array-derived tumor signature has the ability to predict clinical outcome (40). When basal/ErbB2-like (predominantly ER⁻) and the luminal-like (predominantly ER⁺) clusters were compared for outcome of disease, the luminal-like subgroup had a significant advantage over the basal/ErbB2-like subclass for overall relapse-free survival and breast cancer survival (40). These findings in human breast cancer strongly suggest that expression profiling of the primary tumor can predict the clinical course of disease in breast cancer patients (15,16,18,40,41).

3.3. Prediction of Metastasis by Gene Expression Profiling

Because metastasis is a poor prognostic indicator for survival, the question as to how primary tumors gain the ability to metastasize to distant sites remains a critical, but elusive process. The prevailing model for cancer metastasis suggests that acquisition of the metastatic potential by primary tumor cells is a late tumorigenic event that requires important changes in the tumor milieu to enable them to metastasize and seed to distant sites *(42,43)*. Recently, it has been hypothesized by van't Veer and others that the metastatic capacity may be acquired early during tumorigenesis and is intrinsic to the primary tumor, i.e., metastasis is predetermined *(18,43,44)*. Given that metastasis to distant organs is a major cause of death in cancer patients, the ability to predict the event before its occurrence would have great clinical importance. As will be discussed, the use of molecular profiling of primary breast tumors may have predictive power for the future development of metastases *(18,45)*. One may then anticipate that the different tumorigenic stages of breast cancer may share similar features. In support of this notion, Perou et al. reported earlier that primary tumors and metastases share similar patterns of gene expression, suggesting that the molecular program of a primary tumor may generally be maintained in its metastasis *(14)*. Microarray analysis of microdissected epithelium of breast cancers by Ma et al. *(46)* also reveal extensive similarities at the transcriptome level among the premalignant (atypical ductal hyperplasia), preinvasive (DCIS), and invasive (invasive ductal carcinoma) clinical stages of breast cancer. Similarly, chromosomal analysis of DCIS, invasive ductal carcinoma, and LN metastasis by array comparative genomic hybridization and fluorescent *in situ* hybridization revealed consistent chromosomal aberrations shared between the three tumorigenic stages *(47)*. These observations suggest that the potential for invasive and metatastic growth exists in the preinvasive stages of tumor progression.

To further explore the molecular differences between primary solid tumors and metastases, Ramaswamy and colleagues compared gene expression profiles of adenocarcinoma metastases of multiple tumor types (lung, breast, prostate, colorectal, uterus, and ovary) to unmatched primary adenocarcinomas *(45)*. The comparison identified 128 genes that distinguish metastatic adenocarcinomas from the primary tumors. More compelling was that the same gene expression pattern associated with metastasis was present in some primary tumors, thus, suggesting that the gene expression program of metastasis may already exist in primary tumors *(45)*. When lung cancer patients whose primary solid tumors express the metastases-associated gene signature at the time of diagnosis had a significantly poorer clinical outcome, i.e., metastases and shorter survival times, compared to those whose tumor lacked the expression signature. The authors further refined the 128-gene set to a unique 17-gene signature and found that the reduced gene set also recapitulated the observed Kaplan-Meier survival pattern in lung adencarcinoma *(45)*. To investigate whether the refined 17-gene signature could be associated with metastasis of other tumor types, the authors tested 78 small stage I primary breast adenocarcinomas from the van't Veer study *(18)*. The unique metastases-associated signature successful predicted the Kaplan-Meier survival analysis of cluster defined primary tumor subsets for breast cancer *(45)*, suggesting that primary breast tumors bearing the gene expression signature at diagnosis were more likely to develop distant metastases than those lacking this signature.

The refined 17-gene signature, consisting of eight upregulated genes and nine downregulated genes, did not represent any individual metastatic markers *per se*, but taken as a whole, contains predictive information. The genes were predominantly involved in the protein translation apparatus for tumor growth and invasion, chromatid separation during cell division, and angiogenesis and local invasion. More interestingly, the refined metastases-associated gene expression signature also contained genes that were from the nonepithelial component of the tumor, such as genes encoding type I collagens (whose expression is mainly restricted to fibroblasts), actin, myosin heavy chain, myosin light chain kinase, and calponin (markers of smooth muscle), major histocompatibility complex class II DP-β1, and the transcription factor RUNX1 (unique to hematopoietic cells), implicating that the process of metastasis may arise from both malignant and stromal compartments of the primary tumor *(45)*. Based on this study, one can speculate that laser capture microdissection of malignant epithelial cells alone may not provide a complete expression profile of the entire malignant phenotype *(46)*, and that stroma needs to be included in such analysis. Again, these findings not only support the idea that clinical outcome of cancer patients can be predicted using gene expression profiles of primary tumors *(18)*, but also that some primary tumors may already possess a predetermined metastatic program at diagnosis.

To corroborate the notion of a metastatic program mediating breast cancer metastasis, Kang and colleagues elegantly examined the expression profiles of osteolytic bone metastatic lesions that developed in immunodeficient mice following cardiac injection of a human breast cancer cell line, MDA-MB-231 *(48)*. Compared to the parental MDA-MB-231 cell lines, metastatic clones, derived from bone or adrenal medulla lesions, conferred either a high or a weak metastatic potential, respectively. The transcriptome profile from the isolates identified a specific gene expression pattern consisting of 102 genes associated with the formation of metastasis to bone but not to the adrenal medulla. When superimposed with the 70-gene expression signature with predictive capability of metastasis and poor survival in breast cancer patients *(18)*, parental MDA-MB-231 cells and derived metastatic subpopulations both displayed the "poor-prognosis" signature. More importantly, the authors identified a tissue-specific expression profile consisting of genes that encode secretory or cell surface proteins implicated in cellular homing to bone (chemokine C-X-C motif receptor 4), angiogenesis (connective tissue growth factor, fibroblast growth factor-5), invasion (matrix metalloproteinase-1), and osteoclast recruitment (interleukin-11, osteopontin), thereby cooperatively altering the tumor microenvironment to favor bone metastasis *(48)*. Taken together, the studies presented here *(18,45,48)* support the idea that a primary tumor with a poor prognosis profile, as identified by gene expression signatures, has an intrinsic capacity to not only metastasize, but also follow a programmed path of "seed and soil" as hypothesized by Paget *(49)* at distant sites *(44)*.

3.4. Predicting Chemotherapy Response by Gene Expression Profiling

The etiology of breast cancer is complex and involves a wide variety of genomic alterations. Because the disease is further complicated by substantial heterogeneity and the development of drug resistance, therapeutic targeting of the tumor has been a constant challenge. Whereas the ultimate goal behind understanding molecular mechanisms of malignant disease is to discover and implement novel, effective chemotherapeutics with minimum toxicity to the patients, an important objective behind gene expression profiling of tumor specimens is to better predict patients' responsiveness to standard and novel chemotherapeutic agents, as well as ultimately define tailored care for each individual. For example, the status of ERα expression has been an important characteristic in breast cancer and is often a prognostic factor in identifying patients that can benefit from endocrine therapy. Similarly, breast cancer patients who have elevated levels of the HER-2/*neu* proto-oncogene *(50)* may benefit from trastuzumab (Herceptin®) *(51)*.

Whereas a great deal of information has been obtained through gene expression profiling for classification and clinical outcome for breast cancer, its application in predicting sensitivity to chemotherapeutic agents and response to therapy has only begun to be explored. A major limitation, thus far, has been acquiring a large microarray database from enough patients to adequately compare expression profiles of responders with those of nonresponders. Second, many patients have undergone numerous courses of therapy, so their tumor specimens may no longer contain significant predictive value. Nonetheless, molecular profiling is beginning to provide insights into the mechanisms of drug sensitivity and resistance by defining a signature of clinically useful discriminatory genes from responsive and nonresponsive tumors.

Initially, Perou et al. *(14)* demonstrated that gene expression profiles of 15 of the 20 tumors before and after doxorubicin therapy were similar to each other. Interestingly, of the remaining five pairs, three pairs of tumor samples that clinically responded to doxorubicin therapy displayed "normal-like" gene expression profiles, suggesting that a normal breast-like gene expression is a prognostic indicator of a good chemotherapeutic response *(14)*. Although limited by small sample size, Buchholz and colleagues were the first to report global gene expression changes after chemotherapy for breast tumors where good response to treatment, as assessed by histopathology, exhibited gene patterns that clustered distinctly from those of poor responders *(52)*. Recently, Chang et al. defined a set of 92 genes from 24 patients who were either chemosensitive or chemoresistant to neoadjuvant docetaxel therapy *(53)*. Sensitive tumors had higher expression of genes involved in stress response or apoptosis, cell cycle, protein transport and modification, cytoskeletal support, adhesion, and transcription. Resistant tumors, however, had increased expression of some transcriptional and signal transduction genes. Although validation of these findings is required using a larger patient cohort, the discriminatory 92-gene set correctly predicted six out of six independent samples as responders. Such studies have significant clinical implications in that (1) gene signatures can distinguish tumors that are responsive or resistant to any chemotherapeutic treatment, and (2) mechanisms of resistance can be identified for each chemotherapeutic agent.

Whereas additional prospective studies are performed to predict clinical response, the use of in vitro tumor cell culture systems is an alternative approach to approximate pharmacogenomic events in vivo. Although cell lines are not truly representative of cancer cells in vivo, prediction of response based on in vitro studies may be translated and validated based on clinical response *(54,55)*. Hayashi and colleagues analyzed gene expression profiles of estrogen-responsive genes in several ER$^+$ cancer cell lines and derived a 138-gene signature that distinguished responsiveness and nonresponsiveness to estrogen stimulation *(54)*. In another study, gene expression profiles were obtained from immortalized mammary basal epithelial cell lines (ME16C and HME-CC) and luminal epithelial cell lines (MCF-7 and ZR-75-1) treated with doxorubicin and 5-fluorouracil *(55)* to recapitulate events of basal-like and luminal-like breast carcinoma previously described *(14,15)*. Both cell types induced DNA damage-response genes such as *p21^{waf1}*, but displayed distinct responses to the two chemotherapeutic agents. Luminal cell lines had a profound response through alterations in p53-regulated genes, as well as repression of cell cycle-regulated genes, whereas basal cell lines responded by repressing genes involved in cellular differentiation. Notably, the changes in basal cell lines were subtle and did not cluster distinctly like the luminal cell lines, suggesting that basal cells may already have a complex genetic makeup that makes treatment with chemotherapeutic agents more variable. When the in vitro responses were compared with expression responses in breast tumors sampled before and after treatment with doxorubicin or 5-fluorouracil/ mitomycin C *(56,57)*, the in vivo data strongly correlated with the cell-type-specific in vitro responses to chemotherapeutic agents, such as genes encoding p21^{waf1}, activating protein 1 coactivators Fos and Jun, and other genes involved in wound healing, including connective tissue growth factor and matrix metalloproteinase 9. Other groups are also predicting drug sensitivity and resistance by profiling ATP-binding cassette transporter genes in cancer cells in response to various chemotherapeutic agents so that expression signatures can be identified and drug resistance mechanisms related to other pathways could be established *(58)*.

Because most drug agents interact with either specific target proteins or various pathway targets that differ between cell and tissue type, it seems more feasible to examine first drug response and mechanistic effects in vitro. Albeit, cell culture studies are quite limited in providing reliable drug response information for many reasons, they may help identify important response mechanisms to chemotherapeutic agents that can be further validated in cancer patients.

4. CONCLUSION AND FUTURE CHALLENGES

Although the routine implementation of DNA microarray for diagnosis of breast cancer and prediction of therapeutic outcome may be years away, this technology holds great promise and potential clinical value. Currently, women with breast cancer undergo chemotherapy in hopes of achieving a therapeutic response and cure. The clinical reality, however, is often associated with significant toxicity and no survival benefit in a large proportion of treated patients. More accurate classification and prediction of prognosis could identify appropriate treatments and reduce morbidity.

Molecular profiling may be useful in improving targeted treatments for breast cancer by defining subtypes of cancers that may benefit from particular therapies (*see* Fig. 1). As discussed, microarray technology may define markers or key prognostic genes to predict disease outcome. It may also give insights as to whether the primary tumor has already a predetermined program for metastasis so that appropriate treatment could be initiated. Additionally, if the primary tumor or treated tumor bears a molecular profile that suggests drug resistance for a certain chemotherapeutic target, then an alternative treatment could be started.

The ultimate goal of oncology is to prevent cancer altogether. One can envisage the use of microarray technology on normal tissue to identify an expression signature associated with increased breast cancer risk (*see* Fig. 1). Such individuals could then be followed closely or offered on preventive regimes. Because prevention trials generally require many years to determine efficacy of a compound, analysis of tissue at intermediate time points by microarray might help identify individuals responding to the preventive compound. Thus, array technology may be applied to early stages of cancer prevention.

Microarray analysis in the postgenomic era has resulted in an extraordinary amount of information that can give better insights into disease *(59)*. Refined sampling by laser capture microdissection of normal epithelium and tumor-specific stromal cells, vascular endothelial cells, adipose, and connective tissues may allow us to better understand the molecular mechanisms behind breast cancer progression and further identify more specific therapeutic targets *(60–62)*. Sophisticated statistical methods for comparative metaprofiling are being developed to identify and assess the multiple gene expression signatures derived from a diverse collection of microarray data sets for breast cancer *(63)*.

Thus far, gene expression profiling of breast cancer has provided valuable information for molecular classification of tumors and predicting clinical outcome and response to therapies. However, identification of novel targets for therapy by microarray remains more daunting because of the unknown functional significance of many of the signature genes that have been identified. Although microarray technology has been powerful in determining changes at the level of the transcriptome, it is ultimately protein that dictates the cellular function of a gene. Thus, implementing proteomic analyses of tumors will further define mechanisms of tumor development that may be specifically targeted for therapy or prevention.

REFERENCES

1. Jemal A, Tiwari RC, Murray T, et al. Cancer statistics, 2004. CA Cancer J Clin 2004; 54:8–29.
2. Ketcham AS, Sindelar WF. Risk factors in breast cancer. Prog Clin Cancer 1975; 6:99–114.
3. Russo J, Russo IH. Cellular basis of breast cancer susceptibility. Oncol Res 1999; 11:169–178.
4. Nathanson KL, Wooster R, Weber BL, Nathanson KN. Breast cancer genetics: what we know and what we need. Nat Med 2001; 7:552–556.
5. Lichtenstein P, Holm NV, Verkasalo PK, et al. Environmental and heritable factors in the causation of cancer—analyses of cohorts of twins from Sweden, Denmark, and Finland. N Engl J Med 2000; 343:78–85.
6. Vogelstein B, Fearon ER, Hamilton SR, et al. Genetic alterations during colorectal-tumor development. N Engl J Med 1988; 319:525–532.
7. Fitzgibbons PL, Page DL, Weaver D, et al. Prognostic factors in breast cancer. College of American Pathologists Consensus Statement 1999. Arch Pathol Lab Med 2000; 124:966–978.
8. Rosen PP, Groshen S, Saigo PE, Kinne DW, Hellman S. Pathological prognostic factors in stage I (T1N0M0) and stage II (T1N1M0) breast carcinoma: a study of 644 patients with median follow-up of 18 years. J Clin Oncol 1989; 7:1239–1251.
9. Smart CR, Byrne C, Smith RA, et al. Twenty-year follow-up of the breast cancers diagnosed during the Breast Cancer Detection Demonstration Project. CA Cancer J Clin 1997; 47:134–149.
10. Elston CW, Ellis IO. Pathological prognostic factors in breast cancer. I. The value of histological grade in breast cancer: experience from a large study with long-term follow-up. Histopathology 1991; 19:403–410.
11. DeRisi J, Penland L, Brown PO, et al. Use of a cDNA microarray to analyse gene expression patterns in human cancer. Nat Genet 1996; 14:457–460.
12. Schulze A, Downward J. Navigating gene expression using microarrays—a technology review. Nat Cell Biol 2001; 3:E190–E195.
13. Desai KV, Kavanaugh CJ, Calvo A, Green JE. Chipping away at breast cancer: insights from microarray studies of human and mouse mammary cancer. Endocr Relat Cancer 2002; 9:207–220.
14. Perou CM, Sorlie T, Eisen MB, et al. Molecular portraits of human breast tumours. Nature 2000; 406:747–752.
15. Sorlie T, Perou CM, Tibshirani R, et al. Gene expression patterns of breast carcinomas distinguish tumor subclasses with clinical implications. Proc Natl Acad Sci U S A 2001; 98:10,869–10,874.
16. van de Vijver MJ, He YD, van't Veer LJ, et al. A gene-expression signature as a predictor of survival in breast cancer. N Engl J Med 2002; 347:1999–2009.
17. West M, Blanchette C, Dressman H, et al. Predicting the clinical status of human breast cancer by using gene expression profiles. Proc Natl Acad Sci U S A 2001; 98:11,462–11,467.
18. van't Veer LJ, Dai H, van de Vijver MJ, et al. Gene expression profiling predicts clinical outcome of breast cancer. Nature 2002; 415:530–536.
19. Quackenbush J. Computational analysis of microarray data. Nat Rev Genet 2001; 2:418–427.
20. Simon RM, McShane LM, Wright GW, Korn EL, Radmacher MD, Zhao Y. Design and analysis of DNA microarray investigations. New York: Springer, 2003.
21. Easton DF, Bishop DT, Ford D, Crockford GP. Genetic linkage analysis in familial breast and ovarian cancer: results from 214 families. The Breast Cancer Linkage Consortium. Am J Hum Genet 1993; 52:678–701.
22. Struewing JP, Tarone RE, Brody LC, Li FP, Boice JD Jr. BRCA1 mutations in young women with breast cancer. Lancet 1996; 347:1493.
23. Easton DF, Steele L, Fields P, et al. Cancer risks in two large breast cancer families linked to BRCA2 on chromosome 13q12-13. Am J Hum Genet 1997; 61:120–118.
24. Struewing JP, Hartge P, Wacholder S, et al. The risk of cancer associated with specific mutations of BRCA1 and BRCA2 among Ashkenazi Jews. N Engl J Med 1997; 336:1401–1408.

25. Scully R, Livingston DM. In search of the tumour-suppressor functions of BRCA1 and BRCA2. Nature 2000; 408:429–432.

26. Wooster R, Bignell G, Lancaster J, et al. Identification of the breast cancer susceptibility gene BRCA2. Nature 1995; 378:789–792.

27. Chen JJ, Silver D, Cantor S, Livingston DM, Scully R. BRCA1, BRCA2, and Rad51 operate in a common DNA damage response pathway. Cancer Res 1999; 59 (7 Suppl):1752s–1756s.

28. Connor F, Bertwistle D, Mee PJ, et al. Tumorigenesis and a DNA repair defect in mice with a truncating Brca2 mutation. Nat Genet 1997; 17:423–430.

29. Friedman LS, Thistlethwaite FC, Patel KJ, et al. Thymic lymphomas in mice with a truncating mutation in Brca2. Cancer Res 1998; 58:1338–1343.

30. Patel KJ, Yu VP, Lee H, et al. Involvement of Brca2 in DNA repair. Mol Cell 1998; 1:347–357.

31. Sharan SK, Morimatsu M, Albrecht U, et al. Embryonic lethality and radiation hypersensitivity mediated by Rad51 in mice lacking Brca2. Nature 1997; 386:804–810.

32. Loman N, Johannsson O, Bendahl PO, Borg A, Ferno M, Olsson H. Steroid receptors in hereditary breast carcinomas associated with BRCA1 or BRCA2 mutations or unknown susceptibility genes. Cancer 1998; 83:310–319.

33. Hedenfalk I, Duggan D, Chen Y, et al. Gene-expression profiles in hereditary breast cancer. N Engl J Med 2001; 344:539–548.

34. Hedenfalk I, Ringner M, Ben-Dor A, et al. Molecular classification of familial non-BRCA1/BRCA2 breast cancer. Proc Natl Acad Sci U S A 2003; 100:2532–2537.

35. Welsh JB, Zarrinkar PP, Sapinoso LM, et al. Analysis of gene expression profiles in normal and neoplastic ovarian tissue samples identifies candidate molecular markers of epithelial ovarian cancer. Proc Natl Acad Sci U S A 2001; 98:1176–1781.

36. Gruvberger S, Ringner M, Chen Y, et al. Estrogen receptor status in breast cancer is associated with remarkably distinct gene expression patterns. Cancer Res 2001; 61:5979–5984.

37. Khan J, Wei JS, Ringner M, et al. Classification and diagnostic prediction of cancers using gene expression profiling and artificial neural networks. Nat Med 2001; 7:673–679.

38. Yang GP, Ross DT, Kuang WW, Brown PO, Weigel RJ. Combining SSH and cDNA microarrays for rapid identification of differentially expressed genes. Nucleic Acids Res 1999;2 7:1517–1523.

39. Charpentier AH, Bednarek AK, Daniel RL, et al. Effects of estrogen on global gene expression: identification of novel targets of estrogen action. Cancer Res 2000; 60:5977–5983.

40. Sotiriou C, Neo SY, McShane LM, et al. Breast cancer classification and prognosis based on gene expression profiles from a population-based study. Proc Natl Acad Sci U S A 2003; 100:10,393–10,398.

41. Sorlie T, Tibshirani R, Parker J, et al. Repeated observation of breast tumor subtypes in independent gene expression data sets. Proc Natl Acad Sci U S A 2003; 100:8418–8423.

42. Fidler IJ, Kripke ML. Metastasis results from preexisting variant cells within a malignant tumor. Science 1977; 197:893–895.

43. Bernards R, Weinberg RA. A progression puzzle. Nature 2002; 418:823.

44. Van't Veer LJ, Weigelt B. Road map to metastasis. Nat Med 2003; 9:999–1000.

45. Ramaswamy S, Ross KN, Lander ES, Golub TR. A molecular signature of metastasis in primary solid tumors. Nat Genet 2003; 33:49–54.

46. Ma XJ, Salunga R, Tuggle JT, et al. Gene expression profiles of human breast cancer progression. Proc Natl Acad Sci U S A 2003; 100:5974–5979.

47. Aubele M, Mattis A, Zitzelsberger H, et al. Extensive ductal carcinoma In situ with small foci of invasive ductal carcinoma: evidence of genetic resemblance by CGH. Int J Cancer 2000; 85:82–86.

48. Kang Y, Siegel PM, Shu W, et al. A multigenic program mediating breast cancer metastasis to bone. Cancer Cell 2003; 3:537–549.

49. Paget S. The distribution of secondary growths in cancer of the breast. Lancet 1889; 1:99–101.

50. Slamon DJ, Godolphin W, Jones LA, et al. Studies of the HER-2/neu proto-oncogene in human breast and ovarian cancer. Science 1989; 244:707–712.

51. Carter P, Presta L, Gorman CM, et al. Humanization of an anti-p185/HER2 antibody for human cancer therapy. Proc Natl Acad Sci U S A 1992; 89:4285–4289.

52. Buchholz TA, Stivers DN, Stec J, et al. Global gene expression changes during neoadjuvant chemotherapy for human breast cancer. Cancer J 2002; 8:461–468.

53. Chang JC, Wooten EC, Tsimelzon A, et al. Gene expression profiling for the prediction of therapeutic response to docetaxel in patients with breast cancer. Lancet 2003; 362:362–369.

54. Hayashi S. Prediction of hormone sensitivity by DNA microarray. Biomed Pharmacother 2004; 58:1–9.

55. Troester MA, Hoadley KA, Sorlie T, et al. Cell-type-specific responses to chemotherapeutics in breast cancer. Cancer Res 2004; 64:4218–4226.

56. Geisler S, Lonning PE, Aas T, et al. Influence of TP53 gene alterations and c-erbB-2 expression on the response to treatment with doxorubicin in locally advanced breast cancer. Cancer Res 2001; 61:2505–2512.

57. Geisler S, Borresen-Dale AL, Johnsen H, et al. TP53 gene mutations predict the response to neoadjuvant treatment with 5-fluorouracil and mitomycin in locally advanced breast cancer. Clin Cancer Res 2003; 9:5582–5588.

58. Szakacs G, Annereau JP, Lababidi S, et al. Predicting drug sensitivity and resistance: profiling ABC transporter genes in cancer cells. Cancer Cell 2004; 6:129–137.

59. Simon R, Radmacher MD, Dobbin K. Design of studies using DNA microarrays. Genet Epidemiol 2002; 23:21–36.

60. Emmert-Buck MR, Bonner RF, Smith PD, et al. Laser capture microdissection. Science 1996; 274:998–1001.

61. Bonner RF, Emmert-Buck M, Cole K, et al. Laser capture microdissection: molecular analysis of tissue. Science 1997; 278:1481–1483.

62. Simone NL, Bonner RF, Gillespie JW, Emmert-Buck MR, Liotta LA. Laser-capture microdissection: opening the microscopic frontier to molecular analysis. Trends Genet 1998; 14:272–276.

63. Rhodes DR, Yu J, Shanker K, et al. Large-scale meta-analysis of cancer microarray data identifies common transcriptional profiles of neoplastic transformation and progression. Proc Natl Acad Sci U S A 2004; 101:9309–9314.

31 Tumor Immune Escape Mechanisms

Yi Ting Koh, BSc,
M. Luz García-Hernández, PhD,
and W. Martin Kast, PhD

CONTENTS

SUMMARY

The immunosurveillance theory postulates that the immune system is able to identify transformed cells and eliminate them. The theory predicts that the incidence of cancer would increase, or the latency period of cancer would decrease, in the absence of a functional immune system. However, the fact that the incidence of only some cancers increases in immunosuppressed patients shows that not all cancers abide by this theory. Most cancers escape immunosurveillance because they are fundamentally "self," and autoreactive immune cells are usually deleted or anergized so that they do not attack self. The tumors that do face immune pressure are virus-associated cancers and cancers expressing immunogenic tumor antigens. These tumors have, however, evolved mechanisms to escape immune eradication. An effective way of escaping immune eradication is to prevent detection. The expression of tumor-associated antigens enhances the immunogenicity of a tumor, and if it is able to reduce the presentation of such markers, then the tumor remains relatively invisible to the immune system and escapes detection. If the tumor does not manage to escape detection, then it can evolve to prevent the activation of the immune response. The immunosuppressive effects of cancer cells are mediated by the secretion of soluble factors, by the expression of inhibitory molecules,

From: *Cancer Drug Discovery and Development: Cancer Drug Resistance*
Edited by: B. Teicher © Humana Press Inc., Totowa, NJ

and by turning the cellular infiltrates into tolerizing cells that can in turn suppress other potentially tumor-specific immune cells. Some tumor cells have evolved to become resistant to the death effector mechanisms of the immune system. Finally, some tumors have evolved to turn the immune system against itself by causing the death of the immune cells through an activation-induced cell death mechanism that normally functions to limit the immune response under physiological conditions. These immune escape mechanisms in combination make the tumor a formidable foe for the immune system. Therefore, a well thought out immunotherapy strategy would keep in mind the escape mechanisms the tumor could adopt under immune pressure to direct the most propitious strike.

Key Words: Immunosurveillance; immunogenicity; escape mechanisms; tumor antigens; immunodetection; tumor microenvironment.

1. INTRODUCTION: IMMUNOSURVEILLANCE OF CANCER

The immunosurveillance hypothesis states that a physiologic function of the immune cells is to recognize and destroy transformed cells. The concept of immunosurveillance was first introduced in 1909, when Paul Ehrlich proposed that immunity against cancer was mediated by "cellular forces" that kept tumors in check (1). The theory was later appended by Thomas Lewis and Sir MacFarlane Burnet, who proposed that immunological recognition of transformed cells was a form of homeostatic surveillance that could allow the body to guard against malignancies (2,3). Implicitly, the hypothesis predicts that the incidence of cancer would increase or tumor latency periods would be reduced in the absence of immunosurveillance. Epstein-Barr virus (EBV)-related neoplasms are examples of cancers usually controlled by immunosurveillance that increase in incidence in immunosuppressed individuals. EBV is a lymphotropic herpes virus that affects the majority of individuals (4), and causes little significant disease in a healthy immunocompetent person. It establishes itself within the nucleus of B-lymphocytes expressing the CD21 molecule during the initial infection, and remains in the body in a state of latency for that individual's lifetime. This latent state is associated with the production of viral proteins like Epstein-Barr nuclear antigen and latent membrane proteins that protect the B-cell from apoptosis and allow intermittent low-grade viral replication (5). The viral replication is usually held in check by cytotoxic T-cells (CTLs) driven EBV-specific immunosurveillance in healthy individuals. However, in the immunosuppressed transplant recipient, the impaired EBV-specific CTL response leads to an increase in viral replication and ultimately, to B-cell transformation. EBV-induced posttransplant lymphoproliferative disorder (PTLD) is the most common neoplasm found in pediatric renal transplant recipients (6). The incidence of PTLD is four times higher amongst pediatric than adult transplant recipients (7), possibly because of the fact that a larger proportion of the children are EBV naive pretransplant and therefore have little immunity towards the virus. The significant increase in virus-associated cancers in immunocompromised patients, and the finding that preemptive antiviral therapy in hematopoietic stem cell transplantation prevented EBV-associated PTLD (8) supports that immunosurveillance reduces the incidence of virus-induced tumors in an immunocompetent host.

Additional evidence supporting the role of immunosurveillance comes from studies on the incidence of neoplasms amongst transplant patients under long-term immunosuppression and immunocompromised human immunodeficiency virus (HIV)-infected patients. Skin cancer was noted to be increased in patients receiving long-term immunosuppression because of a solid-organ transplant (9); also, the risk of malignancy in renal transplant patients receiving long-term immunosuppression was considerably higher (10). HIV-associated immunosuppression has been linked to a greater increase in cases of Kaposi sarcoma, non-Hodgkin's lymphoma, and invasive cervical cancer (11,12). Most of the malignancies observed in the immunosuppressed and immunocompromised patients were noted to be associated with viral-infections, such as B-cell lymphomas (EBV), Kaposi sarcoma (human herpes simplex virus 8) and cervical cancers (human papilloma virus). This makes the virus-associated cancers excellent targets for immunotherapy.

1.1. Most Cancers Slip Through the Immunosurveillance Net

It is important to note that the cancers that immunosuppressed patients are at an increased risk of developing are not the same as those that are most commonly found in the general populace. This implies that most cancers are not covered under the immunosurveillance theory, and many cancers develop simply because the immune system does not recognize them as foreign in the first place. Cancer cells are basically "altered self-cells" and may not be very immunologically different from normal cells. In fact, most cancer cells escape immunosurveillance, because they simply do not satisfy the primary condition of the immunosurveillance theory, which requires the distinction of transformed cells from normal cells. Central and peripheral tolerance mechanisms such as the clonal deletion by ubiquitous self-antigens and clonal inactivation by tissue-specific antigens presented in the absence of costimulatory signals ensure that the immune system does not attack self. Apart from the virus-associated cancers, most cancers are not immunogenic, because the antigens that they express are self-antigens against which the immune system has been tolerized. However, this does not mean that immunotherapy cannot work on these cancers; it just has to be achieved by breaking immunological tolerance to self-antigens and at the cost of autoimmunity. Therefore, such immuno-therapy strategies can only be done in tissues that can be spared because all cells of these tissues, including the nontransformed cells will be susceptible to immune destruction.

1.2. Immunotherapy—the Need to Pick the Right Target

The success and specificity of immunotherapy strategies is absolutely contingent on the choice of the target antigen. Focusing the immune response on antigens truly unique to the tumor increases the specificity of the response and reduces the chances of devel-oping autoimmunity. In contrast, directing the immune attack at tumor-associated anti-gens detected in both tumor and normal cells could lead to the immune destruction of the self tissues. Naturally, there exists the probability of tumor escape by various means of downregulating the expression of the target antigen because of the immune pressure exerted on the tumor. Therefore, a greater number of available antigenic targets would allow immunotherapy strategies to cast a wider net to counteract tumor escape mecha-nisms. The academy of cancer immunology has a website that contains links to several databases set up with the purpose of characterizing tumor antigens that elicit immune responses in humans (http://www.cancerimmunity.org/statics/databases.htm). The char-acterization and identification of novel tumor antigens is also fundamental to the design of improved therapeutic or prophylactic cancer vaccination schemes. Although most interest has been focused on identifying antigens that could be good targets for CD8+ CTLs that kill transformed cells expressing antigenic peptides in the context of major histocompatibility complex (MHC) class I molecules, currently however, efforts have been turned to identify antigens recognized by CD4+ T-helper (Th) cells that enhance and amplify the immune response through costimulation and the local production of cytokines. A consensus exists that a combined vaccine based on CD8+ and CD4+ T-cell epitopes would improve the efficacy of therapeutic cancer vaccines substantially.

The cells within any particular tumor may contain their own individual mutations; therefore, the tumor is rather heterogeneous in its susceptibility to any sort of therapy. This accounts for the escape variants that evolve after chemotherapy or immunotherapy. To conduct immunotherapy, in addition to choosing an antigenic target that provides specificity, the knowledge of how cancers react in response to immune pressure would help to make the proposed treatment plan more encompassing so that it does not fail because of tumor escape variants.

2. TUMOR ANTIGENS

2.1. Tumor Antigens: How to Identify the Enemy

Tumor antigens are processed and presented to the adaptive immune system as short peptide fragments known as epitopes on major MHC class I and MHC class II molecules. The MHC class I molecules are expressed by nearly all nucleated cells of the body, and normally present peptides that are generated endogenously in the cells. It is imperative that the cancer cell presents some form of immunogenic antigen in order for the CD8+ CTLs to recognize the tumor cell and destroy it. The CD8+ T-cells are the key effectors of antitumor immunity mediated by the adaptive immune system, and they recognize antigenic epitopes presented in the context of MHC class I molecules. CD4+ Th cells also play an important role in antitumor immunity *(13)*, as they enhance and amplify the immune response through costimulation and the local production of cytokines. Th cells recognize antigens presented in the context of MHC class II molecules whose expression is limited to professional antigen-presenting cells (APCs) such as dendritic cells (DCs). The presentation of antigenic epitopes derived from the tumor cells allows the immune system to distinguish between normal and transformed cells and direct the immune attack based on these antigens. Tumor antigens can be classified into five major groups based on their expression patterns: mutational antigens, shared tumor-specific antigens, differentiation antigens, overexpressed antigens, and viral antigens *(14)*.

2.1.1. Mutational Antigens

Mutational antigens are derived from ubiquitous proteins that are mutated in tumor cells. Point mutations, chromosomal translocations, deletions, or gene insertions can lead to the generation of unique tumor antigens distinct for each tumor. The mutational antigens are highly tumor-specific, and some may also be involved in the transformation process. Chronic myelogenous leukemia is characterized by the presence of Bcr-Abl, a fusion product resulting from the translocation of the of cellular Abelson tyrosine kinase from chromosome 9 to a 5.8-kb breakpoint cluster region on chromosome 22 *(15)*. The detection of Bcr-Abl junctional epitopes that bind to both MHC class I human leukocyte antigen (HLA)-A2 *(16)* and MHC class II DR4 *(17,18)* demonstrate that mutational antigens can potentially induce potent immune responses and may be involved in the natural antitumor response in patients. On the other side of the high specificity of mutational antigens is that their potential value as generic cancer vaccines in immunotherapy is limited, as such mutations may not be shared by many patients.

2.1.2. Shared Tumor-Specific Antigens

Shared tumor-specific antigens are antigens whose expression is usually silenced in normal tissues but are activated in tumors of various histological types. Expression of these antigens on normal tissues has only been detected on placental trophoblasts and testicular germ cells that do not express MHC class I molecules. Hence, these antigens are usually not presented to the immune system and can be considered tumor-specific and are also known as cancer–testis antigens. The prototype shared tumor-specific antigens are the melanoma antigen genes, which are normally expressed in testis and placenta and overexpressed in melanoma, bladder cancer, breast cancer, lung cancer, and prostate cancer (19).

2.1.3. Tissue-Specific Differentiation Antigens

Differentiation antigens lack the specificity of tumor-specific shared antigens, as they are differentiation markers that are expressed not just by the malignant cells, but also by the normal cells of the same origin as the cancer cells. Tyrosinase, for example is expressed by both normal melanocytes and most melanoma cells. Targeting such antigens would also result in the autoimmune destruction of the normal tissue as has been demonstrated by the vitiligo (20) induced after vaccination against tyrosinase in melanoma patients. Immunotherapy strategies based on such antigens should be reserved to tissues that are not vital for survival, as exemplified by the targeting of the prostate-specific antigen that could lead to the destruction of the prostate tissues in prostate cancer.

2.1.4. Overexpressed Antigens

T-cell activation is dependent on a minimum number of T-cell receptor/peptide/MHC contacts (21); therefore, the overexpression of many proteins in cancer cells could lead to the generation of an immune response to these self-proteins. The high levels of mutant or wild-type p53 expressed in many cancers make it a potential immunotherapy target, and it has been used against colorectal cancer without inducing autoimmunity (22). However, because these overexpressed proteins are expressed by many normal tissues, it is difficult to assess the safety threshold for each antigen that does not result in widespread autoimmunity.

2.1.5. Viral Antigens

Viral antigens are foreign and are only found on infected cells, thereby making them ideal targets because of their high specificity. Although viruses have evolved their own set of immune evasion strategies, immunotherapy of virus-associated cancers can be directed against viral-antigens vital for viral replication or growth. The human papilloma virus (HPV) E6 and E7 proteins interfere with normal cell-cycle regulation (23,24) and are required for the viral life cycle (25,26). Diverse immunotherapy strategies directed against HPV E7 and HPV E6 (27) have led to promising results (28).

2.2. Tumor-Associated Antigens Can Induce Tolerance

Qualitative and quantitative changes have been observed in the glycolipids and glycoproteins on the cell surface of tumor cells (29,30). The cell surface location of these antigens make them good candidates for therapeutic and diagnostic purposes, because they are accessible to both the cellular and humoral components of the immune system. The mucins are the most extensively studied group of glycoproteins. Mucins are large glycoproteins with high-carbohydrate content expressed by a variety of normal and malignant epithelial cells. The mucins CA-125 and CA-19-9 have been detected in ovarian carcinomas *(31,32)*, whereas mucin (Muc)-1 has been found in breast carcinomas *(33)*. Under physiological conditions, Muc-1 is expressed on the apical surface of breast ductal epithelium and is inaccessible to the immune system. In ductal carcinomas of the breast however, Muc-1 looses its apical polarization and displays new carbohydrate and peptide epitopes, thereby becoming an accessible target for the immune cells. Muc-1 can be easily detected by monoclonal antibodies, and also contains T-cell epitopes and has been used as a target for tumor vaccination schemes *(34)*. However, it has been shown recently that tumor-derived Muc-1 mucins were responsible for the impaired maturation and function of monocyte-derived DCs. Tumor derived-Muc-1 changed the cytokine repertoire of the DCs and resulted in their development into interleukin (IL)-10^{high} IL-12^{low} regulatory APCs *(35)* as a novel mechanism of tumor immune evasion.

3. IMMUNODETECTION

3.1. Stealth and Camouflage—Escaping Immunodetection

Two arms of the immune system work complementarily in immunodetection. The adaptive immune system detects the presence of a transformed cell by scanning for altered self-cells. The innate immune system detects the presence of a transformed cell by looking out for missing self. Therefore, in order to escape successfully both arms of the immune system, cancer cells have evolved a joint strategy of both stealth and camouflage. They have to hide the tumor antigens they express and disguise themselves as something that the body will not reject. The CTLs of the adaptive immune system recognize antigens bound on MHC class I molecules expressed by nearly all nucleated cells of the body. If the MHC class I molecule on the tumor cells presents a viral or aberrant peptide, then the antigen-specific CTLs eliminate the tumor cell. The fetus is an allograft that survives within the maternal host despite its low expression of allogenic MHC molecules that would usually result in immune destruction by the natural killer (NK) cells of the innate immune system. The same immune evasion strategies utilized by the fetus "camouflage" the cancer cells and enable them to escape the NK cells. Together, this stealth and camouflage strategy described in the following two subheadings enables the cancer cells to evade detection.

3.1.1. EVADING THE CTLs

Tumor cells often have an altered expression pattern of class I molecules, as a consequence of profound defects in the antigen processing pathway. This promotes poor expression or loss of class I peptide presentation, which permits tumor cell escape from CTL killing. Different mechanisms that lead to loss of class I molecules have been described so far *(36)*. Production of immunosuppressive molecules that downregulate the expression of MHC class I on nucleated cells and defects in the antigen processing machinery have been clearly demonstrated by examining tissue samples from several cancers. Recently, by microdissection and reverse transcription-polymerase chain reaction, a problem in the presentation of class I peptide was detected in transformed colon cells *(37,38)*. Profound defects in the processing and presentation of peptides were found to be caused by an accumulation of the HLA class I heavy chain in the cytoplasm of neoplastic cells, biallelic inactivation of the β-2 microglobulin, downregulation of the low-molecular-weight protein (LMP)7, and deregulation of the transporter associated with antigen processing (TAP) 2. All these defects allow the colon carcinoma cells to become "invisible" to the adaptive immune system. In addition, histological samples showed downregulation of the proteosome multicatalytic complex subunits LMP-2 and LMP-7 in prostate and renal carcinoma, small cell lung carcinoma, and non-small cell lung cancer *(39–42)*. All these examples indicate that class I down-regulation is an important mechanism of tumor escape.

3.1.2. TRICKING THE NK CELLS

Despite the reduction in MHC class I expression, tumors are still susceptible to attack from immune cells. Tumor cells that lack MHC class I expression are an attractive target for the NK cells of the innate immune system. NK cells bind to the polymorphic determinants of the MHC class I molecules through killer-cell inhibitory receptors (KIRs) *(43)*. The interaction between KIRs and MHC class I molecules is inhibitory in nature, and on ligation leads to inhibition of NK-cell cytotoxicity, maintaining tolerance towards self-tissue. The downregulation of MHC class I molecules on the cell surface of tumor cells will therefore normally lead to the NK-mediated killing of the tumor cells. Another way the NK cells keep track of MHC class I expression is through the heterodimer CD94-NKG2A, which recognizes nonclassical MHC class I molecules such as HLA-E *(44)*. HLA-E presents the signal peptides from the classical MHC class I molecules (HLA-A, -B, and -C), and downregulation of any haplotype molecule in particular would normally result in a reduction of cell surface HLA-E and an increase of the susceptibility of tumor cells to NK-mediated killing.

In order to escape NK-mediated killing, cancer cells have evolved to establish tolerance using similar mechanisms as those found in fetal–maternal interactions. HLA-G is a nonclassical MHC class I molecule expressed in the placenta and helps to maintain tolerance to the fetus. It is expressed by many cancers like melanoma, renal carcinoma, lung carcinoma, glioblastoma, and ovarian cancer. It is upregulated through the local expression of environmental factors such as cytokines, stress factors, and chemotherapeutic agents *(45,46)*. HLA-G exerts its immunoinhibitory effects through at least three KIRs expressed by nearly all cells of the immune system *(47,48)*, and therefore has powerful immunosuppressive effects *(49,50)*. In renal carcinoma, HLA-G expression on tumor cells blocks the cytolytic activity of lymphocyte activated killer cells and CTLs, promoting the evasion of the immune response *(51)*. Soluble HLA-G has also been detected in the plasma of patients suffering from malignant melanoma, glioma, breast, and ovarian cancer *(52)* and can result in local or systemic immunosuppressive effects. However, the signal peptide for HLA-G also serves as a peptide ligand for HLA-E. The interaction between the CD94-NKG2 and HLA-E presenting a nonamer from the the HLA-G signal peptide can lead to inhibition or activation of NK-cytotoxicity, depending on the inhibitory or activating nature of the CD94–NKG2 heterodimer *(53–55)*.

Stress and cellular transformation causes some malignant cells to express MHC class I chain-related (MIC) molecules and UL16-binding protein 1 that are ligands for the NK-activating NKG2D receptor *(56)*. The triggering of NK-activating receptors can result in NK-mediated cytotoxicity of cell types that still express significant level of MHC class I molecules in vitro. NKG2D is also expressed by CTLs and results in their activation when triggered. To avoid being killed by NK cells, tumor cells can produce soluble MICs (sMICs) that block the activating NKG2D receptor. sMICs bind to NKG2D, inducing its endocytosis and degradation, resulting in a reduced expression of NKG2D on tumor-infiltrating and peripheral blood T-cells in cancer patients *(57)*. In colorectal patients,

NKG2D downregulation by sMICs resulted in the decreased expression of another NK-activating receptor, the natural cytotoxicity receptor, and the CXCR1 and CCR7 chemokine receptors. This resulted in homing defects and inactivation of the NKG2D NK population *(58)*.

4. IMMUNOMODULATORY MECHANISMS

4.1. Immunological Regulatory Processes Exploited by the Tumor Cells

Cancer cells are basically self-cells that are no longer regulated by normal cellular processes and proliferate without control. These aberrant cells are predisposed to accumulating genetic errors that place them in a better position to adapt to changes in their environment. Like organisms predicted by Darwin's Theory of Natural Selection to adapt to the environment or suffer extinction, immune pressure selects for tumor variants that are resistant to immune eradication. Apart from the immune evasion strategies listed, modulation of the immune response to incapacitate the antitumor response is a powerful evolutionary adaptation of the cancer cells. Most of the immunomodulatory mechanisms found in tumors are based on normal homeostatic control processes of the immune response set in place to prevent unbridled proliferation of the immune cells, or to maintain tolerance towards self-tissues.

4.1.1. DISRUPTING CELL–CELL INTERACTION

To establish a strong and productive interaction, immune cells are required to reinforce their cellular communication through the induction of adhesion molecules on their surface. The intercellular adhesion molecule (ICAM)-1 is crucial for the formation of the immunological synapse. ICAM-1 participates in the cell–cell interaction between the NK cell and the malignant cell. Transformed cells have been shown to disrupt this cellular interaction by producing the matrix metalloproteinase 9, which results in ICAM-1 shedding and resistance to NK cell killing *(59)*.

4.1.2. REQUIREMENT FOR A SECOND SIGNAL—A CHANCE TO TURN OFF THE IMMUNE RESPONSE

Recognition is only the first step in triggering an immune response. The productive interaction leading to activation requires a second costimulatory signal. The costimulatory signal is provided by the ligation of B7.1 (CD80) or B7.2 (CD86) molecules on the surface of APCs to CD28 on the T-cells or NK cells *(60)*. Although CD28 plays a vital role in the induction of T-cell activation, other members of the CD28 family such as CTL-associated antigen (CTLA)-4, programmed death (PD)-1, and inducible costimulator (ICOS) have opposite functions. Engagement of B7 family members with CTLA-4, PD-1, and ICOS leads to inhibition instead of activation of T-cells *(60)*. Accumulating data suggest that CTLA-4 functions predominantly to regulate activation of naive T-cells in lymphoid organs; ICOS and PD-1 regulate activation and effector phases within and outside lymphoid organs *(61)*.

PD-1 is a negative regulatory receptor expressed by activated T-cells, B-cells, and macrophages, which binds to B7-H1 or B7-DC *(62,63)* expressed on activated DCs, B-cells and monocytes *(64,65)*. B7.H1 plays an important role in the regulation of the humoral and cellular immune responses, promoting the apoptosis of activated B-cells and T-cells that express the ligand PD-1. B7-H1 has been detected in human lung carcinomas, ovary carcinomas, colon carcinomas, and melanomas *(66)*. The expression of B7-H1 on transfected P815 tumor cells increased the apoptosis of tumor-reactive T-cells and facilitated the growth of highly immunogenic B7.1$^+$ tumors in vivo, demonstrating its role in tumor-mediated immunosuppression *(66)*.

B7-H4 is a recently discovered B7 family member that causes detrimental effects on T-cell immunity: inhibiting T-cell proliferation, cytokine production, and cell cycle progression. The expression of the putative ligand of B7-H4 is inducible on T-cells, but has yet to be identified. B7-H4 is not expressed in normal tissues, but is constitutively expressed in 85 and 31%, respectively, of ovarian cancer and lung cancer tissues *(67)*. B7-H4 may have an important role in the immune evasion of these tumors.

4.1.3. CD40—Providing a "Helping" Hand

Most solid tumors are able to escape immunosurveillance, simply because naive T-cells normally circulate between the blood and the secondary lymphoid organs and do not encounter the tumor cells. Tumor-specific protective CTLs can therefore only be induced if sufficient tumor cells reach the secondary lymphatic organs. Therefore, professional APCs that can prime naive T-cells within the lymphoid organs are indispensable in the activation of natural antitumor response. Immature DCs can pick up antigens derived from apoptotic cells, virus infected cells or neoplastically transformed cells and present them on MHC class I molecules in a process known as crosspresentation. Crosspresentation can either activate or suppress the immune response and has been termed "crosspriming" or "crosstolerance," respectively. Although crosspriming has been demonstrated to be inefficient and insufficient in inducing protective CTLs *(68)* on its own, the ability of DCs to present antigens to CD4$^+$ Th cells through MHC class II molecules remains very important, because the presence of Th cells during the priming phase of CTLs contribute significantly to antitumor immunity. Maturation of DCs is mostly dependent on exposure signals resulting from inflammation such as exposure to necrotic cells *(69)* or Toll-like receptor signaling *(70,71)*. CD4$^+$ T-cells and DCs can provide reciprocal "help" to each other. Immature DCs can present antigens on MHC class II molecules to the CD4$^+$ T-cells that express CD40 ligand (CD40L). The CD40L–CD40 interaction enables the maturation of DCs *(72)*. Mature DCs express high levels of costimulatory molecules that provide the costimulation needed for the naive T-cells to proliferate and differentiate. Like the CTLs, the Th cells also require costimulation in order to be fully activated. Absence of the second costimulatory signal can lead to a state of anergy or tolerance in the CTL and the Th cells *(73)*. CD40 ligation of DCs has the capacity to induce high levels of the cytokine IL-12, which polarizes CD4$^+$ T-cells toward a Th1 type, enhances proliferation of CD8$^+$ T-cells, and activates NK cells *(74,75)*.

CD40 is also expressed by B-cells and rescues low-affinity antigen-binding and autoreactive B-cells in germinal centers from Fas–Fas ligand (L)-mediated apoptosis *(76)*. The apoptotic signal is dependent on the activation of the death-inducing signaling complex (DISC) that can be inhibited by the Fas-associating protein with death domain-like interleukin 1 converting enzyme inhibitory protein (FLIP). CD40 signaling leads to the stabilization of FLIP and to the rescue of Fas-mediated apoptosis *(77)*. CD40 has been detected on a variety of human cancer cells, from various origins such as bladder, ovarian, colorectal, liver, lung, pancreas, prostate, cervical, and breast *(78–80)*. It has been shown that CD40 activation on bladder and human gastric carcinoma cells inhibits apoptosis mediated through Fas using a similar mechanism to the one in the B-cell apoptosis rescue *(81,82)*.

In addition, CD40 activation is able to induce an increase in the motility of gastric carcinoma cells *(83)*, and its expression has been detected in the tumor vasculature of renal and breast carcinoma as well as in Kaposi's sarcoma *(84)*, suggesting a potential role of CD40 in the angiogenesis and metastasis of cancer. Elevated plasma levels of soluble CD40L also correlated with metastatic spread in human lung cancer *(83,85)*. The high serum levels of soluble CD40L have proangiogenic effects *(86)*, as it can induce the increased transcription of vascular endothelial growth factor (VEGF) by endothelial cells expressing CD40 *(87)*.

5. TUMOR MICROENVIRONMENT

5.1. The Effects of the Tumor Microenvironment on the Antitumor Response and Tumor Growth

The pleiotropic effects of cytokines can function to support or suppress the immune system. Tumor cells have evolved to produce cytokines that suppress the immune response and to profit from the proangiogenic effects of some cytokines. Cytokines present in the milieu when naive CD4$^+$ T-cells are activated can skew the balance of development into Th1 or Th2. Th1 and Th2 cytokines have reciprocal inhibition on the development of the type of Th response. IL-12 and interferon (IFN)-γ lead to the development of Th1 cells that augment cell-mediated immune responses crucial for antitumor immunity. IL-4 induces the development of Th2 cells *(88,89)*, which promote humoral responses and inhibit the formation of a Th1 response.

The local production of type 1 cytokines like IFNγ, IL-2, and tumor necrosis factor (TNF)-α favor cell-mediated immunity and is important in the control of tumor growth. Tumor cells have been shown to produce *(90)* or to induce the production of type 2 cytokines through tumor-infiltrating lymphocytes. It has also been suggested that the hypoxic conditions found around tumors may bias the immune response towards a type 2 response *(91)*. Type 2 cytokines downregulate the expression of type 1 cytokines, inactivating the cell-mediated antitumor response. Analysis of the cytokine microenvironment from the fresh pleural effusions and tissue samples from several cancers has revealed the predominant expression of type 2 cytokines like IL-4 or immunosuppressive cytokines such as transforming growth factor (TGF)-β and IL-10 *(92,93)*. TGF-β and IL-10 suppress the type 1 and proinflammatory responses of the immune system *(94,95)*.

5.1.1. INTERLEUKIN 10

IL-10 has potent immunosuppressive effects on APCs and effector T-cells. IL-10 reduces the expression of type 1 cytokines, inhibits antigen-specific T-cell proliferation *(96)*, and inhibits the production of proinflammatory cytokines by macrophages *(97)* and APCs *(98)*. DCs matured in vitro in the presence of IL-10 are impaired in their ability to produce type 1 cytokines, leading to the development of Th2 cells in vivo *(99)*, resulting in the development of a humoral response instead of a cellular response that is more beneficial for antitumor immunity. IL-10 has also been shown to turn DCs into tolerogenic DCs. Pretreatment of DCs with IL-10 induces an antigen-specific anergy in CTLs (100). In tumors, local production of IL-10 has also been associated with an increase in the expression of HLA-G, resulting in the induction of tolerance towards the tumor in addition to general immunosuppression *(101,102)*. The exclusion of APCs from the tumor mass has also been attributed to the local production of IL-10 *(103,104)*.

5.1.2. TRANSFORMING GROWTH FACTOR-β

TGF-β is commonly overexpressed in many cancers and has many immunosuppressive effects, including the inhibition of T-cell proliferation and their development into

CTLs and Th cells *(105)*. TGF-β-overexpressing tumors are particularly aggressive, and have been correlated with a more malignant phenotype. Apart from its role in tumor-mediated immunosuppression, TGF-β also regulates cellular proliferation, differentiation, extracellular matrix production, cell motility, and apoptosis *(106,107)*. Tumor cells have exploited the pleiotropic effects of TGF-β to its full advantage. *Ras* is a commonly activated oncogene and the cooperation of TGF-β receptor and the *Ras* oncogene signaling pathway has been implicated in the oncogenic and metastatic process in a mammary epithelial carcinogenesis model *(108–111)*. TGF-β has also been detected in epithelial compartment and in tumor stroma *(112,113)*, where it may have an important role in controlling stromal formation within a developing tumor by increasing the synthesis of matrix proteins such as collagen, fibronectin, laminin, and tenascin *(114)*. TGF-β is also able to induce integrins production important to mediate adhesion and cell migration through the extracellular matrix and induce angiogenesis by inducing PA-1, which inhibits the conversion of plasminogen into angiogenesis inhibitor; angiostatin *(115)*, thereby contributing to the metastatic ability of tumor cells.

TGF-β also mediates cell cycle arrest and theoretically, should also inhibit tumor growth. Binding of TGF-β to the ternary TGF-β receptor complex activates a cascade of signal transduction pathways regulated by mothers against DPP homolog (SMAD)2, SMAD3, SMAD4, and mitogen-activated protein kinase *(116,117)* that negatively regulate the transcriptional levels of c-Myc and inhibit retinoblastoma protein phosphorylation *(108–120)*, resulting in cell cycle arrest. Tumor escape from TGF-β-mediated cell cycle arrest is accounted for by point mutations, homozygous deletions, gene rearrangements, and aberrant transcripts in the RI and RII *(121–123)* of the TGF-β receptor complex. Deletions and mutations of components of the TGF-β receptor signaling pathway like SMAD3 and SMAD4 *(124)* have also been detected. It is yet unknown what the molecular mechanisms are that allow the tumor cells to become insensitive to TGF-β cell cycle arrest effects while remaining sensitive to its induction of migration/invasion.

5.1.3. EFFECTS OF IFN-γ ON ANTITUMOR IMMUNITY

IFN-γ is important for the generation of an effective Th1 response as well as for NK cell-mediated antitumor immunity *(125)*. IFN-γ is a key mediator of antitumor immunity, as it is able to induce the upregulation of many genes containing the IFN response sequence element. In addition, it has been shown to be essential to tumor rejection mediated by both CD4+ T-cells and CD8+ T-cells through induction of angiostasis *(126,127)*. IFN-γ exposure can sensitize breast cancer cells to apoptosis by upregulation of caspase 8 *(128)*. Expression of the antigen presentation machinery is also regulated by IFN-γ. IFN-γ upregulates the transcription of transporter associated with antigen processing and the proteasome subunits low-molecular-weight protein 2 *(129)*. Tumors may become unresponsive to the effects of IFN-γ through defective IFN-γ signaling, allowing them to gain resistance to IFN-γ-mediated apoptosis *(130)* and maintain low MHC class I expression levels *(131)*. In hepatocellular carcinoma, there is a correlation between the degree of metastasis and the poor expression of IFN-γ receptor on tumor cells. In metastatic cases, the decreased expression of IFN-γ receptor on tumor cells causes a considerable reduction of MHC class I molecules and Fas on these cells, impairing IFN-γ control of tumor growth *(132)*.

IFN-γ secretion can also lead to the suppression of the immune response indirectly through the upregulation of IFN-γ-inducible genes. Indoleamine 2,3-dioxygenase (IDO) is an IFN-γ-inducible enzyme *(133)* that catabolizes tryptophan and causes proliferation arrest of T-lymphocytes because of tryptophan degradation *(134,135)*. IDO-expressing cells create a tryptophan-depleted microenvironment around themselves, as tryptophan crosses the plasma membrane readily through specific transporters to be degraded in the cytosol. Its expression by the placenta is important in the prevention of allorejection of the fetus by maternal T-cells *(136)*. IDO is expressed by DCs following ligation of B7.1/B7.2 *(137)*, and may be a mechanism by which DCs regulate T-cell responses *(138)*. Tumor cells can express IDO, and tumor cell lines transfected with IDO in vitro suppress T-cell proliferation *(139)*, and it has been proposed that tumor cells may be able to recruit APCs and induce tolerogenic IDO-expressing APCs *(140)*. These APCs would then be able to home to draining lymph nodes and tolerize naive T-cells to tumor-derived antigens. The discovery of accumulation of IDO-positively staining cells in immunohistochemistry studies of lymph nodes from melanoma patients supports this hypothesis *(141)*. IFN-γ production is often taken as a favorable indicator in the antitumor response. In a setting where the tumor cells have evolved to become less sensitive to IFN-γ-induced apoptosis, the IFN-γ could simply have a negative effect by inducing IDO production and tolerizing the immune system to the tumor.

Another example of the difficulty in accessing the outcome of IFN-γ production on antitumor immunity is illustrated by the interaction between IFN-γ-inducible chemokines and inducible nitric oxide synthase (iNOS). IFN-inducible CXC chemokines are powerful inhibitors of angiogenesis *(142)*. Intratumoral production of IFN-inducible chemokines like CXCL9 and CXL10 is associated with reduced angiogenesis and increased recruitment of CD8[+] T-cells in renal carcinoma *(143)*. IFN-γ also causes the upregulation of iNOS that leads to the production of nitric oxide. Nitric oxide is able to upregulate the production of angiogenic molecules like IL-8 and VEGF, and downregulate the expression of antiangiogenic chemokines like CXCL9 and CXL10 *(144)*. In hepatocellular carcinoma, iNOS expression was associated with increased microvascular density, resistance to apoptosis mediated by Bcl-2 synthesis, and cell proliferation of malignant cells *(145)*. This illustrates the complexities in trying to predict the outcome of IFN-γ-inducible products on angiogenesis and immune modulation in the tumor microenvironment.

5.1.4. Constitutive Signal Transducer and Activator of Transcription 3 Signaling

Many of the cytokine-activated signaling pathways converge on the signal transducer and activator of transcription (STAT)3 signaling molecule. STAT3 is involved in the regulation of cell differentiation, survival, cytokine, and chemokine production, and is required for DC maturation and activation *(146,147)*. The constitutive activation of STAT3 has been reported in many cancers *(148–150)*. STAT3 signaling in tumor cells has been shown to lead to the tumor immune evasion by inhibiting the activation of proinflammatory cytokines and chemokines, leading to a reduction in the number of inflammatory infiltrates like macrophages and neutrophils in the tumors *(151)*. STAT3 signaling also drives the secretion of factors that lead to the inhibition of DC maturation, thereby preventing the induction of an antitumor T-cell response *(151)*. Constitutive STAT3 activity also confers apoptosis resistance to the tumor cells *(152)* and upregulates VEGF expression to stimulate tumor angiogenesis *(153)*. Constitutive STAT3 signaling in tumors results in tumor immune evasion from both the innate and adaptive immune system, protects tumors from apoptosis, supports tumor growth through activation of angiogenesis, and is a clear example of how the tumors can utilize the pleiotropic functions of cytokines by the simple dysregulation of a key signaling molecule involved in cytokine signaling.

5.2. Cellular Infiltrates in the Tumor: Allies or Enemies?

The quantitative and qualitative analysis of the cellular infiltrates in the tumor microenvironment can lead to a greater understanding of the outcome of the immune modulatory effects of the tumor. A reduction in the number of tumor-infiltrating DCs in advanced malignancies can lead to impaired priming and generation of tumor-specific T-cells in the local environment and can be considered as mechanism of immune evasion (154). High numbers of tumor-infiltrating cells may not necessarily be a favorable indicator of an effective antitumor response. Some of the tumor-infiltrating cells can be tolerogenic cells that can actively downregulate the cellular immune response through the production of immunosuppressive molecules. Among these cells, the regulatory T-cells and NK T-cells are considered key players in the negative regulation of tumor immunity through their production of type 2 and immunosuppressive cytokines like IL-4, IL-10, IL-13, and TGF-β (155). Tumor-infiltrating macrophages in the Lewis lung carcinoma model produce considerable quantities of IDO (156) that suppresses the local T-cell response through antigen-specific anergy.

6. ACQUIRING RESISTANCE TO DEATH EFFECTOR MECHANISMS

The immune eradication of tumor cells is mediated by apoptosis that can be induced by the release of cytotoxic granules or death receptors. Tumors have evolved ways to become resistant to the death effector mechanisms, thereby becoming truly impervious to immune attack. The perforin/granzyme and Fas/FasL pathways are the two main effector mechanisms by which CTLs and NK cells mediate antitumor immunity (157–158). The downstream effects of both pathways are similar, as they both lead to activation of the caspase cascade and mitochondrial-dependent cell death. The caspases and cytochrome c released from the mitochondria further synergize by enhancing each others' activation.

6.1. The Perforin/Granzyme B Pathway

In the granule-mediated pathway, CTLs and NK cells package specialized cytotoxic granules containing pore-forming perforins and granzymes. Perforins polymerize in response to calcium, and are inserted into the target cell membrane to create a channel that results in cellular necrosis through disruption of osmotic stability (159). In addition to the cytolytic effect of the perforins, the granzymes in the granules can also induce cellular apoptosis through the activation of caspases. Human CTLs contain five different granzymes that have different substrate specificities and modes of action to induce cell death (160). Granzyme A-induced apoptosis results from single-strand DNA breaks, independent of caspase activation (161). Granzyme B is able to activate both caspase-dependent and caspase-independent pathways of cell death in the target cell (162). Caspase 3 and caspase 8 are direct substrates of granzyme B, and activation of the caspase cascade leads to apoptosis and activation of caspase-activated deoxyribonuclease (CAD) leading to DNA fragmentation (163–165). CAD is normally found in the cytoplasm in an inactive form bound to its inhibitor ICAD. Caspase 8 cleaves ICAD to release CAD, leading to DNA fragmentation. Granzyme B can also activate the proapoptotic Bcl-2-family member, Bcl-2-interacting domain (Bid) (166,167), through cleavage. Activation of Bid leads to the oligomerization and insertion of proapoptotic Bcl-2-associated X protein (Bax) and Bcl-2 antagonist killer 1 into the pore and outer mitochondrial membrane (168,169). This eventually results in the release of cytochrome c, mitochondrial collapse *(170)*, and subsequent release of mitochondrial-derived activator of caspase that bind to the inhibitors of apoptosis and releases the suppression on caspases for their full activation *(171,172)*. The release of cytochrome *c* can result in the formation of an apoptosome that includes apoptotic protease-activating factor 1 and procaspase 9 *(173)*. The apoptosome is able to activate caspase 9 *(174)* in the presence of andenosine triphosphate and activate more caspase 3, augmenting caspase-mediated apoptosis. Overexpression of a serine protease inhibitor, PI-9/SPI-6, was found in a variety of human and murine tumors. PI-9/SPI-6 inactivates granzyme B and protects cells against CTL-mediated perforin killing *(175)*.

6.2. Fas-Mediated Apoptosis

The interaction between the death receptor, Fas and its ligand, FasL, leads to the trimerization of Fas to bring together death domains (DDs) in the cytoplasmic portion of the molecules. The DDs then recruit adaptor proteins that form a DISC capable of activating initiator caspases like caspase 8 and caspase 10. Caspase 8 activation leads to activation of CAD and activation of the mitochondrial-induced death through Bid cleavage. Mutations in the *fas* gene, leading to a reduction in Fas expression, have been reported in many cancers *(176–178)* as a mechanism of gaining resistance to Fas-mediated apoptosis. Fas can also be secreted by tumor cells to bind to the FasL on tumor-specific CTLs to protect tumor cells from apoptosis *(179)*.

Decoy receptors containing functional extracellular ligand-binding domains but lacking intracellular DD have been found that regulate sensitivity to death-receptor-mediated apoptosis. DcR3 is a soluble decoy receptor secreted by tumor cells *(180,181)* and overexpressed in malignant glioma, pancreatic adenocarcinoma, colon, prostate, lung, and gastrointestinal tumors *(182–186)*. DcR3 binds to FasL and allows tumor cells to gain resistance to Fas/FasL-mediated apoptosis. DcR3 also suppresses the activation and differentiation of DCs *(187)* and macrophages *(188)* and downregulates T-cell proliferation. The FasL signaling pathway also serves as a local chemoattractant, and the production of DcR3 results in defective homing by reducing the recruitment of microglial macrophages, neutrophils, CD4+, and CD8+ T-cells *(189,190)* as a means of immune evasion. DcR3 has proangiogenic effects and is able to promote endothelial cell proliferation, migration, and the expression of matrix metalloproteinases *(191)*. Altogether, the immunosuppressive, antiapoptotic, and angiogenic activities of DcR3 can make it an important player in not just immune evasion but also in tumor growth.

Caspase 8 is the key initiator cell death protease in the death receptors pathway. Its activation is dependent on its recruitment to DISC following death receptor engagement. c-FLIP can bind DISC and prevent the activation of caspase 8 *(192)*. c-FLIP is expressed by many cancer cells and represents yet another way by which cancer cells gain resistance to death-receptor-mediated apoptosis *(193)*.

6.3. Production of Antiapoptotic Molecules

Tumor cells can also gain resistance to apoptosis through the production of antiapoptotic molecules. Members of the Bcl family have either proapoptotic functions or antiapoptotic functions and control the mitochrondrial-component of apoptosis. Bcl-2 and Bcl-X_L are commonly overexpressed in cancers and protect cells against apoptosis by preventing cytochrome *c* release *(194)*. Survivin is involved in the downregulation of apoptosis in malignant cells. In a prostate cancer cell line PC3, the increased production of survivin protects cells against apoptosis mediated by TNF-α by preventing the activation of caspase 9 *(195)*. Survivin was also found to cause the upregulation of FasL in colon cancer cells *(196)*.

7. COUNTERATTACK BY THE TUMOR CELLS

Activation-induced cell death is a homeostatic mechanism that controls the magnitude of the immune response that has been exploited by tumor cells in their counterattack against the immune system. Contraction of the immune response after activation is coordinated Fas-FasL interactions that result in the death of activated cells. FasL expression on tumor cells has been documented in several cancers: hilar cholangiocarcinoma *(197)*, intrahepatic cholangiocarcinoma *(198)*, renal cell carcinoma *(199)*, cervical adenocarcinoma *(200)*, and melanoma *(201)*. The expression of FasL on malignant cells can lead to the *in situ* elimination of tumor-specific T-cells that express Fas on their cell surface *(202)*. TNF-related apoptosis-inducing ligand is another member of the TNF super-family that mediates cell death. TNF-related apoptosis-inducing ligand has been detected in metastatic gastric carcinoma cells from malignant ascites *(203)*, resulting in the death of tumor-infiltrating lymphocytes that bear the counter-receptors DR4 and DR5.

Soluble FasL can be released by tumor cells systemically, inducing the death of circulating lymphocytes in the periphery. Astrocytomas are known to produce high levels of soluble FasL *(204)*, which can be cytotoxic to Fas-expressing T-cells. This particular phenomenon has also been detected in colon cancer cells that shed their membrane associated FasL into the environment *(205)*. Tumors can also combine death-resistance mechanisms with counterattack on the immune system. Renal carcinomas were reported to decrease the expression of membrane-bound Fas, and secrete soluble FasL *(206)*.

8. ANGIOGENIC PROCESSES THAT FACILITATE TUMOR IMMUNE EVASION

Angiogenesis is a vital process in tumor survival. However, some of the angiogenic factors can indirectly facilitate tumor immune evasion because of their immunosuppressive effects. VEGF is a key mediator in both vasculogenesis and angiogenesis *(207)*. VEGF expression is associated with poor prognosis and increased metastatic spreading in ovarian cancer *(208)*. In addition, VEGF also inhibits T-cell development and contributes to tumor-mediated immune suppression *(209)*. Cyclooxygenase (COX)-2 is overexpressed in many cancers *(210,211)*, and is implicated in the angiogenic process *(212)*. COX-2 contributes to the production of prostaglandins by catalyzing the oxygenation of arachidonic acid to the common precursor of all prostanoids. The various prostaglandins are synthesized by distinct synthases in different tissues. The local production of prostaglandin (PG)E2 leads to immunosuppression in the tumor microenvironment through inhibition of T-cell and B-cell proliferation and diminished cytotoxicity of NK cells *(213,214)*. PGE2 is a powerful inhibitor of TNF-α and type 1 cytokine production and causes the downregulation of the cellular antitumor immune response. Another prostaglandin that can negatively affect antitumor immunity is PGD2. PGD2 is the ligand for the PGD2 receptor expressed on effector memory Th2 cells. An increased COX-2 activity and subsequent PGD2 production could promote the trafficking and activation of Th2 cells into tumor, suppressing the production of type 1 cytokines as a form of tumor immune evasion.

9. CONCLUSION

The myriad ways by which cancer cells escape immune eradication could be an indication of the immune pressure it faces. Cancer cells are usually successful in escaping immunodetection, because many of them are not particularly immunogenic. Cancer immunotherapy is therefore most successful in situations where the immune system is able to distinguish the transformed cells from surrounding normal cells with which it shares antigens against which the immune system is tolerant. Tumor antigens therefore serve as the first signals to alert the immune system. Vaccination schemes in cancer immunotherapy are distinctly different from classical vaccination that is prophylactic. Cancer cells may have already modulated the immune response and therefore nullified the potential therapeutic effects of a vaccine. The accumulation of data on immunogenic tumor-derived antigens will increase the arsenal of targets against which efforts can be directed. It is imperative for researchers and physicians venturing into cancer immunotherapy to pick their targets carefully, because no immunization scheme can be successful against an enemy that the immune system cannot "see." The inability of most naive T-cells to encounter tumor cells early enough in the blood and secondary lymphoid organs contributes to the lack of immunosurveillance for most types of cancers. Vaccination allows for the activation of tumor-specific T-cells and lowers their threshold of activation, allowing the activated CTLs to eradicate the tumor cells despite their low MHC class I expression. This argues for cancer immunotherapy, even for cancers that are not covered by the immunosurveillance theory, so long as they express antigens that can be targeted with minimal consequence of autoimmunity. The tumor environment shaped by angiogenic processes, chemokines, cytokines, and cellular infiltrates plays a huge determinant in the eradication of the tumor. The presence of T-lymphocytes specific for tumor antigens may not be a good enough indicator for the success of a potential vaccine. Although every tumor is different in itself, understanding the evasion strategies based on tumor type may enable us to support vaccination strategies with other immune modulators in order to conduct successful immunotherapies. The immune evasion strategies that tumors are able to adopt and their immunomodulatory effects as a direct consequence of immune pressure or as an indirect effect of angiogenesis (Fig. 1), pose as hurdles to existing natural antitumor activity and therapeutic vaccination schemes. An effective cancer vaccine needs to create optimal activation conditions, such as adequate costimulation and a cytokine environment conducive for the Th1 response at the priming phase to prevent antigen-specific anergy or Th2-suppression of the Th1 response. Existing tolerance will have to be broken toward antigens that the immune system is already tolerant. Activation of the immune system is the result of the integration of activating and inhibitory signals. Tolerance can be broken by providing "help" in the form of cytokines and costimulation and by inhibiting tolerogenic stimuli such as immunosuppressive cytokines and inhibitory costimulation. A recent paper outlines strategies to potentiate cancer vaccines by inhibiting the immunosuppressive factors *(215)*. Autoimmune diseases are the proof that low levels of autoreactive cells do exist and can turn into potent antigen-specific killers. With the appropriate adjuvants and vaccination strategies, these cells can be unleashed against the cancer cells to eradicate these altered "self" cells. There is great promise for cancer immunotherapy, but there is a need to pick the right targets and strengthen the immune attack in order to break down the tolerogenic obstacles put up by the tumor cells.

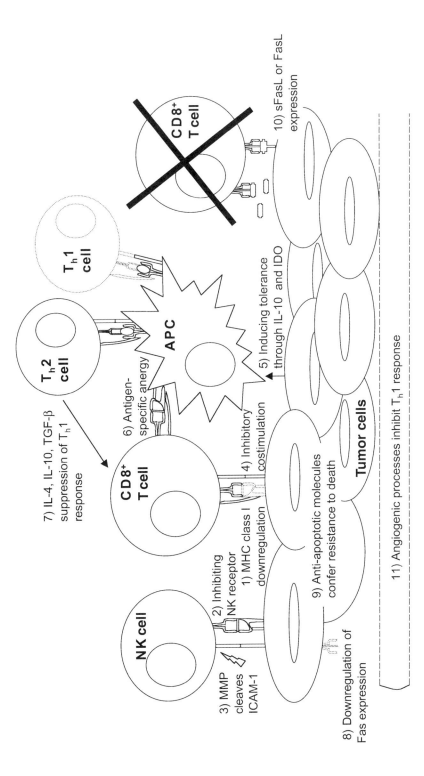

Fig. 1. Tumor immune invasion strategies. Tumor cells can evade immunodetection by (1) downregulation of major histocompatibility complex (MHC) class I molecules and by (2) inhibiting the natural killer (NK) cell receptor. They can inhibit NK cell-mediated killing by (3) disrupting cell–cell interactions. (4) The expression of inhibitory members of the CD28 costimulatory family leads to inhibition of the priming or effector phases of T-cell response. (5) Interleukin (IL)-10 and indoleamine 2,3-dioxygenase (IDO) secreted by tumor cells or by tumor-infiltrating cells can lead to the generation of tolerogenic antigen-presenting cells (APCs) that can (6) induce antigen-specific anergy of T-cells when they home to the lymph nodes, or (7) lead to the development of a type 2 response that suppresses the T-helper (Th) cells response. Tumors can (8) downregulate the expression of Fas and (9) produce antiapoptotic molecules to escape from death effector mechanisms. (10) Soluble (s)Fas and cell surface Fas ligand(L) expression by the tumor cells result in apoptosis of Fas-expressing T-cells. (11) Angiogenesis induced by the tumor cells indirectly results in inhibition of the Th1 response.

ACKNOWLEDGMENTS

M. de la Luz García-Hernández, PhD is supported by the Department of Defense fellowship #PC041078. W. Martin Kast, PhD holds the Walter A. Richter Cancer Research Chair. Yi Ting Koh, BSc is supported by Department of Defense grant #DAMD 17-02-1-0244.

REFERENCES

1. Ehrlich P. Ueber den jetzigen Stand der Karzinomforschung (in German). Ned Tijdschr Geneeskd 1909; 5(Pt 1):273–290.
2. Burnet FM. The concept of immunological surveillance. Prog Exp Tumor Res 1970; 13:1–27.
3. Thomas L. Discussion. In: Lawrence HS, ed. Cellular and humoral aspects of the hypersensitive states. New York: Hoeber-Harper, 1959:529–532.
4. Henle W, Henle G. Epidemiologic aspects of Epstein-Barr virus (EBV)-associated diseases. Ann N Y Acad Sci 1980; 354:326–331.
5. Miyashita EM, Yang B, Lam KM, Crawford DH, Thorley-Lawson DA. A novel form of Epstein-Barr virus latency in normal B-cells in vivo. Cell 1995; 80:593–601.
6. Pinkerton CR, Hann I, Weston CL, et al. Immunodeficiency-related lymphoproliferative disorders: prospective data from the United Kingdom Children's Cancer Study Group Registry. Br J Haematol 2002; 118:456–461.
7. Shapiro R, Nalesnik M, McCauley J, et al. Posttransplant lymphoproliferative disorders in adult and pediatric renal transplant patients receiving tacrolimus-based immunosuppression. Transplantation 1999; 68:1851–1854.
8. Gruhn B, Meerbach A, Hafer R, Zell R, Wutzler P, Zintl F. Pre-emptive therapy with rituximab for prevention of Epstein-Barr virus-associated lymphoproliferative disease after hematopoietic stem cell transplantation. Bone Marrow Transplant 2003; 31:1023–1025.
9. Randle HW. The historical link between solid-organ transplantation, immunosuppression, and skin cancer. Dermatol Surg 2004; 30(Pt 2):595–597.
10. Agraharkar ML, Cinclair RD, Kuo YF, Daller JA, Shahinian VB. Risk of malignancy with long-term immunosuppression in renal transplant recipients. Kidney Int 2004; 66:383–389.
11. Baillargeon J, Pollock BH, Leach CT, Gao SJ. The association of neoplasms and HIV infection in the correctional setting. Int J STD AIDS 2004; 15:348–351.
12. Bellan C, De Falco G, Lazzi S, Leoncini L. Pathologic aspects of AIDS malignancies. Oncogene 2003; 22:6639–6645.
13. Velders MP, Markiewicz MA, Eiben GL, Kast WM. CD4+ T cell matters in tumor immunity. Int Rev Immunol 2003; 22:113–140.
14. van der Bruggen BP, Zhang Y, Chaux P, et al. Tumor-specific shared antigenic peptides recognized by human T cells. Immunol Rev 2002; 188:51–64.
15. Rowley JD. Letter: a new consistent chromosomal abnormality in chronic myelogenous leukaemia identified by quinacrine fluorescence and Giemsa staining. Nature 1973; 243:290–293.
16. Yotnda P, Firat H, Garcia-Pons F, et al. Cytotoxic T cell response against the chimeric p210 BCR-ABL protein in patients with chronic myelogenous leukemia. J Clin Invest 1998; 101:2290–2296.
17. Bosch GJ, Joosten AM, Kessler JH, Melief CJ, Leeksma OC. Recognition of BCR-ABL positive leukemic blasts by human CD4+ T cells elicited by primary in vitro immunization with a BCR-ABL breakpoint peptide. Blood 1996; 88:3522–3527.
18. Makita M, Azuma T, Hamaguchi H, et al. Leukemia-associated fusion proteins, dek-can and bcr-abl, represent immunogenic HLA-DR-restricted epitopes recognized by fusion peptide-specific CD4+ T lymphocytes. Leukemia 2002; 16:2400–2407.
19. Scanlan MJ, Gure AO, Jungbluth AA, Old LJ, Chen YT. Cancer/testis antigens: an expanding family of targets for cancer immunotherapy. Immunol Rev 2002; 188:22–32.
20. Overwijk WW, Lee DS, Surman DR, et al. Vaccination with a recombinant vaccinia virus encoding a "self" antigen induces autoimmune vitiligo and tumor cell destruction in mice: requirement for CD4(+) T lymphocytes. Proc Natl Acad Sci U S A 1999; 96:2982–2987.
21. Viola A, Lanzavecchia A. T cell activation determined by T cell receptor number and tunable thresholds. Science 1996; 273:104–106.

22. Menon AG, Kuppen PJ, Van der Burg SH, et al. Safety of intravenous administration of a canarypox virus encoding the human wild-type *p53* gene in colorectal cancer patients. Cancer Gene Ther 2003; 10:509–517.

23. He W, Staples D, Smith C, Fisher C. Direct activation of cyclin-dependent kinase 2 by human papillomavirus E7. J Virol 2003; 77:10,566–10,574.

24. Mantovani F, Banks L. The human papillomavirus E6 protein and its contribution to malignant progression. Oncogene 2001; 20:7874–7887.

25. Flores ER, Allen-Hoffmann BL, Lee D, Lambert PF. The human papillomavirus type 16 E7 oncogene is required for the productive stage of the viral life cycle. J Virol 2000; 74:6622–6631.

26. McMurray HR, Nguyen D, Westbrook TF, McAnce DJ. Biology of human papillomaviruses. Int J Exp Pathol 2001; 82:15–33.

27. Eiben GL, da Silva DM, Fausch SC, Le Poole IC, Nishimura MI, Kast WM. Cervical cancer vaccines: recent advances in HPV research. Viral Immunol 2003; 16:111–121.

28. Frazer IH. Prevention of cervical cancer through papillomavirus vaccination. Nat Rev Immunol 2004; 4:46–54.

29. Baldus SE, Engelmann K, Hanisch FG. MUC1 and the MUCs: a family of human mucins with impact in cancer biology. Crit Rev Clin Lab Sci 2004; 41:189–231.

30. Carraway KL, Fregien N, Carraway KL, III, Carraway CA. Tumor sialomucin complexes as tumor antigens and modulators of cellular interactions and proliferation. J Cell Sci 1992; 103(Pt 2):299–307.

31. Dietel M, Arps H, Klapdor R, Muller-Hagen S, Sieck M, Hoffmann L. Antigen detection by the monoclonal antibodies CA 19-9 and CA 125 in normal and tumor tissue and patients' sera. J Cancer Res Clin Oncol 1986; 111:257–265.

32. Negishi Y, Furukawa T, Oka T, et al. Clinical use of CA 125 and its combination assay with other tumor marker in patients with ovarian carcinoma. Gynecol Obstet Invest 1987; 23:200–207.

33. Taylor-Papadimitriou J, Burchell JM, et al. MUC1 and the immunobiology of cancer. J Mammary Gland Biol Neoplasia 2002; 7:209–221.

34. Finn OJ, Jerome KR, Henderson RA, et al. MUC-1 epithelial tumor mucin-based immunity and cancer vaccines. Immunol Rev 1995; 145:61–89.

35. Monti P, Leone BE, Zerbi A, et al. Tumor-derived MUC1 mucins interact with differentiating monocytes and induce IL-10^{high}IL-12^{low} regulatory dendritic cell. J Immunol 2004; 172:7341–7349.

36. Garcia-Lora A, Algarra I, Collado A, Garrido F. Tumour immunology, vaccination and escape strategies. Eur J Immunogenet 2003; 30:177–183.

37. Cabrera CM, Jimenez P, Cabrera T, Esparza C, Ruiz-Cabello F, Garrido F. Total loss of MHC class I in colorectal tumors can be explained by two molecular pathways: β2-microglobulin inactivation in MSI-positive tumors and LMP7/TAP2 downregulation in MSI-negative tumors. Tissue Antigens 2003; 61:211–219.

38. Johnsen AK, Templeton DJ, Sy M, Harding CV. Deficiency of transporter for antigen presentation (TAP) in tumor cells allows evasion of immune surveillance and increases tumorigenesis. J Immunol 1999; 163:4224–4231.

39. Sanda MG, Restifo NP, Walsh JC, et al. Molecular characterization of defective antigen processing in human prostate cancer. J Natl Cancer Inst 1995; 87:280–285.

40. Korkolopoulou P, Kaklamanis L, Pezzella F, Harris AL, Gatter KC. Loss of antigen-presenting molecules (MHC class I and TAP-1) in lung cancer. Br J Cancer 1996; 73:148–153.

41. Restifo NP, Esquivel F, Kawakami Y, et al. Identification of human cancers deficient in antigen processing. J Exp Med 1993; 177:265–272.

42. Seliger B, Hohne A, Jung D, et al. Expression and function of the peptide transporters in escape variants of human renal cell carcinomas. Exp Hematol 1997; 25:608–614.

43. Boyington JC, Sun PD. A structural perspective on MHC class I recognition by killer cell immunoglobulin-like receptors. Mol Immunol 2002; 38:1007–1021.

44. Borrego F, Kabat J, Kim DK, et al. Structure and function of major histocompatibility complex (MHC) class I specific receptors expressed on human natural killer (NK) cells. Mol Immunol 2002; 38:637–660.

45. Rouas-Freiss N, Moreau P, Menier C, Carosella ED. HLA-G in cancer: a way to turn off the immune system. Semin Cancer Biol 2003; 13:325–336.

46. Ibrahim EC, Aractingi S, Allory Y, et al. Analysis of HLA antigen expression in benign and malignant melanocytic lesions reveals that upregulation of HLA-G expression correlates with malignant transformation, high inflammatory infiltration and HLA-A1 genotype. Int J Cancer 2004; 108:243–250.

47. Colonna M, Samaridis J, Cella M, et al. Human myelomonocytic cells express an inhibitory receptor for classical and nonclassical MHC class I molecules. J Immunol 1998; 160:3096–3100.

48. Rajagopalan S, Long EO. A human histocompatibility leukocyte antigen (HLA)-G-specific receptor expressed on all natural killer cells. J Exp Med 1999; 189:1093–1100.
49. LeMaoult J, Krawice-Radanne I, Dausset J, Carosella ED. HLA-G1-expressing antigen-presenting cells induce immunosuppressive CD4+ T cells. Proc Natl Acad Sci U S A 2004; 101:7064–7069.
50. Rouas-Freiss N, Moreau P, Menier C, Carosella ED. HLA-G in cancer: a way to turn off the immune system. Semin Cancer Biol 2003; 13:325–336.
51. Bukur J, Rebmann V, Grosse-Wilde H, et al. Functional role of human leukocyte antigen-G up-regulation in renal cell carcinoma. Cancer Res 2003; 63:4107–4111.
52. Rebmann V, Regel J, Stolke D, Grosse-Wilde H. Secretion of sHLA-G molecules in malignancies. Semin Cancer Biol 2003; 13:371–377.
53. Hofmeister V, Weiss EH. HLA-G modulates immune responses by diverse receptor interactions. Semin Cancer Biol 2003; 13:317–323.
54. Llano M, Lee N, Navarro F, et al. HLA-E-bound peptides influence recognition by inhibitory and triggering CD94/NKG2 receptors: preferential response to an HLA-G-derived nonamer. Eur J Immunol 1998; 28:2854–2863.
55. Soderstrom K, Corliss B, Lanier LL, Phillips JH. CD94/NKG2 is the predominant inhibitory receptor involved in recognition of HLA-G by decidual and peripheral blood NK cells. J Immunol 1997; 159:1072–1075.
56. Moretta L, Moretta A. Unravelling natural killer cell function: triggering and inhibitory human NK receptors. EMBO J 2004; 23:255–259.
57. Groh V, Wu J, Yee C, Spies T. Tumour-derived soluble MIC ligands impair expression of NKG2D and T-cell activation. Nature 2002; 419:734–738.
58. Doubrovina ES, Doubrovin MM, Vider E, et al. Evasion from NK cell immunity by MHC class I chain-related molecules expressing colon adenocarcinoma. J Immunol 2003; 171:6891–6899.
59. Fiore E, Fusco C, Romero P, Stamenkovic I. Matrix metalloproteinase 9 (MMP-9/gelatinase B) pro-teolytically cleaves ICAM-1 and participates in tumor cell resistance to natural killer cell-mediated cytotoxicity. Oncogene 2002; 21:5213–5223.
60. Abken H, Hombach A, Heuser C, Kronfeld K, Seliger B. Tuning tumor-specific T-cell activation: a matter of costimulation? Trends Immunol 2002; 23:240–245.
61. Chen L. Co-inhibitory molecules of the B7-CD28 family in the control of T-cell immunity. Nat Rev Immunol 2004; 4:336–347.
62. Blank C, Brown I, Peterson AC, et al. PD-L1/B7H-1 inhibits the effector phase of tumor rejection by T cell receptor (TCR) transgenic CD8+ T cells. Cancer Res 2004; 64:1140–1145.
63. Iwai Y, Ishida M, Tanaka Y, Okazaki T, Honjo T, Minato N. Involvement of PD-L1 on tumor cells in the escape from host immune system and tumor immunotherapy by PD-L1 blockade. Proc Natl Acad Sci U S A 2002; 99:12,293–12,297.
64. Latchman Y, Wood CR, Chernova T, et al. PD-L2 is a second ligand for PD-1 and inhibits T cell activation. Nat Immunol 2001; 2:261–268.
65. Freeman GJ, Long AJ, Iwai Y, et al. Engagement of the PD-1 immunoinhibitory receptor by a novel B7 family member leads to negative regulation of lymphocyte activation. J Exp Med 2000; 192:1027–1034.
66. Dong H, Strome SE, Salomao DR, et al. Tumor-associated B7-H1 promotes T-cell apoptosis: a poten-tial mechanism of immune evasion. Nat Med 2002; 8:793–800.
67. Choi IH, Zhu G, Sica GL, et al. Genomic organization and expression analysis of B7-H4, an immune inhibitory molecule of the B7 family. J Immunol 2003; 171:4650–4654.
68. Ochsenbein AF, Sierro S, Odermatt B, et al. Roles of tumour localization, second signals and cross priming in cytotoxic T-cell induction. Nature 2001; 411:1058–1064.
69. Sauter B, Albert ML, Francisco L, Larsson M, Somersan S, Bhardwaj N. Consequences of cell death: exposure to necrotic tumor cells, but not primary tissue cells or apoptotic cells, induces the maturation of immunostimulatory dendritic cells. J Exp Med 2000; 191:423–434.
70. Kadowaki N, Ho S, Antonenko S, et al. Subsets of human dendritic cell precursors express different toll-like receptors and respond to different microbial antigens. J Exp Med 2001; 194:863–869.
71. Schnare M, Barton GM, Holt AC, Takeda K, Akira S, Medzhitov R. Toll-like receptors control acti-vation of adaptive immune responses. Nat Immunol 2001; 2:947–950.
72. Fujii S, Liu K, Smith C, Bonito AJ, Steinman RM. The linkage of innate to adaptive immunity via maturing dendritic cells in vivo requires CD40 ligation in addition to antigen presentation and CD80/86 costimulation. J Exp Med 2004; 199:1607–1618.
73. Appleman LJ, Boussiotis VA. T cell anergy and costimulation. Immunol Rev 2003; 192:161–180.

74. Cella M, Scheidegger D, Palmer-Lehmann K, Lane P, Lanzavecchia A, Alber G. Ligation of CD40 on dendritic cells triggers production of high levels of interleukin-12 and enhances T cell stimulatory capacity: T-T help via APC activation. J Exp Med 1996; 184:747–752.

75. Lanzavecchia A, Sallusto F. Regulation of T cell immunity by dendritic cells. Cell 2001; 106:263–266.

76. Liu YJ, Joshua DE, Williams GT, Smith CA, Gordon J, MacLennan IC. Mechanism of antigen-driven selection in germinal centres. Nature 1989; 342:929–931.

77. Guzman-Rojas L, Sims-Mourtada JC, Rangel R, Martinez-Valdez H. Life and death within germinal centres: a double-edged sword. Immunology 2002; 107:167–175.

78. Ciaravino G, Bhat M, Manbeian CA, Teng NN. Differential expression of CD40 and CD95 in ovarian carcinoma. Eur J Gynaecol Oncol 2004; 25:27–32.

79. Jakobson E, Jonsson G, Bjorck P, Paulie S. Stimulation of CD40 in human bladder carcinoma cells inhibits anti-Fas/APO-1 (CD95)-induced apoptosis. Int J Cancer 1998; 77:849–853.

80. Loro LL, Ohlsson M, Vintermyr OK, Liavaag PG, Jonsson R, Johannessen AC. Maintained CD40 and loss of polarised CD40 ligand expression in oral squamous cell carcinoma. Anticancer Res 2001; 21(1A):113–117.

81. Jakobson E, Jonsson G, Bjorck P, Paulie S. Stimulation of CD40 in human bladder carcinoma cells inhibits anti-Fas/APO-1 (CD95)-induced apoptosis. Int J Cancer 1998; 77:849–853.

82. Yamaguchi H, Tanaka F, Sadanaga N, Ohta M, Inoue H, Mori M. Stimulation of CD40 inhibits Fas- or chemotherapy-mediated apoptosis and increases cell motility in human gastric carcinoma cells. Int J Oncol 2003; 23:1697–1702.

83. Roselli M, Mineo TC, Basili S, et al. Soluble CD40 ligand plasma levels in lung cancer. Clin Cancer Res 2004; 10:610–614.

84. Pammer J, Plettenberg A, Weninger W, et al. CD40 antigen is expressed by endothelial cells and tumor cells in Kaposi's sarcoma. Am J Pathol 1996; 148:1387–1396.

85. Sabel MS, Yamada M, Kawaguchi Y, Chen FA, Takita H, Bankert RB. CD40 expression on human lung cancer correlates with metastatic spread. Cancer Immunol Immunother 2000; 49:101–108.

86. Reinders ME, Sho M, Robertson SW, Geehan CS, Briscoe DM. Proangiogenic function of CD40 ligand-CD40 interactions. J Immunol 2003; 171:1534–1541.

87. Flaxenburg JA, Melter M, Lapchak PH, Briscoe DM, Pal S. The CD40-induced signaling pathway in endothelial cells resulting in the overexpression of vascular endothelial growth factor involves Ras and phosphatidylinositol 3-kinase. J Immunol 2004; 172:7503–7509.

88. Dong C, Flavell RA. Cell fate decision: T-helper 1 and 2 subsets in immune responses. Arthritis Res 2000; 2:179–188.

89. Reiner SL. Helper T cell differentiation, inside and out. Curr Opin Immunol 2001; 13:351–355.

90. Clerici M, Shearer GM, Clerici E. Cytokine dysregulation in invasive cervical carcinoma and other human neoplasias: time to consider the TH1/TH2 paradigm. J Natl Cancer Inst 1998; 90:261–263.

91. Joon YA, Bazar KA, Lee PY. Tumors may modulate host immunity partly through hypoxia-induced sympathetic bias. Med Hypotheses 2004; 63:352–356.

92. Li R, Ruttinger D, Li R, Si LS, Wang YL. Analysis of the immunological microenvironment at the tumor site in patients with non-small cell lung cancer. Langenbecks Arch Surg 2003; 388:406–412.

93. Kim J, Modlin RL, Moy RL, et al. IL-10 production in cutaneous basal and squamous cell carcinomas. A mechanism for evading the local T cell immune response. J Immunol 1995; 155:2240–2247.

94. Kosiewicz MM, Alard P, Liang S, Clark SL. Mechanisms of tolerance induced by transforming growth factor-β-treated antigen-presenting cells: CD8 regulatory T cells inhibit the effector phase of the immune response in primed mice through a mechanism involving Fas ligand. Int Immunol 2004; 16:697–706.

95. Seo N, Hayakawa S, Takigawa M, Tokura Y. Interleukin-10 expressed at early tumour sites induces subsequent generation of CD4(+) T-regulatory cells and systemic collapse of antitumour immunity. Immunology 2001; 103:449–457.

96. Garcia-Hernandez ML, Hernandez-Pando R, Gariglio P, Berumen J. Interleukin-10 promotes B16-melanoma growth by inhibition of macrophage functions and induction of tumour and vascular cell proliferation. Immunology 2002; 105:231–243.

97. Fiorentino DF, Zlotnik A, Mosmann TR, Howard M, O'Garra A. IL-10 inhibits cytokine production by activated macrophages. J Immunol 1991; 147:3815–3822.

98. Mitra RS, Judge TA, Nestle FO, Turka LA, Nickoloff BJ. Psoriatic skin-derived dendritic cell function is inhibited by exogenous IL-10. Differential modulation of B7-1 (CD80) and B7-2 (CD86) expression. J Immunol 1995; 154:2668–2677.

99. De Smedt T, Van Mechelen M, De Becker G, Urbain J, Leo O, Moser M. Effect of interleukin-10 on dendritic cell maturation and function. Eur J Immunol 1997; 27:1229–1235.

100. Steinbrink K, Jonuleit H, Muller G, Schuler G, Knop J, Enk AH. Interleukin-10-treated human dendritic cells induce a melanoma-antigen-specific anergy in CD8(+) T cells resulting in a failure to lyse tumor cells. Blood 1999; 93:1634–1642.

101. Urosevic M, Dummer R. HLA-G and IL-10 expression in human cancer—different stories with the same message. Semin Cancer Biol 2003; 13:337–342.

102. Mukherjee P, Ginardi AR, Madsen CS, et al. MUC1-specific CTLs are non-functional within a pancreatic tumor microenvironment. Glycoconj J 2001; 18:931–942.

103. Garcia-Hernandez ML, Hernandez-Pando R, Gariglio P, Berumen J. Interleukin-10 promotes B16-melanoma growth by inhibition of macrophage functions and induction of tumour and vascular cell proliferation. Immunology 2002; 105:231–243.

104. Huang S, Xie K, Bucana CD, Ullrich SE, Bar-Eli M. Interleukin 10 suppresses tumor growth and metastasis of human melanoma cells: potential inhibition of angiogenesis. Clin Cancer Res 1996; 2:1969–1979.

105. Luethviksson BR, Gunnlaugsdottir B. Transforming growth factor-β as a regulator of site-specific T-cell inflammatory response. Scand J Immunol 2003; 58:129–138.

106. Roberts AB, Wakefield LM. The two faces of transforming growth factor β in carcinogenesis. Proc Natl Acad Sci U S A 2003; 100:8621–8623.

107. Wakefield LM, Roberts AB. TGF-β signaling: positive and negative effects on tumorigenesis. Curr Opin Genet Dev 2002; 12:22–29.

108. Janda E, Lehmann K, Killisch I, et al. Ras and TGFβ cooperatively regulate epithelial cell plasticity and metastasis: dissection of Ras signaling pathways. J Cell Biol 2002; 156:299–313.

109. Oft M, Peli J, Rudaz C, Schwarz H, Beug H, Reichmann E. TGF-β1 and Ha-Ras collaborate in modulating the phenotypic plasticity and invasiveness of epithelial tumor cells. Genes Dev 1996; 10:2462–2477.

110. Oft M, Heider KH, Beug H. TGFβ signaling is necessary for carcinoma cell invasiveness and metastasis. Curr Biol 1998; 8:1243–1252.

111. Weijzen S, Velders MP, Kast WM. Modulation of the immune response and tumor growth by activated Ras. Leukemia 1999; 13:502–513.

112. Kai T, Taketazu F, Kawakami M, et al. Distribution of transforming growth factor-β and its receptors in gastric carcinoma tissue. Jpn J Cancer Res 1996; 87:296–304.

113. Mizoi T, Ohtani H, Miyazono K, Miyazawa M, Matsuno S, Nagura H. Immunoelectron microscopic localization of transforming growth factor β 1 and latent transforming growth factor β 1 binding protein in human gastrointestinal carcinomas: qualitative difference between cancer cells and stromal cells. Cancer Res 1993; 53:183–190.

114. Roberts AB. Molecular and cell biology of TGF-β. Miner Electrolyte Metab 1998; 24(2–3):111–119.

115. O'Mahony CA, Albo D, Tuszynski GP, Berger DH. Transforming growth factor-β 1 inhibits generation of angiostatin by human pancreatic cancer cells. Surgery 1998; 124:388–393.

116. Tsukazaki T, Chiang TA, Davison AF, Attisano L, Wrana JL. SARA, a FYVE domain protein that recruits Smad2 to the TGFβ receptor. Cell 1998; 95:779–791.

117. Zhang Y, Feng XH, Derynck R. Smad3 and Smad4 cooperate with c-Jun/c-Fos to mediate TGF-β-induced transcription. Nature 1998; 394:909–913.

118. Ewen ME, Sluss HK, Whitehouse LL, Livingston DM. TGF β inhibition of Cdk4 synthesis is linked to cell cycle arrest. Cell 1993; 74:1009–1020.

119. Pietenpol JA, Munger K, Howley PM, Stein RW, Moses HL. Factor-binding element in the human c-myc promoter involved in transcriptional regulation by transforming growth factor β 1 and by the retinoblastoma gene product. Proc Natl Acad Sci U S A 1991; 88:10,227–10,231.

120. Sola S, Ma X, Castro RE, Kren BT, Steer CJ, Rodrigues CM. Ursodeoxycholic acid modulates E2F-1 and p53 expression through a caspase-independent mechanism in transforming growth factor β1-induced apoptosis of rat hepatocytes. J Biol Chem 2003; 278:48,831–48,838.

121. Chen T, Carter D, Garrigue-Antar L, Reiss M. Transforming growth factor β type I receptor kinase mutant associated with metastatic breast cancer. Cancer Res 1998; 58:4805–4810.

122. Goggins M, Shekher M, Turnacioglu K, Yeo CJ, Hruban RH, Kern SE. Genetic alterations of the transforming growth factor β receptor genes in pancreatic and biliary adenocarcinomas. Cancer Res 1998; 58:5329–5332.

123. Kim IY, Ahn HJ, Zelner DJ, et al. Genetic change in transforming growth factor β (TGF-β) receptor type I gene correlates with insensitivity to TGF-β 1 in human prostate cancer cells. Cancer Res 1996; 56:44–48.

124. Zhou S, Buckhaults P, Zawel L, et al. Targeted deletion of Smad4 shows it is required for transforming growth factor β and activin signaling in colorectal cancer cells. Proc Natl Acad Sci U S A 1998; 95:2412–2416.

125. Kelly JM, Takeda K, Darcy PK, Yagita H, Smyth MJ. A role for IFN-γ in primary and secondary immunity generated by NK cell-sensitive tumor-expressing CD80 in vivo. J Immunol 2002; 168:4472–4479.

126. Qin Z, Schwartzkopff J, Pradera F, et al. A critical requirement of interferon γ-mediated angiostasis for tumor rejection by CD8+ T cells. Cancer Res 2003; 63:4095–4100.

127. Qin Z, Blankenstein T. CD4+ T cell-mediated tumor rejection involves inhibition of angiogenesis that is dependent on IFN γ receptor expression by nonhematopoietic cells. Immunity 2000; 12:677–686.

128. Ruiz-Ruiz C, Ruiz dA, Rodriguez A, Ortiz-Ferron G, Redondo JM, Lopez-Rivas A. The up-regulation of human caspase-8 by interferon-γ in breast tumor cells requires the induction and action of the transcription factor interferon regulatory factor-1. J Biol Chem 2004; 279:19,712–19,720.

129. Seliger B, Hammers S, Hohne A, et al. IFN-γ-mediated coordinated transcriptional regulation of the human *TAP-1* and *LMP-2* genes in human renal cell carcinoma. Clin Cancer Res 1997; 3:573–578.

130. Liu K, Abrams SI. Coordinate regulation of IFN consensus sequence-binding protein and caspase-1 in the sensitization of human colon carcinoma cells to Fas-mediated apoptosis by IFN-γ. J Immunol 2003; 170:6329–6337.

131. Dovhey SE, Ghosh NS, Wright KL. Loss of interferon-γ inducibility of TAP1 and LMP2 in a renal cell carcinoma cell line. Cancer Res 2000; 60:5789–5796.

132. Nagao M, Nakajima Y, Kanehiro H, et al. The impact of interferon γ receptor expression on the mechanism of escape from host immune surveillance in hepatocellular carcinoma. Hepatology 2000; 32:491–500.

133. Hassanain HH, Chon SY, Gupta SL. Differential regulation of human indoleamine 2,3-dioxygenase gene expression by interferons-γ and -α. Analysis of the regulatory region of the gene and identification of an interferon-γ-inducible DNA-binding factor. J Biol Chem 1993; 268:5077–5084.

134. Terness P, Bauer TM, Rose L, et al. Inhibition of allogeneic T cell proliferation by indoleamine 2,3-dioxygenase-expressing dendritic cells: mediation of suppression by tryptophan metabolites. J Exp Med 2002; 196:447–457.

135. Fallarino F, Grohmann U, Vacca C, et al. T cell apoptosis by tryptophan catabolism. Cell Death Differ 2002; 9:1069–1077.

136. Munn DH, Zhou M, Attwood JT, et al. Prevention of allogeneic fetal rejection by tryptophan catabolism. Science 1998; 281:1191–1193.

137. Munn DH, Sharma MD, Mellor AL. Ligation of B7-1/B7-2 by human CD4(+) T cells triggers indoleamine 2,3-dioxygenase activity in dendritic cells. J Immunol 2004; 172:4100–4110.

138. Munn DH, Sharma MD, Lee JR, et al. Potential regulatory function of human dendritic cells expressing indoleamine 2,3-dioxygenase. Science 2002; 297:1867–1870.

139. Mellor AL, Keskin DB, Johnson T, Chandler P, Munn DH. Cells expressing indoleamine 2,3-dioxygenase inhibit T cell responses. J Immunol 2002; 168:3771–3776.

140. Munn DH, Mellor AL. IDO and tolerance to tumors. Trends Mol Med 2004; 10:15–18.

141. Lee JR, Dalton RR, Messina JL, et al. Pattern of recruitment of immunoregulatory antigen-presenting cells in malignant melanoma. Lab Invest 2003; 83:1457–1466.

142. Belperio JA, Keane MP, Arenberg DA, et al. CXC chemokines in angiogenesis. J Leukoc Biol 2000; 68:1–8.

143. Kondo T, Ito F, Nakazawa H, Horita S, Osaka Y, Toma H. High expression of chemokine gene as a favorable prognostic factor in renal cell carcinoma. J Urol 2004; 171(Pt 1):2171–2175.

144. Hellmuth M, Paulukat J, Ninic R, Pfeilschifter J, Muhl H. Nitric oxide differentially regulates pro- and anti-angiogenic markers in DLD-1 colon carcinoma cells. FEBS Lett 2004; 563:98–102.

145. Peng JP, Zheng S, Xiao ZX, Zhang SZ. Inducible nitric oxide synthase expression is related to angiogenesis, bcl-2 and cell proliferation in hepatocellular carcinoma. J Zhejiang Univ Sci 2003; 4:221–227.

146. Levy DE, Lee CK. What does Stat3 do? J Clin Invest 2002; 109:1143–1148.

147. Takeda K, Akira S. STAT family of transcription factors in cytokine-mediated biological responses. Cytokine Growth Factor Rev 2000; 11:199–207.

148. Coffer PJ, Koenderman L, de Groot RP. The role of STATs in myeloid differentiation and leukemia. Oncogene 2000; 19:2511–2522.

149. Mora LB, Buettner R, Seigne J, et al. Constitutive activation of Stat3 in human prostate tumors and cell lines: direct inhibition of Stat3 signaling induces apoptosis of prostate cancer cells. Cancer Res 2002; 62:6659–6666.

150. Song JI, Grandis JR. STAT signaling in head and neck cancer. Oncogene 2000; 19:2489–2495.

151. Wang T, Niu G, Kortylewski M, et al. Regulation of the innate and adaptive immune responses by Stat-3 signaling in tumor cells. Nat Med 2004; 10:48–54.

152. Catlett-Falcone R, Landowski TH, Oshiro MM, et al. Constitutive activation of Stat3 signaling confers resistance to apoptosis in human U266 myeloma cells. Immunity 1999; 10:105–115.

153. Niu G, Wright KL, Huang M, et al. Constitutive Stat3 activity up-regulates VEGF expression and tumor angiogenesis. Oncogene 2002; 21:2000–2008.

154. Xiang ST, Zhou SW, Guan W, et al. Tumor infiltrating dendritic cells and Mucin1 gene expression in benign prostatic hyperplasia and prostate cancer (in Chinese). Zhonghua Nan Ke Xue 2003; 9:497–500.

155. Terabe M, Berzofsky JA. Immunoregulatory T cells in tumor immunity. Curr Opin Immunol 2004; 16:157–162.

156. Friberg M, Jennings R, Alsarraj M, et al. Indoleamine 2,3-dioxygenase contributes to tumor cell evasion of T cell-mediated rejection. Int J Cancer 2002; 101:151–155.

157. Kagi D, Vignaux F, Ledermann B, et al. Fas and perforin pathways as major mechanisms of T cell-mediated cytotoxicity. Science 1994; 265:528–530.

158. Smyth MJ, Thia KY, Street SE, MacGregor D, Godfrey DI, Trapani JA. Perforin-mediated cytotoxicity is critical for surveillance of spontaneous lymphoma. J Exp Med 2000; 192:755–760.

159. Trapani JA, Smyth MJ. Functional significance of the perforin/granzyme cell death pathway. Nat Rev Immunol 2002; 2:735–747.

160. Smyth MJ, Kelly JM, Sutton VR, et al. Unlocking the secrets of cytotoxic granule proteins. J Leukoc Biol 2001; 70:18–29.

161. Beresford PJ, Xia Z, Greenberg AH, Lieberman J. Granzyme A loading induces rapid cytolysis and a novel form of DNA damage independently of caspase activation. Immunity 1999; 10:585–594.

162. Trapani JA, Sutton VR. Granzyme B: pro-apoptotic, antiviral and antitumor functions. Curr Opin Immunol 2003; 15:533–543.

163. Sharif-Askari E, Alam A, Rheaume E, et al. Direct cleavage of the human DNA fragmentation factor-45 by granzyme B induces caspase-activated DNase release and DNA fragmentation. EMBO J 2001; 20:3101–3113.

164. Thomas DA, Du C, Xu M, Wang X, Ley TJ. DFF45/ICAD can be directly processed by granzyme B during the induction of apoptosis. Immunity 2000; 12:621–632.

165. Wolf BB, Schuler M, Echeverri F, Green DR. Caspase-3 is the primary activator of apoptotic DNA fragmentation via DNA fragmentation factor-45/inhibitor of caspase-activated DNase inactivation. J Biol Chem 1999; 274:30,651–30,656.

166. Sutton VR, Davis JE, Cancilla M, et al. Initiation of apoptosis by granzyme B requires direct cleavage of bid, but not direct granzyme B-mediated caspase activation. J Exp Med 2000; 192:1403–1414.

167. Heibein JA, Goping IS, Barry M, et al. Granzyme B-mediated cytochrome c release is regulated by the Bcl-2 family members bid and Bax. J Exp Med 2000; 192:1391–1402.

168. Eskes R, Desagher S, Antonsson B, Martinou JC. Bid induces the oligomerization and insertion of Bax into the outer mitochondrial membrane. Mol Cell Biol 2000; 20:929–935.

169. Wei MC, Lindsten T, Mootha VK, et al. tBID, a membrane-targeted death ligand, oligomerizes BAK to release cytochrome c. Genes Dev 2000; 14:2060–2071.

170. Rostovtseva TK, Antonsson B, Suzuki M, Youle RJ, Colombini M, Bezrukov SM. Bid, but not Bax, regulates VDAC channels. J Biol Chem 2004; 279:13,575–13,583.

171. Goping IS, Barry M, Liston P, et al. Granzyme B-induced apoptosis requires both direct caspase activation and relief of caspase inhibition. Immunity 2003; 18:355–365.

172. Verhagen AM, Ekert PG, Pakusch M, et al. Identification of DIABLO, a mammalian protein that promotes apoptosis by binding to and antagonizing IAP proteins. Cell 2000; 102:43–53.

173. Bleackley RC, Heibein JA. Enzymatic control of apoptosis. Nat Prod Rep 2001; 18:431–440.

174. Zou H, Li Y, Liu X, Wang X. An APAF-1.cytochrome c multimeric complex is a functional apoptosome that activates procaspase-9. J Biol Chem 1999; 274:11,549–11,556.

175. Medema JP, de Jong J, Peltenburg LT, et al. Blockade of the granzyme B/perforin pathway through overexpression of the serine protease inhibitor PI-9/SPI-6 constitutes a mechanism for immune escape by tumors. Proc Natl Acad Sci U S A 2001; 98:11,515–11,520.

176. Lee SH, Shin MS, Park WS, et al. Alterations of Fas (*APO-1/CD95*) gene in transitional cell carcinomas of urinary bladder. Cancer Res 1999; 59:3068–3072.

177. Lee SH, Shin MS, Park WS, et al. Alterations of Fas (*Apo-1/CD95*) gene in non-small cell lung cancer. Oncogene 1999; 18:3754–3760.

178. Shin MS, Park WS, Kim SY, et al. Alterations of Fas (*Apo-1/CD95*) gene in cutaneous malignant melanoma. Am J Pathol 1999; 154:1785–1791.

179. Maas S, Warskulat U, Steinhoff C, et al. Decreased Fas expression in advanced-stage bladder cancer is not related to p53 status. Urology 2004; 63:392–397.

180. Pitti RM, Marsters SA, Lawrence DA, et al. Genomic amplification of a decoy receptor for Fas ligand in lung and colon cancer. Nature 1998; 396:699–703.

181. Ashkenazi A, Dixit VM. Apoptosis control by death and decoy receptors. Curr Opin Cell Biol 1999; 11:255–260.

182. Bai C, Connolly B, Metzker ML, et al. Overexpression of M68/DcR3 in human gastrointestinal tract tumors independent of gene amplification and its location in a four-gene cluster. Proc Natl Acad Sci U S A 2000; 97:1230–1235.

183. Pitti RM, Marsters SA, Lawrence DA, et al. Genomic amplification of a decoy receptor for Fas ligand in lung and colon cancer. Nature 1998; 396:699–703.

184. Roth W, Isenmann S, Nakamura M, Platten M, et al. Soluble decoy receptor 3 is expressed by malignant gliomas and suppresses CD95 ligand-induced apoptosis and chemotaxis. Cancer Res 2001; 61:2759–2765.

185. Takahama Y, Yamada Y, Emoto K, et al. The prognostic significance of overexpression of the decoy receptor for Fas ligand (DcR3) in patients with gastric carcinomas. Gastric Cancer 2002; 5:61–68.

186. Tsuji S, Hosotani R, Yonehara S, et al. Endogenous decoy receptor 3 blocks the growth inhibition signals mediated by Fas ligand in human pancreatic adenocarcinoma. Int J Cancer 2003; 106:17–25.

187. Hsu TL, Chang YC, Chen SJ, et al. Modulation of dendritic cell differentiation and maturation by decoy receptor 3. J Immunol 2002; 168:4846–4853.

188. Chang YC, Hsu TL, Lin HH, et al. Modulation of macrophage differentiation and activation by decoy receptor 3. J Leukoc Biol 2004; 75:486–494.

189. Roth W, Isenmann S, Nakamura M, et al. Soluble decoy receptor 3 is expressed by malignant gliomas and suppresses CD95 ligand-induced apoptosis and chemotaxis. Cancer Res 2001; 61:2759–2765.

190. Chen YL, Chen SH, Wang JY, Yang BC. Fas ligand on tumor cells mediates inactivation of neutrophils. J Immunol 2003; 171:1183–1191.

191. Yang CR, Hsieh SL, Teng CM, Ho FM, Su WL, Lin WW. Soluble decoy receptor 3 induces angiogenesis by neutralization of TL1A, a cytokine belonging to tumor necrosis factor superfamily and exhibiting angiostatic action. Cancer Res 2004; 64:1122–1129.

192. MacFarlane M, Harper N, Snowden RT, et al. Mechanisms of resistance to TRAIL-induced apoptosis in primary B cell chronic lymphocytic leukaemia. Oncogene 2002; 21:6809–6818.

193. Dutton A, O'Neil JD, Milner AE, et al. Expression of the cellular FLICE-inhibitory protein (c-FLIP) protects Hodgkin's lymphoma cells from autonomous Fas-mediated death. Proc Natl Acad Sci U S A 2004; 101:6611–6616.

194. Yi X, Yin XM, Dong Z. Inhibition of Bid-induced apoptosis by Bcl-2. tBid insertion, Bax translocation, and Bax/Bak oligomerization suppressed. J Biol Chem 2003; 278:16,992–16,999.

195. Fornaro M, Plescia J, Chheang S, et al. Fibronectin protects prostate cancer cells from tumor necrosis factor-α-induced apoptosis via the AKT/survivin pathway. J Biol Chem 2003; 278:50,402–50,411.

196. Asanuma K, Tsuji N, Endoh T, Yagihashi A, Watanabe N. Survivin enhances Fas ligand expression via up-regulation of specificity protein 1-mediated gene transcription in colon cancer cells. J Immunol 2004; 172:3922–3929.

197. Li ZY, Zou SQ. Fas counterattack in cholangiocarcinoma: a mechanism for immune evasion in human hilar cholangiocarcinomas. World J Gastroenterol 2001; 7:860–863.

198. Shimonishi T, Isse K, Shibata F, et al. Up-regulation of fas ligand at early stages and down-regulation of Fas at progressed stages of intrahepatic cholangiocarcinoma reflect evasion from immune surveillance. Hepatology 2000; 32(Pt 1):761–769.

199. Sejima T, Isoyama T, Miyagawa I. Alteration of apoptotic regulatory molecules expression during carcinogenesis and tumor progression of renal cell carcinoma. Int J Urol 2003; 10:476–484.

200. Kase H, Aoki Y, Tanaka K. Fas ligand expression in cervical adenocarcinoma: relevance to lymph node metastasis and tumor progression. Gynecol Oncol 2003; 90:70–74.

201. Thomas WD, Zhang XD, Franco AV, Nguyen T, Hersey P. TNF-related apoptosis-inducing ligand-induced apoptosis of melanoma is associated with changes in mitochondrial membrane potential and perinuclear clustering of mitochondria. J Immunol 2000; 165:5612–5620.

202. Bennett MW, O'Connell J, O'Sullivan GC, et al. The Fas counterattack in vivo: apoptotic depletion of tumor-infiltrating lymphocytes associated with Fas ligand expression by human esophageal carcinoma. J Immunol 1998; 160:5669–5675.

203. Koyama S, Koike N, Adachi S. Expression of TNF-related apoptosis-inducing ligand (TRAIL) and its receptors in gastric carcinoma and tumor-infiltrating lymphocytes: a possible mechanism of immune evasion of the tumor. J Cancer Res Clin Oncol 2002; 128:73–79.

204. Frankel B, Longo SL, Canute GW. Soluble Fas-ligand (sFasL) in human astrocytoma cyst fluid is cytotoxic to T-cells: another potential means of immune evasion. J Neurooncol 2000; 48:21–26.

205. Song E, Chen J, Ouyang N, Su F, Wang M, Heemann U. Soluble Fas ligand released by colon adeno-carcinoma cells induces host lymphocyte apoptosis: an active mode of immune evasion in colon cancer. Br J Cancer 2001; 85:1047–1054.

206. Gerharz CD, Ramp U, Dejosez M, et al. Resistance to CD95 (APO-1/Fas)-mediated apoptosis in human renal cell carcinomas: an important factor for evasion from negative growth control. Lab Invest 1999; 79:1521–1534.

207. Ferrara N. VEGF: an update on biological and therapeutic aspects. Curr Opin Biotechnol 2000; 11:617–624.

208. Santin AD, Hermonat PL, Ravaggi A, Cannon MJ, Pecorelli S, Parham GP. Secretion of vascular endothelial growth factor in ovarian cancer. Eur J Gynaecol Oncol 1999; 20:177–181.

209. Ohm JE, Gabrilovich DI, Sempowski GD, et al. VEGF inhibits T-cell development and may contribute to tumor-induced immune suppression. Blood 2003; 101:4878–4886.

210. Wang D, Dubois RN. Cyclooxygenase-2: a potential target in breast cancer. Semin Oncol 2004; 31(Suppl 3):S64–S73.

211. Altorki N. COX-2: a target for prevention and treatment of esophageal cancer. J Surg Res 2004; 117:114–120.

212. Rao M, Yang W, Seifalian AM, Winslet MC. Role of cyclooxygenase-2 in the angiogenesis of colorectal cancer. Int J Colorectal Dis 2004; 19:1–11.

213. Eisengart CA, Mestre JR, Naama HA, et al. Prostaglandins regulate melanoma-induced cytokine production in macrophages. Cell Immunol 2000; 204:143–149.

214. Plescia OJ, Smith AH, Grinwich K. Subversion of immune system by tumor cells and role of prostag-landins. Proc Natl Acad Sci U S A 1975; 72:1848–1851.

215. Spaner DE. Amplifying cancer vaccine responses by modifying pathogenic gene programs in tumor cells. J Leukoc Biol 2004; 76:338–351.

Index